MedBooks, 

CENTERS FOR MEDICARE & MED̲ . ̲v̲ ICES (CMS)

2010

HCPCS

(HEALTH CARE PROCEDURE CODING SYSTEM)

Level II National Supply Code Book

Includes:
Alphanumeric Codes
Table of Drugs
Alphanumeric Index
ASC Addendum AA, BB, DD-1, DD-2 and EE
Definitions of all HCPCS Fields

Updated and published annually!
As of October 31, 2009*

copyright 2009 MedBooks, Inc.
ISBN 978-0-9822597-6-4

compiled by Mark Lerner
*Quarterly updates are available at no charge from the CMS website:

http://www.cms.hhs.gov/HCPCSReleaseCodeSets/02_HCPCS_Quarterly_Update.asp#TopOfPage

Quality services from...

MEDBOOKS, Inc.

Serving the Medical, Academic & Professional fields for more than 25 years!

Retroactive Billing Services

Place MedBooks' years of experience to practical use. Let us re-bill and re-file your unpaid claims, thus giving you the money that you have worked for (and not received).

Coding & Reimbursement Seminars

Wide in scope and comprehensive in coverage, our how-to coding seminars uncover the mysteries of:

1. Why physicians lose money,
2. How to help patients pay lower balances,
3. How to obtain payment for supplies and drugs,
4. How to use the fifth digit, and
5. What are the perils of mismatching diagnoses/procedures?

Coding & Reimbursement Audits

MedBooks offers a rare opportunity to sneak an objective and expert peek into what the insurance carriers and Medicare will look for once you have filed your claims. By looking at a broad sampling of your practice's submissions, we evaluate, grade and report back to you how to get paid for the services that you provide, what you may be doing wrong, AND how to stay clear (and safe) in an insurance audit.

Expert Witnessing/Testimony

When you need expert testimony delivered in a way that can be easily understood - MedBooks is your source. Put 23+ years of coding experience on your side.

Superbill/Fee Slip Review

Are you working with an outdated Fee Slip or Superbill? Let MedBooks review what you are currently using, and make the necessary changes.

Physician Fee Analysis Service

Are you billing the correct amount? Let MedBooks review your codes and compare them with the current RBRVS.

2009 HCPCS

TABLE OF CONTENTS

<u>Alpha-Numeric HCPCS File Content</u>

This BOOK contains the Level II alphanumeric HCPCS procedure and modifier codes, their long, and applicable Medicare administrative, coverage, and pricing data. The Level II HCPCS codes, which are established by CMS's Alpha-Numeric Editorial Panel, primarily represent items and supplies and non-physician services not covered by the American Medical Association's Current Procedural Terminology-4 (CPT-4) codes; Medicare, Medicaid, and private health insurers use HCPCS procedure and modifier codes for claims processing. Level II alphanumeric procedure and modifier codes comprise the A to V range.

The Alphanumeric Index and Table of Drugs will be available for download separately at http://www.cms. hhs.gov/HCPCSReleaseCodeSets/ANHCPCS/list.asp.

HCPCS Update Schedule

With the exception of temporary codes, Level II alphanumeric procedure and modifier codes are updated annually on January 1. Temporary codes, which begin with G, K, or Q, are updated on a flow basis throughout the year. Nevertheless, the alphanumeric HCPCS file will only be uploaded to the CMS web site on an annual basis. As a result, temporary coding changes or Medicare administrative, coverage, or pricing data changes that occur outside of the annual update process may not be reflected in the file. In most cases, these temporary coding changes are noted in Program Memoranda (PM) to Medicare carriers and fiscal intermediaries.

Ordering CPT-4 Codes

In light of copyright agreements, this file does not contain the American Medical Association's Level I CPT-4 codes.

Beginning in 2002, the 5-character alphanumeric procedure codes beginning with D are included in the al-phanumeric HCPCS file and are copyright 2007 by the American Dental Association. They are part of the American Dental Association's Current Dental Terminology--Seventh Edition (CDT-07/08). The codes may only be used for purposes directly related to participation in the Medicare program. Permission for any other use must be obtained from the American Dental Association.

The alphanumeric HCPCS file sold by the National Technical Information Service (NTIS) does contain the dental codes. NTIS offers the alphanumeric HCPCS on CD-ROM only. NTIS orders can be submit-ted by phone at 703-487-4650 or by e-mail at orders@ntis.fedworld.gov.

2010
Healthcare Common Procedure Coding System (HCPCS)
Information and Descriptions

Healthcare Common Procedure Coding System Code

The Healthcare Common Procedure Coding System (HCPCS) is a collection of codes that represent procedures, supplies, products and services which may be provided to Medicare beneficiaries and to individuals enrolled in private health insurance programs. The codes are divided into two levels, or groups, as described below:

Level I

Codes and descriptors copyrighted by the American Medical Association's current procedural terminology, fourth edition (CPT-4). These are 5 position numeric codes representing physician and non-physician services.

Level II

Includes codes and descriptors copyrighted by the American Dental Association's current dental terminology, seventh edition (CDT-7/8). These are 5 position alpha-numeric codes comprising the d series. All other level II codes and descriptors are approved and maintained jointly by the alpha-numeric editorial panel (consisting of CMS, the Health Insurance Association of America, and the Blue Cross and Blue Shield Association).

These are 5 position alphanumeric codes representing primarily items and non-physician services that are not represented in the level I codes.

HCPCS Modifier Code

A modifier provides the means by which the reporting physician or provider can indicate that a service or procedure that has been performed has been altered by some specific circumstance but not changed in its definition or code. The judicious application of modifiers obviates the necessity for separate procedure listings that may describe the modifying circumstance. Modifiers may be used to indicate to the recipient of a report that:

- ✓ A service or procedure has both a professional and technical component.
- ✓ A service or procedure was performed by more than one physician and/or in more than one location.
- ✓ A service or procedure has been increased or reduced.
- ✓ Only part of a service was performed.
- ✓ An adjunctive service was performed.
- ✓ A bilateral procedure was performed.
- ✓ A service or procedure was provided more than once.
- ✓ Unusual events occurred.

HCPCS modifier codes are divided into two levels, or groups, as described below:

Level I

Codes and descriptors copyrighted by the American Medical Association's current procedural terminology, fourth edition (CPT-4). These are 2 position numeric codes.

**** NOTE: ****

CPT-4 codes including both long and short descriptions shall be used in accordance with the CMS/AMA agreement. Any other use violates the AMA copyright.

Level II

Codes and descriptors approved and maintained jointly by the alphanumeric editorial panel (consisting of CMS, the Health Insurance Association of America, and the Blue Cross and Blue Shield Association). These are 2 position alpha-numeric codes.

HCPCS Field

This is the area where you will find a particular alphanumeric code or a HCPCS modifier. "HCPCS" is an acronym (a word made out of the first letters of other words) that stands for *Health* Care Financing Administration (now known as CMS or Centers for Medicare and Medicaid Services) *Common Procedure Coding System.* You will see that the codes here mostly describe supplies used by medical providers (e.g., durable medical equipment, drugs for injections, surgical trays), but they also can and do describe some procedures or services (e.g., venipuncture).

HCPCS Long Description

This book contains all text of procedure or modifier long descriptions as of the date of printing. The AMA owns the copyright on the CPT codes and descriptions; CPT codes and descriptions are not public property and must always be used in compliance with copyright law.

HCPCS Coverage Code

This code denotes whether or not Medicare will cover it. 2010 codes include:

D	=	Special coverage instructions apply
I	=	Not payable by Medicare
M	=	Non-covered by Medicare
S	=	Non-covered by Medicare statute
C	=	Carrier judgment

HCPCS Action Code

A code denoting the change made to a procedure or modifier code within the HCPCS system. 2009 codes include:

A	=	Add procedure or modifier code
B	=	Change in both administrative data field and long description of procedure or modifier code
C	=	Change in long description of procedure or modifier code
D	=	Discontinue procedure or modifier code
F	=	Change in administrative data field of procedure or modifier code
N	=	No maintenance for this code
P	=	Payment change (MOG, pricing indicator codes, anesthesia base units, Ambulatory Surgical Centers)

R	=	Re-activate discontinued/deleted procedure or modifier code
S	=	Change in short description of procedure code
T	=	Miscellaneous change (BETOS, type of service)

HCPCS Pricing Indicator Code (PI)

These codes are used to identify the appropriate methodology for developing unique pricing amounts under the Part B portion of the Medicare program. A procedure may have one to four pricing codes. 2009 codes include:

00	=	Service not separately priced by part B (e.g., services not covered, bundled, used by part a only, etc.)

Physician Fee Schedule And Non-Physician Practitioners

Linked To The Physician Fee Schedule

11	=	Price established using national RVU's
12	=	Price established using national anesthesia base units
13	=	Price established by carriers (e.g., not otherwise classified, individual determination, carrier discretion)

Clinical Lab Fee Schedule

21	=	Price subject to national limitation amount
22	=	Price established by carriers (e.g., gap-fills, carrier established panels)

Durable Medical Equipment, Prosthetics, Orthotics, Supplies And Surgical Dressings

31	=	Frequently serviced DME (price subject to floors and ceilings)
32	=	Inexpensive & routinely purchased DME (price subject to floors and ceilings)
33	=	Oxygen and oxygen equipment (price subject to floors and ceilings)
34	=	DME supplies (price subject to floors and ceilings)
35	=	Surgical dressings (price subject to floors and ceilings)
36	=	Capped rental DME (price subject to floors and ceilings)
37	=	Ostomy, tracheostomy and urological supplies (price subject to floors and ceilings)
38	=	Orthotics, prosthetics, prosthetic devices & vision services (price subject to floors and ceilings)
39	=	Parenteral and Enteral Nutrition
45	=	Customized DME items
46	=	Carrier priced (e.g., not otherwise classified, individual determination, carrier discretion, gap-filled amounts)

Other

51	=	Drugs
52	=	Reasonable charge
53	=	Statute
54	=	Vaccinations
55	=	Priced by carriers under clinical psychologist fee schedule (not applicable as of January 1, 1998)
56	=	Priced by carriers under clinical social worker fee schedule (not applicable as of January 1, 1998)
57	=	Other carrier priced
99	=	Value not established

HCPCS Multiple Pricing Indicator Code (MPI)

These codes are used to identify instances where a procedure could be priced under multiple methodologies. 2010 MPI codes include:

9	=	Not applicable as HCPCS not priced separately by part B (pricing indicator is 00) or value is not established (pricing indicator is '99')
A	=	Not applicable as HCPCS priced under one methodology
B	=	Professional component of HCPCS priced using RVU's, while technical component and global service priced by Medicare part B carriers
C	=	Physician interpretation of clinical lab service is priced under physician fee schedule using RVU's, while pricing of lab service is paid under clinical lab fee schedule
D	=	Service performed by physician is priced under physician fee schedule using RVU's, while service performed by clinical psychologist is priced under clinical psychologist fee schedule (not applicable as of January 1, 1998)
E	=	Service performed by physician is priced under physician fee schedule using RVU's, service performed by clinical psychologist is priced under clinical psychologist's fee schedule and service performed by clinical social worker is priced under clinical social worker fee schedule (not applicable as of January 1, 1998)
F	=	Service performed by physician is priced under physician fee schedule by carriers, service performed by clinical psychologist is priced under clinical psychologist's fee schedule and service performed by clinical social worker is priced under clinical social worker fee schedule (not applicable as of January 1, 1998)
G	=	Clinical lab service priced under reasonable charge when service is submitted on claim with blood products, while service is priced under clinical lab fee schedule when there are no blood products on claim.

HCPCS Coverage Issues Manual Reference Section Number (CIM)

Number identifying the reference section of the coverage issues manual.

HCPCS Medicare Carriers Manual Reference Section Number (MCM

Number identifying a section of the Medicare carriers manual.

HCPCS Statute Number

Number identifying a statute reference for coverage or non-coverage of procedure or service.

HCPCS Lab Certification Code

These codes are used to classify laboratory procedures according to the specialty certification categories listed by CMS. Any generally certified laboratory (e.g., 100) may perform any of the tests in its subgroups (e.g., 110, 120, etc.). Lab certicication codes for 2010 include:

010	**Histocompatibility testing**	**300**	**Chemistry**	540	Antibody identification
100	**Microbiology**	310	Routine chemistry	550	Compatibility testing
110	Bacteriology	320	Urinalysis	560	Other immunohematology
115	Mycobacteriology	330	Endocrinology	**600**	**Pathology**
120	Mycology	340	Toxicology	610	Histopathology
130	Parasitology	350	Other chemistry	620	Oral pathology
140	Virology	**400**	**Hematology**	630	Cytology
150	Other microbiology	**500**	**Immunohematology**	**800**	**Radiobioassay**
200	**Diagnostic immunology**	510	Abo group & RH type	**900**	**Clinical cytogenetics**
210	Syphilis serology	520	Antibody detection (transfusion)		
220	General immunology	530	Antibody detection (nontransfusion)		

HCPCS Cross Reference Code (X-Ref)

An explicit reference cross walking a deleted code or a code that is not valid for Medicare to a valid current code (or range of codes).

HCPCS ASC Payment Group Code

The 'YY' indicator represents that this procedure is approved to be performed in an ambulatory surgical center. You must access the ASC tables on the mainframe or CMS website to get the dollar amounts. Please note that if the space is left blank, it is NOT Approved For Ambulatory Surgery Centers.

HCPCS ASC Payment Group Effective Date

The date the procedure is assigned to the ASC payment group.

HCPCS Processing Note Number

Number identifying the processing note contained in Appendix A of the HCPCS manual..

HCPCS Berenson-Eggers Type of Service Code

This field is valid beginning with 2003 data. The Berenson-Eggers Type of Service (BETOS) for the procedure code based on generally agreed upon clinically meaningful groupings of procedures and services.

M1A	Office visits - new	P5A	Ambulatory procedures - skin
M1B	Office visits - established	P5B	Ambulatory procedures - musculoskeletal
M2A	Hospital visit - initial	P5C	Ambulatory procedures - inguinal hernia repair
M2B	Hospital visit - subsequent	P5D	Ambulatory procedures - lithotripsy
M2C	Hospital visit - critical care	P5E	Ambulatory procedures - other
M3	Emergency room visit	P6A	Minor procedures - skin
M4A	Home visit	P6B	Minor procedures - musculoskeletal
M4B	Nursing home visit	P6C	Minor procedures - other (Medicare fee schedule)
M5A	Specialist - pathology	P6D	Minor procedures - other (non-Medicare fee schedule)
M5B	Specialist - psychiatry		
M5C	Specialist - opthamology	P7A	Oncology - radiation therapy
M5D	Specialist - other	P7B	Oncology - other
M6	Consultations	P8A	Endoscopy - arthroscopy
P0	Anesthesia	P8B	Endoscopy - upper gastrointestinal
P1A	Major procedure - breast	P8C	Endoscopy - sigmoidoscopy
P1B	Major procedure - colectomy	P8D	Endoscopy - colonoscopy
P1C	Major procedure - cholecystectomy	P8E	Endoscopy - cystoscopy
P1D	Major procedure - turp	P8F	Endoscopy - bronchoscopy
P1E	Major procedure - hysterectomy	P8G	Endoscopy - laparoscopic cholecystectomy
P1F	Major procedure - explor/decompr/excisdisc	P8H	Endoscopy - laryngoscopy
P1G	Major procedure - Other	P8I	Endoscopy - other
P2A	Major procedure, cardiovascular-CABG	P9A	Dialysis services (medicare fee schedule)
P2B	Major procedure, cardiovascular-Aneurysm repair	P9B	Dialysis services (non-medicare fee schedule)
P2C	Major Procedure, cardiovascular-Thromboendarterectomy	I1A	Standard imaging - chest
		I1B	Standard imaging - musculoskeletal
P2D	Major procedure, cardiovascualr-Coronary angioplasty (PTCA)	I1C	Standard imaging - breast
		I1D	Standard imaging - contrast gastrointestinal
P2E	Major procedure, cardiovascular-Pacemaker insertion	I1E	Standard imaging - nuclear medicine
P2F	Major procedure, cardiovascular-Other	I1F	Standard imaging - other
P3A	Major procedure, orthopedic - Hip fracture repair	I2A	Advanced imaging - CAT/CT/CTA: brain/head/neck
P3B	Major procedure, orthopedic - Hip replacement	I2B	Advanced imaging - CAT/CT/CTA: other
P3C	Major procedure, orthopedic - Knee replacement	I2C	Advanced imaging - MRI/MRA: brain/head/neck
P3D	Major procedure, orthopedic - other	I2D	Advanced imaging - MRI/MRA: other
P4A	Eye procedure - corneal transplant	I3A	Echography/ultrasonography - eye
P4B	Eye procedure - cataract removal/lens insertion	I3B	Echography/ultrasonography - abdomen/pelvis
P4C	Eye procedure - retinal detachment	I3C	Echography/ultrasonography - heart
P4D	Eye procedure - treatment of retinal lesions	I3D	Echography/ultrasonography - carotid arteries
P4E	Eye procedure - other	I3E	Echography/ultrasonography - prostate, transrectal

I3F	Echography/ultrasonography - other	D1B	Hospital beds
I4A	Imaging/procedure - heart including cardiac catheterization	D1C	Oxygen and supplies
		D1D	Wheelchairs
I4B	Imaging/procedure - other	D1E	Other DME
T1A	Lab tests - routine venipuncture (non Medicare fee schedule)	D1F	Prosthetic/Orthotic devices
		D1G	Drugs Administered through DME
T1B	Lab tests - automated general profiles	O1A	Ambulance
T1C	Lab tests - urinalysis	O1B	Chiropractic
T1D	Lab tests - blood counts	O1C	Enteral and parenteral
T1E	Lab tests - glucose	O1D	Chemotherapy
T1F	Lab tests - bacterial cultures	O1E	Other drugs
T1G	Lab tests - other (Medicare fee schedule)	O1F	Hearing and speech services
T1H	Lab tests - other (non-Medicare fee schedule)	O1G	Immunizations/Vaccinations
T2A	Other tests - electrocardiograms	Y1	Other - Medicare fee schedule
T2B	Other tests - cardiovascular stress tests	Y2	Other - non-Medicare fee schedule
T2C	Other tests - EKG monitoring	Z1	Local codes
T2D	Other tests - other	Z2	Undefined codes
D1A	Medical/surgical supplies		

HCPCS Type of Service Code

The carrier assigned CMS type of service which describes the particular kind(s) of   service represented by the procedure code.

1	Medical care	H	Hospice services (discontinued 01/95)
2	Surgery	I	Purchase of DME (installment basis) (discontinued 04/95)
3	Consultation	J	Diabetic shoes (eff. 04/95)
4	Diagnostic radiology	K	Hearing items and services (eff. 04/95)
5	Diagnostic laboratory	L	ESRD supplies (eff. 04/95) (renal supplier in the home before 04/95)
6	Therapeutic radiology		
7	Anesthesia	M	Monthly capitation payment for dialysis
8	Assistant at surgery	N	Kidney donor
9	Other medical items or services	P	Lump sum purchase of DME, prosthetics, orthotics
0	Whole blood only eff. 01/96, whole blood or packed red cells before 01/96	Q	Vision items or services
A	Used durable medical equipment (DME)	R	Rental of DME
B	High risk screening mammography (obsolete 1/1/98)	S	Surgical dressings or other medical supplies (eff. 04/95)
C	Low risk screening mammography (obsolete 1/1/98)	T	Psychological therapy (term. 12/31/97) outpatient mental health limitation (eff. 1/1/98)
D	Ambulance (eff. 04/95)	U	Occupational therapy
E	Enteral/parenteral nutrients/supplies (eff. 04/95)	V	Pneumococcal/flu vaccine (eff. 01/96), Pneumococcal/flu/hepatitis B vaccine (eff. 04/95-12/95), Pneumococcal only before 04/95
F	Ambulatory surgical center (facility usage for surgical services)	W	Physical therapy
G	Immunosuppressive drugs	Y	Second opinion on elective surgery (obsoleted 1/97)
		Z	Third opinion on elective surgery (obsoleted 1/97)

HCPCS Anesthesia Base Unit Quantity

The base unit represents the level of intensity for anesthesia procedure services that reflects all activities except time. These activities include usual preoperative and post-operative visits, the administration of fluids and/or blood incident to anesthesia care, and monitoring procedures.

(Note: the payment amount for anesthesia services is based on a calculation using base unit, time units, and the conversion factor.)

HCPCS Code Added Date

The year the HCPCS code was added to the Healthcare common procedure coding system.

HCPCS Action Effective Date

Effective date of action to a procedure or modifier code

HCPCS Termination Date

Last date for which a procedure or modifier code may be used by Medicare providers.

HCPCS MOG Payment Group Code

Medicare outpatient groups (MOG) payment group code. Please note that this HCPCS book does not contain the MOG payment group codes. For additional information, visit the CMS website.

COMMENTS:

1st digit indicates the body system

2nd digit is sequential numbering within the body system

3rd digit is the level of intensity where:

'1', '2', '3' or '4' represents levels for a given group type

'0' and '9' represent single level for a given group type

000   No MOG applies

Integumentary

102	Level II needle biopsy/aspiration
112	Level II incision and drainage
132	Level II debridement/destruction
142	Level II excision/biopsy
143	Level III excision/biopsy
151	Level I skin repair
152	Level II skin repair
153	Level III skin repair
160	Incision/excision breast
169	Breast reconstruction/mastectomy

Musculoskeletal

201	Level I skull and facial bone procedures
202	Level II skull and facial bone procedures
211	Level I hand musculoskeletal procedures
212	Level II hand musculoskeletal procedures
221	Level I foot musculoskeletal procedures
222	Level II foot musculoskeletal procedures
231	Level I musculoskeletal procedures
232	Level II musculoskeletal procedures
233	Level III musculoskeletal procedures
241	Level I arthroscopy
242	Level II arthroscopy
260	Closed treatment fracture finger/toe/trunk
269	Closed treatment fracture/dislocation/except finger/toe/trunk
270	Open/percutaneous treatment fracture or dislocation
279	Bone/joint manipulation under anesthesia
280	Bunion procedures
289	Arthroplasty
290	Arthroplasty with prosthesis

<u>ENT/Respiratory/Cardiovascular/Lymphatic/Endocrine</u>
302   Level II ENT procedures
303   Level III ENT procedures
304   Level IV ENT procedures
309   Implantation of cochlear device (ASC rate does not include cost of implant)
310   Nasal cauterization/packing
319   Tonsil/adenoid procedures
322   Level II endoscopy upper airway
323   Level III endoscopy upper airway
329   Endoscopy lower airway
330   Thoracentesis/lavage procedures
350   Placement transvenous caths/cutdown
359   Removal/revision, pacemaker/vascular device
360   Vascular ligation
369   Vascular repair/fistula construction
370   Lymph node excisions
379   Thyroid/lymphadenectomy procedures

<u>Digestive</u>
400   Esophageal dilation without endoscopy
410   Esophagoscopy
421   Level I upper GI endoscopy/intubation
422   Level II upper GI endoscopy/intubation
429   Lower GI endoscopy
430   Anoscopy and diagnostic sigmoidoscopy
439   Therapeutic proctosigmoidoscopy
440   Small intestine endoscopy
449   Percutaneous biliary endoscopic procedures
450   Endoscopic retrograde cholangio-pancreatography (ERCP)
460   Hernia/hydrocele procedures
472   Level II anal/rectal procedures
473   Level III anal/rectal procedures
480   Peritoneal and abdominal procedures
490   Tube procedures

<u>Urinary/Genital</u>
501   Level I laparoscopy
502   Level II laparoscopy
509   Lithotripsy
511   Level I cystourethroscopy and other genitourinary procedures
512   Level II cystourethroscopy and other genitourinary procedures
513   Level III cystourethroscopy and other genitourinary procedures
521   Level I urethral procedures
522   Level II urethral procedures
530   Circumcision
539   Penile procedures
540   Insertion of penile prosthesis (ASC rate does include cost of implant)
549   Testes/epididymis procedures
550   Prostrate biopsy
562   Level II female reproductive procedures
563   Level III female reproductive procedures
570   Surgical hysteroscopy
579   D & C
580   Spontaneous abortion
589   Therapeutic abortion

<u>Nervous/Eye</u>
602   Level II nervous system injections
609   Revision/removal neurological device
610   Implantation of neurostimulator electrodes (ASC rate does not include cost of implant)
619   Implantation of neurological devices (asc rate does not include cost of implant)

621   Level I nerve procedures
622   Level II nerve procedures
629   Spinal tap
639   Laser eye procedures except retinal
640   Cataract procedures
649   Cataract procedures with IOL insert (includes $150 insert)
651   Level I anterior segment eye procedures
652   Level II anterior segment eye procedures
659   Corneal transplant (ASC rate includes price of transplant)
660   Posterior segment eye procedures
669   Strabismus/muscle procedures
673   Level III eye procedure
674   Level IV eye procedure
680   Vitrectomy
689   Implantation/replacement of intraitreal drug

HCPCS MOG Payment Policy Indicator

Indicator identifying whether a HCPCS code is subject to payment of an ASC facility fee, to a separate fee under another provision of Medicare, or to no fee at all. Codes for 2009 are listed below. Please note that this HCPCS book does not contain the MOG payment policy indicators. For more information, visit the CMS website.

1   ASC covered procedure
2   Bundled service/no separate payment
3   Excluded from ASC list
4   Invalid code/90 day grace period
6   Separate payment when furnished in an ASC
7   ASC restricted coverage procedure
9   ASC payment not applicable

HCPCS MOG Effective Date

The date the procedure is assigned to the Medicare outpatient group (MOG) payment group. Please note that this HCPCS book does not contain the MOG effective dates. For more information, visit the CMS website.

(CMS)

CENTERS FOR MEDICARE & MEDICAID SERVICES

2010
ALPHANUMERIC
HEALTH CARE PROCEDURE CODING SYSTEM
(HCPCS)

As of October 31, 2009*

*Quarterly updates are available at no charge from the CMS website

Modifiers

HCPCS Code	Long Description	Coverage	Action	PI	MPI	CIM	MCM
A1	DRESSING FOR ONE WOUND	C	N				
A2	DRESSING FOR TWO WOUNDS	C	N				
A3	DRESSING FOR THREE WOUNDS	C	N				
A4	DRESSING FOR FOUR WOUNDS	C	N				
A5	DRESSING FOR FIVE WOUNDS	C	N				
A6	DRESSING FOR SIX WOUNDS	C	N				
A7	DRESSING FOR SEVEN WOUNDS	C	N				
A8	DRESSING FOR EIGHT WOUNDS	C	N				
A9	DRESSING FOR NINE OR MORE WOUNDS	C	N				
AA	ANESTHESIA SERVICES PERFORMED PERSONALLY BY ANESTHESIOLOGIST	D	N				3350.5
AD	MEDICAL SUPERVISION BY A PHYSICIAN: MORE THAN FOUR CONCURRENT ANESTHESIA PROCEDURES	D	N				3350.5
AE	REGISTERED DIETICIAN	C	N				
AF	SPECIALTY PHYSICIAN	C	N				
AG	PRIMARY PHYSICIAN	C	N				
AH	CLINICAL PSYCHOLOGIST	D	N				21,505,112
AI	PRINCIPAL PHYSICIAN OF RECORD	C	A				
AJ	CLINICAL SOCIAL WORKER	D	N				21,525,113
AK	NON PARTICIPATING PHYSICIAN	C	N				
AM	PHYSICIAN, TEAM MEMBER SERVICE	D	N				4105.7
AP	DETERMINATION OF REFRACTIVE STATE WAS NOT PERFORMED IN THE COURSE OF DIAGNOSTIC OPHTHALMOLOGICAL EXAMINATION	C	N				
AQ	PHYSICIAN PROVIDING A SERVICE IN AN UNLISTED HEALTH PROFESSIONAL SHORTAGE AREA (HPSA)	C	N				
AR	PHYSICIAN PROVIDER SERVICES IN A PHYSICIAN SCARCITY AREA	C	N				
AS	PHYSICIAN ASSISTANT, NURSE PRACTITIONER, OR CLINICAL NURSE SPECIALIST SERVICES FOR ASSISTANT AT SURGERY	C	N				
AT	ACUTE TREATMENT (THIS MODIFIER SHOULD BE USED WHEN REPORTING SERVICE 98940, 98941, 98942)	C	N				
AU	ITEM FURNISHED IN CONJUNCTION WITH A UROLOGICAL, OSTOMY, OR TRACHEOSTOMY SUPPLY	C	N				
AV	ITEM FURNISHED IN CONJUNCTION WITH A PROSTHETIC DEVICE, PROSTHETIC OR ORTHOTIC	C	N				
AW	ITEM FURNISHED IN CONJUNCTION WITH A SURGICAL DRESSING	C	N				
AX	ITEM FURNISHED IN CONJUNCTION WITH DIALYSIS SERVICES	C	N				
BA	ITEM FURNISHED IN CONJUNCTION WITH PARENTERAL ENTERAL NUTRITION (PEN) SERVICES	C	N				
BL	SPECIAL ACQUISITION OF BLOOD AND BLOOD PRODUCTS	C	N				
BO	ORALLY ADMINISTERED NUTRITION, NOT BY FEEDING TUBE	C	N				
BP	THE BENEFICIARY HAS BEEN INFORMED OF THE PURCHASE AND RENTAL OPTIONS AND HAS ELECTED TO PURCHASE THE ITEM	C	N				
BR	THE BENEFICIARY HAS BEEN INFORMED OF THE PURCHASE AND RENTAL OPTIONS AND HAS ELECTED TO RENT THE ITEM	C	N				

HCPCS Code	Statute	Lab Cert	X-Ref	ASC Pay Grp	ASC Pay Group Eff. Date	Proc Notes	BETOS	TOS	Anest	Code Add Date	Code Effective Date	Code Term Date
A1									0	20020701	20020701	
A2									0	20020701	20020701	
A3									0	20020701	20020701	
A4									0	20020701	20020701	
A5									0	20020701	20020701	
A6									0	20020701	20020701	
A7									0	20020701	20020701	
A8									0	20020701	20020701	
A9									0	20020701	20020701	
AA									0	19840101	20010101	
AD									0	19840101	20010101	
AE									0	20050101	20050101	
AF									0	20050101	20050101	
AG									0	20050101	20050101	
AH									0	19910101	19970101	
AI									0	20100101	20100101	
AJ									0	19910101	19970101	
AK									0	20050101	20050101	
AM			QM			0069			0	19910101	19970101	
AP									0	19840101	19970101	
AQ									0	20060101	20060101	
AR									0	20050101	20050101	
AS						0069			0	19880101	19990101	
AT									0	19840101	19980101	
AU									0	20030101	20030101	
AV									0	20030101	20030101	
AW									0	20030101	20030101	
AX						0000			0	20030101	20030101	
BA									0	20030101	20030101	
BL									0	20050701	20050701	
BO									0	20030101	20030101	
BP									0	19920101	19970101	
BP												
BR									0	19920101	19970101	
BR												

HCPCS Code	Long Description	Coverage	Action	PI	MPI	CIM	MCM
BU	THE BENEFICIARY HAS BEEN INFORMED OF THE PURCHASE AND RENTAL OPTIONS AND AFTER 30 DAYS HAS NOT INFORMED THE SUPPLIER OF HIS/HER DECISION	C	N				
CA	PROCEDURE PAYABLE ONLY IN THE INPATIENT SETTING WHEN PERFORMED EMERGENTLY ON ANOUTPATIENT WHO EXPIRES PRIOR TO ADMISSION	C	N				
CB	SERVICE ORDERED BY A RENAL DIALYSIS FACILITY (RDF) PHYSICIAN AS PART OF THE ESRD BENEFICIARY'S DIALYSIS BENEFIT, IS NOT PART OF THE COMPOSITE RATE, AND IS SEPARATELY REIMBURSABLE	C	N				
CC	PROCEDURE CODE CHANGE (USE 'CC' WHEN THE PROCEDURE CODE SUBMITTED WAS CHANGED EITHER FOR ADMINISTRATIVE REASONS OR BECAUSE AN INCORRECT CODE WAS FILED)	C	N				
CD	AMCC TEST HAS BEEN ORDERED BY AN ESRD FACILITY OR MCP PHYSICIAN THAT IS PART OF THE COMPOSITE RATE AND IS NOT SEPARATELY BILLABLE	D	N				4270.2
CE	AMCC TEST HAS BEEN ORDERED BY AN ESRD FACILITY OR MCP PHYSICIAN THAT IS A COMPOSITE RATE TEST BUT IS BEYOND THE NORMAL FREQUENCY COVERED UNDER THE RATE AND IS SEPARATELY REIMBURSABLE BASED ON MEDICAL NECESSITY	D	N				4270.2
CF	AMCC TEST HAS BEEN ORDERED BY AN ESRD FACILITY OR MCP PHYSICIAN THAT IS NOT PART OF THE COMPOSITE RATE AND IS SEPARATELY BILLABLE	D	N				4270.2
CG	POLICY CRITERIA APPLIED	C	N				
CR	CATASTROPHE/DISASTER RELATED	C	N				
E1	UPPER LEFT, EYELID	C	N				
E2	LOWER LEFT, EYELID	C	N				
E3	UPPER RIGHT, EYELID	C	N				
E4	LOWER RIGHT, EYELID	C	N				
EA	ERYTHROPOETIC STIMULATING AGENT (ESA) ADMINISTERED TO TREAT ANEMIA DUE TO ANTI-CANCER CHEMOTHERAPY	D	N				
EB	ERYTHROPOETIC STIMULATING AGENT (ESA) ADMINISTERED TO TREAT ANEMIA DUE TO ANTI-CANCER RADIOTHERAPY	D	N				
EC	ERYTHROPOETIC STIMULATING AGENT (ESA) ADMINISTERED TO TREAT ANEMIA NOT DUE TO ANTI-CANCER RADIOTHERAPY OR ANTI-CANCER CHEMOTHERAPY	D	N				
ED	HEMATOCRIT LEVEL HAS EXCEEDED 39% (OR HEMOGLOBIN LEVEL HAS EXCEEDED 13.0 G/DL) FOR 3 OR MORE CONSECUTIVE BILLING CYCLES IMMEDIATELY PRIOR TO AND INCLUDING THE CURRENT CYCLE	D	N				
EE	HEMATOCRIT LEVEL HAS NOT EXCEEDED 39% (OR HEMOGLOBIN LEVEL HAS NOT EXCEEDED 13.0 G/DL) FOR 3 OR MORE CONSECUTIVE BILLING CYCLES IMMEDIATELY PRIOR TO AND INCLUDING THE CURRENT CYCLE	D	N				
EJ	SUBSEQUENT CLAIMS FOR A DEFINED COURSE OF THERAPY, E.G., EPO, SODIUM HYALURONATE, INFLIXIMAB	D	N				4273.2
EM	EMERGENCY RESERVE SUPPLY (FOR ESRD BENEFIT ONLY)	D	N				3045.7

HCPCS Code	Statute	Lab Cert	X-Ref	ASC Pay Grp	ASC Pay Group Eff. Date	Proc Notes	BETOS	TOS	Anest	Code Add Date	Code Effective Date	Code Term Date
BU									0	19920101	19970101	
CA									0	20030101	20030101	
CB									0	20030401	20040101	
CC									0	19900101	19970101	
CD									0	20040101	20040101	
CE									0	20040101	20040101	
CF									0	20040101	20040101	
CG									0	20080701	20080701	
CR									0	20050821	20050821	
E1									0	19950101	19990101	
E2									0	19950101	19990101	
E3									0	19950101	19990101	
E4									0	19950101	19990101	
EA						0147			0	20080101	20080101	
EB						0147			0	20080101	20080101	
EC						0147			0	20080101	20080101	
ED						0145			0	20080101	20080101	
EE						0145			0	20080101	20080101	
EJ									0	19910101	20000101	
EM									0	19910101	19970101	

HCPCS Code	Long Description	Coverage	Action	PI	MPI	CIM	MCM
EP	SERVICE PROVIDED AS PART OF MEDICAID EARLY PERIODIC SCREENING DIAGNOSIS AND TREATMENT (EPSDT) PROGRAM	C	N				
ET	EMERGENCY SERVICES	C	N				
EY	NO PHYSICIAN OR OTHER LICENSED HEALTH CARE PROVIDER ORDER FOR THIS ITEM OR SERVICE	C	N				
F1	LEFT HAND, SECOND DIGIT	C	N				
F2	LEFT HAND, THIRD DIGIT	C	N				
F3	LEFT HAND, FOURTH DIGIT	C	N				
F4	LEFT HAND, FIFTH DIGIT	C	N				
F5	RIGHT HAND, THUMB	C	N				
F6	RIGHT HAND, SECOND DIGIT	C	N				
F7	RIGHT HAND, THIRD DIGIT	C	N				
F8	RIGHT HAND, FOURTH DIGIT	C	N				
F9	RIGHT HAND, FIFTH DIGIT	C	N				
FA	LEFT HAND, THUMB	C	N				
FB	ITEM PROVIDED WITHOUT COST TO PROVIDER, SUPPLIER OR PRACTITIONER, OR FULL CREDIT RECEIVED FOR REPLACED DEVICE (EXAMPLES, BUT NOT LIMITED TO, COVERED UNDER WARRANTY, REPLACED DUE TO DEFECT, FREE SAMPLES)	I	N				
FC	PARTIAL CREDIT RECEIVED FOR REPLACED DEVICE	D	N				
FP	SERVICE PROVIDED AS PART OF FAMILY PLANNING PROGRAM	C	N				
G1	MOST RECENT URR READING OF LESS THAN 60	C	N				
G2	MOST RECENT URR READING OF 60 TO 64.9	C	N				
G3	MOST RECENT URR READING OF 65 TO 69.9	C	N				
G4	MOST RECENT URR READING OF 70 TO 74.9	C	N				
G5	MOST RECENT URR READING OF 75 OR GREATER	C	N				
G6	ESRD PATIENT FOR WHOM LESS THAN SIX DIALYSIS SESSIONS HAVE BEEN PROVIDED IN A MONTH	C	N				
G7	PREGNANCY RESULTED FROM RAPE OR INCEST OR PREGNANCY CERTIFIED BY PHYSICIAN AS LIFE THREATENING	D	N			35-99	2005.1
G8	MONITORED ANESTHESIA CARE (MAC) FOR DEEP COMPLEX, COMPLICATED, OR MARKEDLY INVASIVE SURGICAL PROCEDURE	C	N				
G9	MONITORED ANESTHESIA CARE FOR PATIENT WHO HAS HISTORY OF SEVERE CARDIO-PULMONARY CONDITION	C	N				
GA	WAIVER OF LIABILITY STATEMENT ON FILE	C	N				
GB	CLAIM BEING RE-SUBMITTED FOR PAYMENT BECAUSE IT IS NO LONGER COVERED UNDER A GLOBAL PAYMENT DEMONSTRATION	C	N				
GC	THIS SERVICE HAS BEEN PERFORMED IN PART BY A RESIDENT UNDER THE DIRECTION OF A TEACHING PHYSICIAN	D	N				3350.5, 4116
GD	UNITS OF SERVICE EXCEEDS MEDICALLY UNLIKELY EDIT VALUE AND REPRESENTS REASONABLE AND NECESSARY SERVICES	C	N				
GE	THIS SERVICE HAS BEEN PERFORMED BY A RESIDENT WITHOUT THE PRESENCE OF A TEACHING PHYSICIAN UNDER THE PRIMARY CARE EXCEPTION	D	N				4116

HCPCS Code	Statute	Lab Cert	X-Ref	ASC Pay Grp	ASC Pay Group Eff. Date	Proc Notes	BETOS	TOS	Anest	Code Add Date	Code Effective Date	Code Term Date
EP									0	19870101	19970101	
ET									0	19840101	20020101	
EY									0	20030101	20030101	
F1									0	19950101	19990101	
F2									0	19950101	19990101	
F3									0	19950101	19990101	
F4									0	19950101	19990101	
F5									0	19950101	19990101	
F6									0	19950101	19990101	
F7									0	19950101	19990101	
F8									0	19950101	19990101	
F9									0	19950101	19990101	
FA									0	19950101	19990101	
FB									0	20060101	20080101	
FC						0143			0	20080101	20080101	
FP									0	19870101	20050101	
G1									0	19970101	19980101	
G2									0	19970101	19980101	
G3									0	19970101	19980101	
G4									0	19970101	19970101	
G5									0	19970101	19980101	
G6									0	19980501	19980501	
G7						0084			0	19990701	19990701	
G8						0083			0	19990701	19990701	
G9									0	19990701	19990701	
GA									0	19950101	19970101	
GB									0	20020101	20020101	
GC									0	19970101	20010101	
GC												
GD									0	20080101	20080101	
GE									0	19970101	19970101	

HCPCS Code	Long Description	Coverage	Action	PI	MPI	CIM	MCM
GF	NON-PHYSICIAN (E.G. NURSE PRACTITIONER (NP), CERTIFIED REGISTERED NURSE ANESTHETIST (CRNA), CERTIFIED REGISTERED NURSE (CRN), CLINICAL NURSE SPECIALIST (CNS), PHYSICIAN ASSISTANT (PA)) SERVICES IN A CRITICAL ACCESS HOSPITAL	C	N				
GG	PERFORMANCE AND PAYMENT OF A SCREENING MAMMOGRAM AND DIAGNOSTIC MAMMOGRAM ON THE SAME PATIENT, SAME DAY	C	N				
GH	DIAGNOSTIC MAMMOGRAM CONVERTED FROM SCREENING MAMMOGRAM ON SAME DAY	C	N				
GJ	"OPT OUT" PHYSICIAN OR PRACTITIONER EMERGENCY OR URGENT SERVICE	C	N				
GK	REASONABLE AND NECESSARY ITEM/SERVICE ASSOCIATED WITH A GA OR GZ MODIFIER	C	N				
GL	MEDICALLY UNNECESSARY UPGRADE PROVIDED INSTEAD OF NON-UPGRADED ITEM, NO CHARGE, NO ADVANCE BENEFICIARY NOTICE (ABN)	C	N				
GM	MULTIPLE PATIENTS ON ONE AMBULANCE TRIP	C	N				
GN	SERVICES DELIVERED UNDER AN OUTPATIENT SPEECH LANGUAGE PATHOLOGY PLAN OF CARE	C	N				
GO	SERVICES DELIVERED UNDER AN OUTPATIENT OCCUPATIONAL THERAPY PLAN OF CARE	C	N				
GP	SERVICES DELIVERED UNDER AN OUTPATIENT PHYSICAL THERAPY PLAN OF CARE	C	N				
GQ	VIA ASYNCHRONOUS TELECOMMUNICATIONS SYSTEM	C	N				
GR	THIS SERVICE WAS PERFORMED IN WHOLE OR IN PART BY A RESIDENT IN A DEPARTMENT OF VETERANS AFFAIRS MEDICAL CENTER OR CLINIC, SUPERVISED IN ACCORDANCE WITH VA POLICY	C	N				
GS	DOSAGE OF EPO OR DARBEPOIETIN ALFA HAS BEEN REDUCED AND MAINTAINED IN RESPONSE TO HEMATOCRIT OR HEMOGLOBIN LEVEL	D	N				4273.1
GT	VIA INTERACTIVE AUDIO AND VIDEO TELECOMMUNICATION SYSTEMS	D	N				
GV	ATTENDING PHYSICIAN NOT EMPLOYED OR PAID UNDER ARRANGEMENT BY THE PATIENT'S HOSPICE PROVIDER	D	N				4175-5
GW	SERVICE NOT RELATED TO THE HOSPICE PATIENT'S TERMINAL CONDITION	D	N				4175-5
GY	ITEM OR SERVICE STATUTORILY EXCLUDED, DOES NOT MEET THE DEFINITION OF ANY MEDICARE BENEFIT OR, FOR NON-MEDICARE INSURERS, IS NOT A CONTRACT BENEFIT	S	N				
GZ	ITEM OR SERVICE EXPECTED TO BE DENIED AS NOT REASONABLE AND NECESSARY	M	N				2000
H9	COURT-ORDERED	I	N				
HA	CHILD/ADOLESCENT PROGRAM	I	N				
HB	ADULT PROGRAM, NON GERIATRIC	I	N				
HC	ADULT PROGRAM, GERIATRIC	I	N				
HD	PREGNANT/PARENTING WOMEN'S PROGRAM	I	N				
HE	MENTAL HEALTH PROGRAM	I	N				

HCPCS Code	Statute	Lab Cert	X-Ref	ASC Pay Grp	ASC Pay Group Eff. Date	Proc Notes	BETOS	TOS	Anest	Code Add Date	Code Effective Date	Code Term Date
GF									0	20030401	20030401	
GG									0	20020101	20020101	
GH									0	19981001	19981001	
GJ									0	19981001	19981001	
GK									0	20020101	20080101	
GL									0	20020101	20080101	
GM									0	20020101	20020101	
GN									0	19990101	20030101	
GO									0	19990101	20030101	
GP									0	19990101	20030101	
GQ									0	20011001	20011001	
GR									0	20060101	20060101	
GS									0	20060101	20061001	
GT						0073			0	19990101	19990101	
GV									0	20020101	20020101	
GW									0	20020101	20020101	
GY									0	20020101	20070701	
GZ									0	20020101	20020101	
H9									0	20030101	20030101	
HA									0	20030101	20030101	
HB									0	20030101	20030101	
HC									0	20030101	20030101	
HD									0	20030101	20030101	
HE									0	20030101	20030101	

HCPCS Code	Long Description	Coverage	Action	PI	MPI	CIM	MCM
HF	SUBSTANCE ABUSE PROGRAM	I	N				
HG	OPIOID ADDICTION TREATMENT PROGRAM	I	N				
HH	INTEGRATED MENTAL HEALTH/SUBSTANCE ABUSE PROGRAM	I	N				
HI	INTEGRATED MENTAL HEALTH AND MENTAL RETARDATION/ DEVELOPMENTAL DISABILITIES PROGRAM	I	N				
HJ	EMPLOYEE ASSISTANCE PROGRAM	I	N				
HK	SPECIALIZED MENTAL HEALTH PROGRAMS FOR HIGH-RISK POPULATIONS	I	N				
HL	INTERN	I	N				
HM	LESS THAN BACHELOR DEGREE LEVEL	I	N				
HN	BACHELORS DEGREE LEVEL	I	N				
HO	MASTERS DEGREE LEVEL	I	N				
HP	DOCTORAL LEVEL	I	N				
HQ	GROUP SETTING	I	N				
HR	FAMILY/COUPLE WITH CLIENT PRESENT	I	N				
HS	FAMILY/COUPLE WITHOUT CLIENT PRESENT	I	N				
HT	MULTI-DISCIPLINARY TEAM	I	N				
HU	FUNDED BY CHILD WELFARE AGENCY	I	N				
HV	FUNDED STATE ADDICTIONS AGENCY	I	N				
HW	FUNDED BY STATE MENTAL HEALTH AGENCY	I	N				
HX	FUNDED BY COUNTY/LOCAL AGENCY	I	N				
HY	FUNDED BY JUVENILE JUSTICE AGENCY	I	N				
HZ	FUNDED BY CRIMINAL JUSTICE AGENCY	I	N				
J1	COMPETITIVE ACQUISITION PROGRAM NO-PAY SUBMISSION FOR A PRESCRIPTION NUMBER	C	N				
J2	COMPETITIVE ACQUISITION PROGRAM, RESTOCKING OF EMERGENCY DRUGS AFTER EMERGENCY ADMINISTRATION	C	N				
J3	COMPETITIVE ACQUISITION PROGRAM (CAP), DRUG NOT AVAILABLE THROUGH CAP AS WRITTEN, REIMBURSED UNDER AVERAGE SALES PRICE METHODOLOGY	C	N				
J4	DMEPOS ITEM SUBJECT TO DMEPOS COMPETITIVE BIDDING PROGRAM THAT IS FURNISHED BY A HOSPITAL UPON DISCHARGE	C	A				
JA	ADMINISTERED INTRAVENOUSLY	C	N				
JB	ADMINISTERED SUBCUTANEOUSLY	C	N				
JC	SKIN SUBSTITUTE USED AS A GRAFT	C	N				
JD	SKIN SUBSTITUTE NOT USED AS A GRAFT	C	N				
JW	DRUG AMT. DISCARDED/NOT ADMINISTERED TO ANY PATIENT	C	N				
K0	LOWER EXTREMITY PROSTHESIS FUNCTIONAL LEVEL 0 - DOES NOT HAVE THE ABILITY OR POTENTIAL TO AMBULATE OR TRANSFER SAFELY WITH OR WITHOUT ASSISTANCE AND A PROSTHESIS DOES NOT ENHANCE THEIR QUALITY OF LIFE OR MOBILITY.	C	N				
K1	LOWER EXTREMITY PROSTHESIS FUNCTIONAL LEVEL 1 - HAS THE ABILITY OR POTENTIAL TO USE A PROSTHESIS FOR TRANSFERS OR AMBULATION ON LEVEL SURFACES AT FIXED CADENCE. TYPICAL OF THE LIMITED AND UNLIMITED HOUSEHOLD AMBULATOR.	C	N				

HCPCS Code	Statute	Lab Cert	X-Ref	ASC Pay Grp	ASC Pay Group Eff. Date	Proc Notes	BETOS	TOS	Anest	Code Add Date	Code Effective Date	Code Term Date
HF									0	20030101	20030101	
HG									0	20030101	20030101	
HH									0	20030101	20030101	
HI									0	20030101	20030101	
HJ									0	20030101	20030101	
HK									0	20030101	20030101	
HL									0	20030101	20030101	
HM									0	20030101	20030101	
HN									0	20030101	20030101	
HO									0	20030101	20030101	
HP									0	20030101	20030101	
HQ									0	20030101	20030101	
HR									0	20030101	20030101	
HS									0	20030101	20030101	
HT									0	20030101	20030101	
HU									0	20030101	20030101	
HV									0	20030101	20030101	
HW									0	20030101	20030101	
HX									0	20030101	20030101	
HY									0	20030101	20030101	
HZ									0	20030101	20030101	
J1									0	20060101	20060101	
J2									0	20060101	20060101	
J3									0	20060101	20060101	
J4									0	20100101	20100101	
JA									0	20070101	20070101	
JB									0	20070101	20070101	
JC									0	20090101	20090101	
JD									0	20090101	20090101	
JW									0	20030101	20030101	
K0									0	19930101	20030101	
K1									0	19930101	19970101	

HCPCS Code	Long Description	Coverage	Action	PI	MPI	CIM	MCM
K2	LOWER EXTREMITY PROSTHESIS FUNCTIONAL LEVEL 2 - HAS THE ABILITY OR POTENTIAL FOR AMBULATION WITH THE ABILITY TO TRAVERSE LOW LEVEL ENVIRONMENTAL BARRIERS SUCH AS CURBS, STAIRS OR UNEVEN SURFACES. TYPICAL OF THE LIMITED COMMUNITYAMBULATOR.	C	N				
K3	LOWER EXTREMITY PROSTHESIS FUNCTIONAL LEVEL 3 - HAS THE ABILITY OR POTENTIAL FOR AMBULATION WITH VARIABLE CADENCE. TYPICAL OF THE COMMUNITY AMBULATOR WHO HAS THE ABILITY TO TRANSVERSE MOST ENVIRONMENTAL BARRIERS AND MAY HAVE VOCATIONAL, THERAPEUTIC, OR EXERCISE ACTIVITY THAT DEMANDS PROSTHETICUTILIZATION BEYOND SIMPLE LOCOMOTION.	C	N				
K4	LOWER EXTREMITY PROSTHESIS FUNCTIONAL LEVEL 4 - HAS THE ABILITY OR POTENTIAL FOR PROSTHETIC AMBULATION THAT EXCEEDS THE BASIC AMBULATION SKILLS, EXHIBITING HIGH IMPACT, STRESS, OR ENERGY LEVELS, TYPICAL OF THE PROSTHETIC DEMANDS OF THE CHILD, ACTIVE ADULT, OR ATHLETE.	C	N				
KA	ADD ON OPTION/ACCESSORY FOR WHEELCHAIR	C	N				
KB	BENEFICIARY REQUESTED UPGRADE FOR ABN, MORE THAN 4 MODIFIERS IDENTIFIED ON CLAIM	C	N				
KC	REPLACEMENT OF SPECIAL POWER WHEELCHAIR INTERFACE	C	N				
KD	DRUG OR BIOLOGICAL INFUSED THROUGH DME	C	N				
KE	BID UNDER ROUND ONE OF THE DMEPOS COMPETITIVE BIDDING PROGRAM FOR USE WITH NON-COMPETITIVE BID BASE EQUIPMENT	C	N				
KF	ITEM DESIGNATED BY FDA AS CLASS III DEVICE	C	N				
KG	DMEPOS ITEM SUBJECT TO DMEPOS COMPETITIVE BIDDING PROGRAM NUMBER 1	C	N				
KH	DMEPOS ITEM, INITIAL CLAIM, PURCHASE OR FIRST MONTH RENTAL	C	N				
KI	DMEPOS ITEM, SECOND OR THIRD MONTH RENTAL	C	N				
KJ	DMEPOS ITEM, PARENTERAL ENTERAL NUTRITION (PEN) PUMP OR CAPPED RENTAL, MONTHS FOUR TO FIFTEEN	C	N				
KK	DMEPOS ITEM SUBJECT TO DMEPOS COMPETITIVE BIDDING PROGRAM NUMBER 2	C	N				
KL	DMEPOS ITEM DELIVERED VIA MAIL	C	N				
KM	REPLACEMENT OF FACIAL PROSTHESIS INCLUDING NEW IMPRESSION/MOULAGE	C	N				
KN	REPLACEMENT OF FACIAL PROSTHESIS USING PREVIOUS MASTER MODEL	C	N				
KO	SINGLE DRUG UNIT DOSE FORMULATION	C	N				
KP	FIRST DRUG OF A MULTIPLE DRUG UNIT DOSE FORMULATION	C	N				
KQ	SECOND OR SUBSEQUENT DRUG OF A MULTIPLE DRUG UNIT DOSE FORMULATION	C	N				
KR	RENTAL ITEM, BILLING FOR PARTIAL MONTH	C	N				
KS	GLUCOSE MONITOR SUPPLY FOR DIABETIC BENEFICIARY NOT TREATED WITH INSULIN	D	N				

HCPCS Code	Statute	Lab Cert	X-Ref	ASC Pay Grp	ASC Pay Group Eff. Date	Proc Notes	BETOS	TOS	Anest	Code Add Date	Code Effective Date	Code Term Date
K2									0	19930101	19970101	
K3									0	19930101	19970101	
K4									0	19930101	19970101	
KA									0	19940101	19970101	
KB									0	20030101	20030101	
KC									0	20050101	20050101	
KD									0	20040101	20040101	
KE									0	20090101	20090101	
KF									0	20040401	20040401	
KG									0	20070701	20070701	
KH									0	19940101	19970101	
KI									0	19940101	19970101	
KJ									0	19940101	19970101	
KK									0	20070701	20070701	
KL									0	20070701	20090101	
KM									0	19960101	20010101	
KN									0	19960101	20010101	
KO									0	19970401	19970401	
KP									0	19970401	19970401	
KQ									0	19970401	19970401	
KR									0	20020101	20020101	
KS						0074			0	19981001	19981001	

Modifiers

HCPCS Code	Long Description	Coverage	Action	PI	MPI	CIM	MCM
KT	BENEFICIARY RESIDES IN A COMPETITIVE BIDDING AREA & TRAVELS OUTSIDE THAT COMPETITIVE BIDDING AREA AND RECEIVES A COMPETITIVE BID ITEM	C	N				
KU	DMEPOS ITEM SUBJECT TO DMEPOS COMPETITIVE BIDDING PROGRAM NUMBER 3	C	N				
KV	DMEPOS ITEM SUBJECT TO DMEPOS COMPETITIVE BIDDING PROGRAM THAT IS FURNISHED AS PART OF A PROFESSIONAL SERVICE	C	N				
KW	DMEPOS ITEM SUBJECT TO DMEPOS COMPETITIVE BIDDING PROGRAM NUMBER 4	C	N				
KX	REQUIREMENTS SPECIFIED IN THE MEDICAL POLICY HAVE BEEN MET	C	N				
KY	DMEPOS ITEM SUBJECT TO DMEPOS COMPETITIVE BIDDING PROGRAM NUMBER 5	C	N				
KZ	NEW COVERAGE NOT IMPLEMENTED BY MANAGED CARE	C	N				
LC	LEFT CIRCUMFLEX CORONARY ARTERY	C	N				
LD	LEFT ANTERIOR DESCENDING CORONARY ARTERY	C	N				
LL	LEASE/RENTAL (USE THE 'LL' MODIFIER WHEN DME EQUIPMENT RENTAL IS TO BE APPLIED AGAINST THE PURCHASE PRICE)	C	N				
LR	LABORATORY ROUND TRIP	C	N				
LS	FDA-MONITORED INTRAOCULAR LENS IMPLANT	D	N			65-7	
LT	LEFT SIDE (USED TO IDENTIFY PROCEDURES PERFORMED ON THE LEFT SIDE OF THE BODY)	C	N				
M2	MEDICARE SECONDARY PAYER (MSP)	C	N				
MS	SIX MONTH MAINTENANCE AND SERVICING FEE FOR REASONABLE AND NECESSARY PARTS AND LABOR WHICH ARE NOT COVERED UNDER ANY MANUFACTURER OR SUPPLIER WARRANTY	C	N				
NR	NEW WHEN RENTED (USE THE 'NR' MODIFIER WHEN DME WHICH WAS NEW AT THE TIME OF RENTAL IS SUBSEQUENTLY PURCHASED)	C	N				
NU	NEW EQUIPMENT	C	N				
P1	A NORMAL HEALTHY PATIENT	C	N				
P2	A PATIENT WITH MILD SYSTEMIC DISEASE	C	N				
P3	A PATIENT WITH SEVERE SYSTEMIC DISEASE	C	N				
P4	A PATIENT WITH SEVERE SYSTEMIC DISEASE THAT IS A CONSTANT THREAT TO LIFE	C	N				
P5	A MORIBUND PATIENT WHO IS NOT EXPECTED TO SURVIVE WITHOUT THE OPERATION	C	N				
P6	A DECLARED BRAIN-DEAD PATIENT WHOSE ORGANS ARE BEING REMOVED FOR DONOR PURPOSES	C	N				
PA	SURGICAL OR OTHER INVASIVE PROCEDURE ON WRONG BODY PART	I	A				
PB	SURGICAL OR OTHER INVASIVE PROCEDURE ON WRONG PATIENT	I	A				
PC	WRONG SURGERY OR OTHER INVASIVE PROCEDURE ON PATIENT	I	A				

HCPCS Code	Statute	Lab Cert	X-Ref	ASC Pay Grp	ASC Pay Group Eff. Date	Proc Notes	BETOS	TOS	Anest	Code Add Date	Code Effective Date	Code Term Date
KT									0	20070701	20080401	
KU									0	20070701	20070701	
KV									0	20080101	20080101	
KW									0	20080101	20080101	
KX									0	20020701	20020701	
KY									0	20080101	20080101	
KZ									0	20031001	20031001	
LC									0	19970101	19970101	
LD									0	19970101	19970101	
LL									0	19840101	19970101	
LR									0	19870101	19970101	
LS									0	19910101	19970101	
LT									0	19840101	19970101	
M2									0	20070101	20070101	
MS									0	19890101	19970101	
NR									0	19840101	19970101	
NU									0	19840101	19970101	
P1									0	20060101	20060101	
P2									0	20060101	20060101	
P3									0	20060101	20060101	
P4									0	20060101	20060101	
P5									0	20060101	20060101	
P6									0	20060101	20060101	
PA									0	20090701	20090701	
PB									0	20090701	20090701	
PC									0	20090701	20090701	

HCPCS Code	Long Description	Coverage	Action	PI	MPI	CIM	MCM
PI	POSITRON EMISSION TOMOGRAPHY (PET) OR PET/COMPUTED TOMOGRAPHY (CT) TO INFORM THE INITIAL TREATMENT STRATEGY OF TUMORS THAT ARE BIOPSY PROVEN OR STRONGLY SUSPECTED OF BEING CANCEROUS BASED ON OTHER DIAGNOSTIC TESTING	C	A				
PL	PROGRESSIVE ADDITION LENSES	C	N				
PS	POSITRON EMISSION TOMOGRAPHY (PET) OR PET/COMPUTED TOMOGRAPHY (CT) TO INFORM THE SUBSEQUENT TREATMENT STRATEGY OF CANCEROUS TUMORS WHEN THE BENEFICIARY'S TREATING PHYSICIAN DETERMINES THAT THE PET STUDY IS NEEDED TO INFORM SUBSEQUENT ANTI-TUMOR STRATEGY	C	A				
Q0	INVESTIGATIONAL CLINICAL SERVICE PROVIDED IN A CLINICAL RESEARCH STUDY THAT IS IN AN APPROVED CLINICAL RESEARCH STUDY	D	N				
Q1	ROUTINE CLINICAL SERVICE PROVIDED IN A CLINICAL RESEARCH STUDY THAT IS IN AN APPROVED CLINICAL RESEARCH STUDY	D	N				
Q2	HCFA/ORD DEMONSTRATION PROJECT PROCEDURE/SERVICE	C	N				
Q3	LIVE KIDNEY DONOR SURGERY AND RELATED SERVICES	C	N				
Q4	SERVICE FOR ORDERING/REFERRING PHYSICIAN QUALIFIES AS A SERVICE EXEMPTION	C	N				
Q5	SERVICE FURNISHED BY A SUBSTITUTE PHYSICIAN UNDER A RECIPROCAL BILLING ARRANGEMENT	D	N				3060.6
Q6	SERVICE FURNISHED BY A LOCUM TENENS PHYSICIAN	D	N				3060.7
Q7	ONE CLASS A FINDING	C	N				
Q8	TWO CLASS B FINDINGS	C	N				
Q9	ONE CLASS B AND TWO CLASS C FINDINGS	C	N				
QA	FDA INVESTIGATIONAL DEVICE EXEMPTION	C	N				
QC	SINGLE CHANNEL MONITORING	C	N				
QD	RECORDING AND STORAGE IN SOLID STATE MEMORY BY A DIGITAL RECORDER	C	N				
QE	PRESCRIBED AMOUNT OF OXYGEN IS LESS THAN 1 LITER PER MINUTE (LPM)	C	N				
QF	PRESCRIBED AMOUNT OF OXYGEN EXCEEDS 4 LITERS PER MINUTE (LPM) AND PORTABLE OXYGEN IS PRESCRIBED	C	N				
QG	PRESCRIBED AMOUNT OF OXYGEN IS GREATER THAN 4 LITERS PER MINUTE(LPM)	C	N				
QH	OXYGEN CONSERVING DEVICE IS BEING USED WITH AN OXYGEN DELIVERY SYSTEM	C	N				
QJ	SERVICES/ITEMS PROVIDED TO A PRISONER OR PATIENT IN STATE OR LOCAL CUSTODY, HOWEVER THE STATE OR LOCAL GOVERNMENT, AS APPLICABLE, MEETS THE REQUIREMENTS IN 42 CFR 411.4 (B)	D	N				
QK	MEDICAL DIRECTION OF TWO, THREE, OR FOUR CONCURRENT ANESTHESIA PROCEDURES INVOLVING QUALIFIED INDIVIDUALS	D	N				3350.5
QL	PATIENT PRONOUNCED DEAD AFTER AMBULANCE CALLED	C	N				

HCPCS Code	Statute	Lab Cert	X-Ref	ASC Pay Grp	ASC Pay Group Eff. Date	Proc Notes	BETOS	TOS	Anest	Code Add Date	Code Effective Date	Code Term Date
PI									0	20090701	20090701	
PL									0	19890101	19970101	
PS									0	20090701	20090701	
Q0						0146			0	20080101	20080101	
Q1						0146			0	20080101	20080101	
Q2						0046			0	19920101	19970101	
Q3									0	19950101	20030101	
Q4									0	19940101	19970101	
Q5									0	19930101	19970101	
Q6									0	19930101	19970101	
Q7									0	19950101	19970101	
Q8									0	19950101	19970101	
Q9									0	19950101	19970101	
QA									0	19960101	20080101	20071231
QC									0	19890101	19970101	
QD									0	19890101	19970101	
QE									0	19890101	19970101	
QF									0	19890101	19970101	
QG									0	19890101	19970101	
QH									0	19890101	19970101	
QJ						0111			0	20030101	20030101	
QK									0	19950101	20010101	
QL									0	19990101	19990101	

HCPCS Code	Long Description	Coverage	Action	PI	MPI	CIM	MCM
QM	AMBULANCE SERVICE PROVIDED UNDER ARRANGEMENT BY A PROVIDER OF SERVICES	C	N				
QN	AMBULANCE SERVICE FURNISHED DIRECTLY BY A PROVIDER OF SERVICES	C	N				
QP	DOCUMENTATION IS ON FILE SHOWING THAT THE LABORATORY TEST(S) WAS ORDERED INDIVIDUALLY OR ORDERED AS A CPT-RECOGNIZED PANEL OTHER THAN AUTOMATED PROFILE CODES 80002-80019, G0058, G0059, AND G0060.	D	N				7517.1
QR	ITEM OR SERVICE PROVIDED IN A MEDICARE SPECIFIED STUDY	D	N				
QS	MONITORED ANESTHESIA CARE SERVICE	D	N			15018I	
QT	RECORDING AND STORAGE ON TAPE BY AN ANALOG TAPE RECORDER	C	N				
QV	ITEM OR SERVICE PROVIDED AS ROUTINE CARE IN A MEDICARE QUALIFYING CLINICAL TRIAL	D	N			30-1	
QW	CLIA WAIVED TEST	C	N				
QX	CRNA SERVICE: WITH MEDICAL DIRECTION BY A PHYSICIAN	C	N				
QY	MEDICAL DIRECTION OF ONE CERTIFIED REGISTERED NURSE ANESTHETIST (CRNA) BY AN ANESTHESIOLOGIST	D	N				3350.5
QZ	CRNA SERVICE: WITHOUT MEDICAL DIRECTION BY A PHYSICIAN	C	N				
RA	REPLACEMENT OF A DME ITEM	C	N				
RB	REPLACEMENT OF A PART OF DME FURNISHED AS PART OF A REPAIR	C	N				
RC	RIGHT CORONARY ARTERY	C	N				
RD	DRUG PROVIDED TO BENEFICIARY, BUT NOT ADMINISTERED "INCIDENT-TO"	C	N				
RE	FURNISHED IN FULL COMPLIANCE WITH FDA-MANDATED RISK EVALUATION AND MITIGATION STRATEGY (REMS)	C	N				
RP	REPLACEMENT AND REPAIR -RP MAY BE USED TO INDICATE REPLACEMENT OF DME, ORTHOTIC AND PROSTHETIC DEVICES WHICH HAVE BEEN IN USE FOR SOMETIME. THE CLAIM SHOWS THE CODE FOR THE PART, FOLLOWED BY THE 'RP' MODIFIER AND THE CHARGE FOR THE PART.	C	N				
RR	RENTAL (USE THE 'RR' MODIFIER WHEN DME IS TO BE RENTED)	C	N				
RT	RIGHT SIDE (USED TO IDENTIFY PROCEDURES PERFORMED ON THE RIGHT SIDE OF THE BODY)	C	N				
SA	NURSE PRACTITIONER RENDERING SERVICE IN COLLABORATION WITH A PHYSICIAN	I	N				
SB	NURSE MIDWIFE	I	N				
SC	MEDICALLY NECESSARY SERVICE OR SUPPLY	I	N				
SD	SERVICES PROVIDED BY REGISTERED NURSE WITH SPECIALIZED, HIGHLY TECHNICAL HOME INFUSION TRAINING	I	N				
SE	STATE AND/OR FEDERALLY-FUNDED PROGRAMS/SERVICES	I	N				
SF	SECOND OPINION ORDERED BY A PROFESSIONAL REVIEW ORGANIZATION (PRO) PER SECTION 9401, P.L. 99-272 (100% REIMBURSEMENT - NO MEDICARE DEDUCTIBLE OR COINSURANCE)	C	N				

HCPCS Code	Statute	Lab Cert	X-Ref	ASC Pay Grp	ASC Pay Group Eff. Date	Proc Notes	BETOS	TOS	Anest	Code Add Date	Code Effective Date	Code Term Date
QM									0	19960101	19990101	
QN									0	19960101	19990101	
QP									0	19960101	19960301	
QR						0122			0	20050101	20080101	20071231
QS									0	19900101	19960701	
QT									0	19890101	19970101	
QV									0	20000919	20080101	20071231
QW									0	19960101	19961001	
QX									0	19930101	19970101	
QY									0	19980101	20010101	
QZ									0	19930101	19970101	
RA									0	20090101	20090101	
RB									0	20090101	20090101	
RC									0	19970101	19970101	
RD									0	20040101	20040101	
RE									0	20090101	20090101	
RP									0	19840101	20090101	20081231
RR									0	19840101	19970101	
RT									0	19840101	19970101	
SA									0	20010701	20010701	
SB									0	20010701	20010701	
SC									0	20010701	20010701	
SD									0	20010701	20010701	
SD												
SE									0	20010701	20010701	
SF									0	19870101	19970101	

HCPCS Code	Long Description	Coverage	Action	PI	MPI	CIM	MCM
SG	AMBULATORY SURGICAL CENTER (ASC) FACILITY SERVICE	C	N				
SH	SECOND CONCURRENTLY ADMINISTERED INFUSION THERAPY	I	N				
SJ	THIRD OR MORE CONCURRENTLY ADMINISTERED INFUSION THERAPY	I	N				
SK	MEMBER OF HIGH RISK POPULATION (USE ONLY WITH CODES FOR IMMUNIZATION)	I	N				
SL	STATE SUPPLIED VACCINE	I	N				
SM	SECOND SURGICAL OPINION	I	N				
SN	THIRD SURGICAL OPINION	I	N				
SQ	ITEM ORDERED BY HOME HEALTH	I	N				
SS	HOME INFUSION SERVICES PROVIDED IN THE INFUSION SUITE OF THE IV THERAPY PROVIDER	I	N				
ST	RELATED TO TRAUMA OR INJURY	I	N				
SU	PROCEDURE PERFORMED IN PHYSICIAN'S OFFICE (TO DENOTE USE OF FACILITY AND EQUIPMENT)	I	N				
SV	PHARMACEUTICALS DELIVERED TO PATIENT'S HOME BUT NOT UTILIZED	I	N				
SW	SERVICES PROVIDED BY A CERTIFIED DIABETIC EDUCATOR	C	N				
SY	PERSONS WHO ARE IN CLOSE CONTACT WITH MEMBER OF HIGH-RISK POPULATION (USE ONLY WITH CODES FOR IMMUNIZATION)	I	N				
T1	LEFT FOOT, SECOND DIGIT	C	N				
T2	LEFT FOOT, THIRD DIGIT	C	N				
T3	LEFT FOOT, FOURTH DIGIT	C	N				
T4	LEFT FOOT, FIFTH DIGIT	C	N				
T5	RIGHT FOOT, GREAT TOE	C	N				
T6	RIGHT FOOT, SECOND DIGIT	C	N				
T7	RIGHT FOOT, THIRD DIGIT	C	N				
T8	RIGHT FOOT, FOURTH DIGIT	C	N				
T9	RIGHT FOOT, FIFTH DIGIT	C	N				
TA	LEFT FOOT, GREAT TOE	C	N				
TC	TECHNICAL COMPONENT. UNDER CERTAIN CIRCUMSTANCES, A CHARGE MAY BE MADE FOR THE TECHNICAL COMPONENT ALONE. UNDER THOSE CIRCUMSTANCES THE TECHNICAL COMPONENT CHARGE IS IDENTIFIED BY ADDING MODIFIER 'TC' TO THE USUAL PROCEDURE NUMBER. TECHNICAL COMPONENT CHARGES ARE INSTITUTIONAL CHARGES AND NOT BILLED SEPARATELY BY PHYSICIANS. HOWEVER, PORTABLE X-RAY SUPPLIERS ONLY BILL FOR TECHNICAL COMPONENT AND SHOULD UTILIZE MODIFIER TC. THE CHARGE DATA FROM PORTABLE X-RAY SUPPLIERS WILL THEN BE USED TO BUILD CUSTOMARY AND PREVAILING PROFILES.	C	N				
TD	RN	I	N				
TE	LPN/LVN	I	N				
TF	INTERMEDIATE LEVEL OF CARE	I	N				
TG	COMPLEX/HIGH TECH LEVEL OF CARE	I	N				
TH	OBSTETRICAL TREATMENT/SERVICES, PRENATAL OR POSTPARTUM	I	N				

HCPCS Code	Statute	Lab Cert	X-Ref	ASC Pay Grp	ASC Pay Group Eff. Date	Proc Notes	BETOS	TOS	Anest	Code Add Date	Code Effective Date	Code Term Date
SG									0	19920101	19970101	
SH									0	20010701	20010701	
SJ									0	20010701	20010701	
SK									0	20020401	20020401	
SL									0	20020401	20020401	
SM									0	20020701	20020701	
SN									0	20020701	20020701	
SQ									0	20021001	20021001	
SS									0	20041001	20041001	
ST									0	20030101	20030101	
SU									0	20030101	20030101	
SV									0	20030101	20030101	
SW									0	20040401	20040401	
SY									0	20050101	20050101	
T1									0	19950101	19990101	
T2									0	19950101	19990101	
T3									0	19950101	19990101	
T4									0	19950101	19990101	
T5									0	19950101	19990101	
T6									0	19950101	19990101	
T7									0	19950101	19990101	
T8									0	19950101	19990101	
T9									0	19950101	19990101	
TA									0	19950101	19990101	
TC									0	19840101	19970101	
TD									0	20010701	20010701	
TE									0	20010701	20010701	
TF									0	20010701	20010701	
TG									0	20010701	20010701	
TH									0	20010701	20010701	

HCPCS Code	Long Description	Coverage	Action	PI	MPI	CIM	MCM
TJ	PROGRAM GROUP, CHILD AND/OR ADOLESCENT	I	N				
TK	EXTRA PATIENT OR PASSENGER, NON-AMBULANCE	I	N				
TL	EARLY INTERVENTION/INDIVIDUALIZED FAMILY SERVICE PLAN (IFSP)	I	N				
TM	INDIVIDUALIZED EDUCATION PROGRAM (IEP)	I	N				
TN	RURAL/OUTSIDE PROVIDERS' CUSTOMARY SERVICE AREA	I	N				
TP	"MEDICAL TRANSPORT, UNLOADED VEHICLE"	I	N				
TQ	BASIC LIFE SUPPORT TRANSPORT BY A VOLUNTEER AMBULANCE PROVIDER	I	N				
TR	SCHOOL-BASED INDIVIDUALIZED EDUCATION PROGRAM (IEP) SERVICES PROVIDED OUTSIDE THE PUBLIC SCHOOL DISTRICT RESPONSIBLE FOR THE STUDENT	I	N				
TS	FOLLOW-UP SERVICE	C	N				
TT	INDIVIDUALIZED SERVICE PROVIDED TO MORE THAN ONE PATIENT IN SAME SETTING	I	N				
TU	SPECIAL PAYMENT RATE, OVERTIME	I	N				
TV	SPECIAL PAYMENT RATES, HOLIDAYS/WEEKENDS	I	N				
TW	BACK-UP EQUIPMENT	I	N				
U1	MEDICAID LEVEL OF CARE 1, AS DEFINED BY EACH STATE	I	N				
U2	MEDICAID LEVEL OF CARE 2, AS DEFINED BY EACH STATE	I	N				
U3	MEDICAID LEVEL OF CARE 3, AS DEFINED BY EACH STATE	I	N				
U4	MEDICAID LEVEL OF CARE 4, AS DEFINED BY EACH STATE	I	N				
U5	MEDICAID LEVEL OF CARE 5, AS DEFINED BY EACH STATE	I	N				
U6	MEDICAID LEVEL OF CARE 6, AS DEFINED BY EACH STATE	I	N				
U7	MEDICAID LEVEL OF CARE 7, AS DEFINED BY EACH STATE	I	N				
U8	MEDICAID LEVEL OF CARE 8, AS DEFINED BY EACH STATE	I	N				
U9	MEDICAID LEVEL OF CARE 9, AS DEFINED BY EACH STATE	I	N				
UA	MEDICAID LEVEL OF CARE 10, AS DEFINED BY EACH STATE	I	N				
UB	MEDICAID LEVEL OF CARE 11, AS DEFINED BY EACH STATE	I	N				
UC	MEDICAID LEVEL OF CARE 12, AS DEFINED BY EACH STATE	I	N				
UD	MEDICAID LEVEL OF CARE 13, AS DEFINED BY EACH STATE	I	N				
UE	USED DURABLE MEDICAL EQUIPMENT	C	N				
UF	SERVICES PROVIDED IN THE MORNING	I	N				
UG	SERVICES PROVIDED IN THE AFTERNOON	I	N				
UH	SERVICES PROVIDED IN THE EVENING	I	N				
UJ	SERVICES PROVIDED AT NIGHT	I	N				
UK	SERVICES PROVIDED ON BEHALF OF THE CLIENT TO SOMEONE OTHER THAN THE CLIENT (COLLATERAL RELATIONSHIP)	I	N				
UN	TWO PATIENTS SERVED	C	N				
UP	THREE PATIENTS SERVED	C	N				
UQ	FOUR PATIENTS SERVED	C	N				
UR	FIVE PATIENTS SERVED	C	N				
US	SIX OR MORE PATIENTS SERVED	C	N				
V5	VASCULAR CATHETER	C	A				
V6	ARTERIOVENOUS GRAFT	C	A				
V7	ARTERIOVENOUS FISTULA	C	A				
V8	INFECTION PRESENT	C	A				
V9	NO INFECTION PRESENT	C	A				
VP	APHAKIC PATIENT	C	N				

HCPCS Code	Statute	Lab Cert	X-Ref	ASC Pay Grp	ASC Pay Group Eff. Date	Proc Notes	BETOS	TOS	Anest	Code Add Date	Code Effective Date	Code Term Date
TJ									0	20010701	20010701	
TK									0	20020401	20020401	
TL									0	20020401	20020401	
TM									0	20020401	20020401	
TN									0	20020401	20020401	
TP									0	20020401	20020401	
TQ									0	20020401	20020401	
TR									0	20020701	20020701	
TS									0	20021001	20060101	
TT									0	20021001	20021001	
TU									0	20030101	20030101	
TV									0	20030101	20030101	
TW									0	20030101	20030101	
U1									0	20020701	20020701	
U2									0	20020701	20020701	
U3									0	20020701	20020701	
U4									0	20020701	20020701	
U5									0	20020701	20020701	
U6									0	20020701	20020701	
U7									0	20020701	20020701	
U8									0	20020701	20020701	
U9									0	20020701	20020701	
UA									0	20020701	20020701	
UB									0	20020701	20020701	
UC									0	20020701	20020701	
UD									0	20020701	20020701	
UE									0	19840101	19970101	
UF									0	20030401	20030401	
UG									0	20030401	20030401	
UH									0	20030401	20030401	
UJ									0	20030401	20030401	
UK									0	20030401	20030401	
UN						0114			0	20040101	20040101	
UP						0114			0	20040101	20040101	
UQ						0114			0	20040101	20040101	
UR						0114			0	20040101	20040101	
US						0114			0	20040101	20040101	
V5									0	20100101	20100101	
V6									0	20100101	20100101	
V7									0	20100101	20100101	
V8									0	20100101	20100101	
V9									0	20100101	20100101	
VP									0	19840101	19970101	

HCPCS Code	Long Description	Coverage	Action	PI	MPI	CIM	MCM
A0021	AMBULANCE SERVICE, OUTSIDE STATE PER MILE, TRANSPORT (MEDICAID ONLY)	I	N	00	9		
A0080	NON-EMERGENCY TRANSPORTATION, PER MILE - VEHICLE PROVIDED BY VOLUNTEER (INDIVIDUAL OR ORGANIZATION), WITH NO VESTED INTEREST	I	N	00	9		
A0090	NON-EMERGENCY TRANSPORTATION, PER MILE - VEHICLE PROVIDED BY INDIVIDUAL (FAMILY MEMBER, SELF, NEIGHBOR) WITH VESTED INTEREST	I	N	00	9		
A0100	NON-EMERGENCY TRANSPORTATION; TAXI	I	N	00	9		
A0110	NON-EMERGENCY TRANSPORTATION AND BUS, INTRA OR INTER STATE CARRIER	I	N	00	9		
A0120	NON-EMERGENCY TRANSPORTATION: MINI-BUS, MOUNTAIN AREA TRANSPORTS, OR OTHER TRANSPORTATION SYSTEMS	I	N	00	9		
A0130	NON-EMERGENCY TRANSPORTATION: WHEEL-CHAIR VAN	I	N	00	9		
A0140	NON-EMERGENCY TRANSPORTATION AND AIR TRAVEL (PRIVATE OR COMMERCIAL) INTRA OR INTER STATE	I	N	00	9		
A0160	NON-EMERGENCY TRANSPORTATION: PER MILE - CASE WORKER OR SOCIAL WORKER	I	N	00	9		
A0170	TRANSPORTATION ANCILLARY: PARKING FEES, TOLLS, OTHER	I	N	00	9		
A0180	NON-EMERGENCY TRANSPORTATION: ANCILLARY: LODGING-RECIPIENT	I	N	00	9		
A0190	NON-EMERGENCY TRANSPORTATION: ANCILLARY: MEALS-RECIPIENT	I	N	00	9		
A0200	NON-EMERGENCY TRANSPORTATION: ANCILLARY: LODGING ESCORT	I	N	00	9		
A0210	NON-EMERGENCY TRANSPORTATION: ANCILLARY: MEALS-ESCORT	I	N	00	9		
A0225	AMBULANCE SERVICE, NEONATAL TRANSPORT, BASE RATE, EMERGENCY TRANSPORT, ONE WAY	I	N	00	9		
A0380	BLS MILEAGE (PER MILE)	I	N	00	9		
A0382	BLS ROUTINE DISPOSABLE SUPPLIES	C	N	52	A		
A0384	BLS SPECIALIZED SERVICE DISPOSABLE SUPPLIES; DEFIBRILLATION (USED BY ALS AMBULANCES AND BLS AMBULANCES IN JURISDICTIONS WHERE DEFIBRILLATION IS PERMITTED IN BLS AMBULANCES)	C	N	52	A		
A0390	ALS MILEAGE (PER MILE)	I	N	00	9		
A0392	ALS SPECIALIZED SERVICE DISPOSABLE SUPPLIES; DEFIBRILLATION (TO BE USED ONLY IN JURISDICTIONS WHERE DEFIBRILLATION CANNOT BE PERFORMED IN BLS AMBULANCES)	C	N	52	A		
A0394	ALS SPECIALIZED SERVICE DISPOSABLE SUPPLIES; IV DRUG THERAPY	C	N	52	A		
A0396	ALS SPECIALIZED SERVICE DISPOSABLE SUPPLIES; ESOPHAGEAL INTUBATION	C	N	52	A		
A0398	ALS ROUTINE DISPOSABLE SUPPLIES	C	N	52	A		
A0420	AMBULANCE WAITING TIME (ALS OR BLS), ONE HALF (1/2) HOUR INCREMENTS	C	N	52	A		
A0422	AMBULANCE (ALS OR BLS) OXYGEN AND OXYGEN SUPPLIES, LIFE SUSTAINING SITUATION	C	N	52	A		

HCPCS Code	Statute	Lab Cert	X-Ref	ASC Pay Grp	ASC Pay Group Eff. Date	Proc Notes	BETOS	TOS	Anest	Code Add Date	Code Effective Date	Code Term Date
A0021			A0030				O1A	D	0	19850101	19960910	
A0080							O1A	D	0	19820101	20030101	
A0090							O1A	D	0	19820101	20030101	
A0100							O1A	D	0	19820101	20030101	
A0110							O1A	D	0	19840101	19950101	
A0120							O1A	D	0	19820101	20030101	
A0130							O1A	D	0	19820101	19950101	
A0140							O1A	D	0	19850101	19960910	
A0160							O1A	D	0	19840101	19950101	
A0170							O1A	D	0	19820101	20030101	
A0180							O1A	D	0	19820101	19950101	
A0190							O1A	D	0	19840101	19950101	
A0200							O1A	D	0	19820101	19950101	
A0210							O1A	D	0	19840101	19950101	
A0225							O1A	D	0	19850101	20030401	
A0380			A0425				O1A	D	0	19950101	20030101	
A0382							O1A	D	0	19950101	19950101	
A0384							O1A	D	0	19950101	19950101	
A0390			A0425				O1A	D	0	19950101	20030101	
A0392							O1A	D	0	19950101	19950101	
A0392												
A0394							O1A	D	0	19950101	19950101	
A0396							O1A	D	0	19950101	19950101	
A0398							O1A	D	0	19950101	19950101	
A0420							O1A	D	0	19950101	19950101	
A0422							O1A	D	0	19950101	19950101	

HCPCS Code	Long Description	Coverage	Action	PI	MPI	CIM	MCM
A0424	EXTRA AMBULANCE ATTENDANT, GROUND (ALS OR BLS) OR AIR (FIXED OR ROTARY WINGED);(REQUIRES MEDICAL REVIEW)	C	N	52	A		
A0425	GROUND MILEAGE, PER STATUTE MILE	C	N	52	A		
A0426	AMBULANCE SERVICE, ADVANCED LIFE SUPPORT, NON-EMERGENCY TRANSPORT, LEVEL 1 (ALS 1)	C	N	52	A		
A0427	AMBULANCE SERVICE, ADVANCED LIFE SUPPORT, EMERGENCY TRANSPORT, LEVEL 1 (ALS1-EMERGENCY)	C	N	52	A		
A0428	AMBULANCE SERVICE, BASIC LIFE SUPPORT, NON-EMERGENCY TRANSPORT, (BLS)	C	N	52	A		
A0429	AMBULANCE SERVICE, BASIC LIFE SUPPORT, EMERGENCY TRANSPORT (BLS-EMERGENCY)	C	N	52	A		
A0430	AMBULANCE SERVICE, CONVENTIONAL AIR SERVICES, TRANSPORT, ONE WAY (FIXED WING)	C	N	52	A		
A0431	AMBULANCE SERVICE, CONVENTIONAL AIR SERVICES, TRANSPORT, ONE WAY (ROTARY WING)	C	N	52	A		
A0432	PARAMEDIC INTERCEPT (PI), RURAL AREA, TRANSPORT FURNISHED BY A VOLUNTEER AMBULANCE COMPANY WHICH IS PROHIBITED BY STATE LAW FROM BILLING THIRD PARTY PAYERS	C	N	52	A		
A0433	ADVANCED LIFE SUPPORT, LEVEL 2 (ALS 2)	C	N	52	A		
A0434	SPECIALTY CARE TRANSPORT (SCT)	C	N	52	A		
A0435	FIXED WING AIR MILEAGE, PER STATUTE MILE	C	N	52	A		
A0436	ROTARY WING AIR MILEAGE, PER STATUTE MILE	C	N	52	A		
A0800	AMBULANCE TRANSPORT PROVIDED BETWEEN THE HOURS OF 7PM AND 7AM	I	N	00	9		
A0888	NONCOVERED AMBULANCE MILEAGE, PER MILE (E.G., FOR MILES TRAVELED BEYOND CLOSEST APPROPRIATE FACILITY)	M	N	00	9		2125
A0998	AMBULANCE RESPONSE AND TREATMENT, NO TRANSPORT	I	N	00	9		
A0999	UNLISTED AMBULANCE SERVICE	D	N	57	A		2120.1,2125
A4206	SYRINGE WITH NEEDLE, STERILE, 1 CC OR LESS, EACH	C	N	00	9		
A4207	SYRINGE WITH NEEDLE, STERILE 2CC, EACH	C	N	00	9		
A4208	SYRINGE WITH NEEDLE, STERILE 3CC, EACH	C	N	00	9		
A4209	SYRINGE WITH NEEDLE, STERILE 5CC OR GREATER, EACH	C	N	00	9		
A4210	NEEDLE-FREE INJECTION DEVICE, EACH	M	N	00	9	60-9	
A4211	SUPPLIES FOR SELF-ADMINISTERED INJECTIONS	D	N	00	9		2049
A4212	NON-CORING NEEDLE OR STYLET WITH OR WITHOUT CATHETER	C	N	57	A		
A4213	SYRINGE, STERILE, 20 CC OR GREATER, EACH	C	N	00	9		
A4215	NEEDLE, STERILE, ANY SIZE, EACH	C	N	00	9		
A4216	STERILE WATER, SALINE AND/OR DEXTROSE, DILUENT/FLUSH, 10 ML	D	N	37	A		2049
A4217	STERILE WATER/SALINE, 500 ML	D	N	37	A		2049
A4218	STERILE SALINE OR WATER, METERED DOSE DISPENSER, 10 ML	D	N	51	A		
A4220	REFILL KIT FOR IMPLANTABLE INFUSION PUMP	D	N	57	A	60-14	
A4221	SUPPLIES FOR MAINTENANCE OF DRUG INFUSION CATHETER, PER WEEK (LIST DRUG SEPARATELY)	C	N	34	A		
A4222	INFUSION SUPPLIES FOR EXTERNAL DRUG INFUSION PUMP, PER CASSETTE OR BAG (LIST DRUGS SEPARATELY)	C	N	34	A		

HCPCS Code	Statute	Lab Cert	X-Ref	ASC Pay Grp	ASC Pay Group Eff. Date	Proc Notes	BETOS	TOS	Anest	Code Add Date	Code Effective Date	Code Term Date
A0424							O1A	D	0	19950101	20030101	
A0425							O1A	D	0	20010101	20010101	
A0426							O1A	D	0	20010101	20010101	
A0426												
A0427							O1A	D	0	20010101	20010101	
A0427												
A0428							O1A	D	0	20010101	20010101	
A0429							O1A	D	0	20010101	20010101	
A0430							O1A	D	0	20010101	20010101	
A0431							O1A	D	0	20010101	20010101	
A0432							O1A	D	0	20010101	20010101	
A0433							O1A	D	0	20010101	20010101	
A0434							O1A	D	0	20010101	20010101	
A0435							O1A	D	0	20010101	20010101	
A0436							O1A	D	0	20010101	20010101	
A0800							O1A	D	0	20040101	20070101	20061231
A0888							O1A	D	0	19950101	19950101	
A0998							O1A	D	0	20060101	20060101	
A0999							O1A	D	0	19870101	19980101	
A4206							D1A	S	0	19850101	20080101	
A4207							D1A	S	0	19850101	20070101	
A4208							D1A	S	0	19850101	20070101	
A4209							D1A	S	0	19850101	20070101	
A4210							D1A	S	0	19890101	19960101	
A4211							D1A	S	0	19930101	19970101	
A4212							D1A	S	0	19930101	20000101	
A4213							D1A	S	0	19850101	20070101	
A4215							D1A	L	0	19850101	20070101	
A4216							D1F	1	0	20040101	20070101	
A4217							D1F	1	0	20040101	20040101	
A4218						0127	O1E	1	0	20060101	20060101	
A4220						0050	D1A	P	0	19940101	19980303	
A4221							D1E	P	0	19970101	19970101	
A4221												
A4222							D1E	P	0	19970101	20050101	
A4222												

HCPCS Code	Long Description	Coverage	Action	PI	MPI	CIM	MCM
A4223	INFUSION SUPPLIES NOT USED WITH EXTERNAL INFUSION PUMP, PER CASSETTE OR BAG (LIST DRUGS SEPARATELY)	C	N	00	9		
A4230	INFUSION SET FOR EXTERNAL INSULIN PUMP, NON NEEDLE CANNULA TYPE	D	N	34	A	60-14	
A4231	INFUSION SET FOR EXTERNAL INSULIN PUMP, NEEDLE TYPE	D	N	34	A	60-14	
A4232	SYRINGE WITH NEEDLE FOR EXTERNAL INSULIN PUMP, STERILE, 3CC	I	N	00	9	60-14	
A4233	REPLACEMENT BATTERY, ALKALINE (OTHER THAN J CELL), FOR USE WITH MEDICALLY NECESSARY HOME BLOOD GLUCOSE MONITOR OWNED BY PATIENT, EACH	C	N	36	A		
A4234	REPLACEMENT BATTERY, ALKALINE, J CELL, FOR USE WITH MEDICALLY NECESSARY HOME BLOOD GLUCOSE MONITOR OWNED BY PATIENT, EACH	C	N	36	A		
A4235	REPLACEMENT BATTERY, LITHIUM, FOR USE WITH MEDICALLY NECESSARY HOME BLOOD GLUCOSE MONITOR OWNED BY PATIENT, EACH	C	N	36	A		
A4236	REPLACEMENT BATTERY, SILVER OXIDE, FOR USE WITH MEDICALLY NECESSARY HOME BLOOD GLUCOSE MONITOR OWNED BY PATIENT, EACH	C	N	36	A		
A4244	ALCOHOL OR PEROXIDE, PER PINT	C	N	00	9		
A4245	ALCOHOL WIPES, PER BOX	C	N	00	9		
A4246	BETADINE OR PHISOHEX SOLUTION, PER PINT	C	N	00	9		
A4247	BETADINE OR IODINE SWABS/WIPES, PER BOX	C	N	00	9		
A4248	CHLORHEXIDINE CONTAINING ANTISEPTIC, 1 ML	C	N	52	A		
A4250	URINE TEST OR REAGENT STRIPS OR TABLETS (100 TABLETS OR STRIPS)	M	N	00	9		2100
A4252	BLOOD KETONE TEST OR REAGENT STRIP, EACH	S	N	00	9		
A4253	BLOOD GLUCOSE TEST OR REAGENT STRIPS FOR HOME BLOOD GLUCOSE MONITOR, PER 50 STRIPS	D	N	32	A	60-11	
A4255	PLATFORMS FOR HOME BLOOD GLUCOSE MONITOR, 50 PER BOX	D	N	34	A	60-11	
A4256	NORMAL, LOW AND HIGH CALIBRATOR SOLUTION / CHIPS	D	N	34	A	60-11	
A4257	REPLACEMENT LENS SHIELD CARTRIDGE FOR USE WITH LASER SKIN PIERCING DEVICE, EACH	C	N	34	A		
A4258	SPRING-POWERED DEVICE FOR LANCET, EACH	D	N	34	A	60-11	
A4259	LANCETS, PER BOX OF 100	D	N	34	A	60-11	
A4261	CERVICAL CAP FOR CONTRACEPTIVE USE	S	N	00	9		
A4262	TEMPORARY, ABSORBABLE LACRIMAL DUCT IMPLANT, EACH	D	N	00	9		
A4263	PERMANENT, LONG TERM, NON-DISSOLVABLE LACRIMAL DUCT IMPLANT, EACH	D	N	11	A		15030
A4264	PERMANENT IMPLANTABLE CONTRACEPTIVE INTRATUBAL OCCLUSION DEVICE(S) AND DELIVERY SYSTEM	I	A	00	9		
A4265	PARAFFIN, PER POUND	D	N	34	A	60-9	
A4266	DIAPHRAGM FOR CONTRACEPTIVE USE	I	N	00	9		
A4267	CONTRACEPTIVE SUPPLY, CONDOM, MALE, EACH	I	N	00	9		
A4268	CONTRACEPTIVE SUPPLY, CONDOM, FEMALE, EACH	I	N	00	9		
A4269	CONTRACEPTIVE SUPPLY, SPERMICIDE (E.G., FOAM, GEL), EA.	I	N	00	9		
A4270	DISPOSABLE ENDOSCOPE SHEATH, EACH	C	N	00	9		

HCPCS Code	Statute	Lab Cert	X-Ref	ASC Pay Grp	ASC Pay Group Eff. Date	Proc Notes	BETOS	TOS	Anest	Code Add Date	Code Effective Date	Code Term Date
A4223							D1A	P	0	20050101	20070101	
A4230							D1E	P	0	19960101	20000101	
A4231							D1E	P	0	19960101	20000101	
A4232							D1E	P	0	19960101	20030401	
A4233							D1E	P	0	20060101	20060101	
A4234							D1E	P	0	20060101	20060101	
A4235							D1E	P	0	20060101	20060101	
A4236							D1E	P	0	20060101	20060101	
A4244							D1A	L, S	0	19850101	20070101	
A4245							D1A	L, S	0	19850101	20070101	
A4246							D1A	L, S	0	19850101	20070101	
A4247							D1A	L, S	0	19850101	20070101	
A4248							P9B	L	0	20040101	20040101	
A4250							T1E	9	0	19900101	19970101	
A4252	1861(n)						D1E	P	0	20080101	20080101	
A4253							D1E	P	0	19860101	19980701	
A4255							D1E	P	0	19970101	20020101	
A4256							D1E	P	0	19850101	20020101	
A4257							D1E	P	0	20020101	20020101	
A4258							D1E	P	0	19960101	20020101	
A4259							D1E	P	0	19850101	19960101	
A4261	1862a1						Z2	9	0	19990101	19990101	
A4262						0052	D1A	9	0	19940101	19980101	
A4263							Y1	9	0	19940101	19980101	
A4264							Z2	9	0	20100101	20100101	
A4265							D1E	9	0	19860101	20020101	
A4266							Z2	9	0	20030101	20030101	
A4267							Z2	9	0	20030101	20030101	
A4268							Z2	9	0	20030101	20030101	
A4269							Z2	9	0	20030101	20030101	
A4270							P8D	9	0	19940101	19950401	

HCPCS Code	Long Description	Coverage	Action	PI	MPI	CIM	MCM
A4280	ADHESIVE SKIN SUPPORT ATTACHMENT FOR USE WITH EXTERNAL BREAST PROSTHESIS, EACH	C	N	38	A		
A4281	TUBING FOR BREAST PUMP, REPLACEMENT	C	N	00	9		
A4282	ADAPTER FOR BREAST PUMP, REPLACEMENT	C	N	00	9		
A4283	CAP FOR BREAST PUMP BOTTLE, REPLACEMENT	C	N	00	9		
A4284	BREAST SHIELD AND SPLASH PROTECTOR FOR USE WITH BREAST PUMP, REPLACEMENT	C	N	00	9		
A4285	POLYCARBONATE BOTTLE FOR USE WITH BREAST PUMP, REPLACEMENT	C	N	00	9		
A4286	LOCKING RING FOR BREAST PUMP, REPLACEMENT	C	N	00	9		
A4290	SACRAL NERVE STIMULATION TEST LEAD, EACH	C	N	00	9		
A4300	IMPLANTABLE ACCESS CATHETER, (E.G., VENOUS, ARTERIAL, EPIDURAL SUBARACHNOID, OR PERITONEAL, ETC.) EXTERNAL ACCESS	D	N	11	A		2130
A4301	IMPLANTABLE ACCESS TOTAL CATHETER, PORT/RESERVOIR (E.G., VENOUS, ARTERIAL, EPIDURAL, SUBARACHNOID, PERITONEAL, ETC.)	C	N	00	9		
A4305	DISPOSABLE DRUG DELIVERY SYSTEM, FLOW RATE OF 50 ML OR GREATER PER HOUR	C	N	00	9		
A4306	DISPOSABLE DRUG DELIVERY SYSTEM, FLOW RATE OF LESS THAN 50 ML PER HOUR	C	N	00	9		
A4310	INSERTION TRAY WITHOUT DRAINAGE BAG AND WITHOUT CATHETER (ACCESSORIES ONLY)	D	N	37	A		2130
A4311	INSERTION TRAY WITHOUT DRAINAGE BAG WITH INDWELLING CATHETER, FOLEY TYPE, TWO-WAY LATEX WITH COATING (TEFLON, SILICONE, SILICONE ELASTOMER OR HYDROPHILIC, ETC.)	D	N	37	A		2130
A4312	INSERTION TRAY WITHOUT DRAINAGE BAG WITH INDWELLING CATHETER, FOLEY TYPE, TWO-WAY, ALL SILICONE	D	N	37	A		2130
A4313	INSERTION TRAY WITHOUT DRAINAGE BAG WITH INDWELLING CATHETER, FOLEY TYPE, THREE-WAY, FOR CONTINUOUS IRRIGATION	D	N	37	A		2130
A4314	INSERTION TRAY WITH DRAINAGE BAG WITH INDWELLING CATHETER, FOLEY TYPE, TWO-WAY LATEX WITH COATING (TEFLON, SILICONE, SILICONE ELASTOMER OR HYDROPHILIC, ETC.)	D	N	37	A		2130
A4315	INSERTION TRAY WITH DRAINAGE BAG WITH INDWELLING CATHETER, FOLEY TYPE, TWO-WAY, ALL SILICONE	D	N	37	A		2130
A4316	INSERTION TRAY WITH DRAINAGE BAG WITH INDWELLING CATHETER, FOLEY TYPE, THREE-WAY, FOR CONTINUOUS IRRIGATION	D	N	37	A		2130
A4320	IRRIGATION TRAY WITH BULB OR PISTON SYRINGE, ANY PURPOSE	D	N	37	A		2130
A4321	THERAPEUTIC AGENT FOR URINARY CATHETER IRRIGATION	D	N	37	A		2130
A4322	IRRIGATION SYRINGE, BULB OR PISTON, EACH	D	N	37	A		2130
A4326	MALE EXTERNAL CATHETER WITH INTEGRAL COLLECTION CHAMBER, ANY TYPE, EACH	D	N	37	A		2130

HCPCS Code	Statute	Lab Cert	X-Ref	ASC Pay Grp	ASC Pay Group Eff. Date	Proc Notes	BETOS	TOS	Anest	Code Add Date	Code Effective Date	Code Term Date
A4280							D1F	P	0	20000101	20000101	
A4281							Z2	9	0	20030101	20070101	
A4282							Z2	9	0	20030101	20070101	
A4283							Z2	9	0	20030101	20070101	
A4284							Z2	9	0	20030101	20070101	
A4285							Z2	9	0	20030101	20070101	
A4286							Z2	9	0	20030101	20070101	
A4290							Z2	9	0	20010101	20020101	
A4300							Y1	S	0	19860101	20020101	
A4301							D1A	S	0	19960101	20030101	
A4305							D1A	9	0	19930101	20060101	
A4306							D1A	9	0	19930101	20070101	
A4310							D1F	P	0	19900101	19900101	
A4311							D1F	P	0	19900101	19900101	
A4312							D1F	P	0	19900101	19900101	
A4313							D1F	P	0	19900101	19900101	
A4314							D1F	P	0	19900101	19900101	
A4315							D1F	P	0	19900101	19900101	
A4316							D1F	P	0	19900101	19900101	
A4320							D1A	P	0	19900101	19920101	
A4321							D1F	P	0	19970101	20030101	
A4322							D1F	P	0	19900101	19960101	
A4326							D1F	P	0	19900101	20070101	

HCPCS Code	Long Description	Coverage	Action	PI	MPI	CIM	MCM
A4327	FEMALE EXTERNAL URINARY COLLECTION DEVICE; MEATAL CUP, EACH	D	N	37	A		2130
A4328	FEMALE EXTERNAL URINARY COLLECTION DEVICE; POUCH, EACH	D	N	37	A		2130
A4330	PERIANAL FECAL COLLECTION POUCH WITH ADHESIVE, EA.	D	N	37	A		2130
A4331	EXTENSION DRAINAGE TUBING, ANY TYPE, ANY LENGTH, WITH CONNECTOR/ADAPTOR, FOR USE WITH URINARY LEG BAG OR UROSTOMY POUCH, EACH	D	N	37	A		2130
A4332	LUBRICANT, INDIVIDUAL STERILE PACKET, EACH	D	N	37	A		2130
A4333	URINARY CATHETER ANCHORING DEVICE, ADHESIVE SKIN ATTACHMENT, EACH	D	N	37	A		2130
A4334	URINARY CATHETER ANCHORING DEVICE, LEG STRAP, EACH	D	N	37	A		2130
A4335	INCONTINENCE SUPPLY; MISCELLANEOUS	D	N	46	A		2130
A4336	INCONTINENCE SUPPLY, URETHRAL INSERT, ANY TYPE, EA.	D	A	37	A		
A4338	INDWELLING CATHETER; FOLEY TYPE, TWO-WAY LATEX WITH COATING (TEFLON, SILICONE, SILICONE ELASTOMER, OR HYDROPHILIC, ETC.), EACH	D	N	37	A		2130
A4340	INDWELLING CATHETER; SPECIALTY TYPE, EG; COUDE, MUSHROOM, WING, ETC.), EACH	D	N	37	A		2130
A4344	INDWELLING CATHETER, FOLEY TYPE, TWO-WAY, ALL SILICONE, EACH	D	N	37	A		2130
A4346	INDWELLING CATHETER; FOLEY TYPE, THREE WAY FOR CONTINUOUS IRRIGATION, EACH	D	N	37	A		2130
A4348	MALE EXTERNAL CATHETER WITH INTEGRAL COLLECTION COMPARTMENT, EXTENDED WEAR, EACH (E.G., 2 PER MONTH)	D	N	37	A		2130
A4349	MALE EXTERNAL CATHETER, WITH OR WITHOUT ADHESIVE, DISPOSABLE, EACH	D	N	37	A		2130
A4351	INTERMITTENT URINARY CATHETER; STRAIGHT TIP, WITH OR WITHOUT COATING (TEFLON, SILICONE, SILICONE ELASTOMER, OR HYDROPHILIC, ETC.), EACH	D	N	37	A		2130
A4352	INTERMITTENT URINARY CATHETER; COUDE (CURVED) TIP, WITH OR WITHOUT COATING (TEFLON, SILICONE, SILICONE ELASTOMERIC, OR HYDROPHILIC, ETC.), EACH	D	N	37	A		2130
A4353	INTERMITTENT URINARY CATHETER, WITH INSERTION SUPPLIES	D	N	37	A		2130
A4354	INSERTION TRAY WITH DRAINAGE BAG BUT WITHOUT CATHETER	D	N	37	A		2130
A4355	IRRIGATION TUBING SET FOR CONTINUOUS BLADDER IRRIGATION THROUGH A THREE-WAY INDWELLING FOLEY CATHETER, EACH	D	N	37	A		2130
A4356	EXTERNAL URETHRAL CLAMP OR COMPRESSION DEVICE (NOT TO BE USED FOR CATHETER CLAMP), EACH	D	N	37	A		2130
A4357	BEDSIDE DRAINAGE BAG, DAY OR NIGHT, WITH OR WITHOUT ANTI-REFLUX DEVICE, WITH OR WITHOUT TUBE, EACH	D	N	37	A		2130
A4358	URINARY DRAINAGE BAG, LEG OR ABDOMEN, VINYL, WITH OR WITHOUT TUBE, WITH STRAPS, EACH	D	N	37	A		2130
A4359	URINARY SUSPENSORY WITHOUT LEG BAG, EACH	D	N	37	A		2130
A4360	DISPOSABLE EXTERNAL URETHRAL CLAMP OR COMPRESSION DEVICE, WITH PAD AND/OR POUCH, EACH	D	A	37	A		

HCPCS Code	S t a t u t e	Lab Cert	X-Ref	ASC Pay Grp	ASC Pay Group Eff. Date	Proc Notes	BETOS	TOS	A n e s t	Code Add Date	Code Effective Date	Code Term Date
A4327							D1F	P	0	19900101	19900101	
A4328							D1F	P	0	19900101	19900101	
A4330							D1F	P	0	19900101	19960101	
A4331							D1F	P	0	20010101	20030101	
A4332							D1F	P	0	20010101	20050101	
A4333							D1F	P	0	20010101	20030101	
A4334							D1F	P	0	20010101	20030101	
A4335							D1F	P	0	19900101	19900101	
A4336						0124	D1F	P	0	20100101	20100101	
A4338							D1F	P	0	19900101	19960101	
A4340							D1F	P	0	19900101	19960101	
A4344							D1F	P	0	19830101	19960101	
A4346							D1F	P	0	19830101	19960101	
A4348							D1F	P	0	20010101	20070101	20061231
A4349							D1A	P	0	20050101	20050101	
A4351							D1F	P	0	19900101	20020101	
A4352							D1F	P	0	19900101	20020101	
A4353							D1F	P	0	19970101	20030101	
A4354							D1F	P	0	19860101	19900101	
A4355							D1F	P	0	19840101	19960101	
A4356							D1F	P	0	19850101	19960101	
A4357							D1F	P	0	19850101	19960101	
A4358							D1F	P	0	19850101	20020101	
A4358												
A4359							D1F	P	0	19850101	20070101	20061231
A4360						0124	D1F	9	0	20100101	20100101	
A4360												

HCPCS Code	Long Description	Coverage	Action	PI	MPI	CIM	MCM
A4361	OSTOMY FACEPLATE, EACH	D	N	37	A		2130
A4362	SKIN BARRIER; SOLID, 4 X 4 OR EQUIVALENT; EACH	D	N	37	A		2130
A4363	OSTOMY CLAMP, ANY TYPE, REPLACEMENT ONLY, EACH	D	N	37	A		
A4364	ADHESIVE, LIQUID OR EQUAL, ANY TYPE, PER OZ	D	N	37	A		2130
A4365	ADHESIVE REMOVER WIPES, ANY TYPE, PER 50	D	D	37	A		2130
A4366	OSTOMY VENT, ANY TYPE, EACH	C	N	37	A		
A4367	OSTOMY BELT, EACH	D	N	37	A		2130A
A4368	OSTOMY FILTER, ANY TYPE, EACH	C	N	37	A		
A4369	OSTOMY SKIN BARRIER, LIQUID (SPRAY, BRUSH, ETC), PER OZ	D	N	37	A		2130
A4371	OSTOMY SKIN BARRIER, POWDER, PER OZ	D	N	37	A		2130
A4372	OSTOMY SKIN BARRIER, SOLID 4X4 OR EQUIVALENT, STANDARD WEAR, WITH BUILT-IN CONVEXITY, EACH	D	N	37	A		2130
A4373	OSTOMY SKIN BARRIER, WITH FLANGE (SOLID, FLEXIBLE OR ACCORDIAN), WITH BUILT-IN CONVEXITY, ANY SIZE, EACH	D	N	37	A		2130
A4375	OSTOMY POUCH, DRAINABLE, WITH FACEPLATE ATTACHED, PLASTIC, EACH	D	N	37	A		2130
A4376	OSTOMY POUCH, DRAINABLE, WITH FACEPLATE ATTACHED, RUBBER, EACH	D	N	37	A		2130
A4377	OSTOMY POUCH, DRAINABLE, FOR USE ON FACEPLATE, PLASTIC, EACH	D	N	37	A		2130
A4378	OSTOMY POUCH, DRAINABLE, FOR USE ON FACEPLATE, RUBBER, EACH	D	N	37	A		2130
A4379	OSTOMY POUCH, URINARY, WITH FACEPLATE ATTACHED, PLASTIC, EACH	D	N	37	A		2130
A4380	OSTOMY POUCH, URINARY, WITH FACEPLATE ATTACHED, RUBBER, EACH	D	N	37	A		2130
A4381	OSTOMY POUCH, URINARY, FOR USE ON FACEPLATE, PLASTIC, EACH	D	N	37	A		2130
A4382	OSTOMY POUCH, URINARY, FOR USE ON FACEPLATE, HEAVY PLASTIC, EACH	D	N	37	A		2130
A4383	OSTOMY POUCH, URINARY, FOR USE ON FACEPLATE, RUBBER, EACH	D	N	37	A		2130
A4384	OSTOMY FACEPLATE EQUIVALENT, SILICONE RING, EACH	D	N	37	A		2130
A4385	OSTOMY SKIN BARRIER, SOLID 4X4 OR EQUIVALENT, EXTENDED WEAR, WITHOUT BUILT-IN CONVEXITY, EACH	D	N	37	A		2130
A4387	OSTOMY POUCH, CLOSED, WITH BARRIER ATTACHED, WITH BUILT-IN CONVEXITY (1 PIECE), EACH	D	N	37	A		2130
A4388	OSTOMY POUCH, DRAINABLE, WITH EXTENDED WEAR BARRIER ATTACHED, (1 PIECE), EACH	D	N	37	A		2130
A4389	OSTOMY POUCH, DRAINABLE, WITH BARRIER ATTACHED, WITH BUILT-IN CONVEXITY (1 PIECE), EACH	D	N	37	A		2130
A4390	OSTOMY POUCH, DRAINABLE, WITH EXTENDED WEAR BARRIER ATTACHED, WITH BUILT-IN CONVEXITY (1 PIECE), EA.	D	N	37	A		2130
A4391	OSTOMY POUCH, URINARY, WITH EXTENDED WEAR BARRIER ATTACHED (1 PIECE), EACH	D	N	37	A		2130
A4392	OSTOMY POUCH, URINARY, WITH STANDARD WEAR BARRIER ATTACHED, WITH BUILT-IN CONVEXITY (1 PIECE), EACH	D	N	37	A		2130
A4393	OSTOMY POUCH, URINARY, WITH EXTENDED WEAR BARRIER ATTACHED, WITH BUILT-IN CONVEXITY (1 PIECE), EACH	D	N	37	A		2130

HCPCS Code	Statute	Lab Cert	X-Ref	ASC Pay Grp	ASC Pay Group Eff. Date	Proc Notes	BETOS	TOS	Anest	Code Add Date	Code Effective Date	Code Term Date
A4361							D1F	P	0	19850101	19960101	
A4362							D1F	P	0	19850101	19900101	
A4363						0124	D1F	P	0	20060101	20060101	
A4364							D1F	P	0	19850101	20030101	
A4365							D1F	P	0	19970101	20100101	20091231
A4366							D1F	P	0	20040101	20040101	
A4367							D1F	P	0	19850101	19960101	
A4368							D1F	P	0	19970101	19970101	
A4369							D1F	P	0	20000101	20030101	
A4371							D1F	P	0	20000101	20030101	
A4372							D1F	P	0	20000101	20060101	
A4373							D1F	P	0	20000101	20030101	
A4375							D1F	P	0	20000101	20030101	
A4376							D1F	P	0	20000101	20030101	
A4377							D1F	P	0	20000101	20030101	
A4378							D1F	P	0	20000101	20030101	
A4379							D1F	P	0	20000101	20030101	
A4380							D1F	P	0	20000101	20030101	
A4381							D1F	P	0	20000101	20030101	
A4382							D1F	P	0	20000101	20030101	
A4383							D1F	P	0	20000101	20030101	
A4384							D1F	P	0	20000101	20030101	
A4385							D1F	P	0	20000101	20030101	
A4387							D1F	P	0	20000101	20030101	
A4388							D1F	P	0	20000101	20030101	
A4389							D1F	P	0	20000101	20030101	
A4390							D1F	P	0	20000101	20030101	
A4391							D1F	P	0	20000101	20030101	
A4392							D1F	P	0	20000101	20030101	
A4392												
A4393							D1F	P	0	20000101	20030101	
A4393												

HCPCS Code	Long Description	Coverage	Action	PI	MPI	CIM	MCM
A4394	OSTOMY DEODORANT, WITH OR WITHOUT LUBRICANT, FOR USE IN OSTOMY POUCH, PER FLUID OUNCE	D	N	37	A		2130
A4395	OSTOMY DEODORANT FOR USE IN OSTOMY POUCH, SOLID, PER TABLET	D	N	37	A		2130
A4396	OSTOMY BELT WITH PERISTOMAL HERNIA SUPPORT	D	N	37	A		2130
A4397	IRRIGATION SUPPLY; SLEEVE, EACH	D	N	37	A		2130
A4398	OSTOMY IRRIGATION SUPPLY; BAG, EACH	D	N	37	A		2130
A4399	OSTOMY IRRIGATION SUPPLY; CONE/CATHETER, INCLUDING BRUSH	D	N	37	A		2130
A4400	OSTOMY IRRIGATION SET	D	N	37	A		2130
A4402	LUBRICANT, PER OUNCE	D	N	37	A		2130
A4404	OSTOMY RING, EACH	D	N	37	A		2130
A4405	OSTOMY SKIN BARRIER, NON-PECTIN BASED, PASTE, PER OUNCE	D	N	37	A		2130
A4406	OSTOMY SKIN BARRIER, PECTIN-BASED, PASTE, PER OUNCE	D	N	37	A		2130
A4407	OSTOMY SKIN BARRIER, WITH FLANGE (SOLID, FLEXIBLE, OR ACCORDION), EXTENDED WEAR, WITH BUILT-IN CONVEXITY, 4 X 4 INCHES OR SMALLER, EACH	D	N	37	A		2130
A4408	OSTOMY SKIN BARRIER, WTIH FLANGE (SOLID, FLEXIBLE OR ACCORDION), EXTENDED WEAR, WITH BUILT-IN CONVEXITY, LARGER THAN 4 X 4 INCHES, EACH	D	N	37	A		2130
A4409	OSTOMY SKIN BARRIER, WITH FLANGE (SOLID, FLEXIBLE OR ACCORDION), EXTENDED WEAR, WITHOUT BUILT-IN CONVEXITY, 4 X 4 INCHES OR SMALLER, EACH	D	N	37	A		2130
A4410	OSTOMY SKIN BARRIER, WITH FLANGE (SOLID, FLEXIBLE OR ACCORDION), EXTENDED WEAR, WITHOUT BUILT-IN CONVEXITY, LARGER THAN 4 X 4 INCHES, EACH	D	N	37	A		2130
A4411	OSTOMY SKIN BARRIER, SOLID 4X4 OR EQUIVALENT, EXTENDED WEAR, WITH BUILT-IN CONVEXITY, EACH	D	N	37	A		
A4412	OSTOMY POUCH, DRAINABLE, HIGH OUTPUT, FOR USE ON A BARRIER WITH FLANGE (2 PIECE SYSTEM), WITHOUT FILTER, EACH	D	N	37	A		2130
A4413	OSTOMY POUCH, DRAINABLE, HIGH OUTPUT, FOR USE ON A BARRIER WITH FLANGE (2 PIECE SYSTEM), WITH FILTER, EA.	D	N	37	A		2130
A4414	OSTOMY SKIN BARRIER, WITH FLANGE (SOLID, FLEXIBLE OR ACCORDION), WITHOUT BUILT-IN CONVEXITY, 4 X 4 INCHES OR SMALLER, EACH	D	N	37	A		2130
A4415	OSTOMY SKIN BARRIER, WITH FLANGE (SOLID, FLEXIBLE OR ACCORDION), WITHOUT BUILT-IN CONVEXITY, LARGER THAN 4X4 INCHES, EACH	D	N	37	A		2130
A4416	OSTOMY POUCH, CLOSED, WITH BARRIER ATTACHED, WITH FILTER (1 PIECE), EACH	C	N	37	A		
A4417	OSTOMY POUCH, CLOSED, WITH BARRIER ATTACHED, WITH BUILT-IN CONVEXITY, WITH FILTER (1 PIECE), EACH	C	N	37	A		
A4418	OSTOMY POUCH, CLOSED; WITHOUT BARRIER ATTACHED, WITH FILTER (1 PIECE), EACH	C	N	37	A		
A4419	OSTOMY POUCH, CLOSED; FOR USE ON BARRIER WITH NON-LOCKING FLANGE, WITH FILTER (2 PIECE), EACH	C	N	37	A		

HCPCS Code	Statute	Lab Cert	X-Ref	ASC Pay Grp	ASC Pay Group Eff. Date	Proc Notes	BETOS	TOS	Anest	Code Add Date	Code Effective Date	Code Term Date
A4394							D1F	P	0	20000101	20070101	
A4394												
A4395							D1F	P	0	20000101	20030101	
A4396							D1F	P	0	20010101	20030101	
A4397							D1F	P	0	19900101	19960101	
A4398							D1F	P	0	19890101	19970101	
A4399							D1F	P	0	19890101	19970101	
A4400							D1F	P	0	19820101	19900101	
A4402							D1F	P	0	19850101	19950101	
A4404							D1F	P	0	19850101	19950101	
A4405							D1F	P	0	20030101	20030101	
A4406							D1F	P	0	20030101	20030101	
A4407							D1F	P	0	20030101	20030101	
A4408							D1F	P	0	20030101	20030101	
A4409							D1F	P	0	20030101	20060101	
A4410							D1F	P	0	20030101	20060101	
A4410												
A4411						0124	D1F	P	0	20060101	20060101	
A4412						0124	D1F	P	0	20060101	20060101	
A4413							D1F	P	0	20030101	20030101	
A4414							D1F	P	0	20030101	20060101	
A4415							D1F	P	0	20030101	20060101	
A4416							D1F	P	0	20040101	20040101	
A4417							D1F	P	0	20040101	20040101	
A4418							D1F	P	0	20040101	20040101	
A4419							D1F	P	0	20040101	20040101	

HCPCS Code	Long Description	Coverage	Action	PI	MPI	CIM	MCM
A4420	OSTOMY POUCH, CLOSED; FOR USE ON BARRIER WITH LOCKING FLANGE (2 PIECE), EACH	C	N	37	A		
A4421	OSTOMY SUPPLY; MISCELLANEOUS	C	N	00	9		
A4422	OSTOMY ABSORBENT MATERIAL (SHEET/PAD/CRYSTAL PACKET) FOR USE IN OSTOMY POUCH TO THICKEN LIQUID STOMAL OUTPUT, EACH	D	N	37	A		2130
A4423	OSTOMY POUCH, CLOSED; FOR USE ON BARRIER WITH LOCKING FLANGE, WITH FILTER (2 PIECE), EACH	C	N	37	A		
A4424	OSTOMY POUCH, DRAINABLE, WITH BARRIER ATTACHED, WITH FILTER (1 PIECE), EACH	C	N	37	A		
A4425	OSTOMY POUCH, DRAINABLE; FOR USE ON BARRIER WITH NON-LOCKING FLANGE, WITH FILTER (2 PIECE SYSTEM), EA.	C	N	37	A		
A4426	OSTOMY POUCH, DRAINABLE; FOR USE ON BARRIER WITH LOCKING FLANGE (2 PIECE SYSTEM), EACH	C	N	37	A		
A4427	OSTOMY POUCH, DRAINABLE; FOR USE ON BARRIER WITH LOCKING FLANGE, WITH FILTER (2 PIECE SYSTEM), EACH	C	N	37	A		
A4428	OSTOMY POUCH, URINARY, WITH EXTENDED WEAR BARRIER ATTACHED, WITH FAUCET-TYPE TAP WITH VALVE (1 PIECE), EA.	C	N	37	A		
A4429	OSTOMY POUCH, URINARY, WITH BARRIER ATTACHED, WITH BUILT-IN CONVEXITY, WITH FAUCET-TYPE TAP WITH VALVE (1 PIECE), EACH	C	N	37	A		
A4430	OSTOMY POUCH, URINARY, WITH EXTENDED WEAR BARRIER ATTACHED, WITH BUILT-IN CONVEXITY, WITH FAUCET-TYPE TAP WITH VALVE (1 PIECE), EA.	C	N	37	A		
A4431	OSTOMY POUCH, URINARY; WITH BARRIER ATTACHED, WITH FAUCET-TYPE TAP WITH VALVE (1 PIECE), EACH	C	N	37	A		
A4432	OSTOMY POUCH, URINARY; FOR USE ON BARRIER WITH NON-LOCKING FLANGE, WITH FAUCET-TYPE TAP WITH VALVE (2 PIECE), EACH	C	N	37	A		
A4433	OSTOMY POUCH, URINARY; FOR USE ON BARRIER WITH LOCKING FLANGE (2 PIECE), EACH	C	N	37	A		
A4434	OSTOMY POUCH, URINARY; FOR USE ON BARRIER WITH LOCKING FLANGE, WITH FAUCET-TYPE TAP WITH VALVE (2 PIECE), EACH	C	N	37	A		
A4450	TAPE, NON-WATERPROOF, PER 18 SQUARE INCHES	D	N	37	A		2130
A4452	TAPE, WATERPROOF, PER 18 SQUARE INCHES	D	N	37	A		2130
A4455	ADHESIVE REMOVER OR SOLVENT (FOR TAPE, CEMENT OR OTHER ADHESIVE), PER OUNCE	D	N	37	A		2130
A4456	ADHESIVE REMOVER, WIPES, ANY TYPE, EACH	D	A	37	A		2130
A4458	ENEMA BAG WITH TUBING, REUSABLE	C	N	00	9		
A4461	SURGICAL DRESSING HOLDER, NON-REUSABLE, EACH	C	N	35	A		
A4462	ABDOMINAL DRESSING HOLDER, EACH	D	N	35	A		2079
A4463	SURGICAL DRESSING HOLDER, REUSABLE, EACH	C	N	35	A		
A4465	NON-ELASTIC BINDER FOR EXTREMITY	C	N	00	9		
A4466	GARMENT, BELT, SLEEVE OR OTHER COVERING, ELASTIC OR SIMILAR STRETCHABLE MATERIAL, ANY TYPE, EACH	I	A	00	9		
A4470	GRAVLEE JET WASHER	D	N	00	9	50-4	2320
A4480	VABRA ASPIRATOR	D	N	00	9	50-10	2320
A4481	TRACHEOSTOMA FILTER, ANY TYPE, ANY SIZE, EACH	D	N	37	A		2130

HCPCS Code	S t a t u t e	Lab Cert	X-Ref	ASC Pay Grp	ASC Pay Group Eff. Date	Proc Notes	BETOS	TOS	A n e s t	Code Add Date	Code Effective Date	Code Term Date
A4420							D1F	P	0	20040101	20040101	
A4421							D1F	P	0	19850101	20070101	
A4422							D1F	P	0	20030101	20030101	
A4423							D1F	P	0	20040101	20040101	
A4423												
A4424							D1F	P	0	20040101	20040101	
A4425							D1F	P	0	20040101	20040101	
A4426							D1F	P	0	20040101	20040101	
A4427							D1F	P	0	20040101	20040101	
A4428							D1F	P	0	20040101	20040101	
A4429							D1F	P	0	20040101	20040101	
A4430							D1F	P	0	20040101	20040101	
A4431							D1F	P	0	20040101	20040101	
A4432							D1F	P	0	20040101	20040101	
A4433							D1F	P	0	20040101	20040101	
A4434							D1F	P	0	20040101	20040101	
A4450							D1F	L, P	0	20030101	20030101	
A4452							D1F	L, P	0	20030101	20030101	
A4455							D1F	P	0	19890101	19950101	
A4456							D1F	P	0	20100101	20100101	
A4458							Z2	9	0	20030101	20070101	
A4461							D1A	S	0	20070101	20070101	
A4462							D1A	S	0	19980101	20070101	20061231
A4463							D1A	S	0	20070101	20070101	
A4465							D1A	9	0	19940101	19950101	
A4466							Z2	9	0	20100101	20100101	
A4470							D1A	P	0	19860101	20010101	
A4480							D1A	P	0	19860101	20010101	
A4481							D1F	P	0	19970101	20030101	

HCPCS Code	Long Description	Coverage	Action	PI	MPI	CIM	MCM
A4483	MOISTURE EXCHANGER, DISPOSABLE, FOR USE WITH INVASIVE MECHANICAL VENTILATION	D	N	37	A		2130
A4490	SURGICAL STOCKINGS ABOVE KNEE LENGTH, EACH	M	N	00	9	60-9	2079, 2100
A4495	SURGICAL STOCKINGS THIGH LENGTH, EACH	M	N	00	9	60-9	2079, 2100
A4500	SURGICAL STOCKINGS BELOW KNEE LENGTH, EACH	M	N	00	9	60-9	2079, 2100
A4510	SURGICAL STOCKINGS FULL LENGTH, EACH	M	N	00	9	60-9	2079, 2100
A4520	INCONTINENCE GARMENT, ANY TYPE, (E.G. BRIEF, DIAPER), EA.	M	N	00	9	60-9	
A4550	SURGICAL TRAYS	D	N	11	A		15030
A4554	DISPOSABLE UNDERPADS, ALL SIZES	M	N	00	9	60-9	
A4556	ELECTRODES, (E.G., APNEA MONITOR), PER PAIR	C	N	34	A		
A4557	LEAD WIRES, (E.G., APNEA MONITOR), PER PAIR	C	N	34	A		
A4558	CONDUCTIVE GEL OR PASTE, FOR USE WITH ELECTRICAL DEVICE (E.G., TENS, NMES), PER OZ	C	N	34	A		
A4559	COUPLING GEL OR PASTE, FOR USE WITH ULTRASOUND DEVICE, PER OZ	C	N	34	A		
A4561	PESSARY, RUBBER, ANY TYPE	C	N	38	A		
A4562	PESSARY, NON RUBBER, ANY TYPE	C	N	38	A		
A4565	SLINGS	C	N	52	A		
A4570	SPLINT	I	N	52	A		2079
A4575	TOPICAL HYPERBARIC OXYGEN CHAMBER, DISPOSABLE	M	N	00	9	35-10	
A4580	CAST SUPPLIES (E.G. PLASTER)	I	N	00	9		2079
A4590	SPECIAL CASTING MATERIAL (E.G. FIBERGLASS)	I	N	00	9		2079
A4595	ELECTRICAL STIMULATOR SUPPLIES, 2 LEAD, PER MONTH, (E.G. TENS, NMES)	D	N	34	A	45-25	
A4600	SLEEVE FOR INTERMITTENT LIMB COMPRESSION DEVICE, REPLACEMENT ONLY, EACH	C	N	32	A		
A4601	LITHIUM ION BATTERY FOR NON-PROSTHETIC USE, REPLACEMENT	C	N	32	A		
A4604	TUBING WITH INTEGRATED HEATING ELEMENT FOR USE WITH POSITIVE AIRWAY PRESSURE DEVICE	C	N	32	A		
A4605	TRACHEAL SUCTION CATHETER, CLOSED SYSTEM, EACH	C	N	32	A		
A4606	OXYGEN PROBE FOR USE WITH OXIMETER DEVICE, REPLACEMENT	C	N	00	9		
A4608	TRANSTRACHEAL OXYGEN CATHETER, EACH	C	N	00	9		
A4611	BATTERY, HEAVY DUTY; REPLACEMENT FOR PATIENT OWNED VENTILATOR	C	N	32	A		
A4612	BATTERY CABLES; REPLACEMENT FOR PATIENT-OWNED VENTILATOR	C	N	32	A		
A4613	BATTERY CHARGER; REPLACEMENT FOR PATIENT-OWNED VENTILATOR	C	N	32	A		
A4614	PEAK EXPIRATORY FLOW RATE METER, HAND HELD	C	N	46	A		
A4615	CANNULA, NASAL	D	N	00	9	60-4	3312
A4616	TUBING (OXYGEN), PER FOOT	D	N	00	9	60-4	3312
A4617	MOUTH PIECE	D	N	00	9	60-4	3312
A4618	BREATHING CIRCUITS	D	N	32	A	60-4	3312
A4619	FACE TENT	D	N	33	A	60-4	3312
A4620	VARIABLE CONCENTRATION MASK	D	N	00	9	60-4	3312
A4623	TRACHEOSTOMY, INNER CANNULA	D	N	37	A	65-16	2130

HCPCS Code	Statute	Lab Cert	X-Ref	ASC Pay Grp	ASC Pay Group Eff. Date	Proc Notes	BETOS	TOS	Anest	Code Add Date	Code Effective Date	Code Term Date
A4483							D1F	P	0	19990101	20030101	
A4490							D1A	P	0	19860101	20030101	
A4495							D1A	P	0	19860101	20030101	
A4500							D1A	P	0	19860101	20030101	
A4510							D1A	P	0	19860101	20030101	
A4520							D1A	9	0	20050101	20050101	
							Y1	9	0	19820101	20000101	
A4554							D1A	9	0	19860101	20050101	
A4556							D1E	P	0	19840101	20000101	
A4557							D1E	P	0	19840101	20000101	
A4558							D1E	P	0	19850101	20070101	
A4559							D1E	P	0	20070101	20070101	
A4561							D1F	P	0	20010101	20010101	
A4562							D1F	P	0	20010101	20010101	
A4565							D1A	P	0	19830101	19960101	
A4570							D1A	P	0	19820101	20010701	
A4575							D1A	9	0	19960101	19960101	
A4580							D1A	9	0	19820101	20030101	
A4590							D1A	9	0	19840101	20030101	
A4595							D1E	P	0	19960101	20030101	
A4600							D1E	P	0	20070101	20070101	
A4601							D1E	P	0	20070101	20070101	
A4604							D1E	P	0	20060101	20060101	
A4605							D1E	P	0	20050101	20050101	
A4606							D1E	9	0	20030101	20030101	
A4608							D1E	P	0	20010101	20090101	
A4611							D1E	P	0	19900101	19960101	
A4612							D1E	P	0	19900101	19960101	
A4613							D1E	P	0	19900101	19960101	
A4614							Z2	9	0	19990101	19990101	
A4615							D1C	P	0	19900101	20090101	
A4616							D1C	P	0	19900101	20090101	
A4617							D1C	P	0	19900101	20090101	
A4618							D1E	A, P, R	0	19900101	19900101	19930101
A4619							D1C	P	0	19900101	19960101	
A4620							D1C	P	0	19900101	20090101	
A4623							D1F	P	0	19900101	20040101	

HCPCS Code	Long Description	Coverage	Action	PI	MPI	CIM	MCM
A4624	TRACHEAL SUCTION CATHETER, ANY TYPE OTHER THAN CLOSED SYSTEM, EACH	C	N	32	A		
A4625	TRACHEOSTOMY CARE KIT FOR NEW TRACHEOSTOMY	D	N	37	A		2130
A4626	TRACHEOSTOMY CLEANING BRUSH, EACH	D	N	37	A		2130
A4627	SPACER, BAG OR RESERVOIR, WITH OR WITHOUT MASK, FOR USE WITH METERED DOSE INHALER	M	N	00	9		2100
A4628	OROPHARYNGEAL SUCTION CATHETER, EACH	C	N	32	A		
A4629	TRACHEOSTOMY CARE KIT FOR ESTABLISHED TRACHEOSTOMY	D	N	37	A		2130
A4630	REPLACEMENT BATTERIES, MEDICALLY NECESSARY, TRANSCUTANEOUS ELECTRICAL	D	N	32	A	65-8	
A4630	STIMULATOR, OWNED BY PATIENT						
A4632	REPLACEMENT BATTERY FOR EXTERNAL INFUSION PUMP, ANY TYPE, EACH	I	N	00	9		
A4633	REPLACEMENT BULB/LAMP FOR ULTRAVIOLET LIGHT THERAPY SYSTEM, EACH	C	N	32	A		
A4634	REPLACEMENT BULB FOR THERAPEUTIC LIGHT BOX, TABLETOP MODEL	C	N	00	9		
A4635	UNDERARM PAD, CRUTCH, REPLACEMENT, EACH	D	N	32	A	60-9	
A4636	REPLACEMENT, HANDGRIP, CANE, CRUTCH, OR WALKER, EA.	D	N	32	A	60-9	
A4637	REPLACEMENT, TIP, CANE, CRUTCH, WALKER, EACH.	D	N	32	A	60-9	
A4638	REPLACEMENT BATTERY FOR PATIENT-OWNED EAR PULSE GENERATOR, EACH	C	N	32	A		
A4639	REPLACEMENT PAD FOR INFRARED HEATING PAD SYSTEM, EA.	C	N	32	A		
A4640	REPLACEMENT PAD FOR USE WITH MEDICALLY NECESSARY ALTERNATING PRESSURE PAD OWNED BY PATIENT	D	N	32	A	60-9	4107.6
A4641	RADIOPHARMACEUTICAL, DIAGNOSTIC, NOT OTHERWISE CLASSIFIED	C	N	51	A		
A4642	INDIUM IN-111 SATUMOMAB PENDETIDE, DIAGNOSTIC, PER STUDY DOSE, UP TO 6 MILLICURIES	C	N	51	A		
A4648	TISSUE MARKER, IMPLANTABLE, ANY TYPE, EACH	C	N	57	A		
A4649	SURGICAL SUPPLY; MISCELLANEOUS	C	N	46	A		
A4650	IMPLANTABLE RADIATION DOSIMETER, EACH	C	N	57	A		
A4651	CALIBRATED MICROCAPILLARY TUBE, EACH	D	N	52	A		4270
A4652	MICROCAPILLARY TUBE SEALANT	D	N	52	A		4270
A4653	PERITONEAL DIALYSIS CATHETER ANCHORING DEVICE, BELT, EACH	C	N	52	A		
A4657	SYRINGE, WITH OR WITHOUT NEEDLE, EACH	D	N	52	A		4270
A4660	SPHYGMOMANOMETER/BLOOD PRESSURE APPARATUS WITH CUFF AND STETHOSCOPE	D	N	52	A		4270
A4663	BLOOD PRESSURE CUFF ONLY	D	N	52	A		4270
A4670	AUTOMATIC BLOOD PRESSURE MONITOR	M	N	00	9	50-42	4270
A4671	DISPOSABLE CYCLER SET USED WITH CYCLER DIALYSIS MACHINE, EACH	D	N	52	A		4270
A4672	DRAINAGE EXTENSION LINE, STERILE, FOR DIALYSIS, EACH	D	N	52	A		4270
A4673	EXTENSION LINE WITH EASY LOCK CONNECTORS, USED WITH DIALYSIS	D	N	52	A		4270
A4674	CHEMICALS/ANTISEPTICS SOLUTION USED TO CLEAN/ STERILIZE DIALYSIS EQUIPMENT, PER 8 OZ	D	N	52	A		4270

HCPCS Code	Statute	Lab Cert	X-Ref	ASC Pay Grp	ASC Pay Group Eff. Date	Proc Notes	BETOS	TOS	Anest	Code Add Date	Code Effective Date	Code Term Date
A4624							D1E	P	0	19900101	20030101	
A4625							D1F	P	0	19900101	20030101	
A4626							D1F	P	0	19900101	20030101	
A4627							D1A	9	0	19910101	19970101	
A4628							D1E	A,P,R	0	19960101	19960101	
A4629							D1F	P	0	19960101	20030101	
A4630							D1E	A,P,R	0	19910101	20060101	
A4630												
A4632							D1E	A,P,R	0	20030101	20070101	20061231
A4633							D1E	A,P,R	0	20030101	20030101	
A4634							D1E	9	0	20030101	20030101	
A4635							D1E	A,P,R	0	19910101	19960101	
A4636							D1E	A,P,R	0	19910101	19960101	
A4637							D1E	A,P,R	0	19910101	19960101	
A4638							D1E	P	0	20040101	20040101	
A4639							D1E	A,P,R	0	20030101	20030101	
A4640							D1E	A,P,R	0	19910101	19960101	
A4640												
A4641							I1E	4	0	19940101	20060101	
A4642							I1E	4	0	19950101	20060101	
A4642												
A4648							I1E	9, S	0	20080101	20080101	
A4649							D1A	9	0	19820101	19980101	
A4650							I1E	9, S	0	20080101	20080101	
A4651						0017	P9B	L	0	20020101	20020101	
A4652						0017	P9B	L	0	20020101	20020101	
A4653							P9B	L	0	20030101	20030101	
A4657						0017	P9B	L	0	20020101	20030101	
A4660						0017	P9B	L	0	19860101	20030101	
A4663						0017	P9B	L	0	19860101	20030101	
A4670						0017	P9B	L	0	19860101	20030101	
A4671							P9B	L	0	20040101	20040101	
A4672							P9B	L	0	20040101	20040101	
A4673							P9B	L	0	20040101	20040101	
A4674							P9B	L	0	20040101	20040101	

HCPCS Code	Long Description	Coverage	Action	PI	MPI	CIM	MCM
A4680	ACTIVATED CARBON FILTER FOR HEMODIALYSIS, EACH	D	N	52	A	55-1	4270
A4690	DIALYZER (ARTIFICIAL KIDNEYS), ALL TYPES, ALL SIZES, FOR HEMODIALYSIS, EACH	D	N	52	A		4270
A4706	BICARBONATE CONCENTRATE, SOLUTION, FOR HEMODIALYSIS, PER GALLON	D	N	52	A		4270
A4707	BICARBONATE CONCENTRATE, POWDER, FOR HEMODIALYSIS, PER PACKET	D	N	52	A		4270
A4708	ACETATE CONCENTRATE SOLUTION, FOR HEMODIALYSIS, PER GALLON	D	N	52	A		4270
A4709	ACID CONCENTRATE, SOLUTION, FOR HEMODIALYSIS, PER GALLON	D	N	52	A		4270
A4714	TREATED WATER (DEIONIZED, DISTILLED, OR REVERSE OSMOSIS) FOR PERITONEAL DIALYSIS, PER GALLON	D	N	52	A	55-1	4270
A4719	"Y SET" TUBING FOR PERITONEAL DIALYSIS	D	N	52	A		4270
A4720	DIALYSATE SOLUTION, ANY CONCENTRATION OF DEXTROSE, FLUID VOLUME GREATER THAN 249CC, BUT LESS THAN OR EQUAL TO 999CC, FOR PERITONEAL DIALYSIS	D	N	52	A		4270
A4721	DIALYSATE SOLUTION, ANY CONCENTRATION OF DEXTROSE, FLUID VOLUME GREATER THAN 999CC BUT LESS THAN OR EQUAL TO 1999CC, FOR PERITONEAL DIALYSIS	D	N	52	A		4270
A4722	DIALYSATE SOLUTION, ANY CONCENTRATION OF DEXTROSE, FLUID VOLUME GREATER THAN 1999CC BUT LESS THAN OR EQUAL TO 2999CC, FOR PERITONEAL DIALYSIS	D	N	52	A		4270
A4723	DIALYSATE SOLUTION, ANY CONCENTRATION OF DEXTROSE, FLUID VOLUME GREATER THAN 2999CC BUT LESS THAN OR EQUAL TO 3999CC, FOR PERITONEAL DIALYSIS	D	N	52	A		4270
A4724	DIALYSATE SOLUTION, ANY CONCENTRATION OF DEXTROSE, FLUID VOLUME GREATER THAN 3999CC BUT LESS THAN OR EQUAL TO 4999CC, FOR PERITONEAL DIALYSIS	D	N	52	A		4270
A4725	DIALYSATE SOLUTION, ANY CONCENTRATION OF DEXTROSE, FLUID VOLUME GREATER THAN 4999CC BUT LESS THAN OR EQUAL TO 5999CC, FOR PERITONEAL DIALYSIS	D	N	52	A		4270
A4726	DIALYSATE SOLUTION, ANY CONCENTRATION OF DEXTROSE, FLUID VOLUME GREATER THAN 5999CC, FOR PERITONEAL DIALYSIS	D	N	52	A		4270
A4728	DIALYSATE SOLUTION, NON-DEXTROSE CONTAINING, 500 ML	C	N	52	A		
A4730	FISTULA CANNULATION SET FOR HEMODIALYSIS, EACH	D	N	52	A		4270
A4736	TOPICAL ANESTHETIC, FOR DIALYSIS, PER GRAM	D	N	52	A		4270
A4737	INJECTABLE ANESTHETIC, FOR DIALYSIS, PER 10 ML	D	N	52	A		4270
A4740	SHUNT ACCESSORY, FOR HEMODIALYSIS, ANY TYPE, EACH	D	N	52	A		4270
A4750	BLOOD TUBING, ARTERIAL OR VENOUS, FOR HEMODIALYSIS, EA.	D	N	52	A		4270
A4755	BLOOD TUBING, ARTERIAL AND VENOUS COMBINED, FOR HEMODIALYSIS, EACH	D	N	52	A		4270
A4760	DIALYSATE SOLUTION TEST KIT, FOR PERITONEAL DIALYSIS, ANY TYPE, EACH	D	N	52	A		4270
A4765	DIALYSATE CONCENTRATE, POWDER, ADDITIVE FOR PERITONEAL DIALYSIS, PER PACKET	D	N	52	A		4270
A4766	DIALYSATE CONCENTRATE, SOLUTION, ADDITIVE FOR L PERITONEAL DIALYSIS, PER 10 M	D	N	52	A		4270

HCPCS Code	Statute	Lab Cert	X-Ref	ASC Pay Grp	ASC Pay Group Eff. Date	Proc Notes	BETOS	TOS	Anest	Code Add Date	Code Effective Date	Code Term Date
A4680						0017	P9B	L	0	19860101	20020101	
A4690						0017	P9B	L	0	19860101	20020101	
A4706						0017	P9B	L	0	20020101	20020101	
A4707						0017	P9B	L	0	20020101	20020101	
A4708						0017	P9B	L	0	20020101	20020101	
A4709						0017	P9B	L	0	20020101	20020101	
A4714						0017	P9B	L	0	19860101	20020101	
A4714												
A4719						0017	P9B	L	0	20020101	20020101	
A4720						0017	P9B	L	0	20020101	20020101	
A4721						0017	P9B	L	0	20020101	20020101	
A4722						0017	P9B	L	0	20020101	20020101	
A4723						0017	P9B	L	0	20020101	20020101	
A4724						0017	P9B	L	0	20020101	20020101	
A4725						0017	P9B	L	0	20020101	20020101	
A4726						0017	P9B	L	0	20020101	20020101	
A4728							P9B	L	0	20040101	20040101	
A4730						0017	P9B	L	0	19860101	20020101	
A4736						0017	P9B	L	0	20020101	20020101	
A4737						0017	P9B	L	0	20020101	20020101	
A4740						0017	P9B	L	0	19860101	20020101	
A4750						0017	P9B	L	0	19860101	20020101	
A4755						0017	P9B	L	0	19860101	20020101	
A4760						0017	P9B	L	0	19860101	20020101	
A4765						0017	P9B	L	0	19860101	20020101	
A4766						0017	P9B	L	0	20020101	20020101	

HCPCS Code	Long Description	Coverage	Action	PI	MPI	CIM	MCM
A4770	BLOOD COLLECTION TUBE, VACUUM, FOR DIALYSIS, PER 50	D	N	52	A		4270
A4771	SERUM CLOTTING TIME TUBE, FOR DIALYSIS, PER 50	D	N	52	A		4270
A4772	BLOOD GLUCOSE TEST STRIPS, FOR DIALYSIS, PER 50	D	N	52	A		4270
A4773	OCCULT BLOOD TEST STRIPS, FOR DIALYSIS, PER 50	D	N	52	A		4270
A4774	AMMONIA TEST STRIPS, FOR DIALYSIS, PER 50	D	N	52	A		4270
A4802	PROTAMINE SULFATE, FOR HEMODIALYSIS, PER 50 MG	D	N	52	A		4270
A4860	DISPOSABLE CATHETER TIPS FOR PERITONEAL DIALYSIS, PER 10	D	N	52	A		4270
A4870	PLUMBING AND/OR ELECTRICAL WORK FOR HOME HEMODIALYSIS EQUIPMENT	D	N	52	A		4270
A4890	CONTRACTS, REPAIR AND MAINTENANCE, FOR HEMODIALYSIS EQUIPMENT	D	N	52	A		2100.4
A4911	DRAIN BAG/BOTTLE, FOR DIALYSIS, EACH	D	N	52	A		
A4913	MISCELLANEOUS DIALYSIS SUPPLIES, NOT OTHERWISE SPECIFIED	D	N	52	A		
A4918	VENOUS PRESSURE CLAMP, FOR HEMODIALYSIS, EACH	D	N	52	A		
A4927	GLOVES, NON-STERILE, PER 100	D	N	52	A		
A4928	SURGICAL MASK, PER 20	D	N	52	A		
A4929	TOURNIQUET FOR DIALYSIS, EACH	D	N	52	A		
A4930	GLOVES, STERILE, PER PAIR	D	N	52	A		
A4931	ORAL THERMOMETER, REUSABLE, ANY TYPE, EACH	C	N	52	A		
A4932	RECTAL THERMOMETER, REUSABLE, ANY TYPE, EACH	C	N	00	9		
A5051	OSTOMY POUCH, CLOSED; WITH BARRIER ATTACHED (1 PIECE), EACH	D	N	37	A		2130
A5052	OSTOMY POUCH, CLOSED; WITHOUT BARRIER ATTACHED (1 PIECE), EACH	D	N	37	A		2130
A5053	OSTOMY POUCH, CLOSED; FOR USE ON FACEPLATE, EACH	D	N	37	A		2130
A5054	OSTOMY POUCH, CLOSED; FOR USE ON BARRIER WITH FLANGE (2 PIECE), EACH	D	N	37	A		2130
A5055	STOMA CAP	D	N	37	A		2130
A5061	OSTOMY POUCH, DRAINABLE; WITH BARRIER ATTACHED, (1 PIECE), EACH	C	N	37	A		
A5062	OSTOMY POUCH, DRAINABLE; WITHOUT BARRIER ATTACHED (1 PIECE), EACH	D	N	37	A		2130
A5063	OSTOMY POUCH, DRAINABLE; FOR USE ON BARRIER WITH FLANGE (2 PIECE SYSTEM), EACH	D	N	37	A		2130
A5071	OSTOMY POUCH, URINARY; WITH BARRIER ATTACHED (1 PIECE), EACH	D	N	37	A		2130
A5072	OSTOMY POUCH, URINARY; WITHOUT BARRIER ATTACHED (1 PIECE), EACH	D	N	37	A		2130
A5073	OSTOMY POUCH, URINARY; FOR USE ON BARRIER WITH FLANGE (2 PIECE), EACH	D	N	37	A		2130
A5081	CONTINENT DEVICE; PLUG FOR CONTINENT STOMA	D	N	37	A		2130
A5082	CONTINENT DEVICE; CATHETER FOR CONTINENT STOMA	D	N	37	A		2130
A5083	CONTINENT DEVICE, STOMA ABSORPTIVE COVER FOR CONTINENT STOMA	C	N	37	A		
A5093	OSTOMY ACCESSORY; CONVEX INSERT	D	N	37	A		2130
A5102	BEDSIDE DRAINAGE BOTTLE WITH OR WITHOUT TUBING, RIGID OR EXPANDABLE, EACH	D	N	37	A		2130

HCPCS Code	Statute	Lab Cert	X-Ref	ASC Pay Grp	ASC Pay Group Eff. Date	Proc Notes	BETOS	TOS	Anest	Code Add Date	Code Effective Date	Code Term Date
A4770						0017	P9B	L	0	19860101	20020101	
A4771						0017	P9B	L	0	19860101	20020101	
A4772						0017	P9B	L	0	19860101	20020101	
A4773						0017	P9B	L	0	19860101	20020101	
A4774						0017	P9B	L	0	19860101	20020101	
A4802						0017	P9B	L	0	20020101	20020101	
A4860						0017	P9B	L	0	19860101	20020101	
A4870						0017	P9B	L	0	19860101	20020101	
A4890						0017	P9B	L	0	19860101	20020101	
A4911						0017	P9B	L	0	20020101	20020101	
A4913						0017	P9B	L	0	19860101	20020101	
A4918						0017	P9B	L	0	19860101	20020101	
A4927						0017	P9B	L	0	19860101	20030101	
A4928						0017	P9B	L	0	20020101	20030101	
A4929						0017	P9B	L	0	20020101	20020101	
A4930						0017	P9B	L	0	20030101	20030101	
A4931							P9B	L	0	20030101	20030101	
A4932							Z2	9	0	20030101	20070101	
A5051							D1F	P	0	19900101	20030101	
A5052							D1F	P	0	19900101	20030101	
A5053							D1F	P	0	19900101	20030101	
A5054							D1F	P	0	19900101	20030101	
A5055							D1F	P	0	19900101	19900101	
A5061							D1F	P	0	19900101	20030101	
A5062							D1F	P	0	19900101	20030101	
A5063							D1F	P	0	19900101	20030101	
A5071							D1F	P	0	19900101	20030101	
A5072							D1F	P	0	19900101	20030101	
A5073							D1F	P	0	19900101	20030101	
A5081							D1F	P	0	19900101	19900101	
A5082							D1F	P	0	19900101	19900101	
A5083							D1F	P	0	20080101	20080101	
A5093							D1F	P	0	19900101	19900101	
A5102							D1F	P	0	19900101	19970101	

HCPCS Code	Long Description	Coverage	Action	PI	MPI	CIM	MCM
A5105	URINARY SUSPENSORY WITH LEG BAG, WITH OR WITHOUT TUBE, EACH	D	N	37	A		2130
A5112	URINARY LEG BAG; LATEX	D	N	37	A		2130
A5113	LEG STRAP; LATEX, REPLACEMENT ONLY, PER SET	D	N	37	A		2130
A5114	LEG STRAP; FOAM OR FABRIC, REPLACEMENT ONLY, PER SET	D	N	37	A		2130
A5120	SKIN BARRIER, WIPES OR SWABS, EACH	D	N	37	A		2130
A5121	SKIN BARRIER; SOLID, 6 X 6 OR EQUIVALENT, EACH	D	N	37	A		2130
A5122	SKIN BARRIER; SOLID, 8 X 8 OR EQUIVALENT, EACH	D	N	37	A		2130
A5126	ADHESIVE OR NON-ADHESIVE; DISK OR FOAM PAD	D	N	37	A		2130
A5131	APPLIANCE CLEANER, INCONTINENCE AND OSTOMY APPLIANCES, PER 16 OZ.	D	N	37	A		2130
A5200	PERCUTANEOUS CATHETER/TUBE ANCHORING DEVICE, ADHESIVE SKIN ATTACHMENT	D	N	37	A		2130
A5500	FOR DIABETICS ONLY, FITTING (INCLUDING FOLLOW-UP), CUSTOM PREPARATION AND SUPPLY OF OFF-THE-SHELF DEPTH-INLAY SHOE MANUFACTURED TO ACCOMMODATE MULTI-DENSITY INSERT(S), PER SHOE	D	N	38	A		2134
A5501	FOR DIABETICS ONLY, FITTING (INCLUDING FOLLOW-UP), CUSTOM PREPARATION AND SUPPLY OF SHOE MOLDED FROM CAST(S) OF PATIENT'S FOOT (CUSTOM MOLDED SHOE), PER SHOE	D	N	38	A		2134
A5503	FOR DIABETICS ONLY, MODIFICATION (INCLUDING FITTING) OF OFF-THE-SHELF DEPTH-INLAY SHOE OR CUSTOM-MOLDED SHOE WITH ROLLER OR RIGID ROCKER BOTTOM, PER SHOE	D	N	38	A		2134
A5504	FOR DIABETICS ONLY, MODIFICATION (INCLUDING FITTING) OF OFF-THE-SHELF DEPTH-INLAY SHOE OR CUSTOM-MOLDED SHOE WITH WEDGE(S), PER SHOE	D	N	38	A		2134
A5505	FOR DIABETICS ONLY, MODIFICATION (INCLUDING FITTING) OF OFF-THE-SHELF DEPTH-INLAY SHOE OR CUSTOM-MOLDED SHOE WITH METATARSAL BAR, PER SHOE	D	N	38	A		2134
A5506	FOR DIABETICS ONLY, MODIFICATION (INCLUDING FITTING) OF OFF-THE-SHELF DEPTH-INLAY SHOE OR CUSTOM-MOLDED SHOE WITH OFF-SET HEEL(S), PER SHOE	D	N	38	A		2134
A5507	FOR DIABETICS ONLY, NOT OTHERWISE SPECIFIED MODIFICATION (INCLUDING FITTING) OF OFF-THE-SHELF DEPTH-INLAY SHOE OR CUSTOM-MOLDED SHOE, PER SHOE	D	N	38	A		2134
A5508	FOR DIABETICS ONLY, DELUXE FEATURE OF OFF-THE-SHELF DEPTH-INLAY SHOE OR CUSTOM-MOLDED SHOE, PER SHOE	D	N	38	A		2134
A5510	FOR DIABETICS ONLY, DIRECT FORMED, COMPRESSION MOLDED TO PATIENT'S FOOT WITHOUT EXTERNAL HEAT SOURCE, MULTIPLE-DENSITY INSERT(S) PREFABRICATED, PER SHOE	D	N	38	A		2134
A5512	FOR DIABETICS ONLY, MULTIPLE DENSITY INSERT, DIRECT FORMED, MOLDED TO FOOT AFTER EXTERNAL HEAT SOURCE OF 230 DEGREES FAHRENHEIT OR HIGHER, TOTAL CONTACT WITH PATIENT'S FOOT, INCLUDING ARCH, BASE LAYER MINIMUM OF 1/4 INCH MATERIAL OF SHORE A 35 DUROMETER OR 3/16 INCH MATERIAL OF SHORE A 40 DUROMETER (OR HIGHER), PREFABRICATED, EACH	C	P	38	A		

HCPCS Code	Statute	Lab Cert	X-Ref	ASC Pay Grp	ASC Pay Group Eff. Date	Proc Notes	BETOS	TOS	Anest	Code Add Date	Code Effective Date	Code Term Date
A5105							D1F	P	0	19900101	20080101	
A5112							D1F	P	0	19900101	19900101	
A5113							D1F	P	0	19900101	19980101	
A5114							D1F	P	0	19900101	19980101	
A5120							D1F	P	0	20060101	20060101	
A5121							D1F	P	0	19900101	19900101	
A5122							D1F	P	0	19900101	19900101	
A5126							D1F	P	0	19900101	20000101	
A5131							D1F	P	0	19900101	19900101	
A5200							D1F	P	0	19990101	20030101	
A5500							D1F	J	0	19950101	20050101	
A5501							D1F	J	0	19950101	20050101	
A5503							D1F	J	0	19950101	20050101	
A5504							D1F	J	0	19950101	20050101	
A5505							D1F	J	0	19950101	20050101	
A5505												
A5506							D1F	J	0	19950101	20050101	
A5507							D1F	J	0	19950101	20050101	
A5508							D1F	J	0	20000101	20050101	
A5510							D1F	J	0	20020101	20050101	
A5512							D1F	J	0	20060101	20100101	

HCPCS Code	Long Description	Coverage	Action	PI	MPI	CIM	MCM
A5513	FOR DIABETICS ONLY, MULTIPLE DENSITY INSERT, CUSTOM MOLDED FROM MODEL OF PATIENT'S FOOT, TOTAL CONTACT WITH PATIENT'S FOOT, INCLUDING ARCH, BASE LAYER MINIMUM OF 3/16 INCH MATERIAL OF SHORE A 35 DUROMETER OR HIGHER), INCLUDES ARCH FILLER AND OTHER SHAPING MATERIAL, CUSTOM FABRICATED, EACH	C	P	38	A		
A6000	NON-CONTACT WOUND WARMING WOUND COVER FOR USE WITH THE NON-CONTACT WOUND	M	N	00	9		2303
A6000	WARMING DEVICE AND WARMING CARD						
A6010	COLLAGEN BASED WOUND FILLER, DRY FORM, STERILE, PER GRAM OF COLLAGEN	D	N	35	A		2079
A6011	COLLAGEN BASED WOUND FILLER, GEL/PASTE, STERILE, PER GRAM OF COLLAGEN	D	N	35	A		2079
A6021	COLLAGEN DRESSING, STERILE, PAD SIZE 16 SQ. IN. OR LESS, EACH	D	N	35	A		2079
A6022	COLLAGEN DRESSING, STERILE, PAD SIZE MORE THAN 16 SQ. IN. BUT LESS THAN OR EQUAL TO 48 SQ. IN., EACH	D	N	35	A		2079
A6023	COLLAGEN DRESSING, STERILE, PAD SIZE MORE THAN 48 SQ. IN., EACH	D	N	35	A		2079
A6024	COLLAGEN DRESSING WOUND FILLER, STERILE, PER 6 INCHES	D	N	35	A		2079
A6025	GEL SHEET FOR DERMAL OR EPIDERMAL APPLICATION, (E.G., SILICONE, HYDROGEL, OTHER), EACH	C	N	00	9		
A6154	WOUND POUCH, EACH	D	N	35	A		2079
A6196	ALGINATE OR OTHER FIBER GELLING DRESSING, WOUND COVER, STERILE, PAD SIZE 16 SQ. IN. OR LESS, EA. DRESSING	D	N	35	A		2079
A6197	ALGINATE OR OTHER FIBER GELLING DRESSING, WOUND COVER, STERILE, PAD SIZE MORE THAN 16 SQ. IN. BUT LESS THAN OR EQUAL TO 48 SQ. IN., EACH DRESSING	D	N	35	A		2079
A6198	ALGINATE OR OTHER FIBER GELLING DRESSING, WOUND COVER, STERILE, PAD SIZE MORE THAN 48 SQ. IN., EACH DRESSING	D	N	46	A		2079
A6199	ALGINATE OR OTHER FIBER GELLING DRESSING, WOUND FILLER, STERILE, PER 6 INCHES	D	N	35	A		2079
A6200	COMPOSITE DRESSING, PAD SIZE 16 SQ. IN. OR LESS, WITHOUT ADHESIVE BORDER, EACH DRESSING	I	D	00	9		
A6201	COMPOSITE DRESSING, PAD SIZE MORE THAN 16 SQ. IN. BUT LESS THAN OR EQUAL TO 48 SQ. IN., WITHOUT ADHESIVE BORDER, EACH DRESSING	I	D	00	9		
A6202	COMPOSITE DRESSING, PAD SIZE MORE THAN 48 SQ. IN., WITHOUT ADHESIVE BORDER, EACH DRESSING	I	D	00	9		
A6203	COMPOSITE DRESSING, STERILE, PAD SIZE 16 SQ. IN. OR LESS, WITH ANY SIZE ADHESIVE BORDER, EACH DRESSING	D	N	35	A		2079
A6204	COMPOSITE DRESSING, STERILE, PAD SIZE MORE THAN 16 SQ. IN. BUT LESS THAN OR EQUAL TO 48 SQ. IN., WITH ANY SIZE ADHESIVE BORDER, EACH DRESSING	D	N	35	A		2079
A6205	COMPOSITE DRESSING, STERILE, PAD SIZE MORE THAN 48 SQ. IN., WITH ANY SIZE ADHESIVE BORDER, EACH DRESSING	D	N	46	A		2079
A6206	CONTACT LAYER, STERILE, 16 SQ. IN. OR LESS, EACH DRESSING	D	N	46	A		2079

HCPCS Code	Statute	Lab Cert	X-Ref	ASC Pay Grp	ASC Pay Group Eff. Date	Proc Notes	BETOS	TOS	Anest	Code Add Date	Code Effective Date	Code Term Date
A5513							D1F	J	0	20060101	20100101	
A6000							D1E	P	0	20020101	20020701	
A6000												
A6010							D1A	S	0	20020101	20090101	
A6011							D1A	S	0	20030101	20090101	
A6021							D1A	S	0	20010101	20090101	
A6022							D1A	S	0	20010101	20090101	
A6023							D1A	S	0	20010101	20090101	
A6024							D1A	S	0	20010101	20090101	
A6025							D1A	9	0	19970101	20070101	
A6154							D1A	S	0	19970101	20030101	
A6196							D1A	S	0	19970101	20090101	
A6197							D1A	S	0	19970101	20090101	
A6198							D1A	S	0	19970101	20090101	
A6199							D1A	S	0	19970101	20090101	
A6200							D1A	S	0	19990101	20100101	20091231
A6201							D1A	S	0	19990101	20100101	20091231
A6202							D1A	S	0	19990101	20100101	20091231
A6203							D1A	S	0	19970101	20090101	
A6204							D1A	S	0	19970101	20090101	
A6205							D1A	S	0	19970101	20090101	
A6206							D1A	S	0	19970101	20090101	

HCPCS Code	Long Description	Coverage	Action	PI	MPI	CIM	MCM
A6207	CONTACT LAYER, STERILE, MORE THAN 16 SQ. IN. BUT LESS THAN OR EQUAL TO 48 SQ. IN., EACH DRESSING	D	N	35	A		2079
A6208	CONTACT LAYER, STERILE, MORE THAN 48 SQ. IN., EACH DRESSING	D	N	46	A		2079
A6209	FOAM DRESSING, WOUND COVER, STERILE, PAD SIZE 16 SQ. IN. OR LESS, WITHOUT ADHESIVE BORDER, EACH DRESSING	D	N	35	A		2079
A6210	FOAM DRESSING, WOUND COVER, STERILE, PAD SIZE MORE THAN 16 SQ. IN. BUT LESS THAN OR EQUAL TO 48 SQ. IN., WITHOUT ADHESIVE BORDER, EACH DRESSING	D	N	35	A		2079
A6211	FOAM DRESSING, WOUND COVER, STERILE, PAD SIZE MORE THAN 48 SQ. IN., WITHOUT ADHESIVE BORDER, EA. DRESSING	D	N	35	A		2079
A6212	FOAM DRESSING, WOUND COVER, STERILE, PAD SIZE 16 SQ. IN. OR LESS, WITH ANY SIZE ADHESIVE BORDER, EACH DRESSING	D	N	35	A		2079
A6213	FOAM DRESSING, WOUND COVER, STERILE, PAD SIZE MORE THAN 16 SQ. IN. BUT LESS THAN OR EQUAL TO 48 SQ. IN., WITH ANY SIZE ADHESIVE BORDER, EACH DRESSING	D	N	46	A		2079
A6214	FOAM DRESSING, WOUND COVER, STERILE, PAD SIZE MORE THAN 48 SQ. IN., WITH ANY SIZE ADHESIVE BORDER, EACH DRESSING	D	N	35	A		2079
A6215	FOAM DRESSING, WOUND FILLER, STERILE, PER GRAM	D	N	46	A		2079
A6216	GAUZE, NON-IMPREGNATED, NON-STERILE, PAD SIZE 16 SQ. IN. OR LESS, WITHOUT ADHESIVE BORDER, EACH DRESSING	D	N	35	A		2079
A6217	GAUZE, NON-IMPREGNATED, NON-STERILE, PAD SIZE MORE THAN 16 SQ. IN. BUT LESS THAN OR EQUAL TO 48 SQ. IN., WITHOUT ADHESIVE BORDER, EACH DRESSING	D	N	35	A		2079
A6218	GAUZE, NON-IMPREGNATED, NON-STERILE, PAD SIZE MORE THAN 48 SQ. IN., WITHOUT ADHESIVE BORDER, EA. DRESSING	D	N	46	A		2079
A6219	GAUZE, NON-IMPREGNATED, STERILE, PAD SIZE 16 SQ. IN. OR LESS, WITH ANY SIZE ADHESIVE BORDER, EACH DRESSING	D	N	35	A		2079
A6220	GAUZE, NON-IMPREGNATED, STERILE, PAD SIZE MORE THAN 16 SQ. IN. BUT LESS THAN OR EQUAL TO 48 SQ. IN., WITH ANY SIZE ADHESIVE BORDER, EACH DRESSING	D	N	35	A		2079
A6221	GAUZE, NON-IMPREGNATED, STERILE, PAD SIZE MORE THAN 48 SQ. IN., WITH ANY SIZE ADHESIVE BORDER, EA. DRESSING	D	N	46	A		2079
A6222	GAUZE, IMPREGNATED WITH OTHER THAN WATER, NORMAL SALINE, OR HYDROGEL, STERILE, PAD SIZE 16 SQ. IN. OR LESS, WITHOUT ADHESIVE BORDER, EACH DRESSING	D	N	35	A		2079
A6223	GAUZE, IMPREGNATED WITH OTHER THAN WATER, NORMAL SALINE, OR HYDROGEL, STERILE, PAD SIZE MORE THAN 16 SQ. IN., BUT LESS THAN OR EQUAL TO 48 SQ. IN., WITHOUT ADHESIVE BORDER, EACH DRESSING	D	N	35	A		2079
A6224	GAUZE, IMPREGNATED WITH OTHER THAN WATER, NORMAL SALINE, OR HYDROGEL, STERILE, PAD SIZE MORE THAN 48 SQ. IN., WITHOUT ADHESIVE BORDER, EACH DRESSING	D	N	35	A		2079
A6228	GAUZE, IMPREGNATED, WATER OR NORMAL SALINE, STERILE, PAD SIZE 16 SQ. IN. OR LESS, WITHOUT ADHESIVE BORDER, EACH DRESSING	D	N	46	A		2079

HCPCS Code	Statute	Lab Cert	X-Ref	ASC Pay Grp	ASC Pay Group Eff. Date	Proc Notes	BETOS	TOS	Anest	Code Add Date	Code Effective Date	Code Term Date
A6207							D1A	S	0	19970101	20090101	
A6208							D1A	S	0	19970101	20090101	
A6209							D1A	S	0	19970101	20090101	
A6210							D1A	S	0	19970101	20090101	
A6211							D1A	S	0	19970101	20090101	
A6212							D1A	S	0	19970101	20090101	
A6213							D1A	S	0	19970101	20090101	
A6214							D1A	S	0	19970101	20090101	
A6215							D1A	L, S	0	19970101	20090101	
A6216							D1A	S	0	19970101	20030101	
A6217							D1A	S	0	19970101	20030101	
A6218							D1A	S	0	19970101	20030101	
A6219							D1A	S	0	19970101	20090101	
A6220							D1A	S	0	19970101	20090101	
A6221							D1A	S	0	19970101	20090101	
A6222							D1A	S	0	19970101	20090101	
A6223							D1A	S	0	19970101	20090101	
A6224							D1A	S	0	19970101	20090101	
A6228							D1A	S	0	19970101	20090101	

A Codes

HCPCS Code	Long Description	Coverage	Action	PI	MPI	CIM	MCM
A6229	GAUZE, IMPREGNATED, WATER OR NORMAL SALINE, STERILE, PAD SIZE MORE THAN 16 SQ. IN. BUT LESS THAN OR EQUAL TO 48 SQ. IN., WITHOUT ADHESIVE BORDER, EACH DRESSING	D	N	35	A		2079
A6230	GAUZE, IMPREGNATED, WATER OR NORMAL SALINE, STERILE, PAD SIZE MORE THAN 48 SQ. IN., WITHOUT ADHESIVE BORDER, EACH DRESSING	D	N	46	A		2079
A6231	GAUZE, IMPREGNATED, HYDROGEL, FOR DIRECT WOUND CONTACT, STERILE, PAD SIZE 16 SQ. IN. OR LESS, EACH DRESSING	D	N	35	A		2079
A6232	GAUZE, IMPREGNATED, HYDROGEL, FOR DIRECT WOUND CONTACT, STERILE, PAD SIZE GREATER THAN 16 SQ. IN., BUT LESS THAN OR EQUAL TO 48 SQ. IN., EACH DRESSING	D	N	35	A		2079
A6233	GAUZE, IMPREGNATED, HYDROGEL, FOR DIRECT WOUND CONTACT, STERILE, PAD SIZE MORE THAN 48 SQ. IN., EACH DRESSING	D	N	35	A		2079
A6234	HYDROCOLLOID DRESSING, WOUND COVER, STERILE, PAD SIZE 16 SQ. IN. OR LESS, WITHOUT ADHESIVE BORDER, EACH DRESSING	D	N	35	A		2079
A6235	HYDROCOLLOID DRESSING, WOUND COVER, STERILE, PAD SIZE MORE THAN 16 SQ. IN. BUT LESS THAN OR EQUAL TO 48 SQ. IN., WITHOUT ADHESIVE BORDER, EACH DRESSING	D	N	35	A		2079
A6236	HYDROCOLLOID DRESSING, WOUND COVER, STERILE, PAD SIZE MORE THAN 48 SQ. IN., WITHOUT ADHESIVE BORDER, EACH DRESSING	D	N	35	A		2079
A6237	HYDROCOLLOID DRESSING, WOUND COVER, STERILE, PAD SIZE 16 SQ. IN. OR LESS, WITH ANY SIZE ADHESIVE BORDER, EACH DRESSING	D	N	35	A		2079
A6238	HYDROCOLLOID DRESSING, WOUND COVER, STERILE, PAD SIZE MORE THAN 16 SQ. IN. BUT LESS THAN OR EQUAL TO 48 SQ. IN., WITH ANY SIZE ADHESIVE BORDER, EACH DRESSING	D	N	35	A		2079
A6239	HYDROCOLLOID DRESSING, WOUND COVER, STERILE, PAD SIZE MORE THAN 48 SQ. IN., WITH ANY SIZE ADHESIVE BORDER, EACH DRESSING	D	N	46	A		2079
A6240	HYDROCOLLOID DRESSING, WOUND FILLER, PASTE, STERILE, PER OUNCE	D	N	35	A		2079
A6241	HYDROCOLLOID DRESSING, WOUND FILLER, DRY FORM, STERILE, PER GRAM	D	N	35	A		2079
A6242	HYDROGEL DRESSING, WOUND COVER, STERILE, PAD SIZE 16 SQ. IN. OR LESS, WITHOUT ADHESIVE BORDER, EACH DRESSING	D	N	35	A		2079
A6243	HYDROGEL DRESSING, WOUND COVER, STERILE, PAD SIZE MORE THAN 16 SQ. IN. BUT LESS THAN OR EQUAL TO 48 SQ. IN., WITHOUT ADHESIVE BORDER, EACH DRESSING	D	N	35	A		2079
A6244	HYDROGEL DRESSING, WOUND COVER, STERILE, PAD SIZE MORE THAN 48 SQ. IN., WITHOUT ADHESIVE BORDER, EACH DRESSING	D	N	35	A		2079
A6245	HYDROGEL DRESSING, WOUND COVER, STERILE, PAD SIZE 16 SQ. IN. OR LESS, WITH ANY SIZE ADHESIVE BORDER, EACH DRESSING	D	N	35	A		2079

HCPCS Code	Statute	Lab Cert	X-Ref	ASC Pay Grp	ASC Pay Group Eff. Date	Proc Notes	BETOS	TOS	Anest	Code Add Date	Code Effective Date	Code Term Date
A6229							D1A	S	0	19970101	20090101	
A6230							D1A	S	0	19970101	20090101	
A6231							D1A	S	0	20010101	20090101	
A6232							D1A	S	0	20010101	20090101	
A6233							D1A	S	0	20010101	20090101	
A6234							D1A	S	0	19970101	20090101	
A6235							D1A	S	0	19970101	20090101	
A6236							D1A	S	0	19970101	20090101	
A6237							D1A	S	0	19970101	20090101	
A6238							D1A	S	0	19970101	20090101	
A6239							D1A	S	0	19970101	20090101	
A6240							D1A	S	0	19970101	20090101	
A6241							D1A	S	0	19970101	20090101	
A6242							D1A	S	0	19970101	20090101	
A6243							D1A	S	0	19970101	20090101	
A6244							D1A	S	0	19970101	20090101	
A6245							D1A	S	0	19970101	20090101	

HCPCS Code	Long Description	Coverage	Action	PI	MPI	CIM	MCM
A6246	HYDROGEL DRESSING, WOUND COVER, STERILE, PAD SIZE MORE THAN 16 SQ. IN. BUT LESS THAN OR EQUAL TO 48 SQ. IN., WITH ANY SIZE ADHESIVE BORDER, EACH DRESSING	D	N	35	A		2079
A6247	HYDROGEL DRESSING, WOUND COVER, STERILE, PAD SIZE MORE THAN 48 SQ. IN., WITH ANY SIZE ADHESIVE BORDER, EACH DRESSING	D	N	35	A		2079
A6248	HYDROGEL DRESSING, WOUND FILLER, GEL, STERILE, PER FLUID OUNCE	D	N	35	A		2079
A6250	SKIN SEALANTS, PROTECTANTS, MOISTURIZERS, OINTMENTS, ANY TYPE, ANY SIZE	D	N	00	9		2079
A6251	SPECIALTY ABSORPTIVE DRESSING, WOUND COVER, STERILE, PAD SIZE 16 SQ. IN. OR LESS, WITHOUT ADHESIVE BORDER, EACH DRESSING	D	N	35	A		2079
A6252	SPECIALTY ABSORPTIVE DRESSING, WOUND COVER, STERILE, PAD SIZE MORE THAN 16 SQ. IN. BUT LESS THAN OR EQUAL TO 48 SQ. IN., WITHOUT ADHESIVE BORDER, EACH DRESSING	D	N	35	A		2079
A6253	SPECIALTY ABSORPTIVE DRESSING, WOUND COVER, STERILE, PAD SIZE MORE THAN 48 SQ. IN., WITHOUT ADHESIVE BORDER, EACH DRESSING	D	N	35	A		2079
A6254	SPECIALTY ABSORPTIVE DRESSING, WOUND COVER, STERILE, PAD SIZE 16 SQ. IN. OR LESS, WITH ANY SIZE ADHESIVE BORDER, EACH DRESSING	D	N	35	A		2079
A6255	SPECIALTY ABSORPTIVE DRESSING, WOUND COVER, STERILE, PAD SIZE MORE THAN 16 SQ. IN. BUT LESS THAN OR EQUAL TO 48 SQ. IN., WITH ANY SIZE ADHESIVE BORDER, EACH DRESSING	D	N	35	A		2079
A6256	SPECIALTY ABSORPTIVE DRESSING, WOUND COVER, STERILE, PAD SIZE MORE THAN 48 SQ. IN., WITH ANY SIZE ADHESIVE BORDER, EACH DRESSING	D	N	46	A		2079
A6257	TRANSPARENT FILM, STERILE, 16 SQ. IN. OR LESS, EACH DRESSING	D	N	35	A		2079
A6258	TRANSPARENT FILM, STERILE, MORE THAN 16 SQ. IN. BUT LESS THAN OR EQUAL TO 48 SQ. IN., EACH DRESSING	D	N	35	A		2079
A6259	TRANSPARENT FILM, STERILE, MORE THAN 48 SQ. IN., EACH DRESSING	D	N	35	A		2079
A6260	WOUND CLEANSERS, STERILE, ANY TYPE, ANY SIZE	D	N	00	9		2079
A6261	WOUND FILLER, GEL/PASTE, STERILE, PER FLUID OUNCE, NOT OTHERWISE SPECIFIED	D	N	46	A		2079
A6262	WOUND FILLER, DRY FORM, STERILE, PER GRAM, NOT OTHERWISE SPECIFIED	D	N	46	A		2079
A6266	GAUZE, IMPREGNATED, OTHER THAN WATER, NORMAL SALINE, OR ZINC PASTE, STERILE, ANY WIDTH, PER LINEAR YARD	D	N	35	A		2079
A6402	GAUZE, NON-IMPREGNATED, STERILE, PAD SIZE 16 SQ. IN. OR LESS, WITHOUT ADHESIVE BORDER, EACH DRESSING	D	N	35	A		2079
A6403	GAUZE, NON-IMPREGNATED, STERILE, PAD SIZE MORE THAN 16 SQ. IN. LESS THAN OR EQUAL TO 48 SQ. IN., WITHOUT ADHESIVE BORDER, EACH DRESSING	D	N	35	A		2079

HCPCS Code	Statute	Lab Cert	X-Ref	ASC Pay Grp	ASC Pay Group Eff. Date	Proc Notes	BETOS	TOS	Anest	Code Add Date	Code Effective Date	Code Term Date
A6246							D1A	S	0	19970101	20090101	
A6247							D1A	S	0	19970101	20090101	
A6248							D1A	S	0	19970101	20090101	
A6250							D1A	L, S	0	19970101	20030101	
A6251							D1A	S	0	19970101	20090101	
A6252							D1A	S	0	19970101	20090101	
A6253							D1A	S	0	19970101	20090101	
A6254							D1A	S	0	19970101	20090101	
A6255							D1A	S	0	19970101	20090101	
A6256							D1A	S	0	19970101	20090101	
A6257							D1A	S	0	19970101	20090101	
A6258							D1A	S	0	19970101	20090101	
A6259							D1A	S	0	19970101	20090101	
A6260							D1A	L, S	0	19970101	20090101	
A6261							D1A	S	0	19970101	20090101	
A6262							D1A	S	0	19970101	20090101	
A6266							D1A	S	0	19970101	20090101	
A6402							D1A	L, S	0	19970101	20060101	
A6403							D1A	S	0	19970101	20030101	

HCPCS Code	Long Description	Coverage	Action	PI	MPI	CIM	MCM
A6404	GAUZE, NON-IMPREGNATED, STERILE, PAD SIZE MORE THAN 48 SQ. IN., WITHOUT ADHESIVE BORDER, EACH DRESSING	D	N	35	A		2079
A6407	PACKING STRIPS, NON-IMPREGNATED, STERILE, UP TO 2 INCHES IN WIDTH, PER LINEAR YARD	C	N	35	A		
A6410	EYE PAD, STERILE, EACH	D	N	35	A		2079
A6411	EYE PAD, NON-STERILE, EACH	D	N	35	A		2079
A6412	EYE PATCH, OCCLUSIVE, EACH	C	N	00	9		
A6413	ADHESIVE BANDAGE, FIRST-AID TYPE, ANY SIZE, EACH	S	N	00	9		
A6441	PADDING BANDAGE, NON-ELASTIC, NON-WOVEN/ NON-KNITTED, WIDTH GREATER THAN OR EQUAL TO THREE INCHES AND LESS THAN FIVE INCHES, PER YARD	C	N	35	A		
A6442	CONFORMING BANDAGE, NON-ELASTIC, KNITTED/WOVEN, NON-STERILE, WIDTH LESS THAN THREE INCHES, PER YARD	C	N	35	A		
A6443	CONFORMING BANDAGE, NON-ELASTIC, KNITTED/WOVEN, NON-STERILE, WIDTH GREATER THAN OR EQUAL TO THREE INCHES AND LESS THAN FIVE INCHES, PER YARD	C	N	35	A		
A6444	CONFORMING BANDAGE, NON-ELASTIC, KNITTED/WOVEN, NON-STERILE, WIDTH GREATER THAN OR EQUAL TO 5 INCHES, PER YARD	C	N	35	A		
A6445	CONFORMING BANDAGE, NON-ELASTIC, KNITTED/WOVEN, STERILE, WIDTH LESS THAN THREE INCHES, PER YARD	C	N	35	A		
A6446	CONFORMING BANDAGE, NON-ELASTIC, KNITTED/WOVEN, STERILE, WIDTH GREATER THAN OR EQUAL TO THREE INCHES AND LESS THAN FIVE INCHES, PER YARD	C	N	35	A		
A6447	CONFORMING BANDAGE, NON-ELASTIC, KNITTED/WOVEN, STERILE, WIDTH GREATER THAN OR EQUAL TO FIVE INCHES, PER YARD	C	N	35	A		
A6448	LIGHT COMPRESSION BANDAGE, ELASTIC, KNITTED/WOVEN, WIDTH LESS THAN THREE INCHES, PER YARD	C	N	35	A		
A6449	LIGHT COMPRESSION BANDAGE, ELASTIC, KNITTED/WOVEN, WIDTH GREATER THAN OR EQUAL TO THREE INCHES AND LESS THAN FIVE INCHES, PER YARD	C	N	35	A		
A6450	LIGHT COMPRESSION BANDAGE, ELASTIC, KNITTED/WOVEN, WIDTH GREATER THAN OR EQUAL TO FIVE INCHES, PER YARD	C	N	35	A		
A6451	MODERATE COMPRESSION BANDAGE, ELASTIC, KNITTED/ WOVEN, LOAD RESISTANCE OF 1.25 TO 1.34 FOOT POUNDS AT 50% MAXIMUM STRETCH, WIDTH GREATER THAN OR EQUAL TO THREE INCHES AND LESS THAN FIVE INCHES, PER YARD	C	N	35	A		
A6452	HIGH COMPRESSION BANDAGE, ELASTIC, KNITTED/WOVEN, LOAD RESISTANCE GREATER THAN OR EQUAL TO 1.35 FOOT POUNDS AT 50% MAXIMUM STRETCH, WIDTH GREATER THAN OR EQUAL TO THREE INCHES AND LESS THAN FIVE INCHES, PER YARD	C	N	35	A		
A6453	SELF-ADHERENT BANDAGE, ELASTIC, NON-KNITTED/ NON-WOVEN, WIDTH LESS THAN THREE INCHES, PER YARD	C	N	35	A		
A6454	SELF-ADHERENT BANDAGE, ELASTIC, NON-KNITTED/ NON-WOVEN, WIDTH GREATER THAN OR EQUAL TO THREE INCHES AND LESS THAN FIVE INCHES, PER YARD	C	N	35	A		

HCPCS Code	Statute	Lab Cert	X-Ref	ASC Pay Grp	ASC Pay Group Eff. Date	Proc Notes	BETOS	TOS	Anest	Code Add Date	Code Effective Date	Code Term Date
A6404							D1A	S	0	19970101	20030101	
A6407							D1A	S	0	20040101	20090101	
A6410							D1A	S	0	20030101	20030101	
A6411							D1A	S	0	20030101	20030101	
A6412							Z2	S	0	20030101	20070101	
A6413	1861(s)(5)						D1A	P	0	20080101	20080101	
A6441							D1A	S	0	20040101	20040101	
A6442							D1A	S	0	20040101	20040101	
A6443							D1A	S	0	20040101	20040101	
A6444							D1A	S	0	20040101	20040101	
A6445							D1A	S	0	20040101	20040101	
A6446							D1A	S	0	20040101	20040101	
A6447							D1A	S	0	20040101	20040101	
A6448							D1A	S	0	20040101	20040101	
A6449							D1A	S	0	20040101	20040101	
A6450							D1A	S	0	20040101	20040101	
A6451							D1A	S	0	20040101	20040101	
A6452							D1A	S	0	20040101	20040101	
A6453							D1A	S	0	20040101	20040101	
A6454							D1A	S	0	20040101	20040101	

HCPCS Code	Long Description	Coverage	Action	PI	MPI	CIM	MCM
A6455	SELF-ADHERENT BANDAGE, ELASTIC, NON-KNITTED/ NON-WOVEN, WIDTH GREATER THAN OR EQUAL TO FIVE INCHES, PER YARD	C	N	35	A		
A6456	ZINC PASTE IMPREGNATED BANDAGE, NON-ELASTIC, KNITTED/WOVEN, WIDTH GREATER THAN OR EQUAL TO THREE INCHES AND LESS THAN FIVE INCHES, PER YARD	C	N	35	A		
A6457	TUBULAR DRESSING WITH OR WITHOUT ELASTIC, ANY WIDTH, PER LINEAR YARD	C	N	35	A		
A6501	COMPRESSION BURN GARMENT, BODYSUIT (HEAD TO FOOT), CUSTOM FABRICATED	D	N	35	A		2079
A6502	COMPRESSION BURN GARMENT, CHIN STRAP, CUSTOM FABRICATED	D	N	35	A		2079
A6503	COMPRESSION BURN GARMENT, FACIAL HOOD, CUSTOM FABRICATED	D	N	35	A		2079
A6504	COMPRESSION BURN GARMENT, GLOVE TO WRIST, CUSTOM FABRICATED	D	N	35	A		2079
A6505	COMPRESSION BURN GARMENT, GLOVE TO ELBOW, CUSTOM FABRICATED	D	N	35	A		2079
A6506	COMPRESSION BURN GARMENT, GLOVE TO AXILLA, CUSTOM FABRICATED	D	N	35	A		2079
A6507	COMPRESSION BURN GARMENT, FOOT TO KNEE LENGTH, CUSTOM FABRICATED	D	N	35	A		2079
A6508	COMPRESSION BURN GARMENT, FOOT TO THIGH LENGTH, CUSTOM FABRICATED	D	N	35	A		2079
A6509	COMPRESSION BURN GARMENT, UPPER TRUNK TO WAIST INCLUDING ARM OPENINGS (VEST),CUSTOM FABRICATED	D	N	35	A		2079
A6510	COMPRESSION BURN GARMENT, TRUNK, INCLUDING ARMS DOWN TO LEG OPENINGS (LEOTARD),CUSTOM FABRICATED	D	N	35	A		2079
A6511	COMPRESSION BURN GARMENT, LOWER TRUNK INCLUDING LEG OPENINGS (PANTY), CUSTOM FABRICATED	D	N	35	A		2079
A6512	COMPRESSION BURN GARMENT, NOT OTHERWISE CLASSIFIED	D	N	35	A		2079
A6513	COMPRESSION BURN MASK, FACE AND/OR NECK, PLASTIC OR EQUAL, CUSTOM FABRICATED	C	N	00	9		
A6530	GRADIENT COMPRESSION STOCKING, BELOW KNEE, 18-30 MMHG, EACH	M	N	00	9	60-9	
A6531	GRADIENT COMPRESSION STOCKING, BELOW KNEE, 30-40 MMHG, EACH	D	N	35	A		2079
A6532	GRADIENT COMPRESSION STOCKING, BELOW KNEE, 40-50 MMHG, EACH	D	N	35	A		2079
A6533	GRADIENT COMPRESSION STOCKING, THIGH LENGTH, 18-30 MMHG, EACH	M	N	00	9	60-9	2133
A6534	GRADIENT COMPRESSION STOCKING, THIGH LENGTH, 30-40 MMHG, EACH	M	N	00	9	60-9	2133
A6535	GRADIENT COMPRESSION STOCKING, THIGH LENGTH, 40-50 MMHG, EACH	M	N	00	9	60-9	2133
A6536	GRADIENT COMPRESSION STOCKING, FULL LENGTH/CHAP STYLE, 18-30 MMHG, EACH	M	N	00	9	60-9	2133
A6537	GRADIENT COMPRESSION STOCKING, FULL LENGTH/CHAP STYLE, 30-40 MMHG, EACH	M	N	00	9	60-9	2133

A Codes

HCPCS Code	Statute	Lab Cert	X-Ref	ASC Pay Grp	ASC Pay Group Eff. Date	Proc Notes	BETOS	TOS	Anest	Code Add Date	Code Effective Date	Code Term Date
A6455							D1A	S	0	20040101	20040101	
A6456							D1A	S	0	20040101	20040101	
A6457							D1A	S	0	20060101	20060101	
A6501							D1A	S	0	20030101	20030101	
A6502							D1A	S	0	20030101	20030101	
A6503							D1A	S	0	20030101	20030101	
A6504							D1A	S	0	20030101	20030101	
A6505							D1A	S	0	20030101	20030101	
A6506							D1A	S	0	20030101	20030101	
A6507							D1A	S	0	20030101	20030101	
A6508							D1A	S	0	20030101	20030101	
A6509							D1A	S	0	20030101	20030101	
A6510							D1A	S	0	20030101	20030101	
A6511							D1A	S	0	20030101	20030101	
A6512							D1A	S	0	20030101	20030101	
A6513							D1A	P	0	20060101	20060101	
A6530						0072	D1F	P	0	20060101	20060101	
A6531						0072	D1A	P, S	0	20060101	20060101	
A6532						0072	D1A	P, S	0	20060101	20060101	
A6533						0072	D1F	P	0	20060101	20060101	
A6534						0072	D1F	P	0	20060101	20060101	
A6535						0072	D1F	P	0	20060101	20060101	
A6536						0072	D1F	P	0	20060101	20060101	
A6537						0072	D1F	P	0	20060101	20060101	

HCPCS Code	Long Description	Coverage	Action	PI	MPI	CIM	MCM
A6538	GRADIENT COMPRESSION STOCKING, FULL LENGTH/CHAP STYLE, 40-50 MMHG, EACH	M	N	00	9	60-9	2133
A6539	GRADIENT COMPRESSION STOCKING, WAIST LENGTH, 18-30 MMHG, EACH	M	N	00	9	60-9	2133
A6540	GRADIENT COMPRESSION STOCKING, WAIST LENGTH, 30-40 MMHG, EACH	M	N	00	9	60-9	2133
A6541	GRADIENT COMPRESSION STOCKING, WAIST LENGTH, 40-50 MMHG, EACH	M	N	00	9	60-9	2133
A6542	GRADIENT COMPRESSION STOCKING, CUSTOM MADE	M	D	00	9	60-9	2133
A6543	GRADIENT COMPRESSION STOCKING, LYMPHEDEMA	M	D	00	9	60-9	2133
A6544	GRADIENT COMPRESSION STOCKING, GARTER BELT	M	N	00	9	60-9	2133
A6545	GRADIENT COMPRESSION WRAP, NON-ELASTIC, BELOW KNEE, 30-50 MM HG, EACH	D	N	35	A		2079
A6549	GRADIENT COMPRESSION STOCKING/SLEEVE, NOT OTHERWISE SPECIFIED	M	C	00	9	60-9	2133
A6550	WOUND CARE SET, FOR NEGATIVE PRESSURE WOUND THERAPY ELECTRICAL PUMP, INCLUDES ALL SUPPLIES AND ACCESSORIES	C	N	34	A		
A7000	CANISTER, DISPOSABLE, USED WITH SUCTION PUMP, EACH	C	N	32	A		
A7001	CANISTER, NON-DISPOSABLE, USED WITH SUCTION PUMP, EA.	C	N	32	A		
A7002	TUBING, USED WITH SUCTION PUMP, EACH	C	N	32	A		
A7003	ADMINISTRATION SET, WITH SMALL VOLUME NONFILTERED PNEUMATIC NEBULIZER, DISPOSABLE	C	N	32	A		
A7004	SMALL VOLUME NONFILTERED PNEUMATIC NEBULIZER, DISPOSABLE	C	N	32	A		
A7005	ADMINISTRATION SET, WITH SMALL VOLUME NONFILTERED PNEUMATIC NEBULIZER, NON-DISPOSABLE	C	N	32	A		
A7006	ADMINISTRATION SET, WITH SMALL VOLUME FILTERED PNEUMATIC NEBULIZER	C	N	32	A		
A7007	LARGE VOLUME NEBULIZER, DISPOSABLE, UNFILLED, USED WITH AEROSOL COMPRESSOR	C	N	32	A		
A7008	LARGE VOLUME NEBULIZER, DISPOSABLE, PREFILLED, USED WITH AEROSOL COMPRESSOR	C	N	32	A		
A7009	RESERVOIR BOTTLE, NON-DISPOSABLE, USED WITH LARGE VOLUME ULTRASONIC NEBULIZER	C	N	32	A		
A7010	CORRUGATED TUBING, DISPOSABLE, USED WITH LARGE VOLUME NEBULIZER, 100 FEET	C	N	32	A		
A7011	CORRUGATED TUBING, NON-DISPOSABLE, USED WITH LARGE VOLUME NEBULIZER, 10 FEET	C	N	46	A		
A7012	WATER COLLECTION DEVICE, USED WITH LARGE VOLUME NEBULIZER	C	N	32	A		
A7013	FILTER, DISPOSABLE, USED WITH AEROSOL COMPRESSOR	C	N	32	A		
A7014	FILTER, NONDISPOSABLE, USED WITH AEROSOL COMPRESSOR OR ULTRASONIC GENERATOR	C	N	32	A		
A7015	AEROSOL MASK, USED WITH DME NEBULIZER	C	N	32	A		
A7016	DOME AND MOUTHPIECE, USED WITH SMALL VOLUME ULTRASONIC NEBULIZER	C	N	32	A		
A7017	NEBULIZER, DURABLE, GLASS OR AUTOCLAVABLE PLASTIC, BOTTLE TYPE, NOT USED WITH OXYGEN	D	N	32	A	60-9	

HCPCS Code	Statute	Lab Cert	X-Ref	ASC Pay Grp	ASC Pay Group Eff. Date	Proc Notes	BETOS	TOS	Anest	Code Add Date	Code Effective Date	Code Term Date
A6538						0072	D1F	P	0	20060101	20060101	
A6539						0072	D1F	P	0	20060101	20060101	
A6540						0072	D1F	P	0	20060101	20060101	
A6541						0072	D1F	P	0	20060101	20060101	
A6542						0072	D1F	P	0	20060101	20100101	20091231
A6543						0072	D1F	P	0	20060101	20100101	20091231
A6544						0072	D1F	P	0	20060101	20060101	
A6545							D1F	P, S	0	20090101	20090101	
A6549						0072	D1F	P	0	20060101	20100101	
A6550							D1E	P	0	20040101	20060101	
A7000							D1E	A,P,R	0	20000101	20000101	
A7001							D1E	A,P,R	0	20000101	20000101	
A7002							D1E	A,P,R	0	20000101	20000101	
A7003							D1E	P	0	20000101	20000101	
A7004							D1E	P	0	20000101	20000101	
A7005							D1E	A,P,R	0	20000101	20000101	
A7006							D1E	A,P,R	0	20000101	20000101	
A7007							D1E	P	0	20000101	20000101	
A7008							D1E	P	0	20000101	20000101	
A7009							D1E	A,P,R	0	20000101	20000101	
A7010							D1E	P	0	20000101	20000101	
A7011							D1E	P	0	20000101	20000101	
A7012							D1E	A,P,R	0	20000101	20000101	
A7013							D1E	P	0	20000101	20000101	
A7014							D1E	A,P,R	0	20000101	20000101	
A7015							D1E	A,P,R	0	20000101	20000101	
A7016							D1E	A,P,R	0	20000101	20000101	
A7017							D1E	A,P,R	0	20000101	20000101	

HCPCS Code	Long Description	Coverage	Action	PI	MPI	CIM	MCM
A7018	WATER, DISTILLED, USED WITH LARGE VOLUME NEBULIZER, 1000 ML	C	N	32	A		
A7025	HIGH FREQUENCY CHEST WALL OSCILLATION SYSTEM VEST, REPLACEMENT FOR USE WITH PATIENT OWNED EQUIPMENT, EACH	C	N	32	A		
A7026	HIGH FREQUENCY CHEST WALL OSCILLATION SYSTEM HOSE, REPLACEMENT FOR USE WITH PATIENT OWNED EQUIPMENT, EACH	C	N	32	A		
A7027	COMBINATION ORAL/NASAL MASK, USED WITH CONTINUOUS POSITIVE AIRWAY PRESSURE DEVICE, EACH	C	N	32	A		
A7028	ORAL CUSHION FOR COMBINATION ORAL/NASAL MASK, REPLACEMENT ONLY, EACH	C	N	32	A		
A7029	NASAL PILLOWS FOR COMBINATION ORAL/NASAL MASK, REPLACEMENT ONLY, PAIR	C	N	32	A		
A7030	FULL FACE MASK USED WITH POSITIVE AIRWAY PRESSURE DEVICE, EACH	C	N	32	A		
A7031	FACE MASK INTERFACE, REPLACEMENT FOR FULL FACE MASK, EACH	C	N	32	A		
A7032	CUSHION FOR USE ON NASAL MASK INTERFACE, REPLACEMENT ONLY, EACH	C	N	32	A		
A7033	PILLOW FOR USE ON NASAL CANNULA TYPE INTERFACE, REPLACEMENT ONLY, PAIR	C	N	32	A		
A7034	NASAL INTERFACE (MASK OR CANNULA TYPE) USED WITH POSITIVE AIRWAY PRESSURE DEVICE, WITH OR WITHOUT HEAD STRAP	C	N	32	A		
A7035	HEADGEAR USED WITH POSITIVE AIRWAY PRESSURE DEVICE	C	N	32	A		
A7036	CHINSTRAP USED WITH POSITIVE AIRWAY PRESSURE DEVICE	C	N	32	A		
A7037	TUBING USED WITH POSITIVE AIRWAY PRESSURE DEVICE	C	N	32	A		
A7038	FILTER, DISPOSABLE, USED WITH POSITIVE AIRWAY PRESSURE DEVICE	C	N	32	A		
A7039	FILTER, NON DISPOSABLE, USED WITH POSITIVE AIRWAY PRESSURE DEVICE	C	N	32	A		
A7040	ONE WAY CHEST DRAIN VALVE	C	N	38	A		
A7041	WATER SEAL DRAINAGE CONTAINER AND TUBING FOR USE WITH IMPLANTED CHEST TUBE	C	N	38	A		
A7042	IMPLANTED PLEURAL CATHETER, EACH	C	N	38	A		
A7043	VACUUM DRAINAGE BOTTLE AND TUBING FOR USE WITH IMPLANTED CATHETER	C	N	38	A		
A7044	ORAL INTERFACE USED WITH POSITIVE AIRWAY PRESSURE DEVICE, EACH	C	N	32	A		
A7045	EXHALATION PORT WITH OR WITHOUT SWIVEL USED WITH ACCESSORIES FOR POSITIVE AIRWAY DEVICES, REPLACEMENT ONLY	D	N	32	A	60-17	
A7046	WATER CHAMBER FOR HUMIDIFIER, USED WITH POSITIVE AIRWAY PRESSURE DEVICE, REPLACEMENT, EACH	D	N	32	A	60-17	
A7501	TRACHEOSTOMA VALVE, INCLUDING DIAPHRAGM, EACH	D	N	37	A		2130
A7502	REPLACEMENT DIAPHRAGM/FACEPLATE FOR TRACHEOSTOMA VALVE, EACH	D	N	37	A		2130

HCPCS Code	Statute	Lab Cert	X-Ref	ASC Pay Grp	ASC Pay Group Eff. Date	Proc Notes	BETOS	TOS	Anest	Code Add Date	Code Effective Date	Code Term Date
A7018							D1E	P	0	20010101	20010101	
A7025							D1E	A,P,R	0	20030101	20030101	
A7026							D1E	A,P,R	0	20030101	20030101	
A7027							D1E	A,P,R	0	20080101	20080101	
A7028							D1E	A,P,R	0	20080101	20080101	
A7029							D1E	A,P,R	0	20080101	20080101	
A7030							D1E	A,P,R	0	20030101	20030101	
A7031							D1E	A,P,R	0	20030101	20030101	
A7032							D1E	A,P,R	0	20030101	20060101	
A7033							D1E	A,P,R	0	20030101	20060101	
A7034							D1E	A,P,R	0	20030101	20030101	
A7035							D1E	A,P,R	0	20030101	20030101	
A7036							D1E	A,P,R	0	20030101	20030101	
A7037							D1E	A,P,R	0	20030101	20030101	
A7038							D1E	A,P,R	0	20030101	20030101	
A7039							D1E	A,P,R	0	20030101	20030101	
A7040							D1F	P	0	20050101	20050101	
A7041							D1F	P	0	20050101	20050101	
A7042							D1F	P	0	20030101	20030101	
A7043							D1F	P	0	20030101	20030101	
A7044							D1E	A,P,R	0	20030101	20030101	
A7045							D1E	A,P,R	0	20050101	20050101	
A7046							D1E	P	0	20040101	20040101	
A7501							D1F	P	0	20010101	20010101	
A7502							D1F	P	0	20010101	20010101	

HCPCS Code	Long Description	Coverage	Action	PI	MPI	CIM	MCM
A7503	FILTER HOLDER OR FILTER CAP, REUSABLE, FOR USE IN A TRACHEOSTOMA HEAT AND MOISTURE EXCHANGE SYSTEM, EACH	D	N	37	A		2130
A7504	FILTER FOR USE IN A TRACHEOSTOMA HEAT AND MOISTURE EXCHANGE SYSTEM, EACH	D	N	37	A		2130
A7505	HOUSING, REUSABLE WITHOUT ADHESIVE, FOR USE IN A HEAT AND MOISTURE EXCHANGE SYSTEM AND/OR WITH A TRACHEOSTOMA VALVE, EACH	D	N	37	A		2130
A7506	ADHESIVE DISC FOR USE IN A HEAT AND MOISTURE EXCHANGE SYSTEM AND/OR WITH TRACHEOSTOMA VALVE, ANY TYPE EACH	D	N	37	A		2130
A7507	FILTER HOLDER AND INTEGRATED FILTER WITHOUT ADHESIVE, FOR USE IN A TRACHEOSTOMA HEAT AND MOISTURE EXCHANGE SYSTEM, EACH	D	N	37	A		2130
A7508	HOUSING AND INTEGRATED ADHESIVE, FOR USE IN A TRACHEOSTOMA HEAT AND MOISTURE EXCHANGE SYSTEM AND/OR WITH A TRACHEOSTOMA VALVE, EACH	D	N	37	A		2130
A7509	FILTER HOLDER AND INTEGRATED FILTER HOUSING, AND ADHESIVE, FOR USE AS A TRACHEOSTOMA HEAT AND MOISTURE EXCHANGE SYSTEM, EACH	D	N	37	A		2130
A7520	TRACHEOSTOMY/LARYNGECTOMY TUBE, NON-CUFFED, POLYVINYLCHLORIDE (PVC), SILICONE OR EQUAL, EACH	C	N	37	A		
A7521	TRACHEOSTOMY/LARYNGECTOMY TUBE, CUFFED, POLYVINYLCHLORIDE (PVC), SILICONE OR EQUAL, EACH	C	N	37	A		
A7522	TRACHEOSTOMY/LARYNGECTOMY TUBE, STAINLESS STEEL OR EQUAL (STERILIZABLE AND REUSABLE), EACH	C	N	37	A		
A7523	TRACHEOSTOMY SHOWER PROTECTOR, EACH	C	N	37	A		
A7524	TRACHEOSTOMA STENT/STUD/BUTTON, EACH	C	N	37	A		
A7525	TRACHEOSTOMY MASK, EACH	C	N	37	A		
A7526	TRACHEOSTOMY TUBE COLLAR/HOLDER, EACH	C	N	37	A		
A7527	TRACHEOSTOMY/LARYNGECTOMY TUBE PLUG/STOP, EACH	C	N	37	A		
A8000	HELMET, PROTECTIVE, SOFT, PREFABRICATED, INCLUDES ALL COMPONENTS AND ACCESSORIES	C	N	32	A		
A8001	HELMET, PROTECTIVE, HARD, PREFABRICATED, INCLUDES ALL COMPONENTS AND ACCESSORIES	C	N	32	A		
A8002	HELMET, PROTECTIVE, SOFT, CUSTOM FABRICATED, INCLUDES ALL COMPONENTS AND ACCESSORIES	C	N	45	A		
A8003	HELMET, PROTECTIVE, HARD, CUSTOM FABRICATED, INCLUDES ALL COMPONENTS AND ACCESSORIES	C	N	45	A		
A8004	SOFT INTERFACE FOR HELMET, REPLACEMENT ONLY	C	N	32	A		
A9150	NON-PRESCRIPTION DRUGS	D	N	57	A		2050.5
A9152	SINGLE VITAMIN/MINERAL/TRACE ELEMENT, ORAL, PER DOSE, NOT OTHERWISE SPECIFIED	I	N	00	9		
A9153	MULTIPLE VITAMINS, WITH OR WITHOUT MINERALS AND TRACE ELEMENTS, ORAL, PER DOSE, NOT OTHERWISE SPECIFIED	I	N	00	9		
A9155	ARTIFICIAL SALIVA, 30 ML	C	N	57	A		
A9180	PEDICULOSIS (LICE INFESTATION) TREATMENT, TOPICAL, FOR ADMINISTRATION BY PATIENT/CARETAKER	I	N	00	9		

HCPCS Code	Statute	Lab Cert	X-Ref	ASC Pay Grp	ASC Pay Group Eff. Date	Proc Notes	BETOS	TOS	Anest	Code Add Date	Code Effective Date	Code Term Date
A7503							D1F	P	0	20010101	20010101	
A7504							D1F	P	0	20010101	20010101	
A7505							D1F	P	0	20010101	20010101	
A7506							D1F	P	0	20010101	20010101	
A7507							D1F	P	0	20010101	20010101	
A7508							D1F	P	0	20010101	20010101	
A7509							D1F	P	0	20010101	20010101	
A7520							D1F	P	0	20040101	20040101	
A7521							D1F	P	0	20040101	20040101	
A7522							D1F	P	0	20040101	20040101	
A7523							D1F	P	0	20040101	20040101	
A7524							D1F	P	0	20040101	20040101	
A7525							D1F	P	0	20040101	20040101	
A7526							D1F	P	0	20040101	20040101	
A7527							D1A	P	0	20050101	20050101	
A8000							D1E	A,P,R	0	20070101	20070101	
A8001							D1E	A,P,R	0	20070101	20070101	
A8002							D1E	A,P,R	0	20070101	20070101	
A8003							D1E	A,P,R	0	20070101	20070101	
A8004							D1E	A,P,R	0	20070101	20070101	
A9150							O1E	9	0	19860101	19950401	
A9152							Z2	9	0	20050101	20050101	
A9153							Z2	9	0	20050101	20050101	
A9155							Z2	9	0	20080101	20080101	
A9180							Z2	9	0	20050101	20050101	
A9180							D1F	P	0			

HCPCS Code	Long Description	Coverage	Action	PI	MPI	CIM	MCM
A9270	NON-COVERED ITEM OR SERVICE	M	N	00	9		2303
A9274	EXTERNAL AMBULATORY INSULIN DELIVERY SYSTEM, DISPOSABLE, EACH, INCLUDES ALL SUPPLIES AND ACCESSORIES	I	N	00	9		
A9275	HOME GLUCOSE DISPOSABLE MONITOR, INCLUDES TEST STRIPS	M	N	00	9		
A9276	SENSOR; INVASIVE (E.G. SUBCUTANEOUS), DISPOSABLE, FOR USE WITH INTERSTITIAL CONTINUOUS GLUCOSE MONITORING SYSTEM, ONE UNIT = 1 DAY SUPPLY	S	N	00	9		
A9277	TRANSMITTER; EXTERNAL, FOR USE WITH INTERSTITIAL CONTINUOUS GLUCOSE MONITORING SYSTEM	S	N	00	9		
A9278	RECEIVER (MONITOR); EXTERNAL, FOR USE WITH INTERSTITIAL CONTINUOUS GLUCOSE MONITORING SYSTEM	S	N	00	9		
A9279	MONITORING FEATURE/DEVICE, STAND-ALONE OR INTEGRATED, ANY TYPE, INCLUDES ALL ACCESSORIES, COMPONENTS AND ELECTRONICS, NOT OTHERWISE CLASSIFIED	I	N	00	9		
A9280	ALERT OR ALARM DEVICE, NOT OTHERWISE CLASSIFIED	S	N	00	9		
A9281	REACHING/GRABBING DEVICE, ANY TYPE, ANY LENGTH, EA.	S	N	00	9		
A9282	WIG, ANY TYPE, EACH	S	N	00	9		
A9283	FOOT PRESSURE OFF LOADING/SUPPORTIVE DEVICE, ANY TYPE, EACH	S	N	00	9		
A9284	SPIROMETER, NON-ELECTRONIC, INCLUDES ALL ACCESSORIES	D	N	00	9		
A9300	EXERCISE EQUIPMENT	M	N	00	9	60-9	2100.1
A9500	TECHNETIUM TC-99M SESTAMIBI, DIAGNOSTIC, PER STUDY DOSE	C	C	57	A		
A9501	TECHNETIUM TC-99M TEBOROXIME, DIAGNOSTIC, PER STUDY DOSE	C	N	57	A		
A9502	TECHNETIUM TC-99M TETROFOSMIN, DIAGNOSTIC, PER STUDY DOSE	C	N	57	A		
A9503	TECHNETIUM TC-99M MEDRONATE, DIAGNOSTIC, PER STUDY DOSE, UP TO 30 MILLICURIES	C	N	57	A		
A9504	TECHNETIUM TC-99M APCITIDE, DIAGNOSTIC, PER STUDY DOSE, UP TO 20 MILLICURIES	C	N	57	A		
A9505	THALLIUM TL-201 THALLOUS CHLORIDE, DIAGNOSTIC, PER MILLICURIE	C	N	57	A		
A9507	INDIUM IN-111 CAPROMAB PENDETIDE, DIAGNOSTIC, PER STUDY DOSE, UP TO 10 MILLICURIES	C	N	57	A		
A9508	IODINE I-131 IOBENGUANE SULFATE, DIAGNOSTIC, PER 0.5 MILLICURIE	C	N	51	A		
A9509	IODINE I-123 SODIUM IODIDE, DIAGNOSTIC, PER MILLICURIE	C	N	57	A		
A9510	TECHNETIUM TC-99M DISOFENIN, DIAGNOSTIC, PER STUDY DOSE, UP TO 15 MILLICURIES	C	N	51	A		
A9512	TECHNETIUM TC-99M PERTECHNETATE, DIAGNOSTIC, PER MILLICURIE	C	N	57	A		
A9516	IODINE I-123 SODIUM IODIDE, DIAGNOSTIC, PER 100 MICROCURIES, UP TO 999 MICROCURIES	C	N	57	A		
A9517	IODINE I-131 SODIUM IODIDE CAPSULE(S), THERAPEUTIC, PER MILLICURIE	C	N	57	A		

HCPCS Code	Statute	Lab Cert	X-Ref	ASC Pay Grp	ASC Pay Group Eff. Date	Proc Notes	BETOS	TOS	Anest	Code Add Date	Code Effective Date	Code Term Date
A9270						0106	Z2	9	0	19860101	20020101	
A9274							D1A	9	0	20080101	20080101	
A9275						0131	T1E	9	0	20060101	20060101	
A9276	1861(n)						D1E	9	0	20080101	20080101	
A9277	1861(n)						D1E	9	0	20080101	20080101	
A9278	1861(n)						D1E	9	0	20080101	20080101	
A9279							T2D	9	0	20070101	20070101	
A9280	1861						Z2	9	0	20040101	20040101	
A9281	1862 SSA						D1E	A,P,R	0	20060101	20060101	
A9282	1861SSA						Z2	9	0	20060101	20060101	
A9283	1862a(i)13						D1E	P	0	20080101	20080101	
A9284						0156	Z2	A,P,R	0	20090101	20090101	
A9300							Z2	9	0	19930101	19950401	
A9500							I1E	4	0	19960101	20100101	
A9501							I1E	4	0	20080101	20080101	
A9502							I1E	4	0	19980101	20090101	
A9503							I1E	4	0	19970101	20060101	
A9504							I1E	4	0	20000101	20060101	
A9505							I1E	4	0	19960101	20060101	
A9507							I1E	4	0	19990101	20060101	
A9508							I1E	4	0	20010101	20060101	
A9509							I1E	4	0	20080101	20080101	
A9510							I1E	4	0	20010101	20060101	
A9512							I1E	4	0	20030101	20060101	
A9516							I1E	4	0	20030101	20080101	
A9517							I1E	6	0	20030101	20060101	

HCPCS Code	Long Description	Coverage	Action	PI	MPI	CIM	MCM
A9521	TECHNETIUM TC-99M EXAMETAZIME, DIAGNOSTIC, PER STUDY DOSE, UP TO 25 MILLICURIES	C	N	57	A		
A9524	IODINE I-131 IODINATED SERUM ALBUMIN, DIAGNOSTIC, PER 5 MICROCURIES	C	N	57	A		
A9526	NITROGEN N-13 AMMONIA, DIAGNOSTIC, PER STUDY DOSE, UP TO 40 MILLICURIES	C	N	53	A		
A9527	IODINE I-125, SODIUM IODIDE SOLUTION, THERAPEUTIC, PER MILLICURIE	C	N	57	A		
A9528	IODINE I-131 SODIUM IODIDE CAPSULE(S), DIAGNOSTIC, PER MILLICURIE	C	N	57	A		
A9529	IODINE I-131 SODIUM IODIDE SOLUTION, DIAGNOSTIC, PER MILLICURIE	C	N	57	A		
A9530	IODINE I-131 SODIUM IODIDE SOLUTION, THERAPEUTIC, PER MILLICURIE	C	N	57	A		
A9531	IODINE I-131 SODIUM IODIDE, DIAGNOSTIC, PER MICROCURIE (UP TO 100 MICROCURIES)	C	N	57	A		
A9532	IODINE I-125 SERUM ALBUMIN, DIAGNOSTIC, PER 5 MICROCURIES	C	N	57	A		
A9535	INJECTION, METHYLENE BLUE, 1 ML	C	D	51	A		
A9536	TECHNETIUM TC-99M DEPREOTIDE, DIAGNOSTIC, PER STUDY DOSE, UP TO 35 MILLICURIES	C	N	57	A		
A9537	TECHNETIUM TC-99M MEBROFENIN, DIAGNOSTIC, PER STUDY DOSE, UP TO 15 MILLICURIES	C	N	57	A		
A9538	TECHNETIUM TC-99M PYROPHOSPHATE, DIAGNOSTIC, PER STUDY DOSE, UP TO 25 MILLICURIES	C	N	57	A		
A9539	TECHNETIUM TC-99M PENTETATE, DIAGNOSTIC, PER STUDY DOSE, UP TO 25 MILLICURIES	C	N	57	A		
A9540	TECHNETIUM TC-99M MACROAGGREGATED ALBUMIN, DIAGNOSTIC, PER STUDY DOSE, UP TO 10 MILLICURIES	C	N	57	A		
A9541	TECHNETIUM TC-99M SULFUR COLLOID, DIAGNOSTIC, PER STUDY DOSE, UP TO 20 MILLICURIES	C	N	57	A		
A9542	INDIUM IN-111 IBRITUMOMAB TIUXETAN, DIAGNOSTIC, PER STUDY DOSE, UP TO 5 MILLICURIES	C	N	51	A		
A9543	YTTRIUM Y-90 IBRITUMOMAB TIUXETAN, THERAPEUTIC, PER TREATMENT DOSE, UP TO 40 MILLICURIES	C	N	51	A		
A9544	IODINE I-131 TOSITUMOMAB, DIAGNOSTIC, PER STUDY DOSE	C	N	57	A		
A9545	IODINE I-131 TOSITUMOMAB, THERAPEUTIC, PER TREATMENT DOSE	C	N	57	A		
A9546	COBALT CO-57/58, CYANOCOBALAMIN, DIAGNOSTIC, PER STUDY DOSE, UP TO 1 MICROCURIE	C	N	53	A		
A9547	INDIUM IN-111 OXYQUINOLINE, DIAGNOSTIC, PER 0.5 MILLICURIE	C	N	53	A		
A9548	INDIUM IN-111 PENTETATE, DIAGNOSTIC, PER 0.5 MILLICURIE	C	N	53	A		
A9549	TECHNETIUM TC-99M ARCITUMOMAB, DIAGNOSTIC, PER STUDY DOSE, UP TO 25 MILLICURIES	C	N	53	A		
A9550	TECHNETIUM TC-99M SODIUM GLUCEPTATE, DIAGNOSTIC, PER STUDY DOSE, UP TO 25 MILLICURIE	C	N	53	A		
A9551	TECHNETIUM TC-99M SUCCIMER, DIAGNOSTIC, PER STUDY DOSE, UP TO 10 MILLICURIES	C	N	53	A		

HCPCS Code	Statute	Lab Cert	X-Ref	ASC Pay Grp	ASC Pay Group Eff. Date	Proc Notes	BETOS	TOS	Anest	Code Add Date	Code Effective Date	Code Term Date
A9521							I1E	4	0	20030101	20060101	
A9524							I1E	4	0	20030101	20060101	
A9526							I1E	4	0	20040101	20060101	
A9527				YY	20080101		I1E	4	0	20070101	20070101	
A9528							I1E	4	0	20040101	20060101	
A9529							I1E	4	0	20040101	20060101	
A9530							I1E	6	0	20040101	20060101	
A9531							I1E	4	0	20040101	20060101	
A9532							I1E	6	0	20040101	20060101	
A9535							I1E	4	0	20060101	20100101	20091231
A9536							I1E	4	0	20060101	20060101	
A9537							I1E	4	0	20060101	20060101	
A9538							I1E	4	0	20060101	20060101	
A9539							I1E	4	0	20060101	20060101	
A9540							I1E	4	0	20060101	20060101	
A9541							I1E	4	0	20060101	20060101	
A9542							I1E	4	0	20060101	20060101	
A9543							I1E	6	0	20060101	20060101	
A9544							I1E	4	0	20060101	20060101	
A9545							I1E	6	0	20060101	20060101	
A9546							I1E	4	0	20060101	20060101	
A9547							I1E	4	0	20060101	20060101	
A9548							I1E	4	0	20060101	20060101	
A9549							I1E	4	0	20060101	20070101	20061231
A9550							I1E	4	0	20060101	20060101	
A9551							I1E	4	0	20060101	20060101	

HCPCS Code	Long Description	Coverage	Action	PI	MPI	CIM	MCM
A9552	FLUORODEOXYGLUCOSE F-18 FDG, DIAGNOSTIC, PER STUDY DOSE, UP TO 45 MILLICURIES	C	N	53	A		
A9553	CHROMIUM CR-51 SODIUM CHROMATE, DIAGNOSTIC, PER STUDY DOSE, UP TO 250 MICROCURIES	C	N	53	A		
A9554	IODINE I-125 SODIUM IOTHALAMATE, DIAGNOSTIC, PER STUDY DOSE, UP TO 10 MICROCURIES	C	N	53	A		
A9555	RUBIDIUM RB-82, DIAGNOSTIC, PER STUDY DOSE, UP TO 60 MILLICURIES	C	N	99	9		
A9556	GALLIUM GA-67 CITRATE, DIAGNOSTIC, PER MILLICURIE	C	N	57	A		
A9557	TECHNETIUM TC-99M BICISATE, DIAGNOSTIC, PER STUDY DOSE, UP TO 25 MILLICURIES	C	N	57	A		
A9558	XENON XE-133 GAS, DIAGNOSTIC, PER 10 MILLICURIES	C	N	57	A		
A9559	COBALT CO-57 CYANOCOBALAMIN, ORAL, DIAGNOSTIC, PER STUDY DOSE, UP TO 1 MICROCURIE	C	N	57	A		
A9560	TECHNETIUM TC-99M LABELED RED BLOOD CELLS, DIAGNOSTIC, PER STUDY DOSE, UP TO 30 MILLICURIES	C	N	57	A		
A9561	TECHNETIUM TC-99M OXIDRONATE, DIAGNOSTIC, PER STUDY DOSE, UP TO 30 MILLICURIES	C	N	57	A		
A9562	TECHNETIUM TC-99M MERTIATIDE, DIAGNOSTIC, PER STUDY DOSE, UP TO 15 MILLICURIES	C	N	57	A		
A9563	SODIUM PHOSPHATE P-32, THERAPEUTIC, PER MILLICURIE	C	N	57	A		
A9564	CHROMIC PHOSPHATE P-32 SUSPENSION, THERAPEUTIC, PER MILLICURIE	C	N	57	A		
A9565	INDIUM IN-111 PENTETREOTIDE, DIAGNOSTIC, PER MILLICURIE	C	N	57	A		
A9566	TECHNETIUM TC-99M FANOLESOMAB, DIAGNOSTIC, PER STUDY DOSE, UP TO 25 MILLICURIES	C	N	57	A		
A9567	TECHNETIUM TC-99M PENTETATE, DIAGNOSTIC, AEROSOL, PER STUDY DOSE, UP TO 75 MILLICURIES	C	N	57	A		
A9568	TECHNETIUM TC-99M ARCITUMOMAB, DIAGNOSTIC, PER STUDY DOSE, UP TO 45 MILLICURIES	C	N	53	A		
A9569	TECHNETIUM TC-99M EXAMETAZIME LABELED AUTOLOGOUS WHITE BLOOD CELLS, DIAGNOSTIC, PER STUDY DOSE	C	N	57	A		
A9570	INDIUM IN-111 LABELED AUTOLOGOUS WHITE BLOOD CELLS, DIAGNOSTIC, PER STUDY DOSE	C	N	57	A		
A9571	INDIUM IN-111 LABELED AUTOLOGOUS PLATELETS, DIAGNOSTIC, PER STUDY DOSE	C	N	57	A		
A9572	INDIUM IN-111 PENTETREOTIDE, DIAGNOSTIC, PER STUDY DOSE, UP TO 6 MILLICURIES	C	N	57	A		
A9576	INJECTION, GADOTERIDOL, (PROHANCE MULTIPACK), PER ML	C	N	51	A		
A9577	INJECTION, GADOBENATE DIMEGLUMINE (MULTIHANCE), PER ML	C	N	51	A		
A9578	INJECTION, GADOBENATE DIMEGLUMINE (MULTIHANCE MULTIPACK), PER ML	C	N	51	A		
A9579	INJECTION, GADOLINIUM-BASED MAGNETIC RESONANCE CONTRAST AGENT, NOT OTHERWISE SPECIFIED (NOS), PER ML	C	N	51	A		
A9580	SODIUM FLUORIDE F-18, DIAGNOSTIC, PER STUDY DOSE, UP TO 30 MILLICURIES	C	N	57	A		
A9581	INJECTION, GADOXETATE DISODIUM, 1 ML	C	A	51	A		

HCPCS Code	Statute	Lab Cert	X-Ref	ASC Pay Grp	ASC Pay Group Eff. Date	Proc Notes	BETOS	TOS	Anest	Code Add Date	Code Effective Date	Code Term Date
A9552							I1E	4	0	20060101	20060101	
A9553							I1E	4	0	20060101	20060101	
A9554							I1E	4	0	20060101	20060101	
A9555							I1E	4	0	20060101	20060101	
A9556							I1E	4	0	20060101	20060101	
A9557							I1E	4	0	20060101	20060101	
A9558							I1E	4	0	20060101	20060101	
A9559							I1E	4	0	20060101	20060101	
A9560							I1E	4	0	20060101	20060101	
A9561							I1E	4	0	20060101	20060101	
A9562							I1E	4	0	20060101	20060101	
A9563							I1E	6	0	20060101	20060101	
A9564							I1E	6	0	20060101	20060101	
A9565							I1E	4	0	20060101	20080101	20071231
A9566							I1E	4	0	20060101	20060101	
A9567							I1E	4	0	20060101	20060101	
A9568							I1E	4	0	20070101	20070101	
A9569							I1E	4	0	20080101	20080101	
A9570							I1E	4	0	20080101	20080101	
A9571							I1E	4	0	20080101	20080101	
A9572							I1E	4	0	20080101	20080101	
A9576							I1E	4	0	20080101	20080101	
A9577							I1E	4	0	20080101	20080101	
A9578							I1E	4	0	20080101	20080101	
A9579							I1E	4	0	20080101	20080101	
A9580							I1E	4	0	20090101	20090101	
A9581							I2D	1, P	0	20100101	20100101	

HCPCS Code	Long Description	Coverage	Action	PI	MPI	CIM	MCM
A9582	IODINE I-123 IOBENGUANE, DIAGNOSTIC, PER STUDY DOSE, UP TO 15 MILLICURIES	C	A	51	A		
A9583	INJECTION, GADOFOSVESET TRISODIUM, 1 ML	C	A	51	A		
A9600	STRONTIUM SR-89 CHLORIDE, THERAPEUTIC, PER MILLICURIE	C	N	57	A		
A9604	SAMARIUM SM-153 LEXIDRONAM, THERAPEUTIC, PER TREATMENT DOSE, UP TO 150 MILLICURIES	C	A	57	A		
A9605	SAMARIUM SM-153 LEXIDRONAMM, THERAPEUTIC, PER 50 MILLICURIES	C	D	57	A		
A9698	NON-RADIOACTIVE CONTRAST IMAGING MATERIAL, NOT OTHERWISE CLASSIFIED, PER STUDY	D	N	51	A		15022
A9699	RADIOPHARMACEUTICAL, THERAPEUTIC, NOT OTHERWISE CLASSIFIED	C	N	57	A		
A9700	SUPPLY OF INJECTABLE CONTRAST MATERIAL FOR USE IN ECHOCARDIOGRAPHY, PER STUDY	D	N	57	A		15360
A9900	MISCELLANEOUS DME SUPPLY, ACCESSORY, AND/OR SERVICE COMPONENT OF ANOTHER HCPCS CODE	C	N	46	A		
A9901	DME DELIVERY, SET UP, AND/OR DISPENSING SERVICE COMPONENT OF ANOTHER HCPCS CODE	C	N	46	A		
A9999	MISCELLANEOUS DME SUPPLY OR ACCESSORY, NOT OTHERWISE SPECIFIED	C	N	46	A		
A9554	IODINE I-125 SODIUM IOTHALAMATE, DIAGNOSTIC, PER STUDY DOSE, UP TO 10 MICROCURIES	C	N	53	A		
A9555	RUBIDIUM RB-82, DIAGNOSTIC, PER STUDY DOSE, UP TO 60 MILLICURIES	C	N	99	9		
A9556	GALLIUM GA-67 CITRATE, DIAGNOSTIC, PER MILLICURIE	C	N	57	A		
A9557	TECHNETIUM TC-99M BICISATE, DIAGNOSTIC, PER STUDY DOSE, UP TO 25 MILLICURIES	C	N	57	A		
A9558	XENON XE-133 GAS, DIAGNOSTIC, PER 10 MILLICURIES	C	N	57	A		
A9559	COBALT CO-57 CYANOCOBALAMIN, ORAL, DIAGNOSTIC, PER STUDY DOSE, UP TO 1 MICROCURIE	C	N	57	A		
A9560	TECHNETIUM TC-99M LABELED RED BLOOD CELLS, DIAGNOSTIC, PER STUDY DOSE, UP TO 30 MILLICURIES	C	N	57	A		
A9561	TECHNETIUM TC-99M OXIDRONATE, DIAGNOSTIC, PER STUDY DOSE, UP TO 30 MILLICURIES	C	N	57	A		
A9562	TECHNETIUM TC-99M MERTIATIDE, DIAGNOSTIC, PER STUDY DOSE, UP TO 15 MILLICURIES	C	N	57	A		
A9563	SODIUM PHOSPHATE P-32, THERAPEUTIC, PER MILLICURIE	C	N	57	A		
A9564	CHROMIC PHOSPHATE P-32 SUSPENSION, THERAPEUTIC, PER MILLICURIE	C	N	57	A		
A9565	INDIUM IN-111 PENTETREOTIDE, DIAGNOSTIC, PER MILLICURIE	C	N	57	A		
A9566	TECHNETIUM TC-99M FANOLESOMAB, DIAGNOSTIC, PER STUDY DOSE, UP TO 25 MILLICURIES	C	N	57	A		
A9567	TECHNETIUM TC-99M PENTETATE, DIAGNOSTIC, AEROSOL, PER STUDY DOSE, UP TO 75 'MILLICURIES	C	N	57	A		
A9568	TECHNETIUM TC-99M ARCITUMOMAB, DIAGNOSTIC, PER STUDY DOSE, UP TO 45 MILLICURIES	C	N	53	A		
A9569	TECHNETIUM TC-99M EXAMETAZIME LABELED AUTOLOGOUS WHITE BLOOD CELLS, DIAGNOSTIC, PER STUDY DOSE	C	N	57	A		

HCPCS Code	Statute	Lab Cert	X-Ref	ASC Pay Grp	ASC Pay Group Eff. Date	Proc Notes	BETOS	TOS	Anest	Code Add Date	Code Effective Date	Code Term Date
A9582							I1E	4	0	20100101	20100101	
A9583							I1E	4	0	20100101	20100101	
A9600							I1E	6	0	19980101	20060101	
A9604							I1E	6	0	20100101	20100101	
A9605							I1E	6	0	19990101	20100101	20091231
A9698							I1E	4	0	20060101	20060101	
A9699							I1E	6	0	20030101	20060101	
A9700							I1E	9	0	20010101	20010101	
A9900							D1E	9	0	20000101	20010101	
A9901							D1E	9	0	20000101	20010101	
A9999							D1F	9	0	20040101	20040101	
A9554							I1E	4	0	20060101	20060101	
A9555							I1E	4	0	20060101	20060101	
A9556							I1E	4	0	20060101	20060101	
A9557							I1E	4	0	20060101	20060101	
A9558							I1E	4	0	20060101	20060101	
A9559							I1E	4	0	20060101	20060101	
A9560							I1E	4	0	20060101	20060101	
A9561							I1E	4	0	20060101	20060101	
A9562							I1E	4	0	20060101	20060101	
A9563							I1E	6	0	20060101	20060101	
A9564							I1E	6	0	20060101	20060101	
A9565							I1E	4	0	20060101	20080101	20071231
A9566							I1E	4	0	20060101	20060101	
A9567							I1E	4	0	20060101	20060101	
A9568							I1E	4	0	20070101	20070101	
A9569							I1E	4	0	20080101	20080101	

HCPCS Code	Long Description	Coverage	Action	PI	MPI	CIM	MCM
A9570	INDIUM IN-111 LABELED AUTOLOGOUS WHITE BLOOD CELLS, DIAGNOSTIC, PER STUDY DOSE		C	N	57	A	
A9571	INDIUM IN-111 LABELED AUTOLOGOUS PLATELETS, DIAGNOSTIC, PER STUDY DOSE	C	N	57	A		
A9572	INDIUM IN-111 PENTETREOTIDE, DIAGNOSTIC, PER STUDY DOSE, UP TO 6 MILLICURIES	C	N	57	A		
A9576	INJECTION, GADOTERIDOL, (PROHANCE MULTIPACK), PER ML	C	N	51	A		
A9577	INJECTION, GADOBENATE DIMEGLUMINE (MULTIHANCE), PER ML	C	N	51	A		
A9578	INJECTION, GADOBENATE DIMEGLUMINE (MULTIHANCE MULTIPACK), PER ML	C	N	51	A		
A9579	INJECTION, GADOLINIUM-BASED MAGNETIC RESONANCE CONTRAST AGENT, NOT OTHERWISE SPECIFIED (NOS), PER ML	C	N	51	A		
A9580	SODIUM FLUORIDE F-18, DIAGNOSTIC, PER STUDY DOSE, UP TO 30 MILLICURIES	C	N	57	A		
A9581	INJECTION, GADOXETATE DISODIUM, 1 ML	C	A	51	A		
A9582	IODINE I-123 IOBENGUANE, DIAGNOSTIC, PER STUDY DOSE, UP TO 15 MILLICURIES	C	A	51	A		
A9583	INJECTION, GADOFOSVESET TRISODIUM, 1 ML	C	A	51	A		
A9600	STRONTIUM SR-89 CHLORIDE, THERAPEUTIC, PER MILLICURIE	C	N	57	A		
A9604	SAMARIUM SM-153 LEXIDRONAM, THERAPEUTIC, PER TREATMENT DOSE, UP TO 150 MILLICURIES	C	A	57	A		
A9605	SAMARIUM SM-153 LEXIDRONAMM, THERAPEUTIC, PER 50 MILLICURIES	C	D	57	A		
A9698	NON-RADIOACTIVE CONTRAST IMAGING MATERIAL, NOT OTHERWISE CLASSIFIED, PER STUDY	D	N	51	A		15022
A9699	RADIOPHARMACEUTICAL, THERAPEUTIC, NOT OTHERWISE CLASSIFIED	C	N	57	A		
A9700	SUPPLY OF INJECTABLE CONTRAST MATERIAL FOR USE IN ECHOCARDIOGRAPHY, PER STUDY	D	N	57	A		15360
A9900	MISCELLANEOUS DME SUPPLY, ACCESSORY, AND/OR SERVICE COMPONENT OF ANOTHER HCPCS CODE	C	N	46	A		
A9901	DME DELIVERY, SET UP, AND/OR DISPENSING SERVICE COMPONENT OF ANOTHER HCPCS CODE	C	N	46	A		
A9999	MISCELLANEOUS DME SUPPLY OR ACCESSORY, NOT OTHERWISE SPECIFIED	C	N	46	A		
B4034	ENTERAL FEEDING SUPPLY KIT; SYRINGE FED, PER DAY	D	N	39	A	65-10	2130, 4450
B4035	ENTERAL FEEDING SUPPLY KIT; PUMP FED, PER DAY	D	N	39	A	65-10	2130, 4450
B4036	ENTERAL FEEDING SUPPLY KIT; GRAVITY FED, PER DAY	D	N	39	A	65-10	2130, 4450
B4081	NASOGASTRIC TUBING WITH STYLET	D	N	39	A	65-10	2130, 4450
B4082	NASOGASTRIC TUBING WITHOUT STYLET	D	N	39	A	65-10	2130, 4450
B4083	STOMACH TUBE - LEVINE TYPE	D	N	39	A	65-10	2130, 4450
B4086	GASTROSTOMY / JEJUNOSTOMY TUBE, ANY MATERIAL, ANY TYPE, (STANDARD OR LOW PROFILE), EACH	C	N	39	A		
B4087	GASTROSTOMY/JEJUNOSTOMY TUBE, STANDARD, ANY MATERIAL, ANY TYPE, EACH	C	N	39	A		
B4088	GASTROSTOMY/JEJUNOSTOMY TUBE, LOW-PROFILE, ANY MATERIAL, ANY TYPE, EACH	C	N	39	A		
B4100	FOOD THICKENER, ADMINISTERED ORALLY, PER OUNCE	M	N	00	9	60-9	

HCPCS Code	Statute	Lab Cert	X-Ref	ASC Pay Grp	ASC Pay Group Eff. Date	Proc Notes	BETOS	TOS	Anest	Code Add Date	Code Effective Date	Code Term Date
	A9570							I1E	4	0	20080101	20080101
A9571							I1E	4	0	20080101	20080101	
A9572							I1E	4	0	20080101	20080101	
A9576							I1E	4	0	20080101	20080101	
A9577							I1E	4	0	20080101	20080101	
A9578							I1E	4	0	20080101	20080101	
A9579							I1E	4	0	20080101	20080101	
A9580							I1E	4	0	20090101	20090101	
A9581							I2D	1, P	0	20100101	20100101	
A9582							I1E	4	0	20100101	20100101	
A9583							I1E	4	0	20100101	20100101	
A9600							I1E	6	0	19980101	20060101	
A9604							I1E	6	0	20100101	20100101	
A9605							I1E	6	0	19990101	20100101	20091231
A9698							I1E	4	0	20060101	20060101	
A9699							I1E	6	0	20030101	20060101	
A9700							I1E	9	0	20010101	20010101	
A9900							D1E	9	0	20000101	20010101	
A9901							D1E	9	0	20000101	20010101	
A9999							D1F	9	0	20040101	20040101	
B4034							O1C	E	0	19860101	20080101	
B4035							O1C	E	0	19860101	20020101	
B4036							O1C	E	0	19860101	20020101	
B4081							O1C	E	0	19860101	20020101	
B4082							O1C	E	0	19860101	20020101	
B4083							O1C	E	0	19860101	20020101	
B4086							O1C	E	0	20020101	20080101	20071231
B4086												
B4087							O1C	E	0	20080101	20080101	
B4088							O1E	E	0	20080101	20080101	
B4100							Z2	E	0	20030101	20050101	

HCPCS Code	Long Description	Coverage	Action	PI	MPI	CIM	MCM
B4102	ENTERAL FORMULA, FOR ADULTS, USED TO REPLACE FLUIDS AND ELECTROLYTES (E.G. CLEAR LIQUIDS), 500 ML = 1 UNIT	D	N	39	A	65-10	
B4103	ENTERAL FORMULA, FOR PEDIATRICS, USED TO REPLACE FLUIDS & ELECTROLYTES (E.G. CLEAR LIQUIDS), 500 ML = 1 UNIT	D	N	46	A	65-10	
B4104	ADDITIVE FOR ENTERAL FORMULA (E.G. FIBER)	D	N	00	9	65-10	
B4149	ENTERAL FORMULA, MANUFACTURED BLENDERIZED NATURAL FOODS WITH INTACT NUTRIENTS, INCLUDES PROTEINS, FATS, CARBOHYDRATES, VITAMINS AND MINERALS, MAY INCLUDE FIBER, ADMINISTERED THROUGH AN ENTERAL FEEDING TUBE, 100 CALORIES = 1 UNIT	D	N	39	A	65-10	2130, 4450
B4150	ENTERAL FORMULA, NUTRITIONALLY COMPLETE WITH INTACT NUTRIENTS, INCLUDES PROTEINS, FATS, CARBOHYDRATES, VITAMINS AND MINERALS, MAY INCLUDE FIBER, ADMINISTERED THROUGH AN ENTERAL FEEDING TUBE, 100 CALORIES = 1 UNIT	D	N	39	A	65-10	2130, 4450
B4152	ENTERAL FORMULA, NUTRITIONALLY COMPLETE, CALORICALLY DENSE (EQUAL TO OR GREATER THAN 1.5 KCAL/ML) WITH INTACT NUTRIENTS, INCLUDES PROTEINS, FATS, CARBOHYDRATES, VITAMINS AND MINERALS, MAY INCLUDE FIBER, ADMINISTERED THROUGH AN ENTERAL FEEDING TUBE, 100 CALORIES = 1 UNIT	D	N	39	A	65-10	2130, 4450
B4153	ENTERAL FORMULA, NUTRITIONALLY COMPLETE, HYDROLYZED PROTEINS (AMINO ACIDS AND PEPTIDE CHAIN), INCLUDES FATS, CARBOHYDRATES, VITAMINS AND MINERALS, MAY INCLUDE FIBER, ADMINISTERED THROUGH AN ENTERAL FEEDING TUBE, 100 CALORIES = 1 UNIT	D	N	39	A	65-10	2130, 4450
B4154	ENTERAL FORMULA, NUTRITIONALLY COMPLETE, FOR SPECIAL METABOLIC NEEDS, EXCLUDES INHERITED DISEASE OF METABOLISM, INCLUDES ALTERED COMPOSITION OF PROTEINS, FATS, CARBOHYDRATES, VITAMINS AND/OR MINERALS, MAY INCLUDE FIBER, ADMINISTERED THROUGH AN ENTERAL FEEDING TUBE, 100 CALORIES = 1 UNIT	D	N	39	A	65-10	2130, 4450
B4155	ENTERAL FORMULA, NUTRITIONALLY INCOMPLETE/ MODULAR NUTRIENTS, INCLUDES SPECIFIC NUTRIENTS, CARBOHYDRATES (E.G. GLUCOSE POLYMERS), PROTEINS/ AMINO ACIDS (E.G. GLUTAMINE, ARGININE), FAT (E.G. MEDIUM CHAIN TRIGLYCERIDES) OR COMBINATION, ADMINISTERED THROUGH AN ENTERAL FEEDING TUBE, 100 CALORIES = 1 UNIT	D	N	39	A	65-10	2130, 4450
B4157	ENTERAL FORMULA, NUTRITIONALLY COMPLETE, FOR SPECIAL METABOLIC NEEDS FOR INHERITED DISEASE OF METABOLISM, INCLUDES PROTEINS, FATS, CARBOHYDRATES, VITAMINS AND MINERALS, MAY INCLUDE FIBER, ADMINISTERED THROUGH AN ENTERAL FEEDING TUBE, 100 CALORIES = 1 UNIT	D	N	39	A	65-10	
B4158	ENTERAL FORMULA, FOR PEDIATRICS, NUTRITIONALLY COMPLETE WITH INTACT NUTRIENTS, INCLUDES PROTEINS, FATS, CARBOHYDRATES, VITAMINS AND MINERALS, MAY INCLUDE FIBER AND/OR IRON, ADMINISTERED THROUGH AN ENTERAL FEEDING TUBE, 100 CALORIES = 1 UNIT	D	N	46	A	65-10	

HCPCS Code	Statute	Lab Cert	X-Ref	ASC Pay Grp	ASC Pay Group Eff. Date	Proc Notes	BETOS	TOS	Anest	Code Add Date	Code Effective Date	Code Term Date
B4102							O1C	E	0	20050101	20050101	
B4103							O1C	E	0	20050101	20050101	
B4104							O1C	E	0	20050101	20050101	
B4149							O1C	E	0	20050101	20060101	
B4150							O1C	E	0	19860101	20050101	
B4152							O1C	E	0	19840101	20050101	
B4153							O1C	E	0	19860101	20050101	
B4154							O1C	E	0	19840101	20050101	
B4155							O1C	E	0	19860101	20050101	
B4155												
B4157							O1C	E	0	20050101	20050101	
B4158							O1C	E	0	20050101	20050101	

HCPCS Code	Long Description	Coverage	Action	PI	MPI	CIM	MCM
B4159	ENTERAL FORMULA, FOR PEDIATRICS, NUTRITIONALLY COMPLETE SOY BASED WITH INTACT NUTRIENTS, INCLUDES PROTEINS, FATS, CARBOHYDRATES, VITAMINS AND MINERALS, MAY INCLUDE FIBER AND/OR IRON, ADMINISTERED THROUGH AN ENTERAL FEEDING TUBE, 100 CALORIES = 1 UNIT	D	N	46	A	65-10	
B4160	ENTERAL FORMULA, FOR PEDIATRICS, NUTRITIONALLY COMPLETE CALORICALLY DENSE (EQUAL TO OR GREATER THAN 0.7 KCAL/ML) WITH INTACT NUTRIENTS, INCLUDES PROTEINS, FATS, CARBOHYDRATES, VITAMINS AND MINERALS, MAY INCLUDE FIBER, ADMINISTERED THROUGH AN ENTERAL FEEDING TUBE, 100 CALORIES = 1 UNIT	D	N	46	A	65-10	
B4161	ENTERAL FORMULA, FOR PEDIATRICS, HYDROLYZED/AMINO ACIDS AND PEPTIDE CHAIN PROTEINS, INCLUDES FATS, CARBOHYDRATES, VITAMINS AND MINERALS, MAY INCLUDE FIBER, ADMINISTERED THROUGH AN ENTERAL FEEDING TUBE, 100 CALORIES = 1 UNIT	D	N	46	A	65-10	
B4162	ENTERAL FORMULA, FOR PEDIATRICS, SPECIAL METABOLIC NEEDS FOR INHERITED DISEASE OF METABOLISM, INCLUDES PROTEINS, FATS, CARBOHYDRATES, VITAMINS AND MINERALS, MAY INCLUDE FIBER, ADMINISTERED THROUGH AN ENTERAL FEEDING TUBE, 100 CALORIES = 1 UNIT	D	N	46	A	65-10	
B4164	PARENTERAL NUTRITION SOLUTION: CARBOHYDRATES (DEXTROSE), 50% OR LESS (500 ML =1 UNIT) - HOMEMIX	D	N	39	A	65-10	2130, 4450
B4168	PARENTERAL NUTRITION SOLUTION; AMINO ACID, 3.5%, (500 ML = 1 UNIT) - HOMEMIX	D	N	39	A	65-10	2130, 4450
B4172	PARENTERAL NUTRITION SOLUTION; AMINO ACID, 5.5% THROUGH 7%, (500 ML = 1 UNIT) - HOMEMIX	D	N	39	A	65-10	2130, 4450
B4176	PARENTERAL NUTRITION SOLUTION; AMINO ACID, 7% THROUGH 8.5%, (500 ML = 1 UNIT) - HOMEMIX	D	N	39	A	65-10	2130, 4450
B4178	PARENTERAL NUTRITION SOLUTION: AMINO ACID, GREATER THAN 8.5% (500 ML = 1 UNIT) - HOMEMIX	D	N	39	A	65-10	2130, 4450
B4180	PARENTERAL NUTRITION SOLUTION; CARBOHYDRATES (DEXTROSE), GREATER THAN 50% (500 ML=1 UNIT) - HOMEMIX	D	N	39	A	65-10	2130, 4450
B4185	PARENTERAL NUTRITION SOLUTION, PER 10 GRAMS LIPIDS	D	N	39	A		
B4189	PARENTERAL NUTRITION SOLUTION; COMPOUNDED AMINO ACID AND CARBOHYDRATES WITH ELECTROLYTES, TRACE ELEMENTS, AND VITAMINS, INCLUDING PREPARATION, ANY STRENGTH, 10 TO 51 GRAMS OF PROTEIN - PREMIX	D	N	39	A	65-10	2130, 4450
B4193	PARENTERAL NUTRITION SOLUTION; COMPOUNDED AMINO ACID AND CARBOHYDRATES WITH ELECTROLYTES, TRACE ELEMENTS, AND VITAMINS, INCLUDING PREPARATION, ANY STRENGTH, 52 TO 73 GRAMS OF PROTEIN - PREMIX	D	N	39	A	65-10	2130, 4450
B4197	PARENTERAL NUTRITION SOLUTION; COMPOUNDED AMINO ACID AND CARBOHYDRATES WITH ELECTROLYTES, TRACE ELEMENTS AND VITAMINS, INCLUDING PREPARATION, ANY STRENGTH, 74 TO 100 GRAMS OF PROTEIN - PREMIX	D	N	39	A	65-10	2130, 4450

HCPCS Code	Statute	Lab Cert	X-Ref	ASC Pay Grp	ASC Pay Group Eff. Date	Proc Notes	BETOS	TOS	Anest	Code Add Date	Code Effective Date	Code Term Date
B4159							O1C	E	0	20050101	20050101	
B4160							O1C	E	0	20050101	20050101	
B4160 B4161							O1C	E	0	20050101	20050101	
B4162							O1C	E	0	20050101	20050101	
B4164							O1C	E	0	19860101	20020101	
B4168							O1C	E	0	19840101	20020101	
B4172							O1C	E	0	19840101	20020101	
B4176							O1C	E	0	19860101	20020101	
B4178							O1C	E	0	19880101	20020101	
B4180							O1C	E	0	19860101	20020101	
B4185						0126	O1C	E	0	20060101	20060101	
B4189							O1C	E	0	19880101	20020101	
B4193							O1C	E	0	19880101	20020101	
B4197							O1C	E	0	19880101	20020101	

HCPCS Code	Long Description	Coverage	Action	PI	MPI	CIM	MCM
B4199	PARENTERAL NUTRITION SOLUTION; COMPOUNDED AMINO ACID AND CARBOHYDRATES WITH ELECTROLYTES, TRACE ELEMENTS AND VITAMINS, INCLUDING PREPARATION, ANY STRENGTH, OVER 100 GRAMS OF PROTEIN - PREMIX	D	N	39	A	65-10	2130, 4450
B4216	PARENTERAL NUTRITION; ADDITIVES (VITAMINS, TRACE ELEMENTS, HEPARIN, ELECTROLYTES) HOMEMIX PER DAY	D	N	39	A	65-10	2130, 4450
B4220	PARENTERAL NUTRITION SUPPLY KIT; PREMIX, PER DAY	D	N	39	A	65-10	2130, 4450
B4222	PARENTERAL NUTRITION SUPPLY KIT; HOME MIX, PER DAY	D	N	39	A	65-10	2130, 4450
B4224	PARENTERAL NUTRITION ADMINISTRATION KIT, PER DAY	D	N	39	A	65-10	2130, 4450
B5000	PARENTERAL NUTRITION SOLUTION: COMPOUNDED AMINO ACID AND CARBOHYDRATES WITH ELECTROLYTES, TRACE ELEMENTS, AND VITAMINS, INCLUDING PREPARATION, ANY STRENGTH, RENAL - AMIROSYN RF, NEPHRAMINE, RENAMINE - PREMIX	D	N	39	A	65-10	2130, 4450
B5100	PARENTERAL NUTRITION SOLUTION: COMPOUNDED AMINO ACID AND CARBOHYDRATES WITH ELECTROLYTES, TRACE ELEMENTS, AND VITAMINS, INCLUDING PREPARATION, ANY STRENGTH, HEPATIC - FREAMINE HBC, HEPATAMINE - PREMIX	D	N	39	A	65-10	2130, 4450
B5200	PARENTERAL NUTRITION SOLUTION: COMPOUNDED AMINO ACID AND CARBOHYDRATES WITH ELECTROLYTES, TRACE ELEMENTS, AND VITAMINS, INCLUDING PREPARATION, ANY STRENGTH, STRESS - BRANCH CHAIN AMINO ACIDS - PREMIX	D	N	39	A	65-10	2130, 4450
B9000	ENTERAL NUTRITION INFUSION PUMP - WITHOUT ALARM	D	N	39	A	65-10	2130, 4450
B9002	ENTERAL NUTRITION INFUSION PUMP - WITH ALARM	D	N	39	A	65-10	2130, 4450
B9004	PARENTERAL NUTRITION INFUSION PUMP, PORTABLE	D	N	39	A	65-10	2130, 4450
B9006	PARENTERAL NUTRITION INFUSION PUMP, STATIONARY	D	N	39	A	65-10	2130, 4450
B9998	NOC FOR ENTERAL SUPPLIES	D	N	57	A	65-10	2130, 4450
B9999	NOC FOR PARENTERAL SUPPLIES	D	N	57	A	65-10	2130, 4450
C1178	INJECTION, BUSULFAN, PER 6 MG	D	N	51	A		
C1300	HYPERBARIC OXYGEN UNDER PRESSURE, FULL BODY CHAMBER, PER 30 MINUTE INTERVAL	D	N	53	A		
C1713	ANCHOR/SCREW FOR OPPOSING BONE-TO-BONE OR SOFT TISSUE-TO-BONE (IMPLANTABLE)	D	N	53	A		
C1714	CATHETER, TRANSLUMINAL ATHERECTOMY, DIRECTIONAL	D	N	53	A		
C1715	BRACHYTHERAPY NEEDLE	D	N	53	A		
C1716	BRACHYTHERAPY SOURCE, NON-STRANDED, GOLD-198, PER SOURCE	D	N	53	A		
C1717	BRACHYTHERAPY SOURCE, NON-STRANDED, HIGH DOSE RATE IRIDIUM-192, PER SOURCE	D	N	53	A		
C1718	BRACHYTHERAPY SOURCE, IODINE 125, PER SOURCE	D	N	53	A		
C1719	BRACHYTHERAPY SOURCE, NON-STRANDED, NON-HIGH DOSE RATE IRIDIUM-192, PER SOURCE	D	N	53	A		
C1720	BRACHYTHERAPY SOURCE, PALLADIUM 103, PER SOURCE	D	N	53	A		
C1721	CARDIOVERTER-DEFIBRILLATOR, DUAL CHAMBER (IMPLANTABLE)	D	N	53	A		
C1722	CARDIOVERTER-DEFIBRILLATOR, SINGLE CHAMBER (IMPLANTABLE)	D	N	53	A		
C1724	CATHETER, TRANSLUMINAL ATHERECTOMY, ROTATIONAL	D	N	53	A		

HCPCS Code	Statute	Lab Cert	X-Ref	ASC Pay Grp	ASC Pay Group Eff. Date	Proc Notes	BETOS	TOS	Anest	Code Add Date	Code Effective Date	Code Term Date
B4199							O1C	E	0	19880101	20020101	
B4216							O1C	E	0	19840101	20020101	
B4220							O1C	E	0	19840101	20020101	
B4222							O1C	E	0	19860101	20020101	
B4224							O1C	E	0	19860101	20020101	
B5000							O1C	E	0	19880101	20020101	
B5100							O1C	E	0	19880101	20020101	
B5200							O1C	E	0	19880101	20020101	
B5200												
B9000							O1C	A,P,R	0	19880101	20020101	
B9002							O1C	A,P,R	0	19880101	20020101	
B9004							O1C	A,P,R	0	19880101	20020101	
B9006							O1C	A,P,R	0	19880101	20020101	
B9998							O1C	E	0	19850101	19960101	
B9999							O1C	E	0	19850101	19960101	
C1178	1833(T)		J0594			0093	O1D	1, P	0	20000801	20070101	20061231
C1300	1833(T)					0093	P5E	9	0	20000801	20030701	
C1713	1833(T)						D1A	9, S	0	20010401	20040101	
C1714	1833(T)						D1A	9, S	0	20010401	20040101	
C1715	1833(T)						D1A	9, S	0	20010401	20040101	
C1716	1833(T)			YY	20080101		I4B	6	0	20010401	20010401	
C1717	1833(T)			YY	20080101		I4B	6	0	20010401	20010401	
C1718	1833(T)		C2639				D1A	9, S	0	20010401	20070701	20070630
C1719	1833(T)			YY	20080101		I4B	6	0	20010401	20010401	
C1720	1833(T)		C2641				D1A	9, S	0	20010401	20070701	20070630
C1721	1833(T)						D1A	9, S	0	20010401	20040101	
C1722	1833(T)						D1A	9, S	0	20010401	20040101	
C1724	1833(T)						D1A	9, S	0	20010401	20040101	

C Codes

HCPCS Code	Long Description	Coverage	Action	PI	MPI	CIM	MCM
C1725	CATHETER, TRANSLUMINAL ANGIOPLASTY, NON-LASER (MAY INCLUDE GUIDANCE, INFUSION/PERFUSION CAPABILITY)	D	N	53	A		
C1726	CATHETER, BALLOON DILATATION, NON-VASCULAR	D	N	53	A		
C1727	CATHETER, BALLOON TISSUE DISSECTOR, NON-VASCULAR (INSERTABLE)	D	N	53	A		
C1728	CATHETER, BRACHYTHERAPY SEED ADMINISTRATION	D	N	53	A		
C1729	CATHETER, DRAINAGE	D	N	53	A		
C1730	CATHETER, ELECTROPHYSIOLOGY, DIAGNOSTIC, OTHER THAN 3D MAPPING (19 OR FEWER ELECTRODES)	D	N	53	A		
C1731	CATHETER, ELECTROPHYSIOLOGY, DIAGNOSTIC, OTHER THAN 3D MAPPING (20 OR MORE ELECTRODES)	D	N	53	A		
C1732	CATHETER, ELECTROPHYSIOLOGY, DIAGNOSTIC/ABLATION, 3D OR VECTOR MAPPING	D	N	53	A		
C1733	CATHETER, ELECTROPHYSIOLOGY, DIAGNOSTIC/ABLATION, OTHER THAN 3D OR VECTOR MAPPING, OTHER THAN COOL-TIP	D	N	53	A		
C1750	CATHETER, HEMODIALYSIS/PERITONEAL, LONG-TERM	D	N	53	A		
C1751	CATHETER, INFUSION, INSERTED PERIPHERALLY, CENTRALLY OR MIDLINE (OTHER THAN HEMODIALYSIS)	D	N	53	A		
C1752	CATHETER, HEMODIALYSIS/PERITONEAL, SHORT-TERM	D	N	53	A		
C1753	CATHETER, INTRAVASCULAR ULTRASOUND	D	N	53	A		
C1754	CATHETER, INTRADISCAL	D	N	53	A		
C1755	CATHETER, INTRASPINAL	D	N	53	A		
C1756	CATHETER, PACING, TRANSESOPHAGEAL	D	N	53	A		
C1757	CATHETER, THROMBECTOMY/EMBOLECTOMY	D	N	53	A		
C1758	CATHETER, URETERAL	D	N	53	A		
C1759	CATHETER, INTRACARDIAC ECHOCARDIOGRAPHY	D	N	53	A		
C1760	CLOSURE DEVICE, VASCULAR (IMPLANTABLE/INSERTABLE)	D	N	53	A		
C1762	CONNECTIVE TISSUE, HUMAN (INCLUDES FASCIA LATA)	D	N	53	A		
C1763	CONNECTIVE TISSUE, NON-HUMAN (INCLUDES SYNTHETIC)	D	N	53	A		
C1764	EVENT RECORDER, CARDIAC (IMPLANTABLE)	D	N	53	A		
C1765	ADHESION BARRIER	D	N	53	A		
C1766	INTRODUCER/SHEATH, GUIDING, INTRACARDIAC ELECTROPHYSIOLOGICAL, STEERABLE, OTHER THAN PEEL-AWAY	D	N	53	A		
C1767	GENERATOR, NEUROSTIMULATOR (IMPLANTABLE), NON-RECHARGEABLE	D	N	53	A		
C1768	GRAFT, VASCULAR	D	N	53	A		
C1769	GUIDE WIRE	D	N	53	A		
C1770	IMAGING COIL, MAGNETIC RESONANCE (INSERTABLE)	D	N	53	A		
C1771	REPAIR DEVICE, URINARY, INCONTINENCE, WITH SLING GRAFT	D	N	53	A		
C1772	INFUSION PUMP, PROGRAMMABLE (IMPLANTABLE)	D	N	53	A		
C1773	RETRIEVAL DEVICE, INSERTABLE (USED TO RETRIEVE FRACTURED MEDICAL DEVICES)	D	N	53	A		
C1776	JOINT DEVICE (IMPLANTABLE)	D	N	53	A		
C1777	LEAD, CARDIOVERTER-DEFIBRILLATOR, ENDOCARDIAL SINGLE COIL (IMPLANTABLE)	D	N	53	A		
C1778	LEAD, NEUROSTIMULATOR (IMPLANTABLE)	D	N	53	A		
C1779	LEAD, PACEMAKER, TRANSVENOUS VDD SINGLE PASS	D	N	53	A		
C1780	LENS, INTRAOCULAR (NEW TECHNOLOGY)	D	N	53	A		

HCPCS Code	Statute	Lab Cert	X-Ref	ASC Pay Grp	ASC Pay Group Eff. Date	Proc Notes	BETOS	TOS	Anest	Code Add Date	Code Effective Date	Code Term Date
C1725	1833(T)						D1A	9, S	0	20010401	20040101	
C1726	1833(T)						D1A	9, S	0	20010401	20040101	
C1727	1833(T)						D1A	9, S	0	20010401	20040101	
C1728	1833(T)						D1A	9, S	0	20010401	20040101	
C1729	1833(T)						D1A	9, S	0	20010401	20040101	
C1730	1833(T)						D1A	9, S	0	20010401	20040101	
C1731	1833(T)						D1A	9, S	0	20010401	20040101	
C1732	1833(T)						D1A	9, S	0	20010401	20040101	
C1733	1833(T)						D1A	9, S	0	20010401	20040101	
C1750	1833(T)						D1A	9, S	0	20010401	20010401	
C1751	1833(T)						D1A	9, S	0	20010401	20040101	
C1752	1833(T)						D1A	9, S	0	20010401	20010401	
C1753	1833(T)						D1A	9, S	0	20010401	20040101	
C1754	1833(T)						D1A	9, S	0	20010401	20040101	
C1755	1833(T)						D1A	9, S	0	20010401	20040101	
C1756	1833(T)						D1A	9, S	0	20010401	20040101	
C1757	1833(T)						D1A	9, S	0	20010401	20040101	
C1758	1833(T)						D1A	9, S	0	20010401	20040101	
C1759	1833(T)						D1A	9, S	0	20010401	20040101	
C1760	1833(T)						D1A	9, S	0	20010401	20040101	
C1762	1833(T)						D1A	9, S	0	20010401	20040101	
C1763	1833(T)						D1A	9, S	0	20010401	20040101	
C1764	1833(T)						D1A	9, S	0	20010401	20040101	
C1765	1833(T)						D1A	9, S	0	20010701	20010701	
C1766	1833(T)						D1A	9, S	0	20010401	20040101	
C1767	1833(T)						D1A	9, S	0	20010401	20060101	
C1768	1833(T)						D1A	9, S	0	20010401	20040101	
C1769	1833(T)						D1A	9, S	0	20010401	20040101	
C1770	1833(T)						D1A	9, S	0	20010401	20040101	
C1771	1833(T)						D1A	9, S	0	20010401	20040101	
C1772	1833(T)						D1A	9, S	0	20010401	20040101	
C1773	1833(T)						D1A	9, S	0	20010401	20040101	
C1776	1833(T)						D1A	9, S	0	20010401	20040101	
C1777	1833(T)						D1A	9, S	0	20010401	20040101	
C1778	1833(T)						D1A	9, S	0	20010401	20040101	
C1779	1833(T)						D1A	9, S	0	20010401	20040101	
C1780	1833(T)						D1A	9, S	0	20010401	20040101	

C Codes

HCPCS Code	Long Description	Coverage	Action	PI	MPI	CIM	MCM
C1781	MESH (IMPLANTABLE)	D	N	53	A		
C1782	MORCELLATOR	D	N	53	A		
C1783	OCULAR IMPLANT, AQUEOUS DRAINAGE ASSIST DEVICE	D	N	53	A		
C1784	OCULAR DEVICE, INTRAOPERATIVE, DETACHED RETINA	D	N	53	A		
C1785	PACEMAKER, DUAL CHAMBER, RATE-RESPONSIVE (IMPLANTABLE)	D	N	53	A		
C1786	PACEMAKER, SINGLE CHAMBER, RATE-RESPONSIVE (IMPLANTABLE)	D	N	53	A		
C1787	PATIENT PROGRAMMER, NEUROSTIMULATOR	D	N	53	A		
C1788	PORT, INDWELLING (IMPLANTABLE)	D	N	53	A		
C1789	PROSTHESIS, BREAST (IMPLANTABLE)	D	N	53	A		
C1813	PROSTHESIS, PENILE, INFLATABLE	D	N	53	A		
C1814	RETINAL TAMPONADE DEVICE, SILICONE OIL	D	N	53	A		
C1815	PROSTHESIS, URINARY SPHINCTER (IMPLANTABLE)	D	N	53	A		
C1816	RECEIVER AND/OR TRANSMITTER, NEUROSTIMULATOR (IMPLANTABLE)	D	N	53	A		
C1817	SEPTAL DEFECT IMPLANT SYSTEM, INTRACARDIAC	D	N	53	A		
C1818	INTEGRATED KERATOPROSTHESIS	D	N	53	A		
C1819	SURGICAL TISSUE LOCALIZATION AND EXCISION DEVICE (IMPLANTABLE)	D	N	53	A		
C1820	GENERATOR, NEUROSTIMULATOR (IMPLANTABLE), WITH RECHARGEABLE BATTERY AND CHARGING SYSTEM	D	N	53	A		
C1821	INTERSPINOUS PROCESS DISTRACTION DEVICE (IMPLANTABLE)	D	N	53	A		
C1874	STENT, COATED/COVERED, WITH DELIVERY SYSTEM	D	N	53	A		
C1875	STENT, COATED/COVERED, WITHOUT DELIVERY SYSTEM	D	N	53	A		
C1876	STENT, NON-COATED/NON-COVERED, WITH DELIVERY SYSTEM	D	N	53	A		
C1877	STENT, NON-COATED/NON-COVERED, WITHOUT DELIVERY SYSTEM	D	N	53	A		
C1878	MATERIAL FOR VOCAL CORD MEDIALIZATION, SYNTHETIC (IMPLANTABLE)	D	N	53	A		
C1879	TISSUE MARKER (IMPLANTABLE)	D	N	53	A		
C1880	VENA CAVA FILTER	D	N	53	A		
C1881	DIALYSIS ACCESS SYSTEM (IMPLANTABLE)	D	N	53	A		
C1882	CARDIOVERTER-DEFIBRILLATOR, OTHER THAN SINGLE OR DUAL CHAMBER (IMPLANTABLE)	D	N	53	A		
C1883	ADAPTOR/EXTENSION, PACING LEAD OR NEUROSTIMULATOR LEAD (IMPLANTABLE)	D	N	53	A		
C1884	EMBOLIZATION PROTECTIVE SYSTEM	D	N	53	A		
C1885	CATHETER, TRANSLUMINAL ANGIOPLASTY, LASER	D	N	53	A		
C1887	CATHETER, GUIDING (MAY INCLUDE INFUSION/PERFUSION CAPABILITY)	D	N	53	A		
C1888	CATHETER, ABLATION, NON-CARDIAC, ENDOVASCULAR (IMPLANTABLE)	D	N	53	A		
C1891	INFUSION PUMP, NON-PROGRAMMABLE, PERMANENT (IMPLANTABLE)	D	N	53	A		
C1892	INTRODUCER/SHEATH, GUIDING, INTRACARDIAC ELECTROPHYSIOLOGICAL, FIXED-CURVE, PEEL-AWAY	D	N	53	A		

HCPCS Code	Statute	Lab Cert	X-Ref	ASC Pay Grp	ASC Pay Group Eff. Date	Proc Notes	BETOS	TOS	Anest	Code Add Date	Code Effective Date	Code Term Date
C1781	1833(T)						D1A	9, S	0	20010401	20040101	
C1782	1833(T)						D1A	9, S	0	20010401	20040101	
C1783	1833(T)						D1A	9, S	0	20020701	20020701	
C1784	1833(T)						D1A	9, S	0	20010401	20040101	
C1785	1833(T)						D1A	9, S	0	20010401	20040101	
C1786	1833(T)						D1A	9, S	0	20010401	20040101	
C1787	1833(T)						D1A	9, S	0	20010401	20040101	
C1788	1833(T)						D1A	9, S	0	20010401	20040101	
C1789	1833(T)						D1A	9, S	0	20010401	20040101	
C1813	1833(T)						D1A	9, S	0	20010401	20040101	
C1814	1833t						D1A	9, S	0	20030401	20030401	
C1815	1833(T)						D1A	9, S	0	20010401	20040101	
C1816	1833(T)						D1A	9, S	0	20010401	20040101	
C1817	1833(T)						D1A	9, S	0	20010401	20040101	
C1818	1833T						D1A	9, S	0	20030701	20030701	
C1819	1833T					0093	D1A	9, S	0	20040101	20040101	
C1820	1833(T)						D1A	9	0	20060101	20060101	
C1821	1833(T)						D1A	9	0	20070101	20070101	
C1874	1833(T)						D1A	9, S	0	20010401	20040101	
C1875	1833(T)						D1A	9, S	0	20010401	20040101	
C1876	1833(T)						D1A	9, S	0	20010401	20040101	
C1877	1833(T)						D1A	9, S	0	20010401	20040101	
C1878	1833(T)						D1A	9, S	0	20010401	20040101	
C1879	1833(T)						D1A	9, S	0	20010401	20040101	
C1880	1833(T)						D1A	9, S	0	20010401	20040101	
C1881	1833(T)						D1A	9, S	0	20010401	20040101	
C1882	1833(T)						D1A	9, S	0	20010401	20040101	
C1883	1833(T)						D1A	9, S	0	20010401	20040101	
C1884	1833T						D1A	9, S	0	20030101	20030101	
C1885	1833(T)						D1A	9, S	0	20010401	20040101	
C1887	1833(T)						D1A	9, S	0	20010401	20040101	
C1888	1833(T)						D1A	9, S	0	20020701	20020701	
C1891	1833(T)						D1A	9, S	0	20010401	20040101	
C1892	1833(T)						D1A	9, S	0	20010401	20040101	

C Codes

HCPCS Code	Long Description	Coverage	Action	PI	MPI	CIM	MCM
C1893	INTRODUCER/SHEATH, GUIDING, INTRACARDIAC ELECTROPHYSIOLOGICAL, FIXED-CURVE, OTHER THAN PEEL-AWAY	D	N	53	A		
C1894	INTRODUCER/SHEATH, OTHER THAN GUIDING, OTHER THAN INTRACARDIAC ELECTROPHYSIOLOGICAL, NON-LASER	D	N	53	A		
C1895	LEAD, CARDIOVERTER-DEFIBRILLATOR, ENDOCARDIAL DUAL COIL (IMPLANTABLE)	D	N	53	A		
C1896	LEAD, CARDIOVERTER-DEFIBRILLATOR, OTHER THAN ENDOCARDIAL SINGLE OR DUAL COIL (IMPLANTABLE)	D	N	53	A		
C1897	LEAD, NEUROSTIMULATOR TEST KIT (IMPLANTABLE)	D	N	53	A		
C1898	LEAD, PACEMAKER, OTHER THAN TRANSVENOUS VDD SINGLE PASS	D	N	53	A		
C1899	LEAD, PACEMAKER/CARDIOVERTER-DEFIBRILLATOR COMBINATION (IMPLANTABLE)	D	N	53	A		
C1900	LEAD, LEFT VENTRICULAR CORONARY VENOUS SYSTEM	D	N	53	A		
C2614	PROBE, PERCUTANEOUS LUMBAR DISCECTOMY	D	N	53	A		
C2615	SEALANT, PULMONARY, LIQUID	D	N	53	A		
C2616	BRACHYTHERAPY SOURCE, NON-STRANDED, YTTRIUM-90, PER SOURCE	D	N	53	A		
C2617	STENT, NON-CORONARY, TEMPORARY, WITHOUT DELIVERY SYSTEM	D	N	53	A		
C2618	PROBE, CRYOABLATION	D	N	53	A		
C2619	PACEMAKER, DUAL CHAMBER, NON RATE-RESPONSIVE (IMPLANTABLE)	D	N	53	A		
C2620	PACEMAKER, SINGLE CHAMBER, NON RATE-RESPONSIVE (IMPLANTABLE)	D	N	53	A		
C2621	PACEMAKER, OTHER THAN SINGLE OR DUAL CHAMBER (IMPLANTABLE)	D	N	53	A		
C2622	PROSTHESIS, PENILE, NON-INFLATABLE	D	N	53	A		
C2625	STENT, NON-CORONARY, TEMPORARY, WITH DELIVERY SYSTEM	D	N	53	A		
C2626	INFUSION PUMP, NON-PROGRAMMABLE, TEMPORARY (IMPLANTABLE)	D	N	53	A		
C2627	CATHETER, SUPRAPUBIC/CYSTOSCOPIC	D	N	53	A		
C2628	CATHETER, OCCLUSION	D	N	53	A		
C2629	INTRODUCER/SHEATH, OTHER THAN GUIDING, INTRACARDIAC ELECTROPHYSIOLOGICAL, LASER	D	N	53	A		
C2630	CATHETER, ELECTROPHYSIOLOGY, DIAGNOSTIC/ABLATION, OTHER THAN 3D OR VECTOR MAPPING, COOL-TIP	D	N	53	A		
C2631	REPAIR DEVICE, URINARY, INCONTINENCE, WITHOUT SLING GRAFT	D	N	53	A		
C2632	BRACHYTHERAPY SOLUTION, IODINE-125, PER MCI	D	N	53	A		
C2633	BRACHYTHERAPY SOURCE, CESIUM-131, PER SOURCE	D	N	53	A		
C2634	BRACHYTHERAPY SOURCE, NON-STRANDED, HIGH ACTIVITY, IODINE-125, GREATER THAN 1.01 MCI (NIST), PER SOURCE	D	N	53	A		
C2635	BRACHYTHERAPY SOURCE, NON-STRANDED, HIGH ACTIVITY, PALADIUM-103, GREATER THAN 2.2 MCI (NIST), PER SOURCE	D	N	53	A		
C2636	BRACHYTHERAPY LINEAR SOURCE, NON-STRANDED, PALADIUM-103, PER 1 MM	D	N	53	A		

HCPCS Code	Statute	Lab Cert	X-Ref	ASC Pay Grp	ASC Pay Group Eff. Date	Proc Notes	BETOS	TOS	Anest	Code Add Date	Code Effective Date	Code Term Date
C1893	1833(T)						D1A	9, S	0	20010401	20040101	
C1893												
C1894	1833(T)						D1A	9, S	0	20010401	20020701	
C1895	1833(T)						D1A	9, S	0	20010401	20040101	
C1896	1833(T)						D1A	9, S	0	20010401	20040101	
C1897	1833(T)						D1A	9, S	0	20010401	20040101	
C1898	1833(T)						D1A	9, S	0	20010401	20040101	
C1899	1833(T)						D1A	9, S	0	20010401	20040101	
C1900	1833(T)						D1A	9, S	0	20020701	20020701	
C2614	1833(T)					0093	D1A	9, S	0	20030101	20030101	
C2615	1833(T)						D1A	9, S	0	20010401	20040101	
C2616	1833(T)			YY	20080101		I4B	6	0	20010401	20010401	
C2617	1833(T)						D1A	9, S	0	20010401	20040101	
C2618	1833(T)						D1A	9, S	0	20010401	20010401	
C2619	1833(T)						D1A	9, S	0	20010401	20040101	
C2620	1833(T)						D1A	9, S	0	20010401	20010401	
C2621	1833(T)						D1A	9, S	0	20010401	20040101	
C2622	1833(T)						D1A	9, S	0	20010401	20040101	
C2625	1833(T)						D1A	9, S	0	20010401	20040101	
C2626	1833(T)						D1A	9, S	0	20010401	20040101	
C2627	1833(T)						D1A	9, S	0	20010401	20040101	
C2628	1833(T)						D1A	9, S	0	20010401	20040101	
C2629	1833(T)						D1A	9, S	0	20010401	20040101	
C2630	1833(T)						D1A	9, S	0	20010401	20040101	
C2631	1833(T)						D1A	9, S	0	20010401	20040101	
C2632	1833(T)		A9527			0093	D1A	9	0	20030101	20070101	20061231
C2633	1833T		C2643			0093	D1A	9, S	0	20040101	20070701	20070630
C2634	1833(T)			YY	20080101		I4B	9	0	20050101	20070701	
C2635	1833(T)			YY	20080101		I4B	9	0	20050101	20070701	
C2636	1833(T)			YY	20080101		I4B	9	0	20050101	20070701	

HCPCS Code	Long Description	Coverage	Action	PI	MPI	CIM	MCM
C2637	BRACHYTHERAPY SOURCE, NON-STRANDED, YTTERBIUM-169, PER SOURCE	D	N	53	A		
C2638	BRACHYTHERAPY SOURCE, STRANDED, IODINE-125, PER SOURCE	D	N	53	A		
C2639	BRACHYTHERAPY SOURCE, NON-STRANDED, IODINE-125, PER SOURCE	D	N	53	A		
C2640	BRACHYTHERAPY SOURCE, STRANDED, PALLADIUM-103, PER SOURCE	D	N	53	A		
C2641	BRACHYTHERAPY SOURCE, NON-STRANDED, PALLADIUM-103, PER SOURCE	D	N	53	A		
C2642	BRACHYTHERAPY SOURCE, STRANDED, CESIUM-131, PER SOURCE	D	N	53	A		
C2643	BRACHYTHERAPY SOURCE, NON-STRANDED, CESIUM-131, PER SOURCE	D	N	53	A		
C2698	BRACHYTHERAPY SOURCE, STRANDED, NOT OTHERWISE SPECIFIED, PER SOURCE	D	N	53	A		
C2699	BRACHYTHERAPY SOURCE, NON-STRANDED, NOT OTHERWISE SPECIFIED, PER SOURCE	D	N	53	A		
C8900	MAGNETIC RESONANCE ANGIOGRAPHY WITH CONTRAST, ABDOMEN	D	N	53	A		
C8901	MAGNETIC RESONANCE ANGIOGRAPHY WITHOUT CONTRAST, ABDOMEN	D	N	53	A		
C8902	MAGNETIC RESONANCE ANGIOGRAPHY WITHOUT CONTRAST FOLLOWED BY WITH CONTRAST, ABDOMEN	D	N	53	A		
C8903	MAGNETIC RESONANCE IMAGING WITH CONTRAST, BREAST; UNILATERAL	D	N	53	A		
C8904	MAGNETIC RESONANCE IMAGING WITHOUT CONTRAST, BREAST; UNILATERAL	D	N	53	A		
C8905	MAGNETIC RESONANCE IMAGING WITHOUT CONTRAST FOLLOWED BY WITH CONTRAST, BREAST; UNILATERAL	D	N	53	A		
C8906	MAGNETIC RESONANCE IMAGING WITH CONTRAST, BREAST; BILATERAL	D	N	53	A		
C8907	MAGNETIC RESONANCE IMAGING WITHOUT CONTRAST, BREAST; BILATERAL	D	N	53	A		
C8908	MAGNETIC RESONANCE IMAGING WITHOUT CONTRAST FOLLOWED BY WITH CONTRAST, BREAST; BILATERAL	D	N	53	A		
C8909	MAGNETIC RESONANCE ANGIOGRAPHY WITH CONTRAST, CHEST (EXCLUDING MYOCARDIUM)	D	N	53	A		
C8910	MAGNETIC RESONANCE ANGIOGRAPHY WITHOUT CONTRAST, CHEST (EXCLUDING MYOCARDIUM)	D	N	53	A		
C8911	MAGNETIC RESONANCE ANGIOGRAPHY WITHOUT CONTRAST FOLLOWED BY WITH CONTRAST, CHEST (EXCLUDING MYOCARDIUM)	D	N	53	A		
C8912	MAGNETIC RESONANCE ANGIOGRAPHY WITH CONTRAST, LOWER EXTREMITY	D	N	53	A		
C8913	MAGNETIC RESONANCE ANGIOGRAPHY WITHOUT CONTRAST, LOWER EXTREMITY	D	N	53	A		
C8914	MAGNETIC RESONANCE ANGIOGRAPHY WITHOUT CONTRAST, FOLLOWED BY WITH CONTRAST LOWER EXTREMITY	D	N	53	A		

HCPCS Code	Statute	Lab Cert	X-Ref	ASC Pay Grp	ASC Pay Group Eff. Date	Proc Notes	BETOS	TOS	Anest	Code Add Date	Code Effective Date	Code Term Date
C2637	1833(T)						I4B	4	0	20051001	20070701	
C2638	1833(t)(2)			YY	20080101		I4B	6	0	20070701	20070701	
C2639	1833(t)(2)			YY	20080101		I4B	4	0	20070701	20070701	
C2640	1833(t)(2)			YY	20080101		I4B	4	0	20070701	20070701	
C2641	1833(t)(2)			YY	20080101		I4B	4	0	20070701	20070701	
C2642	1833(t)(2)			YY	20080101		I4B	4	0	20070701	20070701	
C2643	1833(t)(2)			YY	20080101		I4B	4	0	20070701	20070701	
C2698	1833(t)(2)			YY	20080101		I4B	4	0	20070701	20070701	
C2699	1833(t)(2)			YY	20080101		I4B	4	0	20070701	20070701	
C8900	1833(t)(2)			YY	20080101		I2D	4	0	20011001	20011001	
C8901	1833(t)(2)			YY	20080101		I2D	4	0	20011001	20011001	
C8902	1833(t)(2)			YY	20080101		I2D	4	0	20011001	20011001	
C8903	1833(t)(2)			YY	20080101		I2D	4	0	20011001	20011001	
C8904	1833(t)(2)			YY	20080101		I2D	4	0	20011001	20011001	
C8905	1833(t)(2)			YY	20080101		I2D	4	0	20011001	20011001	
C8906	1833(t)(2)			YY	20080101		I2D	4	0	20011001	20011001	
C8907	1833(t)(2)			YY	20080101		I2D	4	0	20011001	20011001	
C8908	1833(t)(2)			YY	20080101		I2D	4	0	20011001	20011001	
C8909	1833(t)(2)			YY	20080101		I2D	4	0	20011001	20011001	
C8910	1833(t)(2)			YY	20080101		I2D	4	0	20011001	20011001	
C8911	1833(t)(2)			YY	20080101		I2D	4	0	20011001	20011001	
C8912	1833(t)(2)			YY	20080101		I2D	4	0	20011001	20011001	
C8913	1833(t)(2)			YY	20080101		I2D	4	0	20011001	20011001	
C8914	1833(t)(2)			YY	20080101		I2D	4	0	20011001	20011001	

HCPCS Code	Long Description	Coverage	Action	PI	MPI	CIM	MCM
C8918	MAGNETIC RESONANCE ANGIOGRAPHY WITH CONTRAST, PELVIS	D	N	53	A		
C8919	MAGNETIC RESONANCE ANGIOGRAPHY WITHOUT CONTRAST, PELVIS	D	N	53	A		
C8920	MAGNETIC RESONANCE ANGIOGRAPHY WITHOUT CONTRAST FOLLOWED BY WITH CONTRAST, PELVIS	D	N	53	A		
C8921	TRANSTHORACIC ECHOCARDIOGRAPHY WITH CONTRAST, OR WITHOUT CONTRAST FOLLOWED BY WITH CONTRAST, FOR CONGENITAL CARDIAC ANOMALIES; COMPLETE	D	N	53	A		
C8922	TRANSTHORACIC ECHOCARDIOGRAPHY WITH CONTRAST, OR WITHOUT CONTRAST FOLLOWED BY WITH CONTRAST, FOR CONGENITAL CARDIAC ANOMALIES; FOLLOW-UP OR LIMITED STUDY	D	N	53	A		
C8923	TRANSTHORACIC ECHOCARDIOGRAPHY WITH CONTRAST, OR WITHOUT CONTRAST FOLLOWED BY WITH CONTRAST, REAL-TIME WITH IMAGE DOCUMENTATION (2D) WITH OR WITHOUT M-MODE RECORDING; COMPLETE	D	N	53	A		
C8924	TRANSTHORACIC ECHOCARDIOGRAPHY WITH CONTRAST, OR WITHOUT CONTRAST FOLLOWED BY WITH CONTRAST, REAL-TIME WITH IMAGE DOCUMENTATION (2D) WITH OR WITHOUT M-MODE RECORDING; FOLLOW-UP OR LIMITED STUDY	D	N	53	A		
C8925	TRANSESOPHAGEAL ECHOCARDIOGRAPHY (TEE) WITH CONTRAST, OR WITHOUT CONTRAST FOLLOWED BY WITH CONTRAST, REAL TIME WITH IMAGE DOCUMENTATION (2D) (WITH OR WITHOUT M-MODE RECORDING); INCLUDING PROBE PLACEMENT, IMAGE ACQUISITION, INTERPRETATION AND REPORT	D	N	53	A		
C8926	TRANSESOPHAGEAL ECHOCARDIOGRAPHY (TEE) WITH CONTRAST, OR WITHOUT CONTRAST FOLLOWED BY WITH CONTRAST, FOR CONGENITAL CARDIAC ANOMALIES; INCLUDING PROBE PLACEMENT, IMAGE ACQUISITION, INTERPRETATION AND REPORT	D	N	53	A		
C8927	TRANSESOPHAGEAL ECHOCARDIOGRAPHY (TEE) WITH CONTRAST, OR WITHOUT CONTRAST FOLLOWED BY WITH CONTRAST, FOR MONITORING PURPOSES, INCLUDING PROBE PLACEMENT, REAL TIME 2-DIMENSIONAL IMAGE ACQUISITION AND INTERPRETATION LEADING TO ONGOING (CONTINUOUS) ASSESSMENT OF (DYNAMICALLY CHANGING) CARDIAC PUMPING FUNCTION AND TO THERAPEUTIC MEASURES ON AN IMMEDIATE TIME BASIS	D	N	53	A		
C8928	TRANSTHORACIC ECHOCARDIOGRAPHY WITH CONTRAST, OR WITHOUT CONTRAST FOLLOWED BY WITH CONTRAST, REAL-TIME WITH IMAGE DOCUMENTATION (2D), WITH OR WITHOUT M-MODE RECORDING, DURING REST AND CARDIOVASCULAR STRESS TEST USING TREADMILL, BICYCLE EXERCISE AND/OR PHARMACOLOGICALLY INDUCED STRESS, WITH INTERPRETATION AND REPORT	D	N	53	A		

HCPCS Code	Statute	Lab Cert	X-Ref	ASC Pay Grp	ASC Pay Group Eff. Date	Proc Notes	BETOS	TOS	Anest	Code Add Date	Code Effective Date	Code Term Date
C8918	430 BIPA			YY	20080101		I2D	4	0	20030701	20030701	
C8919	430 BIPA			YY	20080101		I2D	4	0	20030701	20030701	
C8920	430 BIPA			YY	20080101		I2D	4	0	20030701	20030701	
C8921	1833(t)(2)						I3C	4	0	20080101	20080101	
C8922	1833(t)(2)						I3C	4	0	20080101	20090101	
C8923	1833(t)(2)						I3C	4	0	20080101	20080101	
C8924	1833(t)(2)						I3C	4	0	20080101	20080101	
C8925	1833(t)(2)						I3C	4	0	20080101	20080101	
C8926	1833(t)(2)						I3C	4	0	20080101	20080101	
C8927	1833(t)(2)						I3C	4	0	20080101	20080101	
C8928	1833(t)(2)						I3C	4	0	20080101	20080101	

HCPCS Code	Long Description	Coverage	Action	PI	MPI	CIM	MCM
C8929	TRANSTHORACIC ECHOCARDIOGRAPHY WITH CONTRAST, OR WITHOUT CONTRAST FOLLOWED BY WITH CONTRAST, REAL-TIME WITH IMAGE DOCUMENTATION (2D), INCLUDES M-MODE RECORDING, WHEN PERFORMED, COMPLETE, WITH SPECTRAL DOPPLER ECHOCARDIOGRAPHY, AND WITH COLOR FLOW DOPPLER ECHOCARDIOGRAPHY	D	N	53	A		
C8930	TRANSTHORACIC ECHOCARDIOGRAPHY, WITH CONTRAST, OR WITHOUT CONTRAST FOLLOWED BY WITH CONTRAST, REAL-TIME WITH IMAGE DOCUMENTATION (2D), INCLUDES M-MODE RECORDING, WHEN PERFORMED, DURING REST AND CARDIOVASCULAR STRESS TEST USING TREADMILL, BICYCLE EXERCISE AND/OR PHARMACOLOGICALLY INDUCED STRESS, WITH INTERPRETATION AND REPORT; INCLUDING PERFORMANCE OF CONTINUOUS ELECTROCARDIOGRAPHIC MONITORING, WITH PHYSICIAN SUPERVISION	D	N	53	A		
C8950	INTRAVENOUS INFUSION FOR THERAPY/DIAGNOSIS; UP TO 1 HOUR	D	N	99	9		
C8951	INTRAVENOUS INFUSION FOR THERAPY/DIAGNOSIS; EACH ADDITIONAL HOUR (LIST SEPARATELY IN ADDITION TO C8950)	D	N	99	9		
C8952	THERAPEUTIC, PROPHYLACTIC OR DIAGNOSTIC INJECTION; INTRAVENOUS PUSH OF EACH NEW SUBSTANCE/DRUG	D	N	99	9		
C8953	CHEMOTHERAPY ADMINISTRATION, INTRAVENOUS; PUSH TECHNIQUE	D	N	99	9		
C8954	CHEMOTHERAPY ADMINISTRATION, INTRAVENOUS; INFUSION TECHNIQUE, UP TO ONE HOUR	D	N	99	9		
C8955	CHEMOTHERAPY ADMINISTRATION, INTRAVENOUS; INFUSION TECHNIQUE, EACH ADDITIONAL HOUR (LIST SEPARATELY IN ADDITION TO C8954)	D	N	99	9		
C8957	INTRAVENOUS INFUSION FOR THERAPY/DIAGNOSIS; INITIATION OF PROLONGED INFUSION (MORE THAN 8 HOURS), REQUIRING USE OF PORTABLE OR IMPLANTABLE PUMP	D	N	99	9		
C9003	PALIVIZUMAB-RSV-IGM, PER 50 MG	D	N	53	A		
C9113	INJECTION, PANTOPRAZOLE SODIUM, PER VIAL	D	N	53	A		
C9121	INJECTION, ARGATROBAN, PER 5 MG	D	N	53	A		
C9220	SODIUM HYALURONATE PER 30 MG DOSE, FOR INTRA-ARTICULAR INJECTION	D	N	53	A		
C9221	ACELLULAR DERMAL TISSUE MATRIX, PER 16CM2	D	N	53	A		
C9222	DECELLULARIZED SOFT TISSUE SCAFFOLD, PER 1 CC	D	N	53	A		
C9224	INJECTION, GALSULFASE, PER 5 MG	D	N	51	A		
C9225	INJECTION, FLUOCINOLONE ACETONIDE INTRAVITREAL IMPLANT, PER 0.59 MG	D	N	53	A		
C9227	INJECTION, MICAFUNGIN SODIUM, PER 1 MG	D	N	53	A		
C9228	INJECTION, TIGECYCLINE, PER 1 MG	D	N	53	A		
C9229	INJECTION, IBANDRONATE SODIUM, PER 1 MG	D	N	53	A		
C9230	INJECTION, ABATACEPT, PER 10 MG	D	N	53	A		
C9231	INJECTION, DECITABINE, PER 1 MG	D	N	53	A		
C9232	INJECTION, IDURSULFASE, 1 MG	D	N	53	A		
C9233	INJECTION, RANIBIZUMAB, 0.5 MG	D	N	53	A		
C9234	INJECTION, ALGLUCOSIDASE ALFA, 10 MG	D	N	53	A		

HCPCS Code	Statute	Lab Cert	X-Ref	ASC Pay Grp	ASC Pay Group Eff. Date	Proc Notes	BETOS	TOS	Anest	Code Add Date	Code Effective Date	Code Term Date
C8929	1833(t)(2)						I3C	4	0	20090101	20090101	
C8930	1833(t)(2)						I3C	4	0	20090101	20090101	
C8950	1833(T)						P6D	1	0	20060101	20070101	20061231
C8951	1833(t)						P6D	1	0	20060101	20070101	20061231
C8951												
C8952	1883(t)						P6D	1	0	20060101	20070101	20061231
C8953	1833(t)						P7B	1	0	20060101	20070101	20061231
C8954	1833(t)						P7B	1	0	20060101	20070101	20061231
C8955	1833(t)						P7B	1	0	20060101	20070101	20061231
C8957	1833(t)						P6D	1	0	20060101	20060101	
C9003	1833(t)		90378			0093	O1E	1	0	20001001	20090101	20081231
C9113	1833(T)						O1E	9	0	20020101	20020101	
C9121	1833(T)			YY	20080101	0093	O1E	1, P	0	20030101	20030101	
C9220	1833(t)						O1E	9	0	20050101	20070101	20061231
C9221	1833(t)		J7344				D1A	9	0	20050101	20070101	20061231
C9222	1833(t)		J7346				D1A	9	0	20050101	20070101	20061231
C9224	621MMA		J1458				O1E	9	0	20050531	20070101	20061231
C9225	621MMA		J7311				O1E	9	0	20051001	20070101	20061231
C9227	621MMA		J2248				O1E	9	0	20060401	20070101	20061231
C9228	621MMA		J3243				O1E	9	0	20060401	20070101	20061231
C9229	621MMA		J1740				O1E	9	0	20060701	20070101	20061231
C9230	621MMA		J0129				O1E	9	0	20060701	20070101	20061231
C9231	621MMA		J0894				O1E	9	0	20061001	20070101	20061231
C9232	621MMA		J1743				O1E	9	0	20070101	20080101	20071231
C9233	621MMA		J2778				O1E	9	0	20070101	20080101	20071231
C9234	621MMA		J0220				O1E	9	0	20070101	20080101	20071231

HCPCS Code	Long Description	Coverage	Action	PI	MPI	CIM	MCM
C9235	INJECTION, PANITUMUMAB, 10 MG	D	N	53	A		
C9236	INJECTION, ECULIZUMAB, 10 MG	D	N	53	A		
C9237	INJECTION, LANREOTIDE ACETATE, 1 MG	D	N	53	A		
C9238	INJECTION, LEVETIRACETAM, 10 MG	D	N	53	A		
C9239	INJECTION, TEMSIROLIMUS, 1 MG	D	N	53	A		
C9240	INJECTION, IXABEPILONE, 1 MG	D	N	53	A		
C9241	INJECTION, DORIPENEM, 10 MG	D	N	53	A		
C9242	INJECTION, FOSAPREPITANT, 1 MG	D	N	53	A		
C9243	INJECTION, BENDAMUSTINE HCL, 1 MG	D	N	53	A		
C9244	INJECTION, REGADENOSON, 0.4 MG	D	N	53	A		
C9245	INJECTION, ROMIPLOSTIM, 10 MCG	D	D	53	A		
C9246	INJECTION, GADOXETATE DISODIUM, PER ML	D	D	53	A		
C9247	IOBENGUANE, I-123, DIAGNOSTIC, PER STUDY DOSE, UP TO 10 MILLICURIES	D	D	53	A		
C9248	INJECTION, CLEVIDIPINE BUTYRATE, 1 MG	D	C	53	A		
C9249	INJECTION, CERTOLIZUMAB PEGOL, 1 MG	D	D	53	A		
C9250	HUMAN PLASMA FIBRIN SEALANT, VAPOR-HEATED, SOLVENT-DETERGENT (ARTISS), 2ML	D	A	53	A		
C9251	INJECTION, C1 ESTERASE INHIBITOR (HUMAN), 10 UNITS	D	D	53	A		
C9252	INJECTION, PLERIXAFOR, 1 MG	D	D	53	A		
C9253	INJECTION, TEMOZOLOMIDE, 1 MG	D	D	53	A		
C9254	INJECTION, LACOSAMIDE, 1 MG	D	A	53	A		
C9255	INJECTION, PALIPERIDONE PALMITATE, 1 MG	D	A	53	A		
C9256	INJECTION, DEXAMETHASONE INTRAVITREAL IMPLANT, 0.1 MG	D	A	53	A		
C9257	INJECTION, BEVACIZUMAB, 0.25 MG	D	A	53	A		
C9350	MICROPOROUS COLLAGEN TUBE OF NON-HUMAN ORIGIN, PER CENTIMETER LENGTH	D	N	53	A		
C9351	ACELLULAR DERMAL TISSUE MATRIX OF NON-HUMAN ORIGIN, PER SQUARE CENTIMETER (DO NOT REPORT C9351 IN CONJUNCTION WITH J7345)	D	N	53	A		
C9352	MICROPOROUS COLLAGEN IMPLANTABLE TUBE (NEURAGEN NERVE GUIDE), PER CENTIMETER LENGTH	D	N	53	A		
C9353	MICROPOROUS COLLAGEN IMPLANTABLE SLIT TUBE (NEURAWRAP NERVE PROTECTOR), PER CENTIMETER LENGTH	D	N	53	A		
C9354	ACELLULAR PERICARDIAL TISSUE MATRIX OF NON-HUMAN ORIGIN (VERITAS), PER SQUARE CENTIMETER	D	N	53	A		
C9355	COLLAGEN NERVE CUFF (NEUROMATRIX), PER 0.5 CENTIMETER LENGTH	D	N	53	A		
C9356	TENDON, POROUS MATRIX OF CROSS-LINKED COLLAGEN AND GLYCOSAMINOGLYCAN MATRIX (TENOGLIDE TENDON PROTECTOR SHEET), PER SQUARE CENTIMETER	D	N	53	A		
C9357	DERMAL SUBSTITUTE, GRANULATED CROSS-LINKED COLLAGEN AND GLYCOSAMINOGLYCAN MATRIX (FLOWABLE WOUND MATRIX), 1 CC	D	N	53	A		
C9358	DERMAL SUBSTITUTE, NATIVE, NON-DENATURED COLLAGEN, FETAL BOVINE ORIGIN (SURGIMEND COLLAGEN MATRIX), PER 0.5 SQUARE CENTIMETERS	D	C	53	A		

HCPCS Code	Statute	Lab Cert	X-Ref	ASC Pay Grp	ASC Pay Group Eff. Date	Proc Notes	BETOS	TOS	Anest	Code Add Date	Code Effective Date	Code Term Date
C9235	621MMA		J9303				O1D	9	0	20070101	20080101	20071231
C9236	621MMA		J1300				O1E	1, P	0	20071001	20080101	20071231
C9237	621MMA		J1930				O1E	1	0	20080101	20090101	20081231
C9238	621MMA		J1953				O1E	1, P	0	20080101	20090101	20081231
C9239	621MMA		J9330				O1D	1, P	0	20080101	20090101	20081231
C9240	621MMA		J9207				O1D	9	0	20080101	20090101	20081231
C9241	621MMA		J1267				O1E	1, P	0	20080401	20090101	20081231
C9242	621 MMA		J1453				O1E	1, P	0	20080701	20090101	20081231
C9243	1833(T)		J9033				O1D	9	0	20081001	20090101	20081231
C9244	1833(T)		J2785				O1E	9	0	20081001	20090101	20081231
C9245	1833(t)		J2796				O1E	1	0	20090101	20100101	20091231
C9246	1833(t)		A9581				O1E	1	0	20090101	20100101	20091231
C9247	1833(t)		A9582				O1E	1	0	20090101	20100101	20091231
C9248	1833(t)			YY	20090101		O1E	1	0	20090101	20090101	
C9249	621MMA		J0718				O1E	1	0	20090401	20100101	20091231
C9250	621MMA			YY	20090701		O1E	9	0	20090701	20090701	
C9251	621MMA		J0598				O1E	9	0	20090701	20100101	20091231
C9252	621MMA		J2562				O1E	9	0	20090701	20100101	20091231
C9253	621MMA		J9328				O1D	9	0	20090701	20100101	20091231
C9254	621MMA			YY	20100101		O1E	9	0	20100101	20100101	
C9255	621MMA			YY	20100101		O1E	9	0	20100101	20100101	
C9256	621MMA			YY	20100101		O1E	9	0	20100101	20100101	
C9257	1833(t)			YY	20100101		O1E	9	0	20100101	20100101	
C9350	621MMA						D1A	9	0	20070101	20080101	20071231
C9351	621MMA		J7348, J7349				D1A	9	0	20070101	20080101	20071231
C9352	621MMA						D1A	9	0	20080101	20080101	
C9352												
C9353	621MMA						D1A	9	0	20080101	20080101	
C9354	621MMA						D1A	9	0	20080101	20080101	
C9355	621MMA						D1A	9	0	20080101	20080101	
C9356	621 MMA			YY	20080701		D1A	9	0	20080701	20080701	
C9356												
C9357	621 MMA		Q4114				D1A	9	0	20080701	20090101	20081231
C9357												
C9358	621 MMA			YY	20080701		D1A	9	0	20080701	20080701	
C9358												

HCPCS Code	Long Description	Coverage	Action	PI	MPI	CIM	MCM
C9359	POROUS PURIFIED COLLAGEN MATRIX BONE VOID FILLER (INTEGRA MOZAIK OSTEOCONDUCTIVE SCAFFOLD PUTTY, INTEGRA OS OSTEOCONDUCTIVE SCAFFOLD PUTTY), PER 0.5 CC	D	S	53	A		
C9360	DERMAL SUBSTITUTE, NATIVE, NON-DENATURED COLLAGEN, NEONATAL BOVINE ORIGIN (SURGIMEND COLLAGEN MATRIX), PER 0.5 SQUARE CENTIMETERS	D	A	53	A		
C9361	COLLAGEN MATRIX NERVE WRAP (NEUROMEND COLLAGEN NERVE WRAP), PER 0.5 CENTIMETER LENGTH	D	A	53	A		
C9362	POROUS PURIFIED COLLAGEN MATRIX BONE VOID FILLER (INTEGRA MOZAIK OSTEOCONDUCTIVE SCAFFOLD STRIP), PER 0.5 CC	D	A	53	A		
C9363	SKIN SUBSTITUTE, INTEGRA MESHED BILAYER WOUND MATRIX, PER SQUARE CENTIMETER	D	A	53	A		
C9364	PORCINE IMPLANT, PERMACOL, PER SQUARE CENTIMETER	D	A	53	A		
C9399	UNCLASSIFIED DRUGS OR BIOLOGICALS	D	N	53	A		
C9716	CREATIONS OF THERMAL ANAL LESIONS BY RADIOFREQUENCY ENERGY	D	F	53	A		
C9723	DYNAMIC INFRARED BLOOD PERFUSION IMAGING (DIRI)	D	N	53	A		
C9724	ENDOSCOPIC FULL-THICKNESS PLICATION IN THE GASTRIC CARDIA USING ENDOSCOPIC PLICATION SYSTEM (EPS); INCLUDES ENDOSCOPY	D	N	53	A		
C9725	PLACEMENT OF ENDORECTAL INTRACAVITARY APPLICATOR FOR HIGH INTENSITY BRACHYTHERAPY	D	N	53	A		
C9726	PLACEMENT AND REMOVAL (IF PERFORMED) OF APPLICATOR INTO BREAST FOR RADIATION THERAPY	D	N	53	A		
C9727	INSERTION OF IMPLANTS INTO THE SOFT PALATE; MINIMUM OF THREE IMPLANTS	D	N	53	A		
C9728	PLACEMENT OF INTERSTITIAL DEVICE(S) FOR RADIATION THERAPY/SURGERY GUIDANCE (EG, FIDUCIAL MARKERS, DOSIMETER), FOR OTHER THAN THE FOLLOWING SITES (ANY APPROACH): ABDOMEN, PELVIS, PROSTATE, RETROPERITONEUM, THORAX, SINGLE OR MULTIPLE	D	C	53	A		
C9898	RADIOLABELED PRODUCT PROVIDED DURING A HOSPITAL INPATIENT STAY	D	N	00	9		
C9899	IMPLANTED PROSTHETIC DEVICE, PAYABLE ONLY FOR INPATIENTS WHO DO NOT HAVE INPATIENT COVERAGE	D	N	53	A		
D0120	PERIODIC ORAL EVALUATION - ESTABLISHED PATIENT	S	N	00	9		
D0140	LIMITED ORAL EVALUATION - PROBLEM FOCUSED	S	N	00	9		
D0145	ORAL EVALUATION FOR A PATIENT UNDER THREE YEARS OF AGE AND COUNSELING WITH PRIMARY CAREGIVER	S	N	00	9		
D0150	COMPREHENSIVE ORAL EVALUATION - NEW OR ESTABLISHED PATIENT	D	N	13	A	50-26	2136, 2336
D0160	DETAILED AND EXTENSIVE ORAL EVALUATION - PROBLEM FOCUSED, BY REPORT	S	N	00	9		
D0170	RE-EVALUATION-LIMITED, PROBLEM FOCUSED (ESTABLISHED PATIENT; NOT POST-OPERATIVE VISIT)	S	N	00	9		
D0180	COMPREHENSIVE PERIODONTAL EVALUATION - NEW OR ESTABLISHED PATIENT	S	N	00	9		
D0210	INTRAORAL-COMPLETE SERIES (INCLUDING BITEWINGS)	I	N	00	9		

HCPCS Code	Statute	Lab Cert	X-Ref	ASC Pay Grp	ASC Pay Group Eff. Date	Proc Notes	BETOS	TOS	Anest	Code Add Date	Code Effective Date	Code Term Date
C9359	1833(T)			YY	20081001		D1A	9	0	20081001	20081001	
C9360	621MMA			YY	20090701		D1A	9	0	20090701	20090701	
C9361	621MMA			YY	20090701		D1A	9	0	20090701	20090701	
C9362	621MMA			YY	20090701		D1A	9	0	20090701	20090701	
C9363	621MMA			YY	20090701		D1A	9	0	20090701	20090701	
C9364	621MMA			YY	20090701		D1A	9	0	20090701	20090701	
C9399	621MMA			YY	20080101		O1E	1	0	20040101	20040101	
C9716	1833(t)			YY	20080101		P6D	2	0	20040701	20040701	
C9723	1833(T)					0093	I4B	4	0	20050401	20090101	20081231
C9724	1833(T)			YY	20080101		P8I	2	0	20050401	20050401	
C9725	1833(T)			YY	20080101		P7A	6	0	20051001	20051001	
C9726	1833(T)			YY	20080101		P7A	6	0	20060101	20060101	
C9727	1833(T)			YY	20080101		P6D	2	0	20061001	20061001	
C9728	1833(T)			YY	20080101		P5E	2	0	20070701	20100101	
C9898	NA						Z2	1	0	20080101	20080101	
C9899	1833(t)						Z2	1	0	20090101	20090101	
D0120	1862A(12)					0059	Y1	1	0	19820101	20070101	
D0140	1862A(12)						Y1	1	0	19960101	19960101	
D0145	1862a(12)						Y1	1	0	20070101	20070101	
D0150							Y1	1	0	19960101	20030101	
D0160	1862A(12)						Y1	1	0	19960101	19960101	
D0170	1862a(12)						Y1	1	0	20000101	20000101	
D0180	1862a(12)						Y1	1	0	20030101	20030101	
D0210			70320				Y1	4	0	19820101	19960101	

HCPCS Code	Long Description	Coverage	Action	PI	MPI	CIM	MCM
D0220	INTRAORAL-PERIAPICAL-FIRST FILM	I	N	00	9		
D0230	INTRAORAL-PERIAPICAL-EACH ADDITIONAL FILM	I	N	00	9		
D0240	INTRAORAL-0CCLUSAL FILM	D	N	13	A		2136, 2336
D0250	EXTRAORAL-FIRST FILM	D	N	13	A		2136, 2336
D0260	EXTRAORAL-EACH ADDITIONAL FILM	D	N	13	A		2136, 2336
D0270	BITEWING-SINGLE FILM	D	N	13	A		2136, 2336
D0272	BITEWINGS-TWO FILMS	D	N	13	A		2136, 2336
D0273	BITEWINGS - THREE FILMS	S	N	00	9		
D0274	BITEWINGS-FOUR FILMS	D	N	13	A		2136, 2336
D0277	VERTICAL BITEWINGS - 7 TO 8 FILMS	D	N	13	A		2136, 2336
D0290	POSTERIOR-ANTERIOR OR LATERAL SKULL AND FACIAL BONE SURVEY FILM	I	N	00	9		
D0310	SIALOGRAPHY	I	N	00	9		
D0320	TEMPOROMANDIBULAR JOINT ARTHROGRAM, INCLUDING INJECTION	I	N	00	9		
D0321	OTHER TEMPOROMANDIBULAR JOINT FILMS, BY REPORT	I	N	00	9		
D0322	TOMOGRAPHIC SURVEY	I	N	00	9	50-26	
D0330	PANORAMIC FILM	I	N	00	9		
D0340	CEPHALOMETRIC FILM	I	N	00	9		
D0350	ORAL/FACIAL PHOTOGRAPHIC IMAGES	I	N	00	9		
D0360	CONE BEAM CT - CRANIOFACIAL DATA CAPTURE	S	N	00	9		
D0362	CONE BEAM - TWO-DIMENSIONAL IMAGE RECONSTRUCTION USING EXISTING DATA, INCLUDES MULTIPLE IMAGES	S	N	00	9		
D0363	CONE BEAM - THREE-DIMENSIONAL IMAGE RECONSTRUCTION USING EXISTING DATA, INCLUDES MULTIPLE IMAGES	S	N	00	9		
D0415	COLLECTION OF MICROORGANISMS FOR CULTURE AND SENSITIVITY	S	N	00	9		
D0416	VIRAL CULTURE	D	F	00	9		
D0417	COLLECTION AND PREPARATION OF SALIVA SAMPLE FOR LABORATORY DIAGNOSTIC TESTING	M	F	00	9		
D0418	ANALYSIS OF SALIVA SAMPLE	M	F	00	9		
D0421	GENETIC TEST FOR SUSCEPTIBILITY TO ORAL DISEASES	D	F	00	9		
D0425	CARIES SUSCEPTIBILITY TESTS	S	N	00	9		
D0431	ADJUNCTIVE PRE-DIAGNOSTIC TEST THAT AIDS IN DETECTION OF MUCOSAL ABNORMALITIES INCLUDING PREMALIGNANT AND MALIGNANT LESIONS, NOT TO INCLUDE CYTOLOGY OR BIOPSY PROCEDURES	D	F	00	9		
D0460	PULP VITALITY TESTS	D	N	13	A	50-26	2136, 2336
D0470	DIAGNOSTIC CASTS	S	N	00	9		
D0472	ACCESSION OF TISSUE, GROSS EXAMINATION, PREPARATION AND TRANSMISSION OF WRITTEN REPORT	D	N	13	A	50-26	2136, 2336
D0473	ACCESSION OF TISSUE, GROSS AND MICROSCOPIC EXAMINATION, PREPARATION AND TRANSMISSION OF WRITTEN REPORT	D	N	13	A	50-26	2136, 2336
D0474	ACCESSION OF TISSUE, GROSS AND MICROSCOPIC EXAMINATION, INCLUDING ASSESSMENT OF SURGICAL MARGINS FOR PRESENCE OF DISEASE, PREPARATION AND TRANSMISSION OF WRITTEN REPORT	D	N	13	A	50-26	2136, 2336
D0475	DECALCIFICATION PROCEDURE	D	F	00	9		

HCPCS Code	Statute	Lab Cert	X-Ref	ASC Pay Grp	ASC Pay Group Eff. Date	Proc Notes	BETOS	TOS	Anest	Code Add Date	Code Effective Date	Code Term Date
D0220			70300				Y1	4	0	19840101	19960101	
D0230			70310				Y1	4	0	19840101	19960101	
D0240							Y1	4	0	19840101	19930101	
D0250							Y1	4	0	19840101	19930101	
D0260							Y1	4	0	19820101	19930101	
D0270							Y1	4	0	19820101	19930101	
D0272							Y1	4	0	19820101	19930101	
D0273	1862a(12)						Y1	4	0	20070101	20070101	
D0274							Y1	4	0	19820101	19930101	
D0277							Y1	4	0	20000101	20000101	
D0290			70150				Y1	4	0	19820101	19960101	
D0310			70390				Y1	4	0	19860101	19960101	
D0320			70332				Y1	4	0	19860101	19960101	
D0321			76499				Y1	4	0	19840101	19960101	
D0322			CPT				Y1	4	0	19920101	19960101	
D0330			70320				Y1	4	0	19840101	19960101	
D0340			70350				Y1	4	0	19820101	19960101	
D0350						0090	Y1	4	0	20000101	20050101	
D0360	1862a(12)						Y1	4	0	20070101	20070101	
D0362	1862a(12)						Y1	4	0	20070101	20070101	
D0363	1862a(12)						Y1	4	0	20070101	20070101	
D0415	1862 A(12)		D0410			0059	Y1	5	0	19920101	20050101	
D0416						0159	Y1	5	0	20050101	20100101	
D0417						0159	Y1	5	0	20090101	20100101	
D0418						0159	Y1	5	0	20090101	20100101	
D0421						0159	Y1	5	0	20050101	20100101	
D0425	1862 A(12)		D0420			0059	Y1	5	0	19920101	19970101	
D0431						0159	Y1	5	0	20050101	20100101	
D0460							Y1	5	0	19820101	19930101	
D0470	1862 a(12)						Y1	5	0	19820101	19960101	
D0472							Y1	5	0	20000101	20000101	
D0472												
D0473							Y1	5	0	20000101	20000101	
D0474							Y1	5	0	20000101	20000101	
D0474												
D0475						0159	Y1	5	0	20050101	20100101	

HCPCS Code	Long Description	Coverage	Action	PI	MPI	CIM	MCM
D0476	SPECIAL STAINS FOR MICROORGANISMS	D	F	00	9		
D0477	SPECIAL STAINS, NOT FOR MICROORGANISMS	D	F	00	9		
D0478	IMMUNOHISTOCHEMICAL STAINS	D	F	00	9		
D0479	TISSUE IN-SITU HYBRIDIZATION, INCLUDING INTERPRETATION	D	F	00	9		
D0480	ACCESSION OF EXFOLIATIVE CYTOLOGIC SMEARS, MICROSCOPIC EXAMINATION, PREPARATION AND TRANSMISSION OF WRITTEN REPORT	D	N	13	A	50-26	2136, 2336
D0481	ELECTRON MICROSCOPY - DIAGNOSTIC	D	F	00	9		
D0482	DIRECT IMMUNOFLUORESCENCE	D	F	00	9		
D0483	INDIRECT IMMUNOFLUORESCENCE	D	F	00	9		
D0484	CONSULTATION ON SLIDES PREPARED ELSEWHERE	D	F	00	9		
D0485	CONSULTATION, INCLUDING PREPARATION OF SLIDES FROM BIOPSY MATERIAL SUPPLIED BY REFERRING SOURCE	D	F	00	9		
D0486	LABORATORY ACCESSION OF BRUSH BIOPSY SAMPLE, MICROSCOPIC EXAMINATION, PREPARATION AND TRANSMISSION OF WRITTEN REPORT	S	N	00	9		
D0502	OTHER ORAL PATHOLOGY PROCEDURES, BY REPORT	D	N	13	A	50-26	2136, 2336
D0999	UNSPECIFIED DIAGNOSTIC PROCEDURE, BY REPORT	D	N	13	A	50-26	2136, 2336
D1110	PROPHYLAXIS-ADULT	S	N	00	9		
D1120	PROPHYLAXIS-CHILD	S	N	00	9		
D1201	TOPICAL APPLICATION OF FLUORIDE (INCLUDING PROPHYLAXIS)-CHILD	S	N	00	9		
D1203	TOPICAL APPLICATION OF FLUORIDE - CHILD	S	N	00	9		
D1204	TOPICAL APPLICATION OF FLUORIDE - ADULT	S	N	00	9		
D1205	TOPICAL APPLICATION OF FLUORIDE (INCLUDING PROPHYLAXIS)-ADULT	S	N	00	9		
D1206	TOPICAL FLUORIDE VARNISH; THERAPEUTIC APPLICATION FOR MODERATE TO HIGH CARIES RISK PATIENTS	S	N	00	9		
D1310	NUTRITIONAL COUNSELING FOR THE CONTROL OF DENTAL DISEASE	M	N	00	9		2300
D1320	TOBACCO COUNSELING FOR THE CONTROL AND PREVENTION OF ORAL DISEASE	M	N	00	9		2300
D1330	ORAL HYGIENE INSTRUCTION	M	N	00	9		2300
D1351	SEALANT-PER TOOTH	S	N	00	9		
D1510	SPACE MAINTAINER-FIXED UNILATERAL	D	N	13	A		2336
D1515	SPACE MAINTAINER-FIXED BILATERAL	D	N	13	A		2336, 2136
D1520	SPACE MAINTAINER-REMOVABLE UNILATERAL	D	N	13	A		2336, 2136
D1525	SPACE MAINTAINER-REMOVABLE BILATERAL	D	N	13	A		2336, 2136
D1550	RECEMENTATION OF SPACE MAINTAINER	D	N	13	A		2336, 2136
D1555	REMOVAL OF FIXED SPACE MAINTAINER	S	N	00	9		
D2140	AMALGAM-ONE SURFACE, PRIMARY OR PERMANENT	S	N	00	9		
D2150	AMALGAM-TWO SURFACES, PRIMARY OR PERMANENT	S	N	00	9		
D2160	AMALGAM-THREE SURFACES, PRIMARY OR PERMANENT	S	N	00	9		
D2161	AMALGAM-FOUR OR MORE SURFACES, PRIMARY OR PERMANENT	S	N	00	9		
D2330	RESIN-ONE SURFACE, ANTERIOR	S	N	00	9		
D2331	RESIN-TWO SURFACES, ANTERIOR	S	N	00	9		
D2332	RESIN-THREE SURFACES, ANTERIOR	S	N	00	9		

D Codes

HCPCS Code	Statute	Lab Cert	X-Ref	ASC Pay Grp	ASC Pay Group Eff. Date	Proc Notes	BETOS	TOS	Anest	Code Add Date	Code Effective Date	Code Term Date
D0476						0159	Y1	5	0	20050101	20100101	
D0477						0159	Y1	5	0	20050101	20100101	
D0478						0159	Y1	5	0	20050101	20100101	
D0479						0159	Y1	5	0	20050101	20100101	
D0480							Y1	5	0	20000101	20070101	
D0481						0159	Y1	5	0	20050101	20100101	
D0482						0159	Y1	5	0	20050101	20100101	
D0483						0159	Y1	5	0	20050101	20100101	
D0484						0159	Y1	5	0	20050101	20100101	
D0485						0159	Y1	5	0	20050101	20100101	
D0486	1862a(12)						Y1	5	0	20070101	20090101	
D0502							Y1	5	0	19860101	19930101	
D0999							Y1	5	0	19840101	19930101	
D1110	1862 a(12)						Y1	1	0	19840101	19960101	
D1120	1862 a(12)						Y1	1	0	19840101	19960101	
D1201	1862 a(12)						Y1	1	0	19840101	20070101	20061231
D1203	1862 a(12)						Y1	1	0	19860101	20090101	
D1204	1862 a(12)						Y1	1	0	19860101	20090101	
D1205	1862 a(12)	D1202					Y1	1	0	19920101	20070101	20061231
D1206	1862a(12)						Y1	1	0	20070101	20070101	
D1310							Y1	1	0	19820101	19960101	
D1320							Y1	1	0	19960101	19960101	
D1330							Y1	1	0	19820101	19960101	
D1351	1862 a(12)						Y1	1	0	19850101	19960101	
D1510							Y1	9	0	19840101	19930101	
D1515							Y1	9	0	19840101	19930101	
D1520							Y1	9	0	19840101	19930101	
D1525							Y1	9	0	19840101	19930101	
D1550							Y1	1	0	19820101	19930101	
D1555	1862a(12)						Y1	1	0	20070101	20070101	
D2140	1862 a(12)						Y1	1	0	19820101	20030101	
D2150	1862 a(12)						Y1	1	0	19820101	20030101	
D2160	1862 a(12)						Y1	1	0	19820101	20030101	
D2161	1862 a(12)						Y1	1	0	19820101	20030101	
D2330	1862 a(12)						Y1	1	0	19840101	19960101	
D2331	1861 a(12)						Y1	1	0	19840101	19960101	
D2332	1862 a(12)						Y1	1	0	19840101	19960101	

D Codes

HCPCS Code	Long Description	Coverage	Action	PI	MPI	CIM	MCM
D2335	RESIN-FOUR OR MORE SURFACES OR INVOLVING INCISAL ANGLE (ANTERIOR)	S	N	00	9		
D2390	RESIN-BASED COMPOSITE CROWN, ANTERIOR	S	N	00	9		
D2391	RESIN-BASED COMPOSITE - ONE SURFACE, POSTERIOR	S	N	00	9		
D2392	RESIN-BASED COMPOSITE - TWO SURFACES, POSTERIOR	S	N	00	9		
D2393	RESIN-BASED COMPOSITE - THREE SURFACES, POSTERIOR	S	N	00	9		
D2394	RESIN-BASED COMPOSITE - FOUR OR MORE SURFACES, POSTERIOR	S	N	00	9		
D2410	GOLD FOIL-ONE SURFACE	S	N	00	9		
D2420	GOLD FOIL-TWO SURFACES	S	N	00	9		
D2430	GOLD FOIL-THREE SURFACES	S	N	00	9		
D2510	INLAY-METALLIC-ONE SURFACE	S	N	00	9		
D2520	INLAY-METALLIC-TWO SURFACES	S	N	00	9		
D2530	INLAY-METALLIC-THREE OR MORE SURFACES	S	N	00	9		
D2542	ONLAY-METALLIC-TWO SURFACES	S	N	00	9		
D2543	ONLAY - METALLIC - THREE SURFACES	S	N	00	9		
D2544	ONLAY - METALLIC - FOUR OR MORE SURFACES	S	N	00	9		
D2610	INLAY-PORCELAIN/CERAMIC-ONE SURFACE	S	N	00	9		
D2620	INLAY-PORCELAIN/CERAMIC-TWO SURFACES	S	N	00	9		
D2630	INLAY-PORCELAIN/CERAMIC-THREE OR MORE SURFACES	S	N	00	9		
D2642	ONLAY - PORCELAIN/CERAMIC - TWO SURFACES	S	N	00	9		
D2643	ONLAY - PORCELAIN/CERAMIC - THREE SURFACES	S	N	00	9		
D2644	ONLAY - PORCELAIN/CERAMIC - FOUR OR MORE SURFACES	S	N	00	9		
D2650	INLAY - RESIN-BASED COMPOSITE - ONE SURFACE	S	N	00	9		
D2651	INLAY - RESIN-BASED COMPOSITE - TWO SURFACES	S	N	00	9		
D2652	INLAY - RESIN-BASED COMPOSITE - THREE OR MORE SURFACES	S	N	00	9		
D2662	ONLAY - RESIN-BASED COMPOSITE - TWO SURFACES	S	N	00	9		
D2663	ONLAY - RESIN-BASED COMPOSITE - THREE SURFACES	S	N	00	9		
D2664	ONLAY - - RESIN-BASED COMPOSITE - FOUR OR MORE SURFACES	S	N	00	9		
D2710	CROWN - RESIN-BASED COMPOSITE (INDIRECT)	S	N	00	9		
D2712	CROWN - 3/4 RESIN-BASED COMPOSITE (INDIRECT)	S	N	00	9		
D2720	CROWN-RESIN WITH HIGH NOBLE METAL	S	N	00	9		
D2721	CROWN-RESIN WITH PREDOMINANTLY BASE METAL	S	N	00	9		
D2722	CROWN-RESIN WITH NOBLE METAL	S	N	00	9		
D2740	CROWN-PORCELAIN/CERAMIC SUBSTRATE	S	N	00	9		
D2750	CROWN-PORCELAIN FUSED TO HIGH NOBLE METAL	S	N	00	9		
D2751	CROWN-PROCELAIN FUSED TO PREDOMINANTLY BASE METAL	S	N	00	9		
D2752	CROWN-PORCELAIN FUSED TO NOBLE METAL	S	N	00	9		
D2780	CROWN - 3/4 CAST HIGH NOBLE METAL	S	N	00	9		
D2781	CROWN - 3/4 CAST PREDOMINANTLY BASE METAL	S	N	00	9		
D2782	CROWN - 3/4 CAST NOBLE METAL	S	N	00	9		
D2783	CROWN - 3/4 PORCELAIN/CERAMIC	S	N	00	9		
D2790	CROWN-FULL CAST HIGH NOBLE METAL	S	N	00	9		
D2791	CROWN-FULL CAST PREDOMINANTLY BASE METAL	S	N	00	9		
D2792	CROWN-FULL CAST NOBLE METAL	S	N	00	9		
D2794	CROWN-TITANIUM	S	N	00	9		
D2799	PROVISIONAL CROWN	S	N	00	9		
D2910	RECEMENT INLAY, ONLAY OR PARTIAL COVERAGE RESTORATION	S	N	00	9		

HCPCS Code	Statute	Lab Cert	X-Ref	ASC Pay Grp	ASC Pay Group Eff. Date	Proc Notes	BETOS	TOS	Anest	Code Add Date	Code Effective Date	Code Term Date
D2335	1862 a(12)						Y1	1	0	19840101	19960101	
D2390	1862a(12)						Y1	1	0	20030101	20030101	
D2391	1862a(12)						Y1	1	0	20030101	20030101	
D2392	1862a(12)						Y1	1	0	20030101	20030101	
D2393	1862a(12)						Y1	1	0	20030101	20030101	
D2394	1862a(12)						Y1	1	0	20030101	20030101	
D2410	1862 a(12)						Y1	1	0	19820101	19960101	
D2420	1862 a(12)						Y1	1	0	19820101	19960101	
D2430	1862 a(12)						Y1	1	0	19820101	19960101	
D2510	1862 a(12)						Y1	1	0	19840101	19960101	
D2520	1862 a(12)						Y1	1	0	19840101	19960101	
D2530	1862 a(12)						Y1	1	0	19840101	19960101	
D2542	1862a(12)						Y1	1	0	20000101	20000101	
D2543	1862 a(12)						Y1	1	0	19960101	19960101	
D2544	1862 a(12)						Y1	1	0	19960101	19960101	
D2610	1862 a(12)						Y1	1	0	19840101	19960101	
D2620	1862 a(12)						Y1	1	0	19860101	19960101	
D2630	1862 a(12)						Y1	1	0	19860101	19960101	
D2642	1862 a(12)						Y1	1	0	19960101	19960101	
D2643	1862 a(12)						Y1	1	0	19960101	19960101	
D2644	1862 a(12)						Y1	1	0	19960101	19960101	
D2650	1862 a(12)						Y1	1	0	19920101	20000101	
D2651	1862 a(12)						Y1	1	0	19920101	20000101	
D2652	1862 a(12)						Y1	1	0	19920101	20000101	
D2662	1862 a(12)						Y1	1	0	19960101	20000101	
D2663	1862 a(12)						Y1	1	0	19960101	20000101	
D2664	1862 a(12)						Y1	1	0	19960101	20000101	
D2710	1862a(12)						Y1	1	0	19840101	20050101	
D2712	1862a(12)						Y1	9	0	20050101	20050101	
D2720	1862a(12)						Y1	1	0	19840101	19960101	
D2721	1862a(12)						Y1	1	0	19840101	19960101	
D2722	1862a(12)						Y1	1	0	19840101	19960101	
D2740	1862a(12)						Y1	1	0	19840101	19960101	
D2750	1862a(12)						Y1	1	0	19840101	19960101	
D2751	1862a(12)						Y1	1	0	19860101	19960101	
D2752	1862a(12)						Y1	1	0	19840101	19960101	
D2780	1862a(12)						Y1	1	0	20000101	20000101	
D2781	1862a(12)						Y1	1	0	20000101	20000101	
D2782	1862a(12)						Y1	1	0	20000101	20000101	
D2783	1862a(12)						Y1	1	0	20000101	20000101	
D2790	1862a(12)						Y1	1	0	19840101	19960101	
D2791	1862a(12)						Y1	1	0	19840101	19960101	
D2792	1862a(12)						Y1	1	0	19840101	19960101	
D2794	1862a(12)						Y1	9	0	20050101	20050101	
D2799	1862a(12)						Y1	1	0	20000101	20000101	
D2910	1862a(12)						Y1	1	0	19840101	20050101	

HCPCS Code	Long Description	Coverage	Action	PI	MPI	CIM	MCM
D2915	RECEMENT CAST OR PREFABRICATED POST AND CORE	S	N	00	9		
D2920	RECEMENT CROWN	S	N	00	9		
D2930	PREFABRICATED STAINLESS STEEL CROWN-PRIMARY TOOTH	S	N	00	9		
D2931	PREFABRICATED STAINLESS STEEL CROWN-PERMANENT TOOTH	S	N	00	9		
D2932	PREFABRICATED RESIN CROWN	S	N	00	9		
D2933	PREFABRICATED STAINLESS STEEL CROWN WITH RESIN WINDOW	S	N	00	9		
D2934	PREFABRICATED ESTHETIC COATED STAINLESS STEEL CROWN - PRIMARY TOOTH	S	N	00	9		
D2940	SEDATIVE FILLING	S	N	00	9		
D2950	CORE BUILD-UP, INCLUDING ANY PINS	S	N	00	9		
D2951	PIN RETENTION-PER TOOTH, IN ADDITION TO RESTORATION	S	N	00	9		
D2952	POST AND CORE IN ADDITION TO CROWN, INDIRECTLY FABRICATED	S	N	00	9		
D2953	EACH ADDITIONAL INDIRECTLY FABRICATED POST - SAME TOOTH	S	N	00	9		
D2954	PREFABRICATED POST AND CORE IN ADDITION TO CROWN	S	N	00	9		
D2955	POST REMOVAL (NOT IN CONJUCTION WITH ENDODONTIC THERAPY)	S	N	00	9		
D2957	EACH ADDITIONAL PREFABRICATED POST - SAME TOOTH	S	N	00	9		
D2960	LABIAL VENEER (LAMINATE)-CHAIRSIDE	S	N	00	9		
D2961	LABIAL VENEER (RESIN LAMINATE)-LABORATORY	S	N	00	9		
D2962	LABIAL VENEER (PORCELAIN LAMINATE)-LABORATORY	S	N	00	9		
D2970	TEMPORARY CROWN (FRACTURED TOOTH)	D	N	13	A		2136, 2336
D2971	ADDITIONAL PROCEDURES TO CONSTRUCT NEW CROWN UNDER EXISTING PARTIAL DENTURE FRAMEWORK	S	N	00	9		
D2975	COPING	S	N	00	9		
D2980	CROWN REPAIR, BY REPORT	S	N	00	9		
D2999	UNSPECIFIED RESTORATIVE PROCEDURE, BY REPORT	D	N	13	A		2336, 2136
D3110	PULP CAP-DIRECT (EXCLUDING FINAL RESTORATION)	S	N	00	9		
D3120	PULP CAP-INDIRECT (EXCLUDING FINAL RESTORATION)	S	N	00	9		
D3220	THERAPEUTIC PULPOTOMY (EXCLUDING FINAL RESTORATION) REMOVAL OF PULP CORONAL TO THE DENTINOCEMENTAL JUNCTION AND APPLICATION OF MEDICAMENT	S	N	00	9		
D3221	PULPAL DEBRIDEMENT, PRIMARY AND PERMANENT TEETH	S	N	00	9		
D3222	PARTIAL PULPOTOMY FOR APEXOGENESIS - PERMANENT TOOTH WITH INCOMPLETE ROOT DEVELOPMENT	S	N	00	9		
D3230	PULPAL THERAPY (RESORBABLE FILLING)-ANTERIOR, PRIMARY TOOTH (EXCLUDING FINAL RESTORATION)	S	N	00	9		
D3240	PULPAL THERAPY (RESORBABLE FILLING)-POSTERIOR, PRIMARY TOOTH (EXCLUDING FINAL RESTORATION)	S	N	00	9		
D3310	ENDODONTIC THERAPY, ANTERIOR TOOTH (EXCLUDING FINAL RESTORATION)	S	N	00	9		
D3320	ENDODONTIC THERAPY, BICUSPID TOOTH (EXCLUDING FINAL RESTORATION)	S	N	00	9		
D3330	ENDODONTIC THERAPY, MOLAR (EXCLUDING FINAL RESTORATION)	S	N	00	9		
D3331	TREATMENT OF ROOT CANAL OBSTRUCTION; NON-SURGICAL ACCESS	S	N	00	9		

D Codes

HCPCS Code	Statute	Lab Cert	X-Ref	ASC Pay Grp	ASC Pay Group Eff. Date	Proc Notes	BETOS	TOS	Anest	Code Add Date	Code Effective Date	Code Term Date
D2915	1862a(12)						Y1	9	0	20050101	20050101	
D2920	1862a(12)						Y1	1	0	19840101	19960101	
D2930	1862a(12)						Y1	1	0	19860101	19960101	
D2931	1862a(12)						Y1	1	0	19860101	19960101	
D2932	1862a(12)						Y1	1	0	19860101	19960101	
D2933	1862a(12)						Y1	1	0	19920101	19960101	
D2934	1862a(12)						Y1	9	0	20050101	20050101	
D2940	1862a(12)						Y1	1	0	19840101	19960101	
D2950	1862a(12)						Y1	1	0	19860101	19960101	
D2951	1862a(12)						Y1	1	0	19860101	19960101	
D2952	1862a(12)						Y1	1	0	19860101	20070101	
D2953	1862a(12)						Y1	1	0	20000101	20070101	
D2954	1862a(12)						Y1	1	0	19860101	19960101	
D2955	1862a(12)						Y1	1	0	19960101	19960101	
D2957	1862a(12)						Y1	1	0	20000101	20000101	
D2960	1862a(12)						Y1	1	0	19850101	19960101	
D2961	1862a(12)						Y1	1	0	19920101	19960101	
D2962	1862a(12)						Y1	1	0	19920101	19960101	
D2970							Y1	1	0	20041231	20070101	
D2971	1862a(12)						Y1	9	0	20050101	20050101	
D2975	1862a(12)						Y1	9	0	20050101	20050101	
D2980	1862a(12)						Y1	1	0	19860101	19960101	
D2999							Y1	1	0	19860101	19930101	
D3110	1862a(12)						Y1	1	0	19820101	19960101	
D3120	1862a(12)						Y1	1	0	19840101	19960101	
D3220	1862a(12)						Y1	2	0	19840101	20000101	
D3221	1862a(12)						Y1	2	0	20000101	20030101	
D3222	1862a(12)						Y1	2	0	20090101	20090101	
D3230	1862a(12)						Y1	1	0	19960101	19960101	
D3240	1862a(12)						Y1	1	0	19960101	19960101	
D3240												
D3310	1862a(12)						Y1	1	0	19840101	20090101	
D3320	1862a(12)						Y1	1	0	19840101	20090101	
D3330	1862a(12)						Y1	1	0	19840101	20090101	
D3331	1862a(12)						Y1	1	0	20000101	20000101	

HCPCS Code	Long Description	Coverage	Action	PI	MPI	CIM	MCM
D3332	INCOMPLETE ENDODONTIC THERAPY; INOPERABLE, UNRESTORABLE OR FRACTURED TOOTH	S	N	00	9		
D3333	INTERNAL ROOT REPAIR OF PERFORATION DEFECTS	S	N	00	9		
D3346	RETREATMENT OF PREVIOUS ROOT CANAL THERAPY-ANTERIOR	S	N	00	9		
D3347	RETREATMENT OF PREVIOUS ROOT CANAL THERAPY-BICUSPID	S	N	00	9		
D3348	RETREATMENT OF PREVIOUS ROOT CANAL THERAPY-MOLAR	S	N	00	9		
D3351	APEXIFICATION/RECALCIFICATION-INITIAL VISIT (APICAL CLOSURE/CALCIFIC REPAIR OF PERFORATIONS, ROOT RESORPTION, ETC.)	S	N	00	9		
D3352	APEXIFICATION/RECALCIFICATION-INTERIM MEDICATION REPLACEMENT (APICAL CLOSURE/CALCIFIC REPAIR OF PERFORATIONS, ROOT RESORPTION, ETC.)	S	N	00	9		
D3353	APEXIFICATION/RECALCIFICATION-FINAL VISIT (INCLUDES COMPLETED ROOT CANAL THERAPY-APICAL CLOSURE/ CALCIFIC REPAIR OF PERFORATIONS, ROOT RESORPTION, ETC.)	S	N	00	9		
D3410	APICOECTOMY/PERIRADICULAR SURGERY-ANTERIOR	S	N	00	9		
D3421	APICOECTOMY/PERIRADICULAR SURGERY-BICUSPID (FIRST ROOT)	S	N	00	9		
D3425	APICOECTOMY/PERIRADICULAR SURGERY-MOLAR (FIRST ROOT).	S	N	00	9		
D3426	APICOECTOMY/PERIRADICULAR SURGERY (EACH ADDITIONAL ROOT)	S	N	00	9		
D3430	RETROGRADE FILLING-PER ROOT	S	N	00	9		
D3450	ROOT AMPUTATION-PER ROOT	S	N	00	9		
D3460	ENDODONTIC ENDOSSEOUS IMPLANT	D	N	13	A		2336, 2136
D3470	INTENTIONAL REPLANTATION (INCLUDING NECESSARY SPLINTING)	S	N	00	9		
D3910	SURGICAL PROCEDURE FOR ISOLATION OF TOOTH WITH RUBBER DAM	S	N	00	9		
D3920	HEMISECTION (INCLUDING ANY ROOT REMOVAL), NOT INCLUDING ROOT CANAL THERAPY	S	N	00	9		
D3950	CANAL PREPARATION AND FITTING OF PREFORMED DOWEL OR POST	S	N	00	9		
D3999	UNSPECIFIED ENDODONTIC PROCEDURE, BY REPORT	D	N	13	A		2336, 2136
D4210	GINGIVECTOMY OR GINGIVOPLASTY - FOUR OR MORE CONTIGUOUS TEETH OR TOOTH BOUNDED SPACES PER QUADRANT	I	N	00	9		
D4211	GINGIVECTOMY OR GINGIVOPLASTY - ONE TO THREE CONTIGUOUS TEETH OR TOOTH BOUNDED SPACES PER QUADRANT	I	N	00	9		
D4230	ANATOMICAL CROWN EXPOSURE - FOUR OR MORE CONTIGUOUS TEETH PER QUADRANT	S	N	00	9		
D4231	ANATOMICAL CROWN EXPOSURE - ONE TO THREE TEETH PER QUADRANT	S	N	00	9		
D4240	GINGIVAL FLAP PROCEDURE, INCLUDING ROOT PLANING - FOUR OR MORE CONTIGUOUS TEETH OR TOOTH BOUNDED SPACES PER QUADRANT	S	N	00	9		
D4241	GINGIVAL FLAP PROCEDURE, INCLUDING ROOT PLANING - ONE TO THREE CONTIGUOUS TEETH OR TOOTH BOUNDED SPACES PER QUADRANT	S	N	00	9		

HCPCS Code	Statute	Lab Cert	X-Ref	ASC Pay Grp	ASC Pay Group Eff. Date	Proc Notes	BETOS	TOS	Anest	Code Add Date	Code Effective Date	Code Term Date
D3332	1862a(12)						Y1	1	0	20000101	20050101	
D3333	1862a(12)						Y1	1	0	20000101	20000101	
D3346	1862a(12)						Y1	1	0	19920101	19960101	
D3347	1862a(12)						Y1	1	0	19920101	19960101	
D3348	1862a(12)						Y1	1	0	19920101	19960101	
D3351	1862a(12)						Y1	2	0	19920101	19960101	
D3352	1862a(12)						Y1	2	0	19920101	19960101	
D3353	1862a(12)						Y1	2	0	19920101	19960101	
D3410	1862a(12)						Y1	2	0	19840101	19960101	
D3421	1862a(12)						Y1	2	0	19920101	19960101	
D3425	1862a(12)						Y1	2	0	19920101	19960101	
D3426	1862a(12)						Y1	2	0	19920101	19960101	
D3430	1862a(12)						Y1	2	0	19840101	19960101	
D3450	1862a(12)						Y1	2	0	19840101	19960101	
D3460							Y1	2	0	19840101	19930101	
D3470	1862a(12)						Y1	2	0	19920101	19960101	
D3910	1862a(12)						Y1	2	0	19820101	19960101	
D3920	1862a(12)						Y1	2	0	19840101	19960101	
D3950	1862a(12)						Y1	1	0	19820101	19960101	
D3999							Y1	1	0	19840101	19930101	
D4210			41820				Y1	2	0	19850101	20090101	
D4211			CPT			0019	Y1	2	0	19860101	20090101	
D4230	1862a(12)						Y1	2	0	20070101	20070101	
D4231	1862a(12)						Y1	2	0	20070101	20070101	
D4240	1862a(12)						Y1	2	0	19840101	20090101	
D4241	1862a(12)						Y1	2	0	20030101	20090101	

HCPCS Code	Long Description	Coverage	Action	PI	MPI	CIM	MCM
D4245	APICALLY POSITIONED FLAP	S	N	00	9		
D4249	CLINICAL CROWN LENGTHENING-HARD TISSUE	S	N	00	9		
D4260	OSSEOUS SURGERY (INCLUDING FLAP ENTRY AND CLOSURE) - FOUR OR MORE CONTIGUOUSTEETH OR TOOTH BOUNDED SPACES PER QUADRANT	D	N	13	A		2136, 2336
D4261	OSSEOUS SURGERY (INCLUDING FLAP ENTRY AND CLOSURE) - ONE TO THREE CONTIGUOUSTEETH OR TOOTH BOUNDED SPACES PER QUADRANT	S	N	00	9		
D4263	BONE REPLACEMENT GRAFT - FIRST SITE IN QUADRANT	D	N	13	A	50-26	2336, 2136
D4264	BONE REPLACEMENT GRAFT - EACH ADDITIONAL SITE IN QUADRANT	D	N	13	A	50-26	2336, 2136
D4265	BIOLOGIC MATERIALS TO AID IN SOFT AND OSSEOUS TISSUE REGENERATION	S	N	00	9		
D4266	GUIDED TISSUE REGENERATION - RESORBABLE BARRIER, PER SITE	S	N	00	9		
D4267	GUIDED TISSUE REGENERATION - NONRESORBABLE BARRIER, PER SITE, (INCLUDES MEMBRANE REMOVAL)	S	N	00	9		
D4268	SURGICAL REVISION PROCEDURE, PER TOOTH	D	N	00	9		2136, 2336
D4270	PEDICLE SOFT TISSUE GRAFT PROCEDURE	D	N	13	A		2336, 2136
D4271	FREE SOFT TISSUE GRAFT PROCEDURE (INCLUDING DONOR SITE SURGERY)	D	N	13	A		2336, 2136
D4273	SUBEPITHELIAL CONNECTIVE TISSUE GRAFT PROCEDURES, PER TOOTH	D	N	13	A	50-26	2136, 2336
D4274	DISTAL OR PROXIMAL WEDGE PROCEDURE (WHEN NOT PERFORMED IN CONJUCTION WITH SURGICAL PROCEDURES IN THE SAME ANATOMICAL AREA)	S	N	00	9		
D4275	SOFT TISSUE ALLOGRAFT	S	N	00	9		
D4276	COMBINED CONNECTIVE TISSUE AND DOUBLE PEDICLE GRAFT, PER TOOTH	S	N	00	9		
D4320	PROVISIONAL SPLINTING-INTRACORONAL	S	N	00	9		
D4321	PROVISIONAL SPLINTING-EXTRACORONAL	S	N	00	9		
D4341	PERIODONTAL SCALING AND ROOT PLANING - FOUR OR MORE TEETH PER QUADRANT	S	N	00	9		
D4342	PERIODONTAL SCALING AND ROOT PLANING - ONE TO THREE TEETH, PER QUADRANT	S	N	00	9		
D4355	FULL MOUTH DEBRIDEMENT TO ENABLE COMPREHENSIVE EVALUATION AND DIAGNOSIS	D	N	13	A	50-26	2136, 2336
D4381	LOCALIZED DELIVERY OF ANTIMICROBIAL AGENTS VIA A CONTROLLED RELEASE VEHICLE INTO DISEASED CREVICULAR TISSUE, PER TOOTH, BY REPORT	D	N	13	A	50-26	2136, 2336
D4910	PERIODONTAL MAINTENANCE	S	N	00	9		
D4920	UNSCHEDULED DRESSING CHANGE (BY SOMEONE OTHER THAN TREATING DENTIST)	S	N	00	9		
D4999	UNSPECIFIED PERIODONTAL PROCEDURE, BY REPORT	S	N	00	9		
D5110	COMPLETE DENTURE - MAXILLARY	S	N	00	9		
D5120	COMPLETE DENTURE - MANDIBULAR	S	N	00	9		
D5130	IMMEDIATE DENTURE - MAXILLARY	S	N	00	9		
D5140	IMMEDIATE DENTURE - MANDIBULAR	S	N	00	9		

HCPCS Code	Statute	Lab Cert	X-Ref	ASC Pay Grp	ASC Pay Group Eff. Date	Proc Notes	BETOS	TOS	Anest	Code Add Date	Code Effective Date	Code Term Date
D4245	1862a(12)						Y1	2	0	20000101	20000101	
D4249	1862a(12)						Y1	2	0	19920101	19960101	
D4260							Y1	2	0	19850101	20090101	
D4261	1862a(12)						Y1	2	0	20030101	20090101	
D4263							Y1	2	0	19960101	19960101	
D4264							Y1	2	0	19960101	19960101	
D4265	1862a(12)						Y1	2	0	20030101	20030101	
D4266	1862a(12)						Y1	2	0	19960101	20000101	
D4267	1862a(12)						Y1	2	0	19960101	20000101	
D4268							Y1	2	0	20000101	20000101	
D4270							Y1	2	0	19840101	19930101	
D4271							Y1	2	0	19840101	19960101	
D4273							Y1	2	0	19960101	20050101	
D4274	1862a(12)						Y1	2	0	19960101	19960101	
D4275	1862a(12)						Y1	2	0	20030101	20030101	
D4276	1862a(12)						Y1	2	0	20030101	20050101	
D4320	1862a(12)						Y1	1	0	19840101	19960101	
D4321	1862a(12)						Y1	1	0	19840101	19960101	
D4341	1862a(12)						Y1	1	0	19850101	20050101	
D4342	1862a(12)						Y1	1	0	20030101	20030101	
D4355							Y1	1	0	19960101	20030101	
D4381							Y1	1	0	19960101	20050101	
D4910	1862a(12)						Y1	1	0	19840101	20030101	
D4920	1862a(12)						Y1	1	0	19840101	19960101	
D4999	1862a(12)						Y1	1	0	19840101	19960101	
D5110	1862a(12)						Y1	9	0	19820101	19960101	
D5120	1862a(12)						Y1	9	0	19820101	19960101	
D5130	1862a(12)						Y1	9	0	19820101	19960101	
D5140	1862a(12)						Y1	9	0	19820101	19960101	

HCPCS Code	Long Description	Coverage	Action	PI	MPI	CIM	MCM
D5211	UPPER PARTIAL-RESIN BASE (INCLUDING ANY CONVENTIONAL CLASPS, RESTS AND TEETH)	S	N	00	9		
D5212	LOWER PARTIAL-RESIN BASE (INCLUDING ANY CONVENTIONAL CLASPS, RESTS AND TEETH)	S	N	00	9		
D5213	MAXILLARY PARTIAL DENTURE - CAST METAL FRAMEWORK WITH RESIN DENTURE BASES (INCLUDING ANY CONVENTIONAL CLASPS, RESTS AND TEETH)	S	N	00	9		
D5214	MANDIBULAR PARTIAL DENTURE - CAST METAL FRAMEWORK WITH RESIN DENTURE BASES (INCLUDING ANY CONVENTIONAL CLASPS,RESTS AND TEETH)	S	N	00	9		
D5225	MAXILLARY PARTIAL DENTURE - FLEXIBLE BASE (INCLUDING ANY CLASPS, RESTS AND TEETH)	S	N	00	9		
D5226	MANDIBULAR PARTIAL DENTURE - FLEXIBLE BASE (INCLUDING ANY CLASPS, RESTS AND TEETH)	S	N	00	9		
D5281	REMOVABLE UNILATERAL PARTIAL DENTURE-ONE PIECE CAST METAL (INCLUDING CLASPS AND TEETH)	S	N	00	9		
D5410	ADJUST COMPLETE DENTURE - MAXILLARY	S	N	00	9		
D5411	ADJUST COMPLETE DENTURE - MANDIBULAR	S	N	00	9		
D5421	ADJUST PARTIAL DENTURE - MAXILLARY	S	N	00	9		
D5422	ADJUST PARTIAL DENTURE - MANDIBULAR	S	N	00	9		
D5510	REPAIR BROKEN COMPLETE DENTURE BASE	S	N	00	9		
D5520	REPLACE MISSING OR BROKEN TEETH-COMPLETE DENTURE (EACH TOOTH)	S	N	00	9		
D5610	REPAIR RESIN DENTURE BASE	S	N	00	9		
D5620	REPAIR CAST FRAMEWORK	S	N	00	9		
D5630	REPAIR OR REPLACE BROKEN CLASP	S	N	00	9		
D5640	REPLACE BROKEN TEETH-PER TOOTH	S	N	00	9		
D5650	ADD TOOTH TO EXISTING PARTIAL DENTURE	S	N	00	9		
D5660	ADD CLASP TO EXISTING PARTIAL DENTURE	S	N	PI	9		
D5670	REPLACE ALL TEETH AND ACRYLIC ON CAST METAL FRAMEWORK (MAXILLARY)	S	N	00	9		
D5671	REPLACE ALL TEETH AND ACRYLIC ON CAST METAL FRAMEWORK (MANDIBULAR)	S	N	00	9		
D5710	REBASE COMPLETE MAXILLARY DENTURE	S	N	00	9		
D5711	REBASE COMPLETE MANDIBULAR DENTURE	S	N	00	9		
D5720	REBASE MAXILLARY PARTIAL DENTURE	S	N	00	9		
D5721	REBASE MANDIBULAR PARTIAL DENTURE	S	N	00	9		
D5730	RELINE COMPLETE MAXILLARY DENTURE (CHAIRSIDE)	S	N	00	9		
D5731	RELINE LOWER COMPLETE MANDIBULAR DENTURE (CHAIRSIDE)	S	N	00	9		
D5740	RELINE MAXILLARY PARTIAL DENTURE (CHAIRSIDE)	S	N	00	9		
D5741	RELINE MANDIBULAR PARTIAL DENTURE (CHAIRSIDE)	S	N	00	9		
D5750	RELINE COMPLETE MAXILLARY DENTURE (LABORATORY)	S	N	00	9		
D5751	RELINE COMPLETE MANDIBULAR DENTURE (LABORATORY)	S	N	00	9		
D5760	RELINE MAXILLARY PARTIAL DENTURE (LABORATORY)	S	N	00	9		
D5761	RELINE MANDIBULAR PARTIAL DENTURE (LABORATORY)	S	N	00	9		
D5810	INTERIM COMPLETE DENTURE (MAXILLARY)	S	N	00	9		
D5811	INTERIM COMPLETE DENTURE (MANDIBULAR)	S	N	00	9		
D5820	INTERIM PARTIAL DENTURE (MAXILLARY)	S	N	00	9		

HCPCS Code	Statute	Lab Cert	X-Ref	ASC Pay Grp	ASC Pay Group Eff. Date	Proc Notes	BETOS	TOS	Anest	Code Add Date	Code Effective Date	Code Term Date
D5211	1862a(12)						Y1	9	0	19840101	19960101	
D5212	1862a(12)						Y1	9	0	19840101	19960101	
D5213	1862a(12)						Y1	9	0	19840101	19960101	
D5214	1862a(12)						Y1	9	0	19840101	19960101	
D5225	1862a(12)						Y1	9	0	20050101	20050101	
D5226	1862a(12)						Y1	9	0	20050101	20050101	
D5281	1862a(12)						Y1	9	0	19840101	19960101	
D5410	1862a(12)						Y1	1	0	19840101	19960101	
D5411	1862a(12)						Y1	1	0	19860101	19960101	
D5421	1862a(12)						Y1	1	0	19840101	19960101	
D5422	1862a(12)						Y1	1	0	19840101	19960101	
D5510	1862a(12)						Y1	1	0	19860101	19960101	
D5520	1862a(12)						Y1	1	0	19860101	19960101	
D5610	1862a(12)						Y1	1	0	19840101	19960101	
D5620	1862a(12)						Y1	1	0	19840101	19960101	
D5630	1862a(12)						Y1	1	0	19840101	19960101	
D5640	1862a(12)						Y1	1	0	19840101	19960101	
D5650	1862a(12)						Y1	1	0	19840101	19960101	
D5660	1862a(12)						Y1	1	0	19840101	19960101	
D5670	1862a(12)						Y1	1	0	20030101	20030101	
D5671	1862a(12)						Y1	1	0	20030101	20030101	
D5710	1862a(12)						Y1	1	0	19840101	19960101	
D5711	1862a(12)						Y1	1	0	19860101	19960101	
D5720	1862a(12)						Y1	1	0	19840101	19960101	
D5721	1862a(12)						Y1	1	0	19860101	19960101	
D5730	1862a(12)						Y1	1	0	19840101	19960101	
D5731	1862a(12)						Y1	1	0	19860101	19960101	
D5740	1862a(12)						Y1	1	0	19840101	19960101	
D5741	1862a(12)						Y1	1	0	19860101	19960101	
D5750	1862a(12)						Y1	1	0	19840101	19960101	
D5751	1862a(12)						Y1	1	0	19860101	19960101	
D5760	1862a(12)						Y1	1	0	19840101	19960101	
D5761	1862a(12)						Y1	1	0	19860101	19960101	
D5810	1862a(12)						Y1	9	0	19840101	19960101	
D5811	1862a(12)						Y1	9	0	19840101	19960101	
D5820	1862a(12)						Y1	9	0	19840101	19960101	

HCPCS Code	Long Description	Coverage	Action	PI	MPI	CIM	MCM
D5821	INTERIM PARTIAL DENTURE (MANDIBULAR)	S	N	00	9		
D5850	TISSUE CONDITIONING, MAXILLARY	S	N	00	9		
D5851	TISSUE CONDITIONING, MANDIBULAR	S	N	00	9		
D5860	OVERDENTURE-COMPLETE, BY REPORT	S	N	00	9		
D5861	OVERDENTURE-PARTIAL, BY REPORT	S	N	00	9		
D5862	PRECISION ATTACHMENT, BY REPORT	S	N	00	9		
D5867	REPLACEMENT OF REPLACEABLE PART OF SEMI-PRECISION OR PRECISION ATTACHMENT (MALE OR FEMALE COMPONENT)	S	N	00	9		
D5875	MODIFICATION OF REMOVABLE PROSTHESIS FOLLOWING IMPLANT SURGERY	S	N	00	9		
D5899	UNSPECIFIED REMOVABLE PROSTHODONTIC PROCEDURE, BY REPORT	S	N	00	9		
D5911	FACIAL MOULAGE (SECTIONAL)	D	N	13	A		2130 A, 2136
D5912	FACIAL MOULAGE (COMPLETE)	D	N	13	A		2130 A
D5913	NASAL PROSTHESIS	I	N	00	9		
D5914	AURICULAR PROSTHESIS	I	N	00	9		
D5915	ORBITAL PROSTHESIS	I	N	00	9		
D5916	OCULAR PROSTHESIS	I	N	00	9		
D5919	FACIAL PROSTHESIS	I	N	00	9		
D5922	NASAL SEPTAL PROSTHESIS	I	N	00	9		
D5923	OCULAR PROSTHESIS, INTERIM	I	N	00	9		
D5924	CRANIAL PROSTHESIS	I	N	00	9		
D5925	FACIAL AUGMENTATION IMPLANT PROSTHESIS	I	N	00	9		
D5926	NASAL PROSTHESIS, REPLACEMENT	I	N	00	9		
D5927	AURICULAR PROSTHESIS, REPLACEMENT	I	N	00	9		
D5928	ORBITAL PROSTHESIS, REPLACEMENT	I	N	00	9		
D5929	FACIAL PROSTHESIS, REPLACEMENT	I	N	00	9		
D5931	OBTURATOR PROSTHESIS, SURGICAL	I	N	00	9		
D5932	OBTURATOR PROSTHESIS, DEFINITIVE	I	N	00	9		
D5933	OBTURATOR PROSTHESIS, MODIFICATION	I	N	00	9		
D5934	MANDIBULAR RESECTION PROSTHESIS WITH GUIDE FLANGE	I	N	00	9		
D5935	MANDIBULAR RESECTION PROSTHESIS WITHOUT GUIDE FLANGE	I	N	00	9		
D5936	OBTURATOR/PROSTHESIS, INTERIM	I	N	00	9		
D5937	TRISMUS APPLIANCE (NOT FOR TM TREATMENT)	I	N	00	9		2130
D5951	FEEDING AID	D	N	13	A		2336, 2130
D5952	SPEECH AID PROSTHESIS, PEDIATRIC	I	N	00	9		
D5953	SPEECH AID PROSTHESIS, ADULT	I	N	00	9		
D5954	PALATAL AUGMENTATION PROSTHESIS	I	N	00	9		
D5955	PALATAL LIFT PROSTHESIS, DEFINITIVE	I	N	00	9		
D5958	PALATAL LIFT PROSTHESIS, INTERIM	I	N	00	9		
D5959	PALATAL LIFT PROSTHESIS, MODIFICATION	I	N	00	9		
D5960	SPEECH AID PROSTHESIS, MODIFICATION	I	N	00	9		
D5982	SURGICAL STENT	I	N	00	9		
D5983	RADIATION CARRIER	D	N	13	A		2336, 2136
D5984	RADIATION SHIELD	D	N	13	A		2336, 2136
D5985	RADIATION CONE LOCATOR	D	N	13	A		2336, 2136
D5986	FLUORIDE GEL CARRIER	S	N	00	9		
D5987	COMMISSURE SPLINT	D	N	13	A		2136, 2336

HCPCS Code	Statute	Lab Cert	X-Ref	ASC Pay Grp	ASC Pay Group Eff. Date	Proc Notes	BETOS	TOS	Anest	Code Add Date	Code Effective Date	Code Term Date
D5821	1862a(12)						Y1	9	0	19840101	19960101	
D5850	1862a(12)						Y1	9	0	19840101	19960101	
D5851	1862a(12)						Y1	9	0	19920101	19960101	
D5860	1862a(12)						Y1	9	0	19840101	19960101	
D5861	1862a(12)						Y1	9	0	19840101	19960101	
D5862	1862a(12)						Y1	9	0	19860101	19960101	
D5867	1862a(12)						Y1	9	0	20000101	20000101	
D5875	1862a(12)						Y1	9	0	20000101	20000101	
D5899	1862a(12)						Y1	9	0	19860101	19960101	
D5911							Y1	9	0	19850101	19930101	
D5912							Y1	9	0	19850101	19930101	
D5913			21087				Y1	9	0	19850101	19960101	
D5914			21086				Y1	9	0	19850101	19960101	
D5915			L8611				Y1	9	0	19850101	19960101	
D5916			CPT, V2623, V2629				Y1	9	0	19850101	19960101	
D5919			21088				Y1	9	0	19850101	19960101	
D5922			30220				Y1	9	0	19920101	19960101	
D5923			92330				Y1	9	0	19920101	19960101	
D5924			62143				Y1	9	0	19920101	19960101	
D5925			21208				Y1	9	0	19920101	19960101	
D5926			21087				Y1	9	0	19920101	19960101	
D5927			21086				Y1	9	0	19920101	19960101	
D5928			67550				Y1	9	0	19920101	19960101	
D5929			21088				Y1	9	0	19920101	19960101	
D5931			21079				Y1	9	0	19850101	19960101	
D5932			21080				Y1	9	0	19850101	19960101	
D5933			21080				Y1	9	0	19850101	19960101	
D5934			21081				Y1	9	0	19850101	19960101	
D5935			21081				Y1	9	0	19850101	19960101	
D5936			21079				Y1	9	0	19920101	19960101	
D5937							Y1	9	0	19920101	19960101	
D5951							Y1	9	0	19850101	19930101	
D5952			21084				Y1	9	0	19850101	19960101	
D5953			21084				Y1	9	0	19850101	19960101	
D5954			21082				Y1	9	0	19850101	19960101	
D5955			21083				Y1	9	0	19850101	19960101	
D5958			21083				Y1	9	0	19920101	19960101	
D5959			21083				Y1	9	0	19920101	19960101	
D5960			21084				Y1	9	0	19920101	19960101	
D5982			21085				Y1	9	0	19850101	19960101	
D5983							Y1	9	0	19850101	19930101	
D5984							Y1	9	0	19850101	19930101	
D5985							Y1	9	s	19850101	19930101	
D5986	1862a(12)						Y1	9	0	19850101	19960101	
D5987							Y1	9	0	19920101	19960101	

D Codes

HCPCS Code	Long Description	Coverage	Action	PI	MPI	CIM	MCM
D5988	SURGICAL SPLINT	I	N	13	A		
D5991	TOPICAL MEDICAMENT CARRIER	S	N	00	9		
D5999	UNSPECIFIED MAXILLOFACIAL PROSTHESIS, BY REPORT	I	N	00	9		
D6010	SURGICAL PLACEMENT OF IMPLANT BODY: ENDOSTEAL IMPLANT	I	N	00	9		
D6012	SURGICAL PLACEMENT OF INTERIM IMPLANT BODY FOR TRANSITIONAL PROSTHESIS: ENDOSTEAL IMPLANT	S	N	00	9		
D6040	SURGICAL PLACEMENT: EPOSTEAL IMPLANT	I	N	00	9		
D6050	SURGICAL PLACEMENT: TRANSOSTEAL IMPLANT	I	N	00	9		
D6053	IMPLANT/ABUTMENT SUPPORTED REMOVABLE DENTURE FOR COMPLETELY EDENTULOUS ARCH	M	N	00	9		2136
D6054	IMPLANT/ABUTMENT SUPPORTED REMOVABLE DENTURE FOR PARTIALLY EDENTULOUS ARCH	M	N	00	9		2136
D6055	DENTAL IMPLANT SUPPORTED CONNECTING BAR	I	N	00	9		2136
D6056	PREFABRICATED ABUTMENT - INCLUDES PLACEMENT	M	N	00	9		2136
D6057	CUSTOM ABUTMENT - INCLUDES PLACEMENT	M	N	00	9		2136
D6058	ABUTMENT SUPPORTED PORCELAIN/CERAMIC CROWN	M	N	00	9		2136
D6059	ABUTMENT SUPPORTED PORCELAIN FUSED TO METAL CROWN (HIGH NOBLE METAL)	M	N	00	9		2136
D6060	ABUTMENT SUPPORTED PORCELAIN FUSED TO METAL CROWN (PREDOMINANTLY BASE METAL)	M	N	00	9		2136
D6061	ABUTMENT SUPPORTED PORCELAIN FUSED TO METAL CROWN (NOBLE METAL)	M	N	00	9		2136
D6062	ABUTMENT SUPPORTED CAST METAL CROWN (HIGH NOBLE METAL)	M	N	00	9		2136
D6063	ABUTMENT SUPPORTED CAST METAL CROWN (PREDOMINANTLY BASE METAL)	M	N	00	9		2136
D6064	ABUTMENT SUPPORTED CAST METAL CROWN (NOBLE METAL)	M	N	00	9		2136
D6065	IMPLANT SUPPORTED PORCELAIN/CERAMIC CROWN	M	N	00	9		2136
D6066	IMPLANT SUPPORTED PORCELAIN FUSED TO METAL CROWN (TITANIUM, TITANIUM ALLOY, HIGH NOBLE METAL)	M	N	00	9		2136
D6067	IMPLANT SUPPORTED METAL CROWN (TITANIUM, TITANIUM ALLOY, HIGH NOBLE METAL)	M	N	00	9		2136
D6068	ABUTMENT SUPPORTED RETAINER FOR PORCELAIN/CERAMIC FPD	M	N	00	9		2136
D6069	ABUTMENT SUPPORTED RETAINER FOR PORCELAIN FUSED TO METAL FPD (HIGH NOBLE METAL)	M	N	00	9		2136
D6070	ABUTMENT SUPPORTED RETAINER FOR PORCELAIN FUSED TO METAL FPD (PREDOMINANTLY BASE METAL)	M	N	00	9		2136
D6071	ABUTMENT SUPPORTED RETAINER FOR PORCELAIN FUSED TO METAL FPD (NOBLE METAL)	M	N	00	9		2136
D6072	ABUTMENT SUPPORTED RETAINER FOR CAST METAL FPD (HIGH NOBLE METAL)	M	N	00	9		2136
D6073	ABUTMENT SUPPORTED RETAINER FOR CAST METAL FPD (PREDOMINANTLY BASE METAL)	M	N	00	9		2136
D6074	ABUTMENT SUPPORTED RETAINER FOR CAST METAL FPD (NOBLE METAL)	M	N	00	9		2136
D6075	IMPLANT SUPPORTED RETAINER FOR CERAMIC FPD	M	N	00	9		2136

HCPCS Code	Statute	Lab Cert	X-Ref	ASC Pay Grp	ASC Pay Group Eff. Date	Proc Notes	BETOS	TOS	Anest	Code Add Date	Code Effective Date	Code Term Date
D5988			CPT				Y1	9	0	19920101	19960101	
D5991	1862a(12)						Y1	9	0	20090101	20090101	
D5999			CPT				Y1	9	0	19860101	19960101	
D6010			21248				Y1	2	0	19960101	19960101	
D6012	1862a(12)						Y1	2	0	20070101	20070101	
D6040			21245				Y1	2	0	19920101	19960101	
D6050			21244				Y1	2	0	19920101	19960101	
D6053							Y1	9	0	20030101	20030101	
D6054							Y1	9	0	20030101	20030101	
D6055							Y1	9	0	19920101	19960101	
D6056							Y1	9	0	20000101	20050101	
D6057							Y1	9	0	20000101	20050101	
D6058							Y1	9	0	20000101	20000101	
D6059							Y1	9	0	20000101	20000101	
D6060							Y1	9	0	20000101	20000101	
D6061							Y1	9	0	20000101	20000101	
D6062							Y1	9	0	20000101	20000101	
D6063							Y1	9	0	20000101	20000101	
D6064							Y1	9	0	20000101	20000101	
D6065							Y1	9	0	20000101	20000101	
D6066							Y1	9	0	20000101	20000101	
D6067							Y1	9	0	20000101	20000101	
D6068							Y1	9	0	20000101	20000101	
D6069							Y1	9	0	20000101	20000101	
D6070							Y1	9	0	20000101	20000101	
D6071							Y1	9	0	20000101	20000101	
D6072							Y1	9	0	20000101	20000101	
D6073							Y1	9	0	20000101	20000101	
D6074							Y1	9	0	20000101	20000101	
D6075							Y1	9	0	20000101	20000101	

HCPCS Code	Long Description	Coverage	Action	PI	MPI	CIM	MCM
D6076	IMPLANT SUPPORTED RETAINER FOR PORCELAIN FUSED TO METAL FPD (TITANIUM, TITANIUM ALLOY, OR HIGH NOBLE METAL)	M	N	00	9		2136
D6077	IMPLANT SUPPORTED RETAINER FOR CAST METAL FPD (TITANIUM, TITANIUM ALLOY, OR HIGH NOBLE METAL)	M	N	00	9		2136
D6078	IMPLANT/ABUTMENT SUPPORTED FIXED DENTURE FOR COMPLETELY EDENTULOUS ARCH	M	N	00	9		2136
D6079	IMPLANT/ABUTMENT SUPPORTED FIXED DENTURE FOR PARTIALLY EDENTULOUS ARCH	M	N	00	9		2136
D6080	IMPLANT MAINTENANCE PROCEDURES, INCLUDING: REMOVAL OF PROSTHESIS, CLEANSING OF PROSTHESIS AND ABUTMEN REINSERTION OF PROSTHESIS	I	N	00	9		2136
D6090	REPAIR IMPLANTSUPPORTED PROSTHESIS BY REPORT	I	N	00	9		
D6091	REPLACEMENT OF SEMI-PRECISION OR PRECISION ATTACHMENT (MALE OR FEMALE COMPONENT) OF IMPLANT/ABUTMENT SUPPORTED PROSTHESIS, PER ATTACHMENT	S	N	00	9		
D6092	RECEMENT IMPLANT/ABUTMENT SUPPORTED CROWN	S	N	00	9		
D6093	RECEMENT IMPLANT/ABUTMENT SUPPORTED FIXED PARTIAL DENTURE	S	N	00	9		
D6094	ABUTMENT SUPPORTED CROWN - (TITANIUM)	S	N	00	9		
D6095	REPAIR IMPLANT ABUTMENT, BY REPORT	I	N	00	9		
D6100	IMPLANT REMOVAL, BY REPORT	I	N	00	9		
D6190	RADIOGRAPHIC/SURGICAL IMPLANT INDEX, BY REPORT	S	N	00	9		
D6194	ABUTMENT SUPPORTED RETAINER CROWN FOR FPD - (TITANIUM)	S	N	00	9		
D6199	UNSPECIFIED IMPLANT PROCEDURE, BY REPORT	I	N	00	9		
D6205	PONTIC - INDIRECT RESIN BASED COMPOSITE	S	N	00	9		
D6210	PONTIC-CAST HIGH NOBLE METAL	S	N	00	9		
D6211	PONTIC-CAST PREDOMINANTLY BASE METAL	S	N	00	9		
D6212	PONTIC-CAST NOBLE METAL	S	N	00	9		
D6214	PONTIC - TITANIUM	S	N	00	9		
D6240	PONTIC-PORCELAIN FUSED TO HIGH NOBLE METAL	S	N	00	9		
D6241	PONTIC-PORCELAIN FUSED TO PREDOMINANTLY BASE METAL	S	N	00	9		
D6242	PONTIC-PORCELAIN FUSED TO NOBLE METAL	S	N	00	9		
D6245	PONTIC - PORCELAIN/CERAMIC	M	N	00	9		2136
D6250	PONTIC-RESIN WITH HIGH NOBLE METAL	S	N	00	9		
D6251	PONTIC-RESIN WITH PREDOMINANTLY BASE METAL	S	N	00	9		
D6252	PONTIC-RESIN WITH NOBLE METAL	S	N	00	9		
D6253	PROVISIONAL PONTIC	S	N	00	9		
D6545	RETAINER-CAST METAL FOR RESIN BONDED FIXED PROSTHESIS	S	N	00	9		
D6548	RETAINER - PORCELAIN/CERAMIC FOR RESIN BONDED FIXED PROSTHESIS	M	N	00	9		2136
D6600	INLAY-PORCELAIN/CERAMIC, TWO SURFACES	M	N	00	9		2136
D6601	INLAY - PORCELAIN/CERAMIC, THREE OR MORE SURFACES	M	N	00	9		2136
D6602	INLAY - CAST HIGH NOBLE METAL, TWO SURFACES	M	N	00	9		2136
D6603	INLAY - CAST HIGH NOBLE METAL, THREE OR MORE SURFACES	M	N	00	9		2136
D6604	INLAY - CAST PREDOMINANTLY BASE METAL, TWO SURFACES	M	N	00	9		2136
D6605	INLAY - CAST PREDOMINANTLY BASE METAL, THREE OR MORE SURFACES	M	N	00	9		2136

HCPCS Code	Statute	Lab Cert	X-Ref	ASC Pay Grp	ASC Pay Group Eff. Date	Proc Notes	BETOS	TOS	Anest	Code Add Date	Code Effective Date	Code Term Date
D6076							Y1	9	0	20000101	20000101	
D6077							Y1	9	0	20000101	20000101	
D6078							Y1	9	0	20000101	20000101	
D6079							Y1	9	0	20000101	20000101	
D6080							Y1	2	0	19920101	19960101	
D6090			21299				Y1	9	0	19920101	19960101	
D6091	1862a(12)						Y1	9	0	20070101	20070101	
D6092	1862a(12)						Y1	9	0	20070101	20070101	
D6093	1862a(12)						Y1	9	0	20070101	20070101	
D6094	1862a(12)						Y1	9	0	20050101	20050101	
D6095			21299				Y1	9	0	19960101	19960101	
D6100			21299				Y1	9	0	19920101	19960101	
D6190	1862a(12)						Y1	9	0	20050101	20050101	
D6194	1862a(12)						Y1	9	0	20050101	20050101	
D6199			21299				Y1	9	0	19920101	19960101	
D6205	1862a(12)						Y1	9	0	20050101	20050101	
D6210	1862a(12)						Y1	9	0	19840101	19960101	
D6211	1862a(12)						Y1	9	0	19840101	19960101	
D6212	1862a(12)						Y1	9	0	19840101	19960101	
D6214	1862a(12)						Y1	9	0	20050101	20050101	
D6240	1862a(12)						Y1	9	0	19840101	19960101	
D6241	1862a(12)						Y1	9	0	19840101	19960101	
D6242	1862a(12)						Y1	9	0	19840101	19960101	
D6245							Y1	9	0	20000101	20000101	
D6250	1862a(12)						Y1	9	0	19840101	19960101	
D6251	1862a(12)						Y1	9	0	19840101	19960101	
D6252	1862a(12)						Y1	9	0	19840101	19960101	
D6253	1862a(12)						Y1	9	0	20030101	20030101	
D6545	1862a(12)						Y1	9	0	19840101	19960101	
D6548							Y1	9	0	20000101	20000101	
D6600							Y1	9	0	20030101	20030101	
D6601							Y1	9	0	20030101	20030101	
D6602							Y1	9	0	20030101	20030101	
D6603							Y1	9	0	20030101	20030101	
D6604							Y1	9	0	20030101	20030101	
D6605							Y1	9	0	20030101	20030101	

HCPCS Code	Long Description	Coverage	Action	PI	MPI	CIM	MCM
D6606	INLAY - CAST NOBLE METAL, TWO SURFACES	M	N	00	9		2136
D6607	INLAY - CAST NOBLE METAL, THREE OR MORE SURFACES	M	N	00	9		2136
D6608	ONLAY - PORCELAIN/CERAMIC, TWO SURFACES	M	N	00	9		2136
D6609	ONLAY - PORCELAIN/CERAMIC, THREE OR MORE SURFACES	M	N	00	9		2136
D6610	ONLAY - CAST HIGH NOBLE METAL, TWO SURFACES	M	N	00	9		2136
D6611	ONLAY - CAST HIGH NOBLE METAL, THREE OR MORE SURFACES	M	N	00	9		2136
D6612	ONLAY - CAST PREDOMINANTLY BASE METAL, TWO SURFACES	M	N	00	9		2136
D6613	ONLAY - CAST PREDOMINANTLY BASE METAL, THREE OR MORE SURFACES	M	N	00	9		2136
D6614	ONLAY - CAST NOBLE METAL, TWO SURFACES	M	N	00	9		2136
D6615	ONLAY - CAST NOBLE METAL, THREE OR MORE SURFACES	M	N	00	9		2136
D6624	INLAY - TITANIUM	S	N	00	9		
D6634	ONLAY - TITANIUM	S	N	00	9		
D6710	CROWN - INDIRECT RESIN BASED COMPOSITE	S	N	00	9		
D6720	CROWN-RESIN WITH HIGH NOBLE METAL	S	N	00	9		
D6721	CROWN-RESIN WITH PREDOMINANTLY BASE METAL	S	N	00	9		
D6722	CROWN-RESIN WITH NOBLE METAL	S	N	00	9		
D6740	CROWN - PORCELAIN/CERAMIC	M	N	00	9		2136
D6750	CROWN-PORCELAIN FUSED TO HIGH NOBLE METAL	S	N	00	9		
D6751	CROWN-PORCELAIN FUSED TO PREDOMINANTLY BASE METAL	S	N	00	9		
D6752	CROWN-PORCELAIN FUSED TO NOBLE METAL	S	N	00	9		
D6780	CROWN-3/4 CAST HIGH NOBLE METAL	S	N	00	9		
D6781	CROWN - 3/4 CAST PREDOMINANTLY BASED METAL	M	N	00	9		2136
D6782	CROWN - 3/4 CAST NOBLE METAL	M	N	00	9		2136
D6783	CROWN - 3/4 PORCELAIN/CERAMIC	M	N	00	9		2136
D6790	CROWN-FULL CAST HIGH NOBLE METAL	S	N	00	9		
D6791	CROWN-FULL CAST PREDOMINANTLY BASE METAL	S	N	00	9		
D6792	CROWN-FULL CAST NOBLE METAL	S	N	00	9		
D6793	PROVISIONAL RETAINER CROWN	S	N	00	9		
D6794	CROWN - TITANIUM	S	N	00	9		
D6920	CONNECTOR BAR	D	N	13	A	50-26	23,362,136
D6930	RECEMENT BRIDGE	S	N	00	9		
D6940	STRESS BREAKER	S	N	00	9		
D6950	PRECISION ATTACHMENT	S	N	00	9		
D6970	POST AND CORE IN ADDITION TO FIXED PARTIAL DENTURE RETAINER, INDIRECTLY FABRICATED	S	N	00	9		
D6971	CAST POST AS PART OF BRIDGE RETAINER	S	N	00	9		
D6972	PREFABRICATED POST AND CORE IN ADDITION TO BRIDGE RETAINER	S	N	00	9		
D6973	CORE BUILD UP FOR RETAINER, INCLUDING ANY PINS	S	N	00	9		
D6975	COPING-METAL	S	N	00	9		
D6976	EACH ADDITIONAL INDIRECTLY FABRICATED POST - SAME TOOTH	M	N	00	9		2136
D6977	EACH ADDITIONAL PREFABRICATED POST - SAME TOOTH	M	N	00	9		2136
D6980	BRIDGE REPAIR, BY REPORT	S	N	00	9		
D6985	PEDIATRIC PARTIAL DENTURE, FIXED	S	N	00	9		
D6999	UNSPECIFIED FIXED PROSTHODONTIC PROCEDURE, BY REPORT	S	N	00	9		
D7111	EXTRACTION, CORONAL REMNANTS - DECIDUOUS TOOTH	D	N	13	A		2336

HCPCS Code	Statute	Lab Cert	X-Ref	ASC Pay Grp	ASC Pay Group Eff. Date	Proc Notes	BETOS	TOS	Anest	Code Add Date	Code Effective Date	Code Term Date
D6606							Y1	9	0	20030101	20030101	
D6607							Y1	9	0	20030101	20030101	
D6608							Y1	9	0	20030101	20030101	
D6609							Y1	9	0	20030101	20030101	
D6610							Y1	9	0	20030101	20030101	
D6611							Y1	9	0	20030101	20030101	
D6612							Y1	9	0	20030101	20030101	
D6613							Y1	9	0	20030101	20030101	
D6614							Y1	9	0	20030101	20030101	
D6615							Y1	9	0	20030101	20030101	
D6624	1862a(12)						Y1	9	0	20050101	20050101	
D6634	1862a(12)						Y1	9	0	20050101	20050101	
D6710	1862a(12)						Y1	9	0	20050101	20050101	
D6720	1862a(12)						Y1	9	0	19840101	19960101	
D6721	1862a(12)						Y1	9	0	19860101	19960101	
D6722	1862a(12)						Y1	9	0	19840101	19960101	
D6740							Y1	9	0	20000101	20000101	
D6750	1862a(12)						Y1	9	0	19840101	19960101	
D6751	1862a(12)						Y1	9	0	19840101	19960101	
D6752	1862a(12)						Y1	9	0	19840101	19960101	
D6780	1862a(12)						Y1	9	0	19840101	19960101	
D6781							Y1	9	0	20000101	20000101	
D6782							Y1	9	0	20000101	20000101	
D6783							Y1	9	0	20000101	20000101	
D6790	1862a(12)						Y1	9	0	19840101	19960101	
D6791	1862a(12)						Y1	9	0	19840101	19960101	
D6792	1862a(12)						Y1	9	0	19840101	19960101	
D6793	1862a(12)						Y1	9	0	20030101	20030101	
D6794	1862a(12)						Y1	9	0	20050101	20050101	
D6920							Y1	9	0	19960101	19960101	
D6930	1862a(12)						Y1	9	0	19820101	19960101	
D6940	1862a(12)						Y1	9	0	19820101	19960101	
D6950	1862a(12)						Y1	9	0	19820101	19960101	
D6970	1862a(12)						Y1	9	0	19860101	20070101	
D6971	1862a(12)						Y1	9	0	19860101	20070101	20061231
D6972	1862a(12)						Y1	9	0	19860101	19960101	
D6973	1862a(12)						Y1	9	0	19920101	19960101	
D6975	1862a(12)						Y1	9	0	19920101	19960101	
D6976							Y1	9	0	20000101	20070101	
D6977							Y1	9	0	20000101	20000101	
D6980	1862a(12)						Y1	9	0	19860101	19960101	
D6985	1862a(12)						Y1	9	0	20030101	20030101	
D6999	1862a(12)						Y1	9	s	19840101	19960101	
D7111							Y1	2	0	20030101	20050101	

HCPCS Code	Long Description	Coverage	Action	PI	MPI	CIM	MCM
D7140	EXTRACTION, ERUPTED TOOTH OR EXPOSED ROOT (ELEVATION AND/OR FORCEPS REMOVAL)	D	N	13	A		2336
D7210	SURGICAL REMOVAL OF ERUPTED TOOTH REQUIRING ELEVATION OF MUCOPERIOSTEAL FLAP AND REMOVAL OF BONE AND/OR SECTION OF TOOTH	D	N	13	A		2336, 2136
D7220	REMOVAL OF IMPACTED TOOTH-SOFT TISSUE	D	N	13	A		2336, 2136
D7230	REMOVAL OF IMPACTED TOOTH-PARTIALLY BONY	D	N	13	A		2336, 2136
D7240	REMOVAL OF IMPACTED TOOTH-COMPLETELY BONY	D	N	13	A		2336, 2136
D7241	REMOVAL OF IMPACTED TOOTH-COMPLETELY BONY, WITH UNUSUAL SURGICAL COMPLICATIONS	D	N	13	A		2336, 2136
D7250	SURGICAL REMOVAL OF RESIDUAL TOOTH ROOTS (CUTTING PROCEDURE)	D	N	13	A		2336, 2136
D7260	ORAL ANTRAL FISTULA CLOSURE	D	N	13	A		2336, 2136
D7261	PRIMARY CLOSURE OF A SINUS PERFORATION	D	N	13	A		2336
D7270	TOOTH REIMPLANTATION AND/OR STABILIZATION OF ACCIDENTALLY EVULSED OR DISPLACED TOOTH	S	N	00	9		
D7272	TOOTH TRANSPLANTATION (INCLUDES REIMPLANTATION FROM ONE SITE TO ANOTHER AND SPLINTING AND/OR STABILIZATION)	S	N	00	9		
D7280	SURGICAL ACCESS OF AN UNERUPTED TOOTH	S	N	00	9		
D7282	MOBILIZATION OF ERUPTED OR MALPOSITIONED TOOTH TO AID ERUPTION	S	N	00	9		
D7283	PLACEMENT OF DEVICE TO FACILITATE ERUPTION OF IMPACTED TOOTH	D	F	00	9		
D7285	BIOPSY OF ORAL TISSUE - HARD (BONE, TOOTH)	I	N	00	9		
D7286	BIOPSY OF ORAL TISSUE - SOFT	I	N	00	9		
D7287	EXFOLIATIVE CYTOLOGICAL SAMPLE COLLECTION	I	N	00	9		
D7288	BRUSH BIOPSY - TRANSEPITHELIAL SAMPLE COLLECTION	D	F	00	9		
D7290	SURGICAL REPOSITIONING OF TEETH	S	N	00	9		
D7291	TRANSSEPTAL FIBEROTOMY/SUPRA CRESTAL FIBEROTOMY, BY REPORT	D	N	13	A		2136, 2336
D7292	SURGICAL PLACEMENT: TEMPORARY ANCHORAGE DEVICE [SCREW RETAINED PLATE] REQUIRING SURGICAL FLAP	S	N	00	9		
D7293	SURGICAL PLACEMENT: TEMPORARY ANCHORAGE DEVICE REQUIRING SURGICAL FLAP	S	N	00	9		
D7294	SURGICAL PLACEMENT: TEMPORARY ANCHORAGE DEVICE WITHOUT SURGICAL FLAP	S	N	00	9		
D7310	ALVEOLOPLASTY IN CONJUNCTION WITH EXTRACTIONS - FOUR OR MORE TEETH OR TOOTH SPACES, PER QUADRANT	I	N	00	9		
D7311	ALVEOLOPLASTY IN CONJUNCTION WITH EXTRACTIONS - ONE TO THREE TEETH OR TOOTH SPACES, PER QUADRANT	S	N	00	9		
D7320	ALVEOLOPLASTY NOT IN CONJUNCTION WITH EXTRACTIONS - FOUR OR MORE TEETH OR TOOTH SPACES, PER QUADRANT	I	N	00	9		
D7321	ALVEOLOPLASTY NOT IN CONJUNCTION WITH EXTRACTIONS - ONE TO THREE TEETH OR TOOTH SPACES, PER QUADRANT	D	F	00	9		
D7340	VESTIBULOPLASTY-RIDGE EXTENSION (SECOND EPITHELIALIZATION)	I	N	00	9		

HCPCS Code	Statute	Lab Cert	X-Ref	ASC Pay Grp	ASC Pay Group Eff. Date	Proc Notes	BETOS	TOS	Anest	Code Add Date	Code Effective Date	Code Term Date
D7140							Y1	2	0	20030101	20030101	
D7210							Y1	2	0	19840101	19930101	
D7220							Y1	2	0	19840101	19930101	
D7230							Y1	2	0	19840101	19930101	
D7240							Y1	2	0	19840101	19930101	
D7241							Y1	2	0	19840101	19930101	
D7250							Y1	2	0	19840101	19930101	
D7260							Y1	2	0	19840101	19930101	
D7261							Y1	2	0	20030101	20030101	
D7270	1862a(12)						Y1	2	0	19840101	20030101	
D7272	1862a(12)						Y1	2	0	19820101	19960101	
D7280	1862a(12)						Y1	2	0	19840101	20030101	
D7282	1862a(12)						Y1	2	0	20030101	20030101	
D7283						0159	Y1	9	0	20050101	20100101	
D7285			20220, 25, 40, 45				Y1	2	0	19840101	20000101	
D7286			40808				Y1	2	0	19840101	20050101	
D7287							Y1	2	0	20030101	20050101	
D7288						0159	Y1	2	0	20050101	20100101	
D7290	1862a(12)						Y1	2	0	19820101	19960101	
D7291							Y1	2	0	19860101	20030101	
D7292	1862a(12)						Y1	2	0	20070101	20070101	
D7293	1862a(12)						Y1	2	0	20070101	20070101	
D7294	1862a(12)						Y1	2	0	20070101	20070101	
D7310			41874				Y1	2	0	19840101	20070101	
D7311	1862a(12)						Y1	2	0	20050101	20050101	
D7320			41870				Y1	2	0	19840101	20070101	
D7321						0159	Y1	2	0	20050101	20100101	
D7340			40840, 42-44				Y1	2	0	19840101	19960101	

HCPCS Code	Long Description	Coverage	Action	PI	MPI	CIM	MCM
D7350	VESTIBULOPLASTY-RIDGE EXTENSION (INCLUDING SOFT TISSUE GRAFTS, MUSCLE RE-ATTACHMENTS, REVISION OF SOFT TISSUE ATTACHMENT, AND MANAGEMENT OF HYPERTROPHIED AND HYPERPLASTIC TISSUE)	I	N	00	9		
D7410	EXCISION OF BENIGN LESION UP TO 1.25 CM	I	N	00	9		
D7411	EXCISION OF BENIGN LESION GREATER THAN 1.25 CM	I	N	00	9		
D7412	EXCISION OF BENIGN LESION, COMPLICATED	I	N	00	9		
D7413	EXCISION OF MALIGNANT LESION UP TO 1.25 CM	I	N	00	9		
D7414	EXCISION OF MALIGNANT LESION GREATER THAN 1.25 CM	I	N	00	9		
D7415	EXCISION OF MALIGNANT LESION, COMPLICATED	I	N	00	9		
D7440	EXCISION OF MALIGNANT TUMOR-LESION DIAMETER UP TO 1.25 CM	I	N	00	9		
D7441	EXCISION OF MALIGNANT TUMOR-LESION DIAMETER GREATER THAN 1.25 CM	I	N	00	9		
D7450	REMOVAL OF BENIGN ODONTOGENIC CYST OR TUMOR-LESION DIAMETER UP T0 1.25 CM	I	N	00	9		
D7451	REMOVAL OF BENIGN ODONTOGENIC CYST OR TUMOR-LESION DIAMETER GREATER THAN 1.25 CM	I	N	00	9		
D7460	REMOVAL OF BENIGN NONODONTOGENIC CYST OR TUMOR-LESION DIAMETER UP TO 1.25 CM	I	N	00	9		
D7461	REMOVAL OF BENIGN NONODONTOGENIC CYST OR TUMOR-LESION DIAMETER GREATER THAN 1.25 CM	I	N	00	9		
D7465	DESTRUCTION OF LESION(S) BY PHYSICAL OR CHEMICAL METHODS, BY REPORT	I	N	00	9		
D7471	REMOVAL OF LATERAL EXOSTOSIS (MAXILLA OR MANDIBLE)	I	N	00	9		
D7472	REMOVAL OF TORUS PALATINUS	I	N	00	9		
D7473	REMOVAL OF TORUS MANDIBULARIS	I	N	00	9		
D7485	SURGICAL REDUCTION OF OSSEOUS TUBEROSITY	I	N	00	9		
D7490	RADICAL RESECTION OF MAXILLA OR MANDIBLE	I	N	00	9		
D7510	INCISION AND DRAINAGE OF ABSCESS-INTRAORAL SOFT TISSUE	I	N	00	9		
D7511	INCISION AND DRAINAGE OF ABSCESS - INTRAORAL SOFT TISSUE - COMPLICATED (INCLUDES DRAINAGE OF MULTIPLE FASCIAL SPACES)	D	F	00	9		
D7520	INCISION AND DRAINAGE OF ABSCESS-EXTRAORAL SOFT TISSUE	I	N	00	9		
D7521	INCISION AND DRAINAGE OF ABSCESS - EXTRAORAL SOFT TISSUE - COMPLICATED (INCLUDES DRAINAGE OF MULTIPLE FASCIAL SPACES)	D	F	00	9		
D7530	REMOVAL OF FOREIGN BODY FROM MUCOSA, SKIN, OR SUBCUTANEOUS ALVEOLAR TISSUE	I	N	00	9		
D7540	REMOVAL OF REACTION-PRODUCING FOREIGN BODIES-MUSCULOSKELETAL SYSTEM	I	N	00	9		
D7550	PARTIAL OSTECTOMY/SEQUESTRECTOMY FOR REMOVAL OF NON-VITAL BONE	I	N	00	9		
D7560	MAXILLARY SINUSOTOMY FOR REMOVAL OF TOOTH FRAGMENT OR FOREIGN BODY	I	N	00	9		
D7610	MAXILLA-OPEN REDUCTION (TEETH IMMOBILIZED IF PRESENT)	I	N	00	9		
D7620	MAXILLA-CLOSED REDUCTION (TEETH IMMOBILIZED IF PRESENT)	I	N	00	9		
D7630	MANDIBLE-OPEN REDUCTION (TEETH IMMOBILIZED IF PRESENT)	I	N	00	9		

D Codes

HCPCS Code	Statute	Lab Cert	X-Ref	ASC Pay Grp	ASC Pay Group Eff. Date	Proc Notes	BETOS	TOS	Anest	Code Add Date	Code Effective Date	Code Term Date
D7350			40845				Y1	2	0	19840101	19960101	
D7410			CPT			0020	Y1	2	0	19820101	20030101	
D7411							Y1	2	0	20030101	20030101	
D7412							Y1	2	0	20030101	20030101	
D7413							Y1	2	0	20030101	20030101	
D7414							Y1	2	0	20030101	20030101	
D7415							Y1	2	0	20030101	20030101	
D7440			CPT			0021	Y1	2	0	19840101	19960101	
D7441			CPT			0021	Y1	2	0	19840101	19960101	
D7450			CPT			0021	Y1	2	0	19840101	20030101	
D7451			CPT			0021	Y1	2	0	19840101	20030101	
D7460			CPT			0021	Y1	2	0	19840101	20030101	
D7461			CPT			0021	Y1	2	0	19840101	20030101	
D7465			41850				Y1	2	0	19840101	19960101	
D7471			21031, 32				Y1	2	0	20000101	20030101	
D7472							Y1	2	0	20030101	20030101	
D7473							Y1	2	0	20030101	20030101	
D7485							Y1	2	0	20030101	20030101	
D7490			21095				Y1	2	0	19820101	20050101	
D7510			41800				Y1	2	0	19840101	19960101	
D7511						0159	Y1	2	0	20050101	20100101	
D7520			40800				Y1	2	0	19840101	19960101	
D7521						0159	Y1	2	0	20050101	20100101	
D7530			41805, 28				Y1	2	0	19840101	20030101	
D7540			20520, 41800, 06				Y1	2	0	19840101	19960101	
D7550			20999				Y1	2	0	19820101	20030101	
D7560			31020				Y1	2	0	19820101	19960101	
D7610			CPT			0022	Y1	2	0	19840101	19960101	
D7620			CPT			0023	Y1	2	0	19840101	19960101	
D7630			CPT			0024	Y1	2	0	19840101	19960101	

HCPCS Code	Long Description	Coverage	Action	PI	MPI	CIM	MCM
D7640	MANDIBLE-CLOSED REDUCTION (TEETH IMMOBILIZED IF PRESENT)	I	N	00	9		
D7650	MALAR AND/OR ZYGOMATIC ARCH-OPEN REDUCTION	I	N	00	9		
D7660	MALAR AND/OR ZYGOMATIC ARCH-CLOSED REDUCTION	I	N	00	9		
D7670	ALVEOLUS - CLOSED REDUCTION, MAY INCLUDE STABILIZATION OF TEETH	I	N	00	9		
D7671	ALVEOLUS - OPEN REDUCTION, MAY INCLUDE STABILIZATION OF TEETH	I	N	00	9		
D7680	FACIAL BONES-COMPLICATED REDUCTION WITH FIXATION AND MULTIPLE SURGICAL APPROACHES	I	N	00	9		
D7710	MAXILLA-OPEN REDUCTION	I	N	00	9		
D7720	MAXILLA-CLOSED REDUCTION	I	N	00	9		
D7730	MANDIBLE-OPEN REDUCTION	I	N	00	9		
D7740	MANDIBLE-CLOSED REDUCTION	I	N	00	9		
D7750	MALAR AND/OR ZYGOMATIC ARCH-OPEN REDUCTION	I	N	00	9		
D7760	MALAR AND/OR ZYGOMATIC ARCH-CLOSED REDUCTION	I	N	00	9		
D7770	ALVEOLUS - OPEN REDUCTION STABILIZATION OF TEETH	I	N	00	9		
D7771	ALVEOLUS, CLOSED REDUCTION STABILIZATION OF TEETH	I	N	00	9		
D7780	FACIAL BONES-COMPLICATED REDUCTION WITH FIXATION AND MULTIPLE SURGICAL APPROACHES	I	N	00	9		
D7810	OPEN REDUCTION OF DISLOCATION	I	N	00	9		
D7820	CLOSED REDUCTION OF DISLOCATION	I	N	00	9		
D7830	MANIPULATION UNDER ANESTHESIA	I	N	00	9		
D7840	CONDYLECTOMY	I	N	00	9		
D7850	SURGICAL DISCECTOMY; WITH/WITHOUT IMPLANT	I	N	00	9		
D7852	DISC REPAIR	I	N	00	9		
D7854	SYNOVECTOMY	I	N	00	9		
D7856	MYOTOMY	I	N	00	9		
D7858	JOINT RECONSTRUCTION	I	N	00	9		
D7860	ARTHROTOMY	I	N	00	9		2336, 2136
D7865	ARTHROPLASTY	I	N	00	9		
D7870	ARTHROCENTESIS	I	N	00	9		
D7871	NON-ARTHROSCOPIC LYSIS AND LAVAGE	S	N	00	9		
D7872	ARTHROSCOPY-DIAGNOSIS, WITH OR WITHOUT BIOPSY	I	N	00	9		
D7873	ARTHROSCOPY-SURGICAL: LAVAGE AND LYSIS OF ADHESIONS	I	N	00	9		
D7874	ARTHROSCOPY-SURGICAL: DISC REPOSITIONING AND STABILIZATION	I	N	00	9		
D7875	ARTHROSCOPY-SURGICAL: SYNOVECTOMY	I	N	00	9		
D7876	ARTHROSCOPY-SURGICAL: DISCECTOMY	I	N	00	9		
D7877	ARTHROSCOPY-SURGICAL: DEBRIDEMENT	I	N	00	9		
D7880	OCCLUSAL ORTHOTIC APPLIANCE	I	N	00	9		
D7899	UNSPECIFIED TMD THERAPY, BY REPORT	I	N	00	9		
D7910	SUTURE OF RECENT SMALL WOUNDS UP TO 5 CM	I	N	00	9		
D7911	COMPLICATED SUTURE-UP TO 5 CM	I	N	00	9		
D7912	COMPLICATED SUTURE-GREATER THAN 5 CM	I	N	00	9		
D7920	SKIN GRAFT (IDENTIFY DEFECT COVERED, LOCATION, AND TYPE OF GRAFT)	I	N	00	9		
D7940	OSTEOPLASTY-FOR ORTHOGNATHIC DEFORMITIES	D	N	13	A		2336, 2136
D7941	OSTEOTOMY - MANDIBULAR RAMI	I	N	00	9		

HCPCS Code	Statute	Lab Cert	X-Ref	ASC Pay Grp	ASC Pay Group Eff. Date	Proc Notes	BETOS	TOS	Anest	Code Add Date	Code Effective Date	Code Term Date
D7640			CPT			0025	Y1	2	0	19840101	19960101	
D7650			CPT			0026	Y1	2	0	19840101	19960101	
D7660			CPT			0027	Y1	2	0	19840101	19960101	
D7670			CPT			0028	Y1	2	0	19840101	20030101	
D7671							Y1	2	0	20030101	20030101	
D7680			CPT			0029	Y1	2	0	19820101	19960101	
D7710			21346				Y1	2	0	19840101	19960101	
D7720			21345				Y1	2	0	19840101	19960101	
D7730			21461, 62				Y1	2	0	19840101	19960101	
D7740			21455				Y1	2	0	19840101	19960101	
D7750			21360, 65				Y1	2	0	19840101	19960101	
D7760			21355				Y1	2	0	19840101	19960101	
D7770			21422				Y1	2	0	19840101	20030101	
D7771							Y1	2	0	20030101	20030101	
D7780			21433, 35				Y1	2	0	19820101	19960101	
D7810			21490				Y1	2	0	19820101	19960101	
D7820			21480				Y1	2	0	19820101	19960101	
D7830			00190				Y1	2	0	19820101	19960101	
D7840			21050				Y1	2	0	19820101	19960101	
D7850			21060				Y1	2	0	19840101	19960101	
D7852			21299				Y1	2	0	19920101	19960101	
D7854			21299				Y1	2	0	19920101	19960101	
D7856			21299				Y1	2	0	19920101	19960101	
D7858			21242, 43				Y1	2	0	19920101	19960101	
D7860							Y1	2	0	19820101	19960101	
D7865			21240				Y1	2	0	19920101	19960101	
D7870			21060				Y1	2	0	19820101	19960101	
D7871	1862a(12)						Y1	2	0	20000101	20000101	
D7872			29800				Y1	2	0	19920101	19960101	
D7873			29804				Y1	2	0	19920101	19960101	
D7874			29804				Y1	2	0	19920101	19960101	
D7875			29804				Y1	2	0	19920101	19960101	
D7876			29804				Y1	2	0	19920101	19960101	
D7877			29804				Y1	2	0	19920101	19960101	
D7880			21499				Y1	2	0	19860101	19960101	
D7899			21499				Y1	2	0	19920101	19960101	
D7910			12011, 13				Y1	2	0	19840101	19960101	
D7911			12051, 52				Y1	2	0	19840101	19960101	
D7912			13132				Y1	2	0	19840101	19960101	
D7920			CPT			0030	Y1	2	0	19840101	19960101	
D7940							Y1	2	0	19820101	19930101	
D7941			21193, 95, 96				Y1	2	0	19840101	20000101	

HCPCS Code	Long Description	Coverage	Action	PI	MPI	CIM	MCM
D7943	OSTEOTOMY - MANDIBULAR RAMI WITH BONE GRAFT; INCLUDES OBTAINING THE GRAFT	I	N	00	9		
D7944	OSTEOTOMY-SEGMENTED OR SUBAPICAL	I	N	00	9		
D7945	OSTEOTOMY-BODY OF MANDIBLE	I	N	00	9		
D7946	LEFORT I (MAXILLA-TOTAL)	I	N	00	9		
D7947	LEFORT I (MAXILLA-SEGMENTED)	I	N	00	9		
D7948	LEFORT II OR LEFORT III (OSTEOPLASTY OF FACIAL BONES FOR MIDFACE HYPOPLASIA OR RETRUSION)-WITHOUT BONE GRAFT	I	N	00	9		
D7949	LEFORT II OR LEFORT III-WITH BONE GRAFT	I	N	00	9		
D7950	OSSEOUS, OSTEOPERIOSTEAL, OR CARTILAGE GRAFT OF THE MANDIBLE OR MAXILLA -AUTOGENOUS OR NONAUTOGENOUS, BY REPORT	I	N	00	9		
D7951	SINUS AUGMENTATION WITH BONE OR BONE SUBSTITUTES	S	N	00	9		
D7953	BONE REPLACEMENT GRAFT FOR RIDGE PRESERVATION - PER SITE	S	N	00	9		
D7955	REPAIR OF MAXILLOFACIAL SOFT AND/OR HARD TISSUE DEFECT	I	N	00	9		
D7960	FRENULECTOMY (FRENECTOMY OR FRENOTOMY)-SEPARATE PROCEDURE	I	N	00	9		
D7963	FRENULOPLASTY	S	N	00	9		
D7970	EXCISION OF HYPERPLASTIC TISSUE-PER ARCH	I	N	00	9		
D7971	EXCISION OF PERICORONAL GINGIVA	I	N	00	9		
D7972	SURGICAL REDUCTION OF FIBROUS TUBEROSITY	I	N	00	9		
D7980	SIALOLITHOTOMY	I	N	00	9		
D7981	EXCISION OF SALIVARY GLAND, BY REPORT	I	N	00	9		
D7982	SIALODOCHOPLASTY	I	N	00	9		
D7983	CLOSURE OF SALIVARY FISTULA	I	N	00	9		
D7990	EMERGENCY TRACHEOTOMY	I	N	00	9		
D7991	CORONOIDECTOMY	I	N	00	9		
D7995	SYNTHETIC GRAFT-MANDIBLE OR FACIAL BONES, BY REPORT	I	N	00	9		
D7996	IMPLANT-MANDIBLE FOR AUGMENTATION PURPOSES (EXCLUDING ALVEOLAR RIDGE), BY REPORT	I	N	00	9		
D7997	APPLIANCE REMOVAL (NOT BY DENTIST WHO PLACED APPLIANCE), INCLUDES REMOVAL OF ARCHBAR	S	N	00	9		
D7998	INTRAORAL PLACEMENT OF A FIXATION DEVICE NOT IN CONJUNCTION WITH A FRACTURE	S	N	00	9		
D7999	UNSPECIFIED ORAL SURGERY PROCEDURE, BY REPORT	I	N	00	9		
D8010	LIMITED ORTHODONTIC TREATMENT OF THE PRIMARY DENTITION	S	N	00	9		
D8020	LIMITED ORTHODONTIC TREATMENT OF THE TRANSITIONAL DENTITION	S	N	00	9		
D8030	LIMITED ORTHODONTIC TREATMENT OF THE ADOLESCENT DENTITION	S	N	00	9		
D8040	LIMITED ORTHODONTIC TREATMENT OF THE ADULT DENTITION	S	N	00	9		
D8050	INTERCEPTIVE ORTHODONTIC TREATMENT OF THE PRIMARY DENTITION	S	N	00	9		
D8060	INTERCEPTIVE ORTHODONTIC TREATMENT OF THE TRANSITIONAL DENTITION	S	N	00	9		

HCPCS Code	Statute	Lab Cert	X-Ref	ASC Pay Grp	ASC Pay Group Eff. Date	Proc Notes	BETOS	TOS	Anest	Code Add Date	Code Effective Date	Code Term Date
D7943			21194				Y1	2	0	19840101	20000101	
D7944			21198, 21206				Y1	2	0	19840101	20070101	
D7945			21193-96				Y1	2	0	19840101	19960101	
D7946			21147				Y1	2	0	19840101	19960101	
D7947			21145, 46				Y1	2	0	19840101	19960101	
D7948			21150				Y1	2	0	19840101	19960101	
D7949			CPT			0031	Y1	2	0	19840101	19960101	
D7950			21247				Y1	2	0	19840101	20070101	
D7951	1862a(12)						Y1	2	0	20070101	20070101	
D7953	1862a(12)						Y1	2	0	20050101	20050101	
D7955			21299				Y1	2	0	19820101	20050101	
D7960			40819, 41010, 15						Y1	2	0	19840101
D7963	1862a(12)						Y1	2	0	20050101	20050101	
D7970			CPT			0032	Y1	2	0	19840101	19960101	
D7971			41821				Y1	2	0	19860101	19960101	
D7972							Y1	2	0	20030101	20030101	
D7980			42330, 35, 40				Y1	2	0	19820101	19960101	
D7981			42408				Y1	2	0	19820101	19960101	
D7982			42500				Y1	2	0	19840101	19960101	
D7983			42600				Y1	2	0	19820101	19960101	
D7990			31605				Y1	2	0	19820101	19960101	
D7991			21070				Y1	2	0	19850101	19960101	
D7995			21299				Y1	2	0	19960101	19960101	
D7996			21299				Y1	2	0	19960101	19960101	
D7997	1862a(12)						Y1	2	0	20000101	20000101	
D7998	1862a(12)						Y1	2	0	20070101	20070101	
D7999			21299				Y1	2	0	19840101	19960101	
D8010	1862a(12)						Y1	1	0	19960101	19960101	
D8020	1862a(12)						Y1	1	0	19960101	19960101	
D8030	1862a(12)						Y1	1	0	19960101	19960101	
D8040	1862a(12)						Y1	1	0	19960101	19960101	
D8050	1862a(12)						Y1	1	0	19960101	19960101	
D8060	1862a(12)						Y1	1	0	19960101	19960101	

HCPCS Code	Long Description	Coverage	Action	PI	MPI	CIM	MCM
D8070	COMPREHENSIVE ORTHODONTIC TREATMENT OF THE TRANSITIONAL DENTITION	S	N	00	9		
D8080	COMPREHENSIVE ORTHODONTIC TREATMENT OF THE ADOLESCENT DENTITION	S	N	00	9		
D8090	COMPREHENSIVE ORTHODONTIC TREATMENT OF THE ADULT DENTITION	S	N	00	9		
D8210	REMOVABLE APPLIANCE THERAPY	S	N	00	9		
D8220	FIXED APPLIANCE THERAPY	S	N	00	9		
D8660	PRE-ORTHODONTIC VISIT	S	N	00	9		
D8670	PERIODIC ORTHODONTIC TREATMENT VISIT (AS PART OF CONTRACT)	S	N	00	9		
D8680	ORTHODONTIC RETENTION (REMOVAL OF APPLIANCES, CONSTRUCTION AND PLACEMENT OF RETAINER(S))	S	N	00	9		
D8690	ORTHODONTIC TREATMENT (ALTERNATIVE BILLING TO A CONTRACT FEE)	S	N	00	9		
D8691	REPAIR OF ORTHODONTIC APPLIANCE	S	N	00	9		
D8692	REPLACEMENT OF LOST OR BROKEN RETAINER	S	N	00	9		
D8693	REBONDING OR RECEMENTING; AND/OR REPAIR, AS REQUIRED, OF FIXED RETAINERS	S	N	00	9		
D8999	UNSPECIFIED ORTHODONTIC PROCEDURE, BY REPORT	S	N	00	9		
D9110	PALLIATIVE (EMERGENCY) TREATMENT OF DENTAL PAIN-MINOR PROCEDURES	D	N	13	A		2336, 2136
D9120	FIXED PARTIAL DENTURE SECTIONING	S	N	00	9		
D9210	LOCAL ANESTHESIA N0T IN CONJUNCTION WITH OPERATIVE OR SURGICAL PROCEDURES	I	N	00	9		
D9211	REGIONAL BLOCK ANESTHESIA	I	N	00	9		
D9212	TRIGEMINAL DIVISION BLOCK ANESTHESIA	I	N	00	9		
D9215	LOCAL ANESTHESIA	I	N	00	9		
D9220	DEEP SEDATION/GENERAL ANESTHESIA-FIRST 30 MINUTES	I	N	00	9		
D9221	DEEP SEDATION/GENERAL ANESTHESIA-EACH ADDITIONAL 15 MINUTES	I	N	00	9		2136, 2336
D9230	ANALGESIA, ANXIOLYSIS, INHALATION OF NITROUS OXIDE	D	N	13	A		2136, 2336
D9241	INTRAVENOUS CONSCIOUS SEDATION/ANALGESIA - FIRST 30 MINUTES	I	N	00	9		
D9242	INTRAVENOUS CONSCIOUS SEDATION/ANALGESIA - EACH ADDITIONAL 15 MINUTES	I	N	00	9		
D9248	NON-INTRAVENOUS CONSCIOUS SEDATION	D	N	00	9		
D9310	CONSULTATION - DIAGNOSTIC SERVICE PROVIDED BY DENTIST OR PHYSICIAN OTHER THAN REQUESTING DENTIST OR PHYSICIAN	I	N	00	9		
D9410	HOUSE/EXTENDED CARE FACILITY CALL	I	N	00	9		
D9420	HOSPITAL CALL	I	N	00	9		
D9430	OFFICE VISIT FOR OBSERVATION (DURING REGULARLY SCHEDULED HOURS) NO OTHER SERVICES PERFORMED	I	N	00	9		
D9440	OFFICE VISIT-AFTER REGULARLY SCHEDULED HOURS	I	N	00	9		
D9450	CASE PRESENTATION, DETAILED AND EXTENSIVE TREATMENT PLANNING	I	N	00	9		
D9610	THERAPEUTIC PARENTERAL DRUG, SINGLE ADMINISTRATION	I	N	00	9		
D9612	THERAPEUTIC PARENTERAL DRUGS, TWO OR MORE ADMINISTRATIONS, DIFFERENT MEDICATIONS	S	N	00	9		

HCPCS Code	Statute	Lab Cert	X-Ref	ASC Pay Grp	ASC Pay Group Eff. Date	Proc Notes	BETOS	TOS	Anest	Code Add Date	Code Effective Date	Code Term Date
D8070	1862a(12)						Y1	1	0	19960101	19960101	
D8080	1862a(12)						Y1	1	0	19960101	19960101	
D8090	1862a(12)						Y1	1	0	19960101	19960101	
D8210	1862a(12)						Y1	1	0	19820101	19960101	
D8220	1862a(12)						Y1	1	0	19840101	19960101	
D8660	1862a(12)						Y1	1	0	19960101	19960101	
D8670	1862a(12)						Y1	1	0	19960101	19960101	
D8680	1862a(12)						Y1	1	0	19960101	19960101	
D8690	1862a(12)						Y1	1	0	19960101	19960101	
D8691	1862a(12)						Y1	1	0	20000101	20000101	
D8692	1862a(12)						Y1	1	0	20000101	20000101	
D8693	1862a(12)						Y1	1	0	20070101	20070101	
D8999	1862a(12)						Y1	1	0	19840101	19960101	
D9110							Y1	1	0	19840101	19960101	
D9120	1862a(12)						Y1	2	0	20070101	20070101	
D9210			90784				Y1	7	0	19840101	19960101	
D9211			01995				Y1	7	0	19820101	19960101	
D9212			64400				Y1	7	0	19850101	19960101	
D9215			90784				Y1	7	0	19850101	19960101	
D9220			CPT			0034	Y1	7	0	19820101	20030101	
D9221							Y1	7	0	19920101	20030101	
D9230							Y1	7	0	19820101	20000101	
D9241			90784				Y1	7	0	20000101	20030101	
D9242			90784				Y1	7	0	20000101	20030101	
D9248						0052	Y1	7	0	20000101	20000101	
D9310			CPT			0035	Y1	3	0	19820101	20070101	
D9410			CPT			0036	Y1	1	0	19840101	20000101	
D9420			CPT			0037	Y1	1	0	19840101	19960101	
D9430			CPT			0038	Y1	1	0	19840101	19960101	
D9440			99050				Y1	1	0	19840101	19960101	
D9450							Y1	1	0	20030101	20030101	
D9610							Y1	9	0	19840101	20070101	
D9612	1862a(12)						Y1	9	0	20070101	20070101	

HCPCS Code	Long Description	Coverage	Action	PI	MPI	CIM	MCM
D9630	OTHER DRUGS AND/OR MEDICAMENTS, BY REPORT	D	N	13	A		2336, 2136
D9910	APPLICATION OF DESENSITIZING MEDICAMENT	S	N	00	9		
D9911	APPLICATION OF DESENSITIZING RESIN FOR CERVICAL AND/OR ROOT SURFACE, PER TOOTH	S	N	00	9		
D9920	BEHAVIOR MANAGEMENT, BY REPORT	S	N	00	9		
D9930	TREATMENT OF COMPLICATIONS (POSTSURGICAL) - UNUSUAL CIRCUMSTANCES, BY REPORT	D	N	13	A		2336, 2136
D9940	OCCLUSAL GUARDS, BY REPORT	D	N	13	A		2336, 2136
D9941	FABRICATION OF ATHLETIC MOUTHGUARD	S	N	00	9		
D9942	REPAIR AND/OR RELINE OF OCCLUSAL GUARD	S	N	00	9		
D9950	OCCLUSION ANALYSIS-MOUNTED CASE	D	N	13	A		2336, 2136
D9951	OCCLUSAL ADJUSTMENT-LIMITED	D	N	13	A		2336, 2136
D9952	OCCLUSAL ADJUSTMENT-COMPLETE	D	N	13	A		2336, 2136
D9970	ENAMEL MICROABRASION	S	N	00	9		
D9971	ODONTOPLASTY 1 - 2 TEETH; INCLUDES REMOVAL OF ENAMEL PROJECTIONS	S	N	00	9		
D9972	EXTERNAL BLEACHING - PER ARCH	S	N	00	9		
D9973	EXTERNAL BLEACHING - PER TOOTH	S	N	00	9		
D9974	INTERNAL BLEACHING - PER TOOTH	S	N	00	9		
D9999	UNSPECIFIED ADJUNCTIVE PROCEDURE, BY REPORT	I	N	00	9		
E0100	CANE, INCLUDES CANES OF ALL MATERIALS, ADJUSTABLE OR FIXED, WITH TIP	D	N	32	A	60-3,60-9	2100.1
E0105	CANE, QUAD OR THREE PRONG, INCLUDES CANES OF ALL MATERIALS, ADJUSTABLE OR FIXED, WITH TIPS	D	N	32	A	60-15,60-9	2100.1
E0110	CRUTCHES, FOREARM, INCLUDES CRUTCHES OF VARIOUS MATERIALS, ADJUSTABLE OR FIXED, PAIR, COMPLETE WITH TIPS AND HANDGRIPS	D	N	32	A	60-9	2100.1
E0111	CRUTCH FOREARM, INCLUDES CRUTCHES OF VARIOUS MATERIALS, ADJUSTABLE OR FIXED, EACH, WITH TIP AND HANDGRIPS	D	N	32	A	60-9	2100.1
E0112	CRUTCHES UNDERARM, WOOD, ADJUSTABLE OR FIXED, PAIR, WITH PADS, TIPS AND HANDGRIPS	D	N	32	A	60-9	2100.1
E0113	CRUTCH UNDERARM, WOOD, ADJUSTABLE OR FIXED, EACH, WITH PAD, TIP AND HANDGRIP	D	N	32	A	60-9	2100.1
E0114	CRUTCHES UNDERARM, OTHER THAN WOOD, ADJUSTABLE OR FIXED, PAIR, WITH PADS, TIPS AND HANDGRIPS	D	N	32	A	60-9	2100.1
E0116	CRUTCH, UNDERARM, OTHER THAN WOOD, ADJUSTABLE OR FIXED, WITH PAD, TIP, HANDGRIP, WITH OR WITHOUT SHOCK ABSORBER, EACH	D	N	32	A	60-9	2100.1
E0117	CRUTCH, UNDERARM, ARTICULATING, SPRING ASSISTED, EA.	D	N	32	A		2100.1
E0118	CRUTCH SUBSTITUTE, LOWER LEG PLATFORM, WITH OR WITHOUT WHEELS, EACH	C	N	32	A		
E0130	WALKER, RIGID (PICKUP), ADJUSTABLE OR FIXED HEIGHT	D	N	32	A	60-9	2100.1
E0135	WALKER, FOLDING (PICKUP), ADJUSTABLE OR FIXED HEIGHT	D	N	32	A	60-9	2100.1
E0140	WALKER, WITH TRUNK SUPPORT, ADJUSTABLE OR FIXED HEIGHT, ANY TYPE	D	N	32	A	60-9	2100.1
E0141	WALKER, RIGID, WHEELED, ADJUSTABLE OR FIXED HEIGHT	D	N	32	A	60-9	2100.1
E0143	WALKER, FOLDING, WHEELED, ADJUSTABLE OR FIXED HEIGHT	D	N	32	A	60-9	2100.1

HCPCS Code	Statute	Lab Cert	X-Ref	ASC Pay Grp	ASC Pay Group Eff. Date	Proc Notes	BETOS	TOS	Anest	Code Add Date	Code Effective Date	Code Term Date
D9630							Y1	9	0	19840101	19930101	
D9910	1862a(12)						Y1	1	0	19850101	19960101	
D9911	1862a(12)						Y1	1	0	20000101	20000101	
D9920	1862a(12)						Y1	1	0	19860101	19960101	
D9930							Y1	1	0	19840101	19930101	
D9940							Y1	1	0	19860101	19960101	
D9941	1862a(12)		21089				Y1	1	0	19860101	19960101	
D9942	1862a(12)						Y1	1	0	20050101	20050101	
D9950							Y1	1	0	19840101	19930101	
D9951							Y1	1	0	19860101	19930101	
D9952							Y1	1	0	19860101	19930101	
D9970	1862a(12)						Y1	1	0	19960101	19960101	
D9971	1862a(12)						Y1	1	0	20000101	20000101	
D9972	1862a(12)						Y1	1	0	20000101	20000101	
D9973	1862a(12)						Y1	1	0	20000101	20000101	
D9974	1862a(12)						Y1	1	0	20000101	20000101	
D9999			21499				Y1	1	0	19840101	19960101	
E0100							D1E	A,P,R	0	19860101	19960101	
E0105							D1E	A,P,R	0	19860101	19960101	
E0110							D1E	A,P,R	0	19860101	19960101	
E0111							D1E	A,P,R	0	19860101	19960101	
E0112							D1E	A,P,R	0	19860101	19960101	
E0113							D1E	A,P,R	0	19860101	19960101	
E0114							D1E	A,P,R	0	19860101	19970101	
E0116							D1E	A,P,R	0	19860101	20060101	
E0117							D1E	A,P,R	0	20030101	20030101	
E0118							D1E	A,P,R	0	20040101	20040401	
E0130							D1E	A,P,R	0	19860101	19960101	
E0135							D1E	A,P,R	0	19860101	19960101	
E0140							D1E	A,P,R	0	20040101	20040101	
E0141							D1E	A,P,R	0	19860101	20040101	
E0143							D1E	A,P,R	0	19860101	20040101	

HCPCS Code	Long Description	Coverage	Action	PI	MPI	CIM	MCM
E0144	WALKER, ENCLOSED, FOUR SIDED FRAMED, RIGID OR FOLDING, WHEELED WITH POSTERIOR SEAT	D	N	32	A	60-9	2100.1
E0147	WALKER, HEAVY DUTY, MULTIPLE BRAKING SYSTEM, VARIABLE WHEEL RESISTANCE	D	N	32	A	60-15	2100.1
E0148	WALKER, HEAVY DUTY, WITHOUT WHEELS, RIGID OR FOLDING, ANY TYPE, EACH	C	N	32	A		
E0149	WALKER, HEAVY DUTY, WHEELED, RIGID OR FOLDING, ANY TYPE	C	N	32	A		
E0153	PLATFORM ATTACHMENT, FOREARM CRUTCH, EACH	C	N	32	A		
E0154	PLATFORM ATTACHMENT, WALKER, EACH	C	N	32	A		
E0155	WHEEL ATTACHMENT, RIGID PICK-UP WALKER, PER PAIR	C	N	32	A		
E0156	SEAT ATTACHMENT, WALKER	C	N	32	A		
E0157	CRUTCH ATTACHMENT, WALKER, EACH	C	N	32	A		
E0158	LEG EXTENSIONS FOR WALKER, PER SET OF FOUR (4)	C	N	32	A		
E0159	BRAKE ATTACHMENT FOR WHEELED WALKER, REPLACEMENT, EACH	C	N	32	A		
E0160	SITZ TYPE BATH OR EQUIPMENT, PORTABLE, USED WITH OR WITHOUT COMMODE	D	N	32	A	60-9	
E0161	SITZ TYPE BATH OR EQUIPMENT, PORTABLE, USED WITH OR WITHOUT COMMODE, WITH FAUCET ATTACHMENT/S	D	N	32	A	60-9	
E0162	SITZ BATH CHAIR	D	N	32	A	60-9	
E0163	COMMODE CHAIR, MOBILE OR STATIONARY, WITH FIXED ARMS	D	N	32	A	60-9	2100.1
E0164	COMMODE CHAIR, MOBILE, WITH FIXED ARMS	D	N	32	A	60-9	2100.1
E0165	COMMODE CHAIR, MOBILE OR STATIONARY, WITH DETACHABLE ARMS	D	N	36	A	60-9	2100.1
E0166	COMMODE CHAIR, MOBILE, WITH DETACHABLE ARMS	D	N	36	A	60-9	2100.1
E0167	PAIL OR PAN FOR USE WITH COMMODE CHAIR, REPLACEMENT ONLY	D	N	32	A	60-9	
E0168	COMMODE CHAIR, EXTRA WIDE AND/OR HEAVY DUTY, STATIONARY OR MOBILE, WITH OR WITHOUT ARMS, ANY TYPE, EACH	C	N	32	A		
E0170	COMMODE CHAIR WITH INTEGRATED SEAT LIFT MECHANISM, ELECTRIC, ANY TYPE	C	N	36	A		
E0171	COMMODE CHAIR WITH INTEGRATED SEAT LIFT MECHANISM, NON-ELECTRIC, ANY TYPE	C	N	36	A		
E0172	SEAT LIFT MECHANISM PLACED OVER OR ON TOP OF TOILET, ANY TYPE	S	N	00	9		
E0175	FOOT REST, FOR USE WITH COMMODE CHAIR, EACH	C	N	32	A		
E0180	PRESSURE PAD, ALTERNATING WITH PUMP	D	N	36	A	60-9	4107.6
E0181	POWERED PRESSURE REDUCING MATTRESS OVERLAY/PAD, ALTERNATING, WITH PUMP, INCLUDES HEAVY DUTY	D	N	36	A	60-9	4107.6
E0182	PUMP FOR ALTERNATING PRESSURE PAD, FOR REPLACEMENT ONLY	D	N	36	A	60-9	4107.6
E0184	DRY PRESSURE MATTRESS	D	N	32	A	60-9	4107.6
E0185	GEL OR GEL-LIKE PRESSURE PAD FOR MATTRESS, STANDARD MATTRESS LENGTH AND WIDTH	D	N	32	A	60-9	4107.6
E0186	AIR PRESSURE MATTRESS	D	N	36	A	60-9	
E0187	WATER PRESSURE MATTRESS	D	N	36	A	60-9	
E0188	SYNTHETIC SHEEPSKIN PAD	D	N	32	A	60-9	4107.6

HCPCS Code	Statute	Lab Cert	X-Ref	ASC Pay Grp	ASC Pay Group Eff. Date	Proc Notes	BETOS	TOS	Anest	Code Add Date	Code Effective Date	Code Term Date
E0144							D1E	A,P,R	0	20000101	20071005	
E0147							D1E	A,P,R	0	19860101	20040101	
E0148							D1E	A,P,R	0	20010101	20010101	
E0149							D1E	A,P,R	0	20010101	20040101	
E0153							D1E	A,P,R	0	19860101	19960101	
E0154							D1E	A,P,R	0	19860101	19960101	
E0155							D1E	A,P,R	0	19860101	20000101	
E0156							D1E	A,P,R	0	19860101	19960101	
E0157							D1E	A,P,R	0	19860101	19960101	
E0158							D1E	A,P,R	0	19860101	20000101	
E0159							D1E	A,P,R	0	19970101	19980101	
E0160							D1E	A,P,R	0	19860101	19960101	
E0161							D1E	A,P,R	0	19860101	19960101	
E0162							D1E	A,P,R	0	19860101	19960101	
E0163							D1E	A,P,R	0	19860101	20070101	
E0164							D1E	A,P,R	0	19860101	20070101	20061231
E0165							D1E	R	0	19860101	20070101	
E0166							D1E	R	0	19860101	20070101	20061231
E0167							D1E	A,P,R	0	19860101	20070101	
E0168							D1E	A,P,R	0	20010101	20010101	
E0170							D1E	A,P,R	0	20060101	20060101	
E0171							D1E	A,P,R	0	20060101	20060101	
E0172	1861SSA						D1E	A,P,R	0	20060101	20060101	
E0175							D1E	A,P,R	0	19860101	19960101	
E0180							D1E	R	0	19860101	20070101	20061231
E0181							D1E	R	0	19860101	20070101	
E0182							D1E	R	0	19860101	20070101	
E0184							D1E	A,P,R	0	19860101	19960101	
E0185							D1E	A,P,R	0	19860101	19980101	
E0186							D1E	R	0	19860101	19960101	
E0187							D1E	R	0	19860101	19960101	
E0188							D1E	A,P,R	0	19860101	20010101	

HCPCS Code	Long Description	Coverage	Action	PI	MPI	CIM	MCM
E0189	LAMBSWOOL SHEEPSKIN PAD, ANY SIZE	D	N	32	A	60-9	4107.6
E0190	POSITIONING CUSHION/PILLOW/WEDGE, ANY SHAPE OR SIZE, INCLUDES ALL COMPONENTS AND ACCESSORIES	D	N	00	9		2100.1
E0191	HEEL OR ELBOW PROTECTOR, EACH	C	N	32	A		
E0193	POWERED AIR FLOTATION BED (LOW AIR LOSS THERAPY)	C	N	36	A		
E0194	AIR FLUIDIZED BED	D	N	36	A	60-19	
E0196	GEL PRESSURE MATTRESS	D	N	36	A	60-9	
E0197	AIR PRESSURE PAD FOR MATTRESS, STANDARD MATTRESS LENGTH AND WIDTH	D	N	32	A	60-9	
E0198	WATER PRESSURE PAD FOR MATTRESS, STANDARD MATTRESS LENGTH AND WIDTH	D	N	32	A	60-9	
E0199	DRY PRESSURE PAD FOR MATTRESS, STANDARD MATTRESS LENGTH AND WIDTH	D	N	32	A	60-9	
E0200	HEAT LAMP, WITHOUT STAND (TABLE MODEL), INCLUDES BULB, OR INFRARED ELEMENT	D	N	32	A	60-9	2100.1
E0202	PHOTOTHERAPY (BILIRUBIN) LIGHT WITH PHOTOMETER	C	N	36	A		
E0203	THERAPEUTIC LIGHTBOX, MINIMUM 10,000 LUX, TABLE TOP MODEL	M	N	00	9	60-9	
E0205	HEAT LAMP, WITH STAND, INCLUDES BULB, OR INFRARED ELEMENT	D	N	32	A	60-9	2100.1
E0210	ELECTRIC HEAT PAD, STANDARD	D	N	32	A	60-9	
E0215	ELECTRIC HEAT PAD, MOIST	D	N	32	A	60-9	
E0217	WATER CIRCULATING HEAT PAD WITH PUMP	D	N	32	A	60-9	
E0218	WATER CIRCULATING COLD PAD WITH PUMP	D	N	36	A	60-9	
E0220	HOT WATER BOTTLE	C	N	32	A		
E0221	INFRARED HEATING PAD SYSTEM	C	N	00	9		
E0225	HYDROCOLLATOR UNIT, INCLUDES PADS	D	N	32	A	60-9	2210.3
E0230	ICE CAP OR COLLAR	C	N	32	A		
E0231	NON-CONTACT WOUND WARMING DEVICE (TEMPERATURE CONTROL UNIT, AC ADAPTER AND POWER CORD) FOR USE WITH WARMING CARD AND WOUND COVER	M	N	00	9		2303
E0232	WARMING CARD FOR USE WITH THE NON CONTACT WOUND WARMING DEVICE AND NON CONTACT WOUND WARMING WOUND COVER	M	N	00	9		2303
E0235	PARAFFIN BATH UNIT, PORTABLE (SEE MEDICAL SUPPLY CODE A4265 FOR PARAFFIN)	D	N	36	A	60-9	2210.3
E0236	PUMP FOR WATER CIRCULATING PAD	D	N	36	A	60-9	
E0238	NON-ELECTRIC HEAT PAD, MOIST	D	N	32	A	60-9	
E0239	HYDROCOLLATOR UNIT, PORTABLE	D	N	32	A	60-9	2210.3
E0240	BATH/SHOWER CHAIR, WITH OR WITHOUT WHEELS, ANY SIZE	M	N	00	9	60-9	
E0241	BATH TUB WALL RAIL, EACH	M	N	00	9	60-9	2100.1
E0242	BATH TUB RAIL, FLOOR BASE	M	N	00	9	60-9	2100.1
E0243	TOILET RAIL, EACH	M	N	00	9	60-9	2100.1
E0244	RAISED TOILET SEAT	M	N	00	9	60-9	
E0245	TUB STOOL OR BENCH	M	N	00	9	60-9	
E0246	TRANSFER TUB RAIL ATTACHMENT	C	N	00	9		
E0247	TRANSFER BENCH FOR TUB OR TOILET WITH OR WITHOUT COMMODE OPENING	D	N	00	9	60-9	

HCPCS Code	Statute	Lab Cert	X-Ref	ASC Pay Grp	ASC Pay Group Eff. Date	Proc Notes	BETOS	TOS	Anest	Code Add Date	Code Effective Date	Code Term Date
E0189							D1E	A,P,R	0	19860101	20010101	
E0190							D1E	9	0	20040101	20070101	
E0191							D1E	A,P,R	0	19860101	19960101	
E0193							D1E	R	0	19900101	19930101	
E0194						0013	D1E	R	0	19910101	19910101	
E0196							D1E	R	0	19910101	19910101	
E0197							D1E	A,P,R	0	19910101	19980101	
E0198							D1E	A,P,R	0	19910101	19980101	
E0199							D1E	A,P,R	0	19910101	19980101	
E0200							D1E	A,P,R	0	19860101	19960101	
E0202							D1E	R	0	19850101	19960101	
E0203							D1E	9	0	20030101	20050101	
E0205							D1E	A,P,R	0	19860101	19960101	
E0210							D1E	A,L,P,R	0	19860101	20030101	
E0215							D1E	A,P,R	0	19860101	19960101	
E0217							D1E	A,P,R	0	19970101	19970101	
E0218							D1E	A,P,R	0	19970101	19970101	
E0220							D1E	A,P,R	0	19860101	19960101	
E0221							D1E	A,P,R	0	20020101	20070101	
E0225							D1E	A,P,R	0	19860101	19960101	
E0230							D1E	A,P,R	0	19860101	19960101	
E0231							D1E	R	0	20020101	20020701	
E0232							D1E	P	0	20020101	20020701	
E0235							D1E	R	0	19860101	19960101	
E0236							D1E	R	0	19860101	19960101	
E0238							D1E	A,P,R	0	19860101	19960101	
E0239							D1E	A,P,R	0	19860101	19960101	
E0240							D1E	9	0	20040101	20060101	
E0241							D1E	A,P,R	0	19860101	19960101	
E0242							D1E	A,P,R	0	19860101	19960101	
E0243							D1E	A,P,R	0	19860101	19960101	
E0244							D1E	A,P,R	0	19860101	19960101	
E0245							D1E	A,P,R	0	19860101	19960101	
E0246							D1E	A,P,R	0	19860101	19960101	
E0247							D1E	A,P,R	0	20040101	20040101	

HCPCS Code	Long Description	Coverage	Action	PI	MPI	CIM	MCM
E0248	TRANSFER BENCH, HEAVY DUTY, FOR TUB OR TOILET WITH OR WITHOUT COMMODE OPENING	D	N	00	9	60-9	
E0249	PAD FOR WATER CIRCULATING HEAT UNIT, FOR REPLACEMENT ONLY	D	C	32	A	60-9	
E0250	HOSPITAL BED, FIXED HEIGHT, WITH ANY TYPE SIDE RAILS, WITH MATTRESS	D	N	36	A	60-18	2100.1
E0251	HOSPITAL BED, FIXED HEIGHT, WITH ANY TYPE SIDE RAILS, WITHOUT MATTRESS	D	N	36	A	60-18	2100.1
E0255	HOSPITAL BED, VARIABLE HEIGHT, HI-LO, WITH ANY TYPE SIDE RAILS, WITH MATTRESS	D	N	36	A	60-18	2100.1
E0256	HOSPITAL BED, VARIABLE HEIGHT, HI-LO, WITH ANY TYPE SIDE RAILS, WITHOUT MATTRESS	D	N	36	A	60-18	2100.1
E0260	HOSPITAL BED, SEMI-ELECTRIC (HEAD AND FOOT ADJUSTMENT), WITH ANY TYPE SIDE RAILS, WITH MATTRESS	D	N	36	A	60-18	2100.1
E0261	HOSPITAL BED, SEMI-ELECTRIC (HEAD AND FOOT ADJUSTMENT), WITH ANY TYPE SIDE RAILS, WITHOUT MATTRESS	D	N	36	A	60-18	2100.1
E0265	HOSPITAL BED, TOTAL ELECTRIC (HEAD, FOOT AND HEIGHT ADJUSTMENTS), WITH ANY TYPE SIDE RAILS, WITH MATTRESS	D	N	36	A	60-18	2100.1
E0266	HOSPITAL BED, TOTAL ELECTRIC (HEAD, FOOT AND HEIGHT ADJUSTMENTS), WITH ANY TYPE SIDE RAILS, WITHOUT MATTRESS	D	N	36	A	60-18	2100.1
E0270	HOSPITAL BED, INSTITUTIONAL TYPE INCLUDES: OSCILLATING, CIRCULATING AND STRYKER FRAME, WITH MATTRESS	M	N	00	9	60-9	
E0271	MATTRESS, INNERSPRING	D	N	32	A	60-18, 60-9	
E0272	MATTRESS, FOAM RUBBER	D	N	32	A	60-18, 60-9	
E0273	BED BOARD	M	N	00	9	60-9	
E0274	OVER-BED TABLE	M	N	00	9	60-9	
E0275	BED PAN, STANDARD, METAL OR PLASTIC	D	N	32	A	60-9	
E0276	BED PAN, FRACTURE, METAL OR PLASTIC	D	N	32	A	60-9	
E0277	POWERED PRESSURE-REDUCING AIR MATTRESS	D	N	36	A	60-9	
E0280	BED CRADLE, ANY TYPE	C	N	32	A		
E0290	HOSPITAL BED, FIXED HEIGHT, WITHOUT SIDE RAILS, WITH MATTRESS	D	N	36	A	60-18	2100.1
E0291	HOSPITAL BED, FIXED HEIGHT, WITHOUT SIDE RAILS, WITHOUT MATTRESS	D	N	36	A	60-18	2100.1
E0292	HOSPITAL BED, VARIABLE HEIGHT, HI-LO, WITHOUT SIDE RAILS, WITH MATTRESS	D	N	36	A	60-18	2100.1
E0293	HOSPITAL BED, VARIABLE HEIGHT, HI-LO, WITHOUT SIDE RAILS, WITHOUT MATTRESS	D	N	36	A	60-18	2100.1
E0294	HOSPITAL BED, SEMI-ELECTRIC (HEAD AND FOOT ADJUSTMENT), WITHOUT SIDE RAILS, WITH MATTRESS	D	N	36	A	60-18	2100.1
E0295	HOSPITAL BED, SEMI-ELECTRIC (HEAD AND FOOT ADJUSTMENT), WITHOUT SIDE RAILS, WITHOUT MATTRESS	D	N	36	A	60-18	2100.1
E0296	HOSPITAL BED, TOTAL ELECTRIC (HEAD, FOOT AND HEIGHT ADJUSTMENTS). WITHOUT SIDE RAILS, WITH MATTRESS	D	N	36	A	60-18	2100.1
E0297	HOSPITAL BED, TOTAL ELECTRIC (HEAD, FOOT AND HEIGHT ADJUSTMENTS), WITHOUT SIDE RAILS, WITHOUT MATTRESS	D	N	36	A	60-18	2100.1
E0300	PEDIATRIC CRIB, HOSPITAL GRADE, FULLY ENCLOSED	C	N	32	A		

HCPCS Code	Statute	Lab Cert	X-Ref	ASC Pay Grp	ASC Pay Group Eff. Date	Proc Notes	BETOS	TOS	Anest	Code Add Date	Code Effective Date	Code Term Date
E0248							D1E	A,P,R	0	20040101	20040101	
E0249							D1E	A,P,R	0	19860101	20100101	
E0250							D1B	R	0	19860101	19910101	
E0251							D1B	R	0	19860101	19910101	
E0255							D1B	R	0	19860101	19910101	
E0256							D1B	R	0	19910101	19910101	
E0260							D1B	R	0	19860101	19910101	
E0261							D1B	R	0	19910101	19910101	
E0265							D1B	R	0	19860101	19910101	
E0266							D1B	R	0	19860101	19910101	
E0270							D1B	R	0	19860101	19930101	
E0271							D1B	A,P,R	0	19860101	19930101	
E0272							D1B	A,P,R	0	19860101	19930101	
E0273							D1B	A,P,R	0	19860101	19890101	
E0274							D1B	A,P,R	0	19860101	19890101	
E0275							D1E	A,P,R	0	19860101	19960101	
E0276							D1E	A,P,R	0	19860101	19960101	
E0277							D1E	R	0	19920101	19980101	
E0280							D1B	A,P,R	0	19860101	19890101	
E0290							D1B	R	0	19910101	19910101	
E0291							D1B	R	0	19910101	19910101	
E0292							D1B	R	0	19910101	19910101	
E0293							D1B	R	0	19910101	19910101	
E0294							D1B	R	0	19910101	19910101	
E0295							D1B	R	0	19910101	19910101	
E0296							D1B	R	0	19910101	19920101	
E0297							D1B	R	0	19910101	19910101	
E0300							D1B	A,P,R	0	20040101	20040101	

HCPCS Code	Long Description	Coverage	Action	PI	MPI	CIM	MCM
E0301	HOSPITAL BED, HEAVY DUTY, EXTRA WIDE, WITH WEIGHT CAPACITY GREATER THAN 350 POUNDS, BUT LESS THAN OR EQUAL TO 600 POUNDS, WITH ANY TYPE SIDE RAILS, WITHOUT MATTRESS	D	N	36	A	60-18	
E0302	HOSPITAL BED, EXTRA HEAVY DUTY, EXTRA WIDE, WITH WEIGHT CAPACITY GREATER THAN 600 POUNDS, WITH ANY TYPE SIDE RAILS, WITHOUT MATTRESS	D	N	36	A	60-18	
E0303	HOSPITAL BED, HEAVY DUTY, EXTRA WIDE, WITH WEIGHT CAPACITY GREATER THAN 350 POUNDS, BUT LESS THAN OR EQUAL TO 600 POUNDS, WITH ANY TYPE SIDE RAILS, WITH MATTRESS	D	N	36	A	60-18	
E0304	HOSPITAL BED, EXTRA HEAVY DUTY, EXTRA WIDE, WITH WEIGHT CAPACITY GREATER THAN 600 POUNDS, WITH ANY TYPE SIDE RAILS, WITH MATTRESS	D	N	36	A	60-18	
E0305	BED SIDE RAILS, HALF LENGTH	D	N	36	A	60-18	
E0310	BED SIDE RAILS, FULL LENGTH	D	N	32	A	60-18	
E0315	BED ACCESSORY: BOARD, TABLE, OR SUPPORT DEVICE, ANY TYPE	M	N	00	9	60-9	
E0316	SAFETY ENCLOSURE FRAME/CANOPY FOR USE WITH HOSPITAL BED, ANY TYPE	C	N	36	A		
E0325	URINAL; MALE, JUG-TYPE, ANY MATERIAL	D	N	32	A	60-9	
E0326	URINAL; FEMALE, JUG-TYPE, ANY MATERIAL	D	N	32	A	60-9	
E0328	HOSPITAL BED, PEDIATRIC, MANUAL, 360 DEGREE SIDE ENCLOSURES, TOP OF HEADBOARD, FOOTBOARD AND SIDE RAILS UP TO 24 INCHES ABOVE THE SPRING, INCLUDES MATTRESS	C	N	36	A		
E0329	HOSPITAL BED, PEDIATRIC, ELECTRIC OR SEMI-ELECTRIC, 360 DEGREE SIDE ENCLOSURES, TOP OF HEADBOARD, FOOTBOARD AND SIDE RAILS UP TO 24 INCHES ABOVE THE SPRING, INCLUDES MATTRESS	C	N	36	A		
E0350	CONTROL UNIT FOR ELECTRONIC BOWEL IRRIGATION/ EVACUATION SYSTEM	C	N	57	A		
E0352	DISPOSABLE PACK (WATER RESERVOIR BAG, SPECULUM, VALVING MECHANISM AND COLLECTION BAG/BOX) FOR USE WITH THE ELECTRONIC BOWEL IRRIGATION/EVACUATION SYSTEM	C	N	57	A		
E0370	AIR PRESSURE ELEVATOR FOR HEEL	C	N	00	9		
E0371	NONPOWERED ADVANCED PRESSURE REDUCING OVERLAY FOR MATTRESS, STANDARD MATTRESS LENGTH AND WIDTH	C	N	36	A		
E0372	POWERED AIR OVERLAY FOR MATTRESS, STANDARD MATTRESS LENGTH AND WIDTH	C	N	36	A		
E0373	NONPOWERED ADVANCED PRESSURE REDUCING MATTRESS	C	N	36	A		
E0424	STATIONARY COMPRESSED GASEOUS OXYGEN SYSTEM, RENTAL; INCLUDES CONTAINER, CONTENTS, REGULATOR, FLOWMETER, HUMIDIFIER, NEBULIZER, CANNULA OR MASK, AND TUBING	D	N	33	A	60-4	4107.9
E0425	STATIONARY COMPRESSED GAS SYSTEM, PURCHASE; INCLUDES REGULATOR, FLOWMETER, HUMIDIFIER, NEBULIZER, CANNULA OR MASK, AND TUBING	D	N	00	9	60-4	4107.9

HCPCS Code	Statute	Lab Cert	X-Ref	ASC Pay Grp	ASC Pay Group Eff. Date	Proc Notes	BETOS	TOS	Anest	Code Add Date	Code Effective Date	Code Term Date
E0301							D1B	R	0	20040101	20040101	
E0302							D1B	R	0	20040101	20040101	
E0303							D1B	R	0	20040101	20040101	
E0304							D1B	R	0	20040101	20040101	
E0305							D1B	R	0	19860101	19900101	
E0310							D1B	A,P,R	0	19860101	19900101	
E0315							D1B	A,P,R	0	19860101	19970101	
E0316							D1B	A,P,R	0	20020101	20020101	
E0325							D1E	A,P,R	0	19860101	19960101	
E0326							D1E	A,P,R	0	19860101	19960101	
E0328							D1B	R	0	20080101	20080101	
E0329							D1B	R	0	20080101	20080101	
E0350							Z2	9	0	19950101	19950101	
E0352							Z2	9	0	19950101	19950101	
E0370							D1E	A,P,R	0	19970101	19980101	
E0371							D1E	A,P,R	0	19980101	19980101	
E0372							D1E	A,P,R	0	19980101	19980101	
E0373							D1E	A,P,R	0	19980101	19980101	
E0424							D1C	R	0	19930101	20010101	
E0424 E0425							D1C	R	0	19860101	19930101	

HCPCS Code	Long Description	Coverage	Action	PI	MPI	CIM	MCM
E0430	PORTABLE GASEOUS OXYGEN SYSTEM, PURCHASE; INCLUDES REGULATOR, FLOWMETER, HUMIDIFIER, CANNULA OR MASK, AND TUBING	D	N	00	9	60-4	4107.9
E0431	PORTABLE GASEOUS OXYGEN SYSTEM, RENTAL; INCLUDES PORTABLE CONTAINER, REGULATOR, FLOWMETER, HUMIDIFIER, CANNULA OR MASK, AND TUBING	D	N	33	A	60-4	4107.9
E0433	PORTABLE LIQUID OXYGEN SYSTEM, RENTAL; HOME LIQUEFIER USED TO FILL PORTABLE LIQUID OXYGEN CONTAINERS, INCLUDES PORTABLE CONTAINERS, REGULATOR, FLOWMETER, HUMIDIFIER, CANNULA OR MASK AND TUBING, WITH OR WITHOUT SUPPLY RESERVOIR AND CONTENTS GAUGE	C	A	33	A		
E0434	PORTABLE LIQUID OXYGEN SYSTEM, RENTAL; INCLUDES PORTABLE CONTAINER, SUPPLY RESERVOIR, HUMIDIFIER, FLOWMETER, REFILL ADAPTOR, CONTENTS GAUGE, CANNULA OR MASK, AND TUBING	D	N	33	A	60-4	4107.9
E0435	PORTABLE LIQUID OXYGEN SYSTEM, PURCHASE; INCLUDES PORTABLE CONTAINER, SUPPLY RESERVOIR, FLOWMETER, HUMIDIFIER, CONTENTS GAUGE, CANNULA OR MASK, TUBING AND REFILL ADAPTOR	D	N	00	9	60-4	4107.9
E0439	STATIONARY LIQUID OXYGEN SYSTEM, RENTAL; INCLUDES CONTAINER, CONTENTS, REGULATOR, FLOWMETER, HUMIDIFIER, NEBULIZER, CANNULA OR MASK, & TUBING	D	N	33	A	60-4	4107.9
E0440	STATIONARY LIQUID OXYGEN SYSTEM, PURCHASE; INCLUDES USE OF RESERVOIR, CONTENTS INDICATOR, REGULATOR, FLOWMETER, HUMIDIFIER, NEBULIZER, CANNULA OR MASK, AND TUBING	D	N	00	9	60-4	4107.9
E0441	STATIONARY OXYGEN CONTENTS, GASEOUS, 1 MONTH'S SUPPLY = 1 UNIT	D	C	33	A	60-4	4107.9
E0442	STATIONARY OXYGEN CONTENTS, LIQUID, 1 MONTH'S SUPPLY = 1 UNIT	D	C	33	A	60-4	4107.9
E0443	PORTABLE OXYGEN CONTENTS, GASEOUS, 1 MONTH'S SUPPLY = 1 UNIT	D	C	33	A	60-4	4107.9
E0444	PORTABLE OXYGEN CONTENTS, LIQUID, 1 MONTH'S SUPPLY = 1 UNIT	D	C	33	A	60-4	4107.9
E0445	OXIMETER DEVICE FOR MEASURING BLOOD OXYGEN LEVELS NON-INVASIVELY	C	N	00	9		
E0450	VOLUME CONTROL VENTILATOR, WITHOUT PRESSURE SUPPORT MODE, MAY INCLUDE PRESSURE CONTROL MODE, USED WITH INVASIVE INTERFACE (E.G., TRACHEOSTOMY TUBE)	D	N	31	A	60-9	
E0455	OXYGEN TENT, EXCLUDING CROUP OR PEDIATRIC TENTS	D	N	33	A	60-4	4107.9
E0457	CHEST SHELL (CUIRASS)	C	N	32	A		
E0459	CHEST WRAP	C	N	36	A		
E0460	NEGATIVE PRESSURE VENTILATOR; PORTABLE OR STATIONARY	D	N	31	A	60-9	
E0461	VOLUME CONTROL VENTILATOR, WITHOUT PRESSURE SUPPORT MODE, MAY INCLUDE PRESSURE CONTROL MODE, USED WITH NON-INVASIVE INTERFACE (E.G. MASK)	D	N	31	A	60-9	
E0462	ROCKING BED WITH OR WITHOUT SIDE RAILS	C	N	36	A		

HCPCS Code	Statute	Lab Cert	X-Ref	ASC Pay Grp	ASC Pay Group Eff. Date	Proc Notes	BETOS	TOS	Anest	Code Add Date	Code Effective Date	Code Term Date
E0430							D1C	R	0	19860101	19930101	
E0431							D1C	R	0	19930101	20010101	
E0433							D1C	A,P,R	0	20100101	20100101	
E0434							D1C	R	0	19930101	19930101	
E0435							D1C	R	0	19860101	19930101	
E0439							D1C	R	0	19930101	20010101	
E0440							D1C	R	0	19860101	19930101	
E0441							D1C	P	0	19930101	20100101	
E0442							D1C	P	0	19930101	20100101	
E0443							D1C	P	0	19930101	20100101	
E0444							D1C	P	0	19930101	20100101	
E0445							Z2	9	0	20030101	20030101	
E0450							D1E	R	0	19850101	20050101	
E0455							D1C	R	0	19860101	19900101	
E0457							D1E	A,P,R	0	19900101	20010101	
E0459							D1E	R	0	19900101	19960101	
E0460							D1E	R	0	19900101	19960101	
E0461							D1E	R	0	20030101	20050101	
E0462							D1B	R	0	19900101	19960101	

HCPCS Code	Long Description	Coverage	Action	PI	MPI	CIM	MCM
E0463	PRESSURE SUPPORT VENTILATOR WITH VOLUME CONTROL MODE, MAY INCLUDE PRESSURE CONTROL MODE, USED WITH INVASIVE INTERFACE (E.G. TRACHEOSTOMY TUBE)	C	N	31	A		
E0464	PRESSURE SUPPORT VENTILATOR WITH VOLUME CONTROL MODE, MAY INCLUDE PRESSURE CONTROL MODE, USED WITH NON-INVASIVE INTERFACE (E.G. MASK)	C	N	31	A		
E0470 E0470	RESPIRATORY ASSIST DEVICE, BI-LEVEL PRESSURE CAPABILITY, WITHOUT BACKUP RATE FEATURE, USED WITH NONINVASIVE INTERFACE, E.G., NASAL OR FACIAL MASK (INTERMITTENT ASSIST DEVICE WITH CONTINUOUS POSITIVE AIRWAY PRESSURE DEVICE)	D	N	36	A	60-9	
E0471	RESPIRATORY ASSIST DEVICE, BI-LEVEL PRESSURE CAPABILITY, WITH BACK-UP RATE FEATURE, USED WITH NONINVASIVE INTERFACE, E.G., NASAL OR FACIAL MASK (INTERMITTENT ASSIST DEVICE WITH CONTINUOUS POSITIVE AIRWAY PRESSURE DEVICE)	D	N	36	A	60-9	
E0472	RESPIRATORY ASSIST DEVICE, BI-LEVEL PRESSURE CAPABILITY, WITH BACKUP RATE FEATURE, USED WITH INVASIVE INTERFACE, E.G., TRACHEOSTOMY TUBE (INTERMITTENT ASSIST DEVICE WITH CONTINUOUS POSITIVE AIRWAY PRESSURE DEVICE)	D	N	36	A	60-9	
E0480	PERCUSSOR, ELECTRIC OR PNEUMATIC, HOME MODEL	D	N	36	A	60-9	
E0481	INTRAPULMONARY PERCUSSIVE VENTILATION SYSTEM AND RELATED ACCESSORIES	M	N	00	9	60-21	
E0482	COUGH STIMULATING DEVICE, ALTERNATING POSITIVE AND NEGATIVE AIRWAY PRESSURE	C	N	36	A		
E0483	HIGH FREQUENCY CHEST WALL OSCILLATION AIR-PULSE GENERATOR SYSTEM, (INCLUDES HOSES AND VEST), EACH	C	N	36	A		
E0484	OSCILLATORY POSITIVE EXPIRATORY PRESSURE DEVICE, NON-ELECTRIC, ANY TYPE, EACH	C	N	32	A		
E0485	ORAL DEVICE/APPLIANCE USED TO REDUCE UPPER AIRWAY COLLAPSIBILITY, ADJUSTABLE OR NON-ADJUSTABLE, PREFABRICATED, INCLUDES FITTING AND ADJUSTMENT	C	N	32	A		
E0486	ORAL DEVICE/APPLIANCE USED TO REDUCE UPPER AIRWAY COLLAPSIBILITY, ADJUSTABLE OR NON-ADJUSTABLE, CUSTOM FABRICATED, INCLUDES FITTING AND ADJUSTMENT	C	N	32	A		
E0487	SPIROMETER, ELECTRONIC, INCLUDES ALL ACCESSORIES	D	N	00	9		
E0500	IPPB MACHINE, ALL TYPES, WITH BUILT-IN NEBULIZATION; MANUAL OR AUTOMATIC VALVES; INTERNAL OR EXTERNAL POWER SOURCE	D	N	31	A	60-9	
E0550	HUMIDIFIER, DURABLE FOR EXTENSIVE SUPPLEMENTAL HUMIDIFICATION DURING IPPB TREATMENTS OR OXYGEN DELIVERY	D	N	33	A	60-9	
E0555	HUMIDIFIER, DURABLE, GLASS OR AUTOCLAVABLE PLASTIC BOTTLE TYPE, FOR USE WITH REGULATOR OR FLOWMETER	D	N	33	A	60-9	4107.9
E0560	HUMIDIFIER, DURABLE FOR SUPPLEMENTAL HUMIDIFICATION DURING IPPB TREATMENT OR OXYGEN DELIVERY	D	N	33	A	60-9	
E0561	HUMIDIFIER, NON-HEATED, USED WITH POSITIVE AIRWAY PRESSURE DEVICE	C	N	32	A		

HCPCS Code	Statute	Lab Cert	X-Ref	ASC Pay Grp	ASC Pay Group Eff. Date	Proc Notes	BETOS	TOS	Anest	Code Add Date	Code Effective Date	Code Term Date
E0463							D1E	R	0	20050101	20050101	
E0464							D1E	R	0	20050101	20050101	
E0470							D1E	R	0	20040101	20040101	
E0471							D1E	R	0	20040101	20060401	
E0472							D1E	R	0	20040101	20060401	
E0480							D1E	R	0	19860101	19960101	
E0481							D1E	A,P,R	0	20020101	20020701	
E0482							D1E	R	0	20020101	20020101	
E0483							D1E	R	0	20030101	20030101	
E0484							D1E	A,P,R	0	20030101	20030101	
E0485							D1E	P	0	20060101	20060101	
E0486							D1E	P	0	20060101	20060101	
E0487						0156	Z2	A,P,R	0	20090101	20090101	
E0500							D1E	R	0	19860101	19960101	
E0550							D1E	R	0	19860101	20050701	
E0555							D1C	P	0	19860101	19960101	
E0560							D1E	A,P,R	0	19860101	20050701	
E0561							D1E	A,P,R	0	20040101	20040101	

HCPCS Code	Long Description	Coverage	Action	PI	MPI	CIM	MCM
E0562	HUMIDIFIER, HEATED, USED WITH POSITIVE AIRWAY PRESSURE DEVICE	C	N	32	A		
E0565	COMPRESSOR, AIR POWER SOURCE FOR EQUIPMENT WHICH IS NOT SELF- CONTAINED OR CYLINDER DRIVEN	C	N	36	A		
E0570	NEBULIZER, WITH COMPRESSOR	D	N	36	A	60-9	4107.9
E0571	AEROSOL COMPRESSOR, BATTERY POWERED, FOR USE WITH SMALL VOLUME NEBULIZER	D	N	36	A	60-9	
E0572	AEROSOL COMPRESSOR, ADJUSTABLE PRESSURE, LIGHT DUTY FOR INTERMITTENT USE	C	N	36	A		
E0574	ULTRASONIC/ELECTRONIC AEROSOL GENERATOR WITH SMALL VOLUME NEBULIZER	C	N	36	A		
E0575	NEBULIZER, ULTRASONIC, LARGE VOLUME	D	N	31	A	60-9	
E0580	NEBULIZER, DURABLE, GLASS OR AUTOCLAVABLE PLASTIC, BOTTLE TYPE, FOR USE WITH REGULATOR OR FLOWMETER	D	N	32	A	60-9	4107.9
E0585	NEBULIZER, WITH COMPRESSOR AND HEATER	D	N	36	A	60-9	4107.9
E0600	RESPIRATORY SUCTION PUMP, HOME MODEL, PORTABLE OR STATIONARY, ELECTRIC	D	N	36	A	60-9	E0600
E0601	CONTINUOUS AIRWAY PRESSURE (CPAP) DEVICE	D	N	36	A	60-17	
E0602	BREAST PUMP, MANUAL, ANY TYPE	C	N	32	A		
E0603	BREAST PUMP, ELECTRIC (AC AND/OR DC), ANY TYPE	C	N	00	9		
E0604	BREAST PUMP, HOSPITAL GRADE, ELECTRIC (AC AND / OR DC), ANY TYPE	C	N	00	9		
E0605	VAPORIZER, ROOM TYPE	D	N	32	A	60-9	
E0606	POSTURAL DRAINAGE BOARD	D	N	36	A	60-9	
E0607	HOME BLOOD GLUCOSE MONITOR	D	N	32	A	60-11	
E0610	PACEMAKER MONITOR, SELF-CONTAINED, (CHECKS BATTERY DEPLETION, INCLUDES AUDIBLE & VISIBLE CHECK SYSTEMS)	D	N	32	A	60-7, 50-1	
E0615	PACEMAKER MONITOR, SELF CONTAINED, CHECKS BATTERY DEPLETION AND OTHER PACEMAKER	D	N	32	A	60-7, 50-1	
E0615	COMPONENTS, INCLUDES DIGITAL/VISIBLE CHECK SYSTEMS						
E0616	IMPLANTABLE CARDIAC EVENT RECORDER WITH MEMORY, ACTIVATOR AND PROGRAMMER	C	N	00	9		
E0617	EXTERNAL DEFIBRILLATOR WITH INTEGRATED ELECTROCARDIOGRAM ANALYSIS	C	N	36	A		
E0618	APNEA MONITOR, WITHOUT RECORDING FEATURE	C	N	00	9		
E0619	APNEA MONITOR, WITH RECORDING FEATURE	C	N	00	9		
E0620	SKIN PIERCING DEVICE FOR COLLECTION OF CAPILLARY BLOOD, LASER, EACH	C	N	32	A		
E0621	SLING OR SEAT, PATIENT LIFT, CANVAS OR NYLON	D	N	32	A	60-9	
E0625	PATIENT LIFT, BATHROOM OR TOILET, NOT OTHERWISE CLASSIFIED	M	N	00	9	60-9	
E0627	SEAT LIFT MECHANISM INCORPORATED INTO A COMBINATION LIFT-CHAIR MECHANISM	D	N	32	A	60-8	4107.8
E0628	SEPARATE SEAT LIFT MECHANISM FOR USE WITH PATIENT OWNED FURNITURE-ELECTRIC	D	N	32	A	60-8	4107.8
E0629	SEPARATE SEAT LIFT MECHANISM FOR USE WITH PATIENT OWNED FURNITURE-NON-ELECTRIC	D	N	32	A		4107.8
E0630	PATIENT LIFT, HYDRAULIC OR MECHANICAL, INCLUDES ANY SEAT, SLING, STRAP(S) OR PAD(S)	D	N	36	A	60-9	

HCPCS Code	Statute	Lab Cert	X-Ref	ASC Pay Grp	ASC Pay Group Eff. Date	Proc Notes	BETOS	TOS	Anest	Code Add Date	Code Effective Date	Code Term Date
E0562							D1E	A,P,R	0	20040101	20040101	
E0565							D1E	R	0	19820101	19960101	
E0565												
E0570							D1E	R	0	19860101	19960101	
E0571							D1E	A,P,R	0	20010101	20010101	
E0572							D1E	A,P,R	0	20010101	20010101	
E0574							D1E	A,P,R	0	20010101	20030101	
E0575							D1E	R	0	19860101	20010101	
E0580							D1E	P, R	0	19860101	19980101	
E0585							D1E	R	0	19860101	19960101	
							D1E	R	0	19860101	20020101	
E0601							D1E	R	0	19880101	19960101	
E0602							D1E	9	0	20000101	20020101	
E0603							Z2	9	0	20020101	20020101	
E0604							Z2	9	0	20020101	20080101	
E0605							D1E	A,P,R	0	19860101	19960101	
E0606							D1E	R	0	19860101	19960101	
E0607							D1E	A,P,R	0	19860101	19960101	
E0610							D1E	A,P,R	0	19860101	19960101	
E0615							D1E	A,P,R	0	19860101	19960101	
E0615												
E0616							D1E	9	0	20000101	20050401	
E0617							D1E	9, R	0	20010101	20010101	
E0618							D1E	R	0	20030101	20030101	
E0619							D1E	R	0	20030101	20030101	
E0620							D1E	A,P,R	0	20020101	20020101	
E0621							D1E	A,P,R	0	19860101	19960101	
E0625							D1E	A,P,R	0	19860101	20050101	
E0627			Q0080				D1E	A,P,R	0	19920101	19960101	
E0628			Q0078				D1E	A,P,R	0	19920101	19960101	
E0629			Q0079				D1E	A,P,R	0	19920101	19960101	
E0630							D1E	R	0	19860101	20080101	

HCPCS Code	Long Description	Coverage	Action	PI	MPI	CIM	MCM
E0635	PATIENT LIFT, ELECTRIC WITH SEAT OR SLING	D	N	36	A	60-9	
E0636	MULTIPOSITIONAL PATIENT SUPPORT SYSTEM, WITH INTEGRATED LIFT, PATIENT ACCESSIBLE CONTROLS	C	N	36	A		
E0637	COMBINATION SIT TO STAND SYSTEM, ANY SIZE INCLUDING PEDIATRIC, WITH SEATLIFT FEATURE, WITH OR WITHOUT WHEELS	D	N	32	A	60-9	
E0638	STANDING FRAME SYSTEM, ONE POSITION (E.G. UPRIGHT, SUPINE OR PRONE STANDER),ANY SIZE INCLUDING PEDIATRIC, WITH OR WITHOUT WHEELS	M	N	00	9	60-9	
E0639	PATIENT LIFT, MOVEABLE FROM ROOM TO ROOM WITH DISASSEMBLY AND REASSEMBLY, INCLUDES ALL COMPONENTS/ACCESSORIES	C	N	00	9		
E0640	PATIENT LIFT, FIXED SYSTEM, INCLUDES ALL COMPONENTS/ ACCESSORIES	C	N	00	9		
E0641	STANDING FRAME SYSTEM, MULTI-POSITION (E.G. THREE-WAY STANDER), ANY SIZE INCLUDING PEDIATRIC, WITH OR WITHOUT WHEELS	M	N	00	9	60-9	
E0642	STANDING FRAME SYSTEM, MOBILE (DYNAMIC STANDER), ANY SIZE INCLUDING PEDIATRIC	M	N	00	9	60-9	
E0650	PNEUMATIC COMPRESSOR, NON-SEGMENTAL HOME MODEL	D	N	32	A	60-16	
E0651	PNEUMATIC COMPRESSOR, SEGMENTAL HOME MODEL WITHOUT CALIBRATED GRADIENT PRESSURE	D	N	32	A	60-16	
E0652	PNEUMATIC COMPRESSOR, SEGMENTAL HOME MODEL WITH CALIBRATED GRADIENT PRESSURE	D	N	32	A	60-16	
E0655	NON-SEGMENTAL PNEUMATIC APPLIANCE FOR USE WITH PNEUMATIC COMPRESSOR, HALF ARM	D	N	32	A	60-16	
E0656	SEGMENTAL PNEUMATIC APPLIANCE FOR USE WITH PNEUMATIC COMPRESSOR, TRUNK	D	N	32	A		
E0657	SEGMENTAL PNEUMATIC APPLIANCE FOR USE WITH PNEUMATIC COMPRESSOR, CHEST	D	N	32	A		
E0660	NON-SEGMENTAL PNEUMATIC APPLIANCE FOR USE WITH PNEUMATIC COMPRESSOR, FULL LEG	D	N	32	A	60-16	
E0665	NON-SEGMENTAL PNEUMATIC APPLIANCE FOR USE WITH PNEUMATIC COMPRESSOR, FULL ARM	D	N	32	A	60-16	
E0666	NON-SEGMENTAL PNEUMATIC APPLIANCE FOR USE WITH PNEUMATIC COMPRESSOR, HALF LEG	D	N	32	A	60-16	
E0667	SEGMENTAL PNEUMATIC APPLIANCE FOR USE WITH PNEUMATIC COMPRESSOR, FULL LEG	D	N	32	A	60-16	
E0668	SEGMENTAL PNEUMATIC APPLIANCE FOR USE WITH PNEUMATIC COMPRESSOR, FULL ARM	D	N	32	A	60-16	
E0669	SEGMENTAL PNEUMATIC APPLIANCE FOR USE WITH PNEUMATIC COMPRESSOR, HALF LEG	D	N	32	A	60-16	
E0671	SEGMENTAL GRADIENT PRESSURE PNEUMATIC APPLIANCE, FULL LEG	D	N	32	A	60-16	
E0672	SEGMENTAL GRADIENT PRESSURE PNEUMATIC APPLIANCE, FULL ARM	D	N	32	A	60-16	
E0673	SEGMENTAL GRADIENT PRESSURE PNEUMATIC APPLIANCE, HALF LEG	D	N	32	A	60-16	

HCPCS Code	Statute	Lab Cert	X-Ref	ASC Pay Grp	ASC Pay Group Eff. Date	Proc Notes	BETOS	TOS	Anest	Code Add Date	Code Effective Date	Code Term Date
E0635							D1E	R	0	19860101	19960101	
E0636							D1E	R	0	20030101	20030101	
E0637							D1E	A,P,R	0	20040101	20060101	
E0638							D1E	A,P,R	0	20040101	20060101	
E0639							Y2	9	0	20050101	20070101	
E0640							Y2	9	0	20050101	20070101	
E0641							D1E	A,P,R	0	20060101	20060101	
E0642							D1E	A,P,R	0	20060101	20060101	
E0650							D1E	A,P,R	0	19860101	19960101	
E0651							D1E	A,P,R	0	19880101	19960101	
E0652							D1E	A,P,R	0	19880101	19960101	
E0655							D1E	A,P,R	0	19860101	19960101	
E0656						0125	D1E	A,P,R	0	20090101	20090101	
E0657						0125	D1E	A,P,R	0	20090101	20090101	
E0660							D1E	A,P,R	0	19860101	19960101	
E0665							D1E	A,P,R	0	19860101	19960101	
E0666							D1E	A,P,R	0	19860101	19960101	
E0667							D1E	A,P,R	0	19880101	19960101	
E0668							D1E	A,P,R	0	19880101	19960101	
E0669							D1E	A,P,R	0	19940101	19940101	
E0671							D1E	A,P,R	0	19950101	19950101	
E0672							D1E	A,P,R	0	19950101	19950101	
E0673							D1E	A,P,R	0	19950101	19950101	

HCPCS Code	Long Description	Coverage	Action	PI	MPI	CIM	MCM
E0675	PNEUMATIC COMPRESSION DEVICE, HIGH PRESSURE, RAPID INFLATION/DEFLATION CYCLE, FOR ARTERIAL INSUFFICIENCY (UNILATERAL OR BILATERAL SYSTEM)	C	N	36	A		
E0676	INTERMITTENT LIMB COMPRESSION DEVICE (INCLUDES ALL ACCESSORIES), NOT OTHERWISE SPECIFIED	C	N	00	9		
E0691	ULTRAVIOLET LIGHT THERAPY SYSTEM PANEL, INCLUDES BULBS/LAMPS, TIMER AND EYE PROTECTION; TREATMENT AREA 2 SQUARE FEET OR LESS	C	N	32	A		
E0692	ULTRAVIOLET LIGHT THERAPY SYSTEM PANEL, INCLUDES BULBS/LAMPS, TIMER AND EYE PROTECTION, 4 FOOT PANEL	C	N	32	A		
E0693	ULTRAVIOLET LIGHT THERAPY SYSTEM PANEL, INCLUDES BULBS/LAMPS, TIMER AND EYE PROTECTION, 6 FOOT PANEL	C	N	32	A		
E0694	ULTRAVIOLET MULTIDIRECTIONAL LIGHT THERAPY SYSTEM IN 6 FOOT CABINET, INCLUDES BULBS/LAMPS, TIMER AND EYE PROTECTION	C	N	32	A		
E0700	SAFETY EQUIPMENT, DEVICE OR ACCESSORY, ANY TYPE	C	C	00	9		
E0701	HELMET WITH FACE GUARD AND SOFT INTERFACE MATERIAL, PREFABRICATED	C	N	32	A		
E0705	TRANSFER DEVICE, ANY TYPE, EACH	D	N	32	A		
E0710	RESTRAINTS, ANY TYPE (BODY, CHEST, WRIST OR ANKLE)	C	N	57	A		
E0720	TRANSCUTANEOUS ELECTRICAL NERVE STIMULATION (TENS) DEVICE, TWO LEAD, LOCALIZED STIMULATION	D	N	32	A	35-20, 35-46	4107.6
E0730	TRANSCUTANEOUS ELECTRICAL NERVE STIMULATION (TENS) DEVICE, FOUR OR MORE LEADS, FOR MULTIPLE NERVE STIMULATION	D	N	32	A	35-20, 35-46	4107.6
E0731	FORM FITTING CONDUCTIVE GARMENT FOR DELIVERY OF TENS OR NMES (WITH CONDUCTIVE FIBERS SEPARATED FROM THE PATIENT'S SKIN BY LAYERS OF FABRIC)	D	N	34	A	45-25	
E0740	INCONTINENCE TREATMENT SYSTEM, PELVIC FLOOR STIMULATOR, MONITOR, SENSOR AND/OR TRAINER	D	N	32	A	60.24	
E0744	NEUROMUSCULAR STIMULATOR FOR SCOLIOSIS	C	N	36	A		
E0745	NEUROMUSCULAR STIMULATOR, ELECTRONIC SHOCK UNIT	D	N	36	A	35-77	
E0746	ELECTROMYOGRAPHY (EMG), BIOFEEDBACK DEVICE	D	N	52	A	35-27	
E0747	OSTEOGENESIS STIMULATOR, ELECTRICAL, NON-INVASIVE, OTHER THAN SPINAL APPLICATIONS	D	N	32	A	35-48	
E0748	OSTEOGENESIS STIMULATOR, ELECTRICAL, NON-INVASIVE, SPINAL APPLICATIONS	D	N	32	A	35-48	
E0749	OSTEOGENESIS STIMULATOR, ELECTRICAL, SURGICALLY IMPLANTED	D	N	36	A	35-48	
E0755	ELECTRONIC SALIVARY REFLEX STIMULATOR (INTRA-ORAL/NON-INVASIVE)	C	N	52	A		
E0760	OSTEOGENESIS STIMULATOR, LOW INTENSITY ULTRASOUND, NON-INVASIVE	C	N	32	A		35-48
E0761	NON-THERMAL PULSED HIGH FREQUENCY RADIOWAVES, HIGH PEAK POWER ELECTROMAGNETIC ENERGY TREATMENT DEVICE	D	N	00	9	35-102	
E0762	TRANSCUTANEOUS ELECTRICAL JOINT STIMULATION DEVICE SYSTEM, INCLUDES ALL ACCESSORIES	C	N	36	A		

HCPCS Code	Statute	Lab Cert	X-Ref	ASC Pay Grp	ASC Pay Group Eff. Date	Proc Notes	BETOS	TOS	Anest	Code Add Date	Code Effective Date	Code Term Date
E0675							D1E	R	0	20040101	20040101	
E0676							D1E	A,P,R	0	20070101	20070101	
E0691							D1E	A,P,R	0	20030101	20030101	
E0692							D1E	A,P,R	0	20030101	20030101	
E0693							D1E	A,P,R	0	20030101	20030101	
E0694							D1E	A,P,R	0	20030101	20030101	
E0700							D1E	A,P,R	0	19860101	20100101	
E0701							D1E	A,P,R	0	20030101	20070101	20061231
E0705						0125	D1E	A,P,R	0	20060101	20080101	
E0710							Z2	A,P,R	0	19860101	19960101	
E0720							D1E	A,P,R	0	19860101	20070101	
E0720												
E0730							D1E	A,P,R	0	19860101	20070101	
E0730												
E0731							D1E	A,P,R	0	19890101	19960101	
E0740							D1E	A,P,R	0	19860101	20010401	
E0744							D1E	R	0	19890101	19960101	
E0745							D1E	R	0	19860101	19960101	
E0746							D1E	A,P,R	0	19890101	19960101	
E0747							D1E	A,P,R	0	19860101	19970101	
E0748							D1E	A,P,R	0	19960101	19970101	
E0749							D1E	9	0	19860101	20000701	
E0755							Z2	A,P,R	0	19900101	19950401	
E0760							D1E	A,P,R	0	19970101	20010101	
E0761							D1E	9	0	20030101	20050101	
E0762							D1E	A,P,R	0	20060101	20060101	

HCPCS Code	Long Description	Coverage	Action	PI	MPI	CIM	MCM
E0764	FUNCTIONAL NEUROMUSCULAR STIMULATION, TRANSCUTANEOUS STIMULATION OF SEQUENTIAL MUSCLE GROUPS OF AMBULATION WITH COMPUTER CONTROL, USED FOR WALKING BY SPINAL CORD INJURED, ENTIRE SYSTEM, AFTER COMPLETION OF TRAINING PROGRAM	D	N	32	A	35-77	
E0765	FDA APPROVED NERVE STIMULATOR, WITH REPLACEABLE BATTERIES, FOR TREATMENT OF NAUSEA AND VOMITING	C	N	32	A		
E0769	ELECTRICAL STIMULATION OR ELECTROMAGNETIC WOUND TREATMENT DEVICE, NOT OTHERWISE CLASSIFIED	D	N	00	9	35-102	
E0770	FUNCTIONAL ELECTRICAL STIMULATOR, TRANSCUTANEOUS STIMULATION OF NERVE AND/OR MUSCLE GROUPS, ANY TYPE, COMPLETE SYSTEM, NOT OTHERWISE SPECIFIED	D	N	46	A		
E0776	IV POLE	C	N	32	A		
E0779	AMBULATORY INFUSION PUMP, MECHANICAL, REUSABLE, FOR INFUSION 8 HOURS OR GREATER	C	N	36	A		
E0780	AMBULATORY INFUSION PUMP, MECHANICAL, REUSABLE, FOR INFUSION LESS THAN 8 HOURS	C	N	32	A		
E0781	AMBULATORY INFUSION PUMP, SINGLE OR MULTIPLE CHANNELS, ELECTRIC OR BATTERY OPERATED, WITH ADMINISTRATIVE EQUIPMENT, WORN BY PATIENT	D	N	36	A	60-14	
E0782	INFUSION PUMP, IMPLANTABLE, NON-PROGRAMMABLE (INCLUDES ALL COMPONENTS, E.G., PUMP, CATHETER, CONNECTORS, ETC.)	D	N	32	A	60-14	
E0783	INFUSION PUMP SYSTEM, IMPLANTABLE, PROGRAMMABLE (INCLUDES ALL COMPONENTS, E.G., PUMP, CATHETER, CONNECTORS, ETC.)	D	N	32	A	60-14	
E0784	EXTERNAL AMBULATORY INFUSION PUMP, INSULIN	D	N	36	A	60-14	
E0785	IMPLANTABLE INTRASPINAL (EPIDURAL/INTRATHECAL) CATHETER USED WITH IMPLANTABLE INFUSION PUMP, REPLACEMENT	D	N	32	A		60-14
E0786	IMPLANTABLE PROGRAMMABLE INFUSION PUMP, REPLACEMENT (EXCLUDES IMPLANTABLE INTRASPINAL CATHETER)	D	N	32	A	60-14	
E0791	PARENTERAL INFUSION PUMP, STATIONARY, SINGLE OR MULTI-CHANNEL	D	N	36	A	65-10	2130, 4550
E0830	AMBULATORY TRACTION DEVICE, ALL TYPES, EACH	D	N	00	9	60-9	
E0840	TRACTION FRAME, ATTACHED TO HEADBOARD, CERVICAL TRACTION	D	N	32	A	60-9	
E0849	TRACTION EQUIPMENT, CERVICAL, FREE-STANDING STAND/FRAME, PNEUMATIC, APPLYING TRACTION FORCE TO OTHER THAN MANDIBLE	C	N	32	A		
E0850	TRACTION STAND, FREE STANDING, CERVICAL TRACTION	D	N	32	A	60-9	
E0855	CERVICAL TRACTION EQUIPMENT NOT REQUIRING ADDITIONAL STAND OR FRAME	C	N	32	A		
E0856	CERVICAL TRACTION DEVICE, CERVICAL COLLAR WITH INFLATABLE AIR BLADDER	C	N	32	A		
E0860	TRACTION EQUIPMENT, OVERDOOR, CERVICAL	D	N	32	A	60-9	
E0870	TRACTION FRAME, ATTACHED TO FOOTBOARD, EXTREMITY TRACTION, (E.G. BUCK'S)	D	N	32	A	60-9	

HCPCS Code	Statute	Lab Cert	X-Ref	ASC Pay Grp	ASC Pay Group Eff. Date	Proc Notes	BETOS	TOS	Anest	Code Add Date	Code Effective Date	Code Term Date
E0764							D1F	A,P,R	0	20060101	20090101	
E0765							D1E	A, P	0	20010101	20010101	
E0769							Y2	9	0	20050101	20050101	
E0770						0152	D1E	A,P,R	0	20090101	20090101	
E0776							D1E	A,E,P,R	0	19850101	19950401	
E0779							D1E	A,P,R	0	20000101	20000101	
E0780							D1E	A,P,R	0	20000101	20000101	
E0781							D1E	9, R	0	19870101	20000701	
E0782							D1E	A,P,R	0	19860101	20030101	
E0783							D1E	A,P,R	0	19950101	19980101	
E0784							D1E	R	0	19960101	20000701	
E0785							D1E	P	0	19990101	19990101	
E0786							D1E	9	0	20010101	20010101	
E0791							D1E	R	0	19890101	19960101	
E0830							D1E	P	0	20010101	20010101	
E0840							D1E	A,P,R	0	19840101	19940101	
E0849							D1E	A,P,R	0	20050101	20050101	
E0850							D1E	A,P,R	0	19820101	19940101	
E0855							D1E	A,P,R	0	19980101	19980101	
E0856							D1E	A,P,R	0	20080101	20080101	
E0860							D1E	A,P,R	0	19860101	19890101	
E0870							D1E	A,P,R	0	19860101	19940101	

HCPCS Code	Long Description	Coverage	Action	PI	MPI	CIM	MCM
E0880	TRACTION STAND, FREE STANDING, EXTREMITY TRACTION, (E.G., BUCK'S)	D	N	32	A	60-9	
E0890	TRACTION FRAME, ATTACHED TO FOOTBOARD, PELVIC TRACTION	D	N	32	A	60-9	
E0900	TRACTION STAND, FREE STANDING, PELVIC TRACTION, (E.G., BUCK'S)	D	N	32	A	60-9	
E0910	TRAPEZE BARS, A/K/A PATIENT HELPER, ATTACHED TO BED, WITH GRAB BAR	D	N	36	A	60-9	
E0911	TRAPEZE BAR, HEAVY DUTY, FOR PATIENT WEIGHT CAPACITY GREATER THAN 250 POUNDS, ATTACHED TO BED, WITH GRAB BAR	D	N	36	A	60-9	
E0912	TRAPEZE BAR, HEAVY DUTY, FOR PATIENT WEIGHT CAPACITY GREATER THAN 250 POUNDS, FREE STANDING, COMPLETE WITH GRAB BAR	D	N	36	A	60-9	
E0920	FRACTURE FRAME, ATTACHED TO BED, INCLUDES WEIGHTS	D	N	36	A	60-9	
E0930	FRACTURE FRAME, FREE STANDING, INCLUDES WEIGHTS	D	N	36	A	60-9	
E0935	CONTINUOUS PASSIVE MOTION EXERCISE DEVICE FOR USE ON KNEE ONLY	D	N	31	A	60-9	
E0936	CONTINUOUS PASSIVE MOTION EXERCISE DEVICE FOR USE OTHER THAN KNEE	M	N	00	9		
E0940	TRAPEZE BAR, FREE STANDING, COMPLETE WITH GRAB BAR	D	N	36	A	60-9	
E0941	GRAVITY ASSISTED TRACTION DEVICE, ANY TYPE	D	N	36	A	60-9	
E0942	CERVICAL HEAD HARNESS/HALTER	C	N	32	A		
E0944	PELVIC BELT/HARNESS/BOOT	C	N	32	A		
E0945	EXTREMITY BELT/HARNESS	C	N	32	A		
E0946	FRACTURE, FRAME, DUAL WITH CROSS BARS, ATTACHED TO BED, (E.G. BALKEN, 4 POSTER)	D	N	36	A	60-9	
E0947	FRACTURE FRAME, ATTACHMENTS FOR COMPLEX PELVIC TRACTION	D	N	32	A	60-9	
E0948	FRACTURE FRAME, ATTACHMENTS FOR COMPLEX CERVICAL TRACTION	D	N	32	A	60-9	
E0950	WHEELCHAIR ACCESSORY, TRAY, EACH	D	N	00	9	60-9	
E0951	HEEL LOOP/HOLDER, ANY TYPE, WITH OR WITHOUT ANKLE STRAP, EACH	C	N	00	9		
E0952	TOE LOOP/HOLDER, ANY TYPE, EACH	D	N	00	9	60-9	
E0955	WHEELCHAIR ACCESSORY, HEADREST, CUSHIONED, ANY TYPE, INCLUDING FIXED MOUNTING HARDWARE, EACH	C	N	32	A		
E0956	WHEELCHAIR ACCESSORY, LATERAL TRUNK OR HIP SUPPORT, ANY TYPE, INCLUDING FIXED MOUNTING HARDWARE, EACH	C	N	32	A		
E0957	WHEELCHAIR ACCESSORY, MEDIAL THIGH SUPPORT, ANY TYPE, INCLUDING FIXED MOUNTING HARDWARE, EACH	C	N	32	A		
E0958	MANUAL WHEELCHAIR ACCESSORY, ONE-ARM DRIVE ATTACHMENT, EACH	D	N	00	9	60-9	
E0959	MANUAL WHEELCHAIR ACCESSORY, ADAPTER FOR AMPUTEE, EACH	C	N	00	9	60-9	
E0960	WHEELCHAIR ACCESSORY, SHOULDER HARNESS/STRAPS OR CHEST STRAP, INCLUDING ANY TYPE MOUNTING HARDWARE	C	N	32	A		
E0961	MANUAL WHEELCHAIR ACCESSORY, WHEEL LOCK BRAKE EXTENSION (HANDLE), EACH	C	N	00	9	60-9	

HCPCS Code	Statute	Lab Cert	X-Ref	ASC Pay Grp	ASC Pay Group Eff. Date	Proc Notes	BETOS	TOS	Anest	Code Add Date	Code Effective Date	Code Term Date
E0880							D1E	A,P,R	0	19860101	19940101	
E0890							D1E	A,P,R	0	19860101	19940101	
E0900							D1E	A,P,R	0	19860101	19940101	
E0910							D1E	R	0	19860101	19840101	
E0911							D1B	R	0	20060101	20060101	
E0912							D1B	R	0	20060101	20060101	
E0920							D1E	R	0	19860101	19890101	
E0930							D1E	R	0	19860101	19890101	
E0935							D1E	R	0	19860101	20060101	
E0936						0137	D1E	R	0	20070101	20070101	
E0940							D1B	R	0	19860101	19890101	
E0941							D1E	R	0	19860101	19890101	
E0942							D1E	A,P,R	0	19860101	19860101	
E0944							D1E	A,P,R	0	19850101	19960101	
E0945							D1E	A,P,R	0	19850101	19960101	
E0946							D1E	R	0	19860101	19890101	
E0947							D1E	A,P,R	0	19860101	19890101	
E0948							D1E	A,P,R	0	19860101	19890101	
E0950							D1D	A,P,R	0	19860101	20040101	
E0951							D1D	A,P,R	0	19860101	20050101	
E0952							D1D	A,P,R	0	19860101	20050101	
E0955							D1D	A,P,R	0	20040101	20050101	
E0956							D1D	A,P,R	0	20040101	20050101	
E0957							D1D	A,P,R	0	20040101	20050101	
E0958							D1D	R	0	19860101	20040101	
E0959							D1D	A,P,R	0	19860101	20040101	
E0960							D1D	A,P,R	0	20040101	20040101	
E0961							D1D	A,P,R	0	19860101	20040101	

HCPCS Code	Long Description	Coverage	Action	PI	MPI	CIM	MCM
E0966	MANUAL WHEELCHAIR ACCESSORY, HEADREST EXTENSION, EA.	C	N	00	9	60-9	
E0967	MANUAL WHEELCHAIR ACCESSORY, HAND RIM WITH PROJECTIONS, ANY TYPE, EACH	D	N	32	A	60-9	
E0968	COMMODE SEAT, WHEELCHAIR	D	N	36	A	60-9	
E0969	NARROWING DEVICE, WHEELCHAIR	D	N	32	A	60-9	
E0970	NO.2 FOOTPLATES, EXCEPT FOR ELEVATING LEG REST	I	N	00	9	60-9	
E0971	MANUAL WHEELCHAIR ACCESSORY, ANTI-TIPPING DEVICE, EA.	C	N	00	9	60-9	
E0973	WHEELCHAIR ACCESSORY, ADJUSTABLE HEIGHT, DETACHABLE ARMREST, COMPLETE ASSEMBLY, EACH	D	N	00	9	60-9	
E0974	MANUAL WHEELCHAIR ACCESSORY, ANTI-ROLLBACK DEVICE, EACH	D	N	00	9	60-9	
E0977	WEDGE CUSHION, WHEELCHAIR	C	N	32	A		
E0978	WHEELCHAIR ACCESSORY, POSITIONING BELT/SAFETY BELT/PELVIC STRAP, EACH	C	N	00	9		
E0980	SAFETY VEST, WHEELCHAIR	C	N	32	A		
E0981	WHEELCHAIR ACCESSORY, SEAT UPHOLSTERY, REPLACEMENT ONLY, EACH	C	N	32	A		
E0982	WHEELCHAIR ACCESSORY, BACK UPHOLSTERY, REPLACEMENT ONLY, EACH	C	N	32	A		
E0983	MANUAL WHEELCHAIR ACCESSORY, POWER ADD-ON TO CONVERT MANUAL WHEELCHAIR TO MOTORIZED WHEELCHAIR, JOYSTICK CONTROL	C	N	36	A		
E0984	MANUAL WHEELCHAIR ACCESSORY, POWER ADD-ON TO CONVERT MANUAL WHEELCHAIR TO MOTORIZED WHEELCHAIR, TILLER CONTROL	C	N	32	A		
E0985	WHEELCHAIR ACCESSORY, SEAT LIFT MECHANISM	C	N	32	A		
E0986	MANUAL WHEELCHAIR ACCESSORY, PUSH ACTIVATED POWER ASSIST, EACH	C	N	32	A		
E0990	WHEELCHAIR ACCESSORY, ELEVATING LEG REST, COMPLETE ASSEMBLY, EACH	C	N	00	9	60-9	
E0992	MANUAL WHEELCHAIR ACCESSORY, SOLID SEAT INSERT	C	N	32	A		
E0994	ARM REST, EACH	D	N	32	A	60-9	
E0995	WHEELCHAIR ACCESSORY, CALF REST/PAD, EACH	C	N	00	9	60-9	
E0997	CASTER WITH A FORK	I	N	00	9		
E0998	CASTER WITHOUT FORK	I	N	00	9		
E0999	PNEUMATIC TIRE WITH WHEEL	I	N	00	9		
E1002	WHEELCHAIR ACCESSORY, POWER SEATING SYSTEM, TILT ONLY	C	N	32	A		
E1003	WHEELCHAIR ACCESSORY, POWER SEATING SYSTEM, RECLINE ONLY, WITHOUT SHEAR REDUCTION	C	N	32	A		
E1004	WHEELCHAIR ACCESSORY, POWER SEATING SYSTEM, RECLINE ONLY, WITH MECHANICAL SHEAR REDUCTION	C	N	32	A		
E1005	WHEELCHAIR ACCESSORY, POWER SEATNG SYSTEM, RECLINE ONLY, WITH POWER SHEAR REDUCTION	C	N	32	A		
E1006	WHEELCHAIR ACCESSORY, POWER SEATING SYSTEM, COMBI-NATION TILT AND RECLINE, WITHOUT SHEAR REDUCTION	C	N	32	A		
E1007	WHEELCHAIR ACCESSORY, POWER SEATING SYSTEM, COMBI-NATION TILT AND RECLINE, WITH MECHANICAL SHEAR REDUCTION	C	N	32	A		

HCPCS Code	Statute	Lab Cert	X-Ref	ASC Pay Grp	ASC Pay Group Eff. Date	Proc Notes	BETOS	TOS	Anest	Code Add Date	Code Effective Date	Code Term Date
E0966							D1D	A,P,R	0	19860101	20040101	
E0967							D1D	A,P,R	0	19860101	20070101	
E0968							D1D	R	0	19860101	19890101	
E0969							D1D	A,P,R	0	19860101	19890101	
E0970			K0037, 42				D1D	A,P,R	0	19860101	20010401	
E0971			K0021				D1D	A,P,R	0	19860101	20060101	
E0973							D1D	A,P,R	0	19860101	20040101	
E0974							D1D	A,P,R	0	19860101	20040101	
E0977							D1D	A,P,R	0	19860101	20070101	20061231
E0978							D1D	A,P,R	0	19860101	20050101	
E0980							D1D	A,P,R	0	19860101	19890101	
E0981							D1D	A,P,R	0	20040101	20040101	
E0982							D1D	A,P,R	0	20040101	20040101	
E0983							D1D	R	0	20040101	20040101	
E0984							D1D	A,P,R	0	20040101	20040101	
E0985							D1D	A,P,R	0	20040101	20040101	
E0986							D1D	A,P,R	0	20040101	20050101	
E0990							D1D	A,P,R	0	19860101	20040101	
E0992							D1D	A,P,R	0	19860101	20040101	
E0994							D1D	A,P,R	0	19860101	19890101	
E0995							D1D	A,P,R	0	19860101	20040101	
E0997							D1D	A,P,R	0	19860101	20070101	20061231
E0998							D1D	A,P,R	0	19860101	20070101	20061231
E0999							D1D	A,P,R	0	19860101	20070101	20061231
E1002							D1D	A,P,R	0	20040101	20040101	
E1003							D1D	A,P,R	0	20040101	20040101	
E1004							D1D	A,P,R	0	20040101	20040101	
E1005							D1D	A,P,R	0	20040101	20040101	
E1006							D1D	A,P,R	0	20040101	20040101	
E1007							D1D	A,P,R	0	20040101	20040101	

HCPCS Code	Long Description	Coverage	Action	PI	MPI	CIM	MCM
E1008	WHEELCHAIR ACCESSORY, POWER SEATING SYSTEM, COMBINATION TILT AND RECLINE, WITH POWER SHEAR REDUCTION	C	N	32	A		
E1009	WHEELCHAIR ACCESSORY, ADDITION TO POWER SEATING SYSTEM, MECHANICALLY LINKED LEG ELEVATION SYSTEM, INCLUDING PUSHROD AND LEG REST, EACH	C	N	32	A		
E1010	WHEELCHAIR ACCESSORY, ADDITION TO POWER SEATING SYSTEM, POWER LEG ELEVATION SYSTEM, INCLUDING LEG REST, PAIR	C	N	32	A		
E1011	MODIFICATION TO PEDIATRIC SIZE WHEELCHAIR, WIDTH ADJUSTMENT PACKAGE (NOT TO BE DISPENSED WITH INITIAL CHAIR)	D	N	32	A	60-9	
E1014	RECLINING BACK, ADDITION TO PEDIATRIC SIZE WHEELCHAIR	D	N	32	A	60-9	
E1015	SHOCK ABSORBER FOR MANUAL WHEELCHAIR, EACH	D	N	32	A		60.9
E1016	SHOCK ABSORBER FOR POWER WHEELCHAIR, EACH	D	N	32	A		60.9
E1017	HEAVY DUTY SHOCK ABSORBER FOR HEAVY DUTY OR EXTRA HEAVY DUTY MANUAL WHEELCHAIR, EACH	D	N	32	A		60.9
E1018	HEAVY DUTY SHOCK ABSORBER FOR HEAVY DUTY OR EXTRA HEAVY DUTY POWER WHEELCHAIR, EACH	D	N	32	A		60.9
E1020	RESIDUAL LIMB SUPPORT SYSTEM FOR WHEELCHAIR	D	N	32	A		60-6
E1028	WHEELCHAIR ACCESSORY, MANUAL SWINGAWAY, RETRACTABLE OR REMOVABLE MOUNTING HARDWARE FOR JOYSTICK, OTHER CONTROL INTERFACE OR POSITIONING ACCESSORY	C	N	32	A		
E1029	WHEELCHAIR ACCESSORY, VENTILATOR TRAY, FIXED	C	N	32	A		
E1030	WHEELCHAIR ACCESSORY, VENTILATOR TRAY, GIMBALED	C	N	32	A		
E1031	ROLLABOUT CHAIR, ANY AND ALL TYPES WITH CASTORS 5" OR GREATER	D	N	36	A	60-9	
E1035	MULTI-POSITIONAL PATIENT TRANSFER SYSTEM, WITH INTEGRATED SEAT, OPERATED BY CARE GIVER, PATIENT WEIGHT CAPACITY UP TO AND INCLUDING 300 LBS	D	C	36	A		2100
E1036	MULTI-POSITIONAL PATIENT TRANSFER SYSTEM, EXTRA-WIDE, WITH INTEGRATED SEAT, OPERATED BY CAREGIVER, PATIENT WEIGHT CAPACITY GREATER THAN 300 LBS	C	A	36	A		
E1037	TRANSPORT CHAIR, PEDIATRIC SIZE	D	N	36	A	60-9	
E1038	TRANSPORT CHAIR, ADULT SIZE, PATIENT WEIGHT CAPACITY UP TO AND INCLUDING 300 POUNDS	D	N	36	A	60-9	
E1039	TRANSPORT CHAIR, ADULT SIZE, HEAVY DUTY, PATIENT WEIGHT CAPACITY GREATER THAN 300 POUNDS	C	N	36	A		
E1050	FULLY-RECLINING WHEELCHAIR, FIXED FULL LENGTH ARMS, SWING AWAY DETACHABLE ELEVATING LEG RESTS	D	N	36	A	60-9	
E1060	FULLY-RECLINING WHEELCHAIR, DETACHABLE ARMS, DESK OR FULL LENGTH, SWING AWAY DETACHABLE ELEVATING LEGRESTS	D	N	36	A	60-9	
E1070	FULLY-RECLINING WHEELCHAIR, DETACHABLE ARMS (DESK OR FULL LENGTH) SWING AWAY DETACHABLE FOOTREST	D	N	36	A	60-9	
E1083	HEMI-WHEELCHAIR, FIXED FULL LENGTH ARMS, SWING AWAY DETACHABLE ELEVATING LEG REST	D	N	36	A	60-9	

HCPCS Code	Statute	Lab Cert	X-Ref	ASC Pay Grp	ASC Pay Group Eff. Date	Proc Notes	BETOS	TOS	Anest	Code Add Date	Code Effective Date	Code Term Date
E1008							D1D	A,P,R	0	20040101	20040101	
E1009							D1D	A,P,R	0	20040101	20040101	
E1010							D1D	A,P,R	0	20040101	20050101	
E1011							D1D	A,P,R	0	20030101	20050101	
E1014							D1D	A,P,R	0	20030101	20050101	
E1015							D1D	A,P,R	0	20030101	20030101	
E1016							D1D	A,P,R	0	20030101	20030101	
E1017							D1D	A,P,R	0	20030101	20030101	
E1018							D1D	A,P,R	0	20030101	20030101	
E1020							D1D	A,P,R	0	20030101	20030101	
E1028							D1D	A,P,R	0	20040101	20040101	
E1029							D1D	A,P,R	0	20040101	20040101	
E1030							D1D	A,P,R	0	20040101	20040101	
E1031							D1D	R	0	19900101	19900101	
E1035							D1D	R	0	20010101	20100101	
E1036							D1D	R	0	20100101	20100101	
E1037							D1D	R	0	20030101	20030101	
E1038							D1D	R	0	20030101	20060101	
E1039							D1D	R	0	20050101	20060101	
E1050							D1D	R	0	19860101	19840101	
E1060							D1D	R	0	19860101	19890101	
E1070							D1D	R	0	19860101	19890101	
E1083							D1D	R	0	19860101	19890101	

HCPCS Code	Long Description	Coverage	Action	PI	MPI	CIM	MCM
E1084	HEMI-WHEELCHAIR, DETACHABLE ARMS DESK OR FULL LENGTH ARMS, SWING AWAY DETACHABLE ELEVATING LEG RESTS	D	N	36	A	60-9	
E1085	HEMI-WHEELCHAIR, FIXED FULL LENGTH ARMS, SWING AWAY DETACHABLE FOOT RESTS	I	N	00	9	60-9	
E1086	HEMI-WHEELCHAIR DETACHABLE ARMS DESK OR FULL LENGTH, SWING AWAY DETACHABLE FOOTRESTS	I	N	00	9	60-9	
E1087	HIGH STRENGTH LIGHTWEIGHT WHEELCHAIR, FIXED FULL LENGTH ARMS, SWING AWAY DETACHABLE ELEVATING LEG RESTS	D	N	36	A	60-9	
E1088	HIGH STRENGTH LIGHTWEIGHT WHEELCHAIR, DETACHABLE ARMS DESK OR FULL LENGTH, SWING AWAY DETACHABLE ELEVATING LEG RESTS	D	N	36	A	60-9	
E1089	HIGH STRENGTH LIGHTWEIGHT WHEELCHAIR, FIXED LENGTH ARMS, SWING AWAY DETACHABLE FOOTREST	I	N	00	9	60-9	
E1090	HIGH STRENGTH LIGHTWEIGHT WHEELCHAIR, DETACHABLE ARMS DESK OR FULL LENGTH, SWING AWAY DETACHABLE FOOT RESTS	I	N	00	9	60-9	
E1092	WIDE HEAVY DUTY WHEEL CHAIR, DETACHABLE ARMS (DESK OR FULL LENGTH), SWING AWAY DETACHABLE ELEVATING LEG RESTS	D	N	36	A	60-9	
E1093	WIDE HEAVY DUTY WHEELCHAIR, DETACHABLE ARMS DESK OR FULL LENGTH ARMS, SWING AWAY DETACHABLE FOOTRESTS	D	N	36	A	60-9	
E1100	SEMI-RECLINING WHEELCHAIR, FIXED FULL LENGTH ARMS, SWING AWAY DETACHABLE ELEVATING LEG RESTS	D	N	36	A	60-9	
E1110	SEMI-RECLINING WHEELCHAIR, DETACHABLE ARMS (DESK OR FULL LENGTH) ELEVATING LEG REST	D	N	36	A	60-9	
E1130	STANDARD WHEELCHAIR, FIXED FULL LENGTH ARMS, FIXED OR SWING AWAY DETACHABLE FOOTRESTS	I	N	00	9	60-9	
E1140	WHEELCHAIR, DETACHABLE ARMS, DESK OR FULL LENGTH, SWING AWAY DETACHABLE FOOTRESTS	I	N	00	9	60-9	
E1150	WHEELCHAIR, DETACHABLE ARMS, DESK OR FULL LENGTH SWING AWAY DETACHABLE ELEVATING LEGRESTS	D	N	36	A	60-9	
E1160	WHEELCHAIR, FIXED FULL LENGTH ARMS, SWING AWAY DETACHABLE ELEVATING LEGRESTS	D	N	36	A	60-9	
E1161	MANUAL ADULT SIZE WHEELCHAIR, INCLUDES TILT IN SPACE	C	N	36	A		
E1170	AMPUTEE WHEELCHAIR, FIXED FULL LENGTH ARMS, SWING AWAY DETACHABLE ELEVATING LEGRESTS	D	N	36	A	60-9	
E1171	AMPUTEE WHEELCHAIR, FIXED FULL LENGTH ARMS, WITHOUT FOOTRESTS OR LEGREST	D	N	36	A	60-9	
E1172	AMPUTEE WHEELCHAIR, DETACHABLE ARMS (DESK OR FULL LENGTH) WITHOUT FOOTRESTS OR LEGREST	D	N	36	A	60-9	
E1180	AMPUTEE WHEELCHAIR, DETACHABLE ARMS (DESK OR FULL LENGTH) SWING AWAY DETACHABLE FOOTRESTS	D	N	36	A	60-9	
E1190	AMPUTEE WHEELCHAIR, DETACHABLE ARMS (DESK OR FULL LENGTH) SWING AWAY DETACHABLE ELEVATING LEGRESTS	D	N	36	A	60-9	
E1195	HEAVY DUTY WHEELCHAIR, FIXED FULL LENGTH ARMS, SWING AWAY DETACHABLE ELEVATING LEGRESTS	D	N	36	A	60-9	

HCPCS Code	Statute	Lab Cert	X-Ref	ASC Pay Grp	ASC Pay Group Eff. Date	Proc Notes	BETOS	TOS	Anest	Code Add Date	Code Effective Date	Code Term Date
E1084							D1D	R	0	19860101	19890101	
E1085			K0002				D1D	R	0	19860101	20010401	
E1086			K0002				D1D	R	0	19860101	20010401	
E1087							D1D	R	0	19860101	19890101	
E1088							D1D	R	0	19860101	19890101	
E1089			K0004				D1D	R	0	19860101	20010401	
E1090			K0004				D1D	R	0	19860101	20010401	
E1092							D1D	R	0	19860101	19890101	
E1093							D1D	R	0	19860101	19890101	
E1100							D1D	R	0	19860101	19880101	
E1110							D1D	R	0	19860101	19890101	
E1130			K0001				D1D	R	0	19860101	20010401	
E1140			K0001				D1D	R	0	19860101	20010401	
E1150							D1D	R	0	19860101	19890101	
E1160							D1D	R	0	19860101	19890101	
E1161							D1D	A,P,R	0	20030101	20030101	
E1170							D1D	R	0	19860101	19890101	
E1171							D1D	R	0	19860101	19890101	
E1172							D1D	R	0	19860101	19890101	
E1180							D1D	R	0	19860101	19890101	
E1190							D1D	R	0	19860101	19890101	
E1195							D1D	R	0	19860101	19890101	

HCPCS Code	Long Description	Coverage	Action	PI	MPI	CIM	MCM
E1200	AMPUTEE WHEELCHAIR, FIXED FULL LENGTH ARMS, SWING AWAY DETACHABLE FOOTREST	D	N	36	A	60-9	
E1220	WHEELCHAIR; SPECIALLY SIZED OR CONSTRUCTED, (INDICATE BRAND NAME, MODEL NUMBER, IF ANY) AND JUSTIFICATION	D	N	45	A	60-6	
E1221	WHEELCHAIR WITH FIXED ARM, FOOTRESTS	D	N	36	A	60-6	
E1222	WHEELCHAIR WITH FIXED ARM, ELEVATING LEGRESTS	D	N	36	A	60-6	
E1223	WHEELCHAIR WITH DETACHABLE ARMS, FOOTRESTS	D	N	36	A	60-6	
E1224	WHEELCHAIR WITH DETACHABLE ARMS, ELEVATING LEGRESTS	D	N	36	A	60-6	
E1225	WHEELCHAIR ACCESSORY, MANUAL SEMI-RECLINING BACK, (RECLINE GREATER THAN 15 DEGREES, BUT LESS THAN 80 DEGREES), EACH	D	N	36	A	60-6	
E1226	WHEELCHAIR ACCESSORY, MANUAL FULLY RECLINING BACK, (RECLINE GREATER THAN 80 DEGREES), EACH	D	N	00	9	60-9	
E1227	SPECIAL HEIGHT ARMS FOR WHEELCHAIR	D	N	32	A	60-6	
E1228	SPECIAL BACK HEIGHT FOR WHEELCHAIR	D	N	36	A	60-6	
E1229	WHEELCHAIR, PEDIATRIC SIZE, NOT OTHERWISE SPECIFIED	C	N	32	A		
E1230	POWER OPERATED VEHICLE (THREE OR FOUR WHEEL NONHIGHWAY) SPECIFY BRAND NAME AND MODEL NUMBER	D	N	32	A	60-5	4107.6
E1231	WHEELCHAIR, PEDIATRIC SIZE, TILT-IN-SPACE, RIGID, ADJUSTABLE, WITH SEATING SYSTEM	D	N	32	A	60-9	
E1232	WHEELCHAIR, PEDIATRIC SIZE, TILT-IN-SPACE, FOLDING, ADJUSTABLE, WITH SEATING SYSTEM	D	N	32	A	60-9	
E1233	WHEELCHAIR, PEDIATRIC SIZE, TILT-IN-SPACE, RIGID, ADJUSTABLE, WITHOUT SEATING SYSTEM	D	N	32	A	60-9	
E1234	WHEELCHAIR, PEDIATRIC SIZE, TILT-IN-SPACE, FOLDING, ADJUSTABLE, WITHOUT SEATING SYSTEM	D	N	32	A	60-9	
E1235	WHEELCHAIR, PEDIATRIC SIZE, RIGID, ADJUSTABLE, WITH SEATING SYSTEM	D	N	32	A	60-9	
E1236	WHEELCHAIR, PEDIATRIC SIZE, FOLDING, ADJUSTABLE, WITH SEATING SYSTEM	D	N	32	A	60-9	
E1237	WHEELCHAIR, PEDIATRIC SIZE, RIGID, ADJUSTABLE, WITHOUT SEATING SYSTEM	D	N	32	A	60-9	
E1238	WHEELCHAIR, PEDIATRIC SIZE, FOLDING, ADJUSTABLE, WITHOUT SEATING SYSTEM	D	N	32	A	60-9	
E1239	POWER WHEELCHAIR, PEDIATRIC SIZE, NOT OTHERWISE SPECIFIED	C	N	36	A		
E1240	LIGHTWEIGHT WHEELCHAIR, DETACHABLE ARMS, (DESK OR FULL LENGTH) SWING AWAY DETACHABLE, ELEVATING LEGREST	D	N	36	A	60-9	
E1250	LIGHTWEIGHT WHEELCHAIR, FIXED FULL LENGTH ARMS, SWING AWAY DETACHABLE FOOTREST	I	N	00	9	60-9	
E1260	LIGHTWEIGHT WHEELCHAIR, DETACHABLE ARMS (DESK OR FULL LENGTH) SWING AWAY DETACHABLE FOOTREST	I	N	00	9	60-9	
E1270	LIGHTWEIGHT WHEELCHAIR, FIXED FULL LENGTH ARMS, SWING AWAY DETACHABLE ELEVATING LEGRESTS	D	N	36	A	60-9	
E1280	HEAVY DUTY WHEELCHAIR, DETACHABLE ARMS (DESK OR FULL LENGTH) ELEVATING LEGRESTS	D	N	36	A	60-9	

HCPCS Code	Statute	Lab Cert	X-Ref	ASC Pay Grp	ASC Pay Group Eff. Date	Proc Notes	BETOS	TOS	Anest	Code Add Date	Code Effective Date	Code Term Date
E1200							D1D	R	0	19860101	19890101	
E1220							D1D	P	0	19860101	19900101	
E1221							D1D	R	0	19860101	19900101	
E1222							D1D	R	0	19860101	19900101	
E1223							D1D	R	0	19860101	19900101	
E1224							D1D	R	0	19860101	19900101	
E1225							D1D	R	0	19860101	20050101	
E1225												
E1226							D1D	A,P,R	0	19860101	20050101	
E1227							D1D	A,P,R	0	19860101	19900101	
E1228							D1D	R	0	19860101	19900101	
E1229							D1D	A,P,R	0	20050101	20050101	
E1230							D1D	AA,P,R	0	19860101	19910101	
E1231							D1D	A,P,R	0	20030101	20090101	
E1232							D1D	A,P,R	0	20030101	20090101	
E1233							D1D	A,P,R	0	20030101	20090101	
E1234							D1D	A,P,R	0	20030101	20090101	
E1235							D1D	A,P,R	0	20030101	20090101	
E1236							D1D	A,P,R	0	20030101	20090101	
E1237							D1D	A,P,R	0	20030101	20090101	
E1238							D1D	A,P,R	0	20030101	20090101	
E1239							D1D	A,P,R	0	20050101	20050101	
E1240							D1D	R	0	19860101	19890101	
E1250			K0003				D1D	R	0	19860101	20010401	
E1260			K0003				D1D	R	0	19860101	20010401	
E1270							D1D	R	0	19860101	19890101	
E1280							D1D	R	0	19860101	19890101	

HCPCS Code	Long Description	Coverage	Action	PI	MPI	CIM	MCM
E1285	HEAVY DUTY WHEELCHAIR, FIXED FULL LENGTH ARMS, SWING AWAY DETACHABLE FOOTREST	I	N	00	9	60-9	
E1290	HEAVY DUTY WHEELCHAIR, DETACHABLE ARMS (DESK OR FULL LENGTH) SWING AWAY DETACHABLE FOOTREST	I	N	00	9	60-9	
E1295	HEAVY DUTY WHEELCHAIR, FIXED FULL LENGTH ARMS, ELEVATING LEGREST	D	N	36	A	60-9	
E1296	SPECIAL WHEELCHAIR SEAT HEIGHT FROM FLOOR	D	N	32	A	60-6	
E1297	SPECIAL WHEELCHAIR SEAT DEPTH, BY UPHOLSTERY	D	N	32	A	60-6	
E1298	SPECIAL WHEELCHAIR SEAT DEPTH AND/OR WIDTH, BY CONSTRUCTION	D	N	32	A	60-6	
E1300	WHIRLPOOL, PORTABLE (OVERTUB TYPE)	M	N	00	9	60-9	
E1310	WHIRLPOOL, NON-PORTABLE (BUILT-IN TYPE)	D	N	32	A	60-9	
E1340	REPAIR OR NONROUTINE SERVICE FOR DURABLE MEDICAL EQUIPMENT REQUIRING THE SKILL OF A TECHNICIAN, LABOR COMPONENT, PER 15 MINUTES	I	D	00	9		
E1353	REGULATOR	D	N	00	9	60-4	4107.9
E1354	OXYGEN ACCESSORY, WHEELED CART FOR PORTABLE CYLINDER OR PORTABLE CONCENTRATOR, ANY TYPE, REPLACEMENT ONLY, EACH	C	N	00	9		
E1355	STAND/RACK	D	N	00	9	60-4	
E1356	OXYGEN ACCESSORY, BATTERY PACK/CARTRIDGE FOR PORTABLE CONCENTRATOR, ANY TYPE, REPLACEMENT ONLY, EACH	C	N	00	9		
E1357	OXYGEN ACCESSORY, BATTERY CHARGER FOR PORTABLE CONCENTRATOR, ANY TYPE, REPLACEMENT ONLY, EACH	C	N	00	9		
E1358	OXYGEN ACCESSORY, DC POWER ADAPTER FOR PORTABLE CONCENTRATOR, ANY TYPE, REPLACEMENT ONLY, EACH	I	N	00	9		
E1372	IMMERSION EXTERNAL HEATER FOR NEBULIZER	D	N	32	A	60-4	
E1390	OXYGEN CONCENTRATOR, SINGLE DELIVERY PORT, CAPABLE OF DELIVERING 85 PERCENT OR GREATER OXYGEN CONCENTRATION AT THE PRESCRIBED FLOW RATE	D	N	33	A	60-4	
E1391	OXYGEN CONCENTRATOR, DUAL DELIVERY PORT, CAPABLE OF DELIVERING 85 PERCENT OR GREATER OXYGEN CONCENTRATION AT THE PRESCRIBED FLOW RATE, EACH	D	N	33	A	60-4	
E1392	PORTABLE OXYGEN CONCENTRATOR, RENTAL	D	N	33	A	60-4	
E1399	DURABLE MEDICAL EQUIPMENT, MISCELLANEOUS	C	N	46	A		
E1405	OXYGEN AND WATER VAPOR ENRICHING SYSTEM WITH HEATED DELIVERY	D	N	33	A	60-4	4107
E1406	OXYGEN AND WATER VAPOR ENRICHING SYSTEM WITHOUT HEATED DELIVERY	D	N	33	A	60-4	4107
E1500	CENTRIFUGE, FOR DIALYSIS	D	N	52	A		
E1510	KIDNEY, DIALYSATE DELIVERY SYST. KIDNEY MACHINE, PUMP RECIRCULAT- ING, AIR REMOVAL SYST, FLOWRATE METER, POWER OFF, HEATER AND TEMPERATURE CONTROL WITH ALARM, I.V.POLES, PRESSURE GAUGE, CONCENTRATE CONTAINER	D	N	52	A		
E1520	HEPARIN INFUSION PUMP FOR HEMODIALYSIS	D	N	52	A		
E1530	AIR BUBBLE DETECTOR FOR HEMODIALYSIS, EA., REPLACEMENT	D	N	52	A		
E1540	PRESSURE ALARM FOR HEMODIALYSIS, EACH, REPLACEMENT	D	N	52	A		

HCPCS Code	Statute	Lab Cert	X-Ref	ASC Pay Grp	ASC Pay Group Eff. Date	Proc Notes	BETOS	TOS	Anest	Code Add Date	Code Effective Date	Code Term Date
E1285			K0006				D1D	R	0	19860101	20010401	
E1290			K0006				D1D	R	0	19860101	20010401	
E1295							D1D	R	0	19860101	19890101	
E1296							D1D	A,P,R	0	19860101	19890101	
E1297							D1D	A,P,R	0	19860101	19890101	
E1298							D1D	A,P,R	0	19860101	19890101	
E1300							D1E	A,P,R	0	19860101	19960101	
E1310							D1E	A,P,R	0	19860101	19960101	
E1340							D1E	9	0	19970101	20100101	20091231
E1340												
E1353							D1C	R	0	19860101	20090101	
E1354							D1C	A,P,R	0	20090101	20090101	
E1355							D1C	R	0	19860101	20090101	
E1356							D1C	A,P,R	0	20090101	20090101	
E1357							D1C	A,P,R	0	20090101	20090101	
E1357												
E1358							D1C	A,P,R	0	20090101	20090101	
E1372							D1E	A,P,R	0	19860101	19960101	
E1390							D1C	R	t	20000101	20040101	
E1391							D1C	R	0	20040101	20040101	
E1392							D1C	R	0	20060101	20060101	
E1399							D1E	A,P,R	0	19860101	19960101	
E1405							D1C	R	0	19880101	19900101	
E1406							D1C	R	0	19880101	19900101	
E1500						0017	P9B	L	0	20020101	20020101	
E1510						0017	P9B	L	0	19860101	20020101	
E1520						0017	P9B	L	0	19860101	20020101	
E1530						0017	P9B	L	0	19860101	20020101	
E1540						0017	P9B	L	0	19860101	20020101	

HCPCS Code	Long Description	Coverage	Action	PI	MPI	CIM	MCM
E1550	BATH CONDUCTIVITY METER FOR HEMODIALYSIS, EACH	D	N	52	A		
E1560	BLOOD LEAK DETECTOR FOR HEMODIALYSIS, EA., REPLACEMENT	D	N	52	A		
E1570	ADJUSTABLE CHAIR, FOR ESRD PATIENTS	D	N	52	A		
E1575	TRANSDUCER PROTECTORS/FLUID BARRIERS, FOR HEMODIALYSIS, ANY SIZE, PER 10	D	N	52	A		
E1580	UNIPUNCTURE CONTROL SYSTEM FOR HEMODIALYSIS	D	N	52	A		
E1590	HEMODIALYSIS MACHINE	D	N	52	A		
E1592	AUTOMATIC INTERMITTENT PERITONEAL DIALYSIS SYSTEM	D	N	52	A		
E1594	CYCLER DIALYSIS MACHINE FOR PERITONEAL DIALYSIS	D	N	52	A		
E1600	DELIVERY AND/OR INSTALLATION CHARGES FOR HEMODIALYSIS EQUIPMENT	D	N	52	A		
E1610	REVERSE OSMOSIS WATER PURIFICATION SYSTEM, FOR HEMODIALYSIS	D	N	52	A	55-1A	
E1615	DEIONIZER WATER PURIFICATION SYSTEM, FOR HEMODIALYSIS	D	N	52	A	55-1A	
E1620	BLOOD PUMP FOR HEMODIALYSIS, REPLACEMENT	D	N	52	A		
E1625	WATER SOFTENING SYSTEM, FOR HEMODIALYSIS	D	N	52	A	55-1B	
E1630	RECIPROCATING PERITONEAL DIALYSIS SYSTEM	C	N	52	A		
E1632	WEARABLE ARTIFICIAL KIDNEY, EACH	D	N	52	A		
E1634	PERITONEAL DIALYSIS CLAMPS, EACH	D	N	52	A		4270
E1635	COMPACT (PORTABLE) TRAVEL HEMODIALYZER SYSTEM	D	N	52	A		
E1636	SORBENT CARTRIDGES, FOR HEMODIALYSIS, PER 10	D	N	52	A		
E1637	HEMOSTATS, EACH	D	N	52	A		
E1639	SCALE, EACH	D	N	52	A		
E1699	DIALYSIS EQUIPMENT, NOT OTHERWISE SPECIFIED	D	N	52	A		
E1700	JAW MOTION REHABILITATION SYSTEM	C	N	32	A		
E1701	REPLACEMENT CUSHIONS FOR JAW MOTION REHABILITATION SYSTEM, PKG. OF 6	C	N	34	A		
E1702	REPLACEMENT MEASURING SCALES FOR JAW MOTION REHABILITATION SYSTEM, PKG. OF 200	C	N	34	A		
E1800	DYNAMIC ADJUSTABLE ELBOW EXTENSION/FLEXION DEVICE, INCLUDES SOFT INTERFACE MATERIAL	C	N	36	A		
E1801	STATIC PROGRESSIVE STRETCH ELBOW DEVICE, EXTENSION AND/OR FLEXION, WITH OR WITHOUT RANGE OF MOTION ADJUSTMENT, INCLUDES ALL COMPONENTS & ACCESSORIES	C	N	36	A		
E1802	DYNAMIC ADJUSTABLE FOREARM PRONATION/SUPINATION DEVICE, INCLUDES SOFT INTERFACE MATERIAL	C	N	36	A		
E1805	DYNAMIC ADJUSTABLE WRIST EXTENSION / FLEXION DEVICE, INCLUDES SOFT INTERFACE MATERIAL	C	N	36	A		
E1806	STATIC PROGRESSIVE STRETCH WRIST DEVICE, FLEXION AND/OR EXTENSION, WITH OR WITHOUT RANGE OF MOTION ADJUSTMENT, INCLUDES ALL COMPONENTS & ACCESSORIES	C	N	36	A		
E1810	DYNAMIC ADJUSTABLE KNEE EXTENSION / FLEXION DEVICE, INCLUDES SOFT INTERFACE MATERIAL	C	N	36	A		
E1811	STATIC PROGRESSIVE STRETCH KNEE DEVICE, EXTENSION AND/OR FLEXION, WITH OR WITHOUT RANGE OF MOTION ADJUSTMENT, INCLUDES ALL COMPONENTS & ACCESSORIES	C	N	36	A		
E1812	DYNAMIC KNEE, EXTENSION/FLEXION DEVICE WITH ACTIVE RESISTANCE CONTROL	C	N	36	A		

HCPCS Code	Statute	Lab Cert	X-Ref	ASC Pay Grp	ASC Pay Group Eff. Date	Proc Notes	BETOS	TOS	Anest	Code Add Date	Code Effective Date	Code Term Date
E1550						0017	P9B	L	0	19860101	20020101	
E1560						0017	P9B	L	0	19860101	20020101	
E1570						0017	P9B	L	0	19860101	20020101	
E1575						0017	P9B	L	0	19860101	20020101	
E1580						0017	P9B	L	0	19860101	20020101	
E1590						0017	P9B	L	0	19860101	20020101	
E1592						0017	P9B	L	0	19860101	20020101	
E1594						0017	P9B	L	0	19860101	20020101	
E1600						0017	P9B	L	0	19860101	20020101	
E1610						0017	P9B	L	0	19860101	20020101	
E1615						0017	P9B	L	0	19860101	20020101	
E1620						0017	P9B	L	0	19860101	20020101	
E1625						0017	P9B	L	0	19860101	20020101	
E1630						0017	P9B	L	0	19860101	20020101	
E1632						0017	P9B	L	0	19860101	20020101	
E1634							P9B	L	0	20040101	20040101	
E1635						0017	P9B	L	0	19860101	20020101	
E1636						0017	P9B	L	0	19860101	20020101	
E1637						0017	P9B	L	0	20020101	20030101	
E1639						0017	P9B	L	0	20020101	20030101	
E1699						0017	P9B	L	0	19860101	20020101	
E1700							D1E	A,P,R	0	19930101	19971020	
E1701							D1E	P	0	19930101	19960101	
E1702							D1E	P	0	19930101	19960101	
E1800							D1E	P, R	0	19960101	20020101	
E1801							D1E	P, R	0	20020101	20080101	
E1802							D1E	R	0	20030101	20030101	
E1805							D1E	P, R	0	19960101	20020101	
E1806							D1E	P, R	0	20020101	20080101	
E1810							D1E	P, R	0	19960101	20020101	
E1811							D1E	P, R	0	20020101	20080101	
E1812							D1E	P, R	0	20060101	20060101	

HCPCS Code	Long Description	Coverage	Action	PI	MPI	CIM	MCM
E1815	DYNAMIC ADJUSTABLE ANKLE EXTENSION/FLEXION DEVICE, INCLUDES SOFT INTERFACE MATERIAL	C	N	36	A		
E1816	STATIC PROGRESSIVE STRETCH ANKLE DEVICE, FLEXION AND/OR EXTENSION, WITH OR WITHOUT RANGE OF MOTION ADJUSTMENT, INCLUDES ALL COMPONENTS & ACCESSORIES	C	N	36	A		
E1818	STATIC PROGRESSIVE STRETCH FOREARM PRONATION / SUPINATION DEVICE, WITH OR WITHOUT RANGE OF MOTION ADJUSTMENT, INCLUDES ALL COMPONENTS & ACCESSORIES	C	N	36	A		
E1820	REPLACEMENT SOFT INTERFACE MATERIAL, DYNAMIC ADJUSTABLE EXTENSION/FLEXION DEVICE	C	N	32	A		
E1821	REPLACEMENT SOFT INTERFACE MATERIAL/CUFFS FOR BI-DIRECTIONAL STATIC PROGRESSIVE STRETCH DEVICE	C	N	32	A		
E1825	DYNAMIC ADJUSTABLE FINGER EXTENSION/FLEXION DEVICE, INCLUDES SOFT INTERFACE MATERIAL	C	N	36	A		
E1830	DYNAMIC ADJUSTABLE TOE EXTENSION/FLEXION DEVICE, INCLUDES SOFT INTERFACE MATERIAL	C	N	36	A		
E1840	DYNAMIC ADJUSTABLE SHOULDER FLEXION / ABDUCTION / ROTATION DEVICE, INCLUDES SOFT INTERFACE MATERIAL	C	N	36	A		
E1841	STATIC PROGRESSIVE STRETCH SHOULDER DEVICE, WITH OR WITHOUT RANGE OF MOTION ADJUSTMENT, INCLUDES ALL COMPONENTS AND ACCESSORIES	C	N	36	A		
E1902	COMMUNICATION BOARD, NON-ELECTRONIC AUGMENTATIVE OR ALTERNATIVE COMMUNICATION DEVICE	C	N	00	9		
E2000	GASTRIC SUCTION PUMP, HOME MODEL, PORTABLE OR STATIONARY, ELECTRIC	C	N	36	A		
E2100	BLOOD GLUCOSE MONITOR WITH INTEGRATED VOICE SYNTHESIZER	D	N	32	A	60-11	
E2101	BLOOD GLUCOSE MONITOR WITH INTEGRATED LANCING/BLOOD SAMPLE	D	N	32	A	60-11	
E2120	PULSE GENERATOR SYSTEM FOR TYMPANIC TREATMENT OF INNER EAR ENDOLYMPHATIC FLUID	C	N	36	A		
E2201	MANUAL WHEELCHAIR ACCESSORY, NONSTANDARD SEAT FRAME, WIDTH GREATER THAN OR EQUAL TO 20 INCHES AND LESS THAN 24 INCHES	C	N	32	A		
E2202	MANUAL WHEELCHAIR ACCESSORY, NONSTANDARD SEAT FRAME WIDTH, 24-27 INCHES	C	N	32	A		
E2203	MANUAL WHEELCHAIR ACCESSORY, NONSTANDARD SEAT FRAME DEPTH, 20 TO LESS THAN 22 INCHES	C	N	32	A		
E2204	MANUAL WHEELCHAIR ACCESSORY, NONSTANDARD SEAT FRAME DEPTH, 22 TO 25 INCHES	C	N	32	A		
E2205	MANUAL WHEELCHAIR ACCESSORY, HANDRIM WITHOUT PROJECTIONS (INCLUDES ERGONOMIC OR CONTOURED), ANY TYPE, REPLACEMENT ONLY, EACH	C	N	32	A		
E2206	MANUAL WHEELCHAIR ACCESSORY, WHEEL LOCK ASSEMBLY, COMPLETE, EACH	C	N	32	A		
E2207	WHEELCHAIR ACCESSORY, CRUTCH AND CANE HOLDER, EA.	C	N	32	A		
E2208	WHEELCHAIR ACCESSORY, CYLINDER TANK CARRIER, EACH	C	N	32	A		
E2209	ACCESSORY, ARM TROUGH, WITH OR WITHOUT HAND SUPPORT, EACH	C	N	32	A		

HCPCS Code	Statute	Lab Cert	X-Ref	ASC Pay Grp	ASC Pay Group Eff. Date	Proc Notes	BETOS	TOS	Anest	Code Add Date	Code Effective Date	Code Term Date
E1815							D1E	P, R	0	19960101	20020101	
E1816							D1E	P, R	0	20020101	20080101	
E1818							D1E	P, R	0	20020101	20080101	
E1820							D1E	P, R	0	19960101	20020101	
E1821							D1E	P, R	0	20020101	20020101	
E1825							D1E	P, R	0	19960101	20020101	
E1830							D1E	P, R	0	19960101	20020101	
E1840							D1E	P, R	0	20020101	20020101	
E1841							D1E	R	0	20050101	20080101	
E1902							Z2	A,P,R	0	20020101	20020101	
E2000							D1E	R	0	20020101	20020101	
E2100							D1E	A,P,R	0	20020101	20020101	
E2101							D1E	A,P,R	0	20020101	20020101	
E2120							D1E	R	0	20040101	20040101	
E2201							D1D	A,P,R	0	20040101	20040101	
E2202							D1D	A,P,R	0	20040101	20040101	
E2203							D1D	A,P,R	0	20040101	20040101	
E2204							D1D	A,P,R	0	20040101	20040101	
E2205							D1D	A,P,R	0	20050101	20080101	
E2206							D1D	A,P,R	0	20050101	20050101	
E2207							D1D	A,P,R	0	20060101	20060101	
E2208							D1D	A,P,R	0	20060101	20060101	
E2209							D1D	A,P,R	0	20060101	20070101	

HCPCS Code	Long Description	Coverage	Action	PI	MPI	CIM	MCM
E2210	WHEELCHAIR ACCESSORY, BEARINGS, ANY TYPE, REPLACEMENT ONLY, EACH	C	N	32	A		
E2211	MANUAL WHEELCHAIR ACCESSORY, PNEUMATIC PROPULSION TIRE, ANY SIZE, EACH	C	N	32	A		
E2212	MANUAL WHEELCHAIR ACCESSORY, TUBE FOR PNEUMATIC PROPULSION TIRE, ANY SIZE, EACH	C	N	32	A		
E2213	MANUAL WHEELCHAIR ACCESSORY, INSERT FOR PNEUMATIC PROPULSION TIRE (REMOVABLE),ANY TYPE, ANY SIZE, EACH	C	N	32	A		
E2214	MANUAL WHEELCHAIR ACCESSORY, PNEUMATIC CASTER TIRE, ANY SIZE, EACH	C	N	32	A		
E2215	MANUAL WHEELCHAIR ACCESSORY, TUBE FOR PNEUMATIC CASTER TIRE, ANY SIZE, EACH	C	N	32	A		
E2216	MANUAL WHEELCHAIR ACCESSORY, FOAM FILLED PROPULSION TIRE, ANY SIZE, EACH	C	N	32	A		
E2217	MANUAL WHEELCHAIR ACCESSORY, FOAM FILLED CASTER TIRE, ANY SIZE, EACH	C	N	32	A		
E2218	MANUAL WHEELCHAIR ACCESSORY, FOAM PROPULSION TIRE, ANY SIZE, EACH	C	N	32	A		
E2219	MANUAL WHEELCHAIR ACCESSORY, FOAM CASTER TIRE, ANY SIZE, EACH	C	N	32	A		
E2220	MANUAL WHEELCHAIR ACCESSORY, SOLID (RUBBER/PLASTIC) PROPULSION TIRE, ANY SIZE, EACH	C	N	32	A		
E2221	MANUAL WHEELCHAIR ACCESSORY, SOLID (RUBBER/PLASTIC) CASTER TIRE (REMOVABLE),ANY SIZE, EACH	C	N	32	A		
E2222	MANUAL WHEELCHAIR ACCESSORY, SOLID (RUBBER/PLASTIC) CASTER TIRE WITH INTEGRATED WHEEL, ANY SIZE, EACH	C	N	32	A		
E2223	MANUAL WHEELCHAIR ACCESSORY, VALVE, ANY TYPE, REPLACEMENT ONLY, EACH	C	D	32	A		
E2224	MANUAL WHEELCHAIR ACCESSORY, PROPULSION WHEEL EXCLUDES TIRE, ANY SIZE, EACH	C	N	32	A		
E2225	MANUAL WHEELCHAIR ACCESSORY, CASTER WHEEL EXCLUDES TIRE, ANY SIZE, REPLACEMENT ONLY, EACH	C	N	32	A		
E2226	MANUAL WHEELCHAIR ACCESSORY, CASTER FORK, ANY SIZE, REPLACEMENT ONLY, EACH	C	N	32	A		
E2227	MANUAL WHEELCHAIR ACCESSORY, GEAR REDUCTION DRIVE WHEEL, EACH	C	N	32	A		
E2228	MANUAL WHEELCHAIR ACCESSORY, WHEEL BRAKING SYSTEM AND LOCK, COMPLETE, EACH	C	N	32	A		
E2230	MANUAL WHEELCHAIR ACCESSORY, MANUAL STANDING SYSTEM	I	N	00	9		
E2231	MANUAL WHEELCHAIR ACCESSORY, SOLID SEAT SUPPORT BASE (REPLACES SLING SEAT),INCLUDES ANY TYPE MOUNTING HARDWARE	C	N	32	A		
E2291	BACK, PLANAR, FOR PEDIATRIC SIZE WHEELCHAIR INCLUDING FIXED ATTACHING HARDWARE	C	N	32	A		
E2292	SEAT, PLANAR, FOR PEDIATRIC SIZE WHEELCHAIR INCLUDING FIXED ATTACHING HARDWARE	C	N	32	A		
E2293	BACK, CONTOURED, FOR PEDIATRIC SIZE WHEELCHAIR INCLUDING FIXED ATTACHING HARDWARE	C	N	32	A		

HCPCS Code	Statute	Lab Cert	X-Ref	ASC Pay Grp	ASC Pay Group Eff. Date	Proc Notes	BETOS	TOS	Anest	Code Add Date	Code Effective Date	Code Term Date
E2210							D1D	A,P,R	0	20060101	20060101	
E2211							D1D	A,P,R	0	20060101	20060101	
E2212							D1D	A,P,R	0	20060101	20060101	
E2213							D1D	A,P,R	0	20060101	20060101	
E2213 E2214							D1D	A,P,R	0	20060101	20060101	
E2215							D1D	A,P,R	0	20060101	20060101	
E2216							D1D	A,P,R	0	20060101	20060101	
E2217							D1D	A,P,R	0	20060101	20060101	
E2218							D1D	A,P,R	0	20060101	20060101	
E2219							D1D	A,P,R	0	20060101	20060101	
E2220							D1D	A,P,R	0	20060101	20060101	
E2221							D1D	A,P,R	0	20060101	20060101	
E2222							D1D	A,P,R	0	20060101	20060101	
E2223							D1D	A,P,R	0	20060101	20100101	20091231
E2224							D1D	A,P,R	0	20060101	20060101	
E2225							D1D	A,P,R	0	20060101	20060101	
E2226							D1D	A,P,R	0	20060101	20060101	
E2227							D1D	A,P,R	0	20080101	20080101	
E2228							D1D	A,P,R	0	20080101	20080101	
E2230							D1D	A,P,R	0	20090101	20090101	
E2231							D1D	A,P,R	0	20090101	20090101	
E2291							D1D	A,P,R	0	20050101	20060101	
E2292							D1D	A,P,R	0	20050101	20060101	
E2293							D1D	A,P,R	0	20050101	20060101	

HCPCS Code	Long Description	Coverage	Action	PI	MPI	CIM	MCM
E2294	SEAT, CONTOURED, FOR PEDIATRIC SIZE WHEELCHAIR INCLUDING FIXED ATTACHING HARDWARE	C	N	32	A		
E2295	MANUAL WHEELCHAIR ACCESSORY, FOR PEDIATRIC SIZE WHEELCHAIR, DYNAMIC SEATING FRAME, ALLOWS COORDINATED MOVEMENT OF MULTIPLE POSITIONING FEATURES	C	N	32	A		
E2300	POWER WHEELCHAIR ACCESSORY, POWER SEAT ELEVATION SYSTEM	C	N	32	A		
E2301	POWER WHEELCHAIR ACCESSORY, POWER STANDING SYSTEM	C	N	00	9		
E2310	POWER WHEELCHAIR ACCESSORY, ELECTRONIC CONNECTION BETWEEN WHEELCHAIR CONTROLLER AND ONE POWER SEATING SYSTEM MOTOR, INCLUDING ALL RELATED ELECTRONICS, INDICATOR FEATURE, MECHANICAL FUNCTION SELECTION SWITCH, AND FIXED MOUNTING HARDWARE	C	N	32	A		
E2311	POWER WHEELCHAIR ACCESSORY, ELECTRONIC CONNECTION BETWEEN WHEELCHAIR CONTROLLER AND TWO OR MORE POWER SEATING SYSTEM MOTORS, INCLUDING ALL RELATED ELECTRONICS, INDICATOR FEATURE, MECHANICAL FUNCTION SELECTION SWITCH, AND FIXED MOUNTING HARDWARE	C	N	32	A		
E2312	POWER WHEELCHAIR ACCESSORY, HAND OR CHIN CONTROL INTERFACE, MINI-PROPORTIONAL REMOTE JOYSTICK, PROPORTIONAL, INCLUDING FIXED MOUNTING HARDWARE	C	N	32	A		
E2313	POWER WHEELCHAIR ACCESSORY, HARNESS FOR UPGRADE TO EXPANDABLE CONTROLLER, INCLUDING ALL FASTENERS, CONNECTORS AND MOUNTING HARDWARE, EACH	C	N	32	A		
E2320	POWER WHEELCHAIR ACCESSORY, HAND OR CHIN CONTROL INTERFACE, REMOTE JOYSTICK OR TOUCHPAD, PROPORTIONAL, INCLUDING ALL RELATED ELECTRONICS, AND FIXED MOUNTING HARDWARE	C	N	32	A		
E2321	POWER WHEELCHAIR ACCESSORY, HAND CONTROL INTERFACE, REMOTE JOYSTICK, NONPROPORTIONAL, INCLUDING ALL RELATED ELECTRONICS, MECHANICAL STOP SWITCH, AND FIXED MOUNTING HARDWARE	C	N	32	A		
E2322	POWER WHEELCHAIR ACCESSORY, HAND CONTROL INTERFACE, MULTIPLE MECHANICAL SWITCHES, NONPROPORTIONAL, INCLUDING ALL RELATED ELECTRONICS, MECHANICAL STOP SWITCH, AND FIXED MOUNTING HARDWARE	C	N	32	A		
E2323	POWER WHEELCHAIR ACCESSORY, SPECIALTY JOYSTICK HANDLE FOR HAND CONTROL INTERFACE, PREFABRICATED	C	N	32	A		
E2324	POWER WHEELCHAIR ACCESSORY, CHIN CUP FOR CHIN CONTROL INTERFACE	C	N	32	A		
E2325	POWER WHEELCHAIR ACCESSORY, SIP AND PUFF INTERFACE, NONPROPORTIONAL, INCLUDING ALL RELATED ELECTRONICS, MECHANICAL STOP SWITCH, AND MANUAL SWINGAWAY MOUNTING HARDWARE	C	N	32	A		
E2326	POWER WHEELCHAIR ACCESSORY, BREATH TUBE KIT FOR SIP AND PUFF INTERFACE	C	N	32	A		

HCPCS Code	Statute	Lab Cert	X-Ref	ASC Pay Grp	ASC Pay Group Eff. Date	Proc Notes	BETOS	TOS	Anest	Code Add Date	Code Effective Date	Code Term Date
E2294							D1D	A,P,R	0	20050101	20060101	
E2295							D1D	A,P,R	0	20090101	20090101	
E2300							D1D	A,P,R	0	20040101	20040101	
E2301							D1D	A,P,R	0	20040101	20090101	
E2310							D1D	A,P,R	0	20040101	20040101	
E2310												
E2311							D1D	A,P,R	0	20040101	20040101	
E2312							D1D	A,P,R	0	20080101	20080101	
E2313							D1D	A,P,R	0	20080101	20080101	
E2320							D1D	A,P,R	0	20040101	20070101	20061231
E2321							D1D	A,P,R	0	20040101	20040101	
E2322							D1D	A,P,R	0	20040101	20040101	
E2323							D1D	A,P,R	0	20040101	20040101	
E2324							D1D	A,P,R	0	20040101	20040101	
E2325							D1D	A,P,R	0	20040101	20040101	
E2326							D1D	A,P,R	0	20040101	20040101	

HCPCS Code	Long Description	Coverage	Action	PI	MPI	CIM	MCM
E2327	POWER WHEELCHAIR ACCESSORY, HEAD CONTROL INTERFACE, MECHANICAL, PROPORTIONAL, INCLUDING ALL RELATED ELECTRONICS, MECHANICAL DIRECTION CHANGE SWITCH, AND FIXED MOUNTING HARDWARE	C	N	32	A		
E2328	POWER WHEELCHAIR ACCESSORY, HEAD CONTROL OR EXTREMITY CONTROL INTERFACE, ELECTRONIC, PROPORTIONAL, INCLUDING ALL RELATED ELECTRONICS AND FIXED MOUNTING HARDWARE	C	N	32	A		
E2329	POWER WHEELCHAIR ACCESSORY, HEAD CONTROL INTERFACE, CONTACT SWITCH MECHANISM, NONPROPORTIONAL, INCLUDING ALL RELATED ELECTRONICS, MECHANICAL STOP SWITCH, MECHANICAL DIRECTION CHANGE SWITCH, HEAD ARRAY, AND FIXED MOUNTING HARDWARE	C	N	32	A		
E2330	POWER WHEELCHAIR ACCESSORY, HEAD CONTROL INTERFACE, PROXIMITY SWITCH MECHANISM, NONPROPORTIONAL, INCLUDING ALL RELATED ELECTRONICS, MECHANICAL STOP SWITCH, MECHANICAL DIRECTION CHANGE SWITCH, HEAD ARRAY, AND FIXED MOUNTING HARDWARE	C	N	32	A		
E2331	POWER WHEELCHAIR ACCESSORY, ATTENDANT CONTROL, PROPORTIONAL, INCLUDING ALL RELATED ELECTRONICS AND FIXED MOUNTING HARDWARE	C	N	32	A		
E2340	POWER WHEELCHAIR ACCESSORY, NONSTANDARD SEAT FRAME WIDTH, 20-23 INCHES	C	N	32	A		
E2341	POWER WHEELCHAIR ACCESSORY, NONSTANDARD SEAT FRAME WIDTH, 24-27 INCHES	C	N	32	A		
E2342	POWER WHEELCHAIR ACCESSORY, NONSTANDARD SEAT FRAME DEPTH, 20 OR 21 INCHES	C	N	32	A		
E2343	POWER WHEELCHAIR ACCESSORY, NONSTANDARD SEAT FRAME DEPTH, 22-25 INCHES	C	N	32	A		
E2351	POWER WHEELCHAIR ACCESSORY, ELECTRONIC INTERFACE TO OPERATE SPEECH GENERATING DEVICE USING POWER WHEELCHAIR CONTROL INTERFACE	C	N	32	A		
E2360	POWER WHEELCHAIR ACCESSORY, 22 NF NON-SEALED LEAD ACID BATTERY, EACH	C	N	32	A		
E2361	POWER WHEELCHAIR ACCESSORY, 22NF SEALED LEAD ACID BATTERY, EACH, (E.G. GEL CELL, ABSORBED GLASSMAT)	C	N	32	A		
E2362	POWER WHEELCHAIR ACCESSORY, GROUP 24 NON-SEALED LEAD ACID BATTERY, EACH	C	N	32	A		
E2363	POWER WHEELCHAIR ACCESSORY, GROUP 24 SEALED LEAD ACID BATTERY, EACH (E.G. GEL CELL, ABSORBED GLASSMAT)	C	N	32	A		
E2364	POWER WHEELCHAIR ACCESSORY, U-1 NON-SEALED LEAD ACID BATTERY, EACH	C	N	32	A		
E2365	POWER WHEELCHAIR ACCESSORY, U-1 SEALED LEAD ACID, BATTERY, EACH (E.G. GEL CELL ABSORBED GLASSMAT)	C	N	32	A		
E2366	POWER WHEELCHAIR ACCESSORY, BATTERY CHARGER, SINGLE MODE, FOR USE WITH ONLY ONE BATTERY TYPE, SEALED OR NON-SEALED, EACH	C	N	32	A		

HCPCS Code	Statute	Lab Cert	X-Ref	ASC Pay Grp	ASC Pay Group Eff. Date	Proc Notes	BETOS	TOS	Anest	Code Add Date	Code Effective Date	Code Term Date
E2327							D1D	A,P,R	0	20040101	20040101	
E2328							D1D	A,P,R	0	20040101	20040101	
E2329							D1D	A,P,R	0	20040101	20040101	
E2330							D1D	A,P,R	0	20040101	20040101	
E2331							D1D	A,P,R	0	20040101	20040101	
E2340							D1D	A,P,R	0	20040101	20040101	
E2341							D1D	A,P,R	0	20040101	20040101	
E2342							D1D	A,P,R	0	20040101	20040101	
E2343							D1D	A,P,R	0	20040101	20040101	
E2351							D1D	A,P,R	0	20040101	20040101	
E2360							D1D	A,P,R	0	20040101	20040101	
E2361							D1D	A,P,R	0	20040101	20040101	
E2362							D1D	A,P,R	0	20040101	20040101	
E2363							D1D	A,P,R	0	20040101	20040101	
E2364							D1D	A,P,R	0	20040101	20040101	
E2365							D1D	A,P,R	0	20040101	20040101	
E2366							D1D	A,P,R	0	20040101	20040101	

HCPCS Code	Long Description	Coverage	Action	PI	MPI	CIM	MCM
E2367	POWER WHEELCHAIR ACCESSORY, BATTERY CHARGER, DUAL MODE, FOR USE WITH EITHER BATTERY TYPE, SEALED OR NON-SEALED, EACH	C	N	32	A		
E2368	POWER WHEELCHAIR COMPONENT, MOTOR, REPLACEMENT ONLY	C	N	32	A		
E2369	POWER WHEELCHAIR COMPONENT, GEAR BOX, REPLACEMENT ONLY	C	N	32	A		
E2370	POWER WHEELCHAIR COMPONENT, MOTOR AND GEAR BOX COMBINATION, REPLACEMENT ONLY	C	N	32	A		
E2371	POWER WHEELCHAIR ACCESSORY, GROUP 27 SEALED LEAD ACID BATTERY, (E.G. GEL CELL, ABSORBED GLASSMAT), EA.	C	N	32	A		
E2372	POWER WHEELCHAIR ACCESSORY, GROUP 27 NON-SEALED LEAD ACID BATTERY, EACH	C	N	32	A		
E2373	POWER WHEELCHAIR ACCESSORY, HAND OR CHIN CONTROL INTERFACE, COMPACT REMOTE JOYSTICK, PROPORTIONAL, INCLUDING FIXED MOUNTING HARDWARE	C	N	32	A		
E2374	POWER WHEELCHAIR ACCESSORY, HAND OR CHIN CONTROL INTERFACE, STANDARD REMOTE JOYSTICK (NOT INCLUDING CONTROLLER), PROPORTIONAL, INCLUDING ALL RELATED ELECTRONICS AND FIXED MOUNTING HARDWARE, REPLACEMENT ONLY	D	N	32	A		
E2375	POWER WHEELCHAIR ACCESSORY, NON-EXPANDABLE CONTROLLER, INCLUDING ALL RELATED ELECTRONICS AND MOUNTING HARDWARE, REPLACEMENT ONLY	D	N	32	A		
E2376	POWER WHEELCHAIR ACCESSORY, EXPANDABLE CONTROLLER, INCLUDING ALL RELATED ELECTRONICS AND MOUNTING HARDWARE, REPLACEMENT ONLY	D	N	32	A		
E2377	POWER WHEELCHAIR ACCESSORY, EXPANDABLE CONTROLLER, INCLUDING ALL RELATED ELECTRONICS AND MOUNTING HARDWARE, UPGRADE PROVIDED AT INITIAL ISSUE	D	N	32	A		
E2381	POWER WHEELCHAIR ACCESSORY, PNEUMATIC DRIVE WHEEL TIRE, ANY SIZE, REPLACEMENT ONLY, EACH	D	N	32	A		
E2382	POWER WHEELCHAIR ACCESSORY, TUBE FOR PNEUMATIC DRIVE WHEEL TIRE, ANY SIZE, REPLACEMENT ONLY, EACH	D	N	32	A		
E2383	POWER WHEELCHAIR ACCESSORY, INSERT FOR PNEUMATIC DRIVE WHEEL TIRE (REMOVABLE),ANY TYPE, ANY SIZE, REPLACEMENT ONLY, EACH	D	N	32	A		
E2384	POWER WHEELCHAIR ACCESSORY, PNEUMATIC CASTER TIRE, ANY SIZE, REPLACEMENT ONLY, EACH	D	N	32	A		
E2385	POWER WHEELCHAIR ACCESSORY, TUBE FOR PNEUMATIC CASTER TIRE, ANY SIZE, REPLACEMENT ONLY, EACH	D	N	32	A		
E2386	POWER WHEELCHAIR ACCESSORY, FOAM FILLED DRIVE WHEEL TIRE, ANY SIZE, REPLACEMENT ONLY, EACH	D	N	32	A		
E2387	POWER WHEELCHAIR ACCESSORY, FOAM FILLED CASTER TIRE, ANY SIZE, REPLACEMENT ONLY, EACH	D	N	32	A		
E2388	POWER WHEELCHAIR ACCESSORY, FOAM DRIVE WHEEL TIRE, ANY SIZE, REPLACEMENT ONLY, EACH	D	N	32	A		
E2389	POWER WHEELCHAIR ACCESSORY, FOAM CASTER TIRE, ANY SIZE, REPLACEMENT ONLY, EACH	D	N	32	A		

HCPCS Code	Statute	Lab Cert	X-Ref	ASC Pay Grp	ASC Pay Group Eff. Date	Proc Notes	BETOS	TOS	Anest	Code Add Date	Code Effective Date	Code Term Date
E2367							D1D	A,P,R	0	20040101	20040101	
E2368							D1D	A,P,R	0	20050101	20050101	
E2369							D1D	A,P,R	0	20050101	20050101	
E2370							D1D	A,P,R	0	20050101	20050101	
E2371							D1D	A,P,R	0	20060101	20060101	
E2371 E2372							D1D	A,P,R	0	20060101	20060101	
E2373							D1D	A,P,R	0	20070101	20080101	
E2374						0125	D1D	A,P,R	0	20070101	20070101	
E2375						0125	D1D	A,P,R	0	20070101	20070101	
E2376						0125	D1D	A,P,R	00	20070101	20070101	
E2376 E2377						0125	D1D	A,P,R	0	20070101	20070101	
E2381						0125	D1D	A,P,R	0	20070101	20070101	
E2382						0125	D1D	A,P,R	0	20070101	20070101	
E2383						0125	D1D	A,P,R	0	20070101	20070101	
E2384						0125	D1D	A,P,R	0	20070101	20070101	
E2385						0125	D1D	A,P,R	0	20070101	20070101	
E2386						0125	D1D	A,P,R	0	20070101	20070101	
E2387						0125	D1D	A,P,R	0	20070101	20070101	
E2388						0125	D1D	A,P,R	0	20070101	20070101	
E2389						0125	D1D	A,P,R	0	20070101	20070101	

HCPCS Code	Long Description	Coverage	Action	PI	MPI	CIM	MCM
E2390	POWER WHEELCHAIR ACCESSORY, SOLID (RUBBER/PLASTIC) DRIVE WHEEL TIRE, ANY SIZE, REPLACEMENT ONLY, EACH	D	N	32	A		
E2391	POWER WHEELCHAIR ACCESSORY, SOLID (RUBBER/PLASTIC) CASTER TIRE (REMOVABLE), ANY SIZE, REPLACEMENT ONLY, EACH	D	N	32	A		
E2392	POWER WHEELCHAIR ACCESSORY, SOLID (RUBBER/PLASTIC) CASTER TIRE WITH INTEGRATED WHEEL, ANY SIZE, REPLACEMENT ONLY, EACH	D	N	32	A		
E2393	POWER WHEELCHAIR ACCESSORY, VALVE FOR PNEUMATIC TIRE TUBE, ANY TYPE, REPLACEMENT ONLY, EACH	D	D	32	A		
E2394	POWER WHEELCHAIR ACCESSORY, DRIVE WHEEL EXCLUDES TIRE, ANY SIZE, REPLACEMENT ONLY, EACH	D	N	32	A		
E2395	POWER WHEELCHAIR ACCESSORY, CASTER WHEEL EXCLUDES TIRE, ANY SIZE, REPLACEMENT ONLY, EACH	D	N	32	A		
E2396	POWER WHEELCHAIR ACCESSORY, CASTER FORK, ANY SIZE, REPLACEMENT ONLY, EACH	D	N	32	A		
E2397	POWER WHEELCHAIR ACCESSORY, LITHIUM-BASED BATTERY, EACH	C	N	32	A		
E2399	POWER WHEELCHAIR ACCESSORY, NOT OTHERWISE CLASSIFIED INTERFACE, INCLUDING ALL RELATED ELECTRONICS AND ANY TYPE MOUNTING HARDWARE	C	D	32	A		
E2402	NEGATIVE PRESSURE WOUND THERAPY ELECTRICAL PUMP, STATIONARY OR PORTABLE	C	N	36	A		
E2500	SPEECH GENERATING DEVICE, DIGITIZED SPEECH, USING PRE-RECORDED MESSAGES, LESS THAN OR EQUAL TO 8 MINUTES RECORDING TIME	D	N	32	A	60-23	
E2502	SPEECH GENERATING DEVICE, DIGITIZED SPEECH, USING PRE-RECORDED MESSAGES, GREATER THAN 8 MINUTES BUT LESS THAN OR EQUAL TO 20 MINUTES RECORDING TIME	D	N	32	A	60-23	
E2504	SPEECH GENERATING DEVICE, DIGITIZED SPEECH, USING PRE-RECORDED MESSAGES, GREATER THAN 20 MINUTES BUT LESS THAN OR EQUAL TO 40 MINUTES RECORDING TIME	D	N	32	A	60-23	
E2506	SPEECH GENERATING DEVICE, DIGITIZED SPEECH, USING PRE-RECORDED MESSAGES, GREATER THAN 40 MINUTES RECORDING TIME	D	N	32	A	60-23	
E2508	SPEECH GENERATING DEVICE, SYNTHESIZED SPEECH, REQUIRING MESSAGE FORMULATION BY SPELLING AND ACCESS BY PHYSICAL CONTACT WITH THE DEVICE	D	N	32	A	60-23	
E2510	SPEECH GENERATING DEVICE, SYNTHESIZED SPEECH, PERMITTING MULTIPLE METHODS OF MESSAGE FORMULATION AND MULTIPLE METHODS OF DEVICE ACCESS	D	N	32	A	60-23	
E2511	SPEECH GENERATING SOFTWARE PROGRAM, FOR PERSONAL COMPUTER OR PERSONAL DIGITAL ASSISTANT	D	N	32	A	60-23	
E2512	ACCESSORY FOR SPEECH GENERATING DEVICE, MOUNTING SYSTEM	D	N	32	A	60-23	
E2599	ACCESSORY FOR SPEECH GENERATING DEVICE, NOT OTHERWISE CLASSIFIED	D	N	32	A	60-23	
E2601	GENERAL USE WHEELCHAIR SEAT CUSHION, WIDTH LESS THAN 22 INCHES, ANY DEPTH	C	N	32	A		

HCPCS Code	Statute	Lab Cert	X-Ref	ASC Pay Grp	ASC Pay Group Eff. Date	Proc Notes	BETOS	TOS	Anest	Code Add Date	Code Effective Date	Code Term Date
E2390						0125	D1D	A,P,R	0	20070101	20070101	
E2391						0125	D1D	A,P,R	0	20070101	20070101	
E2392						0125	D1D	A,P,R	0	20070101	20070101	
E2393						0125	D1D	A,P,R	0	20070101	20100101	20091231
E2394						0125	D1D	A,P,R	0	20070101	20070101	
E2395						0125	D1D	A,P,R	0	20070101	20070101	
E2396						0125	D1D	A,P,R	0	20070101	20070101	
E2397							D1D	P	0	20080101	20080101	
E2399							D1D	A,P,R	0	20040101	20100101	20091231
E2402							D1E	R	0	20040101	20040101	
E2500							D1E	A,P,R	0	20040101	20040101	
E2502							D1E	A,P,R	0	20040101	20040101	
E2504							D1E	A,P,R	0	20040101	20040101	
E2506							D1E	A,P,R	0	20040101	20040101	
E2508							D1E	A,P,R	0	20040101	20040101	
E2510							D1E	A,P,R	0	20040101	20040101	
E2511							D1E	A,P,R	0	20040101	20040101	
E2512							D1E	A, P, R	0		20040101	20040101
E2599							D1E	A,P,R	0	20040101	20040101	
E2601							D1D	A,P,R	0	20050101	20050101	

HCPCS Code	Long Description	Coverage	Action	PI	MPI	CIM	MCM
E2602	GENERAL USE WHEELCHAIR SEAT CUSHION, WIDTH 22 INCHES OR GREATER, ANY DEPTH	C	N	32	A		
E2603	SKIN PROTECTION WHEELCHAIR SEAT CUSHION, WIDTH LESS THAN 22 INCHES, ANY DEPTH	C	N	32	A		
E2604	SKIN PROTECTION WHEELCHAIR SEAT CUSHION, WIDTH 22 INCHES OR GREATER, ANY DEPTH	C	N	32	A		
E2605	POSITIONING WHEELCHAIR SEAT CUSHION, WIDTH LESS THAN 22 INCHES, ANY DEPTH	C	N	32	A		
E2606	POSITIONING WHEELCHAIR SEAT CUSHION, WIDTH 22 INCHES OR GREATER, ANY DEPTH	C	N	32	A		
E2607	SKIN PROTECTION AND POSITIONING WHEELCHAIR SEAT CUSHION, WIDTH LESS THAN 22 INCHES, ANY DEPTH	C	N	32	A		
E2608	SKIN PROTECTION AND POSITIONING WHEELCHAIR SEAT CUSHION, WIDTH 22 INCHES OR GREATER, ANY DEPTH	C	N	32	A		
E2609	CUSTOM FABRICATED WHEELCHAIR SEAT CUSHION, ANY SIZE	C	N	32	A		
E2610	WHEELCHAIR SEAT CUSHION, POWERED	C	N	32	A		
E2611	GENERAL USE WHEELCHAIR BACK CUSHION, WIDTH LESS THAN 22 INCHES, ANY HEIGHT, INCLUDING ANY TYPE MOUNTING HARDWARE	C	N	32	A		
E2612	GENERAL USE WHEELCHAIR BACK CUSHION, WIDTH 22 INCHES OR GREATER, ANY HEIGHT, INCLUDING ANY TYPE MOUNTING HARDWARE	C	N	32	A		
E2613	POSITIONING WHEELCHAIR BACK CUSHION, POSTERIOR, WIDTH LESS THAN 22 INCHES, ANY HEIGHT, INCLUDING ANY TYPE MOUNTING HARDWARE	C	N	32	A		
E2614	POSITIONING WHEELCHAIR BACK CUSHION, POSTERIOR, WIDTH 22 INCHES OR GREATER, ANY HEIGHT, INCLUDING ANY TYPE MOUNTING HARDWARE	C	N	32	A		
E2615	POSITIONING WHEELCHAIR BACK CUSHION, POSTERIOR-LATERAL, WIDTH LESS THAN 22 INCHES, ANY HEIGHT, INCLUDING ANY TYPE MOUNTING HARDWARE	C	N	32	A		
E2616	POSITIONING WHEELCHAIR BACK CUSHION, POSTERIOR-LATERAL, WIDTH 22 INCHES OR GREATER, ANY HEIGHT, INCLUDING ANY TYPE MOUNTING HARDWARE	C	N	32	A		
E2617	CUSTOM FABRICATED WHEELCHAIR BACK CUSHION, ANY SIZE, INCLUDING ANY TYPE MOUNTING HARDWARE	C	N	32	A		
E2618	WHEELCHAIR ACCESSORY, SOLID SEAT SUPPORT BASE (REPLACES SLING SEAT), FOR USE WITH MANUAL WHEELCHAIR OR LIGHTWEIGHT POWER WHEELCHAIR, INCLUDES ANY TYPE MOUNTING HARDWARE	C	N	32	A		
E2619	REPLACEMENT COVER FOR WHEELCHAIR SEAT CUSHION OR BACK CUSHION, EACH	C	N	32	A		
E2620	POSITIONING WHEELCHAIR BACK CUSHION, PLANAR BACK WITH LATERAL SUPPORTS, WIDTH LESS THAN 22 INCHES, ANY HEIGHT, INCLUDING ANY TYPE MOUNTING HARDWARE	C	N	32	A		
E2621	POSITIONING WHEELCHAIR BACK CUSHION, PLANAR BACK WITH LATERAL SUPPORTS, WIDTH 22 INCHES OR GREATER, ANY HEIGHT, INCLUDING ANY TYPE MOUNTING HARDWARE	C	N	32	A		

E Codes

HCPCS Code	Statute	Lab Cert	X-Ref	ASC Pay Grp	ASC Pay Group Eff. Date	Proc Notes	BETOS	TOS	Anest	Code Add Date	Code Effective Date	Code Term Date
E2602							D1D	A,P,R	0	20050101	20050101	
E2603							D1D	A,P,R	0	20050101	20050101	
E2604							D1D	A,P,R	0	20050101	20050101	
E2605							D1D	A,P,R	0	20050101	20050101	
E2606							D1D	A,P,R	0	20050101	20050101	
E2607							D1D	A,P,R	0	20050101	20050101	
E2608							D1D	A,P,R	0	20050101	20050101	
E2609							D1D	A, P, R	0	20050101	20050101	20050101
E2610							D1D	A, P, R	0	20050101	20050101	20050101
E2611							D1D	A,P,R	0	20050101	20050101	
E2612							D1D	A,P,R	0	20050101	20050101	
E2613							D1D	A,P,R	0	20050101	20050101	
E2614							D1D	A,P,R	0	20050101	20050101	
E2615							D1D	A,P,R	0	20050101	20050101	
E2616							D1D	A,P,R	0	20050101	20050101	
E2617							D1D	A,P,R	0	20050101	20050101	
E2618							D1D	A,P,R	0	20050101	20080101	20071231
E2619							D1D	A,P,R	0	20050101	20050101	
E2620							D1D	A,P,R	0	20050101	20050101	
E2621							D1D	A,P,R	0	20050101	20050101	

HCPCS Code	Long Description	Coverage	Action	PI	MPI	CIM	MCM
E8000	GAIT TRAINER, PEDIATRIC SIZE, POSTERIOR SUPPORT, INCLUDES ALL ACCESSORIES AND COMPONENTS	I	N	00	9		
E8001	GAIT TRAINER, PEDIATRIC SIZE, UPRIGHT SUPPORT, INCLUDES ALL ACCESSORIES AND COMPONENTS	I	N	00	9		
E8002	GAIT TRAINER, PEDIATRIC SIZE, ANTERIOR SUPPORT, INCLUDES ALL ACCESSORIES AND COMPONENTS	I	N	00	9		
G0008	ADMINISTRATION OF INFLUENZA VIRUS VACCINE	C	N	54	A		
G0009	ADMINISTRATION OF PNEUMOCOCCAL VACCINE	C	N	54	A		
G0010	ADMINISTRATION OF HEPATITIS B VACCINE	C	N	54	A		
G0027	SEMEN ANALYSIS; PRESENCE AND/OR MOTILITY OF SPERM EXCLUDING HUHNER	C	N	21	A		
G0101	CERVICAL OR VAGINAL CANCER SCREENING; PELVIC AND CLINICAL BREAST EXAMINATION	D	N	11	A		
G0102	PROSTATE CANCER SCREENING; DIGITAL RECTAL EXAMINATION	D	N	11	A	50-55	4182
G0103	PROSTATE CANCER SCREENING; PROSTATE SPECIFIC ANTIGEN TEST (PSA)	D	N	21	A	50-55	4182
G0104	COLORECTAL CANCER SCREENING; FLEXIBLE SIGMOIDOSCOPY	D	N	11	A		
G0105	COLORECTAL CANCER SCREENING; COLONOSCOPY ON INDIVIDUAL AT HIGH RISK	D	N	11	A		
G0106	COLORECTAL CANCER SCREENING; ALTERNATIVE TO G0104, SCREENING SIGMOIDOSCOPY, BARIUM ENEMA	D	N	11	A		
G0107	COLORECTAL CANCER SCREENING; FECAL-OCCULT BLOOD TEST, 1-3 SIMULTANEOUS DETERMINATIONS	D	N	21	A		
G0108	DIABETES OUTPATIENT SELF-MANAGEMENT TRAINING SERVICES, INDIVIDUAL, PER 30 MINUTES	C	N	11	A		
G0109	DIABETES OUTPATIENT SELF-MANAGEMENT TRAINING SERVICES, GROUP SESSION (2 OR MORE), PER 30 MINUTES	C	N	11	A		
G0117	GLAUCOMA SCREENING FOR HIGH RISK PATIENTS FURNISHED BY AN OPTOMETRIST OR OPHTHALMOLOGIST	C	N	11	A		
G0118	GLAUCOMA SCREENING FOR HIGH RISK PATIENT FURNISHED UNDER THE DIRECT SUPERVISION OF AN OPTOMETRIST OR OPHTHALOMOLOGIST	C	N	11	A		
G0120	COLORECTAL CANCER SCREENING; ALTERNATIVE TO G0105, SCREENING COLONOSCOPY, BARIUM ENEMA.	D	N	11	A		
G0121	COLORECTAL CANCER SCREENING; COLONOSCOPY ON INDIVIDUAL NOT MEETING CRITERIA FOR HIGH RISK	D	N	11	A		
G0122	COLORECTAL CANCER SCREENING; BARIUM ENEMA	M	N	00	9		
G0123	SCREENING CYTOPATHOLOGY, CERVICAL OR VAGINAL (ANY REPORTING SYSTEM), COLLECTED IN PRESERVATIVE FLUID, AUTOMATED THIN LAYER PREPARATION, SCREENING BY CYTOTECHNOLOGIST UNDER PHYSICIAN SUPERVISION	D	N	21	A	50-20	
G0124	SCREENING CYTOPATHOLOGY, CERVICAL OR VAGINAL (ANY REPORTING SYSTEM), COLLECTED IN PRESERVATIVE FLUID, AUTOMATED THIN LAYER PREPARATION, REQUIRING INTERPRETATION BY PHYSICIAN	D	N	11, 21	A	C	50-20
G0127	TRIMMING OF DYSTROPHIC NAILS, ANY NUMBER	D	N	11	A		2323, 4120

HCPCS Code	Statute	Lab Cert	X-Ref	ASC Pay Grp	ASC Pay Group Eff. Date	Proc Notes	BETOS	TOS	Anest	Code Add Date	Code Effective Date	Code Term Date
E8000							Z2	9	0	20050101	20050101	
E8001							Z2	9	0	20050101	20050101	
E8002							Z2	9	0	20050101	20050101	
G0008							O1G	V	0	19940101	19960101	
G0009							O1G	V	0	19940101	19960101	
G0010							O1G	1	0	19940101	19960101	
G0027		400					T1H	5	0	19950101	20031001	
G0101						0064	M1A	1	0	19980101	19980101	
G0102						0079	Y1	1	0	20000101	20000101	
G0103		310				0064	T1H	5	0	20000101	20070101	
G0104				YY	20080101	0064	P8C	2	0	19980101	19980101	
G0105				YY	19980101	0064	P8D	2	0	19980101	19980101	
G0106						0064	I1D	4	0	19980101	19980101	
G0107						0064	T1H	5	0	19980101	20070101	20061231
G0108						0071	Y1	1	0	19980701	20010101	
G0109						0071	Y1	1	0	19980701	20010101	
G0117							T2D	Q	0	20020101	20031001	
G0117 G0118							T2D	Q	0	20020101	20031001	
G0120						0064	I1D	4	0	19980101	19980101	
G0121				YY	20010701	0064	I1D	2	0	19980101	20010701	
G0122						0064	I1D	4	0	19980101	19980101	
G0123		630				0045	T1H	5	0	19980401	19980401	
G0124		630				0045	T1H	5	0	19980401	19980401	
G0127				YY	20080101		P5A	2	0	19980101	19980101	

HCPCS Code	Long Description	Coverage	Action	PI	MPI	CIM	MCM
G0128	DIRECT (FACE-TO-FACE WITH PATIENT) SKILLED NURSING SERVICES OF A REGISTERED NURSE PROVIDED IN A COMPREHENSIVE OUTPATIENT REHABILITATION FACILITY, EACH 10 MINUTES BEYOND THE FIRST 5 MINUTES	D	N	99	9		
G0129	OCCUPATIONAL THERAPY SERVICES REQUIRING THE SKILLS OF A QUALIFIED OCCUPATIONAL THERAPIST, FURNISHED AS A COMPONENT OF A PARTIAL HOSPITALIZATION TREATMENT PROGRAM, PER SESSION (45 MINUTES OR MORE)	C	N	00	9		
G0130	SINGLE ENERGY X-RAY ABSORPTIOMETRY (SEXA) BONE DENSITY STUDY, ONE OR MORE SITES; APPENDICULAR SKELETON (PERIPHERAL) (EG, RADIUS, WRIST, HEEL)	D	N	11	A	50-44	
G0141	SCREENING CYTOPATHOLOGY SMEARS, CERVICAL OR VAGINAL, PERFORMED BY AUTOMATED SYSTEM, WITH MANUAL RESCREENING, REQUIRING INTERPRETATION BY PHYSICIAN	C	N	11	A		
G0143	SCREENING CYTOPATHOLOGY, CERVICAL OR VAGINAL (ANY REPORTING SYSTEM), COLLECTED IN PRESERVATIVE FLUID, AUTOMATED THIN LAYER PREPARATION, WITH MANUAL SCREENING AND RESCREENING BY CYTOTECHNOLOGIST UNDER PHYSICIAN SUPERVISION	C	N	21	A		
G0144	SCREENING CYTOPATHOLOGY, CERVICAL OR VAGINAL (ANY REPORTING SYSTEM), COLLECTED IN PRESERVATIVE FLUID, AUTOMATED THIN LAYER PREPARATION, WITH SCREENING BY AUTOMATED SYSTEM, UNDER PHYSICIAN SUPERVISION	C	N	21	A		
G0145	SCREENING CYTOPATHOLOGY, CERVICAL OR VAGINAL (ANY REPORTING SYSTEM), COLLECTED IN PRESERVATIVE FLUID, AUTOMATED THIN LAYER PREPARATION, WITH SCREENING BY AUTOMATED SYSTEM AND MANUAL RESCREENING UNDER PHYSICIAN SUPERVISION	C	N	21	A		
G0147	SCREENING CYTOPATHOLOGY SMEARS, CERVICAL OR VAGINAL, PERFORMED BY AUTOMATED SYSTEM UNDER PHYSICIAN SUPERVISION	C	N	21	A		
G0148	SCREENING CYTOPATHOLOGY SMEARS, CERVICAL OR VAGINAL, PERFORMED BY AUTOMATED SYSTEM WITH MANUAL RESCREENING	C	N	21	A		
G0151	SERVICES OF A PHYSICAL THERAPIST IN HOME HEALTH OR HOSPICE SETTINGS, EACH 15 MINUTES	C	C	00	9		
G0152	SERVICES OF AN OCCUPATIONAL THERAPIST IN HOME HEALTH OR HOSPICE SETTINGS, EACH 15 MINUTES	C	C	00	9		
G0153	SERVICES OF A SPEECH AND LANGUAGE PATHOLOGIST IN HOME HEALTH OR HOSPICE SETTINGS, EACH 15 MINUTES	C	C	00	9		
G0154	SERVICES OF SKILLED NURSE IN HOME HEALTH, OR NURSE IN HOSPICE SETTINGS, EACH 15 MINUTES	C	C	00	9		
G0155	SERVICES OF CLINICAL SOCIAL WORKER IN HOME HEALTH OR HOSPICE SETTINGS, EACH 15 MINUTES	C	C	00	9		
G0156	SERVICES OF HOME HEALTH/HOSPICE AIDE IN HOME HEALTH OR HOSPICE SETTINGS, EACH 15 MINUTES	C	C	00	9		
G0166	EXTERNAL COUNTERPULSATION, PER TREATMENT SESSION	D	N	11	A	35-74	
G0168	WOUND CLOSURE UTILIZING TISSUE ADHESIVE(S) ONLY	C	N	00	9		

HCPCS Code	Statute	Lab Cert	X-Ref	ASC Pay Grp	ASC Pay Group Eff. Date	Proc Notes	BETOS	TOS	Anest	Code Add Date	Code Effective Date	Code Term Date
G0128	1833(a)					0070	Y2	1	0	19980401	19980401	
G0129						0087	Y1	U	0	20000401	20080401	
G0130				YY	20080101		I4B	4	0	19980701	19980701	
G0141		630				0045	T1H	5	0	19990101	19990101	
G0143		630				0045	T1H	5	0	19990101	19990101	
G0144		630				0045	T1H	5	0	19990101	20030101	
G0145		630				0045	T1H	5	0	19990101	20030101	
G0147		630				0045	T1H	5	0	19990101	19990101	
G0148		630				0045	T1H	5	0	19990101	19990101	
G0151						0082	Y2	1	0	19990701	20100101	
G0152						0082	Y2	1	0	19990701	20100101	
G0153						0082	Y2	1	0	19990701	20100101	
G0154						0082	Y2	1	0	19990701	20100101	
G0155						0082	Y2	1	0	19990701	20100101	
G0156						0082	Y2	1	0	19990701	20100101	
G0166						0078	P6C	1	0	20000101	20000101	
G0168							P6C	1	0	20000101	20000101	

HCPCS Code	Long Description	Coverage	Action	PI	MPI	CIM	MCM
G0173	LINEAR ACCELERATOR BASED STEREOTACTIC RADIOSURGERY, COMPLETE COURSE OF THERAPY IN ONE SESSION	D	N	00	9		
G0175	SCHEDULED INTERDISCIPLINARY TEAM CONFERENCE (MINIMUM OF THREE EXCLUSIVE OF PATIENT CARE NURSING STAFF) WITH PATIENT PRESENT	C	N	00	9		
G0176	ACTIVITY THERAPY, SUCH AS MUSIC, DANCE, ART OR PLAY THERAPIES NOT FOR RECREATION, RELATED TO THE CARE AND TREATMENT OF PATIENT'S DISABLING MENTAL HEALTH PROBLEMS, PER SESSION (45 MINUTES OR MORE)	D	N	00	9		
G0177	TRAINING AND EDUCATIONAL SERVICES RELATED TO THE CARE AND TREATMENT OF PATIENT'S DISABLING MENTAL HEALTH PROBLEMS PER SESSION (45 MINUTES OR MORE)	D	N	00	9		
G0179	PHYSICIAN RE-CERTIFICATION FOR MEDICARE-COVERED HOME HEALTH SERVICES UNDER A HOME HEALTH PLAN OF CARE (PATIENT NOT PRESENT), INCLUDING CONTACTS WITH HOME HEALTH AGENCY AND REVIEW OF REPORTS OF PATIENT STATUS REQUIRED BY PHYSICIANS TO AFFIRM THE INITIAL IMPLEMENTATION OF THE PLAN OF CARE THAT MEETS PATIENT'S NEEDS, PER RE-CERTIFICATION PERIOD	C	N	11	A		
G0180	PHYSICIAN CERTIFICATION FOR MEDICARE-COVERED HOME HEALTH SERVICES UNDER A HOME HEALTH PLAN OF CARE (PATIENT NOT PRESENT), INCLUDING CONTACTS WITH HOME HEALTH AGENCY AND REVIEW OF REPORTS OF PATIENT STATUS REQUIRED BY PHYSICIANS TO AFFIRM THE INITIAL IMPLEMENTATION OF THE PLAN OF CARE THAT MEETS PATIENT'S NEEDS, PER CERTIFICATION PERIOD	C	N	11	A		
G0181	PHYSICIAN SUPERVISION OF A PATIENT RECEIVING MEDICARE-COVERED SERVICES PROVIDED BY A PARTICIPATING HOME HEALTH AGENCY (PATIENT NOT PRESENT) REQUIRING COMPLEX AND MULTIDISCIPLINARY CARE MODALITIES INVOLVING REGULAR PHYSICIAN DEVELOPMENT AND/OR REVISION OF CARE PLANS, REVIEW OF SUBSEQUENT REPORTS OF PATIENT STATUS, REVIEW OF LABORATORY AND OTHER STUDIES, COMMUNICATION (INCLUDING TELEPHONE CALLS) WITH OTHER HEALTH CARE PROFESSIONALS INVOLVED IN THE PATIENT'S CARE, INTEGRATION OF NEW INFORMATION INTO THE MEDICAL TREATMENT PLAN AND/OR ADJUSTMENT OF MEDICAL THERAPY, WITHIN A CALENDAR MONTH, 30 MINUTES OR MORE	C	N	11	A		

HCPCS Code	Statute	Lab Cert	X-Ref	ASC Pay Grp	ASC Pay Group Eff. Date	Proc Notes	BETOS	TOS	Anest	Code Add Date	Code Effective Date	Code Term Date
G0173				YY	20080101	0094	P5E	2	0	20000801	20050101	
G0175						0101	M6	1	0	20000701	20000701	
G0176						0102	Y2	U	0	20010101	20010101	
G0177						0102	Y2	U	0	20010101	20010101	
G0179							Y1	1	0	20010101	20010101	
G0180						0100	Y1	1	0	20001001	20001001	
G0181							Y1	1	0	20010101	20010101	

HCPCS Code	Long Description	Coverage	Action	PI	MPI	CIM	MCM
G0182	PHYSICIAN SUPERVISION OF A PATIENT UNDER A MEDICARE-APPROVED HOSPICE (PATIENT NOT PRESENT) REQUIRING COMPLEX AND MULTIDISCIPLINARY CARE MODALITIES INVOLVING REGULAR PHYSICIAN DEVELOPMENT AND/OR REVISION OF CARE PLANS, REVIEW OF SUBSEQUENT REPORTS OF PATIENT STATUS, REVIEW OF LABORATORY AND OTHER STUDIES, COMMUNICATION (INCLUDING TELEPHONE CALLS) WITH OTHER HEALTH CARE PROFESSIONALS INVOLVED IN THE PATIENT'S CARE, INTEGRATION OF NEW INFORMATION INTO THE MEDICAL TREATMENT PLAN AND/OR ADJUSTMENT OF MEDICAL THERAPY, WITHIN A CALENDAR MONTH, 30 MINUTES OR MORE	C	N	11	A		
G0186	DESTRUCTION OF LOCALIZED LESION OF CHOROID (FOR EXAMPLE, CHOROIDAL NEOVASCULARIZATION); PHOTOCOAGULATION, FEEDER VESSEL TECHNIQUE (ONE OR MORE SESSIONS)	C	N	00	9		
G0202	SCREENING MAMMOGRAPHY, PRODUCING DIRECT DIGITAL IMAGE, BILATERAL, ALL VIEWS	C	N	11	A		
G0204	DIAGNOSTIC MAMMOGRAPHY, PRODUCING DIRECT DIGITAL IMAGE, BILATERAL, ALL VIEWS	C	N	11	A		
G0206	DIAGNOSTIC MAMMOGRAPHY, PRODUCING DIRECT DIGITAL IMAGE, UNILATERAL, ALL VIEWS	C	N	11	A		
G0219	PET IMAGING WHOLE BODY; MELANOMA FOR NON-COVERED INDICATIONS	M	N	00	9	50-36	4173
G0235	PET IMAGING, ANY SITE, NOT OTHERWISE SPECIFIED	M	N	00	9	50-36	
G0237	THERAPEUTIC PROCEDURES TO INCREASE STRENGTH OR ENDURANCE OF RESPIRATORY MUSCLES, FACE TO FACE, ONE ON ONE, EACH 15 MINUTES (INCLUDES MONITORING)	C	N	11	A		
G0238	THERAPEUTIC PROCEDURES TO IMPROVE RESPIRATORY FUNCTION, OTHER THAN DESCRIBED BY G0237, ONE ON ONE, FACE TO FACE, PER 15 MINUTES (INCLUDES MONITORING)	C	N	11	A		
G0239	THERAPEUTIC PROCEDURES TO IMPROVE RESPIRATORY FUNCTION OR INCREASE STRENGTH OR ENDURANCE OF RESPIRATORY MUSCLES, TWO OR MORE INDIVIDUALS (INCLUDES MONITORING)	C	N	11	A		
G0243	MULTI-SOURCE PHOTON STEREOTACTIC RADIOSURGERY, DELIVERY INCLUDING COLLIMATOR CHANGES AND CUSTOM PLUGGING, COMPLETE COURSE OF TREATMENT, ALL LESIONS	D	N	00	9		
G0245	INITIAL PHYSICIAN EVALUATION AND MANAGEMENT OF A DIABETIC PATIENT WITH DIABETIC SENSORY NEUROPATHY RESULTING IN A LOSS OF PROTECTIVE SENSATION (LOPS) WHICH MUST INCLUDE: (1) THE DIAGNOSIS OF LOPS, (2) A PATIENT HISTORY, (3) A PHYSICAL EXAMINATION THAT CONSISTS OF AT LEAST THE FOLLOWING ELEMENTS: (A) VISUAL INSPECTION OF THE FOREFOOT, HINDFOOT AND TOE WEB SPACES, (B)EVALUATION OF A PROTECTIVE SENSATION, (C) EVALUATION OF FOOT STRUCTURE AND BIOMECHANICS, (D) EVALUATION OF VASCULAR STATUS AND SKIN INTEGRITY, AND (E) EVALUATION AND RECOMMENDATION OF FOOTWEAR AND (4) PATIENT EDUCATION	D	N	11	A	50.81	

G Codes

HCPCS Code	Statute	Lab Cert	X-Ref	ASC Pay Grp	ASC Pay Group Eff. Date	Proc Notes	BETOS	TOS	Anest	Code Add Date	Code Effective Date	Code Term Date
G0182							Y1	1	0	20010101	20010101	
G0186				YY	20080101	0099	P4D	2	0	20010101	20010101	
G0202							I1C	1	0	20010401	20010401	
G0204							I1C	4	0	20010401	20030101	
G0206							I1C	4	0	20010401	20030101	
G0219							I4B	4	0	20010701	20010701	
G0235							T2D	1	0	20060101	20060101	
G0237							P6C	1,U,W	0	20020101	20041001	
G0238							P6C	1,U,W	0	20020101	20041001	
G0239							P6C	1,U,W	0	20020101	20041001	
G0243						0094	P5E	2	0	20020101	20070101	20061231
G0243												
G0245							M1A	1	0	20020701	20020701	
G0245							Y1	1	0			

HCPCS Code	Long Description	Coverage	Action	PI	MPI	CIM	MCM
G0246	FOLLOW-UP PHYSICIAN EVALUATION AND MANAGEMENT OF A DIABETIC PATIENT WITH DIABETIC SENSORY NEUROPATHY RESULTING IN A LOSS OF PROTECTIVE SENSATION (LOPS) TO INCLUDE AT LEAST THE FOLLOWING: (1) A PATIENT HISTORY, (2) A PHYSICAL EXAMINATION THAT INCLUDES: (A) VISUAL INSPECTION OF THE FOREFOOT, HINDFOOT AND TOE WEB SPACES, (B) EVALUATION OF PROTECTIVE SENSATION, (C) EVALUATION OF FOOT STRUCTURE AND BIOMECHANICS, (D) EVALUATION OF VASCULAR STATUS AND SKIN INTEGRITY, AND (E) EVALUATION AND RECOMMENDATION OF FOOTWEAR, AND (3) PATIENT EDUCATION	D	N	11	A	50.81	
G0247	ROUTINE FOOT CARE BY A PHYSICIAN OF A DIABETIC PATIENT WITH DIABETIC SENSORY NEUROPATHY RESULTING IN A LOSS OF PROTECTIVE SENSATION (LOPS) TO INCLUDE, THE LOCAL CARE OF SUPERFICIAL WOUNDS (I.E. SUPERFICIAL TO MUSCLE AND FASCIA) AND AT LEAST THE FOLLOWING IF PRESENT: (1) LOCAL CARE OF SUPERFICIAL WOUNDS, (2) DEBRIDEMENT OF CORNS AND CALLUSES, AND (3) TRIMMING AND DEBRIDEMENT OF NAILS	D	N	11	A	50.81	
G0248	DEMONSTRATION, PRIOR TO INITIATION OF HOME INR MONITORING, FOR PATIENT WITH EITHER MECHANICAL HEART VALVE(S), CHRONIC ATRIAL FIBRILLATION, OR VENOUS THROMBOEMBOLISM WHO MEETS MEDICARE COVERAGE CRITERIA, UNDER THE DIRECTION OF A PHYSICIAN; INCLUDES: FACE-TO-FACE DEMONSTRATION OF USE AND CARE OF THE INR MONITOR, OBTAINING AT LEAST ONE BLOOD SAMPLE, PROVISION OF INSTRUCTIONS FOR REPORTING HOME INR TEST RESULTS, AND DOCUMENTATION OF PATIENT'S ABILITY TO PERFORM TESTING AND REPORT RESULTS	D	N	11	A	50.55	
G0249	PROVISION OF TEST MATERIALS AND EQUIPMENT FOR HOME INR MONITORING OF PATIENT WITH EITHER MECHANICAL HEART VALVE(S), CHRONIC ATRIAL FIBRILLATION, OR VENOUS THROMBOEMBOLISM WHO MEETS MEDICARE COVERAGE CRITERIA; INCLUDES: PROVISION OF MATERIALS FOR USE IN THE HOME AND REPORTING OF TEST RESULTS TO PHYSICIAN; TESTING NOT OCCURRING MORE FREQUENTLY THAN ONCE A WEEK; TESTING MATERIALS, BILLING UNITS OF SERVICE INCLUDE 4 TESTS	D	N	11	A	50.55	
G0250	PHYSICIAN REVIEW, INTERPRETATION, AND PATIENT MANAGEMENT OF HOME INR TESTING FOR PATIENT WITH EITHER MECHANICAL HEART VALVE(S), CHRONIC ATRIAL FIBRILLATION, OR VENOUS THROMBOEMBOLISM WHO MEETS MEDICARE COVERAGE CRITERIA; TESTING NOT OCCURRING MORE FREQUENTLY THAN ONCE A WEEK; BILLING UNITS OF SERVICE INCLUDE 4 TESTS	D	N	11	A	50.55	
G0251	LINEAR ACCELERATOR BASED STEREOTACTIC RADIOSURGERY, DELIVERY INCLUDING COLLIMATOR CHANGES AND CUSTOM PLUGGING, FRACTIONATED TREATMENT, ALL LESIONS, PER SESSION, MAXIMUM FIVE SESSIONS PER COURSE OF TREATMENT	D	N	00	9		

HCPCS Code	Statute	Lab Cert	X-Ref	ASC Pay Grp	ASC Pay Group Eff. Date	Proc Notes	BETOS	TOS	Anest	Code Add Date	Code Effective Date	Code Term Date
G0246							M1B	1	0	20020701	20020701	
G0246 G0247				YY	20080101		M1B	1	0	20020701	20030701	
G0247 G0248							M1A	5	0	20020701	20080319	
G0249							Y1	5	0	20020701	20080319	
G0250							M1B	1	0	20020701	20080319	
G0251				YY	20080101	0107	I1F	4	0	20020401	20020401	

HCPCS Code	Long Description	Coverage	Action	PI	MPI	CIM	MCM
G0252	PET IMAGING, FULL AND PARTIAL-RING PET SCANNERS ONLY, FOR INITIAL DIAGNOSIS OF BREAST CANCER AND/OR SURGICAL PLANNING FOR BREAST CANCER (E.G. INITIAL STAGING OF AXILLARY LYMPH NODES)	M	N	00	9	50-36	
G0255	CURRENT PERCEPTION THRESHOLD/SENSORY NERVE CONDUCTION TEST, (SNCT) PER LIMB, ANY NERVE	M	N	00	9	50-57	
G0257	UNSCHEDULED OR EMERGENCY DIALYSIS TREATMENT FOR AN ESRD PATIENT IN A HOSPITAL OUTPATIENT DEPARTMENT THAT IS NOT CERTIFIED AS AN ESRD FACILITY	D	N	00	9		
G0259	INJECTION PROCEDURE FOR SACROILIAC JOINT; ARTHROGRAPY	D	N	00	9		
G0260	INJECTION PROCEDURE FOR SACROILIAC JOINT; PROVISION OF ANESTHETIC, STEROID AND/OR OTHER THERAPEUTIC AGENT, WITH OR WITHOUT ARTHROGRAPHY	D	N	00	9		
G0265	CRYOPRESERVATION, FREEZING AND STORAGE OF CELLS FOR THERAPEUTIC USE, EACH CELL LINE	C	N	13	A		
G0266	THAWING AND EXPANSION OF FROZEN CELLS FOR THERAPEUTIC USE, EACH ALIQUOT	C	N	11	A		
G0267	BONE MARROW OR PERIPHERAL STEM CELL HARVEST, MODIFICATION OR TREATMENT TO ELIMINATE CELL TYPE(S) (E.G. T-CELLS, METASTATIC CARCINOMA)	C	N	11	A		
G0268	REMOVAL OF IMPACTED CERUMEN (ONE OR BOTH EARS) BY PHYSICIAN ON SAME DATE OF SERVICE AS AUDIOLOGIC FUNCTION TESTING	C	N	11	A		
G0269	PLACEMENT OF OCCLUSIVE DEVICE INTO EITHER A VENOUS OR ARTERIAL ACCESS SITE, POST SURGICAL OR INTERVENTIONAL PROCEDURE (E.G. ANGIOSEAL PLUG, VASCULAR PLUG)	D	N	00	9		
G0270	MEDICAL NUTRITION THERAPY; REASSESSMENT AND SUBSEQUENT INTERVENTION(S) FOLLOWING SECOND REFERRAL IN SAME YEAR FOR CHANGE IN DIAGNOSIS, MEDICAL CONDITION OR TREATMENT REGIMEN (INCLUDING ADDITIONAL HOURS NEEDED FOR RENAL DISEASE), INDIVIDUAL, FACE TO FACE WITH THE PATIENT, EACH 15 MINUTES	C	N	11	A		
G0271	MEDICAL NUTRITION THERAPY, REASSESSMENT AND SUBSEQUENT INTERVENTION(S) FOLLOWING SECOND REFERRAL IN SAME YEAR FOR CHANGE IN DIAGNOSIS, MEDICAL CONDITION, OR TREATMENT REGIMEN (INCLUDING ADDITIONAL HOURS NEEDED FOR RENAL DISEASE), GROUP (2 OR MORE INDIVIDUALS), EACH 30 MINUTES	C	N	11	A		
G0275	RENAL ANGIOGRAPHY, NON-SELECTIVE, ONE OR BOTH KIDNEYS, PERFORMED AT THE SAME TIME AS CARDIAC CATHETERIZATION AND/OR CORONARY ANGIOGRAPHY, INCLUDES POSITIONING OR PLACEMENT OF ANY CATHETER IN THE ABDOMINAL AORTA AT OR NEAR THE ORIGINS (OSTIA) OF THE RENAL ARTERIES, INJECTION OF DYE, FLUSH AORTOGRAM, PRODUCTION OF PERMANENT IMAGES, AND RADIOLOGIC SUPERVISION AND INTERPRETATION (LIST SEPARATELY IN ADDITION TO PRIMARY PROCEDURE)	C	N	11	A		

HCPCS Code	Statute	Lab Cert	X-Ref	ASC Pay Grp	ASC Pay Group Eff. Date	Proc Notes	BETOS	TOS	Anest	Code Add Date	Code Effective Date	Code Term Date
G0252							I2D	4	0	20021001	20021001	
G0255							T2D	4	0	20021001	20021001	
G0257						0107	P6D	1	0	20030101	20030101	
G0259						0107	O1E	1	0	20030101	20030101	
G0260				YY	20030101	0107	O1E	F	0	20030101	20041001	
G0265							T1H	5	0	20030101	20080101	20071231
G0266							T1H	5	0	20030101	20080101	20071231
G0267							T1H	5	0	20030101	20080101	20071231
G0268							P6C	2	0	20030101	20030101	
G0269						0108	P6D	1	0	20030101	20030101	
G0270							M5D	1	0	20030101	20030101	
G0271							M5D	1	0	20030101	20030101	
G0275							I4A	2	0	20030101	20080101	

HCPCS Code	Long Description	Coverage	Action	PI	MPI	CIM	MCM
G0278	ILIAC AND/OR FEMORAL ARTERY ANGIOGRAPHY, NON-SELECTIVE, BILATERAL OR IPSILATERAL TO CATHETER INSERTION, PERFORMED AT THE SAME TIME AS CARDIAC CATHETERIZATION AND/OR CORONARY ANGIOGRAPHY, INCLUDES POSITIONING OR PLACEMENT OF THE CATHETER IN THE DISTAL AORTA OR IPSILATERAL FEMORAL OR ILIAC ARTERY, INJECTION OF DYE, PRODUCTION OF PERMANENT IMAGES, AND RADIOLOGIC SUPERVISION & INTERPRETATION (LIST SEPARATELY IN ADDITION TO PRIMARY PROCEDURE)	C	N	11	A		
G0281	ELECTRICAL STIMULATION, (UNATTENDED), TO ONE OR MORE AREAS, FOR CHRONIC STAGE III AND STAGE IV PRESSURE ULCERS, ARTERIAL ULCERS, DIABETIC ULCERS, AND VENOUS STATSIS ULCERS NOT DEMONSTRATING MEASURABLE SIGNS OF HEALING AFTER 30 DAYS OF CONVENTIONAL CARE, AS PART OF A THERAPY PLAN OF CARE	C	N	11	A		
G0282	ELECTRICAL STIMULATION, (UNATTENDED), TO ONE OR MORE AREAS, FOR WOUND CARE OTHER THAN DESCRIBED IN G0281	M	N	00	9		35-98
G0283	ELECTRICAL STIMULATION (UNATTENDED), TO ONE OR MORE AREAS FOR INDICATION(S) OTHER THAN WOUND CARE, AS PART OF A THERAPY PLAN OF CARE	C	N	11	A		
G0288	RECONSTRUCTION, COMPUTED TOMOGRAPHIC ANGIOGRAPHY OF AORTA FOR SURGICAL PLANNING FOR VASCULAR SURGERY	C	N	11	A		
G0289	ARTHROSCOPY, KNEE, SURGICAL, FOR REMOVAL OF LOOSE BODY, FOREIGN BODY, DEBRIDEMENT/SHAVING OF ARTICULAR CARTILAGE (CHRONDROPLASTY) AT THE TIME OF OTHER SURGICAL KNEE ARTHROSCOPY IN A DIFFERENT COMPARTMENT OF THE SAME KNEE	C	N	11	A		
G0290	TRANSCATHETER PLACEMENT OF A DRUG ELUTING INTRACORONARY STENT(S), PERCUTANEOUS, WITH OR WITHOUT OTHER THERAPEUTIC INTERVENTION, ANY METHOD; SINGLE VESSEL	D	N	00	9		
G0291	TRANSCATHETER PLACEMENT OF A DRUG ELUTING INTRACORONARY STENT(S), PERCUTANEOUS, WITH OR WITHOUT OTHER THERAPEUTIC INTERVENTION, ANY METHOD; EACH ADDITIONAL VESSEL	D	N	00	9		
G0293	NONCOVERED SURGICAL PROCEDURE(S) USING CONSCIOUS SEDATION, REGIONAL, GENERAL OR SPINAL ANESTHESIA IN A MEDICARE QUALIFYING CLINICAL TRIAL, PER DAY	D	N	00	9		
G0294	NONCOVERED PROCEDURE(S) USING EITHER NO ANESTHESIA OR LOCAL ANESTHESIA ONLY, IN A MEDICARE QUALIFYING CLINICAL TRIAL, PER DAY	D	N	00	9		
G0295	ELECTROMAGNETIC THERAPY, TO ONE OR MORE AREAS, FOR WOUND CARE OTHER THAN DESCRIBED IN G0329 OR FOR OTHER USES	M	N	00	9	35-98	
G0297	INSERTION OF SINGLE CHAMBER PACING CARDIOVERTER DEFIBRILLATOR PULSE GENERATOR	C	N	00	9		
G0298	INSERTION OF DUAL CHAMBER PACING CARDIOVERTER DEFIBRILLATOR PULSE GENERATOR	C	N	00	9		

HCPCS Code	Statute	Lab Cert	X-Ref	ASC Pay Grp	ASC Pay Group Eff. Date	Proc Notes	BETOS	TOS	Anest	Code Add Date	Code Effective Date	Code Term Date
G0278							I4A	2	0	20030101	20080101	
G0278												
G0281							P5E	1, U, W	0		20030401	20030401
G0282							P5E	1, U, W	0		20030401	20030401
G0283							P5E	1, U, W	0		20030101	20030101
G0288							I2B	4	0	20030101	20060101	
G0289							P8A	2	0	20030101	20030101	
G0290						0107	P2D	2	0	20030101	20030101	
G0291						0107	P2D	2	0	20030101	20030101	
G0293						0107	Y2	2	0	20030101	20030101	
G0294						0109	Y2	2	0	20030101	20030101	
G0295							I2B	1,U,W	0	20030401	20040701	
G0297							P2B	2	0	20031001	20080101	20071231
G0298			33240				P2B	2	0	20031001	20080101	20071231
							I4A	2	0			

HCPCS Code	Long Description	Coverage	Action	PI	MPI	CIM	MCM
G0299	INSERTION OR REPOSITIONING OF ELECTRODE LEAD FOR SINGLE CHAMBER PACING CARDIOVERTER DEFIBRILLATOR AND INSERTION OF PULSE GENERATOR	C	N	00	9		
G0300	INSERTION OR REPOSITIONING OF ELECTRODE LEAD(S) FOR DUAL CHAMBER PACING CARDIOVERTER DEFIBRILLATOR AND INSERTION OF PULSE GENERATOR	C	N	00	9		
G0302	PRE-OPERATIVE PULMONARY SURGERY SERVICES FOR PREPARATION FOR LVRS, COMPLETE COURSE OF SERVICES, TO INCLUDE A MINIMUM OF 16 DAYS OF SERVICES	C	N	00	9		
G0303	PRE-OPERATIVE PULMONARY SURGERY SERVICES FOR PREPARATION FOR LVRS, 10 TO 15 DAYS OF SERVICES	C	N	00	9		
G0304	PRE-OPERATIVE PULMONARY SURGERY SERVICES FOR PREPARATION FOR LVRS, 1 TO 9 DAYS OF SERVICES	C	N	00	9		
G0305	POST-DISCHARGE PULMONARY SURGERY SERVICES AFTER LVRS, MINIMUM OF 6 DAYS OF SERVICES	C	N	00	9		
G0306	COMPLETE CBC, AUTOMATED (HGB, HCT, RBC, WBC, WITHOUT PLATELET COUNT) & AUTOMATED WBC DIFFERENTIAL COUNT	C	N	00	9		
G0307	COMPLETE (CBC), AUTOMATED (HGB, HCT, RBC, WBC; WITHOUT PLATELET COUNT)	C	N	00	9		
G0308	END STAGE RENAL DISEASE (ESRD) RELATED SERVICES DURING THE COURSE OF TREATMENT, FOR PATIENTS UNDER 2 YEARS OF AGE TO INCLUDE MONITORING FOR THE ADEQUACY OF NUTRITION, ASSESSMENT OF GROWTH AND DEVELOPMENT, AND COUNSELING OF PARENTS; WITH 4 OR MORE FACE-TO-FACE PHYSICIAN VISITS PER MONTH	D	N	11	A		2230
G0309	END STAGE RENAL DISEASE (ESRD) RELATED SERVICES DURING THE COURSE OF TREATMENT FOR PATIENTS UNDER 2 YEARS OF AGE TO INCLUDE MONITORING FOR THE ADEQUACY OF NUTRITION, ASSESSMENT OF GROWTH AND DEVELOPMENT, AND COUNSELING OF PARENTS; WITH 2 OR 3 FACE-TO-FACE PHYSICIAN VISITS PER MONTH	D	N	11	A		2230
G0310	END STAGE RENAL DISEASE (ESRD) RELATED SERVICES DURING THE COURSE OF TREATMENT, FOR PATIENTS UNDER 2 YEARS OF AGE TO INCLUDE MONITORING FOR THE ADEQUACY OF NUTRITION, ASSESSMENT OF GROWTH AND DEVELOPMENT, AND COUNSELING OF PARENTS; WITH 1 FACE-TO-FACE PHYSICIAN VISIT PER MONTH	D	N	11	A		2230
G0311	END STAGE RENAL DISEASE (ESRD) RELATED SERVICES DURING THE COURSE OF TREATMENT, FOR PATIENTS BETWEEN 2 AND 11 YEARS OF AGE TO INCLUDE MONITORING FOR THE ADEQUACY OF NUTRITION, ASSESSMENT OF GROWTH AND DEVELOPMENT, AND COUNSELING OF PARENTS; WITH 4 OR MORE FACE-TO-FACE PHYSICIAN VISITS PER MONTH	D	N	11	A		2230
G0312	END STAGE RENAL DISEASE (ESRD) RELATED SERVICES DURING THE COURSE OF TREATMENT, FOR PATIENTS BETWEEN 2 AND 11 YEARS OF AGE TO INCLUDE MONITORING FOR THE ADEQUACY OF NUTRITION, ASSESSMENT OF GROWTH AND DEVELOPMENT, AND COUNSELING OF PARENTS; WITH 2 OR 3 FACE-TO-FACE PHYSICIAN VISITS PER MONTH	D	N	11	A		2230

HCPCS Code	Statute	Lab Cert	X-Ref	ASC Pay Grp	ASC Pay Group Eff. Date	Proc Notes	BETOS	TOS	Anest	Code Add Date	Code Effective Date	Code Term Date
G0299			33249				P2B	2	0	20031001	20080101	20071231
G0300							P2B	2	0	20031001	20080101	20071231
G0302							T2D	1	0	20040101	20040101	
G0303							T2D	1	0	20040101	20040101	
G0304							T2D	1	0	20040101	20040101	
G0305							T2D	1	0	20040101	20040101	
G0306		400					T1D	5	0	20040101	20040101	
G0307		400					T1D	5	0	20040101	20040101	
G0308							P9B	M	0	20040101	20090101	20081231
G0309							P9B	M	0	20040101	20090101	20081231
G0309												
G0310							P9B	M	0	20040101	20090101	20081231
G0311							P9B	M	0	20040101	20090101	20081231
G0311												
G0312							P9B	M	0	20040101	20090101	20081231

HCPCS Code	Long Description	Coverage	Action	PI	MPI	CIM	MCM
G0313	END STAGE RENAL DISEASE (ESRD) RELATED SERVICES DURING THE COURSE OF TREATMENT, FOR PATIENTS BETWEEN 2 AND 11 YEARS OF AGE TO INCLUDE MONITORING FOR THE ADEQUACY OF NUTRITION, ASSESSMENT OF GROWTH & DEVELOPMENT, AND COUNSELING OF PARENTS; WITH 1 FACE-TO-FACE PHYSICIAN VISIT PER MONTH	D	N	11	A		2230
G0314	END STAGE RENAL DISEASE (ESRD) RELATED SERVICES, DURING THE COURSE OF TREATMENT, FOR PATIENTS BETWEEN 12 & 19 YEARS OF AGE TO INCLUDE MONITORING FOR THE ADEQUACY OF NUTRITION, ASSESSMENT OF GROWTH & DEVELOPMENT, & COUNSELING OF PARENTS; WITH 4 OR MORE FACE-TO-FACE PHYSICIAN VISITS PER MONTH	D	N	11	A		2230
G0315	END STAGE RENAL DISEASE (ESRD) RELATED SERVICES DURING THE COURSE OF TREATMENT, FOR PATIENTS BETWEEN 12 & 19 YEARS OF AGE TO INCLUDE MONITORING FOR THE ADEQUACY OF NUTRITION, ASSESSMENT OF GROWTH & DEVELOPMENT, AND COUNSELING OF PARENTS; WITH 2 OR 3 FACE-TO-FACE PHYSICIAN VISITS PER MONTH	D	N	11	A		2230
G0316	END STAGE RENAL DISEASE (ESRD) RELATED SERVICES DURING THE COURSE OF TREATMENT, FOR PATIENTS BETWEEN 12 & 19 YEARS OF AGE TO INCLUDE MONITORING FOR THE ADEQUACY OF NUTRITION, ASSESSMENT OF GROWTH & DEVELOPMENT, AND COUNSELING OF PARENTS; WITH 1 FACE-TO-FACE PHYSICIAN VISIT PER MONTH	D	N	11	A		2230
G0317	END STAGE RENAL DISEASE (ESRD) RELATED SERVICES DURING THE COURSE OF TREATMENT, FOR PATIENTS 20 YEARS OF AGE AND OVER; WITH 4 OR MORE FACE-TO-FACE PHYSICIAN VISITS PER MONTH	D	N	11	A		2230
G0318	END STAGE RENAL DISEASE (ESRD) RELATED SERVICES DURING THE COURSE OF TREATMENT, FOR PATIENTS 20 YEARS OF AGE AND OVER; WITH 2 OR 3 FACE-TO-FACE PHYSICIAN VISITS PER MONTH	D	N	11	A		2230
G0319	END STAGE RENAL DISEASE (ESRD) RELATED SERVICES DURING THE COURSE OF TREATMENT, FOR PATIENTS 20 YEARS OF AGE & OVER; WITH 1 FACE-TO-FACE PHYSICIAN VISIT PER MONTH	D	N	11	A		2230
G0320	END STAGE RENAL DISEASE (ESRD) RELATED SERVICES FOR HOME DIALYSIS PATIENTS PER FULL MONTH; FOR PATIENTS UNDER TWO YEARS OF AGE TO INCLUDE MONITORING FOR ADEQUACY OF NUTRITION, ASSESSMENT OF GROWTH AND DEVELOPMENT, AND COUNSELING OF PARENTS	D	N	11	A		2230
G0321	END STAGE RENAL DISEASE (ESRD) RELATED SERVICES FOR HOME DIALYSIS PATIENTS PER FULL MONTH; FOR PATIENTS TWO TO ELEVEN YEARS OF AGE TO INCLUDE MONITORING FOR ADEQUACY OF NUTRITION, ASSESSMENT OF GROWTH AND DEVELOPMENT, AND COUNSELING OF PARENTS	D	N	11	A		2230

HCPCS Code	Statute	Lab Cert	X-Ref	ASC Pay Grp	ASC Pay Group Eff. Date	Proc Notes	BETOS	TOS	Anest	Code Add Date	Code Effective Date	Code Term Date
G0313							P9B	M	0	20040101	20090101	20081231
G0314							P9B	M	0	20040101	20090101	20081231
G0315							P9B	M	0	20040101	20090101	20081231
G0316							P9B	M	0	20040101	20090101	20081231
G0317							P9B	M	0	20040101	20090101	20081231
G0318							P9B	M	0	20040101	20090101	20081231
G0319							P9B	M	0	20040101	20090101	20081231
G0320							P9B	M	0	20040101	20090101	20081231
G0321							P9B	M	0	20040101	20090101	20081231

HCPCS Code	Long Description	Coverage	Action	PI	MPI	CIM	MCM
G0322	END STAGE RENAL DISEASE (ESRD) RELATED SERVICES FOR HOME DIALYSIS PATIENTS PER FULL MONTH; FOR PATIENTS TWELVE TO NINETEEN YEARS OF AGE TO INCLUDE MONITORING FOR ADEQUACY OF NUTRITION, ASSESSMENT OF GROWTH AND DEVELOPMENT, AND COUNSELING OF PARENTS	D	N	11	A		2230
G0323	END STAGE RENAL DISEASE (ESRD) RELATED SERVICES FOR HOME DIALYSIS PATIENTS PER FULL MONTH; FOR PATIENTS TWENTY YEARS OF AGE AND OLDER	D	N	11	A		2230
G0324	END STAGE RENAL DISEASE (ESRD) RELATED SERVICES LESS THAN FULL MONTH, PER DAY; FOR PATIENTS UNDER TWO YEARS OF AGE	D	N	11	A		2230
G0325	END STAGE RENAL DISEASE (ESRD) RELATED SERVICES LESS THAN FULL MONTH, PER DAY; FOR PATIENTS BETWEEN TWO AND ELEVEN YEARS OF AGE	D	N	11	A		2230
G0326	END STAGE RENAL DISEASE (ESRD) RELATED SERVICES LESS THAN FULL MONTH, PER DAY; FOR PATIENTS BETWEEN TWELVE AND NINETEEN YEARS OF AGE	D	N	11	A		2230
G0327	END STAGE RENAL DISEASE (ESRD) RELATED SERVICES LESS THAN FULL MONTH, PER DAY; FOR PATIENTS TWENTY YEARS OF AGE AND OVER	D	N	11	A		2230
G0328	COLORECTAL CANCER SCREENING; FECAL OCCULT BLOOD TEST, IMMUNOASSAY, 1-3 SIMULTANEOUS	D	N	21	A		
G0329	ELECTROMAGNETIC THERAPY, TO ONE OR MORE AREAS FOR CHRONIC STAGE III & STAGE IV PRESSURE ULCERS, ARTERIAL ULCERS, DIABETIC ULCERS AND VENOUS STASIS ULCERS NOT DEMONSTRATING MEASURABLE SIGNS OF HEALING AFTER 30 DAYS OF CONVENTIONAL CARE AS PART OF A THERAPY PLAN OF CARE	C	N	00	9		
G0332	SERVICES FOR INTRAVENOUS INFUSION OF IMMUNOGLOBULIN PRIOR TO ADMINISTRATION (THIS SERVICE IS TO BE BILLED IN CONJUNCTION WITH ADMINISTRATION OF IMMUNOGLOBULIN)	C	N	13	A		
G0333	PHARMACY DISPENSING FEE FOR INHALATION DRUG(S); INITIAL 30-DAY SUPPLY AS A BENEFICIARY	D	N	46	A		
G0337	HOSPICE EVALUATION AND COUNSELING SERVICES, PRE-ELECTION	C	N	11	A		
G0339	IMAGE-GUIDED ROBOTIC LINEAR ACCELERATOR-BASED STEREOTACTIC RADIOSURGERY, COMPLETE COURSE OF THERAPY IN ONE SESSION OR FIRST SESSION OF FRACTIONATED TREATMENT	C	N	00	9		
G0340	IMAGE-GUIDED ROBOTIC LINEAR ACCELERATOR-BASED STEREOTACTIC RADIOSURGERY, DELIVERY INCLUDING COLLIMATOR CHANGES AND CUSTOM PLUGGING, FRACTIONATED TREATMENT, ALL LESIONS, PER SESSION, SECOND THROUGH FIFTH SESSIONS, MAXIMUM FIVE SESSIONS PER COURSE OF TREATMENT	C	N	00	9		
G0341	PERCUTANEOUS ISLET CELL TRANSPLANT, INCLUDES PORTAL VEIN CATHETERIZATION AND INFUSION	D	N	13	A	260.3, 35-82	

HCPCS Code	Statute	Lab Cert	X-Ref	ASC Pay Grp	ASC Pay Group Eff. Date	Proc Notes	BETOS	TOS	Anest	Code Add Date	Code Effective Date	Code Term Date
G0322							P9B	M	0	20040101	20090101	20081231
G0323							P9B	M	0	20040101	20090101	20081231
G0324							P9B	1	0	20040101	20090101	20081231
G0325							P9B	1	0	20040101	20090101	20081231
G0326							P9B	1	0	20040101	20090101	20081231
G0327							P9B	1	0	20040101	20090101	20081231
G0328		310				0064	T1H	1	0	20040101	20040101	
G0329							I2B	1,U,W	0	20040701	20040701	
G0332							P7B	1	0	20060101	20090101	20081231
G0333						0121	D1E	9	0	20060101	20060101	
G0337							M5D	1	0	20050101	20050101	
G0339				YY	20080101		P5E	1	0	20040101	20040101	
G0340				YY	20080101		P5E	1	0	20040101	20040101	
G0341							P1G	2	0	20041001	20041001	
G0341												

HCPCS Code	Long Description	Coverage	Action	PI	MPI	CIM	MCM
G0342	LAPAROSCOPY FOR ISLET CELL TRANSPLANT, INCLUDES PORTAL VEIN CATHETERIZATION AND INFUSION	D	N	13	A	35-82	
G0343	LAPAROTOMY FOR ISLET CELL TRANSPLANT, INCLUDES PORTAL VEIN CATHETERIZATION AND INFUSION	D	N	13	A	35-82	
G0344	INITIAL PREVENTIVE PHYSICAL EXAMINATION; FACE-TO-FACE VISIT, SERVICES LIMITED TO A NEW BENEFICIARY DURING THE FIRST 12 MONTHS OF MEDICARE ENROLLMENT	C	N	11	A		
G0364	BONE MARROW ASPIRATION PERFORMED WITH BONE MARROW BIOPSY THROUGH THE SAME INCISION ON THE SAME DATE OF SERVICE	C	N	11	A		
G0365	VESSEL MAPPING OF VESSELS FOR HEMODIALYSIS ACCESS (SERVICES FOR PREOPERATIVE VESSEL MAPPING PRIOR TO CREATION OF HEMODIALYSIS ACCESS USING AN AUTOGENOUS HEMODIALYSIS CONDUIT, INCLUDING ARTERIAL INFLOW AND VENOUS OUTFLOW)	C	N	11	A		
G0366	ELECTROCARDIOGRAM, ROUTINE ECG WITH 12 LEADS; PERFORMED AS A COMPONENT OF THE INITIAL PREVENTIVE EXAMINATION WITH INTERPRETATION AND REPORT	C	N	11	A		
G0367	TRACING ONLY, WITHOUT INTERPRETATION AND REPORT, PERFORMED AS A COMPONENT OF THE INITIAL PREVENTIVE EXAMINATION	C	N	11	A		
G0368	INTERPRETATION AND REPORT ONLY, PERFORMED AS A COMPONENT OF THE INITIAL PREVENTIVE EXAMINATION	C	N	11	A		
G0372	PHYSICIAN SERVICE REQUIRED TO ESTABLISH AND DOCUMENT THE NEED FOR A POWER MOBILITY DEVICE	D	N	13	A		
G0375	SMOKING AND TOBACCO USE CESSATION COUNSELING VISIT; INTERMEDIATE, GREATER THAN 3 MINUTES UP TO 10 MINUTES	C	N	13	A		
G0376	SMOKING AND TOBACCO USE CESSATION COUNSELING VISIT; INTENSIVE, GREATER THAN 10 MINUTES	C	N	13	A		
G0377	ADMINISTRATION OF VACCINE FOR PART D DRUG	C	N	11	A		
G0378	HOSPITAL OBSERVATION SERVICE, PER HOUR	D	N	00	9		
G0379	DIRECT ADMISSION OF PATIENT FOR HOSPITAL OBSERVATION CARE	D	S	00	9		
G0380	LEVEL 1 HOSPITAL EMERGENCY DEPARTMENT VISIT PROVIDED IN A TYPE B EMERGENCY DEPARTMENT; (THE ED MUST MEET AT LEAST ONE OF THE FOLLOWING REQUIREMENTS: (1) IT IS LICENSED BY THE STATE IN WHICH IT IS LOCATED UNDER APPLICABLE STATE LAW AS AN EMERGENCY ROOM OR EMERGENCY DEPARTMENT; (2) IT IS HELD OUT TO THE PUBLIC (BY NAME, POSTED SIGNS, ADVERTISING, OR OTHER MEANS) AS A PLACE THAT PROVIDES CARE FOR EMERGENCY MEDICAL CONDITIONS ON AN URGENT BASIS WITHOUT REQUIRING A PREVIOUSLY SCHEDULED APPOINTMENT; OR (3) DURING THE CALENDAR YEAR IMMEDIATELY PRECEDING THE CALENDAR YEAR IN WHICH A DETERMINATION UNDER 42 CFR °489.24 IS BEING MADE, BASED ON A REPRESENTATIVE SAMPLE OF PATIENT VISITS THAT OCCURRED DURING THAT CALENDAR YEAR, IT PROVIDES AT LEAST ONE-THIRD OF ALL OF ITS OUTPATIENT VISITS FOR THE TREATMENT OF EMERGENCY MEDICAL CONDITIONS ON AN URGENT BASIS WITHOUT REQUIRING A PREVIOUSLY SCHEDULED APPOINTMENT)	C	N	00	9		

HCPCS Code	Statute	Lab Cert	X-Ref	ASC Pay Grp	ASC Pay Group Eff. Date	Proc Notes	BETOS	TOS	Anest	Code Add Date	Code Effective Date	Code Term Date
G0342							P1G	2	0	20041001	20041001	
G0343							P1G	2	0	20041001	20041001	
G0344							M1A	1	0	20050101	20090101	20081231
G0364				YY	20080101		P6C	2	0	20050101	20050101	
G0365							P9A	5	0	20050101	20050101	
G0366							T2C	5	0	20050101	20090101	20081231
G0367							T2C	5	0	20050101	20090101	20081231
G0368							T2C	5	0	20050101	20090101	20081231
G0372						0128	M5D	1	0	20051025	20051025	
G0375						0150	M6	9	0	20050323	20080101	20071231
G0376						0150	M6	9	0	20050323	20080101	20071231
G0377	1861s10B						O1E	1	0	20070101	20080101	20071231
G0378						0107	M2A	1	0	20060101	20060101	
G0379						0107	M2A	1	0	20060101	20100101	
G0380							M3	1	0	20070101	20080101	

HCPCS Code	Long Description	Coverage	Action	PI	MPI	CIM	MCM
G0381	LEVEL 2 HOSPITAL EMERGENCY DEPARTMENT VISIT PROVIDED IN A TYPE B EMERGENCY DEPARTMENT; (THE ED MUST MEET AT LEAST ONE OF THE FOLLOWING REQUIREMENTS: (1) IT IS LICENSED BY THE STATE IN WHICH IT IS LOCATED UNDER APPLICABLE STATE LAW AS AN EMERGENCY ROOM OR EMERGENCY DEPARTMENT; (2) IT IS HELD OUT TO THE PUBLIC (BY NAME, POSTED SIGNS, ADVERTISING, OR OTHER MEANS) AS A PLACE THAT PROVIDES CARE FOR EMERGENCY MEDICAL CONDITIONS ON AN URGENT BASIS WITHOUT REQUIRING A PREVIOUSLY SCHEDULED APPOINTMENT; OR (3) DURING THE CALENDAR YEAR IMMEDIATELY PRECEDING THE CALENDAR YEAR IN WHICH A DETERMINATION UNDER 42 CFR °489.24 IS BEING MADE, BASED ON A REPRESENTATIVE SAMPLE OF PATIENT VISITS THAT OCCURRED DURING THAT CALENDAR YEAR, IT PROVIDES AT LEAST ONE-THIRD OF ALL OF ITS OUTPATIENT VISITS FOR THE TREATMENT OF EMERGENCY MEDICAL CONDITIONS ON AN URGENT BASIS WITHOUT REQUIRING A PREVIOUSLY SCHEDULED APPOINTMENT)	C	N	00	9		
G0382	LEVEL 3 HOSPITAL EMERGENCY DEPARTMENT VISIT PROVIDED IN A TYPE B EMERGENCY DEPARTMENT; (THE ED MUST MEET AT LEAST ONE OF THE FOLLOWING REQUIREMENTS: (1) IT IS LICENSED BY THE STATE IN WHICH IT IS LOCATED UNDER APPLICABLE STATE LAW AS AN EMERGENCY ROOM OR EMERGENCY DEPARTMENT; (2) IT IS HELD OUT TO THE PUBLIC (BY NAME, POSTED SIGNS, ADVERTISING, OR OTHER MEANS) AS A PLACE THAT PROVIDES CARE FOR EMERGENCY MEDICAL CONDITIONS ON AN URGENT BASIS WITHOUT REQUIRING A PREVIOUSLY SCHEDULED APPOINTMENT; OR (3) DURING THE CALENDAR YEAR IMMEDIATELY PRECEDING THE CALENDAR YEAR IN WHICH A DETERMINATION UNDER 42 CFR °489.24 IS BEING MADE, BASED ON A REPRESENTATIVE SAMPLE OF PATIENT VISITS THAT OCCURRED DURING THAT CALENDAR YEAR, IT PROVIDES AT LEAST ONE-THIRD OF ALL OF ITS OUTPATIENT VISITS FOR THE TREATMENT OF EMERGENCY MEDICAL CONDITIONS ON AN URGENT BASIS WITHOUT REQUIRING A PREVIOUSLY SCHEDULED APPOINTMENT)	C	N	00	9		
G0383	LEVEL 4 HOSPITAL EMERGENCY DEPARTMENT VISIT PROVIDED IN A TYPE B EMERGENCY DEPARTMENT; (THE ED MUST MEET AT LEAST ONE OF THE FOLLOWING REQUIREMENTS: (1) IT IS LICENSED BY THE STATE IN WHICH IT IS LOCATED UNDER APPLICABLE STATE LAW AS AN EMERGENCY ROOM OR EMERGENCY DEPARTMENT; (2) IT IS HELD OUT TO THE PUBLIC (BY NAME, POSTED SIGNS, ADVERTISING, OR OTHER MEANS) AS A PLACE THAT PROVIDES CARE FOR EMERGENCY MEDICAL CONDITIONS ON AN URGENT BASIS WITHOUT REQUIRING A PREVIOUSLY SCHEDULED APPOINTMENT; OR (3) DURING THE CALENDAR YEAR IMMEDIATELY PRECEDING THE CALENDAR YEAR IN WHICH A DETERMINATION UNDER 42 CFR °489.24 IS BEING MADE, BASED ON A REPRESENTATIVE SAMPLE OF PATIENT VISITS THAT OCCURRED DURING THAT CALENDAR YEAR, IT PROVIDES AT LEAST ONE-THIRD OF ALL OF ITS OUTPATIENT VISITS FOR THE TREATMENT OF EMERGENCY MEDICAL CONDITIONS ON ANURGENT BASIS WITHOUT REQUIRING A PREVIOUSLY SCHEDULED APPOINTMENT)	C	N	00	9		

HCPCS Code	Statute	Lab Cert	X-Ref	ASC Pay Grp	ASC Pay Group Eff. Date	Proc Notes	BETOS	TOS	Anest	Code Add Date	Code Effective Date	Code Term Date
G0381							M3	1	0	20070101	20080101	
G0382							M3	1	0	20070101	20080101	
G0383							M3	1	0	20070101	20080101	

HCPCS Code	Long Description	Coverage	Action	PI	MPI	CIM	MCM
G0384	LEVEL 5 HOSPITAL EMERGENCY DEPARTMENT VISIT PROVIDED IN A TYPE B EMERGENCY DEPARTMENT; (THE ED MUST MEET AT LEAST ONE OF THE FOLLOWING REQUIREMENTS: (1) IT IS LICENSED BY THE STATE IN WHICH IT IS LOCATED UNDER APPLICABLE STATE LAW AS AN EMERGENCY ROOM OR EMERGENCY DEPARTMENT; (2) IT IS HELD OUT TO THE PUBLIC (BY NAME, POSTED SIGNS, ADVERTISING, OR OTHER MEANS) AS A PLACE THAT PROVIDES CARE FOR EMERGENCY MEDICAL CONDITIONS ON AN URGENT BASIS WITHOUT REQUIRING A PREVIOUSLY SCHEDULED APPOINTMENT; OR (3) DURING THE CALENDAR YEAR IMMEDIATELY PRECEDING THE CALENDAR YEAR IN WHICH A DETERMINATION UNDER 42 CFR °489.24 IS BEING MADE, BASED ON A REPRESENTATIVE SAMPLE OF PATIENT VISITS THAT OCCURRED DURING THAT CALENDAR YEAR, IT PROVIDES AT LEAST ONE-THIRD OF ALL OF ITS OUT-PATIENT VISITS FOR THE TREATMENT OF EMERGENCY MEDICAL CONDITIONS ON AN URGENT BASIS WITHOUT REQUIRING A PREVIOUSLY SCHEDULED APPOINTMENT)	C	N	00	9		
G0389	ULTRASOUND B-SCAN AND/OR REAL TIME WITH IMAGE DOCUMENTATION; FOR ABDOMINAL AORTIC ANEURYSM (AAA) SCREENING	D	N	13	A		
G0390	TRAUMA RESPONSE TEAM ASSOCIATED WITH HOSPITAL CRITICAL CARE SERVICE	D	N	00	9		
G0392	TRANSLUMINAL BALLOON ANGIOPLASTY, PERCUTANEOUS; FOR MAINTENANCE OF HEMODIALYSIS ACCESS, ARTERIOVENOUS FISTULA OR GRAFT; ARTERIAL	C	D	13	A		
G0393	TRANSLUMINAL BALLOON ANGIOPLASTY, PERCUTANEOUS; FOR MAINTENANCE OF HEMODIALYSIS ACCESS, ARTERIOVENOUS FISTULA OR GRAFT; VENOUS	C	D	13	A		
G0394	BLOOD OCCULT TEST (E.G., GUAIAC), FECES, FOR SINGLE DETERMINATION FOR COLORECTAL NEOPLASM (I.E., PATIENT WAS PROVIDED THREE CARDS OR SINGLE TRIPLE CARD FOR CONSECUTIVE COLLECTION)	C	N	21	A		
G0396	ALCOHOL AND/OR SUBSTANCE (OTHER THAN TOBACCO) ABUSE STRUCTURED ASSESSMENT (E.G., AUDIT, DAST), AND BRIEF INTERVENTION 15 TO 30 MINUTES	C	N	11	A		
G0397	ALCOHOL AND/OR SUBSTANCE (OTHER THAN TOBACCO) ABUSE STRUCTURED ASSESSMENT (E.G., AUDIT, DAST), AND INTERVENTION, GREATER THAN 30 MINUTES	C	N	11	A		
G0398	HOME SLEEP STUDY TEST (HST) WITH TYPE II PORTABLE MONITOR, UNATTENDED; MINIMUM OF 7 CHANNELS: EEG, EOG, EMG, ECG/HEART RATE, AIRFLOW, RESPIRATORY EFFORT AND OXYGEN SATURATION	C	N	13	A		
G0399	HOME SLEEP TEST (HST) WITH TYPE III PORTABLE MONITOR, UNATTENDED; MINIMUM OF 4 CHANNELS: 2 RESPIRATORY MOVEMENT/AIRFLOW, 1 ECG/HEART RATE AND 1 OXYGEN SATURATION	C	N	13	A		
G0400	HOME SLEEP TEST (HST) WITH TYPE IV PORTABLE MONITOR, UNATTENDED; MINIMUM OF 3 CHANNELS	C	N	13	A		

HCPCS Code	Statute	Lab Cert	X-Ref	ASC Pay Grp	ASC Pay Group Eff. Date	Proc Notes	BETOS	TOS	Anest	Code Add Date	Code Effective Date	Code Term Date
G0384							M3	1	0	20070101	20080101	
G0389						0134	I3B	4	0	20070101	20070101	
G0390						0136	M5D	1	0	20070101	20070101	
G0392							P1G	2	0	20070101	20100101	20091231
G0393							P1G	2	0	20070101	20100101	20091231
G0394							T1H	5	0	20070101	20090101	20081231
G0396							M5D	1	0	20080101	20080101	
G0397							M5D	1	0	20080101	20080101	
G0398							T2D	5	0	20080313	20080313	
G0399							T2D	5	0	20080313	20080313	
G0400							T2D	5	0	20080313	20080313	

HCPCS Code	Long Description	Coverage	Action	PI	MPI	CIM	MCM
G0402	INITIAL PREVENTIVE PHYSICAL EXAMINATION; FACE-TO-FACE VISIT, SERVICES LIMITED TO NEW BENEFICIARY DURING THE FIRST 12 MONTHS OF MEDICARE ENROLLMENT	C	N	11	A		
G0403	ELECTROCARDIOGRAM, ROUTINE ECG WITH 12 LEADS; PERFORMED AS A SCREENING FOR THE INITIAL PREVENTIVE PHYSICAL EXAMINATION WITH INTERPRETATION AND REPORT	C	N	11	A		
G0404	ELECTROCARDIOGRAM, ROUTINE ECG WITH 12 LEADS; TRACING ONLY, WITHOUT INTERPRETATION AND REPORT, PERFORMED AS A SCREENING FOR THE INITIAL PREVENTIVE PHYSICAL EXAMINATION	C	N	11	A		
G0405	ELECTROCARDIOGRAM, ROUTINE ECG WITH 12 LEADS; INTERPRETATION AND REPORT ONLY, PERFORMED AS A SCREENING FOR THE INITIAL PREVENTIVE PHYSICAL EXAMINATION	C	N	11	A		
G0406	FOLLOW-UP INPATIENT TELEHEALTH CONSULTATION, LIMITED, PHYSICIANS TYPICALLY SPEND 15 MINUTES COMMUNICATING WITH THE PATIENT VIA TELEHEALTH	C	N	13	A		
G0407	FOLLOW-UP INPATIENT TELEHEALTH CONSULTATION, INTERMEDIATE, PHYSICIANS TYPICALLY SPEND 25 MINUTES COMMUNICATING WITH THE PATIENT VIA TELEHEALTH	C	N	11	A		
G0408	FOLLOW-UP INPATIENT TELEHEALTH CONSULTATION, COMPLEX, PHYSICIANS TYPICALLY SPEND 35 MINUTES OR MORE COMMUNICATING WITH THE PATIENT VIA TELEHEALTH	C	N	11	A		
G0409	SOCIAL WORK AND PSYCHOLOGICAL SERVICES, DIRECTLY RELATING TO AND/OR FURTHERING THE PATIENT'S REHABIL-ITATION GOALS, EACH 15 MINUTES, FACE-TO-FACE; INDIVIDUAL (SERVICES PROVIDED BY A CORF-QUALIFIED SOCIAL WORKER OR PSYCHOLOGIST IN A CORF)	C	N	13	A		
G0410	GROUP PSYCHOTHERAPY OTHER THAN OF A MULTIPLE-FAMILY GROUP, IN A PARTIAL HOSPITALIZATION SETTING, APPROXIMATELY 45 TO 50 MINUTES	C	N	13	A		
G0411	INTERACTIVE GROUP PSYCHOTHERAPY, IN A PARTIAL HOSPITALIZATION SETTING, APPROXIMATELY 45 TO 50 MINUTES	C	N	13	A		
G0412	OPEN TREATMENT OF ILIAC SPINE(S), TUBEROSITY AVULSION, OR ILIAC WING FRACTURE(S), UNILATERAL OR BILATERAL FOR PELVIC BONE FRACTURE PATTERNS WHICH DO NOT DISRUPT THE PELVIC RING INCLUDES INTERNAL FIXATION, WHEN PERFORMED	C	N	13	A		
G0413	PERCUTANEOUS SKELETAL FIXATION OF POSTERIOR PELVIC BONE FRACTURE AND/OR DISLOCATION, FOR FRACTURE OR PATTERNS WHICH DISRUPT THE PELVIC RING, UNILATERAL BILATERAL, (INCLUDES ILIUM, SACROILIAC JOINT AND/OR SACRUM)	C	N	13	A		
G0414	OPEN TREATMENT OF ANTERIOR PELVIC BONE FRACTURE AND/OR DISLOCATION FOR FRACTURE PATTERNS WHICH DISRUPT THE PELVIC RING, UNILATERAL OR BILATERAL, INCLUDES INTERNAL FIXATION WHEN PERFORMED (INCLUDES PUBIC SYMPHYSIS AND/OR SUPERIOR/INFERIOR RAMI)	C	N	13	A		

HCPCS Code	Statute	Lab Cert	X-Ref	ASC Pay Grp	ASC Pay Group Eff. Date	Proc Notes	BETOS	TOS	Anest	Code Add Date	Code Effective Date	Code Term Date
G0402						0153	M1A	1	0	20090101	20090101	
G0403						0153	T2C	5	0	20090101	20090101	
G0404						0153	T2C	5	0	20090101	20090101	
G0405						0153	T2C	5	0	20090101	20090101	
G0406							M6	3	0	20090101	20090101	
G0407							M6	3	0	20090101	20090101	
G0408							M6	3	0	20090101	20090101	
G0409							M5D	1	0	20090101	20090101	
G0410							P6D	1	0	20090101	20090101	
G0411							P6D	1	0	20090101	20090101	
G0412						0155	P3D	2	0	20090101	20090101	
G0413						0155	P3D	2	0	20090101	20090101	
G0414						0155	P3D	2	0	20090101	20090101	

HCPCS Code	Long Description	Coverage	Action	PI	MPI	CIM	MCM
G0415	OPEN TREATMENT OF POSTERIOR PELVIC BONE FRACTURE AND/OR DISLOCATION, FOR FRACTURE PATTERNS WHICH DISRUPT THE PELVIC RING, UNILATERAL OR BILATERAL, INCLUDES INTERNAL FIXATION, WHEN PERFORMED (INCLUDES ILIUM, SACROILIAC JOINT AND/OR SACRUM)	C	N	13	A		
G0416	SURGICAL PATHOLOGY, GROSS AND MICROSCOPIC EXAMINATION FOR PROSTATE NEEDLE SATURATION BIOPSY SAMPLING, 1-20 SPECIMENS	C	F	13	A		
G0417	SURGICAL PATHOLOGY, GROSS AND MICROSCOPIC EXAMINATION FOR PROSTATE NEEDLE SATURATION BIOPSY SAMPLING, 21-40 SPECIMENS	C	F	13	A		
G0418	SURGICAL PATHOLOGY, GROSS AND MICROSCOPIC EXAMINATION FOR PROSTATE NEEDLE SATURATION BIOPSY SAMPLING, 41-60 SPECIMENS	C	F	13	A		
G0419	SURGICAL PATHOLOGY, GROSS AND MICROSCOPIC EXAMINATION FOR PROSTATE NEEDLE SATURATION BIOPSY SAMPLING, GREATER THAN 60 SPECIMENS	C	F	13	A		
G0420	FACE-TO-FACE EDUCATIONAL SERVICES RELATED TO THE CARE OF CHRONIC KIDNEY DISEASE; INDIVIDUAL, PER SESSION, PER ONE HOUR	C	A	11	A		
G0421	FACE-TO-FACE EDUCATIONAL SERVICES RELATED TO THE CARE OF CHRONIC KIDNEY DISEASE; GROUP, PER SESSION, PER ONE HOUR	C	A	11	A		
G0422	INTENSIVE CARDIAC REHABILITATION; WITH OR WITHOUT CONTINUOUS ECG MONITORING WITH EXERCISE, PER SESSION	C	A	11	A		
G0423	INTENSIVE CARDIAC REHABILITATION; WITH OR WITHOUT CONTINUOUS ECG MONITORING; WITHOUT EXERCISE, PER SESSION	C	A	11	A		
G0424	PULMONARY REHABILITATION, INCLUDING EXERCISE (INCLUDES MONITORING), ONE HOUR, PER SESSION, UP TO TWO SESSIONS PER DAY	C	A	11	A		
G0425	INITIAL INPATIENT TELEHEALTH CONSULTATION, TYPICALLY 30 MINUTES COMMUNICATING WITH THE PATIENT VIA TELEHEALTH	C	A	13	A		
G0426	INITIAL INPATIENT TELEHEALTH CONSULTATION, TYPICALLY 50 MINUTES COMMUNICATING WITH THE PATIENT VIA TELEHEALTH	C	A	13	A		
G0427	INITIAL INPATIENT TELEHEALTH CONSULTATION, TYPICALLY 70 MINUTES OR MORE COMMUNICATING WITH THE PATIENT VIA TELEHEALTH	C	A	13	A		
G0430	DRUG SCREEN, QUALITATIVE; MULTIPLE DRUG CLASSES OTHER THAN CHROMATOGRAPHIC METHOD, EA. PROCEDURE	C	A	13	A		
G0431	DRUG SCREEN, QUALITATIVE; SINGLE DRUG CLASS METHOD (E.G., IMMUNOASSAY, ENZYME ASSAY), EACH DRUG CLASS	C	A	13	A		
G3001	ADMINISTRATION AND SUPPLY OF TOSITUMOMAB, 450 MG	C	N	13	A		
G8006	ACUTE MYOCARDIAL INFARCTION: PATIENT DOCUMENTED TO HAVE RECEIVED ASPIRIN AT ARRIVAL	C	N	00	9		
G8007	ACUTE MYOCARDIAL INFARCTION: PATIENT NOT DOCUMENTED TO HAVE RECEIVED ASPIRIN AT ARRIVAL	C	N	00	9		

HCPCS Code	Statute	Lab Cert	X-Ref	ASC Pay Grp	ASC Pay Group Eff. Date	Proc Notes	BETOS	TOS	Anest	Code Add Date	Code Effective Date	Code Term Date
G0415						0155	P3D	2	0	20090101	20090101	
G0416		610					T1G	5	0	20090101	20100101	
G0416 G0417		610					T1G	5	0	20090101	20100101	
G0418		610					T1G	5	0	20090101	20100101	
G0419		610					T1G	5	0	20090101	20100101	
G0420							M1B	1	0	20100101	20100101	
G0421							M1B	1	0	20100101	20100101	
G0422							M5D	1	0	20100101	20100101	
G0423							M5D	1	0	20100101	20100101	
G0424							M5D	1	0	20100101	20100101	
G0425							M6	3	0	20100101	20100101	
G0426							M6	3	0	20100101	20100101	
G0427							M6	3	0	20100101	20100101	
G0430		340					T1H	5	0	20100101	20100101	
G0431		340					T1H	5	0	20100101	20100101	
G3001							T2D	1	0	20030701	20030701	
G8006							M5D	1	0	20060101	20060101	
G8007							M5D	1	0	20060101	20060101	

HCPCS Code	Long Description	Coverage	Action	PI	MPI	CIM	MCM
G8008	CLINICIAN DOCUMENTED THAT ACUTE MYOCARDIAL INFARCTION PATIENT WAS NOT AN ELIGIBLE CANDIDATE TO RECEIVE ASPIRIN AT ARRIVAL MEASURE	C	N	00	9		
G8009	ACUTE MYOCARDIAL INFARCTION: PATIENT DOCUMENTED TO HAVE RECEIVED BETA-BLOCKER AT ARRIVAL	C	N	00	9		
G8010	ACUTE MYOCARDIAL INFARCTION: PATIENT NOT DOCUMENTED TO HAVE RECEIVED BETA-BLOCKER AT ARRIVAL	C	N	00	9		
G8011	CLINICIAN DOCUMENTED THAT ACUTE MYOCARDIAL INFARCTION PATIENT WAS NOT AN ELIGIBLE CANDIDATE FOR BETA-BLOCKER AT ARRIVAL MEASURE	C	N	00	9		
G8012	PNEUMONIA: PATIENT DOCUMENTED TO HAVE RECEIVED ANTIBIOTIC WITHIN 4 HOURS OF PRESENTATION	C	N	00	9		
G8013	PNEUMONIA: PATIENT NOT DOCUMENTED TO HAVE RECEIVED ANTIBIOTIC WITHIN 4 HOURS OF PRESENTATION	C	N	00	9		
G8014	CLINICIAN DOCUMENTED THAT PNEUMONIA PATIENT WAS R NOT AN ELIGIBLE CANDIDATE FOANTIBIOTIC WITHIN 4 HOURS OF PRESENTATION MEASURE	C	N	00	9		
G8015	DIABETIC PATIENT WITH MOST RECENT HEMOGLOBIN A1C LEVEL (WITHIN THE LAST 6 MONTHS) DOCUMENTED AS GREATER THAN 9%	C	N	00	9		
G8016	DIABETIC PATIENT WITH MOST RECENT HEMOGLOBIN A1C LEVEL (WITHIN THE LAST 6 MONTHS) DOCUMENTED AS LESS THAN OR EQUAL TO 9%	C	N	00	9		
G8017	CLINICIAN DOCUMENTED THAT DIABETIC PATIENT WAS NOT ELIGIBLE CANDIDATE FOR HEMOGLOBIN A1C MEASURE	C	N	00	9		
G8018	CLINICIAN HAS NOT PROVIDED CARE FOR THE DIABETIC PATIENT FOR THE REQUIRED TIME FOR HEMOGLOBIN A1C MEASURE (6 MONTHS)	C	N	00	9		
G8019	DIABETIC PATIENT WITH MOST RECENT LOW-DENSITY LIPOPROTEIN (WITHIN THE LAST 12 MONTHS) DOCUMENTED AS GREATER THAN OR EQUAL TO 100 MG/DL	C	N	00	9		
G8020	DIABETIC PATIENT WITH MOST RECENT LOW-DENSITY LIPOPROTEIN (WITHIN THE LAST 12 MONTHS) DOCUMENTED AS LESS THAN 100 MG/DL	C	N	00	9		
G8021	CLINICIAN DOCUMENTED THAT DIABETIC PATIENT WAS NOT ELIGIBLE CANDIDATE FOR LOW-DENSITY LIPOPROTEIN MEASURE	C	N	00	9		
G8022	CLINICIAN HAS NOT PROVIDED CARE FOR THE DIABETIC PATIENT FOR THE REQUIRED TIME FOR LOW-DENSITY LIPOPROTEIN MEASURE (12 MONTHS)	C	N	00	9		
G8023	DIABETIC PATIENT WITH MOST RECENT BLOOD PRESSURE (WITHIN THE LAST 6 MONTHS) DOCUMENTED AS EQUAL TO OR GREATER THAN 140 SYSTOLIC OR EQUAL TO OR GREATER THAN 80 MMHG DIASTOLIC	C	N	00	9		
G8024	DIABETIC PATIENT WITH MOST RECENT BLOOD PRESSURE (WITHIN THE LAST 6 MONTHS) DOCUMENTED AS LESS THAN 140 SYSTOLIC AND LESS THAN 80 DIASTOLIC	C	N	00	9		
G8025	CLINICIAN DOCUMENTED THAT THE DIABETIC PATIENT WAS NOT ELIGIBLE CANDIDATE FOR BLOOD PRESSURE MEASURE	C	N	00	9		

HCPCS Code	Statute	Lab Cert	X-Ref	ASC Pay Grp	ASC Pay Group Eff. Date	Proc Notes	BETOS	TOS	Anest	Code Add Date	Code Effective Date	Code Term Date
G8008							M5D	1	0	20060101	20060101	
G8009							M5D	1	0	20060101	20060101	
G8010							M5D	1	0	20060101	20060101	
G8011							M5D	1	0	20060101	20060101	
G8012							M5D	1	0	20060101	20060101	
G8013							M5D	1	0	20060101	20060101	
G8014							M5D	1	0	20060101	20060101	
G8015							M5D	1	0	20060101	20060101	
G8016							M5D	1	0	20060101	20060101	
G8017							M5D	1	0	20060101	20060101	
G8018							M5D	1	0	20060101	20060101	
G8019							M5D	1	0	20060101	20060101	
G8020							M5D	1	0	20060101	20060101	
G8021							M5D	1	0	20060101	20060101	
G8022							M5D	1	0	20060101	20060101	
G8023							M5D	1	0	20060101	20060101	
G8024							M5D	1	0	20060101	20060101	
G8025							M5D	1	0	20060101	20060101	

HCPCS Code	Long Description	Coverage	Action	PI	MPI	CIM	MCM
G8026	CLINICIAN HAS NOT PROVIDED CARE FOR THE DIABETIC PATIENT FOR THE REQUIRED TIME FOR BLOOD PRESSURE MEASURE (WITHIN THE LAST 6 MONTHS)	C	N	00	9		
G8027	HEART FAILURE PATIENT WITH LEFT VENTRICULAR SYSTOLIC DYSFUNCTION (LVSD) DOCUMENTED TO BE ON EITHER ANGIOTENSIN-CONVERTING ENZYME INHIBITOR OR ANGIOTENSIN-RECEPTOR BLOCKER (ACE-I OR ARB) THERAPY	C	N	00	9		
G8028	HEART FAILURE PATIENT WITH LEFT VENTRICULAR SYSTOLIC DYSFUNCTION (LVSD) NOT DOCUMENTED TO BE ON EITHER ANGIOTENSIN-CONVERTING ENZYME INHIBITOR OR ANGIOTENSIN-RECEPTOR BLOCKER (ACE-I OR ARB) THERAPY	C	N	00	9		
G8029	CLINICIAN DOCUMENTED THAT HEART FAILURE PATIENT WAS NOT AN ELIGIBLE CANDIDATE FOR EITHER ANGIOTENSIN-CONVERTING ENZYME INHIBITOR OR ANGIOTENSIN-RECEPTOR BLOCKER (ACE-I OR ARB) THERAPY MEASURE	C	N	00	9		
G8030	HEART FAILURE PATIENT WITH LEFT VENTRICULAR SYSTOLIC DYSFUNCTION (LVSD) DOCUMENTED TO BE ON BETA-BLOCKER THERAPY	C	N	00	9		
G8031	HEART FAILURE PATIENT WITH LEFT VENTRICULAR SYSTOLIC DYSFUNCTION (LVSD) NOT DOCUMENTED TO BE ON BETA-BLOCKER THERAPY	C	N	00	9		
G8032	CLINICIAN DOCUMENTED THAT HEART FAILURE PATIENT WAS NOT ELIGIBLE CANDIDATE FOR BETA-BLOCKER THERAPY MEASURE	C	N	00	9		
G8033	PRIOR MYOCARDIAL INFARCTION - CORONARY ARTERY DISEASE PATIENT DOCUMENTED TO BE ON BETA-BLOCKER THERAPY	C	N	00	9		
G8034	PRIOR MYOCARDIAL INFARCTION - CORONARY ARTERY DISEASE PATIENT NOT DOCUMENTED TO BE ON BETA-BLOCKER THERAPY	C	N	00	9		
G8035	CLINICIAN DOCUMENTED THAT PRIOR MYOCARDIAL INFARCTION - CORONARY ARTERY DISEASE PATIENT WAS NOT ELIGIBLE CANDIDATE FOR BETA-BLOCKER THERAPY MEASURE	C	N	00	9		
G8036	CORONARY ARTERY DISEASE PATIENT DOCUMENTED TO BE ON ANTIPLATELET THERAPY	C	N	00	9		
G8037	CORONARY ARTERY DISEASE PATIENT NOT DOCUMENTED TO BE ON ANTIPLATELET THERAPY	C	N	00	9		
G8038	CLINICIAN DOCUMENTED THAT CORONARY ARTERY DISEASE PATIENT WAS NOT ELIGIBLE CANDIDATE FOR ANTIPLATELET THERAPY MEASURE	C	N	00	9		
G8039	CORONARY ARTERY DISEASE - PATIENT WITH LOW-DENSITY LIPOPROTEIN DOCUMENTED TO BE GREATER THAN 100MG/DL	C	N	00	9		
G8040	CORONARY ARTERY DISEASE - PATIENT WITH LOW-DENSITY LIPOPROTEIN DOCUMENTED TO BE LESS THAN OR EQUAL TO 100MG/DL	C	N	00	9		
G8041	CLINICIAN DOCUMENTED THAT CORONARY ARTERY DISEASE PATIENT WAS NOT ELIGIBLE CANDIDATE FOR LOW-DENSITY LIPOPROTEIN MEASURE	C	N	00	9		

HCPCS Code	Statute	Lab Cert	X-Ref	ASC Pay Grp	ASC Pay Group Eff. Date	Proc Notes	BETOS	TOS	Anest	Code Add Date	Code Effective Date	Code Term Date
G8026							M5D	1	0	20060101	20060101	
G8027							M5D	1	0	20060101	20060101	
G8028							M5D	1	0	20060101	20060101	
G8029							M5D	1	0	20060101	20060101	
G8030							M5D	1	0	20060101	20060101	
G8031							M5D	1	0	20060101	20060101	
G8032							M5D	1	0	20060101	20060101	
G8033							M5D	1	0	20060101	20060101	
G8034							M5D	1	0	20060101	20060101	
G8035							M5D	1	0	20060101	20060101	
G8036							M5D	1	0	20060101	20060101	
G8037							M5D	1	0	20060101	20060101	
G8038							M5D	1	0	20060101	20060101	
G8039							M5D	1	0	20060101	20060101	
G8040							M5D	1	0	20060101	20060101	
G8041							M5D	1	0	20060101	20060101	

HCPCS Code	Long Description	Coverage	Action	PI	MPI	CIM	MCM
G8051	PATIENT (FEMALE) DOCUMENTED TO HAVE BEEN ASSESSED FOR OSTEOPOROSIS	C	N	00	9		
G8052	PATIENT (FEMALE) NOT DOCUMENTED TO HAVE BEEN ASSESSED FOR OSTEOPOROSIS	C	N	00	9		
G8053	CLINICIAN DOCUMENTED THAT (FEMALE) PATIENT WAS NOT AN ELIGIBLE CANDIDATE FOR OSTEOPOROSIS ASSESSMENT MEASURE	C	N	00	9		
G8054	PATIENT NOT DOCUMENTED FOR THE ASSESSMENT FOR FALLS WITHIN LAST 12 MONTHS	C	N	00	9		
G8055	PATIENT DOCUMENTED FOR THE ASSESSMENT FOR FALLS WITHIN LAST 12 MONTHS	C	N	00	9		
G8056	CLINICIAN DOCUMENTED THAT PATIENT WAS NOT AN ELIGIBLE CANDIDATE FOR THE FALLS ASSESSMENT MEASURE WITHIN THE LAST 12 MONTHS	C	N	00	9		
G8057	PATIENT DOCUMENTED TO HAVE RECEIVED HEARING ASSESSMENT	C	N	00	9		
G8058	PATIENT NOT DOCUMENTED TO HAVE RECEIVED HEARING ASSESSMENT	C	N	00	9		
G8059	CLINICIAN DOCUMENTED THAT PATIENT WAS NOT AN ELIGIBLE CANDIDATE FOR HEARING ASSESSMENT MEASURE	C	N	00	9		
G8060	PATIENT DOCUMENTED FOR THE ASSESSMENT OF URINARY INCONTINENCE	C	N	00	9		
G8061	PATIENT NOT DOCUMENTED FOR THE ASSESSMENT OF URINARY INCONTINENCE	C	N	00	9		
G8062	CLINICIAN DOCUMENTED THAT PATIENT WAS NOT AN ELIGIBLE CANDIDATE FOR URINARY INCONTINENCE ASSESSMENT MEASURE	C	N	00	9		
G8075	END STAGE RENAL DISEASE PATIENT WITH DOCUMENTED DIALYSIS DOSE OF URR GREATER THAN OR EQUAL TO 65% (OR KT/V GREATER THAN OR EQUAL TO 1.2)	C	N	00	9		
G8076	END STAGE RENAL DISEASE PATIENT WITH DOCUMENTED DIALYSIS DOSE OF URR LESS THAN65% (OR KT/V LESS THAN 1.2)	C	N	00	9		
G8077	CLINICIAN DOCUMENTED THAT END STAGE RENAL DISEASE PATIENT WAS NOT AN ELIGIBLE CANDIDATE FOR URR OR KT/V MEASURE	C	N	00	9		
G8078	END STAGE RENAL DISEASE PATIENT WITH DOCUMENTED HEMATOCRIT GREATER THAN OR EQUAL TO 33 (OR HEMOGLOBIN GREATER THAN OR EQUAL TO 11)	C	N	00	9		
G8079	END STAGE RENAL DISEASE PATIENT WITH DOCUMENTED HEMATOCRIT LESS THAN 33 (OR HEMOGLOBIN LESS THAN 11)	C	N	00	9		
G8080	CLINICIAN DOCUMENTED THAT END STAGE RENAL DISEASE PATIENT WAS NOT AN ELIGIBLE CANDIDATE FOR HEMATOCRIT (HEMOGLOBIN) MEASURE	C	N	00	9		
G8081	END STAGE RENAL DISEASE PATIENT REQUIRING HEMODIALYSIS VASCULAR ACCESS DOCUMENTED TO HAVE RECEIVED AUTOGENOUS AV FISTULA	C	N	00	9		
G8082	END STAGE RENAL DISEASE PATIENT REQUIRING HEMODIALYSIS DOCUMENTED TO HAVE RECEIVED VASCULAR ACCESS OTHER THAN AUTOGENOUS AV FISTULA	C	N	00	9		

HCPCS Code	Statute	Lab Cert	X-Ref	ASC Pay Grp	ASC Pay Group Eff. Date	Proc Notes	BETOS	TOS	Anest	Code Add Date	Code Effective Date	Code Term Date
G8051							M5D	1	0	20060101	20060101	
G8052							M5D	1	0	20060101	20060101	
G8053							M5D	1	0	20060101	20060101	
G8054							M5D	1	0	20060101	20060101	
G8055							M5D	1	0	20060101	20060101	
G8056							M5D	1	0	20060101	20060101	
G8057							M5D	1	0	20060101	20060101	
G8058							M5D	1	0	20060101	20060101	
G8059							M5D	1	0	20060101	20060101	
G8060							M5D	1	0	20060101	20060101	
G8061							M5D	1	0	20060101	20060101	
G8062							M5D	1	0	20060101	20060101	
G8075							M5D	1	0	20060101	20060101	
G8076							M5D	1	0	20060101	20060101	
G8077							M5D	1	0	20060101	20060101	
G8078							M5D	1	0	20060101	20060101	
G8079							M5D	1	0	20060101	20060101	
G8080							M5D	1	0	20060101	20060101	
G8081							M5D	1	0	20060101	20060101	
G8082							M5D	1	0	20060101	20060101	

HCPCS Code	Long Description	Coverage	Action	PI	MPI	CIM	MCM
G8085	END-STAGE RENAL DISEASE PATIENT REQUIRING HEMODIALYSIS VASCULAR ACCESS WAS NOT AN ELIGIBLE CANDIDATE FOR AUTOGENOUS AV FISTULA	C	N	00	9		
G8093	NEWLY DIAGNOSED CHRONIC OBSTRUCTIVE PULMONARY DISEASE (COPD) PATIENT DOCUMENTED TO HAVE RECEIVED SMOKING CESSATION INTERVENTION, WITHIN 3 MONTHS OF DIAGNOSIS	C	N	00	9		
G8094	NEWLY DIAGNOSED CHRONIC OBSTRUCTIVE PULMONARY DISEASE (COPD) PATIENT NOT DOCUMENTED TO HAVE RECEIVED SMOKING CESSATION INTERVENTION, WITHIN 3 MONTHS OF DIAGNOSIS	C	N	00	9		
G8099	OSTEOPOROSIS PATIENT DOCUMENTED TO HAVE BEEN PRESCRIBED CALCIUM AND VITAMIN D SUPPLEMENTS	C	N	00	9		
G8100	CLINICIAN DOCUMENTED THAT OSTEOPOROSIS PATIENT WAS NOT AN ELIGIBLE CANDIDATE FOR CALCIUM AND VITAMIN D SUPPLEMENT MEASURE	C	N	00	9		
G8103	NEWLY DIAGNOSED OSTEOPOROSIS PATIENTS DOCUMENTED TO HAVE BEEN TREATED WITH ANTIRESORPTIVE THERAPY AND/OR PTH WITHIN 3 MONTHS OF DIAGNOSIS	C	N	00	9		
G8104	CLINICIAN DOCUMENTED THAT NEWLY DIAGNOSED OSTEOPOROSIS PATIENT WAS NOT AN ELIGIBLE CANDIDATE FOR ANTIRESORPTIVE THERAPY AND/OR PTH TREATMENT MEASURE WITHIN 3 MONTHS OF DIAGNOSIS	C	N	00	9		
G8106	WITHIN 6 MONTHS OF SUFFERING A NONTRAUMATIC FRACTURE, FEMALE PATIENT 65 YEARS OF AGE OR OLDER DOCUMENTED TO HAVE UNDERGONE BONE MINERAL DENSITY TESTING OR TO HAVE BEEN PRESCRIBED A DRUG TO TREAT OR PREVENT OSTEOPOROSIS	C	N	00	9		
G8107	CLINICIAN DOCUMENTED THAT FEMALE PATIENT 65 YEARS OF AGE OR OLDER WHO SUFFERED A NONTRAUMATIC FRACTURE WITHIN THE LAST 6 MONTHS WAS NOT AN ELIGIBLE CANDIDATE FOR MEASURE TO TEST BONE MINERAL DENSITY OR DRUG TO TREAT OR PREVENT OSTEOPOROSIS	C	N	00	9		
G8108	PATIENT DOCUMENTED TO HAVE RECEIVED INFLUENZA VACCINATION DURING INFLUENZA SEASON	C	N	00	9		
G8109	PATIENT NOT DOCUMENTED TO HAVE RECEIVED INFLUENZA VACCINATION DURING INFLUENZA SEASON	C	N	00	9		
G8110	CLINICIAN DOCUMENTED THAT PATIENT WAS NOT AN ELIGIBLE CANDIDATE FOR INFLUENZA VACCINATION MEASURE	C	N	00	9		
G8111	PATIENT (FEMALE) DOCUMENTED TO HAVE RECEIVED A MAMMOGRAM DURING THE MEASUREMENT YEAR OR PRIOR YEAR TO THE MEASUREMENT YEAR	C	N	00	9		
G8112	PATIENT (FEMALE) NOT DOCUMENTED TO HAVE RECEIVED A MAMMOGRAM DURING THE MEASUREMENT YEAR OR PRIOR YEAR TO THE MEASUREMENT YEAR	C	N	00	9		
G8113	CLINICIAN DOCUMENTED THAT FEMALE PATIENT WAS NOT AN ELIGIBLE CANDIDATE FOR MAMMOGRAPHY MEASURE	C	N	00	9		

HCPCS Code	Statute	Lab Cert	X-Ref	ASC Pay Grp	ASC Pay Group Eff. Date	Proc Notes	BETOS	TOS	Anest	Code Add Date	Code Effective Date	Code Term Date
G8085							M5D	1	0	20060101	20060101	
G8093							M5D	1	0	20060101	20060101	
G8094							M5D	1	0	20060101	20060101	
G8099							M5D	1	0	20060101	20060101	
G8100							M5D	1	0	20060101	20060101	
G8103							M5D	1	0	20060101	20060101	
G8104							M5D	1	0	20060101	20060101	
G8106							M5D	1	0	20060101	20060101	
G8107							M5D	1	0	20060101	20060101	
G8108							M5D	1	0	20060101	20060101	
G8109							M5D	1	0	20060101	20060101	
G8110							M5D	1	0	20060101	20060101	
G8111							M5D	1	0	20060101	20060101	
G8112							M5D	1	0	20060101	20060101	
G8113							M5D	1	0	20060101	20060101	

HCPCS Code	Long Description	Coverage	Action	PI	MPI	CIM	MCM
G8114	CLINICIAN DID NOT PROVIDE CARE TO PATIENT FOR THE REQUIRED TIME OF MAMMOGRAPHY MEASURE (I.E., MEASUREMENT YEAR OR PRIOR YEAR)	C	N	00	9		
G8115	PATIENT DOCUMENTED TO HAVE RECEIVED PNEUMOCOCCAL VACCINATION	C	N	00	9		
G8116	PATIENT NOT DOCUMENTED TO HAVE RECEIVED PNEUMOCOCCAL VACCINATION	C	N	00	9		
G8117	CLINICIAN DOCUMENTED THAT PATIENT WAS NOT AN ELIGIBLE CANDIDATE FOR PNEUMOCOCCAL VACCINATION MEASURE	C	N	00	9		
G8126	PATIENT DOCUMENTED AS BEING TREATED WITH ANTIDEPRESSANT MEDICATION DURING THE ENTIRE 12 WEEK ACUTE TREATMENT PHASE	C	N	00	9		
G8127	PATIENT NOT DOCUMENTED AS BEING TREATED WITH ANTIDEPRESSANT MEDICATION DURING THE ENTIRE 12 WEEKS ACUTE TREATMENT PHASE	C	N	00	9		
G8128	CLINICIAN DOCUMENTED THAT PATIENT WAS NOT AN ELIGIBLE CANDIDATE FOR ANTIDEPRESSANT MEDICATION DURING THE ENTIRE 12 WEEK ACUTE TREATMENT PHASE MEASURE	C	N	00	9		
G8129	PATIENT DOCUMENTED AS BEING TREATED WITH ANTIDEPRESSANT MEDICATION FOR AT LEAST 6 MONTHS CONTINUOUS TREATMENT PHASE	C	N	00	9		
G8130	PATIENT NOT DOCUMENTED AS BEING TREATED WITH ANTIDEPRESSANT MEDICATION FOR AT LEAST 6 MONTHS CONTINUOUS TREATMENT PHASE	C	N	00	9		
G8131	CLINICIAN DOCUMENTED THAT PATIENT WAS NOT AN ELIGIBLE CANDIDATE FOR ANTIDEPRESSANT MEDICATION FOR CONTINUOUS TREATMENT PHASE	C	N	00	9		
G8152	PATIENT DOCUMENTED TO HAVE RECEIVED ANTIBIOTIC PROPHYLAXIS ONE HOUR PRIOR TO INCISION TIME (TWO HOURS FOR VANCOMYCIN)	C	N	00	9		
G8153	PATIENT NOT DOCUMENTED TO HAVE RECEIVED ANTIBIOTIC PROPHYLAXIS ONE HOUR PRIOR TO INCISION TIME (TWO HOURS FOR VANCOMYCIN)	C	N	00	9		
G8154	CLINICIAN DOCUMENTED THAT PATIENT WAS NOT AN ELIGIBLE CANDIDATE FOR ANTIBIOTIC PROPHYLAXIS ONE HOUR PRIOR TO INCISION TIME (TWO HOURS FOR VANCOMYCIN) MEASURE	C	N	00	9		
G8155	PATIENT WITH DOCUMENTED RECEIPT OF THROMBOEMBOLISM PROPHYLAXIS	C	N	00	9		
G8156	PATIENT WITHOUT DOCUMENTED RECEIPT OF THROMBOEMBOLISM PROPHYLAXIS	C	N	00	9		
G8157	CLINICIAN DOCUMENTED THAT PATIENT WAS NOT AN ELIGIBLE CANDIDATE FOR THROMBOEMBOLISM PROPHYLAXIS MEASURE	C	N	00	9		
G8158	PATIENT DOCUMENTED TO HAVE RECEIVED CORONARY ARTERY BYPASS GRAFT WITH USE OF INTERNAL MAMMARY ARTERY	C	N	00	9		

HCPCS Code	Statute	Lab Cert	X-Ref	ASC Pay Grp	ASC Pay Group Eff. Date	Proc Notes	BETOS	TOS	Anest	Code Add Date	Code Effective Date	Code Term Date
G8114							M5D	1	0	20060101	20060101	
G8115							M5D	1	0	20060101	20060101	
G8116							M5D	1	0	20060101	20060101	
G8117							M5D	1	0	20060101	20060101	
G8126							M5D	1	0	20060101	20060101	
G8127							M5D	1	0	20060101	20060101	
G8128							M5D	1	0	20060101	20060101	
G8129							M5D	1	0	20060101	20060101	
G8130							M5D	1	0	20060101	20060101	
G8131							M5D	1	0	20060101	20060101	
G8152							M5D	1	0	20060101	20060101	
G8153							M5D	1	0	20060101	20060101	
G8154							M5D	1	0	20060101	20060101	
G8155							M5D	1	0	20060101	20060101	
G8156							M5D	1	0	20060101	20060101	
G8157							M5D	1	0	20060101	20060101	
G8158							M5D	1	0	20060101	20070701	20070630

HCPCS Code	Long Description	Coverage	Action	PI	MPI	CIM	MCM
G8159	PATIENT DOCUMENTED TO HAVE RECEIVED CORONARY ARTERY BYPASS GRAFT WITHOUT USE OF INTERNAL MAMMARY ARTERY	C	N	00	9		
G8160	CLINICIAN DOCUMENTED THAT PATIENT WAS NOT AN ELIGIBLE CANDIDATE FOR CORONARY ARTERY BYPASS GRAFT WITH USE OF INTERNAL MAMMARY ARTERY MEASURE	C	N	00	9		
G8161	PATIENT WITH ISOLATED CORONARY ARTERY BYPASS GRAFT DOCUMENTED TO HAVE RECEIVED PRE-OPERATIVE BETA-BLOCKADE	C	N	00	9		
G8162	PATIENT WITH ISOLATED CORONARY ARTERY BYPASS GRAFT NOT DOCUMENTED TO HAVE RECEIVED PRE-OPERATIVE BETA-BLOCKADE	C	N	00	9		
G8163	CLINICIAN DOCUMENTED THAT PATIENT WITH ISOLATED CORONARY ARTERY BYPASS GRAFT WAS NOT AN ELIGIBLE CANDIDATE FOR PRE-OPERATIVE BETA-BLOCKADE MEASURE	C	N	00	9		
G8164	PATIENT WITH ISOLATED CORONARY ARTERY BYPASS GRAFT DOCUMENTED TO HAVE PROLONGED INTUBATION	C	N	00	9		
G8165	PATIENT WITH ISOLATED CORONARY ARTERY BYPASS GRAFT NOT DOCUMENTED TO HAVE PROLONGED INTUBATION	C	N	00	9		
G8166	PATIENT WITH ISOLATED CORONARY ARTERY BYPASS GRAFT DOCUMENTED TO HAVE REQUIRED SURGICAL RE-EXPLORATION	C	N	00	9		
G8167	PATIENT WITH ISOLATED CORONARY ARTERY BYPASS GRAFT DID NOT REQUIRE SURGICAL RE-EXPLORATION	C	N	00	9		
G8170	PATIENT WITH ISOLATED CORONARY ARTERY BYPASS GRAFT DOCUMENTED TO HAVE BEEN DISCHARGED ON ASPIRIN OR CLOPIDOGREL	C	N	00	9		
G8171	PATIENT WITH ISOLATED CORONARY ARTERY BYPASS GRAFT NOT DOCUMENTED TO HAVE BEEN DISCHARGED ON ASPIRIN OR CLOPIDOGREL	C	N	00	9		
G8172	CLINICIAN DOCUMENTED THAT PATIENT WITH ISOLATED CORONARY ARTERY BYPASS GRAFT WAS NOT AN ELIGIBLE CANDIDATE FOR ANTIPLATELET THERAPY AT DISCHARGE MEASURE	C	N	00	9		
G8182	CLINICIAN HAS NOT PROVIDED CARE FOR THE CARDIAC PATIENT FOR THE REQUIRED TIME FOR LOW-DENSITY LIPOPROTEIN MEASURE (6 MONTHS)	C	N	00	9		
G8183	PATIENT WITH HEART FAILURE AND ATRIAL FIBRILLATION DOCUMENTED TO BE ON WARFARIN THERAPY	C	N	00	9		
G8184	CLINICIAN DOCUMENTED THAT PATIENT WITH HEART FAILURE AND ATRIAL FIBRILLATION WAS NOT AN ELIGIBLE CANDIDATE FOR WARFARIN THERAPY MEASURE	C	N	00	9		
G8185	PATIENTS DIAGNOSED WITH SYMPTOMATIC OSTEOARTHRITIS WITH DOCUMENTED ANNUAL ASSESSMENT OF FUNCTION AND PAIN	C	N	00	9		
G8186	CLINICIAN DOCUMENTED THAT SYMPTOMATIC OSTEOARTHRITIS PATIENT WAS NOT AN ELIGIBLE CANDIDATE FOR ANNUAL ASSESSMENT OF FUNCTION AND PAIN MEASURE	C	N	00	9		

G Codes

HCPCS Code	Statute	Lab Cert	X-Ref	ASC Pay Grp	ASC Pay Group Eff. Date	Proc Notes	BETOS	TOS	Anest	Code Add Date	Code Effective Date	Code Term Date
G8159							M5D	1	0	20060101	20060101	
G8160							M5D	1	0	20060101	20070701	20070630
G8161							M5D	1	0	20060101	20070701	20070630
G8162							M5D	1	0	20060101	20060101	
G8163							M5D	1	0	20060101	20070701	20070630
G8163												
G8164							M5D	1	0	20060101	20060101	
G8165							M5D	1	0	20060101	20060101	
G8166							M5D	1	0	20060101	20060101	
G8167							M5D	1	0	20060101	20060101	
G8170							M5D	1	0	20060101	20060101	
G8171							M5D	1	0	20060101	20060101	
G8171												
G8172							M5D	1	0	20060101	20060101	
G8182							M5D	1	0	20060101	20060101	
G8183							M5D	1	0	20060101	20060101	
G8184							M5D	1	0	20060101	20060101	
G8185							M5D	1	0	20060101	20060101	
G8186							M5D	1	0	20060101	20060101	

HCPCS Code	Long Description	Coverage	Action	PI	MPI	CIM	MCM
G8191	CLINICIAN DOCUMENTED TO HAVE GIVEN ORDER FOR PROPHYLACTIC ANTIBIOTIC TO BE GIVEN WITHIN ONE HOUR (IF VANCOMYCIN, TWO HOURS) PRIOR TO SURGICAL INCISION (OR START OF PROCEDURE WHEN NO INCISION IS REQUIRED)	C	N	00	9		
G8192	CLINICIAN DOCUMENTED TO HAVE GIVEN THE PROPHYLACTIC ANTIBIOTIC WITHIN ONE HOUR (IF VANCOMYCIN, TWO HOURS) PRIOR TO THE SURGICAL INCISION (OR START OF PROCEDURE WHEN NO INCISION IS REQUIRED)	C	N	00	9		
G8193	CLINICIAN DID NOT DOCUMENT THAT AN ORDER FOR PROPHYLACTIC ANTIBIOTIC TO BE GIVEN WITHIN ONE HOUR (IF VANCOMYCIN, TWO HOURS) PRIOR TO SURGICAL INCISION (OR START OF PROCEDURE WHEN NO INCISION IS REQUIRED) WAS GIVEN	C	N	00	9		
G8194	CLINICIAN DOCUMENTED THAT PATIENT WAS NOT AN ELIGIBLE CANDIDATE FOR PROPHYLACTIC ANTIBIOTIC	C	N	00	9		
G8195	CLINICIAN DOCUMENTED TO HAVE GIVEN THE PROPHYLACTIC ANTIBIOTIC WITHIN ONE HOUR (IF VANCOMYCIN, TWO HOURS) PRIOR TO THE SURGICAL INCISION (OR START OF PROCEDURE WHEN NO INCISION IS REQUIRED)	C	N	00	9		
G8196	CLINICIAN DID NOT DOCUMENT A PROPHYLACTIC ANTIBIOTIC WAS ADMINISTERED WITHIN ONE HOUR (IF VANCOMYCIN, TWO HOURS) PRIOR TO SURGICAL INCISION (OR START OF PROCEDURE WHEN NO INCISION IS REQUIRED)	C	N	00	9		
G8197	PATIENT DOCUMENTED TO HAVE ORDER FOR PROPHYLACTIC ANTIBIOTIC TO BE GIVEN WITHIN ONE HOUR (IF VANCOMYCIN, TWO HOURS) PRIOR TO SURGICAL INCISION (OR START OF PROCEDURE WHEN NO INCISION IS REQUIRED)	C	N	00	9		
G8198	PATIENT DOCUMENTED TO HAVE ORDER FOR CEFAZOLIN OR CEFUROXIME FOR ANTIMICROBIAL PROPHYLAXIS	C	N	00	9		
G8199	CLINICIAN DOCUMENTED TO HAVE GIVEN CEFAZOLIN OR CEFUROXIME FOR ANTIMICROBIAL PROPHYLAXIS	C	N	00	9		
G8200	ORDER FOR CEFAZOLIN OR CEFUROXIME FOR ANTIMICROBIAL PROPHYLAXIS NOT DOCUMENTED	C	N	00	9		
G8201	PATIENT WAS NOT AN ELIGIBLE CANDIDATE FOR CEFAZOLIN OR CEFUROXIME FOR ANTIMICROBIAL PROPHYLAXIS	C	N	00	9		
G8202	CLINICIAN DOCUMENTED AN ORDER WAS GIVEN TO DISCONTINUE PROPHYLACTIC ANTIBIOTICS WITHIN 24 HOURS OF SURGICAL END TIME	C	N	00	9		
G8203	CLINICIAN DOCUMENTED THAT PROPHYLACTIC ANTIBIOTICS WERE DISCONTINUED WITHIN 24 HOURS OF SURGICAL END TIME	C	N	00	9		
G8204	CLINICIAN DID NOT DOCUMENT AN ORDER WAS GIVEN TO DISCONTINUE PROPHYLACTIC ANTIBIOTICS WITHIN 24 HOURS OF SURGICAL END TIME	C	N	00	9		
G8205	CLINICIAN DOCUMENTED THAT PATIENT WAS NOT AN ELIGIBLE CANDIDATE FOR PROPHYLACTIC ANTIBIOTIC DISCONTINUATION WITHIN 24 HOURS OF SURGICAL END TIME	C	N	00	9		
G8206	CLINICIAN DOCUMENTED THAT PROPHYLACTIC ANTIBIOTIC WAS GIVEN	C	N	00	9		

HCPCS Code	Statute	Lab Cert	X-Ref	ASC Pay Grp	ASC Pay Group Eff. Date	Proc Notes	BETOS	TOS	Anest	Code Add Date	Code Effective Date	Code Term Date
G8191							M5D	1	0	20070101	20070701	20070630
G8192							M5D	1	0	20070101	20070701	20070630
G8193							M5D	1	0	20070101	20070101	
G8194							M5D	1	0	20070101	20070701	20070630
G8195							M5D	1	0	20070101	20070701	20070630
G8196							M5D	1	0	20070101	20070101	
G8197							M5D	1	0	20070101	20070701	20070630
G8198							M5D	1	0	20070101	20070701	20070630
G8199							M5D	1	0	20070101	20070701	20070630
G8200							M5D	1	0	20070101	20070101	
G8201							M5D	1	0	20070101	20070701	20070630
G8202							M5D	1	0	20070101	20070701	20070630
G8203							M5D	1	0	20070101	20070701	20070630
G8204							M5D	1	0	20070101	20070101	
G8205							M5D	1	0	20070101	20070701	20070630
G8206							M5D	1	0	20070101	20070701	20070630

HCPCS Code	Long Description	Coverage	Action	PI	MPI	CIM	MCM
G8207	CLINICIAN DOCUMENTED AN ORDER WAS GIVEN TO DISCONTINUE PROPHYLACTIC ANTIBIOTICS WITHIN 48 HOURS OF SURGICAL END TIME	C	N	00	9		
G8208	CLINICIAN DOCUMENTED THAT PROPHYLACTIC ANTIBIOTICS WERE DISCONTINUED WITHIN 48 HOURS OF SURGICAL END TIME	C	N	00	9		
G8209	CLINICIAN DID NOT DOCUMENT AN ORDER WAS GIVEN TO DISCONTINUE PROPHYLACTIC ANTIBIOTICS WITHIN 48 HOURS OF SURGICAL END TIME	C	N	00	9		
G8210	CLINICIAN DOCUMENTED PATIENT WAS NOT AN ELIGIBLE CANDIDATE FOR DISCONTINUATION OF PROPHYLACTIC ANTIBIOTIC DISCONTINUATION WITHIN 48 HOURS OF SURGICAL END TIME	C	N	00	9		
G8211	CLINICIAN DOCUMENTED THAT PROPHYLACTIC ANTIBIOTIC WAS GIVEN	C	N	00	9		
G8212	CLINICIAN DOCUMENTED AN ORDER WAS GIVEN FOR APPROPRIATE VENOUS THROMBOEMBOLISM (VTE) PROPHYLAXIS TO BE GIVEN WITHIN 24 HRS PRIOR TO INCISION TIME OR 24 HOURS AFTER SURGERY END TIME	C	N	00	9		
G8213	CLINICIAN DOCUMENTED TO HAVE GIVEN VTE PROPHYLAXIS WITHIN 24 HRS PRIOR TO INCISION TIME OR 24 HOURS AFTER SURGERY END TIME	C	N	00	9		
G8214	CLINICIAN DID NOT DOCUMENT AN ORDER WAS GIVEN FOR APPROPRIATE VENOUS THROMBOEMBOLISM (VTE) PROPHYLAXIS TO BE GIVEN WITHIN 24 HRS PRIOR TO INCISION TIME OR 24 HOURS AFTER SURGERY END TIME	C	N	00	9		
G8215	CLINICIAN DOCUMENTED THAT PATIENT WAS NOT AN ELIGIBLE CANDIDATE FOR VENOUS THROMBOEMBOLISM (VTE) PROPHYLAXIS TO BE GIVEN WITHIN 24 HOURS PRIOR TO INCISION	C	N	00	9		
G8215	TIME OR 24 HOURS AFTER SURGERY END TIME						
G8216	PATIENT DOCUMENTED TO HAVE RECEIVED DVT PROPHYLAXIS BY END OF HOSPITAL DAY TWO	C	N	00	9		
G8217	PATIENT NOT DOCUMENTED TO HAVE RECEIVED DVT PROPHYLAXIS BY END OF HOSPITAL DAY 2	C	N	00	9		
G8218	PATIENT WAS NOT AN ELIGIBLE CANDIDATE FOR DVT PROPHYLAXIS BY END OF HOSPITAL DAY 2, INCLUDING PHYSICIAN DOCUMENTATION THAT PATIENT IS AMBULATORY	C	N	00	9		
G8219	PATIENT DOCUMENTED TO HAVE RECEIVED DVT PROPHYLAXIS BY END OF HOSPITAL DAY 2	C	N	00	9		
G8220	PATIENT NOT DOCUMENTED TO HAVE RECEIVED DVT PROPHYLAXIS BY END OF HOSPITAL DAY 2	C	N	00	9		
G8221	CLINICIAN DOCUMENTED THAT PATIENT WAS NOT AN ELIGIBLE CANDIDATE FOR DVT PROPHYLAXIS BY THE END OF HOSPITAL DAY 2, INCLUDING PHYSICIAN DOCUMENTATION THAT PATIENT IS AMBULATORY	C	N	00	9		
G8222	PATIENT DOCUMENTED TO HAVE BEEN PRESCRIBED ANTIPLATELET THERAPY AT DISCHARGE	C	N	00	9		
G8223	PATIENT NOT DOCUMENTED TO HAVE RECEIVED PRESCRIPTION FOR ANTIPLATELET THERAPY AT DISCHARGE	C	N	00	9		

HCPCS Code	Statute	Lab Cert	X-Ref	ASC Pay Grp	ASC Pay Group Eff. Date	Proc Notes	BETOS	TOS	Anest	Code Add Date	Code Effective Date	Code Term Date
G8207							M5D	1	0	20070101	20070701	20070630
G8208							M5D	1	0	20070101	20070701	20070630
G8209							M5D	1	0	20070101	20070101	
G8210							M5D	1	0	20070101	20070701	20070630
G8211							M5D	1	0	20070101	20070701	20070630
G8212							M5D	1	0	20070101	20070701	20070630
G8213							M5D	1	0	20070101	20070701	20070630
G8214							M5D	1	0	20070101	20070101	
G8215							M5D	1	0	20070101	20070701	20070630
G8215												
G8216							M5D	1	0	20070101	20070701	20070630
G8217							M5D	1	0	20070101	20070101	
G8218							M5D	1	0	20070101	20070701	20070630
G8219							M5D	1	0	20070101	20070101	
G8220							M5D	1	0	20070101	20070101	
G8221							M5D	1	0	20070101	20070101	
G8222							M5D	1	0	20070101	20070701	20070630
G8223							M5D	1	0	20070101	20070101	

HCPCS Code	Long Description	Coverage	Action	PI	MPI	CIM	MCM
G8224	CLINICIAN DOCUMENTED THAT PATIENT WAS NOT AN ELIGIBLE CANDIDATE FOR ANTIPLATELET THERAPY AT DISCHARGE, INCLUDING IDENTIFICATION FROM MEDICAL RECORD THAT PATIENT IS ON ANTICOAGULATION THERAPY	C	N	00	9		
G8225	PATIENT DOCUMENTED TO HAVE BEEN PRESCRIBED AN ANTICOAGULANT AT DISCHARGE	C	N	00	9		
G8226	PATIENT NOT DOCUMENTED TO HAVE RECEIVED PRESCRIPTION FOR ANTICOAGULANT THERAPY AT DISCHARGE	C	N	00	9		
G8227	PATIENT NOT DOCUMENTED TO HAVE PERMANENT, PERSISTENT, OR PAROXYSMAL ATRIAL FIBRILLATION	C	N	00	9		
G8228	CLINICIAN DOCUMENTED THAT PATIENT WAS NOT AN ELIGIBLE CANDIDATE FOR ANTICOAGULANT THERAPY AT DISCHARGE	C	N	00	9		
G8229	PATIENT DOCUMENTED TO HAVE BEEN ADMINISTERED OR CONSIDERED FOR T-PA	C	N	00	9		
G8230	PATIENT NOT ELIGIBLE FOR T-PA ADMINISTRATION, ISCHEMIC STROKE SYMPTOM ONSET OF MORE THAN 3 HOURS	C	N	00	9		
G8231	PATIENT NOT DOCUMENTED TO HAVE RECEIVED T-PA OR NOT DOCUMENTED TO HAVE BEEN CONSIDERED A CANDIDATE FOR T-PA ADMINISTRATION	C	N	00	9		
G8232	PATIENT DOCUMENTED TO HAVE RECEIVED DYSPHAGIA SCREENING PRIOR TO TAKING ANY FOODS, FLUIDS OR MEDICATION BY MOUTH	C	N	00	9		
G8234	PATIENT NOT DOCUMENTED TO HAVE RECEIVED DYSPHAGIA SCREENING	C	N	00	9		
G8235	PATIENT NOT RECEIVING OR INELIGIBLE TO RECEIVE FOOD, FLUIDS OR MEDICATION BY MOUTH, OR DOCUMENTATION OF NPO (NOTHING BY MOUTH) ORDER	C	N	00	9		
G8236	CLINICIAN DOCUMENTED THAT PATIENT WAS NOT AN ELIGIBLE CANDIDATE FOR DYSPHAGIA SCREENING PRIOR TO TAKING ANY FOODS, FLUIDS OR MEDICATION BY MOUTH	C	N	00	9		
G8237	PATIENT DOCUMENTED TO HAVE RECEIVED ORDER FOR REHABILITATION SERVICES OR DOCUMENTATION OF CONSIDERATION FOR REHABILITATION SERVICES	C	N	00	9		
G8238	PATIENT NOT DOCUMENTED TO HAVE RECEIVED ORDER FOR OR CONSIDERATION FOR REHABILITATION SERVICES	C	N	00	9		
G8239	INTERNAL CAROTID STENOSIS PATIENT BELOW 30%, REFERENCE TO MEASUREMENTS OF DISTAL INTERNAL CAROTID DIAMETER AS THE DENOMINATOR FOR STENOSIS MEASUREMENT NOT NECESSARY	C	N	00	9		
G8240	INTERNAL CAROTID STENOSIS PATIENT IN THE 30-99% RANGE, AND NO DOCUMENTATION OF REFERENCE TO MEASUREMENTS OF DISTAL INTERNAL CAROTID DIAMETER AS THE DENOMINATOR FOR STENOSIS MEASUREMENT	C	N	00	9		
G8241	CLINICIAN DOCUMENTED THAT PATIENT WHOSE FINAL REPORT OF THE CAROTID IMAGING STUDY PERFORMED (NECK MRA, NECK CTA, NECK DUPLEX ULTRASOUND, CAROTID ANGIOGRAM), WITH CHARACTERIZATION OF AN INTERNAL CAROTID STENOSIS IN THE 30-99% RANGE, WAS NOT AN ELIGIBLE CANDIDATE FOR REFERENCE TO MEASUREMENTS OF DISTAL INTERNAL CAROTID DIAMETER AS THE DENOMINATOR FOR STENOSIS MEASUREMENT	C	N	00	9		

HCPCS Code	Statute	Lab Cert	X-Ref	ASC Pay Grp	ASC Pay Group Eff. Date	Proc Notes	BETOS	TOS	Anest	Code Add Date	Code Effective Date	Code Term Date
G8224							M5D	1	0	20070101	20070701	20070630
G8225							M5D	1	0	20070101	20070701	20070630
G8226							M5D	1	0	20070101	20070101	
G8226												
G8227							M5D	1	0	20070101	20070701	20070630
G8228							M5D	1	0	20070101	20070701	20070630
G8229							M5D	1	0	20070101	20070701	20070630
G8230							M5D	1	0	20070101	20070701	20070630
G8231							M5D	1	0	20070101	20070101	
G8232							M5D	1	0	20070101	20070701	20070630
G8234							M5D	1	0	20070101	20070101	
G8235							M5D	1	0	20070101	20070701	20070630
G8236							M5D	1	0	20070101	20070701	20070630
G8237							M5D	1	0	20070101	20070701	20070630
G8238							M5D	1	0	20070101	20070101	
G8239							M5D	1	0	20070101	20070701	20070630
G8240							M5D	1	0	20070101	20070101	
G8241							M5D	1	0	20070101	20070701	20070630

HCPCS Code	Long Description	Coverage	Action	PI	MPI	CIM	MCM
G8242	PATIENT DOCUMENTED TO HAVE RECEIVED CT OR MRI WITH PRESENCE OR ABSENCE OF HEMORRHAGE, MASS LESION & ACUTE INFARCTION DOCUMENTED IN THE FINAL REPORT	C	N	00	9		
G8243	PATIENT NOT DOCUMENTED TO HAVE RECEIVED CT OR MRI AND THE PRESENCE OR ABSENCE OF HEMORRHAGE, MASS LESION AND ACUTE INFARCTION NOT DOCUMENTED IN THE FINAL REPORT	C	N	00	9		
G8245	CLINICIAN DOCUMENTED PRESENCE OR ABSENCE ALARM SYMPTOMS	C	N	00	9		
G8246	PATIENT WAS NOT AN ELIGIBLE CANDIDATE FOR MEDICAL HISTORY REVIEW WITH ASSESSMENT OF NEW OR CHANGING MOLES	C	N	00	9		
G8247	PATIENT WITH ALARM SYMPTOM(S) DOCUMENTED TO HAVE HAD UPPER ENDOSCOPY PERFORMED OR REFERRAL FOR UPPER ENDOSCOPY	C	N	00	9		
G8248	PATIENT WITH AT LEAST ONE ALARM SYMPTOM NOT DOCUMENTED TO HAVE HAD UPPER ENDOSCOPY OR REFERRAL FOR UPPER ENDOSCOPY	C	N	00	9		
G8249	CLINICIAN DOCUMENTED THAT PATIENT WAS NOT AN ELIGIBLE CANDIDATE FOR UPPER ENDOSCOPY	C	N	00	9		
G8250	PATIENT WITH SUSPICION OF BARRETT'S ESOPHAGUS IN ENDOSCOPY REPORT AND DOCUMENTED TO HAVE RECEIVED AN ESOPHAGEAL BIOPSY	C	N	00	9		
G8251	PATIENT NOT DOCUMENTED TO HAVE RECEIVED AN ESOPHAGEAL BIOPSY WHEN SUSPICION OF BARRETT'S ESOPHAGUS IS INDICATED IN THE ENDOSCOPY REPORT	C	N	00	9		
G8252	CLINICIAN DOCUMENTED THAT PATIENT WAS NOT AN ELIGIBLE CANDIDATE FOR ESOPHAGEAL BIOPSY	C	N	00	9		
G8253	PATIENT DOCUMENTED TO HAVE RECEIVED AN ORDER FOR A BARIUM SWALLOW TEST	C	N	00	9		
G8254	PATIENT WITH NO DOCUMENTATION ORDER FOR BARIUM SWALLOW TEST	C	N	00	9		
G8255	CLINICIAN DOCUMENTATION THAT PATIENT WAS AN ELIGIBLE CANDIDATE FOR BARIUM SWALLOW TEST	C	N	00	9		
G8256	CLINICIAN DOCUMENTED RECONCILIATION OF DISCHARGE MEDICATIONS WITH CURRENT MEDICATION LIST IN MEDICAL RECORD	C	N	00	9		
G8257	CLINICIAN HAS NOT DOCUMENTED RECONCILIATION OF DISCHARGE MEDICATIONS WITH CURRENT MEDICATION LIST IN MEDICAL RECORD	C	N	00	9		
G8258	PATIENT WAS NOT AN ELIGIBLE CANDIDATE FOR DISCHARGE MEDICATIONS REVIEW	C	N	00	9		
G8259	PATIENT DOCUMENTED TO HAVE SURROGATE DECISION MAKER OR ADVANCE CARE PLAN IN MEDICAL RECORD	C	N	00	9		
G8260	PATIENT NOT DOCUMENTED TO HAVE SURROGATE DECISION MAKER OR ADVANCE CARE PLAN IN MEDICAL RECORD	C	N	00	9		
G8261	CLINICIAN DOCUMENTED THAT PATIENT WAS NOT AN ELIGIBLE CANDIDATE FOR SURROGATE DECISION MAKER OR ADVANCE CARE PLAN	C	N	00	9		

HCPCS Code	Statute	Lab Cert	X-Ref	ASC Pay Grp	ASC Pay Group Eff. Date	Proc Notes	BETOS	TOS	Anest	Code Add Date	Code Effective Date	Code Term Date
G8242							M5D	1	0	20070101	20070701	20070630
G8243							M5D	1	0	20070101	20070101	
G8245							M5D	1	0	20070101	20070701	20070630
G8246							M5D	1	0	20070101	20070101	
G8247							M5D	1	0	20070101	20070701	20070630
G8248							M5D	1	0	20070101	20070101	
G8249							M5D	1	0	20070101	20070701	20070630
G8250							M5D	1	0	20070101	20070701	20070630
G8251							M5D	1	0	20070101	20070101	
G8252							M5D	1	0	20070101	20070701	20070630
G8253							M5D	1	0	20070101	20070701	20070630
G8254							M5D	1	0	20070101	20070101	
G8255							M5D	1	0	20070101	20070701	20070630
G8256							M5D	1	0	20070101	20070701	20070630
G8257							M5D	1	0	20070101	20070101	
G8258							M5D	1	0	20070101	20070701	20070630
G8259							M5D	1	0	20070101	20070701	20070630
G8260							M5D	1	0	20070101	20070101	
G8261							M5D	1	0	20070101	20070701	20070630

HCPCS Code	Long Description	Coverage	Action	PI	MPI	CIM	MCM
G8262	PATIENT DOCUMENTED TO HAVE BEEN ASSESSED FOR PRESENCE OR ABSENCE OF URINARY INCONTINENCE	C	N	00	9		
G8263	PATIENT NOT DOCUMENTED TO HAVE BEEN ASSESSED FOR PRESENCE OR ABSENCE OF URINARY INCONTINENCE	C	N	00	9		
G8264	CLINICIAN DOCUMENTED THAT PATIENT WAS NOT AN ELIGIBLE CANDIDATE FOR AN ASSESSMENT OF THE PRESENCE OR ABSENCE OF URINARY INCONTINENCE	C	N	00	9		
G8265	PATIENT DOCUMENTED TO HAVE RECEIVED CHARACTERIZATION OF URINARY INCONTINENCE	C	N	00	9		
G8266	PATIENT NOT DOCUMENTED TO HAVE RECEIVED CHARACTERIZATION OF URINARY INCONTINENCE	C	N	00	9		
G8267	PATIENT DOCUMENTED TO HAVE RECEIVED A PLAN OF CARE FOR URINARY INCONTINENCE	C	N	00	9		
G8268	PATIENT NOT DOCUMENTED TO HAVE RECEIVED PLAN OF CARE FOR URINARY INCONTINENCE	C	N	00	9		
G8269	CLINICIAN HAS NOT PROVIDED CARE FOR THE PATIENT FOR THE REQUIRED TIME TO DEVELOP PLAN OF CARE FOR URINARY INCONTINENCE	C	N	00	9		
G8270	PATIENT DOCUMENTED TO HAVE RECEIVED SCREENING FOR FALL RISK (2 OR MORE FALLS IN THE PAST YEAR OR ANY FALL WITH INJURY IN THE PAST YEAR)	C	N	00	9		
G8271	PATIENT WITH NO DOCUMENTATION OF SCREENING FOR FALL RISKS (2 OR MORE FALLS IN THE PAST YEAR OR ANY FALL WITH INJURY IN THE PAST YEAR)	C	N	00	9		
G8272	CLINICIAN DOCUMENTATION THAT PATIENT WAS NOT AN ELIGIBLE CANDIDATE FOR FALL RISK SCREENING	C	N	00	9		
G8273	CLINICIAN HAS NOT PROVIDED CARE FOR THE PATIENT FOR THE REQUIRED TIME TO SCREEN FOR FALL RISK	C	N	00	9		
G8274	CLINICIAN HAS NOT DOCUMENTED PRESENCE OR ABSENCE OF ALARM SYMPTOMS	C	N	00	9		
G8275	PATIENT DOCUMENTED TO HAVE MEDICAL HISTORY TAKEN WHICH INCLUDED ASSESSMENT OF NEW OR CHANGING MOLES	C	N	00	9		
G8276	PATIENT NOT DOCUMENTED TO HAVE RECEIVED MEDICAL HISTORY WITH ASSESSMENT OF NEW OR CHANGING MOLES	C	N	00	9		
G8277	PATIENT WAS NOT AN ELIGIBLE CANDIDATE FOR MEDICAL HISTORY REVIEW WITH ASSESSMENT OF NEW OR CHANGING MOLES	C	N	00	9		
G8278	PATIENT DOCUMENTED TO HAVE RECEIVED COMPLETE PHYSICAL SKIN EXAM	C	N	00	9		
G8279	PATIENT NOT DOCUMENTED TO HAVE RECEIVED A COMPLETE PHYSICAL SKIN EXAM	C	N	00	9		
G8280	PATIENT WAS NOT AN ELIGIBLE CANDIDATE FOR COMPLETE PHYSICAL SKIN EXAM DURING THE REPORTING YEAR	C	N	00	9		
G8281	PATIENT DOCUMENTED TO HAVE RECEIVED COUNSELING TO PERFORM A SELF-EXAMINATION	C	N	00	9		
G8282	PATIENT NOT DOCUMENTED TO HAVE RECEIVED COUNSELING TO PERFORM A SELF-EXAMINATION	C	N	00	9		
G8283	PATIENT WAS NOT AN ELIGIBLE CANDIDATE FOR COUNSELING TO PERFORM SELF-EXAMINATION	C	N	00	9		

HCPCS Code	Statute	Lab Cert	X-Ref	ASC Pay Grp	ASC Pay Group Eff. Date	Proc Notes	BETOS	TOS	Anest	Code Add Date	Code Effective Date	Code Term Date
G8262							M5D	1	0	20070101	20070701	20070630
G8263							M5D	1	0	20070101	20070101	
G8264							M5D	1	0	20070101	20070701	20070630
G8265							M5D	1	0	20070101	20070701	20070630
G8266							M5D	1	0	20070101	20070101	
G8267							M5D	1	0	20070101	20070701	20070630
G8268							M5D	1	0	20070101	20070101	
G8269							M5D	1	0	20070101	20070701	20070630
G8270							M5D	1	0	20070101	20070701	20070630
G8271							M5D	1	0	20070101	20070101	
G8272							M5D	1	0	20070101	20070701	20070630
G8273							M5D	1	0	20070101	20070701	20070630
G8274							M5D	1	0	20070101	20070101	
G8275							M5D	1	0	20070101	20070701	20070630
G8276							M5D	1	0	20070101	20070101	
G8277							M5D	1	0	20070101	20070701	20070630
G8278							M5D	1	0	20070101	20070701	20070630
G8279							M5D	1	0	20070101	20070101	
G8280							M5D	1	0	20070101	20070701	20070630
G8281							M5D	1	0	20070101	20070701	20070630
G8282							M5D	1	0	20070101	20070101	
G8283							M5D	1	0	20070101	20070701	20070630

HCPCS Code	Long Description	Coverage	Action	PI	MPI	CIM	MCM
G8284	PATIENT DOCUMENTED TO HAVE RECEIVED A PRESCRIPTION FOR PHARMACOLOGIC THERAPY FOR OSTEOPOROSIS	C	N	00	9		
G8285	PATIENT NOT DOCUMENTED TO HAVE RECEIVED PHARMACOLOGIC THERAPY	C	N	00	9		
G8286	CLINICIAN DOCUMENTED THAT PATIENT WAS NOT AN ELIGIBLE CANDIDATE FOR PHARMACOLOGIC THERAPY	C	N	00	9		
G8287	CLINICIAN HAS NOT PROVIDED CARE FOR THE PATIENT FOR THE REQUIRED TIME FOR THE PHARMACOLOGIC THERAPY MEASURE	C	N	00	9		
G8288	PATIENT DOCUMENTED TO HAVE RECEIVED CALCIUM AND VITAMIN D OR COUNSELING ON BOTH CALCIUM AND VITAMIN D USE, AND EXERCISE	C	N	00	9		
G8289	PATIENT WITH NO DOCUMENTATION OF CALCIUM AND VITAMIN D USE OR COUNSELING REGARDING BOTH CALCIUM AND VITAMIN D USE, OR EXERCISE	C	N	00	9		
G8290	CLINICIAN DOCUMENTATION THAT PATIENT WAS NOT AN ELIGIBLE CANDIDATE FOR CALCIUM AND VITAMIN D, AND EXERCISE DURING THE REPORTING YEAR	C	N	00	9		
G8291	CLINICIAN HAS NOT PROVIDED CARE FOR THE PATIENT FOR THE REQUIRED TIME FOR THE CALCIUM, VITAMIN D, AND EXERCISE MEASURE	C	N	00	9		
G8292	COPD PATIENT WITH SPIROMETRY RESULTS DOCUMENTED	C	N	00	9		
G8293	COPD PATIENT WITHOUT SPIROMETRY RESULTS DOCUMENTED	C	N	00	9		
G8294	COPD PATIENT WAS NOT ELIGIBLE FOR SPIROMETRY RESULTS	C	N	00	9		
G8295	COPD PATIENT DOCUMENTED TO HAVE RECEIVED INHALED BRONCHODILATOR THERAPY	C	N	00	9		
G8296	COPD PATIENT NOT DOCUMENTED TO HAVE INHALED BRONCHODILATOR THERAPY PRESCRIBED	C	N	00	9		
G8297	COPD PATIENT WAS NOT ELIGIBLE FOR INHALED BRONCHODILATOR THERAPY	C	N	00	9		
G8298	PATIENT DOCUMENTED TO HAVE RECEIVED OPTIC NERVE HEAD EVALUATION	C	N	00	9		
G8299	PATIENT NOT DOCUMENTED TO HAVE RECEIVED OPTIC NERVE HEAD EVALUATION	C	N	00	9		
G8300	CLINICIAN DOCUMENTED THAT PATIENT WAS NOT AN ELIGIBLE CANDIDATE FOR OPTIC NERVE HEAD EVALUATION DURING THE REPORTING YEAR	C	N	00	9		
G8301	CLINICIAN HAS NOT PROVIDED CARE FOR THE PRIMARY OPEN-ANGLE GLAUCOMA PATIENT FOR THE REQUIRED TIME FOR OPTIC NERVE HEAD EVALUATION MEASURE	C	N	00	9		
G8302	PATIENT DOCUMENTED TO HAVE A SPECIFIC TARGET INTRAOCULAR PRESSURE RANGE GOAL	C	N	00	9		
G8303	PATIENT NOT DOCUMENTED TO HAVE A SPECIFIC TARGET INTRAOCULAR PRESSURE RANGE GOAL	C	N	00	9		
G8304	CLINICIAN DOCUMENTED THAT PATIENT WAS NOT AN ELIGIBLE CANDIDATE FOR A SPECIFIC TARGET INTRAOCULAR PRESSURE RANGE GOAL	C	N	00	9		

HCPCS Code	Statute	Lab Cert	X-Ref	ASC Pay Grp	ASC Pay Group Eff. Date	Proc Notes	BETOS	TOS	Anest	Code Add Date	Code Effective Date	Code Term Date
G8284							M5D	1	0	20070101	20070701	20070630
G8285							M5D	1	0	20070101	20070101	
G8286							M5D	1	0	20070101	20070701	20070630
G8287							M5D	1	0	20070101	20070701	20070630
G8288							M5D	1	0	20070101	20070701	20070630
G8289							M5D	1	0	20070101	20070101	
G8290							M5D	1	0	20070101	20070701	20070630
G8291							M5D	1	0	20070101	20070701	20070630
G8292							M5D	1	0	20070101	20070701	20070630
G8293							M5D	1	0	20070101	20070101	
G8294							M5D	1	0	20070101	20070701	20070630
G8295							M5D	1	0	20070101	20070701	20070630
G8296							M5D	1	0	20070101	20070101	
G8297							M5D	1	0	20070101	20070701	20070630
G8298							M5D	1	0	20070101	20070101	
G8299							M5D	1	0	20070101	20070101	
G8300							M5D	1	0	20070101	20070701	20070630
G8301							M5D	1	0	20070101	20070701	20070630
G8302							M5D	1	0	20070101	20070101	
G8303							M5D	1	0	20070101	20070101	
G8304							M5D	1	0	20070101	20070101	

HCPCS Code	Long Description	Coverage	Action	PI	MPI	CIM	MCM
G8305	CLINICIAN HAS NOT PROVIDED CARE FOR THE PRIMARY OPEN-ANGLE GLAUCOMA PATIENT FOR THE REQUIRED TIME FOR TREATMENT RANGE GOAL DOCUMENTATION MEASUREMENT	C	N	00	9		
G8306	PRIMARY OPEN-ANGLE GLAUCOMA PATIENT WITH INTRAOCULAR PRESSURE ABOVE THE TARGET RANGE GOAL DOCUMENTED TO HAVE RECEIVED PLAN OF CARE	C	N	00	9		
G8307	PRIMARY OPEN-ANGLE GLAUCOMA PATIENT WITH INTRAOCULAR PRESSURE AT OR BELOW GOAL, NO PLAN OF CARE NECESSARY	C	N	00	9		
G8308	PRIMARY OPEN-ANGLE GLAUCOMA PATIENT WITH INTRAOCULAR PRESSURE ABOVE THE TARGET RANGE GOAL, AND NOT DOCUMENTED TO HAVE RECEIVED PLAN OF CARE DURING THE REPORTING YEAR	C	N	00	9		
G8309	PATIENT DOCUMENTED TO HAVE BEEN PRESCRIBED/ RECOMMENDED ANTIOXIDANT VITAMIN OR MINERAL SUPPLEMENT	C	N	00	9		
G8310	PATIENT NOT DOCUMENTED TO HAVE BEEN PRESCRIBED/ RECOMMENDED AT LEAST ONE ANTIOXIDANT VITAMIN OR MINERAL SUPPLEMENT DURING THE REPORTING YEAR	C	N	00	9		
G8311	CLINICIAN DOCUMENTATION THAT PATIENT WAS NOT AN ELIGIBLE CANDIDATE FOR ANTIOXIDANT VITAMIN OR MINERAL SUPPLEMENT DURING THE REPORTING YEAR	C	N	00	9		
G8312	CLINICIAN HAS NOT PROVIDED CARE FOR THE AGE-RELATED MACULAR DEGENERATION PATIENT FOR THE REQUIRED TIME FOR ANTIOXIDANT SUPPLEMENT PRESCRIPTION/ RECOMMENDED MEASURE	C	N	00	9		
G8313	PATIENT DOCUMENTED TO HAVE RECEIVED MACULAR EXAM, INCLUDING DOCUMENTATION OF THE PRESENCE OR ABSENCE OF MACULAR THICKENING OR HEMORRHAGE AND THE LEVEL OF MACULAR DEGENERATION SEVERITY	C	N	00	9		
G8314	PATIENT NOT DOCUMENTED TO HAVE RECEIVED MACULAR EXAM WITH DOCUMENTATION OF PRESENCE OR ABSENCE OF MACULAR THICKENING OR HEMORRHAGE AND NO DOCUMENTATION OF LEVEL OF MACULAR DEGENERATION SEVERITY	C	N	00	9		
G8315	CLINICIAN DOCUMENTATION THAT PATIENT WAS NOT AN ELIGIBLE CANDIDATE FOR MACULAR EXAMINATION DURING THE REPORTING YEAR	C	N	00	9		
G8316	CLINICIAN HAS NOT PROVIDED CARE FOR THE AGE-RELATED MACULAR DEGENERATION PATIENT FOR THE REQUIRED TIME FOR MACULAR EXAMINATION MEASUREMENT	C	N	00	9		
G8317	PATIENT DOCUMENTED TO HAVE VISUAL FUNCTIONAL STATUS ASSESSED	C	N	00	9		
G8318	PATIENT DOCUMENTED NOT TO HAVE VISUAL FUNCTIONAL STATUS ASSESSED	C	N	00	9		
G8319	CLINICIAN DOCUMENTED THAT PATIENT WAS NOT AN ELIGIBLE CANDIDATE FOR ASSESSMENT OF VISUAL FUNCTIONAL STATUS	C	N	00	9		

HCPCS Code	Statute	Lab Cert	X-Ref	ASC Pay Grp	ASC Pay Group Eff. Date	Proc Notes	BETOS	TOS	Anest	Code Add Date	Code Effective Date	Code Term Date
G8305							M5D	1	0	20070101	20070101	
G8306							M5D	1	0	20070101	20070101	
G8307							M5D	1	0	20070101	20070101	
G8308							M5D	1	0	20070101	20070101	
G8309							M5D	1	0	20070101	20070701	20070630
G8310							M5D	1	0	20070101	20070101	
G8311							M5D	1	0	20070101	20070701	20070630
G8312							M5D	1	0	20070101	20070701	20070630
G8313							M5D	1	0	20070101	20070701	20070630
G8313 G8314							M5D	1	0	20070101	20070101	
G8315							M5D	1	0	20070101	20070701	20070630
G8316							M5D	1	0	20070101	20070701	20070630
G8317							M5D	1	0	20070101	20070701	20070630
G8318							M5D	1	0	20070101	20070101	
G8319							M5D	1	0	20070101	20070701	20070630

HCPCS Code	Long Description	Coverage	Action	PI	MPI	CIM	MCM
G8320	CLINICIAN HAS NOT PROVIDED CARE FOR THE CATARACT PATIENT FOR THE REQUIRED TIME FOR ASSESSMENT OF VISUAL FUNCTIONAL STATUS MEASUREMENT	C	N	00	9		
G8321	PATIENT DOCUMENTED TO HAVE HAD PRE-SURGICAL AXIAL LENGTH, CORNEAL POWER MEASUREMENT AND METHOD OF INTRAOCULAR LENS POWER CALCULATION	C	N	00	9		
G8322	PATIENT NOT DOCUMENTED TO HAVE HAD PRE-SURGICAL AXIAL LENGTH, CORNEAL POWER MEASUREMENT AND METHOD OF INTRAOCULAR LENS POWER CALCULATION	C	N	00	9		
G8323	CLINICIAN DOCUMENTATION THAT PATIENT WAS NOT AN ELIGIBLE CANDIDATE FOR PRE-SURGICAL AXIAL LENGTH, CORNEAL POWER MEASUREMENT AND METHOD OF INTRAOCULAR LENS POWER CALCULATION	C	N	00	9		
G8324	CLINICIAN HAS NOT PROVIDED CARE FOR THE CATARACT PATIENT FOR THE REQUIRED TIME FOR PRE-SURGICAL MEASUREMENT AND INTRAOCULAR LENS POWER CALCULATION MEASURE	C	N	00	9		
G8325	PATIENT DOCUMENTED TO HAVE RECEIVED FUNDUS EVALUATION WITHIN SIX MONTHS PRIOR TO CATARACT SURGERY	C	N	00	9		
G8326	PATIENT NOT DOCUMENTED TO HAVE RECEIVED FUNDUS EVALUATION WITHIN SIX MONTHS PRIOR TO CATARACT SURGERY	C	N	00	9		
G8327	PATIENT WAS NOT AN ELIGIBLE CANDIDATE FOR PRE-SURGICAL FUNDUS EVALUATION	C	N	00	9		
G8328	CLINICIAN HAS NOT PROVIDED CARE FOR THE CATARACT PATIENT FOR THE REQUIRED TIME FOR FUNDUS EVALUATION MEASUREMENT	C	N	00	9		
G8329	PATIENT DOCUMENTED TO HAVE RECEIVED DILATED MACULAR OR FUNDUS EXAM WITH LEVEL OF SEVERITY OF RETINOPATHY AND THE PRESENCE OR ABSENCE OF MACULAR EDEMA DOCUMENTED	C	N	00	9		
G8330	PATIENT NOT DOCUMENTED TO HAVE RECEIVED DILATED MACULAR OR FUNDUS EXAM WITH LEVEL OF SEVERITY OF RETINOPATHY AND THE PRESENCE OR ABSENCE OF MACULAR EDEMA NOT DOCUMENTED	C	N	00	9		
G8331	CLINICIAN DOCUMENTATION THAT PATIENT WAS NOT AN ELIGIBLE CANDIDATE FOR DILATED MACULAR OR FUNDUS EXAM DURING THE REPORTING YEAR	C	N	00	9		
G8332	CLINICIAN HAS NOT PROVIDED CARE FOR THE DIABETIC RETINOPATHY PATIENT FOR THE REQUIRED TIME FOR MACULAR EDEMA AND RETINOPATHY MEASUREMENT	C	N	00	9		
G8333	PATIENT DOCUMENTED TO HAVE HAD FINDINGS OF MACULAR OR FUNDUS EXAM COMMUNICATED TO THE PHYSICIAN MANAGING THE DIABETES CARE	C	N	00	9		
G8334	DOCUMENTATION OF FINDINGS OF MACULAR OR FUNDUS EXAM NOT COMMUNICATED TO THE PHYSICIAN MANAGING THE PATIENT'S ONGOING DIABETES CARE	C	N	00	9		

HCPCS Code	Statute	Lab Cert	X-Ref	ASC Pay Grp	ASC Pay Group Eff. Date	Proc Notes	BETOS	TOS	Anest	Code Add Date	Code Effective Date	Code Term Date
G8320							M5D	1	0	20070101	20070701	20070630
G8321							M5D	1	0	20070101	20070701	20070630
G8322							M5D	1	0	20070101	20070101	
G8323							M5D	1	0	20070101	20070701	20070630
G8324							M5D	1	0	20070101	20070701	20070630
G8325							M5D	1	0	20070101	20070701	20070630
G8326							M5D	1	0	20070101	20070101	
G8327							M5D	1	0	20070101	20070701	20070630
G8328							M5D	1	0	20070101	20070701	20070630
G8329							M5D	1	0	20070101	20070701	20070630
G8330							M5D	1	0	20070101	20070101	
G8331							M5D	1	0	20070101	20070701	20070630
G8332							M5D	1	0	20070101	20070701	20070630
G8333							M5D	1	0	20070101	20070701	20070630
G8334							M5D	1	0	20070101	20070101	

HCPCS Code	Long Description	Coverage	Action	PI	MPI	CIM	MCM
G8335	CLINICIAN DOCUMENTATION THAT PATIENT WAS NOT AN ELIGIBLE CANDIDATE FOR THE FINDINGS OF THEIR MACULAR OR FUNDUS EXAM BEING COMMUNICATED TO THE PHYSICIAN MANAGING THEIR DIABETES CARE DURING THE REPORTING YEAR	C	N	00	9		
G8336	CLINICIAN HAS NOT PROVIDED CARE FOR THE DIABETIC RETINOPATHY PATIENT FOR THE REQUIRED TIME FOR PHYSICIAN COMMUNICATION MEASUREMENT	C	N	00	9		
G8337	CLINICIAN DOCUMENTED THAT COMMUNICATION WAS SENT TO THE PHYSICIAN MANAGING ONGOING CARE OF PATIENT THAT A FRACTURE OCCURRED AND THAT THE PATIENT WAS OR SHOULD BE TESTED OR TREATED FOR OSTEOPOROSIS	C	N	00	9		
G8338	CLINICIAN HAS NOT DOCUMENTED THAT COMMUNICATION WAS SENT TO THE PHYSICIAN MANAGING ONGOING CARE OF PATIENT THAT A FRACTURE OCCURRED AND THAT THE PATIENT WAS OR SHOULD BE TESTED OR TREATED FOR OSTEOPOROSIS	C	N	00	9		
G8339	PATIENT WAS NOT AN ELIGIBLE CANDIDATE FOR COMMUNICATION WITH THE PHYSICIAN MANAGING THE PATIENT'S ONGOING CARE THAT A FRACTURE OCCURRED & THAT THE PATIENT WAS OR SHOULD BE TESTED OR TREATED FOR OSTEOPOROSIS	C	N	00	9		
G8340	PATIENT DOCUMENTED TO HAVE HAD CENTRAL DEXA PERFORMED AND RESULTS DOCUMENTED OR CENTRAL DEXA ORDERED OR PHARMACOLOGIC THERAPY PRESCRIBED	C	N	00	9		
G8341	PATIENT NOT DOCUMENTED TO HAVE HAD CENTRAL DEXA MEASUREMENT OR PHARMACOLOGIC THERAPY	C	N	00	9		
G8342	CLINICIAN DOCUMENTED THAT PATIENT WAS NOT AN ELIGIBLE CANDIDATE FOR CENTRAL DEXA MEASUREMENT OR PRESCRIBING PHARMACOLOGIC	C	N	00	9		
G8343	CLINICIAN HAS NOT PROVIDED CARE FOR THE PATIENT FOR THE REQUIRED TIME FOR CENTRAL DEXA MEASUREMENT OR PHARMACOLOGICAL THERAPY MEASURE	C	N	00	9		
G8344	PATIENT DOCUMENTED TO HAVE HAD CENTRAL DEXA ORDERED OR PERFORMED AND RESULTS DOCUMENTED OR PHARMACOLOGICAL THERAPY PRESCRIBED	C	N	00	9		
G8345	PATIENT NOT DOCUMENTED TO HAVE HAD CENTRAL DEXA MEASUREMENT ORDERED OR PERFORMED OR PHARMACOLOGIC THERAPY	C	N	00	9		
G8346	CLINICIAN DOCUMENTED THAT PATIENT WAS NOT AN ELIGIBLE CANDIDATE FOR CENTRAL DEXA MEASUREMENT OR PHARMACOLOGIC THERAPY	C	N	00	9		
G8347	CLINICIAN HAS NOT PROVIDED CARE FOR THE PATIENT FOR THE REQUIRED TIME FOR CENTRAL DEXA MEASUREMENT OR PHARMACOLOGICAL THERAPY MEASURE	C	N	00	9		
G8348	INTERNAL CAROTID STENOSIS PATIENT IN THE 30-99% RANGE DOCUMENTED TO HAVE REFERENCE TO MEASUREMENTS OF DISTAL INTERNAL CAROTID DIAMETER AS THE DENOMINATOR FOR STENOSIS MEASUREMENT	C	N	00	9		

HCPCS Code	Statute	Lab Cert	X-Ref	ASC Pay Grp	ASC Pay Group Eff. Date	Proc Notes	BETOS	TOS	Anest	Code Add Date	Code Effective Date	Code Term Date
G8335							M5D	1	0	20070101	20070701	20070630
G8336							M5D	1	0	20070101	20070701	20070630
G8337							M5D	1	0	20070101	20070701	20070630
G8338							M5D	1	0	20070101	20070101	
G8339							M5D	1	0	20070101	20070701	20070630
G8340							M5D	1	0	20070101	20070701	20070630
G8341							M5D	1	0	20070101	20070101	
G8342							M5D	1	0	20070101	20070701	20070630
G8343							M5D	1	0	20070101	20070701	20070630
G8344							M5D	1	0	20070101	20070701	20070630
G8345							M5D	1	0	20070101	20070101	
G8346							M5D	1	0	20070101	20070701	20070630
G8347							M5D	1	0	20070101	20070701	20070630
G8348							M5D	1	0	20070101	20070701	20070630

HCPCS Code	Long Description	Coverage	Action	PI	MPI	CIM	MCM
G8349	PATIENT WAS NOT AN ELIGIBLE CANDIDATE FOR DOCUMENTATION OF PRESENCE OR ABSENCE OF ALARM SYMPTOMS	C	N	00	9		
G8350	PATIENT DOCUMENTED TO HAVE HAD 12-LEAD ECG PERFORMED	C	N	00	9		
G8351	PATIENT NOT DOCUMENTED TO HAVE HAD ECG	C	N	00	9		
G8352	CLINICIAN DOCUMENTED THAT PATIENT WAS NOT AN ELIGIBLE CANDIDATE FOR ECG	C	N	00	9		
G8353	PATIENT DOCUMENTED TO HAVE RECEIVED OR TAKEN ASPIRIN 24 HOURS BEFORE EMERGENCY DEPARTMENT ARRIVAL OR DURING EMERGENCY DEPARTMENT STAY	C	N	00	9		
G8354	PATIENT NOT DOCUMENTED TO HAVE RECEIVED OR TAKEN ASPIRIN 24 HOURS BEFORE EMERGENCY DEPARTMENT ARRIVAL OR DURING EMERGENCY DEPARTMENT STAY	C	N	00	9		
G8355	CLINICIAN DOCUMENTED THAT PATIENT WAS NOT AN ELIGIBLE CANDIDATE TO RECEIVE ASPIRIN	C	N	00	9		
G8356	PATIENT DOCUMENTED TO HAVE HAD ECG PERFORMED	C	N	00	9		
G8357	PATIENT NOT DOCUMENTED TO HAVE HAD ECG	C	N	00	9		
G8358	CLINICIAN DOCUMENTED THAT PATIENT WAS NOT AN ELIGIBLE CANDIDATE FOR ECG	C	N	00	9		
G8359	PATIENT DOCUMENTED TO HAVE HAD VITAL SIGNS RECORDED AND REVIEWED	C	N	00	9		
G8360	PATIENT NOT DOCUMENTED TO HAVE VITAL SIGNS RECORDED AND REVIEWED	C	N	00	9		
G8361	PATIENT DOCUMENTED TO HAVE OXYGEN SATURATION ASSESSED	C	N	00	9		
G8362	PATIENT NOT DOCUMENTED TO HAVE OXYGEN SATURATION ASSESSED	C	N	00	9		
G8363	CLINICIAN DOCUMENTED THAT PATIENT WAS NOT AN ELIGIBLE CANDIDATE FOR OXYGEN SATURATION ASSESSMENT	C	N	00	9		
G8364	PATIENT DOCUMENTED TO HAVE MENTAL STATUS ASSESSED	C	N	00	9		
G8365	PATIENT NOT DOCUMENTED TO HAVE MENTAL STATUS ASSESSED	C	N	00	9		
G8366	PATIENT DOCUMENTED TO HAVE APPROPRIATE EMPIRIC ANTIBIOTIC PRESCRIBED	C	N	00	9		
G8367	PATIENT NOT DOCUMENTED TO HAVE APPROPRIATE EMPIRIC ANTIBIOTIC PRESCRIBED	C	N	00	9		
G8368	CLINICIAN DOCUMENTED THAT PATIENT WAS NOT AN ELIGIBLE CANDIDATE FOR APPROPRIATE EMPIRIC ANTIBIOTIC	C	N	00	9		
G8370	ASTHMA PATIENTS WITH NUMERIC FREQUENCY OF SYMPTOMS OR PATIENT COMPLETION OF AN ASTHMA ASSESSMENT TOOL/SURVEY/QUESTIONNAIRE NOT DOCUMENTED	C	N	00	9		
G8371	CHEMOTHERAPY DOCUMENTED AS NOT RECEIVED OR PRESCRIBED FOR STAGE III COLON CANCER PATIENTS	C	N	00	9		
G8372	CHEMOTHERAPY DOCUMENTED AS RECEIVED OR PRESCRIBED FOR STAGE III COLON CANCER PATIENTS	C	N	00	9		
G8373	CHEMOTHERAPY PLAN DOCUMENTED PRIOR TO CHEMOTHERAPY ADMINISTRATION	C	N	00	9		
G8374	CHEMOTHERAPY PLAN NOT DOCUMENTED PRIOR TO CHEMOTHERAPY ADMINISTRATION	C	N	00	9		

HCPCS Code	Statute	Lab Cert	X-Ref	ASC Pay Grp	ASC Pay Group Eff. Date	Proc Notes	BETOS	TOS	Anest	Code Add Date	Code Effective Date	Code Term Date
G8349							M5D	1	0	20070101	20070701	20070630
G8350							M5D	1	0	20070101	20070701	20070630
G8351							M5D	1	0	20070101	20070101	
G8352							M5D	1	0	20070101	20070701	20070630
G8353							M5D	1	0	20070101	20070701	20070630
G8354							M5D	1	0	20070101	20070101	
G8355							M5D	1	0	20070101	20070701	20070630
G8356							M5D	1	0	20070101	20070701	20070630
G8357							M5D	1	0	20070101	20070101	
G8358							M5D	1	0	20070101	20070701	20070630
G8359							M5D	1	0	20070101	20070701	20070630
G8360							M5D	1	0	20070101	20070101	
G8361							M5D	1	0	20070101	20070701	20070630
G8362							M5D	1	0	20070101	20070101	
G8363							M5D	1	0	20070101	20070701	20070630
G8364							M5D	1	0	20070101	20070701	20070630
G8365							M5D	1	0	20070101	20070101	
G8366							M5D	1	0	20070101	20070701	20070630
G8367							M5D	1	0	20070101	20070101	
G8368							M5D	1	0	20070101	20070701	20070630
G8370							M5D	1	0	20070701	20070701	
G8371							M5D	1	0	20070701	20070701	
G8372							M5D	1	0	20070701	20070701	
G8373							M5D	1	0	20070701	20070701	
G8374							M5D	1	0	20070701	20070701	

HCPCS Code	Long Description	Coverage	Action	PI	MPI	CIM	MCM
G8375	CHRONIC LYMPHOCYTIC LEUKEMIA (CLL) PATIENT WITH NO DOCUMENTATION OF BASELINE FLOW CYTOMETRY PERFORMED	C	N	00	9		
G8376	CLINICIAN DOCUMENTATION THAT BREAST CANCER PATIENT WAS NOT ELIGIBLE FOR TAMOXIFEN OR AROMATASE INHIBITOR THERAPY MEASURE	C	N	00	9		
G8377	CLINICIAN DOCUMENTATION THAT COLON CANCER PATIENT IS NOT ELIGIBLE FOR CHEMOTHERAPY MEASURE	C	N	00	9		
G8378	CLINICIAN DOCUMENTATION THAT PATIENT WAS NOT AN ELIGIBLE CANDIDATE FOR RADIATION THERAPY MEASURE	C	N	00	9		
G8379	DOCUMENTATION OF RADIATION THERAPY RECOMMENDED WITHIN 12 MONTHS OF FIRST OFFICE VISIT	C	N	00	9		
G8380	FOR PATIENTS WITH ER OR PR POSITIVE, STAGE IC-III BREAST CANCER, CLINICIAN DID NOT DOCUMENT THAT THE PATIENT RECEIVED OR WAS PRESCRIBED TAMOXIFEN OR AROMATASE INHIBITOR	C	N	00	9		
G8381	FOR PATIENTS WITH ER OR PR POSITIVE, STAGE IC-III BREAST CANCER, CLINICIAN DOCUMENTED OR PRESCRIBED THAT THE PATIENT IS RECEIVING TAMOXIFEN OR AROMATASE INHIBITOR	C	N	00	9		
G8382	MULTIPLE MYELOMA PATIENTS WITH NO DOCUMENTATION OF PRESCRIBED OR RECEIVED INTRAVENOUS BISPHOSPHONATE THERAPY	C	N	00	9		
G8383	NO DOCUMENTATION OF RADIATION THERAPY RECOMMENDED WITHIN 12 MONTHS OF FIRST OFFICE VISIT	C	N	00	9		
G8384	BASELINE CYTOGENETIC TESTING NOT PERFORMED IN PATIENTS WITH MYELODYSPLASTIC SYNDROME (MDS) OR ACUTE LEUKEMIAS	C	N	00	9		
G8385	DIABETIC PATIENTS WITH NO DOCUMENTATION OF HEMOGLOBIN A1C LEVEL (WITHIN THE LAST 12 MONTHS)	C	N	00	9		
G8386	DIABETIC PATIENTS WITH NO DOCUMENTATION OF LOW-DENSITY LIPOPROTEIN (WITHIN THE LAST 12 MONTHS)	C	N	00	9		
G8387	END-STAGE RENAL DISEASE PATIENT WITH A HEMATOCRIT OR HEMOGLOBIN NOT DOCUMENTED	C	N	00	9		
G8388	END-STAGE RENAL DISEASE PATIENT WITH URR OR KT/V VALUE NOT DOCUMENTED, BUT OTHERWISE ELIGIBLE FOR MEASURE	C	N	00	9		
G8389	MYELODYSPLASTIC SYNDROME (MDS) PATIENTS WITH NO DOCUMENTATION OF IRON STORES PRIOR TO RECEIVING ERYTHROPOIETIN THERAPY	C	N	00	9		
G8390	DIABETIC PATIENTS WITH NO DOCUMENTATION OF BLOOD PRESSURE MEASUREMENT (WITHIN THE LAST 12 MONTHS)	C	N	00	9		
G8391	PATIENTS WITH PERSISTENT ASTHMA, NO DOCUMENTATION OF PREFERRED LONG TERM CONTROL MEDICATION OR ACCEPTABLE ALTERNATIVE TREATMENT PRESCRIBED	C	N	00	9		
G8395	LEFT VENTRICULAR EJECTION FRACTION (LVEF) >= 40% OR DOCUMENTATION AS NORMAL OR MILDLY DEPRESSED LEFT VENTRICULAR SYSTOLIC FUNCTION	C	N	00	9		

HCPCS Code	Statute	Lab Cert	X-Ref	ASC Pay Grp	ASC Pay Group Eff. Date	Proc Notes	BETOS	TOS	Anest	Code Add Date	Code Effective Date	Code Term Date
G8375							M5D	1	0	20070701	20070701	
G8376							M5D	1	0	20070701	20070701	
G8377							M5D	1	0	20070701	20070701	
G8378							M5D	1	0	20070701	20070701	
G8379							M5D	1	0	20070701	20070701	
G8380							M5D	1	0	20070701	20070701	
G8381							M5D	1	0	20070701	20070701	
G8382							M5D	1	0	20070701	20070701	
G8383							M5D	1	0	20070701	20070701	
G8384							M5D	1	0	20070701	20070701	
G8385							M5D	1	0	20070701	20070701	
G8386							M5D	1	0	20070701	20070701	
G8387							M5D	1	0	20070701	20070701	
G8388							M5D	1	0	20070701	20070701	
G8389							M5D	1	0	20070701	20070701	
G8390							M5D	1	0	20070701	20070701	
G8391							M5D	1	0	20070701	20070701	
G8395							M5D	1	0	20080101	20080101	

HCPCS Code	Long Description	Coverage	Action	PI	MPI	CIM	MCM
G8396	LEFT VENTRICULAR EJECTION FRACTION (LVEF) NOT PERFORMED OR DOCUMENTED	C	N	00	9		
G8397	DILATED MACULAR OR FUNDUS EXAM PERFORMED, INCLUDING DOCUMENTATION OF THE PRESENCE OR ABSENCE OF MACULAR EDEMA AND LEVEL OF SEVERITY OF RETINOPATHY	C	N	00	9		
G8398	DILATED MACULAR OR FUNDUS EXAM NOT PERFORMED	C	N	00	9		
G8399	PATIENT WITH CENTRAL DUAL-ENERGY X-RAY ABSORPTIOMETRY (DXA) RESULTS DOCUMENTED OR ORDERED OR PHARMACOLOGIC THERAPY (OTHER THAN MINERALS/VITAMINS) FOR OSTEOPOROSIS PRESCRIBED)	C	N	00	9		
G8400	PATIENT WITH CENTRAL DUAL-ENERGY X-RAY ABSORPTIOMETRY (DXA) RESULTS NOT DOCUMENTED OR NOT ORDERED OR PHARMACOLOGIC THERAPY (OTHER THAN MINERALS/VITAMINS) FOR OSTEOPOROSIS NOT PRESCRIBED	C	N	00	9		
G8401	CLINICIAN DOCUMENTED THAT PATIENT WAS NOT AN ELIGIBLE CANDIDATE FOR SCREENING OR THERAPY FOR OSTEOPOROSIS FOR WOMEN MEASURE	C	N	00	9		
G8402	TOBACCO (SMOKE) USE CESSATION INTERVENTION, COUNSELING	C	N	00	9		
G8403	TOBACCO (SMOKE) USE CESSATION INTERVENTION NOT COUNSELED	C	N	00	9		
G8404	LOWER EXTREMITY NEUROLOGICAL EXAM PERFORMED AND DOCUMENTED	C	N	00	9		
G8405	LOWER EXTREMITY NEUROLOGICAL EXAM NOT PERFORMED	C	N	00	9		
G8406	CLINICIAN DOCUMENTED THAT PATIENT WAS NOT AN ELIGIBLE CANDIDATE FOR LOWER EXTREMITY NEUROLOGICAL EXAM MEASURE	C	N	00	9		
G8407	ABI MEASURED AND DOCUMENTED	C	N	00	9		
G8408	ABI MEASUREMENT WAS NOT OBTAINED	C	N	00	9		
G8409	CLINICIAN DOCUMENTED THAT PATIENT WAS NOT AN ELIGIBLE CANDIDATE FOR ABI MEASUREMENT MEASURE	C	N	00	9		
G8410	FOOTWEAR EVALUATION PERFORMED AND DOCUMENTED	C	N	00	9		
G8415	FOOTWEAR EVALUATION WAS NOT PERFORMED	C	N	00	9		
G8416	CLINICIAN DOCUMENTED THAT PATIENT WAS NOT AN ELIGIBLE CANDIDATE FOR FOOTWEAR EVALUATION MEASURE	C	N	00	9		
G8417	CALCULATED BMI ABOVE THE UPPER PARAMETER AND A FOLLOW-UP PLAN WAS DOCUMENTED IN THE MEDICAL RECORD	C	N	00	9		
G8418	CALCULATED BMI BELOW THE LOWER PARAMETER AND A FOLLOW-UP PLAN WAS DOCUMENTED IN THE MEDICAL RECORD	C	N	00	9		
G8419	CALCULATED BMI OUTSIDE NORMAL PARAMETERS, NO FOLLOW-UP PLAN WAS DOCUMENTED IN THE MEDICAL RECORD	C	N	00	9		
G8420	CALCULATED BMI WITHIN NORMAL PARAMETERS & DOCUMENTED	C	N	00	9		
G8421	BMI NOT CALCULATED	C	N	00	9		
G8422	PATIENT NOT ELIGIBLE FOR BMI CALCULATION	C	N	00	9		
G8423	DOCUMENTED THAT PATIENT WAS SCREENED AND EITHER INFLUENZA VACCINATION STATUS IS CURRENT OR PATIENT WAS COUNSELED	C	N	00	9		

HCPCS Code	Statute	Lab Cert	X-Ref	ASC Pay Grp	ASC Pay Group Eff. Date	Proc Notes	BETOS	TOS	Anest	Code Add Date	Code Effective Date	Code Term Date
G8396							M5D	1	0	20080101	20080101	
G8397							M5D	1	0	20080101	20080101	
G8398							M5D	1	0	20080101	20080101	
G8399							M5D	1	0	20080101	20080101	
G8400							M5D	1	0	20080101	20080101	
G8401							M5D	1	0	20080101	20080101	
G8402							M5D	1	0	20080101	20080101	
G8403							M5D	1	0	20080101	20080101	
G8404							M5D	1	0	20080101	20080101	
G8405							M5D	1	0	20080101	20080101	
G8406							M5D	1	0	20080101	20080101	
G8407							M5D	1	0	20080101	20080101	
G8408							M5D	1	0	20080101	20080101	
G8409							M5D	1	0	20080101	20080101	
G8410							M5D	1	0	20080101	20080101	
G8415							M5D	1	0	20080101	20080101	
G8416							M5D	1	0	20080101	20080101	
G8417							M5D	1	0	20080101	20090101	
G8418							M5D	1	0	20080101	20090101	
G8419							M5D	1	0	20080101	20090101	
G8420							M5D	1	0	20080101	20090101	
G8421							M5D	1	0	20080101	20080101	
G8422							M5D	1	0	20080101	20080101	
G8423							M5D	1	0	20080101	20080101	

HCPCS Code	Long Description	Coverage	Action	PI	MPI	CIM	MCM
G8424	INFLUENZA VACCINE STATUS WAS NOT SCREENED	C	N	00	9		
G8425	INFLUENZA VACCINE STATUS SCREENED, PATIENT NOT CURRENT AND COUNSELING WAS NOT PROVIDED	C	N	00	9		
G8426	DOCUMENTED THAT PATIENT WAS NOT APPROPRIATE FOR SCREENING AND/OR COUNSELING ABOUT THE INFLUENZA VACCINE (E.G., ALLERGY TO EGGS)	C	N	00	9		
G8427	LIST OF CURRENT MEDICATIONS WITH DOSAGES (INCLUDES PRESCRIPTION, OVER-THE-COUNTER, HERBALS, VITAMIN/MINERAL/DIETARY [NUTRITIONAL] SUPPLEMENTS) AND VERIFICATION WITH THE PATIENT OR AUTHORIZED REPRESENTATIVE DOCUMENTED BY THE PROVIDER	C	N	00	9		
G8428	PROVIDER DOCUMENTATION OF CURRENT MEDICATIONS WITH DOSAGES (INCLUDES PRESCRIPTION, OVER-THE-COUNTER, HERBALS, VITAMIN/MINERAL/DIETARY [NUTRITIONAL] SUPPLEMENTS) WITHOUT DOCUMENTED PATIENT VERIFICATION	C	N	00	9		
G8429	INCOMPLETE OR NO PROVIDER DOCUMENTATION THAT PATIENT'S CURRENT MEDICATIONS WITH DOSAGES (INCLUDES PRESCRIPTION, OVER-THE-COUNTER, HERBALS, VITAMIN/MINERAL/DIETARY [NUTRITIONAL] SUPPLEMENTS) WERE ASSESSED	C	N	00	9		
G8430	PROVIDER DOCUMENTATION THAT PATIENT IS NOT ELIGIBLE FOR MEDICATION ASSESSMENT	C	N	00	9		
G8431	POSITIVE SCREEN FOR CLINICAL DEPRESSION USING A STANDARDIZED TOOL & A FOLLOW-UP PLAN DOCUMENTED	C	N	00	9		
G8432	NO DOCUMENTATION OF CLINICAL DEPRESSION SCREENING USING A STANDARDIZED TOOL	C	N	00	9		
G8433	SCREENING FOR CLINICAL DEPRESSION USING A STANDARDIZED TOOL NOT DOCUMENTED, PATIENT NOT ELIGIBLE/APPROPRIATE	C	N	00	9		
G8434	DOCUMENTATION OF COGNITIVE IMPAIRMENT SCREENING USING A STANDARDIZED TOOL	C	N	00	9		
G8435	NO DOCUMENTATION OF COGNITIVE IMPAIRMENT SCREENING USING A STANDARDIZED TOOL	C	N	00	9		
G8436	PATIENT NOT ELIGIBLE/NOT APPROPRIATE FOR COGNITIVE IMPAIRMENT SCREENING	C	N	00	9		
G8437	DOCUMENTATION OF CLINICIAN AND PATIENT INVOLVEMENT WITH THE DEVELOPMENT OF A PLAN OF CARE INCLUDING SIGNATURE BY THE PRACTITIONER/THERAPIST AND EITHER A CO-SIGNATURE BY THE PATIENT OR DOCUMENTED VERBAL AGREEMENT OBTAINED FROM THE PATIENT OR, WHEN NECESSARY, AN AUTHORIZED REPRESENTATIVE	C	N	00	9		
G8438	NO DOCUMENTATION OF CLINICIAN AND PATIENT INVOLVEMENT WITH THE DEVELOPMENT OF A PLAN OF CARE INCLUDING SIGNATURE BY THE PRACTITIONER/THERAPIST AND EITHER A CO-SIGNATURE BY THE PATIENT OR DOCUMENTED VERBAL AGREEMENT OBTAINED FROM THE PATIENT OR, WHEN NECESSARY, AN AUTHORIZED REPRESENTATIVE	C	N	00	9		

HCPCS Code	Statute	Lab Cert	X-Ref	ASC Pay Grp	ASC Pay Group Eff. Date	Proc Notes	BETOS	TOS	Anest	Code Add Date	Code Effective Date	Code Term Date
G8424							M5D	1	0	20080101	20080101	
G8425							M5D	1	0	20080101	20080101	
G8426							M5D	1	0	20080101	20080101	
G8427							M5D	1	0	20080101	20090101	
G8428							M5D	1	0	20080101	20090101	
G8429							M5D	1	0	20080101	20090101	
G8430							M5D	1	0	20080101	20090101	
G8431							M5D	1	0	20080101	20090101	
G8432							M5D	1	0	20080101	20080101	
G8433							M5D	1	0	20080101	20090101	
G8434							M5D	1	0	20080101	20080101	
G8435							M5D	1	0	20080101	20080101	
G8436							M5D	1	0	20080101	20080101	
G8437							M5D	1	0	20080101	20090101	
G8438							M5D	1	0	20080101	20090101	

HCPCS Code	Long Description	Coverage	Action	PI	MPI	CIM	MCM
G8439	DOCUMENTATION THAT PATIENT IS NOT ELIGIBLE FOR CO-DEVELOPING A PLAN OF CARE INCLUDING SIGNATURE BY THE PRACTITIONER/THERAPIST AND EITHER A CO-SIGNATURE BY THE PATIENT OR DOCUMENTED VERBAL AGREEMENT OBTAINED FROM THE PATIENT OR, WHEN NECESSARY, AN AUTHORIZED REPRESENTATIVE	C	N	00	9		
G8440	DOCUMENTATION OF PAIN ASSESSMENT (INCLUDING LOCATION, INTENSITY AND DESCRIPTION) PRIOR TO INITIATION OF TREATMENT OR DOCUMENTATION OF THE ABSENCE OF PAIN AS A RESULT OF ASSESSMENT THROUGH DISCUSSION WITH THE PATIENT INCLUDING THE USE OF A STANDARDIZED TOOL & A FOLLOW-UP PLAN IS DOCUMENTED	C	N	00	9		
G8441	NO DOCUMENTATION OF PAIN ASSESSMENT (INCLUDING LOCATION, INTENSITY AND DESCRIPTION) PRIOR TO INITIATION OF TREATMENT	C	N	00	9		
G8442	DOCUMENTATION THAT PATIENT IS NOT ELIGIBLE FOR PAIN ASSESSMENT	C	N	00	9		
G8443	ALL PRESCRIPTIONS CREATED DURING THE ENCOUNTER WERE GENERATED USING A QUALIFIED E-PRESCRIBING SYSTEM	C	N	00	9		
G8445	NO PRESCRIPTIONS WERE GENERATED DURING THE ENCOUNTER, PROVIDER DOES HAVE ACCESS TO A QUALIFIED E-PRESCRIBING SYSTEM	C	N	00	9		
G8446	PROVIDER DOES HAVE ACCESS TO A QUALIFIED E-PRESCRIBING SYSTEM AND SOME OR ALL OF THE PRESCRIPTIONS GENERATED DURING THE ENCOUNTER WERE PRINTED OR PHONED IN AS REQUIRED BY STATE OR FEDERAL LAW OR REGULATIONS, PATIENT REQUEST OR PHARMACY SYSTEM BEING UNABLE TO RECEIVE ELECTRONIC TRANSMISSION; OR BECAUSE THEY WERE FOR NARCOTICS OR OTHER CONTROLLED SUBSTANCES	C	N	00	9		
G8447	PATIENT ENCOUNTER WAS DOCUMENTED USING A CCHIT CERTIFIED EHR	C	N	00	9		
G8448	PATIENT ENCOUNTER WAS DOCUMENTED USING A QUALIFIED (NON-CCHIT CERTIFIED) EHR	C	N	00	9		
G8449	PATIENT ENCOUNTER WAS NOT DOCUMENTED USING AN EMR DUE TO SYSTEM REASONS SUCH AS, THE SYSTEM BEING INOPERABLE AT THE TIME OF THE VISIT; USE OF THIS CODE IMPLIES THAT AN EMR IS IN PLACE AND GENERALLY AVAILABLE	C	N	00	9		
G8450	BETA-BLOCKER THERAPY PRESCRIBED FOR PATIENTS WITH LEFT VENTRICULAR EJECTION FRACTION (LVEF) <40% OR DOCUMENTATION AS MODERATELY OR SEVERELY DEPRESSED LEFT VENTRICULAR SYSTOLIC FUNCTION	C	N	00	9		
G8451	CLINICIAN DOCUMENTED PATIENT WITH LEFT VENTRICULAR EJECTION FRACTION (LVEF) <40% OR DOCUMENTATION AS MODERATELY OR SEVERELY DEPRESSED LEFT VENTRICULAR SYSTOLIC FUNCTION WAS NOT ELIGIBLE CANDIDATE FOR BETA-BLOCKER THERAPY	C	N	00	9		

G Codes

HCPCS Code	Statute	Lab Cert	X-Ref	ASC Pay Grp	ASC Pay Group Eff. Date	Proc Notes	BETOS	TOS	Anest	Code Add Date	Code Effective Date	Code Term Date
G8439							M5D	1	0	20080101	20090101	
G8440							M5D	1	0	20080101	20090101	
G8441							M5D	1	0	20080101	20080101	
G8442							M5D	1	0	20080101	20080101	
G8443							M5D	1	0	20080101	20080101	
G8445							M5D	1	0	20080101	20080101	
G8446							M5D	1	0	20080101	20090101	
G8447							M5D	1	0	20080101	20090101	
G8448							M5D	1	0	20080101	20090101	
G8449							M5D	1	0	20080101	20080101	
G8450							M5D	1	0	20080101	20080101	
G8451							M5D	1	0	20080101	20080101	

HCPCS Code	Long Description	Coverage	Action	PI	MPI	CIM	MCM
G8452	BETA-BLOCKER THERAPY NOT PRESCRIBED FOR PATIENTS WITH LEFT VENTRICULAR EJECTION FRACTION (LVEF) <40% OR DOCUMENTATION AS MODERATELY OR SEVERELY DEPRESSED LEFT VENTRICULAR SYSTOLIC FUNCTION	C	N	00	9		
G8453	TOBACCO USE CESSATION INTERVENTION, COUNSELING	C	N	00	9		
G8454	TOBACCO USE CESSATION INTERVENTION NOT COUNSELED, REASON NOT SPECIFIED	C	N	00	9		
G8455	CURRENT TOBACCO SMOKER	C	N	00	9		
G8456	CURRENT SMOKELESS TOBACCO USER	C	S	00	9		
G8457	CURRENT TOBACCO NON-USER	C	N	00	9		
G8458	CLINICIAN DOCUMENTED THAT PATIENT IS NOT AN ELIGIBLE CANDIDATE FOR GENOTYPE TESTING; PATIENT NOT RECEIVING ANTIVIRAL TREATMENT FOR HEPATITIS C	C	N	00	9		
G8459	CLINICIAN DOCUMENTED THAT PATIENT IS RECEIVING ANTIVIRAL TREATMENT FOR HEPATITIS C	C	N	00	9		
G8460	CLINICIAN DOCUMENTED THAT PATIENT IS NOT AN ELIGIBLE CANDIDATE FOR QUANTITATIVE RNA TESTING AT WEEK 12; PATIENT NOT RECEIVING ANTIVIRAL TREATMENT FOR HEPATITIS C	C	N	00	9		
G8461	PATIENT RECEIVING ANTIVIRAL TREATMENT FOR HEPATITIS C	C	N	00	9		
G8462	CLINICIAN DOCUMENTED THAT PATIENT IS NOT AN ELIGIBLE CANDIDATE FOR COUNSELING REGARDING CONTRACEPTION PRIOR TO ANTIVIRAL TREATMENT; PATIENT NOT RECEIVING ANTIVIRAL TREATMENT FOR HEPATITIS C	C	N	00	9		
G8463	PATIENT RECEIVING ANTIVIRAL TREATMENT FOR HEPATITIS C DOCUMENTED	C	N	00	9		
G8464	CLINICIAN DOCUMENTED THAT PROSTATE CANCER PATIENT IS NOT AN ELIGIBLE CANDIDATE FOR ADJUVANT HORMONAL THERAPY; LOW OR INTERMEDIATE RISK OF RECURRENCE OR RISK OF RECURRENCE NOT DETERMINED	C	N	00	9		
G8465	HIGH RISK OF RECURRENCE OF PROSTATE CANCER	C	N	00	9		
G8466	CLINICIAN DOCUMENTED THAT PATIENT IS NOT AN ELIGIBLE CANDIDATE FOR SUICIDE RISK ASSESSMENT; MAJOR DEPRESSIVE DISORDER, IN REMISSION	C	N	00	9		
G8467	DOCUMENTATION OF NEW DIAGNOSIS OF INITIAL OR RECURRENT EPISODE OF MAJOR DEPRESSIVE DISORDER	C	N	00	9		
G8468	ANGIOTENSIN CONVERTING ENZYME (ACE) INHIBITOR OR ANGIOTENSIN RECEPTOR BLOCKER (ARB) THERAPY PRESCRIBED FOR PATIENTS WITH A LEFT VENTRICULAR EJECTION FRACTION (LVEF) <40% OR DOCUMENTATION OF MODERATELY OR SEVERELY DEPRESSED LEFT VENTRICULAR SYSTOLIC FUNCTION	C	N	00	9		
G8469	CLINICIAN DOCUMENTED THAT PATIENT WITH A LEFT VENTRICULAR EJECTION FRACTION (LVEF) <40% OR DOCUMENTATION OF MODERATELY OR SEVERELY DEPRESSED LEFT VENTRICULAR SYSTOLIC FUNCTION WAS NOT AN ELIGIBLE CANDIDATE FOR ANGIOTENSIN CONVERTING ENZYME (ACE) INHIBITOR OR ANGIOTENSIN RECEPTOR BLOCKER (ARB) THERAPY	C	N	00	9		

HCPCS Code	Statute	Lab Cert	X-Ref	ASC Pay Grp	ASC Pay Group Eff. Date	Proc Notes	BETOS	TOS	Anest	Code Add Date	Code Effective Date	Code Term Date
G8452							M5D	1	0	20080101	20080101	
G8453							M5D	1	0	20080101	20080101	
G8454							M5D	1	0	20080101	20080101	
G8455							M5D	1	0	20080101	20080101	
G8456							M5D	1	0	20080101	20100101	
G8457							M5D	1	0	20080101	20090101	
G8458							M5D	1	0	20080101	20080101	
G8458												
G8459							M5D	1	0	20080101	20080101	
G8460							M5D	1	0	20080101	20080101	
G8461							M5D	1	0	20080101	20080101	
G8462							M5D	1	0	20080101	20080101	
G8463							M5D	1	0	20080101	20080101	
G8464							M5D	1	0	20080101	20080101	
G8465							M5D	1	0	20080101	20080101	
G8466							M5D	1	0	20080101	20080101	
G8467							M5D	1	0	20080101	20080101	
G8468							M5D	1	0	20080101	20080101	
G8469							M5D	1	0	20080101	20080101	

HCPCS Code	Long Description	Coverage	Action	PI	MPI	CIM	MCM
G8470	PATIENT WITH LEFT VENTRICULAR EJECTION FRACTION (LVEF) >=40% OR DOCUMENTATION AS NORMAL OR MILDLY DEPRESSED LEFT VENTRICULAR SYSTOLIC FUNCTION	C	N	00	9		
G8471	LEFT VENTRICULAR EJECTION FRACTION (LVEF) WAS NOT PERFORMED OR DOCUMENTED	C	N	00	9		
G8472	ANGIOTENSIN CONVERTING ENZYME (ACE) INHIBITOR OR ANGIOTENSIN RECEPTOR BLOCKER (ARB) THERAPY NOT PRESCRIBED FOR PATIENTS WITH A LEFT VENTRICULAR EJECTION FRACTION (LVEF) <40% OR DOCUMENTATION OF MODERATELY OR SEVERELY DEPRESSED LEFT VENTRICULAR SYSTOLIC FUNCTION, REASON NOT SPECIFIED	C	N	00	9		
G8473	ANGIOTENSIN CONVERTING ENZYME (ACE) INHIBITOR OR ANGIOTENSIN RECEPTOR BLOCKER (ARB) THERAPY PRESCRIBED	C	N	00	9		
G8474	ANGIOTENSIN CONVERTING ENZYME (ACE) INHIBITOR OR ANGIOTENSIN RECEPTOR BLOCKER (ARB) THERAPY NOT PRESCRIBED FOR REASONS DOCUMENTED BY THE CLINICIAN	C	N	00	9		
G8475	ANGIOTENSIN CONVERTING ENZYME (ACE) INHIBITOR OR ANGIOTENSIN RECEPTOR BLOCKER (ARB) THERAPY NOT PRESCRIBED, REASON NOT SPECIFIED	C	N	00	9		
G8476	MOST RECENT BLOOD PRESSURE HAS A SYSTOLIC MEASUREMENT OF <130 MM/HG AND A DIASTOLIC MEASUREMENT OF <80 MM/HG	C	N	00	9		
G8477	MOST RECENT BLOOD PRESSURE HAS A SYSTOLIC MEASUREMENT OF >=130 MM/HG AND/OR A DIASTOLIC MEASUREMENT OF >=80 MM/HG	C	N	00	9		
G8478	BLOOD PRESSURE MEASUREMENT NOT PERFORMED OR DOCUMENTED, REASON NOT SPECIFIED	C	N	00	9		
G8479	CLINICIAN PRESCRIBED ANGIOTENSIN CONVERTING ENZYME (ACE) INHIBITOR OR ANGIOTENSIN RECEPTOR BLOCKER (ARB) THERAPY	C	N	00	9		
G8480	CLINICIAN DOCUMENTED THAT PATIENT WAS NOT AN ELIGIBLE CANDIDATE FOR ANGIOTENSIN CONVERTING ENZYME (ACE) INHIBITOR OR ANGIOTENSIN RECEPTOR BLOCKER (ARB) THERAPY	C	N	00	9		
G8481	CLINICIAN DID NOT PRESCRIBE ANGIOTENSIN CONVERTING ENZYME (ACE) INHIBITOR OR ANGIOTENSIN RECEPTOR BLOCKER (ARB) THERAPY, REASON NOT SPECIFIED	C	N	00	9		
G8482	INFLUENZA IMMUNIZATION WAS ORDERED OR ADMINISTERED	C	N	00	9		
G8483	INFLUENZA IMMUNIZATION WAS NOT ORDERED OR ADMINISTERED FOR REASONS DOCUMENTED BY CLINICIAN	C	N	00	9		
G8484	INFLUENZA IMMUNIZATION WAS NOT ORDERED OR ADMINISTERED, REASON NOT SPECIFIED	C	N	00	9		
G8485	I INTEND TO REPORT THE DIABETES MELLITUS MEASURES GROUP	C	N	00	9		
G8486	I INTEND TO REPORT THE PREVENTIVE CARE MEASURES GROUP	C	N	00	9		
G8487	I INTEND TO REPORT THE CHRONIC KIDNEY DISEASE (CKD) MEASURES GROUP	C	N	00	9		

HCPCS Code	Statute	Lab Cert	X-Ref	ASC Pay Grp	ASC Pay Group Eff. Date	Proc Notes	BETOS	TOS	Anest	Code Add Date	Code Effective Date	Code Term Date
G8470							M5D	1	0	20080101	20080101	
G8471							M5D	1	0	20080101	20080101	
G8472							M5D	1	0	20080101	20080101	
G8473							M5D	1	0	20080101	20080101	
G8474							M5D	1	0	20080101	20080101	
G8475							M5D	1	0	20080101	20080101	
G8476							M5D	1	0	20080101	20080101	
G8477							M5D	1	0	20080101	20080101	
G8478							M5D	1	0	20080101	20080101	
G8479							M5D	1	0	20080101	20080101	
G8480							M5D	1	0	20080101	20080101	
G8481							M5D	1	0	20080101	20080101	
G8482							M5D	1	0	20080101	20080101	
G8483							M5D	1	0	20080101	20080101	
G8484							M5D	1	0	20080101	20080101	
G8485							M5D	1	0	20080701	20080701	
G8486							M5D	1	0	20080701	20080701	
G8487							M5D	1	0	20080701	20080701	

HCPCS Code	Long Description	Coverage	Action	PI	MPI	CIM	MCM
G8488	CLINICIAN INTENDS TO REPORT THE END STAGE RENAL DISEASE (ESRD) MEASURE GROUP	C	N	00	9		
G8489	I INTEND TO REPORT THE CORONARY ARTERY DISEASE (CAD) MEASURES GROUP	C	N	00	9		
G8490	I INTEND TO REPORT THE RHEUMATOID ARTHRITIS MEASURES GROUP	C	N	00	9		
G8491	I INTEND TO REPORT THE HIV/AIDS MEASURES GROUP	C	N	00	9		
G8492	I INTEND TO REPORT THE PERIOPERATIVE CARE MEASURES GROUP	C	S	00	9		
G8493	I INTEND TO REPORT THE BACK PAIN MEASURES GROUP	C	N	00	9		
G8494	ALL QUALITY ACTIONS FOR THE APPLICABLE MEASURES IN THE DIABETES MELLITUS MEASURES GROUP HAVE BEEN PERFORMED FOR THIS PATIENT	C	N	00	9		
G8495	ALL QUALITY ACTIONS FOR THE APPLICABLE MEASURES IN THE CKD MEASURES GROUP HAVE BEEN PERFORMED FOR THIS PATIENT	C	N	00	9		
G8496	ALL QUALITY ACTIONS FOR THE APPLICABLE MEASURES IN THE PREVENTIVE CARE MEASURES GROUP HAVE BEEN PERFORMED FOR THIS PATIENT	C	S	00	9		
G8497	ALL QUALITY ACTIONS FOR THE APPLICABLE MEASURES IN THE CORONARY ARTERY BYPASS GRAFT (CABG) MEASURES GROUP HAVE BEEN PERFORMED FOR THIS PATIENT	C	N	00	9		
G8498	ALL QUALITY ACTIONS FOR THE APPLICABLE MEASURES IN THE CORONARY ARTERY DISEASE (CAD) MEASURES GROUP HAVE BEEN PERFORMED FOR THIS PATIENT	C	N	00	9		
G8499	ALL QUALITY ACTIONS FOR THE APPLICABLE MEASURES IN THE RHEUMATOID ARTHRITIS MEASURES GROUP HAVE BEEN PERFORMED FOR THIS PATIENT	C	N	00	9		
G8500	ALL QUALITY ACTIONS FOR THE APPLICABLE MEASURES IN THE HIV/AIDS MEASURES GROUP HAVE BEEN PERFORMED FOR THIS PATIENT	C	N	00	9		
G8501	ALL QUALITY ACTIONS FOR THE APPLICABLE MEASURES IN THE PERIOPERATIVE CARE MEASURES GROUP HAVE BEEN PERFORMED FOR THIS PATIENT	C	N	00	9		
G8502	ALL QUALITY ACTIONS FOR THE APPLICABLE MEASURES IN THE BACK PAIN MEASURES GROUP HAVE BEEN PERFORMED FOR THIS PATIENT	C	S	00	9		
G8503	DOCUMENTATION THAT PROPHYLACTIC ANTIBIOTIC WAS GIVEN WITHIN ONE HOUR (IF FLUOROQUINOLONE OR VANCOMYCIN, TWO HOURS) PRIOR TO SURGICAL INCISION (OR START OF PROCEDURE WHEN NO INCISION IS REQUIRED)	C	D	00	9		
G8504	DOCUMENTATION OF ORDER FOR PROPHYLACTIC ANTIBIOTICS TO BE GIVEN WITHIN ONE HOUR (IF FLUOROQUINOLONE OR VANCOMYCIN, TWO HOURS) PRIOR TO SURGICAL INCISION (OR START OF PROCEDURE WHEN NO INCISION IS REQUIRED)	C	D	00	9		

HCPCS Code	S t a t u t e	Lab Cert	X-Ref	ASC Pay Grp	ASC Pay Group Eff. Date	Proc Notes	BETOS	TOS	A n e s t	Code Add Date	Code Effective Date	Code Term Date
G8488							M5D	1	0	20080701	20080701	
G8489							M5D	1	0	20090101	20090101	
G8490							M5D	1	0	20090101	20090101	
G8491							M5D	1	0	20090101	20090101	
G8492							M5D	1	0	20090101	20100101	
G8493							M5D	1	0	20090101	20090101	
G8494							M5D	1	0	20090101	20090101	
G8495							M5D	1	0	20090101	20090101	
G8496							M5D	1	0	20090101	20100101	
G8497							M5D	1	0	20090101	20090101	
G8498							M5D	1	0	20090101	20090101	
G8499							M5D	1	0	20090101	20090101	
G8500							M5D	1	0	20090101	20090101	
G8501							M5D	1	0	20090101	20090101	
G8502							M5D	1	0	20090101	20100101	
G8503							M5D	1	0	20090101	20100101	20091231
G8504							M5D	1	0	20090101	20100101	20091231

HCPCS Code	Long Description	Coverage	Action	PI	MPI	CIM	MCM
G8505	DOCUMENTATION THAT PROPHYLACTIC ANTIBIOTIC WAS NOT GIVEN WITHIN ONE HOUR (IF FLUOROQUINOLONE OR VANCOMYCIN, TWO HOURS) PRIOR TO SURGICAL INCISION (OR START OF PROCEDURE WHEN NO INCISION IS REQUIRED), REASON NOT SPECIFIED	C	D	00	9		
G8506	PATIENT RECEIVING ANGIOTENSIN CONVERTING ENZYME (ACE) INHIBITOR OR ANGIOTENSIN RECEPTOR BLOCKER (ARB) THERAPY	C	N	00	9		
G8507	PROVIDER DOCUMENTATION THAT PATIENT IS NOT ELIGIBLE FOR PATIENT VERIFICATION OF CURRENT MEDICATIONS	C	N	00	9		
G8508	DOCUMENTATION OF PAIN ASSESSMENT (INCLUDING LOCATION, INTENSITY AND DESCRIPTION) PRIOR TO INITIATION OF TREATMENT OR DOCUMENTATION OF THE ABSENCE OF PAIN AS A RESULT OF ASSESSMENT THROUGH DISCUSSION WITH THE PATIENT INCLUDING THE USE OF A STANDARDIZED TOOL; NO DOCUMENTATION OF A FOLLOW-UP PLAN, PATIENT NOT ELIGIBLE	C	N	00	9		
G8509	DOCUMENTATION OF PAIN ASSESSMENT (INCLUDING LOCATION, INTENSITY AND DESCRIPTION) PRIOR TO INITIATION OF TREATMENT OR DOCUMENTATION OF THE ABSENCE OF PAIN AS A RESULT OF ASSESSMENT THROUGH DISCUSSION WITH THE PATIENT INCLUDING THE USE OF A STANDARDIZED TOOL; NO DOCUMENTATION OF A FOLLOW-UP PLAN, REASON NOT SPECIFIED	C	N	00	9		
G8510	NEGATIVE SCREEN FOR CLINICAL DEPRESSION USING A STANDARDIZED TOOL, PATIENT NOT ELIGIBLE/APPROPRIATE FOR FOLLOW-UP PLAN DOCUMENTED	C	N	00	9		
G8511	SCREEN FOR CLINICAL DEPRESSION USING A STANDARDIZED TOOL DOCUMENTED, FOLLOW UP PLAN NOT DOCUMENTED, REASON NOT SPECIFIED	C	N	00	9		
G8512	PAIN SEVERITY QUANTIFIED; PAIN PRESENT	C	D	00	9		
G8513	ABI MEASURED AND DOCUMENTED	C	D	00	9		
G8514	CLINICIAN DOCUMENTED THAT PATIENT WAS NOT AN ELIGIBLE CANDIDATE FOR ABI MEASUREMENT MEASURE	C	D	00	9		
G8515	ABI MEASUREMENT WAS NOT OBTAINED	C	D	00	9		
G8516	PATIENT SCREENED FOR FUTURE FALLS RISK; DOCUMENTATION OF TWO OR MORE FALLS IN THE PAST YEAR OR ANY FALL WITH INJURY IN THE PAST YEAR	C	D	00	9		
G8517	PATIENT SCREENED FOR FUTURE FALL RISK; DOCUMENTATION OF NO FALLS IN THE PAST YEAR OR ONLY ONE FALL WITHOUT INJURY IN THE PAST YEAR	C	D	00	9		
G8518	CLINICAL STAGE PRIOR TO SURGERY FOR LUNG CANCER AND ESOPHAGEAL CANCER RESECTION WAS RECORDED	C	N	00	9		
G8519	CLINICIAN DOCUMENTED THAT PATIENT WAS NOT ELIGIBLE FOR CLINICAL STAGE PRIOR TO SURGERY FOR LUNG CANCER AND ESOPHAGEAL CANCER RESECTION MEASURE	C	N	00	9		
G8520	CLINICIAN STAGE PRIOR TO SURGERY FOR LUNG CANCER AND ESOPHAGEAL CANCER RESECTION WAS NOT RECORDED, REASON NOT SPECIFIED	C	N	00	9		

HCPCS Code	Statute	Lab Cert	X-Ref	ASC Pay Grp	ASC Pay Group Eff. Date	Proc Notes	BETOS	TOS	Anest	Code Add Date	Code Effective Date	Code Term Date
G8505							M5D	1	0	20090101	20100101	20091231
G8506							M5D	1	0	20090101	20090101	
G8507							M5D	1	0	20090101	20090101	
G8508							M5D	1	0	20090101	20090101	
G8509							M5D	1	0	20090101	20090101	
G8510							M5D	1	0	20090101	20090101	
G8511							M5D	1	0	20090101	20090101	
G8512							M5D	1	0	20090101	20100101	20091231
G8513							M5D	1	0	20090101	20100101	20091231
G8514							M5D	1	0	20090101	20100101	20091231
G8515							M5D	1	0	20090101	20100101	20091231
G8516							M5D	1	0	20090101	20100101	20091231
G8517							M5D	1	0	20090101	20100101	20091231
G8518							M5D	1	0	20090101	20090101	
G8519							M5D	1	0	20090101	20090101	
G8520							M5D	1	0	20090101	20090101	

HCPCS Code	Long Description	Coverage	Action	PI	MPI	CIM	MCM
G8521	ANTIPLATELET THERAPY RECEIVED (ASA [81-325 MG/DAY] AND/OR CLOPIDOGREL [75 MG/DAY]) WITHIN 48 HOURS OF THE INITIATION OF SURGERY AND AT DISCHARGE	C	D	00	9		
G8522	CLINICIAN DOCUMENTED THAT PATIENT WAS NOT AN ELIGIBLE CANDIDATE FOR ANTIPLATELET THERAPY	C	D	00	9		
G8523	ANTIPLATELET THERAPY NOT RECEIVED 48 HOURS PRIOR TO CEA AND AT DISCHARGE, REASON NOT SPECIFIED	C	D	00	9		
G8524	PATCH CLOSURE USED FOR PATIENT UNDERGOING CONVENTIONAL CEA	C	N	00	9		
G8525	CLINICIAN DOCUMENTED THAT PATIENT DID NOT RECEIVE CONVENTIONAL CEA	C	N	00	9		
G8526	PATCH CLOSURE NOT USED FOR PATIENT UNDERGOING CONVENTIONAL CEA, REASON NOT SPECIFIED	C	N	00	9		
G8527	DOCUMENTATION OF ORDER FOR CEFAZOLIN OR CEFUROXIME FOR ANTIMICROBIAL PROPHYLAXIS	C	D	00	9		
G8528	CLINICIAN DOCUMENTED THAT PATIENT WAS INELIGIBLE FOR PROPHYLACTIC ANTIBIOTIC SELECTION MEASURE	C	D	00	9		
G8529	ORDER FOR CEFAZOLIN OR CEFUROXIME FOR ANTIMICROBIAL PROPHYLAXIS NOT DOCUMENTED, REASON NOT SPECIFIED	C	D	00	9		
G8530	AUTOGENOUS AV FISTULA RECEIVED	C	N	00	9		
G8531	CLINICIAN DOCUMENTED THAT PATIENT WAS NOT AN ELIGIBLE CANDIDATE FOR AUTOGENOUS AV FISTULA	C	N	00	9		
G8532	CLINICIAN DOCUMENTED THAT PATIENT RECEVIED VASCULAR ACCESS OTHER THAN AUTOGENOUS AV FISTULA, REASON NOT SPECIFIED	C	N	00	9		
G8533	PARTICIPATION BY A PHYSICIAN OR OTHER CLINICIAN IN SYSTEMATIC CLINICAL DATABASE REGISTRY THAT I NCLUDES CONSENSUS-ENDORSED QUALITY MEASURES	C	D	00	9		
G8534	DOCUMENTATION OF AN ELDER MALTREATMENT SCREEN AND FOLLOW-UP PLAN	C	N	00	9		
G8535	NO DOCUMENTATION OF AN ELDER MALTREATMENT SCREEN, PATIENT NOT ELIGIBLE	C	N	00	9		
G8536	NO DOCUMENTATION OF AN ELDER MALTREATMENT SCREEN, REASON NOT SPECIFIED	C	N	00	9		
G8537	ELDER MALTREATMENT SCREEN DOCUMENTED, FOLLOW-UP PLAN NOT DOCUMENTED, PATIENT NOT ELIGIBLE	C	N	00	9		
G8538	ELDER MALTREATMENT SCREEN DOCUMENTED, FOLLOW-UP PLAN NOT DOCUMENTED, REASON NOT SPECIFIED	C	N	00	9		
G8539	DOCUMENTATION OF A CURRENT FUNCTIONAL OUTCOME ASSESSMENT USING A STANDARDIZED TOOL AND CARE PLAN BASED ON IDENTIFIED DEFICIENCIES	C	N	00	9		
G8540	DOCUMENTATION THAT THE PATIENT IS NOT ELIGIBLE FOR A FUNCTIONAL OUTCOME ASSESSMENT USING A STANDARDIZED TOOL	C	N	00	9		
G8541	NO DOCUMENTATION OF A CURRENT FUNCTIONAL OUTCOME ASSESSMENT USING A STANDARDIZED TOOL, REASON NOT SPECIFIED	C	N	00	9		
G8542	DOCUMENTATION OF A CURRENT FUNCTIONAL OUTCOME ASSESSMENT USING A STANDARDIZED TOOL; NO DOCUMENTATION OF A CARE PLAN, PATIENT NOT ELIGIBLE	C	N	00	9		

HCPCS Code	Statute	Lab Cert	X-Ref	ASC Pay Grp	ASC Pay Group Eff. Date	Proc Notes	BETOS	TOS	Anest	Code Add Date	Code Effective Date	Code Term Date
G8521							M5D	1	0	20090101	20100101	20091231
G8522							M5D	1	0	20090101	20100101	20091231
G8523							M5D	1	0	20090101	20100101	20091231
G8524							M5C	1	0	20090101	20090101	
G8525							M5D	1	0	20090101	20090101	
G8526							M5D	1	0	20090101	20090101	
G8527							M5D	1	0	20090101	20100101	20091231
G8528							M5D	1	0	20090101	20100101	20091231
G8529							M5D	1	0	20090101	20100101	20091231
G8530							M5D	1	0	20090101	20090101	
G8531							M5D	1	0	20090101	20090101	
G8532							M5D	1	0	20090101	20090101	
G8533							M5D	1	0	20090101	20100101	20091231
G8534							M5D	1	0	20090101	20090101	
G8535							M5D	1	0	20090101	20090101	
G8536							M5D	1	0	20090101	20090101	
G8537							M5D	1	0	20090101	20090101	
G8538							M5D	1	0	20090101	20090101	
G8539							M5D	1	0	20090101	20090101	
G8540							M5D	1	0	20090101	20090101	
G8541							M5D	1	0	20090101	20090101	
G8542							M5D	1	0	20090101	20090101	

HCPCS Code	Long Description	Coverage	Action	PI	MPI	CIM	MCM
G8543	DOCUMENTATION OF A CURRENT FUNCTIONAL OUTCOME ASSESSMENT USING A STANDARDIZED TOOL; NO DOCUMENTATION OF A CARE PLAN, REASON NOT SPECIFIED	C	N	00	9		
G8544	I INTEND TO REPORT THE CORONARY ARTERY BYPASS GRAFT (CABG) MEASURES GROUP	C	N	00	9		
G8545	I INTEND TO REPORT THE HEPATITIS C MEASURES GROUP	C	A	00	9		
G8546	I INTEND TO REPORT THE COMMUNITY-ACQUIRED PNEUMONIA (CAP) MEASURES GROUP	C	A	00	9		
G8547	I INTEND TO REPORT THE ISCHEMIC VASCULAR DISEASE (IVD) MEASURES GROUP	C	A	00	9		
G8548	I INTEND TO REPORT THE HEART FAILURE (HF) MEASURES GROUP	C	A	00	9		
G8549	ALL QUALITY ACTIONS FOR THE APPLICABLE MEASURES IN THE HEPATITIS C MEASURES GROUP HAVE BEEN PERFORMED FOR THIS PATIENT	C	A	00	9		
G8550	ALL QUALITY ACTIONS FOR THE APPLICABLE MEASURES IN THE COMMUNITY-ACQUIRED PNEUMONIA (CAP) MEASURES GROUP HAVE BEEN PERFORMED FOR THIS PATIENT	C	A	00	9		
G8551	ALL QUALITY ACTIONS FOR THE APPLICABLE MEASURES IN THE HEART FAILURE (HF) MEASURES GROUP HAVE BEEN PERFORMED FOR THIS PATIENT	C	A	00	9		
G8552	ALL QUALITY ACTIONS FOR THE APPLICABLE MEASURES IN THE ISCHEMIC VASCULAR DISEASE (IVD) MEASURES GROUP HAVE BEEN PERFORMED FOR THIS PATIENT	C	A	00	9		
G8553	AT LEAST ONE PRESCRIPTION CREATED DURING THE ENCOUNTER WAS GENERATED AND TRANSMITTED ELECTRONICALLY USING A QUALIFIED ERX SYSTEM	C	A	00	9		
G8556	REFERRED TO A PHYSICIAN (PREFERABLY A PHYSICIAN WITH TRAINING IN DISORDERS OF THE EAR) FOR AN OTOLOGIC EVALUATION	C	A	00	9		
G8557	PATIENT IS NOT ELIGIBLE FOR THE REFERRAL FOR OTOLOGIC EVALUATION MEASURE	C	A	00	9		
G8558	NOT REFERRED TO A PHYSICIAN (PREFERABLY A PHYSICIAN WITH TRAINING IN DISORDERS OF THE EAR) FOR AN OTOLOGIC EVALUATION, REASON NOT SPECIFIED	C	A	00	9		
G8559	PATIENT REFERRED TO A PHYSICIAN (PREFERABLY A PHYSICIAN WITH TRAINING IN DISORDERS OF THE EAR) FOR AN OTOLOGIC EVALUATION	C	A	00	9		
G8560	PATIENT HAS A HISTORY OF ACTIVE DRAINAGE FROM THE EAR WITHIN THE PREVIOUS 90 DAYS	C	A	00	9		
G8561	PATIENT IS NOT ELIGIBLE FOR THE REFERRAL FOR OTOLOGIC EVALUATION FOR PATIENTS WITH A HISTORY OF ACTIVE DRAINAGE MEASURE	C	A	00	9		
G8562	PATIENT DOES NOT HAVE A HISTORY OF ACTIVE DRAINAGE FROM THE EAR WITHIN THE PREVIOUS 90 DAYS	C	A	00	9		
G8563	PATIENT NOT REFERRED TO A PHYSICIAN (PREFERABLY A PHYSICIAN WITH TRAINING IN DISORDERS OF THE EAR) FOR AN OTOLOGIC EVALUATION, REASON NOT SPECIFIED	C	A	00	9		

HCPCS Code	Statute	Lab Cert	X-Ref	ASC Pay Grp	ASC Pay Group Eff. Date	Proc Notes	BETOS	TOS	Anest	Code Add Date	Code Effective Date	Code Term Date
G8543							M5D	1	0	20090101	20090101	
G8544							M5D	1	0	20090101	20090101	
G8545							M5D	1	0	20100101	20100101	
G8546							M5D	1	0	20100101	20100101	
G8547							M5D	1	0	20100101	20100101	
G8548							M5D	1	0	20100101	20100101	
G8549							M5D	1	0	20100101	20100101	
G8550							M5D	1	0	20100101	20100101	
G8551							M5D	1	0	20100101	20100101	
G8552							M5D	1	0	20100101	20100101	
G8553							M5D	1	0	20100101	20100101	
G8556							M5D	1	0	20100101	20100101	
G8557							M5D	1	0	20100101	20100101	
G8558							M5D	1	0	20100101	20100101	
G8559							M5D	1	0	20100101	20100101	
G8560							M5D	1	0	20100101	20100101	
G8561							M5D	1	0	20100101	20100101	
G8562							M5D	1	0	20100101	20100101	
G8563							M5D	1	0	20100101	20100101	

HCPCS Code	Long Description	Coverage	Action	PI	MPI	CIM	MCM
G8564	PATIENT WAS REFERRED TO A PHYSICIAN (PREFERABLY A PHYSICIAN WITH TRAINING IN DISORDERS OF THE EAR) FOR AN OTOLOGIC EVALUATION, REASON NOT SPECIFIED)	C	A	00	9		
G8565	VERIFICATION AND DOCUMENTATION OF SUDDEN OR RAPIDLY PROGRESSIVE HEARING LOSS	C	A	00	9		
G8566	PATIENT IS NOT ELIGIBLE FOR THE "REFERRAL FOR OTOLOGIC EVALUATION FOR SUDDEN OR RAPIDLY PROGRESSIVE HEARING LOSS" MEASURE	C	A	00	9		
G8567	PATIENT DOES NOT HAVE VERIFICATION AND DOCUMENTATION OF SUDDEN OR RAPIDLY PROGRESSIVE HEARING LOSS	C	A	00	9		
G8568	PATIENT WAS NOT REFERRED TO A PHYSICIAN (PREFERABLY A PHYSICIAN WITH TRAINING IN DISORDERS OF THE EAR) FOR AN OTOLOGIC EVALUATION, REASON NOT SPECIFIED)	C	A	00	9		
G8569	PROLONGED INTUBATION (>24 HRS) REQUIRED	C	A	00	9		
G8570	PROLONGED INTUBATION (>24 HRS) NOT REQUIRED	C	A	00	9		
G8571	DEVELOPMENT OF DEEP STERNAL WOUND INFECTION WITHIN 30 DAYS POSTOPERATIVELY	C	A	00	9		
G8572	NO DEEP STERNAL WOUND INFECTION	C	A	00	9		
G8573	STROKE/CBA FOLLOWING ISOLATED CABG SURGERY	C	A	00	9		
G8574	NO STROKE/CVA FOLLOWING ISOLATED CABG SURGERY	C	A	00	9		
G8575	DEVELOPED POSTOPERATIVE RENAL INSUFFICIENCY OR REQUIRED DIALYSIS	C	A	00	9		
G8576	NO POSTOPERATIVE RENAL INSUFFICIENCY/DIALYSIS NOT REQUIRED	C	A	00	9		
G8577	REOPERATION REQUIRED DUE TO BLEEDING/TAMPONADE, GRAFT OCCLUSION OR OTHER CARDIAC REASON	C	A	00	9		
G8578	REOPERATION NOT REQUIRED DUE TO BLEEDING/TAMPONADE, GRAFT OCCLUSION OR OTHER CARDIAC REASON	C	A	00	9		
G8579	ANTIPLATELET MEDICATION AT DISCHARGE	C	A	00	9		
G8580	ANTIPLATELET MEDICATION CONTRAINDICATED/NOT INDICATED	C	A	00	9		
G8581	NO ANTIPLATELET MEDICATION AT DISCHARGE	C	A	00	9		
G8582	BETA-BLOCKER AT DISCHARGE	C	A	00	9		
G8583	BETA-BLOCKER CONTRAINDICATED/NOT INDICATED	C	A	00	9		
G8584	NO BETA-BLOCKER AT DISCHARGE	C	A	00	9		
G8585	ANTI-LIPID TREATMENT AT DISCHARGE	C	A	00	9		
G8586	ANTI-LIPID TREATMENT CONTRAINDICATED/NOT INDICATED	C	A	00	9		
G8587	NO ANTI-LIPID TREATMENT AT DISCHARGE	C	A	00	9		
G8588	MOST RECENT SYSTOLIC BLOOD PRESSURE < 140 MMHG	C	A	00	9		
G8589	MOST RECENT SYSTOLIC BLOOD PRESSURE >= 140 MMHG	C	A	00	9		
G8590	MOST RECENT DIASTOLIC BLOOD PRESSURE < 90 MMHG	C	A	00	9		
G8591	MOST RECENT DIASTOLIC BLOOD PRESSURE >= 90 MMHG	C	A	00	9		
G8592	NO DOCUMENTATION OF BLOOD PRESSURE MEASUREMENT	C	A	00	9		
G8593	LIPID PROFILE RESULTS DOCUMENTED AND REVIEWED (MUST INCLUDE TOTAL CHOLESTEROL, HDL-C, TRIGLYCERIDES AND CALCULATED LDL-C)	C	A	00	9		
G8594	LIPID PROFILE NOT PERFORMED, REASON NOT OTHERWISE SPECIFIED	C	A	00	9		
G8595	MOST RECENT LDL-C < 100 MG/DL	C	A	00	9		

HCPCS Code	Statute	Lab Cert	X-Ref	ASC Pay Grp	ASC Pay Group Eff. Date	Proc Notes	BETOS	TOS	Anest	Code Add Date	Code Effective Date	Code Term Date
G8564							M5D	1	0	20100101	20100101	
G8565							M5D	1	0	20100101	20100101	
G8566							M5D	1	0	20100101	20100101	
G8567							M5D	1	0	20100101	20100101	
G8568							M5D	1	0	20100101	20100101	
G8569							M5D	1	0	20100101	20100101	
G8570							M5D	1	0	20100101	20100101	
G8571							M5D	1	0	20100101	20100101	
G8572							M5D	1	0	20100101	20100101	
G8573							M5D	1	0	20100101	20100101	
G8574							M5D	1	0	20100101	20100101	
G8575							M5D	1	0	20100101	20100101	
G8576							M5D	1	0	20100101	20100101	
G8577							M5D	1	0	20100101	20100101	
G8578							M5D	1	0	20100101	20100101	
G8579							M5D	1	0	20100101	20100101	
G8580							M5D	1	0	20100101	20100101	
G8581							M5D	1	0	20100101	20100101	
G8582							M5D	1	0	20100101	20100101	
G8583							M5D	1	0	20100101	20100101	
G8584							M5D	1	0	20100101	20100101	
G8585							M5D	1	0	20100101	20100101	
G8586							M5D	1	0	20100101	20100101	
G8587							M5D	1	0	20100101	20100101	
G8588							M5D	1	0	20100101	20100101	
G8589							M5D	1	0	20100101	20100101	
G8590							M5D	1	0	20100101	20100101	
G8591							M5D	1	0	20100101	20100101	
G8592							M5D	1	0	20100101	20100101	
G8593							M5D	1	0	20100101	20100101	
G8594							M5D	1	0	20100101	20100101	
G8595							M5D	1	0	20100101	20100101	

HCPCS Code	Long Description	Coverage	Action	PI	MPI	CIM	MCM
G8596	LDL-C WAS NOT PERFORMED	C	A	00	9		
G8597	MOST RECENT LDL-C >= 100 MG/DL	C	A	00	9		
G8598	ASPIRIN OR ANOTHER ANTITHROMBOTIC THERAPY USED	C	A	00	9		
G8599	ASPIRIN OR ANOTHER ANTITHROMBOTIC THERAPY NOT USED, REASON NOT OTHERWISE SPECIFIED	C	A	00	9		
G8600	IV T-PA INITIATED WITHIN THREE HOURS (<= 180 MINUTES) OF TIME LAST KNOWN WELL	C	A	00	9		
G8601	IV T-PA NOT INITIATED WITHIN THREE HOURS (<= 180 MINUTES) OF TIME LAST KNOWN WELL FOR REASONS DOCUMENTED BY CLINICIAN	C	A	00	9		
G8602	IV T-PA NOT INITIATED WITHIN THREE HOURS (<= 180 MINUTES) OF TIME LAST KNOWN WELL, REASON NOT SPECIFIED	C	A	00	9		
G8603	SCORE ON THE SPOKEN LANGUAGE COMPREHENSION FUNCTIONAL COMMUNICATION MEASURE AT DISCHARGE WAS HIGHER THAN AT ADMISSION	C	A	00	9		
G8604	SCORE ON THE SPOKEN LANGUAGE COMPREHENSION FUNCTIONAL COMMUNICATION MEASURE AT DISCHARGE WAS NOT HIGHER THAN AT ADMISSION, REASON NOT SPECIFIED	C	A	00	9		
G8605	PATIENT WAS NOT SCORED ON THE SPOKEN LANGUAGE COMPREHENSION FUNCTIONAL COMMUNICATION MEASURE EITHER AT ADMISSION OR AT DISCHARGE	C	A	00	9		
G8606	SCORE ON THE ATTENTION FUNCTIONAL COMMUNICATION MEASURE AT DISCHARGE WAS HIGHER THAN AT ADMISSION	C	A	00	9		
G8607	SCORE ON THE ATTENTION FUNCTIONAL COMMUNICATION MEASURE AT DISCHARGE WAS NOT HIGHER THAN AT ADMISSION, REASON NOT SPECIFIED	C	A	00	9		
G8608	PATIENT WAS NOT SCORED ON THE ATTENTION FUNCTIONAL COMMUNICATION MEASURE EITHER AT ADMISSION OR AT DISCHARGE	C	A	00	9		
G8609	SCORE ON THE MEMORY FUNCTIONAL COMMUNICATION MEASURE AT DISCHARGE WAS HIGHER THAN AT ADMISSION	C	A	00	9		
G8610	SCORE ON THE MEMORY FUNCTIONAL COMMUNICATION MEASURE AT DISCHARGE WAS NOT HIGHER THAN AT ADMISSION, REASON NOT SPECIFIED	C	A	00	9		
G8611	PATIENT WAS NOT SCORED ON THE MEMORY FUNCTIONAL COMMUNICATION MEASURE AT EITHER ADMISSION OR AT DISCHARGE	C	A	00	9		
G8612	SCORE ON THE MOTOR SPEECH FUNCTIONAL COMMUNICATION MEASURE AT DISCHARGE WAS HIGHER THAN AT ADMISSION	C	A	00	9		
G8613	SCORE ON THE MOTOR SPEECH FUNCTIONAL COMMUNICATION MEASURE AT DISCHARGE WAS NOT HIGHER THAN AT ADMISSION, REASON NOT SPECIFIED	C	A	00	9		
G8614	PATIENT WAS NOT SCORED ON THE MOTOR SPEECH FUNCTIONAL COMMUNICATION MEASURE EITHER AT ADMISSION OR AT DISCHARGE	C	A	00	9		
G8615	SCORE ON THE READING FUNCTIONAL COMMUNICATION MEASURE AT DISCHARGE WAS HIGHER THAN AT ADMISSION	C	A	00	9		

HCPCS Code	Statute	Lab Cert	X-Ref	ASC Pay Grp	ASC Pay Group Eff. Date	Proc Notes	BETOS	TOS	Anest	Code Add Date	Code Effective Date	Code Term Date
G8596							M5D	1	0	20100101	20100101	
G8597							M5D	1	0	20100101	20100101	
G8598							M5D	1	0	20100101	20100101	
G8599							M5D	1	0	20100101	20100101	
G8600							M5D	1	0	20100101	20100101	
G8601							M5D	1	0	20100101	20100101	
G8602							M5D	1	0	20100101	20100101	
G8603							M5D	1	0	20100101	20100101	
G8604							M5D	1	0	20100101	20100101	
G8605							M5D	1	0	20100101	20100101	
G8606							M5D	1	0	20100101	20100101	
G8607							M5D	1	0	20100101	20100101	
G8608							M5D	1	0	20100101	20100101	
G8609							M5D	1	0	20100101	20100101	
G8610							M5D	1	0	20100101	20100101	
G8611							M5D	1	0	20100101	20100101	
G8612							M5D	1	0	20100101	20100101	
G8613							M5D	1	0	20100101	20100101	
G8614							M5D	1	0	20100101	20100101	
G8615							M5D	1	0	20100101	20100101	

HCPCS Code	Long Description	Coverage	Action	PI	MPI	CIM	MCM
G8616	SCORE ON THE READING FUNCTIONAL COMMUNICATION MEASURE AT DISCHARGE WAS NOT HIGHER THAN AT ADMISSION, REASON NOT SPECIFIED	C	A	00	9		
G8617	PATIENT WAS NOT SCORED ON THE READING FUNCTIONAL COMMUNICATION MEASURE EITHER AT ADMISSION OR AT DISCHARGE	C	A	00	9		
G8618	SCORE ON THE SPOKEN LANGUAGE EXPRESSION FUNCTIONAL COMMUNICATION MEASURE AT DISCHARGE WAS HIGHER THAN AT ADMISSION	C	A	00	9		
G8619	SCORE ON THE SPOKEN LANGUAGE EXPRESSION FUNCTIONAL COMMUNICATION MEASURE AT DISCHARGE WAS NOT HIGHER THAN AT ADMISSION, REASON NOT SPECIFIED	C	A	00	9		
G8620	PATIENT WAS NOT SCORED ON THE SPOKEN LANGUAGE EXPRESSION FUNCTIONAL COMMUNICATION MEASURE EITHER AT ADMISSION OR AT DISCHARGE	C	A	00	9		
G8621	SCORE ON THE WRITING FUNCTIONAL COMMUNICATION MEASURE AT DISCHARGE WAS HIGHER THAN AT ADMISSION	C	A	00	9		
G8622	SCORE ON THE WRITING FUNCTIONAL COMMUNICATION MEASURE AT DISCHARGE WAS NOT HIGHER THAN AT ADMISSION, REASON NOT SPECIFIED	C	A	00	9		
G8623	PATIENT WAS NOT SCORED ON THE WRITING FUNCTIONAL COMMUNICATION MEASURE EITHER AT ADMISSION OR AT DISCHARGE	C	A	00	9		
G8624	SCORE ON THE SWALLOWING FUNCTIONAL COMMUNICATION MEASURE AT DISCHARGE WAS HIGHER THAN AT ADMISSION	C	A	00	9		
G8625	SCORE ON THE SWALLOWING FUNCTIONAL COMMUNICATION MEASURE AT DISCHARGE WAS NOT HIGHER THAN AT ADMISSION, REASON NOT SPECIFIED	C	A	00	9		
G8626	PATIENT WAS NOT SCORED ON THE SWALLOWING FUNCTIONAL COMMUNICATION MEASURE AT ADMISSION OR AT DISCHARGE	C	A	00	9		
G8627	SURGICAL PROCEDURE PERFORMED WITHIN 30 DAYS FOLLOWING CATARACT SURGERY FOR MAJOR COMPLICATIONS (E.G. RETAINED NUCLEAR FRAGMENTS, ENDOPHTHALMITIS, DISLOCATED OR WRONG POWER IOL, RETINAL DETACHMENT, OR WOUND DEHISCENCE)	C	A	00	9		
G8628	SURGICAL PROCEDURE NOT PERFORMED WITHIN 30 DAYS FOLLOWING CATARACT SURGERY FOR MAJOR COMPLICATIONS (E.G. RETAINED NUCLEAR FRAGMENTS, ENDOPHTHALMITIS, DISLOCATED OR WRONG POWER IOL, RETINAL DETACHMENT, OR WOUND DEHISCENCE)	C	A	00	9		
G9001	COORDINATED CARE FEE, INITIAL RATE	D	N	00	9		
G9002	COORDINATED CARE FEE, MAINTENANCE RATE	D	N	00	9		
G9003	COORDINATED CARE FEE, RISK ADJUSTED HIGH, INITIAL	D	N	00	9		
G9004	COORDINATED CARE FEE, RISK ADJUSTED LOW, INITIAL	D	N	00	9		
G9005	COORDINATED CARE FEE, RISK ADJUSTED MAINTENANCE	D	N	00	9		
G9006	COORDINATED CARE FEE, HOME MONITORING	D	N	00	9		
G9007	COORDINATED CARE FEE, SCHEDULED TEAM CONFERENCE	D	N	00	9		
G9008	COORDINATED CARE FEE, PHYSICIAN COORDINATED CARE OVERSIGHT SERVICES	D	N	00	9		

HCPCS Code	Statute	Lab Cert	X-Ref	ASC Pay Grp	ASC Pay Group Eff. Date	Proc Notes	BETOS	TOS	Anest	Code Add Date	Code Effective Date	Code Term Date
G8616							M5D	1	0	20100101	20100101	
G8617							M5D	1	0	20100101	20100101	
G8618							M5D	1	0	20100101	20100101	
G8619							M5D	1	0	20100101	20100101	
G8620							M5D	1	0	20100101	20100101	
G8621							M5D	1	0	20100101	20100101	
G8622							M5D	1	0	20100101	20100101	
G8623							M5D	1	0	20100101	20100101	
G8624							M5D	1	0	20100101	20100101	
G8625							M5D	1	0	20100101	20100101	
G8626							M5D	1	0	20100101	20100101	
G8627							M5D	1	0	20100101	20100101	
G8628							M5D	1	0	20100101	20100101	
G9001						0097	Y2	1	0	20001001	20001001	
G9002						0097	Y2	1	0	20001001	20001001	
G9003						0097	Y2	1	0	20001001	20001001	
G9004						0097	Y2	1	0	20001001	20001001	
G9005						0097	Y2	1	0	20001001	20001001	
G9006						0097	Y2	1	0	20001001	20001001	
G9007						0097	Y2	1	0	20001001	20001001	
G9008						0097	Y2	1	0	20001001	20001001	

HCPCS Code	Long Description	Coverage	Action	PI	MPI	CIM	MCM
G9009	COORDINATED CARE FEE, RISK ADJUSTED MAINTENANCE, LEVEL 3	D	N	00	9		
G9010	COORDINATED CARE FEE, RISK ADJUSTED MAINTENANCE, LEVEL 4	D	N	00	9		
G9011	COORDINATED CARE FEE, RISK ADJUSTED MAINTENANCE, LEVEL 5	D	N	00	9		
G9012	OTHER SPECIFIED CASE MANAGEMENT SERVICE NOT ELSEWHERE CLASSIFIED	D	N	00	9		
G9013	ESRD DEMO BASIC BUNDLE LEVEL I	M	N	00	9		
G9014	ESRD DEMO EXPANDED BUNDLE INCLUDING VENOUS ACCESS AND RELATED SERVICES	M	N	00	9		
G9016	SMOKING CESSATION COUNSELING, INDIVIDUAL, IN THE ABSENCE OF OR IN ADDITION TO ANY OTHER EVALUATION AND MANAGEMENT SERVICE, PER SESSION (6-10 MINUTES) [DEMO PROJECT CODE ONLY]	M	N	00	9		
G9017	AMANTADINE HYDROCHLORIDE, ORAL, PER 100 MG (FOR USE IN A MEDICARE-APPROVED DEMONSTRATION PROJECT)	C	N	13	A		
G9018	ZANAMIVIR, INHALATION POWDER, ADMINISTERED THROUGH INHALER, PER 10 MG (FOR USE IN A MEDICARE-APPROVED DEMONSTRATION PROJECT)	C	N	13	A		
G9019	OSELTAMIVIR PHOSPHATE, ORAL, PER 75 MG (FOR USE IN A MEDICARE-APPROVED DEMONSTRATION PROJECT)	C	N	13	A		
G9020	RIMANTADINE HYDROCHLORIDE, ORAL, PER 100 MG (FOR USE IN A MEDICARE-APPROVED DEMONSTRATION PROJECT)	C	N	13	A		
G9033	AMANTADINE HYDROCHLORIDE, ORAL BRAND, PER 100 MG (FOR USE IN AMEDICARE-APPROVED DEMONSTRATION PROJECT)	C	N	13	A		
G9034	ZANAMIVIR, INHALATION POWDER, ADMINISTERED THROUGH INHALER, BRAND, PER 10 MG (FOR USE IN A MEDICARE-APPROVED DEMONSTRATION PROJECT)	C	N	00	9		
G9035	OSELTAMIVIR PHOSPHATE, ORAL, BRAND, PER 75 MG (FOR USE IN A MEDICARE-APPROVED DEMONSTRATION PROJECT)	C	N	00	9		
G9036	RIMANTADINE HYDROCHLORIDE, ORAL, BRAND, PER 100 MG (FOR USE IN AMEDICARE-APPROVED DEMONSTRATION PROJECT)	C	N	00	9		
G9041	REHABILITATION SERVICES FOR LOW VISION BY QUALIFIED OCCUPATIONAL THERAPIST, DIRECT ONE-ON-ONE CONTACT, EACH 15 MINUTES	C	N	00	9		
G9042	REHABILITATION SERVICES FOR LOW VISION BY CERTIFIED ORIENTATION AND MOBILITY SPECIALISTS, DIRECT ONE-ON-ONE CONTACT, EACH 15 MINUTES	C	N	00	9		
G9043	REHABILITATION SERVICES FOR LOW VISION BY CERTIFIED LOW VISION REHABILITATION THERAPIST, DIRECT ONE-ON-ONE CONTACT, EACH 15 MINUTES	C	N	00	9		
G9044	REHABILITATION SERVICES FOR LOW VISION BY CERTIFIED LOW VISION REHABILITATION TEACHER, DIRECT ONE-ON-ONE CONTACT, EACH 15 MINUTES	C	N	00	9		

HCPCS Code	Statute	Lab Cert	X-Ref	ASC Pay Grp	ASC Pay Group Eff. Date	Proc Notes	BETOS	TOS	Anest	Code Add Date	Code Effective Date	Code Term Date
G9009						0096	Y2	1	0	20011001	20011001	
G9010						0096	Y2	1	0	20011001	20011001	
G9011						0096	Y2	1	0	20011001	20011001	
G9012						0096	Y2	1	0	20011001	20011001	
G9013						0096	Y2	1	0	20040701	20040701	
G9014						0096	Y2	1	0	20040701	20040701	
G9016						0096	Y2	1	0	20010101	20010101	
G9017							O1E	1	0	20041201	20041201	
G9018							O1E	1	0	20041201	20041201	
G9019							O1E	1	0	20041201	20041201	
G9020							O1E	1	0	20041201	20041201	
G9033							O1E	1	0	20041201	20041201	
G9034							O1E	1	0	20041201	20041201	
G9035							O1E	1	0	20041201	20041201	
G9036							O1E	1	0	20041201	20041201	
G9041							T2D	1	0	20060101	20060101	
G9042							T2D	1	0	20060101	20060101	
G9043							T2D	1	0	20060101	20060101	
G9044							T2D	1	0	20060101	20060101	

HCPCS Code	Long Description	Coverage	Action	PI	MPI	CIM	MCM
G9050	ONCOLOGY; PRIMARY FOCUS OF VISIT; WORK-UP, EVALUATION, OR STAGING AT THE TIME OF CANCER DIAGNOSIS OR RECURRENCE (FOR USE IN A MEDICARE-APPROVED DEMONSTRATION PROJECT)	I	N	00	9		
G9051	ONCOLOGY; PRIMARY FOCUS OF VISIT; TREATMENT DECISION-MAKING AFTER DISEASE IS STAGED OR RESTAGED, DISCUSSION OF TREATMENT OPTIONS, SUPERVISING/COORDINATING ACTIVE CANCER DIRECTED THERAPY OR MANAGING CONSEQUENCES OF CANCER DIRECTED THERAPY (FOR USE IN A MEDICARE-APPROVED DEMONSTRATION PROJECT)	I	N	00	9		
G9052	ONCOLOGY; PRIMARY FOCUS OF VISIT; SURVEILLANCE FOR DISEASE RECURRENCE FOR PATIENT WHO HAS COMPLETED DEFINITIVE CANCER-DIRECTED THERAPY AND CURRENTLY LACKS EVIDENCE OF RECURRENT DISEASE; CANCER DIRECTED THERAPY MIGHT BE CONSIDERED IN THE FUTURE (FOR USE IN A MEDICARE-APPROVED DEMONSTRATION PROJECT)	I	N	00	9		
G9053	ONCOLOGY; PRIMARY FOCUS OF VISIT; EXPECTANT MANAGEMENT OF PATIENT WITH EVIDENCE OF CANCER FOR WHOM NO CANCER DIRECTED THERAPY IS BEING ADMINISTERED OR ARRANGED AT PRESENT; CANCER DIRECTED THERAPY MIGHT BE CONSIDERED IN THE FUTURE (FOR USE IN A MEDICARE-APPROVED DEMONSTRATION PROJECT)	I	N	00	9		
G9054	ONCOLOGY; PRIMARY FOCUS OF VISIT; SUPERVISING, COORDINATING OR MANAGING CARE OF PATIENT WITH TERMINAL CANCER OR FOR WHOM OTHER MEDICAL ILLNESS PREVENTS FURTHER CANCER TREATMENT; INCLUDES SYMPTOM MANAGEMENT, END-OF-LIFE CARE PLANNING, MANAGEMENT OF PALLIATIVE THERAPIES (FOR USE IN A MEDICARE-APPROVED DEMONSTRATION PROJECT)	I	N	00	9		
G9055	ONCOLOGY; PRIMARY FOCUS OF VISIT; OTHER, UNSPECIFIED SERVICE NOT OTHERWISE LISTED (FOR USE IN A MEDICARE-APPROVED DEMONSTRATION PROJECT)	I	N	00	9		
G9056	ONCOLOGY; PRACTICE GUIDELINES; MANAGEMENT ADHERES TO GUIDELINES (FOR USE IN A MEDICARE-APPROVED DEMONSTRATION PROJECT)	I	N	00	9		
G9057	ONCOLOGY; PRACTICE GUIDELINES; MANAGEMENT DIFFERS FROM GUIDELINES AS A RESULT OF PATIENT ENROLLMENT IN AN INSTITUTIONAL REVIEW BOARD APPROVED CLINICAL TRIAL (FOR USE IN A MEDICARE-APPROVED DEMONSTRATION PROJECT)	I	N	00	9		
G9058	ONCOLOGY; PRACTICE GUIDELINES; MANAGEMENT DIFFERS FROM GUIDELINES BECAUSE THE TREATING PHYSICIAN DISAGREES WITH GUIDELINE RECOMMENDATIONS (FOR USE IN A MEDICARE-APPROVED DEMONSTRATION PROJECT)	I	N	00	9		

HCPCS Code	Statute	Lab Cert	X-Ref	ASC Pay Grp	ASC Pay Group Eff. Date	Proc Notes	BETOS	TOS	Anest	Code Add Date	Code Effective Date	Code Term Date
G9050							P7B	1	0	20060101	20070101	
G9051							P7B	1	0	20060101	20070101	
G9052							P7B	1	0	20060101	20070101	
G9053							P7B	1	0	20060101	20070101	
G9054							P7B	1	0	20060101	20070101	
G9055							P7B	1	0	20060101	20070101	
G9056							P7B	1	0	20060101	20070101	
G9057							P7B	1	0	20060101	20070101	
G9058							P7B	1	0	20060101	20070101	

HCPCS Code	Long Description	Coverage	Action	PI	MPI	CIM	MCM
G9059	ONCOLOGY; PRACTICE GUIDELINES; MANAGEMENT DIFFERS FROM GUIDELINES BECAUSE THE PATIENT, AFTER BEING OFFERED TREATMENT CONSISTENT WITH GUIDELINES, HAS OPTED FOR ALTERNATIVE TREATMENT OR MANAGEMENT, INCLUDING NO TREATMENT (FOR USE IN A MEDICARE-APPROVED DEMONSTRATION PROJECT)	I	N	00	9		
G9060	ONCOLOGY; PRACTICE GUIDELINES; MANAGEMENT DIFFERS FROM GUIDELINES FOR REASON(S) ASSOCIATED WITH PATIENT COMORBID ILLNESS OR PERFORMANCE STATUS NOT FACTORED INTO GUIDELINES (FOR USE IN A MEDICARE-APPROVED DEMONSTRATION PROJECT)	I	N	00	9		
G9061	ONCOLOGY; PRACTICE GUIDELINES; PATIENT'S CONDITION NOT ADDRESSED BY AVAILABLE GUIDELINES (FOR USE IN A MEDICARE-APPROVED DEMONSTRATION PROJECT)	I	N	00	9		
G9062	ONCOLOGY; PRACTICE GUIDELINES; MANAGEMENT DIFFERS FROM GUIDELINES FOR OTHER REASON(S) NOT LISTED (FOR USE IN A MEDICARE-APPROVED DEMONSTRATION PROJECT)	I	N	00	9		
G9063	ONCOLOGY; DISEASE STATUS; LIMITED TO NON-SMALL CELL LUNG CANCER; EXTENT OF DISEASE INITIALLY ESTABLISHED AS STAGE I (PRIOR TO NEO-ADJUVANT THERAPY, IF ANY) WITH NO EVIDENCE OF DISEASE PROGRESSION, RECURRENCE, OR METASTASES (FOR USE IN A MEDICARE-APPROVED DEMONSTRATION PROJECT)	C	N	00	9		
G9064	ONCOLOGY; DISEASE STATUS; LIMITED TO NON-SMALL CELL LUNG CANCER; EXTENT OF DISEASE INITIALLY ESTABLISHED AS STAGE II (PRIOR TO NEO-ADJUVANT THERAPY, IF ANY) WITH NO EVIDENCE OF DISEASE PROGRESSION, RECURRENCE, OR METASTASES (FOR USE IN A MEDICARE-APPROVED DEMONSTRATION PROJECT)	C	N	00	9		
G9065	ONCOLOGY; DISEASE STATUS; LIMITED TO NON-SMALL CELL LUNG CANCER; EXTENT OF DISEASE INITIALLY ESTABLISHED AS STAGE III A (PRIOR TO NEO-ADJUVANT THERAPY, IF ANY) WITH NO EVIDENCE OF DISEASE PROGRESSION, RECURRENCE, OR METASTASES (FOR USE IN A MEDICARE-APPROVED DEMONSTRATION PROJECT)	C	N	00	9		
G9066	ONCOLOGY; DISEASE STATUS; LIMITED TO NON-SMALL CELL LUNG CANCER; STAGE III B-IV AT DIAGNOSIS, METASTATIC, LOCALLY RECURRENT, OR PROGRESSIVE (FOR USE IN A MEDICARE-APPROVED DEMONSTRATION PROJECT)	C	N	00	9		
G9067	ONCOLOGY; DISEASE STATUS; LIMITED TO NON-SMALL CELL LUNG CANCER; EXTENT OF DISEASE UNKNOWN, STAGING IN PROGRESS, OR NOT LISTED (FOR USE IN A MEDICARE-APPROVED DEMONSTRATION PROJECT)	C	N	00	9		
G9068	ONCOLOGY; DISEASE STATUS; LIMITED TO SMALL CELL AND COMBINED SMALL CELL/NON-SMALL CELL; EXTENT OF DISEASE INITIALLY ESTABLISHED AS LIMITED WITH NO EVIDENCE OF DISEASE PROGRESSION, RECURRENCE, OR METASTASES (FOR USE IN A MEDICARE-APPROVED DEMONSTRATION PROJECT)	C	N	00	9		

HCPCS Code	Statute	Lab Cert	X-Ref	ASC Pay Grp	ASC Pay Group Eff. Date	Proc Notes	BETOS	TOS	Anest	Code Add Date	Code Effective Date	Code Term Date
G9059							P7B	1	0	20060101	20070101	
G9060							P7B	1	0	20060101	20070101	
G9061							P7B	1	0	20060101	20070101	
G9062							P7B	1	0	20060101	20070101	
G9063							P7B	1	0	20060101	20070101	
G9064							P7B	1	0	20060101	20070101	
G9065							P7B	1	0	20060101	20070101	
G9066							P7B	1	0	20060101	20070101	
G9067							P7B	1	0	20060101	20070101	
G9068							P7B	1	0	20060101	20070101	

HCPCS Code	Long Description	Coverage	Action	PI	MPI	CIM	MCM
G9069	ONCOLOGY; DISEASE STATUS; SMALL CELL LUNG CANCER, LIMITED TO SMALL CELL AND COMBINED SMALL CELL/NON-SMALL CELL; EXTENSIVE STAGE AT DIAGNOSIS, METASTATIC, LOCALLY RECURRENT, OR PROGRESSIVE (FOR USE IN A MEDICARE-APPROVED DEMONSTRATION PROJECT)	C	N	00	9		
G9070	ONCOLOGY; DISEASE STATUS; SMALL CELL LUNG CANCER, LIMITED TO SMALL CELL AND COMBINED SMALL CELL/NON-SMALL; EXTENT OF DISEASE UNKNOWN, STAGING IN PROGRESS, OR NOT LISTED (FOR USE IN A MEDICARE-APPROVED DEMONSTRATION PROJECT)	C	N	00	9		
G9071	ONCOLOGY; DISEASE STATUS; INVASIVE FEMALE BREAST CANCER (DOES NOT INCLUDE DUCTAL CARCINOMA IN SITU); ADENOCARCINOMA AS PREDOMINANT CELL TYPE; STAGE I OR STAGE IIA-IIB; OR T3, N1, M0; AND ER AND/OR PR POSITIVE; WITH NO EVIDENCE OF DISEASE PROGRESSION, RECURRENCE, OR METASTASES (FOR USE IN A MEDICARE-APPROVED DEMONSTRATION PROJECT)	C	N	00	9		
G9072	ONCOLOGY; DISEASE STATUS; INVASIVE FEMALE BREAST CANCER (DOES NOT INCLUDE DUCTAL CARCINOMA IN SITU); ADENOCARCINOMA AS PREDOMINANT CELL TYPE; STAGE I, OR STAGE IIA-IIB; OR T3, N1, M0; AND ER AND PR NEGATIVE; WITH NO EVIDENCE OF DISEASE PROGRESSION, RECURRENCE, OR METASTASES (FOR USE IN A MEDICARE-APPROVED DEMONSTRATION PROJECT)	C	N	00	9		
G9073	ONCOLOGY; DISEASE STATUS; INVASIVE FEMALE BREAST CANCER (DOES NOT INCLUDE DUCTAL CARCINOMA IN SITU); ADENOCARCINOMA AS PREDOMINANT CELL TYPE; STAGE IIIA-IIIB; AND NOT T3, N1, M0; AND ER AND/OR PR POSITIVE; WITH NO EVIDENCE OF DISEASE PROGRESSION, RECURRENCE, OR METASTASES (FOR USE IN A MEDICARE-APPROVED DEMONSTRATION PROJECT)	C	N	00	9		
G9074	ONCOLOGY; DISEASE STATUS; INVASIVE FEMALE BREAST CANCER (DOES NOT INCLUDE DUCTAL CARCINOMA IN SITU); ADENOCARCINOMA AS PREDOMINANT CELL TYPE; STAGE IIIA-IIIB; AND NOT T3, N1, M0; AND ER AND PR NEGATIVE; WITH NO EVIDENCE OF DISEASE PROGRESSION, RECURRENCE, OR METASTASES (FOR USE IN A MEDICARE-APPROVED DEMONSTRATION PROJECT)	C	N	00	9		
G9075	ONCOLOGY; DISEASE STATUS; INVASIVE FEMALE BREAST CANCER (DOES NOT INCLUDE DUCTAL CARCINOMA IN SITU); ADENOCARCINOMA AS PREDOMINANT CELL TYPE; M1 AT DIAGNOSIS, METASTATIC, LOCALLY RECURRENT, OR PROGRESSIVE (FOR USE IN A MEDICARE-APPROVED DEMONSTRATION PROJECT)	C	N	00	9		
G9076	ONCOLOGY; DISEASE STATUS; INVASIVE FEMALE BREAST CANCER (DOES NOT INCLUDE DUCTAL CARCINOMA IN SITU); ADENOCARCINOMA AS PREDOMINANT CELL TYPE; EXTENT OF DISEASE UNKNOWN, UNDER EVALUATION, PRE-SURGICAL OR NOT LISTED (FOR USE IN A MEDICARE-APPROVED DEMONSTRATION PROJECT)	C	N	13	A		

HCPCS Code	Statute	Lab Cert	X-Ref	ASC Pay Grp	ASC Pay Group Eff. Date	Proc Notes	BETOS	TOS	Anest	Code Add Date	Code Effective Date	Code Term Date
G9069							P7B	1	0	20060101	20070101	
G9070							P7B	1	0	20060101	20070101	
G9071							P7B	1	0	20060101	20070101	
G9072							P7B	1	0	20060101	20070101	
G9073							P7B	1	0	20060101	20070101	
G9074							P7B	1	0	20060101	20070101	
G9075							P7B	1	0	20060101	20070101	
G9076							P7B	1	0	20060101	20070101	20061231

HCPCS Code	Long Description	Coverage	Action	PI	MPI	CIM	MCM
G9077	ONCOLOGY; DISEASE STATUS; PROSTATE CANCER, LIMITED TO ADENOCARCINOMA AS PREDOMINANT CELL TYPE; T1-T2C & GLEASON 2-7 AND PSA < OR EQUAL TO 20 AT DIAGNOSIS WITH NO EVIDENCE OF DISEASE PROGRESSION, RECURRENCE, OR METASTASES (FOR USE IN A MEDICARE-APPROVED DEMONSTRATION PROJECT)	C	N	00	9		
G9078	ONCOLOGY; DISEASE STATUS; PROSTATE CANCER, LIMITED TO ADENOCARCINOMA AS PREDOMINANT CELL TYPE; T2 OR T3A GLEASON 8-10 OR PSA > 20 AT DIAGNOSIS WITH NO EVIDENCE OF DISEASE PROGRESSION, RECURRENCE, OR METASTASES (FOR USE IN A MEDICARE-APPROVED DEMONSTRATION PROJECT)	C	N	00	9		
G9079	ONCOLOGY; DISEASE STATUS; PROSTATE CANCER, LIMITED TO ADENOCARCINOMA AS PREDOMINANT CELL TYPE; T3B-T4, ANY N; ANY T, N1 AT DIAGNOSIS WITH NO EVIDENCE OF DISEASE PROGRESSION, RECURRENCE, OR METASTASES (FOR USE IN A MEDICARE-APPROVED DEMONSTRATION PROJECT)	C	N	00	9		
G9080	ONCOLOGY; DISEASE STATUS; PROSTATE CANCER, LIMITED TO ADENOCARCINOMA; AFTER INITIAL TREATMENT WITH RISING PSA OR FAILURE OF PSA DECLINE (FOR USE IN A MEDICARE-APPROVED DEMONSTRATION PROJECT)	C	N	00	9		
G9081	ONCOLOGY; DISEASE STATUS; PROSTATE CANCER, LIMITED TO ADENOCARCINOMA; NON-CASTRATE, INCOMPLETELY CASTRATE; CLINICAL METASTASES OR M1 AT DIAGNOSIS (FOR USE IN A MEDICARE-APPROVED DEMONSTRATION PROJECT)	C	N	13	A		
G9082	ONCOLOGY; DISEASE STATUS; PROSTATE CANCER, LIMITED TO ADENOCARCINOMA; CASTRATE; CLINICAL METASTASES OR M1 AT DIAGNOSIS (FOR USE IN A MEDICARE-APPROVED DEMONSTRATION PROJECT)	C	N	13	A		
G9083	ONCOLOGY; DISEASE STATUS; PROSTATE CANCER, LIMITED TO ADENOCARCINOMA; EXTENT OF DISEASE UNKNOWN, STAGING IN PROGRESS, OR NOT LISTED (FOR USE IN A MEDICARE-APPROVED DEMONSTRATION PROJECT)	C	N	00	9		
G9084	ONCOLOGY; DISEASE STATUS; COLON CANCER, LIMITED TO INVASIVE CANCER, ADENOCARCINOMA AS PREDOMINANT CELL TYPE; EXTENT OF DISEASE INITIALLY ESTABLISHED AS T1-3, N0, M0 WITH NO EVIDENCE OF DISEASE PROGRESSION, RECURRENCE, OR METASTASES (FOR USE IN A MEDICARE-APPROVED DEMONSTRATION PROJECT)	C	N	00	9		
G9085	ONCOLOGY; DISEASE STATUS; COLON CANCER, LIMITED TO INVASIVE CANCER, ADENOCARCINOMA AS PREDOMINANT CELL TYPE; EXTENT OF DISEASE INITIALLY ESTABLISHED AS T4, N0, M0 WITH NO EVIDENCE OF DISEASE PROGRESSION, RECURRENCE, OR METASTASES (FOR USE IN A MEDICARE-APPROVED DEMONSTRATION PROJECT)	C	N	00	9		

G Codes

HCPCS Code	Statute	Lab Cert	X-Ref	ASC Pay Grp	ASC Pay Group Eff. Date	Proc Notes	BETOS	TOS	Anest	Code Add Date	Code Effective Date	Code Term Date
G9077							P7B	1	0	20060101	20070101	
G9078							P7B	1	0	20060101	20070101	
G9079							P7B	1	0	20060101	20070101	
G9080							P7B	1	0	20060101	20070101	
G9081							P7B	1	0	20060101	20070101	20061231
G9082							P7B	1	0	20060101	20070101	20061231
G9083							P7B	1	0	20060101	20070101	
G9084							P7B	1	0	20060101	20070101	
G9085							P7B	1	0	20060101	20070101	

HCPCS Code	Long Description	Coverage	Action	PI	MPI	CIM	MCM
G9086	ONCOLOGY; DISEASE STATUS; COLON CANCER, LIMITED TO INVASIVE CANCER, ADENOCARCINOMA AS PREDOMINANT CELL TYPE; EXTENT OF DISEASE INITIALLY ESTABLISHED AS T1-4, N1-2, M0 WITH NO EVIDENCE OF DISEASE PROGRESSION, RECURRENCE, OR METASTASES (FOR USE IN A MEDICARE-APPROVED DEMONSTRATION PROJECT)	C	N	00	9		
G9087	ONCOLOGY; DISEASE STATUS; COLON CANCER, LIMITED TO INVASIVE CANCER, ADENOCARCINOMA AS PREDOMINANT CELL TYPE; M1 AT DIAGNOSIS, METASTATIC, LOCALLY RECURRENT, OR PROGRESSIVE WITH CURRENT CLINICAL, RADIOLOGIC, OR BIOCHEMICAL EVIDENCE OF DISEASE (FOR USE IN A MEDICARE-APPROVED DEMONSTRATION PROJECT)	C	N	00	9		
G9088	ONCOLOGY; DISEASE STATUS; COLON CANCER, LIMITED TO INVASIVE CANCER, ADENOCARCINOMA AS PREDOMINANT CELL TYPE; M1 AT DIAGNOSIS, METASTATIC, LOCALLY RECURRENT, OR PROGRESSIVE WITHOUT CURRENT CLINICAL, RADIOLOGIC, OR BIOCHEMICAL EVIDENCE OF DISEASE (FOR USE IN A MEDICARE-APPROVED DEMONSTRATION PROJECT)	C	N	00	9		
G9089	ONCOLOGY; DISEASE STATUS; COLON CANCER, LIMITED TO INVASIVE CANCER, ADENOCARCINOMA AS PREDOMINANT CELL TYPE; EXTENT OF DISEASE UNKNOWN, STAGING IN PROGRESS, OR NOT LISTED (FOR USE IN A MEDICARE-APPROVED DEMONSTRATION PROJECT)	C	N	00	9		
G9090	ONCOLOGY; DISEASE STATUS; RECTAL CANCER, LIMITED TO INVASIVE CANCER, ADENOCARCINOMA AS PREDOMINANT CELL TYPE; EXTENT OF DISEASE INITIALLY ESTABLISHED AS T1-2, N0, M0 (PRIOR TO NEO-ADJUVANT THERAPY, IF ANY) WITH NO EVIDENCE OF DISEASE PROGRESSION, RECURRENCE, OR METASTASES (FOR USE IN A MEDICARE-APPROVED DEMONSTRATION PROJECT)	C	N	00	9		
G9091	ONCOLOGY; DISEASE STATUS; RECTAL CANCER, LIMITED TO INVASIVE CANCER, ADENOCARCINOMA AS PREDOMINANT CELL TYPE; EXTENT OF DISEASE INITIALLY ESTABLISHED AS T3, N0, M0 (PRIOR TO NEO-ADJUVANT THERAPY, IF ANY) WITH NO EVIDENCE OF DISEASE PROGRESSION, RECURRENCE, OR METASTASES (FOR USE IN A MEDICARE-APPROVED DEMONSTRATION PROJECT)	C	N	00	9		
G9092	ONCOLOGY; DISEASE STATUS; RECTAL CANCER, LIMITED TO INVASIVE CANCER, ADENOCARCINOMA AS PREDOMINANT CELL TYPE; EXTENT OF DISEASE INITIALLY ESTABLISHED AS T1-3, N1-2, M0 (PRIOR TO NEO-ADJUVANT THERAPY, IF ANY) WITH NO EVIDENCE OF DISEASE PROGRESSION, RECURRENCE OR METASTASES (FOR USE IN A MEDICARE-APPROVED DEMONSTRATION PROJECT)	C	N	00	9		

HCPCS Code	Statute	Lab Cert	X-Ref	ASC Pay Grp	ASC Pay Group Eff. Date	Proc Notes	BETOS	TOS	Anest	Code Add Date	Code Effective Date	Code Term Date
G9086							P7B	1	0	20060101	20070101	
G9087							P7B	1	0	20060101	20070101	
G9088							P7B	1	0	20060101	20070101	
G9089							P7B	1	0	20060101	20070101	
G9090							P7B	1	0	20060101	20070101	
G9091							P7B	1	0	20060101	20070101	
G9092							P7B	1	0	20060101	20070101	
G9092							P7B	1	0			

HCPCS Code	Long Description	Coverage	Action	PI	MPI	CIM	MCM
G9093	ONCOLOGY; DISEASE STATUS; RECTAL CANCER, LIMITED TO INVASIVE CANCER, ADENOCARCINOMA AS PREDOMINANT CELL TYPE; EXTENT OF DISEASE INITIALLY ESTABLISHED AS T4, ANY N, M0 (PRIOR TO NEO-ADJUVANT THERAPY, IF ANY) WITH NO EVIDENCE OF DISEASE PROGRESSION, RECURRENCE, OR METASTASES (FOR USE IN A MEDICARE-APPROVED DEMONSTRATION PROJECT)	C	N	00	9		
G9094	ONCOLOGY; DISEASE STATUS; RECTAL CANCER, LIMITED TO INVASIVE CANCER, ADENOCARCINOMA AS PREDOMINANT CELL TYPE; M1 AT DIAGNOSIS, METASTATIC, LOCALLY RECURRENT, OR PROGRESSIVE (FOR USE IN A MEDICARE-APPROVED DEMONSTRATION PROJECT)	C	N	00	9		
G9095	ONCOLOGY; DISEASE STATUS; RECTAL CANCER, LIMITED TO INVASIVE CANCER, ADENOCARCINOMA AS PREDOMINANT CELL TYPE; EXTENT OF DISEASE UNKNOWN, STAGING IN PROGRESS, OR NOT LISTED (FOR USE IN A MEDICARE-APPROVED DEMONSTRATION PROJECT)	C	N	00	9		
G9096	ONCOLOGY; DISEASE STATUS; ESOPHAGEAL CANCER, LIMITED TO ADENOCARCINOMA OR SQUAMOUS CELL CARCINOMA AS PREDOMINANT CELL TYPE; EXTENT OF DISEASE INITIALLY ESTABLISHED AS T1-T3, N0-N1 OR NX (PRIOR TO NEO-ADJUVANT THERAPY, IF ANY) WITH NO EVIDENCE OF DISEASE PROGRESSION, RECURRENCE, OR METASTASES (FOR USE IN A MEDICARE-APPROVED DEMONSTRATION PROJECT)	C	N	00	9		
G9097	ONCOLOGY; DISEASE STATUS; ESOPHAGEAL CANCER, LIMITED TO ADENOCARCINOMA OR SQUAMOUS CELL CARCINOMA AS PREDOMINANT CELL TYPE; EXTENT OF DISEASE INITIALLY ESTABLISHED AS T4, ANY N, M0 (PRIOR TO NEO-ADJUVANT THERAPY, IF ANY) WITH NO EVIDENCE OF DISEASE PROGRESSION, RECURRENCE, OR METASTASES (FOR USE IN A MEDICARE-APPROVED DEMONSTRATION PROJECT)	C	N	00	9		
G9098	ONCOLOGY; DISEASE STATUS; ESOPHAGEAL CANCER, LIMITED TO ADENOCARCINOMA OR SQUAMOUS CELL CARCINOMA AS PREDOMINANT CELL TYPE; M1 AT DIAGNOSIS, METASTATIC, LOCALLY RECURRENT, OR PROGRESSIVE (FOR USE IN A MEDICARE-APPROVED DEMONSTRATION PROJECT)	C	N	00	9		
G9099	ONCOLOGY; DISEASE STATUS; ESOPHAGEAL CANCER, LIMITED TO ADENOCARCINOMA OR SQUAMOUS CELL CARCINOMA AS PREDOMINANT CELL TYPE; EXTENT OF DISEASE UNKNOWN, STAGING IN PROGRESS, OR NOT LISTED (FOR USE IN A MEDICARE-APPROVED DEMONSTRATION PROJECT)	C	N	00	9		
G9100	ONCOLOGY; DISEASE STATUS; GASTRIC CANCER, LIMITED TO ADENOCARCINOMA AS PREDOMINANT CELL TYPE; POST R0 RESECTION (WITH OR WITHOUT NEOADJUVANT THERAPY) WITH NO EVIDENCE OF DISEASE RECURRENCE, PROGRESSION, OR METASTASES (FOR USE IN A MEDICARE-APPROVED DEMONSTRATION PROJECT)	C	N	00	9		

HCPCS Code	Statute	Lab Cert	X-Ref	ASC Pay Grp	ASC Pay Group Eff. Date	Proc Notes	BETOS	TOS	Anest	Code Add Date	Code Effective Date	Code Term Date
G9093							P7B	1	0	20060101	20070101	
G9093 G9094							P7B	1	0	20060101	20070101	
G9095							P7B	1	0	20060101	20070101	
G9096							P7B	1	0	20060101	20070101	
G9097							P7B	1	0	20060101	20070101	
G9098							P7B	1	0	20060101	20070101	
G9099							P7B	1	0	20060101	20070101	
G9100							P7B	1	0	20060101	20070101	
G9100												

HCPCS Code	Long Description	Coverage	Action	PI	MPI	CIM	MCM
G9101	ONCOLOGY; DISEASE STATUS; GASTRIC CANCER, LIMITED TO ADENOCARCINOMA AS PREDOMINANT CELL TYPE; POST R1 OR R2 RESECTION (WITH OR WITHOUT NEOADJUVANT THERAPY) WITH NO EVIDENCE OF DISEASE PROGRESSION, OR METASTASES (FOR USE IN A MEDICARE-APPROVED DEMONSTRATION PROJECT)	C	N	00	9		
G9102	ONCOLOGY; DISEASE STATUS; GASTRIC CANCER, LIMITED TO ADENOCARCINOMA ASPREDOMINANT CELL TYPE; CLINICAL OR PATHOLOGIC M0, UNRESECTABLE WITH NO EVIDENCE OF DISEASE PROGRESSION, OR METASTASES (FOR USE IN A MEDICARE-APPROVED DEMONSTRATION PROJECT)	C	N	00	9		
G9103	ONCOLOGY; DISEASE STATUS; GASTRIC CANCER, LIMITED TO ADENOCARCINOMA AS PREDOMINANT CELL TYPE; CLINICAL OR PATHOLOGIC M1 AT DIAGNOSIS, METASTATIC, LOCALLY RECURRENT, OR PROGRESSIVE (FOR USE IN A MEDICARE-APPROVED DEMONSTRATION PROJECT)	C	N	00	9		
G9104	ONCOLOGY; DISEASE STATUS; GASTRIC CANCER, LIMITED TO ADENOCARCINOMA AS PREDOMINANT CELL TYPE; EXTENT OF DISEASE UNKNOWN, STAGING IN PROGRESS, OR NOT LISTED (FOR USE IN A MEDICARE-APPROVED DEMONSTRATION PROJECT)	C	N	00	9		
G9105	ONCOLOGY; DISEASE STATUS; PANCREATIC CANCER, LIMITED TO ADENOCARCINOMA AS PREDOMINANT CELL TYPE; POST R0 RESECTION WITHOUT EVIDENCE OF DISEASE PROGRESSION, RECURRENCE, OR METASTASES (FOR USE IN A MEDICARE-APPROVED DEMONSTRATION PROJECT)	C	N	00	9		
G9106	ONCOLOGY; DISEASE STATUS; PANCREATIC CANCER, LIMITED TO ADENOCARCINOMA; POST R1 OR R2 RESECTION WITH NO EVIDENCE OF DISEASE PROGRESSION, OR METASTASES (FOR USE IN A MEDICARE-APPROVED DEMONSTRATION PROJECT)	C	N	00	9		
G9107	ONCOLOGY; DISEASE STATUS; PANCREATIC CANCER, LIMITED TO ADENOCARCINOMA; UNRESECTABLE AT DIAGNOSIS, M1 AT DIAGNOSIS, METASTATIC, LOCALLY RECURRENT, OR PROGRESSIVE (FOR USE IN A MEDICARE-APPROVED DEMONSTRATION PROJECT)	C	N	00	9		
G9108	ONCOLOGY; DISEASE STATUS; PANCREATIC CANCER, LIMITED TO ADENOCARCINOMA; EXTENT OF DISEASE UNKNOWN, STAGING IN PROGRESS, OR NOT LISTED (FOR USE IN A MEDICARE-APPROVED DEMONSTRATION PROJECT)	C	N	00	9		
G9109	ONCOLOGY; DISEASE STATUS; HEAD AND NECK CANCER, LIMITED TO CANCERS OF ORAL CAVITY, PHARYNX AND LARYNX WITH SQUAMOUS CELL AS PREDOMINANT CELL TYPE; EXTENT OF DISEASE INITIALLY ESTABLISHED AS T1-T2 AND N0, M0 (PRIOR TO NEO-ADJUVANT THERAPY, IF ANY) WITH NO EVIDENCE OF DISEASE PROGRESSION, RECURRENCE, OR METASTASES (FOR USE IN A MEDICARE-APPROVED DEMONSTRATION PROJECT)	C	N	00	9		

HCPCS Code	Statute	Lab Cert	X-Ref	ASC Pay Grp	ASC Pay Group Eff. Date	Proc Notes	BETOS	TOS	Anest	Code Add Date	Code Effective Date	Code Term Date
G9101							P7B	1	0	20060101	20070101	
G9102							P7B	1	0	20060101	20070101	
G9103							P7B	1	0	20060101	20070101	
G9104							P7B	1	0	20060101	20070101	
G9105							P7B	1	0	20060101	20070101	
G9106							P7B	1	0	20060101	20070101	
G9107							P7B	1	0	20060101	20070101	
G9108							P7B	1	0	20060101	20070101	
G9109							P7B	1	0	20060101	20070101	

HCPCS Code	Long Description	Coverage	Action	PI	MPI	CIM	MCM
G9110	ONCOLOGY; DISEASE STATUS; HEAD AND NECK CANCER, LIMITED TO CANCERS OF ORAL CAVITY, PHARYNX AND LARYNX WITH SQUAMOUS CELL AS PREDOMINANT CELL TYPE; EXTENT OF DISEASE INITIALLY ESTABLISHED AS T3-4 AND/OR N1-3, M0 (PRIOR TO NEO-ADJUVANT THERAPY, IF ANY) WITH NO EVIDENCE OF DISEASE PROGRESSION, RECURRENCE, OR METASTASES (FOR USE IN A MEDICARE-APPROVED DEMONSTRATION PROJECT)	C	N	00	9		
G9111	ONCOLOGY; DISEASE STATUS; HEAD AND NECK CANCER, LIMITED TO CANCERS OF ORAL CAVITY, PHARYNX AND LARYNX WITH SQUAMOUS CELL AS PREDOMINANT CELL TYPE; M1 AT DIAGNOSIS, METASTATIC, LOCALLY RECURRENT, OR PROGRESSIVE (FOR USE IN A MEDICARE-APPROVED DEMONSTRATION PROJECT)	C	N	00	9		
G9112	ONCOLOGY; DISEASE STATUS; HEAD AND NECK CANCER, LIMITED TO CANCERS OF ORAL CAVITY, PHARYNX AND LARYNX WITH SQUAMOUS CELL AS PREDOMINANT CELL TYPE; EXTENT OF DISEASE UNKNOWN, STAGING IN PROGRESS, OR NOT LISTED (FOR USE IN A MEDICARE-APPROVED DEMONSTRATION PROJECT)	C	N	00	9		
G9113	ONCOLOGY; DISEASE STATUS; OVARIAN CANCER, LIMITED TO EPITHELIAL CANCER; PATHOLOGIC STAGE IA-B (GRADE 1) WITHOUT EVIDENCE OF DISEASE PROGRESSION, RECURRENCE, OR METASTASES (FOR USE IN A MEDICARE-APPROVED DEMONSTRATION PROJECT)	C	N	00	9		
G9114	ONCOLOGY; DISEASE STATUS; OVARIAN CANCER, LIMITED TO EPITHELIAL CANCER; PATHOLOGIC STAGE IA-B (GRADE 2-3); OR STAGE IC (ALL GRADES); OR STAGE II; WITHOUT EVIDENCE OF DISEASE PROGRESSION, RECURRENCE, OR METASTASES (FOR USE IN A MEDICARE-APPROVED DEMONSTRATION PROJECT)	C	N	00	9		
G9115	ONCOLOGY; DISEASE STATUS; OVARIAN CANCER, LIMITED TO EPITHELIAL CANCER; PATHOLOGIC STAGE III-IV; WITHOUT EVIDENCE OF PROGRESSION, RECURRENCE, OR METASTASES (FOR USE IN A MEDICARE-APPROVED DEMONSTRATION PROJECT)	C	N	00	9		
G9116	ONCOLOGY; DISEASE STATUS; OVARIAN CANCER, LIMITED TO EPITHELIAL CANCER; EVIDENCE OF DISEASE PROGRESSION, OR RECURRENCE, AND/OR PLATINUM RESISTANCE (FOR USE IN A MEDICARE-APPROVED DEMONSTRATION PROJECT)	C	N	00	9		
G9117	ONCOLOGY; DISEASE STATUS; OVARIAN CANCER, LIMITED TO EPITHELIAL CANCER; EXTENT OF DISEASE UNKNOWN, STAGING IN PROGRESS, OR NOT LISTED (FOR USE IN A MEDICARE-APPROVED DEMONSTRATION PROJECT)	C	N	00	9		
G9118	ONCOLOGY; DISEASE STATUS; NON-HODGKIN'S LYMPHOMA, LIMITED TO FOLLICULAR LYMPHOMA, MANTLE CELL LYMPHOMA, DIFFUSE LARGE B-CELL LYMPHOMA, SMALL LYMPHOCYTIC LYMPHOMA; STAGE I, II AT DIAGNOSIS, NOT RELAPSED, NOT REFRACTORY (FOR USE IN A MEDICARE-APPROVED DEMONSTRATION PROJECT)	C	N	13	A		

HCPCS Code	Statute	Lab Cert	X-Ref	ASC Pay Grp	ASC Pay Group Eff. Date	Proc Notes	BETOS	TOS	Anest	Code Add Date	Code Effective Date	Code Term Date
G9110							P7B	1	0	20060101	20070101	
G9111							P7B	1	0	20060101	20070101	
G9112							P7B	1	0	20060101	20070101	
G9113							P7B	1	0	20060101	20070101	
G9114							P7B	1	0	20060101	20070101	
G9115							P7B	1	0	20060101	20070101	
G9116							P7B	1	0	20060101	20070101	
G9117							P7B	1	0	20060101	20070101	
G9118							P7B	1	0	20060101	20070101	20061231

HCPCS Code	Long Description	Coverage	Action	PI	MPI	CIM	MCM
G9119	ONCOLOGY; DISEASE STATUS; NON-HODGKIN'S LYMPHOMA, LIMITED TO FOLLICULAR LYMPHOMA, MANTLE CELL LYMPHOMA, DIFFUSE LARGE B-CELL LYMPHOMA, SMALL LYMPHOCYTIC LYMPHOMA; STAGE III, IV NOT RELAPSED, NOT REFRACTORY (FOR USE IN A MEDICARE-APPROVED DEMONSTRATION PROJECT)	C	N	13	A		
G9120	ONCOLOGY; DISEASE STATUS; NON-HODGKIN'S LYMPHOMA; TRANSFORMED FROM FOLLICULAR LYMPHOMA TO DIFFUSE LARGE B-CELL LYMPHOMA (FOR USE IN A MEDICARE-APPROVED DEMONSTRATION PROJECT)	C	N	13	A		
G9121	ONCOLOGY; DISEASE STATUS; NON-HODGKIN'S LYMPHOMA, LIMITED TO FOLLICULAR LYMPHOMA, MANTLE CELL LYMPHOMA, DIFFUSE LARGE B-CELL LYMPHOMA, SMALL LYMPHOCYTIC LYMPHOMA; RELAPSED/REFRACTORY (FOR USE IN A MEDICARE-APPROVED DEMONSTRATION PROJECT)	C	N	13	A		
G9122	ONCOLOGY; DISEASE STATUS; NON-HODGKIN'S LYMPHOMA, LIMITED TO FOLLICULAR LYMPHOMA, MANTLE CELL LYMPHOMA, DIFFUSE LARGE B-CELL LYMPHOMA, SMALL LYMPHOCYTIC LYMPHOMA; DIAGNOSTIC EVALUATION, STAGE NOT DETERMINED, EVALUATION OF POSSIBLE RELAPSE OR NON-RESPONSE TO THERAPY, OR NOT LISTED (FOR USE IN A MEDICARE-APPROVED DEMONSTRATION PROJECT)	C	N	13	A		
G9123	ONCOLOGY; DISEASE STATUS; CHRONIC MYELOGENOUS LEUKEMIA, LIMITED TO PHILADELPHIA CHROMOSOME POSITIVE AND/OR BCR-ABL POSITIVE; CHRONIC PHASE NOT IN HEMATOLOGIC, CYTOGENETIC, OR MOLECULAR REMISSION (FOR USE IN A MEDICARE-APPROVED DEMONSTRATION PROJECT)	C	N	00	9		
G9124	ONCOLOGY; DISEASE STATUS; CHRONIC MYELOGENOUS LEUKEMIA, LIMITED TO PHILADELPHIA CHROMOSOME POSITIVE AND/OR BCR-ABL POSITIVE; ACCELERATED PHASE NOT IN HEMATOLOGIC CYTOGENETIC, OR MOLECULAR REMISSION (FOR USE IN A MEDICARE-APPROVED DEMONSTRATION PROJECT)	C	N	00	9		
G9125	ONCOLOGY; DISEASE STATUS; CHRONIC MYELOGENOUS LEUKEMIA, LIMITED TO PHILADELPHIA CHROMOSOME POSITIVE AND/OR BCR-ABL POSITIVE; BLAST PHASE NOT IN HEMATOLOGIC, CYTOGENETIC, OR MOLECULAR REMISSION (FOR USE IN A MEDICARE-APPROVED DEMONSTRATION PROJECT)	C	N	00	9		
G9126	ONCOLOGY; DISEASE STATUS; CHRONIC MYELOGENOUS LEUKEMIA, LIMITED TO PHILADELPHIA CHROMOSOME POSITIVE AND/OR BCR-ABL POSITIVE; IN HEMATOLOGIC, CYTOGENETIC, OR MOLECULAR REMISSION (FOR USE IN A MEDICARE-APPROVED DEMONSTRATION PROJECT)	C	N	00	9		
G9127	ONCOLOGY; DISEASE STATUS; CHRONIC MYELOGENOUS LEUKEMIA, LIMITED TO PHILADELPHIA CHROMOSOME POSITIVE AND/OR BCR-ABL POSITIVE; EXTENT OF DISEASE UNKNOWN, UNDER EVALUATION, NOT LISTED (FOR USE IN A MEDICARE-APPROVED DEMONSTRATION PROJECT)	C	N	13	A		

HCPCS Code	Statute	Lab Cert	X-Ref	ASC Pay Grp	ASC Pay Group Eff. Date	Proc Notes	BETOS	TOS	Anest	Code Add Date	Code Effective Date	Code Term Date
G9119							P7B	1	0	20060101	20070101	20061231
G9120							P7B	1	0	20060101	20070101	20061231
G9121							P7B	1	0	20060101	20070101	20061231
G9122							P7B	1	0	20060101	20070101	20061231
G9123							P7B	1	0	20060101	20070101	
G9124							P7B	1	0	20060101	20070101	
G9125							P7B	1	0	20060101	20070101	
G9126							P7B	1	0	20060101	20070101	
G9127							P7B	1	0	20060101	20070101	20061231
G9127												

HCPCS Code	Long Description	Coverage	Action	PI	MPI	CIM	MCM
G9128	ONCOLOGY; DISEASE STATUS; LIMITED TO MULTIPLE MYELOMA, SYSTEMIC DISEASE; SMOLDERING, STAGE I (FOR USE IN A MEDICARE-APPROVED DEMONSTRATION PROJECT)	C	N	00	9		
G9129	ONCOLOGY; DISEASE STATUS; LIMITED TO MULTIPLE MYELOMA, SYSTEMIC DISEASE; STAGE II OR HIGHER (FOR USE IN A MEDICARE-APPROVED DEMONSTRATION PROJECT)	C	N	00	9		
G9130	ONCOLOGY; DISEASE STATUS; LIMITED TO MULTIPLE MYELOMA, SYSTEMIC DISEASE; EXTENT OF DISEASE UNKNOWN, STAGING IN PROGRESS, OR NOT LISTED (FOR USE IN A MEDICARE-APPROVED DEMONSTRATION PROJECT)	C	N	00	9		
G9131	ONCOLOGY; DISEASE STATUS; INVASIVE FEMALE BREAST CANCER (DOES NOT INCLUDE DUCTAL CARCINOMA IN SITU); ADENOCARCINOMA AS PREDOMINANT CELL TYPE; EXTENT OF DISEASE UNKNOWN, STAGING IN PROGRESS, OR NOT LISTED (FOR USE IN A MEDICARE-APPROVED DEMONSTRATION PROJECT)	C	N	00	9		
G9132	ONCOLOGY; DISEASE STATUS; PROSTATE CANCER, LIMITED TO ADENOCARCINOMA; HORMONE-REFRACTORY/ ANDROGEN-INDEPENDENT (E.G., RISING PSA ON ANTI-ANDROGEN THERAPY OR POST-ORCHIECTOMY); CLINICAL METASTASES (FOR USE IN A MEDICARE-APPROVED DEMONSTRATION PROJECT)	C	N	00	9		
G9133	ONCOLOGY; DISEASE STATUS; PROSTATE CANCER, LIMITED TO ADENOCARCINOMA; HORMONE-RESPONSIVE; CLINICAL METASTASES OR M1 AT DIAGNOSIS (FOR USE IN A MEDICARE-APPROVED DEMONSTRATION PROJECT)	C	N	00	9		
G9134	ONCOLOGY; DISEASE STATUS; NON-HODGKIN'S LYMPHOMA, ANY CELLULAR CLASSIFICATION; STAGE I, II AT DIAGNOSIS, NOT RELAPSED, NOT REFRACTORY (FOR USE IN A MEDICARE-APPROVED DEMONSTRATION PROJECT)	C	N	00	9		
G9135	ONCOLOGY; DISEASE STATUS; NON-HODGKIN'S LYMPHOMA, ANY CELLULAR CLASSIFICATION; STAGE III, IV, NOT RELAPSED, NOT REFRACTORY (FOR USE IN A MEDICARE-APPROVED DEMONSTRATION PROJECT)	C	N	00	9		
G9136	ONCOLOGY; DISEASE STATUS; NON-HODGKIN'S LYMPHOMA, TRANSFORMED FROM ORIGINAL CELLULAR DIAGNOSIS TO A SECOND CELLULAR CLASSIFICATION (FOR USE IN A MEDICARE-APPROVED DEMONSTRATION PROJECT)	C	N	00	9		
G9137	ONCOLOGY; DISEASE STATUS; NON-HODGKIN'S LYMPHOMA, ANY CELLULAR CLASSIFICATION; RELAPSED/REFRACTORY (FOR USE IN A MEDICARE-APPROVED DEMONSTRATION PROJECT)	C	N	00	9		
G9138	ONCOLOGY; DISEASE STATUS; NON-HODGKIN'S LYMPHOMA, ANY CELLULAR CLASSIFICATION; DIAGNOSTIC EVALUATION, STAGE NOT DETERMINED, EVALUATION OF POSSIBLE RELAPSE OR NON-RESPONSE TO THERAPY, OR NOT LISTED (FOR USE IN A MEDICARE-APPROVED DEMONSTRATION PROJECT)	C	N	00	9		

HCPCS Code	Statute	Lab Cert	X-Ref	ASC Pay Grp	ASC Pay Group Eff. Date	Proc Notes	BETOS	TOS	Anest	Code Add Date	Code Effective Date	Code Term Date
G9128							P7B	1	0	20060101	20070101	
G9129							P7B	1	0	20060101	20070101	
G9130							P7B	1	0	20060101	20070101	
G9131							P7B	1	0	20070101	20070101	
G9132							P7B	1	0	20070101	20070101	
G9133							P7B	1	0	20070101	20070101	
G9134							P7B	1	0	20070101	20070101	
G9135							P7B	1	0	20070101	20070101	
G9136							P7B	1	0	20070101	20070101	
G9137							P7B	1	0	20070101	20070101	
G9138							P7B	1	0	20070101	20070101	
G9138												

HCPCS Code	Long Description	Coverage	Action	PI	MPI	CIM	MCM
G9139	ONCOLOGY; DISEASE STATUS; CHRONIC MYELOGENOUS LEUKEMIA, LIMITED TO PHILADELPHIA CHROMOSOME POSITIVE AND/OR BCR-ABL POSITIVE; EXTENT OF DISEASE UNKNOWN, STAGING IN PROGRESS, NOT LISTED (FOR USE IN A MEDICARE-APPROVED DEMONSTRATION PROJECT)	C	N	00	9		
G9140	FRONTIER EXTENDED STAY CLINIC DEMONSTRATION; FOR A PATIENT STAY IN A CLINIC APPROVED FOR THE CMS DEMONSTRATION PROJECT; THE FOLLOWING MEASURES SHOULD BE PRESENT: THE STAY MUST BE EQUAL TO OR GREATER THAN 4 HOURS; WEATHER OR OTHER CONDITIONS MUST PREVENT TRANSFER OR THE CASE FALLS INTO A CATEGORY OF MONITORING AND OBSERVATION CASES THAT ARE PERMITTED BY THE RULES OF THE DEMONSTRATION; THERE IS A MAXIMUM FRONTIER EXTENDED STAY CLINIC (FESC) VISIT OF 48 HOURS, EXCEPT IN THE CASE WHEN WEATHER OR OTHER CONDITIONS PREVENT TRANSFER; PAYMENT IS MADE ON EACH PERIOD UP TO 4 HOURS, AFTER THE FIRST 4 HOURS	C	N	00	9		
G9141	INFLUENZA A (H1N1) IMMUNIZATION ADMINISTRATION (INCLUDES THE PHYSICIAN COUNSELING THE PATIENT/FAMILY)	C	A	13	A		
G9142	INFLUENZA A (H1N1) VACCINE, ANY ROUTE OF ADMINISTRATION	C	A	13	A		
G9143	WARFARIN RESPONSIVENESS TESTING BY GENETIC TECHNIQUE USING ANY METHOD, ANY NUMBER OF SPECIMEN(S)	C	A	13	A		
H0001	ALCOHOL AND/OR DRUG ASSESSMENT	I	N	00	9		
H0002	BEHAVIORAL HEALTH SCREENING TO DETERMINE ELIGIBILITY FOR ADMISSION TO TREATMENT PROGRAM	I	N	00	9		
H0003	ALCOHOL AND/OR DRUG SCREENING; LABORATORY ANALYSIS OF SPECIMENS FOR PRESENCE OF ALCOHOL AND/OR DRUGS	I	N	00	9		
H0004	BEHAVIORAL HEALTH COUNSELING AND THERAPY, PER 15 MINUTES	I	N	00	9		
H0005	ALCOHOL AND/OR DRUG SERVICES; GROUP COUNSELING BY A CLINICIAN	I	N	00	9		
H0006	ALCOHOL AND/OR DRUG SERVICES; CASE MANAGEMENT	I	N	00	9		
H0007	ALCOHOL AND/OR DRUG SERVICES; CRISIS INTERVENTION (OUTPATIENT)	I	N	00	9		
H0008	ALCOHOL AND/OR DRUG SERVICES; SUB-ACUTE DETOXIFICATION (HOSPITAL INPATIENT)	I	N	00	9		
H0009	ALCOHOL AND/OR DRUG SERVICES; ACUTE DETOXIFICATION (HOSPITAL INPATIENT)	I	N	00	9		
H0010	ALCOHOL AND/OR DRUG SERVICES; SUB-ACUTE DETOXIFICATION (RESIDENTIAL ADDICTION PROGRAM INPATIENT)	I	N	00	9		
H0011	ALCOHOL AND/OR DRUG SERVICES; ACUTE DETOXIFICATION (RESIDENTIAL ADDICTION PROGRAM INPATIENT)	I	N	00	9		
H0012	ALCOHOL AND/OR DRUG SERVICES; SUB-ACUTE DETOXIFICATION (RESIDENTIAL ADDICTION PROGRAM OUTPATIENT)	I	N	00	9		

HCPCS Code	Statute	Lab Cert	X-Ref	ASC Pay Grp	ASC Pay Group Eff. Date	Proc Notes	BETOS	TOS	Anest	Code Add Date	Code Effective Date	Code Term Date
G9139							P7B	1	0	20070101	20070101	
G9140							Z2	1	0	20071001	20071001	
G9141							O1G	1	0	20090901	20090901	
G9142							O1G	1	0	20090901	20090901	
G9143							M5D	1	0	20090803	20090803	
H0001							Z2	9	0	20010101	20010101	
H0002							Z2	9	0	20010101	20030101	
H0003							Z2	9	0	20010101	20010101	
H0004							Z2	9	0	20010101	20030101	
H0005							Z2	9	0	20010101	20010101	
H0006							Z2	9	0	20010101	20010101	
H0007							Z2	9	0	20010101	20010101	
H0008							Z2	9	0	20010101	20010101	
H0009							Z2	9	0	20010101	20010101	
H0010							Z2	9	0	20010101	20010101	
H0011							Z2	9	0	20010101	20010101	
H0012							Z2	9	0	20010101	20010101	

HCPCS Code	Long Description	Coverage	Action	PI	MPI	CIM	MCM
H0013	ALCOHOL AND/OR DRUG SERVICES; ACUTE DETOXIFICATION (RESIDENTIAL ADDICTION PROGRAM OUTPATIENT)	I	N	00	9		
H0014	ALCOHOL AND/OR DRUG SERVICES; AMBULATORY DETOXIFICATION	I	N	00	9		
H0015	ALCOHOL AND/OR DRUG SERVICES; INTENSIVE OUTPATIENT (TREATMENT PROGRAM THAT OPERATES AT LEAST 3 HOURS/DAY AND AT LEAST 3 DAYS/WEEK AND IS BASED ON AN INDIVIDUALIZED TREATMENT PLAN), INCLUDING ASSESSMENT, COUNSELING; CRISIS INTERVENTION, AND ACTIVITY THERAPIES OR EDUCATION	I	N	00	9		
H0016	ALCOHOL AND/OR DRUG SERVICES; MEDICAL/SOMATIC (MEDICAL INTERVENTION IN AMBULATORY SETTING)	I	N	00	9		
H0017	BEHAVIORAL HEALTH; RESIDENTIAL (HOSPITAL RESIDENTIAL TREATMENT PROGRAM),WITHOUT ROOM AND BOARD, PER DIEM	I	N	00	9		
H0018	BEHAVIORAL HEALTH; SHORT-TERM RESIDENTIAL (NON-HOSPITAL RESIDENTIAL TREATMENT PROGRAM), WITHOUT ROOM AND BOARD, PER DIEM	I	N	00	9		
H0019	BEHAVIORAL HEALTH; LONG-TERM RESIDENTIAL (NON-MEDICAL, NON-ACUTE CARE IN A RESIDENTIAL TREATMENT PROGRAM WHERE STAY IS TYPICALLY LONGER THAN 30 DAYS), WITHOUT ROOM AND BOARD, PER DIEM	I	N	00	9		
H0020	ALCOHOL AND/OR DRUG SERVICES; METHADONE ADMINISTRATION AND/OR SERVICE (PROVISION OF THE DRUG BY A LICENSED PROGRAM)	I	N	00	9		
H0021	ALCOHOL AND/OR DRUG TRAINING SERVICE (FOR STAFF AND PERSONNEL NOT EMPLOYED BY PROVIDERS)	I	N	00	9		
H0022	ALCOHOL AND/OR DRUG INTERVENTION SERVICE (PLANNED FACILITATION)	I	N	00	9		
H0023	BEHAVIORAL HEALTH OUTREACH SERVICE (PLANNED APPROACH TO REACH A TARGETED POPULATION)	I	N	00	9		
H0024	BEHAVIORAL HEALTH PREVENTION INFORMATION DISSEMINATION SERVICE (ONE-WAY DIRECT OR NON-DIRECT CONTACT WITH SERVICE AUDIENCES TO AFFECT KNOWLEDGE AND ATTITUDE)	I	N	00	9		
H0025	BEHAVIORAL HEALTH PREVENTION EDUCATION SERVICE (DELIVERY OF SERVICES WITH TARGET POPULATION TO AFFECT KNOWLEDGE, ATTITUDE AND/OR BEHAVIOR)	I	N	00	9		
H0026	ALCOHOL AND/OR DRUG PREVENTION PROCESS SERVICE, COMMUNITY-BASED (DELIVERY OF SERVICES TO DEVELOP SKILLS OF IMPACTORS)	I	N	00	9		
H0027	ALCOHOL AND/OR DRUG PREVENTION ENVIRONMENTAL SERVICE (BROAD RANGE OF EXTERNAL ACTIVITIES GEARED TOWARD MODIFYING SYSTEMS IN ORDER TO MAINSTREAM PREVENTION THROUGH POLICY AND LAW)	I	N	00	9		
H0028	ALCOHOL AND/OR DRUG PREVENTION PROBLEM IDENTIFICATION AND REFERRAL SERVICE (E.G. STUDENT ASSISTANCE AND EMPLOYEE ASSISTANCE PROGRAMS), DOES NOT INCLUDE ASSESSMENT	I	N	00	9		

HCPCS Code	Statute	Lab Cert	X-Ref	ASC Pay Grp	ASC Pay Group Eff. Date	Proc Notes	BETOS	TOS	Anest	Code Add Date	Code Effective Date	Code Term Date
H0013							Z2	9	0	20010101	20010101	
H0014							Z2	9	0	20010101	20010101	
H0015							Z2	9	0	20010101	20010101	
H0016							Z2	9	0	20010101	20010101	
H0017							Z2	9	0	20010101	20030101	
H0018							Z2	9	0	20010101	20030101	
H0019							Z2	9	0	20010101	20030101	
H0020							Z2	9	0	20010101	20010101	
H0021							Z2	9	0	20010101	20010101	
H0022							Z2	9	0	20010101	20010101	
H0023							Z2	9	0	20010101	20030101	
H0024							Z2	9	0	20010101	20030101	
H0025							Z2	9	0	20010101	20030101	
H0026							Z2	9	0	20010101	20010101	
H0027							Z2	9	0	20010101	20010101	
H0028							Z2	9	0	20010101	20010101	
H0028							Z2	9	0			

HCPCS Code	Long Description	Coverage	Action	PI	MPI	CIM	MCM
H0029	ALCOHOL AND/OR DRUG PREVENTION ALTERNATIVES SERVICE (SERVICES FOR POPULATIONS THAT EXCLUDE ALCOHOL AND OTHER DRUG USE E.G. ALCOHOL FREE SOCIAL EVENTS)	I	N	00	9		
H0030	BEHAVIORAL HEALTH HOTLINE SERVICE	I	N	00	9		
H0031	MENTAL HEALTH ASSESSMENT, BY NON-PHYSICIAN	I	N	00	9		
H0032	MENTAL HEALTH SERVICE PLAN DEVELOPMENT BY NON-PHYSICIAN	I	N	00	9		
H0033	ORAL MEDICATION ADMINISTRATION, DIRECT OBSERVATION	I	N	00	9		
H0034	MEDICATION TRAINING AND SUPPORT, PER 15 MINUTES	I	N	00	9		
H0035	MENTAL HEALTH PARTIAL HOSPITALIZATION, TREATMENT, LESS THAN 24 HOURS	I	N	00	9		
H0036	COMMUNITY PSYCHIATRIC SUPPORTIVE TREATMENT, FACE-TO-FACE, PER 15 MINUTES	I	N	00	9		
H0037	COMMUNITY PSYCHIATRIC SUPPORTIVE TREATMENT PROGRAM, PER DIEM	I	N	00	9		
H0038	SELF-HELP/PEER SERVICES, PER 15 MINUTES	I	N	00	9		
H0039	ASSERTIVE COMMUNITY TREATMENT, FACE-TO-FACE, PER 15 MINUTES	I	N	00	9		
H0040	ASSERTIVE COMMUNITY TREATMENT PROGRAM, PER DIEM	I	N	00	9		
H0041	FOSTER CARE, CHILD, NON-THERAPEUTIC, PER DIEM	I	N	00	9		
H0042	FOSTER CARE, CHILD, NON-THERAPEUTIC, PER MONTH	I	N	00	9		
H0043	SUPPORTED HOUSING, PER DIEM	I	N	00	9		
H0044	SUPPORTED HOUSING, PER MONTH	I	N	00	9		
H0045	RESPITE CARE SERVICES, NOT IN THE HOME, PER DIEM	I	N	00	9		
H0046	MENTAL HEALTH SERVICES, NOT OTHERWISE SPECIFIED	I	N	00	9		
H0047	ALCOHOL AND/OR OTHER DRUG ABUSE SERVICES, NOT OTHERWISE SPECIFIED	I	N	00	9		
H0048	ALCOHOL AND/OR OTHER DRUG TESTING: COLLECTION AND HANDLING ONLY, SPECIMENS OTHER THAN BLOOD	I	N	00	9		
H0049	ALCOHOL AND/OR DRUG SCREENING	I	N	00	9		
H0050	ALCOHOL AND/OR DRUG SERVICES, BRIEF INTERVENTION, PER 15 MINUTES	I	N	00	9		
H1000	PRENATAL CARE, AT-RISK ASSESSMENT	I	N	00	9		
H1001	PRENATAL CARE, AT-RISK ENHANCED SERVICE; ANTEPARTUM MANAGEMENT	I	N	00	9		
H1002	PRENATAL CARE, AT RISK ENHANCED SERVICE; CARE COORDINATION	I	N	00	9		
H1003	PRENATAL CARE, AT-RISK ENHANCED SERVICE; EDUCATION	I	N	00	9		
H1004	PRENATAL CARE, AT-RISK ENHANCED SERVICE; FOLLOW-UP HOME VISIT	I	N	00	9		
H1005	PRENATAL CARE, AT-RISK ENHANCED SERVICE PACKAGE (INCLUDES H1001-H1004)	I	N	00	9		
H1010	NON-MEDICAL FAMILY PLANNING EDUCATION, PER SESSION	I	N	00	9		
H1011	FAMILY ASSESSMENT BY LICENSED BEHAVIORAL HEALTH PROFESSIONAL FOR STATE DEFINED PURPOSES	I	N	00	9		
H2000	COMPREHENSIVE MULTIDISCIPLINARY EVALUATION	I	N	00	9		
H2001	REHABILITATION PROGRAM, PER 1/2 DAY	I	N	00	9		
H2010	COMPREHENSIVE MEDICATION SERVICES, PER 15 MINUTES	I	N	00	9		

HCPCS Code	S t a t u t e	Lab Cert	X-Ref	ASC Pay Grp	ASC Pay Group Eff. Date	Proc Notes	BETOS	TOS	A n e s t	Code Add Date	Code Effective Date	Code Term Date
H0029							Z2	9	0	20010101	20010101	
H0030							Z2	9	0	20010101	20030101	
H0031							Z2	9	0	20030101	20030101	
H0032							Z2	9	0	20030101	20030101	
H0033							Z2	9	0	20030101	20030101	
H0034							Z2	9	0	20030101	20030101	
H0035							Z2	9	0	20030101	20030101	
H0036							Z2	9	0	20030101	20030101	
H0037							Z2	9	0	20030101	20030101	
H0038							Z2	9	0	20030101	20030101	
H0039							Z2	9	0	20030101	20030101	
H0040							Z2	9	0	20030101	20030101	
H0041							Z2	9	0	20030101	20030101	
H0042							Z2	9	0	20030101	20030101	
H0043							Z2	9	0	20030101	20030101	
H0044							Z2	9	0	20030101	20030101	
H0045							Z2	9	0	20030101	20030101	
H0046							Z2	9	0	20030101	20030101	
H0047							Z2	9	0	20030101	20030101	
H0048							Z2	9	0	20030101	20030101	
H0049							Z2	9	0	20070101	20070101	
H0050							Z2	9	0	20070101	20070101	
H1000							Z2	9	0	20020101	20020101	
H1001							Z2	9	0	20020101	20020101	
H1002							Z2	9	0	20020101	20020101	
H1003							Z2	9	0	20020101	20020101	
H1004							Z2	9	0	20020101	20020101	
H1005							Z2	9	0	20020101	20020101	
H1010							Z2	9	0	20030101	20030101	
H1011							Z2	9	0	20030101	20030101	
H2000							Z2	9	0	20030101	20030101	
H2001							Z2	9	0	20030101	20030101	
H2010							Z2	9	0	20030401	20030401	

HCPCS Code	Long Description	Coverage	Action	PI	MPI	CIM	MCM
H2011	CRISIS INTERVENTION SERVICE, PER 15 MINUTES	I	N	00	9		
H2012	BEHAVIORAL HEALTH DAY TREATMENT, PER HOUR	I	N	00	9		
H2013	PSYCHIATRIC HEALTH FACILITY SERVICE, PER DIEM	I	N	00	9		
H2014	SKILLS TRAINING AND DEVELOPMENT, PER 15 MINUTES	I	N	00	9		
H2015	COMPREHENSIVE COMMUNITY SUPPORT SERVICES, PER 15 MINUTES	I	N	00	9		
H2016	COMPREHENSIVE COMMUNITY SUPPORT SERVICES, PER DIEM	I	N	00	9		
H2017	PSYCHOSOCIAL REHABILITATION SERVICES, PER 15 MINUTES	I	N	00	9		
H2018	PSYCHOSOCIAL REHABILITATION SERVICES, PER DIEM	I	N	00	9		
H2019	THERAPEUTIC BEHAVIORAL SERVICES, PER 15 MINUTES	I	N	00	9		
H2020	THERAPEUTIC BEHAVIORAL SERVICES, PER DIEM	I	N	00	9		
H2021	COMMUNITY-BASED WRAP-AROUND SERVICES, PER 15 MINUTES	I	N	00	9		
H2022	COMMUNITY-BASED WRAP-AROUND SERVICES, PER DIEM	I	N	00	9		
H2023	SUPPORTED EMPLOYMENT, PER 15 MINUTES	I	N	00	9		
H2024	SUPPORTED EMPLOYMENT, PER DIEM	I	N	00	9		
H2025	ONGOING SUPPORT TO MAINTAIN EMPLOYMENT, PER 15 MINUTES	I	N	00	9		
H2026	ONGOING SUPPORT TO MAINTAIN EMPLOYMENT, PER DIEM	I	N	00	9		
H2027	PSYCHOEDUCATIONAL SERVICE, PER 15 MINUTES	I	N	00	9		
H2028	SEXUAL OFFENDER TREATMENT SERVICE, PER 15 MINUTES	I	N	00	9		
H2029	SEXUAL OFFENDER TREATMENT SERVICE, PER DIEM	I	N	00	9		
H2030	MENTAL HEALTH CLUBHOUSE SERVICES, PER 15 MINUTES	I	N	00	9		
H2031	MENTAL HEALTH CLUBHOUSE SERVICES, PER DIEM	I	N	00	9		
H2032	ACTIVITY THERAPY, PER 15 MINUTES	I	N	00	9		
H2033	MULTISYSTEMIC THERAPY FOR JUVENILES, PER 15 MINUTES	I	N	00	9		
H2034	ALCOHOL AND/OR DRUG ABUSE HALFWAY HOUSE SERVICES, PER DIEM	I	N	00	9		
H2035	ALCOHOL AND/OR OTHER DRUG TREATMENT PROGRAM, PER HOUR	I	N	00	9		
H2036	ALCOHOL AND/OR OTHER DRUG TREATMENT PROGRAM, PER DIEM	I	N	00	9		
H2037	DEVELOPMENTAL DELAY PREVENTION ACTIVITIES, DEPENDENT CHILD OF CLIENT, PER 15 MINUTES	I	N	00	9		
J0120	INJECTION, TETRACYCLINE, UP TO 250 MG	D	N	51	A		2049
J0128	INJECTION, ABARELIX, 10 MG	C	N	51	A		
J0129	INJECTION, ABATACEPT, 10 MG	C	N	51	A		
J0130	INJECTION ABCIXIMAB, 10 MG	D	N	51	A		2049
J0132	INJECTION, ACETYLCYSTEINE, 100 MG	C	N	51	A		
J0133	INJECTION, ACYCLOVIR, 5 MG	C	N	51	A		
J0135	INJECTION, ADALIMUMAB, 20 MG	C	N	51	A		
J0150	INJECTION, ADENOSINE FOR THERAPEUTIC USE, 6 MG (NOT TO BE USED TO REPORT ANY ADENOSINE PHOSPHATE COMPOUNDS, INSTEAD USE A9270)	D	N	51	A		2049
J0152	INJECTION, ADENOSINE FOR DIAGNOSTIC USE, 30 MG (NOT TO BE USED TO REPORT ANY ADENOSINE PHOSPHATE COMPOUNDS; INSTEAD USE A9270)	C	N	51	A		
J0170	INJECTION, ADRENALIN, EPINEPHRINE, UP TO 1 ML AMPULE	D	N	51	A		2049
J0180	INJECTION, AGALSIDASE BETA, 1 MG	C	N	51	A		

HCPCS Code	Statute	Lab Cert	X-Ref	ASC Pay Grp	ASC Pay Group Eff. Date	Proc Notes	BETOS	TOS	Anest	Code Add Date	Code Effective Date	Code Term Date
H2011							Z2	9	0	20030401	20030401	
H2012							Z2	9	0	20030401	20030401	
H2013							Z2	9	0	20030401	20030401	
H2014							Z2	9	0	20030401	20030401	
H2015							Z2	9	0	20030401	20030401	
H2016							Z2	9	0	20030401	20030401	
H2017							Z2	9	0	20030401	20030401	
H2018							Z2	9	0	20030401	20030401	
H2019							Z2	9	0	20030401	20030401	
H2020							Z2	9	0	20030401	20030401	
H2021							Z2	9	0	20030401	20030401	
H2022							Z2	9	0	20030401	20030401	
H2023							Z2	9	0	20030401	20030401	
H2024							Z2	9	0	20030401	20030401	
H2025							Z2	9	0	20030401	20030401	
H2026							Z2	9	0	20030401	20030401	
H2027							Z2	9	0	20030401	20030401	
H2028							Z2	9	0	20030401	20030401	
H2029							Z2	9	0	20030401	20030401	
H2030							Z2	9	0	20030401	20030401	
H2031							Z2	9	0	20030401	20030401	
H2032							Z2	9	0	20030401	20030401	
H2033							Z2	9	0	20030401	20030401	
H2034							Z2	9	0	20030401	20030401	
H2035							Z2	9	0	20030401	20030401	
H2036							Z2	9	0	20030401	20030401	
H2037							Z2	9	0	20030401	20030401	
J0120							O1E	1, P	0	19860101	19970101	
J0128							O1E	1, P	0	20050101	20050101	
J0129				YY	20080101		O1E	1, P	0	20070101	20070101	
J0130				YY	20080101		O1E	1, P	0	19990101	19990101	
J0132				YY	20090101		O1E	1, P	0	20060101	20060101	
J0133							O1E	1, P	0	20060101	20060101	
J0135				YY	20080101		O1E	1, P	0	20050101	20050101	
J0150				YY	20080101		O1E	1, P	0	19940101	20050101	
J0152				YY	20080101		O1E	1, P	0	20040101	20050101	
J0170							O1E	1, P	0	19860101	19970101	
J0180				YY	20080101		O1E	1, P	0	20050101	20050101	

HCPCS Code	Long Description	Coverage	Action	PI	MPI	CIM	MCM
J0190	INJECTION, BIPERIDEN LACTATE, PER 5 MG	D	N	51	A		2049
J0200	INJECTION, ALATROFLOXACIN MESYLATE, 100 MG	D	N	51	A		2049.5
J0205	INJECTION, ALGLUCERASE, PER 10 UNITS	D	N	51	A		2049
J0207	INJECTION, AMIFOSTINE, 500 MG	D	N	51	A		2049
J0210	INJECTION, METHYLDOPATE HCL, UP TO 250 MG	D	N	51	A		2049
J0215	INJECTION, ALEFACEPT, 0.5 MG	C	N	51	A		
J0220	INJECTION, ALGLUCOSIDASE ALFA, 10 MG	C	N	51	A		
J0256	INJECTION, ALPHA 1 - PROTEINASE INHIBITOR - HUMAN, 10 MG	D	N	51	A		2049
J0270	INJECTION, ALPROSTADIL, 1.25 MCG (CODE MAY BE USED FOR MEDICARE WHEN DRUG ADMINISTERED UNDER THE DIRECT SUPERVISION OF A PHYSICIAN, NOT FOR USE WHEN DRUG IS SELF ADMINISTERED)	D	N	51	A		2049
J0275	ALPROSTADIL URETHRAL SUPPOSITORY (CODE MAY BE USED FOR MEDICARE WHEN DRUG ADMINISTERED UNDER THE DIRECT SUPERVISION OF A PHYSICIAN, NOT FOR USE WHEN DRUG IS SELF ADMINISTERED)	D	N	51	A		2049
J0278	INJECTION, AMIKACIN SULFATE, 100 MG	C	N	51	A		
J0280	INJECTION, AMINOPHYLLIN, UP TO 250 MG	D	N	51	A		2049
J0282	INJECTION, AMIODARONE HYDROCHLORIDE, 30 MG	D	N	51	A		2049
J0285	INJECTION, AMPHOTERICIN B, 50 MG	D	N	51	A		2049
J0287	INJECTION, AMPHOTERICIN B LIPID COMPLEX, 10 MG	D	N	51	A		2049
J0288	INJECTION, AMPHOTERICIN B CHOLESTERYL SULFATE COMPLEX, 10 MG	D	N	51	A		2049
J0289	INJECTION, AMPHOTERICIN B LIPOSOME, 10 MG	D	N	51	A		2049
J0290	INJECTION, AMPICILLIN SODIUM, 500 MG	D	N	51	A		2049
J0295	INJECTION, AMPICILLIN SODIUM/SULBACTAM SODIUM, PER 1.5 GM	D	N	51	A		2049
J0300	INJECTION, AMOBARBITAL, UP TO 125 MG	D	N	51	A		2049
J0330	INJECTION, SUCCINYLCHOLINE CHLORIDE, UP TO 20 MG	D	N	51	A		2049
J0348	INJECTION, ANIDULAFUNGIN, 1 MG	C	N	51	A		
J0350	INJECTION, ANISTREPLASE, PER 30 UNITS	D	N	51	A		2049
J0360	INJECTION, HYDRALAZINE HCL, UP TO 20 MG	D	N	51	A		2049
J0364	INJECTION, APOMORPHINE HYDROCHLORIDE, 1 MG	C	N	51	A		
J0365	INJECTION, APROTONIN, 10,000 KIU	D	N	51	A		2049
J0380	INJECTION, METARAMINOL BITARTRATE, PER 10 MG	D	N	51	A		2049
J0390	INJECTION, CHLOROQUINE HYDROCHLORIDE, UP TO 250 MG	D	N	51	A		2049
J0395	INJECTION, ARBUTAMINE HCL, 1 MG	D	N	51	A		2049
J0400	INJECTION, ARIPIPRAZOLE, INTRAMUSCULAR, 0.25 MG	C	N	51	A		
J0456	INJECTION, AZITHROMYCIN, 500 MG	D	N	51	A		2049.5
J0460	INJECTION, ATROPINE SULFATE, UP TO 0.3 MG	D	D	51	A		2049
J0461	INJECTION, ATROPINE SULFATE, 0.01 MG	D	A	51	A		2049
J0470	INJECTION, DIMERCAPROL, PER 100 MG	D	N	51	A		2049
J0475	INJECTION, BACLOFEN, 10 MG	D	N	51	A		2049
J0476	INJECTION, BACLOFEN, 50 MCG FOR INTRATHECAL TRIAL	D	N	51	A		2049
J0480	INJECTION, BASILIXIMAB, 20 MG	D	N	51	A		2049
J0500	INJECTION, DICYCLOMINE HCL, UP TO 20 MG	D	N	51	A		2049
J0515	INJECTION, BENZTROPINE MESYLATE, PER 1 MG	D	N	51	A		2049
J0520	INJECTION, BETHANECHOL CHLORIDE, MYOTONACHOL OR URECHOLINE, UP TO 5 MG	D	N	51	A		2049

HCPCS Code	Statute	Lab Cert	X-Ref	ASC Pay Grp	ASC Pay Group Eff. Date	Proc Notes	BETOS	TOS	Anest	Code Add Date	Code Effective Date	Code Term Date
J0190							O1E	1, P	0	19820101	19970101	
J0200							O1E	1, P	0	20000101	20000101	
J0205				YY	20080101		O1E	1, P	0	19930101	19970101	
J0207				YY	20080101		O1D	1, P	0	19980101	19980101	
J0210				YY	20080101		O1E	1, P	0	19840101	19970101	
J0215				YY	20080101		O1E	1, P	0	20040101	20040101	
J0220				YY	20080101		O1E	1, P	0	20080101	20080101	
J0256				YY	20080101		O1E	1, P	0	19890101	19990101	
J0270							O1E	1	0	19970101	20000101	
J0275							O1E	1	0	19990101	20000101	
J0278							O1E	1, P	0	20060101	20060101	
J0280							O1E	1, P	0	19840101	19970101	
J0282							O1E	1, P	0	20010101	20010101	
J0285							O1E	1, P	0	19990101	19990101	
J0287				YY	20080101		O1E	1, P	0	20030101	20030101	
J0288				YY	20080101		O1E	1, P	0	20030101	20030101	
J0289				YY	20080101		O1E	1, P	0	20030101	20030101	
J0290							O1E	1, P	0	19840101	20000101	
J0295							O1E	1, P	0	19950101	19970101	
J0300							O1E	1, P	0	19820101	19970101	
J0330							O1E	1, P	0	19860101	19970101	
J0348				YY	20080101		O1E	1, P	0	20070101	20090101	
J0350							O1E	1, P	0	19860101	19970101	
J0360							O1E	1, P	0	19860101	19970101	
J0364							O1E	1, P	0	20070101	20070101	
J0365				YY	20080101	0095	O1E	1, P	0	20060101	20060101	
J0380							O1E	1, P	0	19820101	19970101	
J0390							O1E	1, P	0	19860101	19970101	
J0395							O1E	1, P	0	19990101	20090101	
J0400							O1E	1, P	0	20080101	20080101	
J0456							O1E	1, P	0	20000101	20000101	
J0460							O1E	1, P	0	19820101	20100101	20091231
J0461							O1E	1, P	0	20100101	20100101	
J0470				YY	20090101		O1E	1, P	0	19820101	19970101	
J0475				YY	20080101		O1E	1, P	0	19940101	19970101	
J0476				YY	20080101		O1E	1, P	0	19990101	19990101	
J0480				YY	20080101	0095	O1E	1, G	0	20060101	20060101	
J0500							O1E	1, P	0	19860101	19970101	
J0515							O1E	1, P	0	19820101	19970101	
J0520							O1E	1, P	0	19840101	19970101	

HCPCS Code	Long Description	Coverage	Action	PI	MPI	CIM	MCM
J0530	INJECTION, PENICILLIN G BENZATHINE AND PENICILLIN G PROCAINE, UP TO 600,000 UNITS	D	D	51	A		2049
J0540	INJECTION, PENICILLIN G BENZATHINE AND PENICILLIN G PROCAINE, UP TO 1,200,000 UNITS	D	D	51	A		2049
J0550	INJECTION, PENICILLIN G BENZATHINE AND PENICILLIN G PROCAINE, UP TO 2,400,000 UNITS	D	D	51	A		2049
J0559	INJECTION, PENICILLIN G BENZATHINE AND PENICILLIN G PROCAINE, 2500 UNITS	D	A	51	A		2049
J0560	INJECTION, PENICILLIN G BENZATHINE, UP TO 600,000 UNITS	D	N	51	A		2049
J0570	INJECTION, PENICILLIN G BENZATHINE, UP TO 1,200,000 UNITS	D	N	51	A		2049
J0580	INJECTION, PENICILLIN G BENZATHINE, UP TO 2,400,000 UNITS	D	N	51	A		2049
J0583	INJECTION, BIVALIRUDIN, 1 MG	C	N	51	A		
J0585	INJECTION, ONABOTULINUMTOXINA, 1 UNIT	D	C	51	A		2049
J0586	INJECTION, ABOBOTULINUMTOXINA, 5 UNITS	C	A	51	A		
J0587	INJECTION, RIMABOTULINUMTOXINB, 100 UNITS	D	C	51	A		2049
J0592	INJECTION, BUPRENORPHINE HYDROCHLORIDE, 0.1 MG	D	N	51	A		2049
J0594	INJECTION, BUSULFAN, 1 MG	C	N	51	A		
J0595	INJECTION, BUTORPHANOL TARTRATE, 1 MG	C	N	51	A		
J0598	INJECTION, C1 ESTERASE INHIBITOR (HUMAN), 10 UNITS	C	A	51	A		
J0600	INJECTION, EDETATE CALCIUM DISODIUM, UP TO 1000 MG	D	N	51	A		2049
J0610	INJECTION, CALCIUM GLUCONATE, PER 10 ML	D	N	51	A		2049
J0620	INJECTION, CALCIUM GLYCEROPHOSPHATE AND CALCIUM LACTATE, PER 10 ML	D	N	51	A		2049
J0630	INJECTION, CALCITONIN SALMON, UP TO 400 UNITS	D	N	51	A		2049
J0636	INJECTION, CALCITRIOL, 0.1 MCG	D	N	51	A		2049
J0637	INJECTION, CASPOFUNGIN ACETATE, 5 MG	C	N	51	A		
J0640	INJECTION, LEUCOVORIN CALCIUM, PER 50 MG	D	N	51	A		2049
J0641	INJECTION, LEVOLEUCOVORIN CALCIUM, 0.5 MG	D	N	51	A		
J0670	INJECTION, MEPIVACAINE HYDROCHLORIDE, PER 10 ML	D	N	51	A		2049
J0690	INJECTION, CEFAZOLIN SODIUM, 500 MG	D	N	51	A		2049
J0692	INJECTION, CEFEPIME HYDROCHLORIDE, 500 MG	C	N	51	A		
J0694	INJECTION, CEFOXITIN SODIUM, 1 GM	D	N	51	A		2049
J0696	INJECTION, CEFTRIAXONE SODIUM, PER 250 MG	D	N	51	A		2049
J0697	INJECTION, STERILE CEFUROXIME SODIUM, PER 750 MG	D	N	51	A		2049
J0698	INJECTION, CEFOTAXIME SODIUM, PER GM	D	N	51	A		2049
J0702	INJECTION, BETAMETHASONE ACETATE 3MG AND BETAMETHASONE SODIUM PHOSPHATE 3MG	D	N	51	A		2049
J0704	INJECTION, BETAMETHASONE SODIUM PHOSPHATE, PER 4 MG	D	N	51	A		2049
J0706	INJECTION, CAFFEINE CITRATE, 5MG	C	N	51	A		
J0710	INJECTION, CEPHAPIRIN SODIUM, UP TO 1 GM	D	N	51	A		2049
J0713	INJECTION, CEFTAZIDIME, PER 500 MG	D	N	51	A		2049
J0715	INJECTION, CEFTIZOXIME SODIUM, PER 500 MG	D	N	51	A		2049
J0718	INJECTION, CERTOLIZUMAB PEGOL, 1 MG	C	A	51	A		
J0720	INJECTION, CHLORAMPHENICOL SODIUM SUCCINATE, UP TO 1 GM	D	N	51	A		2049
J0725	INJECTION, CHORIONIC GONADOTROPIN, PER 1,000 USP UNITS	D	N	51	A		2049
J0735	INJECTION, CLONIDINE HYDROCHLORIDE, 1 MG	D	N	51	A		2049
J0740	INJECTION, CIDOFOVIR, 375 MG	D	N	51	A		2049
J0743	INJECTION, CILASTATIN SODIUM; IMIPENEM, PER 250 MG	D	N	51	A		2049

HCPCS Code	Statute	Lab Cert	X-Ref	ASC Pay Grp	ASC Pay Group Eff. Date	Proc Notes	BETOS	TOS	Anest	Code Add Date	Code Effective Date	Code Term Date
J0530							O1E	1, P	0	19820101	20100101	20091231
J0540							O1E	1, P	0	19820101	20100101	20091231
J0550							O1E	1, P	0	19820101	20100101	20091231
J0559							O1E	1, P	0	20100101	20100101	
J0560							O1E	1, P	0	19820101	19970101	
J0570							O1E	1, P	0	19820101	19970101	
J0580							O1E	1, P	0	19820101	19970101	
J0583				YY	20080101		O1E	1, P	0	20040101	20040101	
J0585				YY	20080101		O1E	1, P	0	19910101	20100101	
J0586				YY	20100101		O1E	1, P	0	20100101	20100101	
J0587				YY	20080101		O1E	1, P	0	20020101	20100101	
J0592							O1E	1, P	0	20030101	20030101	
J0594				YY	20080101		O1E	1, P	0	20070101	20070101	
J0595							O1E	1	0	20040101	20040101	
J0598				YY	20100101		O1E	1, P	0	20100101	20100101	
J0600				YY	20080101		O1E	1, P	0	19820101	19970101	
J0610							O1E	1, P	0	19820101	19970101	
J0620							O1E	1, P	0	19820101	19970101	
J0630				YY	20090101		O1E	1, P	0	19820101	19970101	
J0636							O1E	1, P	0	20030101	20030101	
J0637				YY	20080101		O1E	1, P	0	20030101	20030101	
J0640							O1E	1, P	0	19820101	19970101	
J0641				YY	20090101	0127	O1E	1, P	0	20090101	20090101	
J0670							O1E	1, P	0	19860101	19970101	
J0690							O1E	1, P	0	19820101	20000101	
J0692							O1E	1, P	0	20020101	20020101	
J0694			Q0090				O1E	1, P	0	19920101	19970101	
J0696							O1E	1, P	0	19900101	19970101	
J0697							O1E	1, P	0	19900101	19970101	
J0698							O1E	1, P	0	19910101	19970101	
J0702							O1E	1, P	0	19950101	20080101	
J0704							O1E	1, P	0	19950101	19970101	
J0706							O1E	1, P	0	20020101	20020101	
J0710							O1E	1, P	0	19820101	19970101	
J0713							O1E	1, P	0	19960101	19970101	
J0715							O1E	1, P	0	19950101	19970101	
J0718				YY	20100101		O1E	1, P	0	20100101	20100101	
J0720							O1E	1, P	0	19820101	19970101	
J0725							O1E	1, P	0	19860101	19970101	
J0735				YY	20080101		O1E	1, P	0	19980101	19980101	
J0740				YY	20080101		O1E	1, P	0	19980101	19980101	
J0743							O1E	1, P	0	19930101	19970101	

HCPCS Code	Long Description	Coverage	Action	PI	MPI	CIM	MCM
J0744	INJECTION, CIPROFLOXACIN FOR INTRAVENOUS INFUSION, 200 MG	C	N	51	A		
J0745	INJECTION, CODEINE PHOSPHATE, PER 30 MG	D	N	51	A		2049
J0760	INJECTION, COLCHICINE, PER 1MG	D	N	51	A		2049
J0770	INJECTION, COLISTIMETHATE SODIUM, UP TO 150 MG	D	N	51	A		2049
J0780	INJECTION, PROCHLORPERAZINE, UP TO 10 MG	D	N	51	A		2049
J0795	INJECTION, CORTICORELIN OVINE TRIFLUTATE, 1 MICROGRAM	D	N	51	A		2049
J0800	INJECTION, CORTICOTROPIN, UP TO 40 UNITS	D	N	51	A		2049
J0833	INJECTION, COSYNTROPIN, NOT OTHERWISE SPECIFIED, 0.25 MG	C	A	51	A		
J0834	INJECTION, COSYNTROPIN (CORTROSYN), 0.25 MG	C	A	51	A		
J0835	INJECTION, COSYNTROPIN, PER 0.25 MG	D	D	51	A		2049
J0850	INJECTION, CYTOMEGALOVIRUS IMMUNE GLOBULIN INTRAVENOUS (HUMAN), PER VIAL	D	N	51	A		2049
J0878	INJECTION, DAPTOMYCIN, 1 MG	C	N	51	A		
J0881	INJECTION, DARBEPOETIN ALFA, 1 MICROGRAM (NON-ESRD USE)	D	N	51	A		
J0882	INJECTION, DARBEPOETIN ALFA, 1 MICROGRAM (FOR ESRD ON DIALYSIS)	D	N	57	A		4273.1
J0885	INJECTION, EPOETIN ALFA, (FOR NON-ESRD USE), 1000 UNITS	D	N	51	A		2049
J0886	INJECTION, EPOETIN ALFA, 1000 UNITS (FOR ESRD ON DIALYSIS)	D	N	57	A		4273.1
J0894	INJECTION, DECITABINE, 1 MG	C	N	51	A		
J0895	INJECTION, DEFEROXAMINE MESYLATE, 500 MG	D	N	51	A		2049
J0900	INJECTION, TESTOSTERONE ENANTHATE AND ESTRADIOL VALERATE, UP TO 1 CC	D	N	51	A		2049
J0945	INJECTION, BROMPHENIRAMINE MALEATE, PER 10 MG	D	N	51	A		2049
J0970	INJECTION, ESTRADIOL VALERATE, UP TO 40 MG	D	N	51	A		2049
J1000	INJECTION, DEPO-ESTRADIOL CYPIONATE, UP TO 5 MG	D	N	51	A		2049
J1020	INJECTION, METHYLPREDNISOLONE ACETATE, 20 MG	D	N	51	A		2049
J1030	INJECTION, METHYLPREDNISOLONE ACETATE, 40 MG	D	N	51	A		2049
J1040	INJECTION, METHYLPREDNISOLONE ACETATE, 80 MG	D	N	51	A		2049
J1051	INJECTION, MEDROXYPROGESTERONE ACETATE, 50 MG	D	N	51	A		2049
J1055	INJECTION, MEDROXYPROGESTERONE ACETATE FOR CONTRACEPTIVE USE, 150 MG	S	N	00	9		
J1056	INJECTION, MEDROXYPROGESTERONE ACETATE / ESTRADIOL CYPIONATE, 5MG / 25MG	C	N	51	A		
J1060	INJECTION, TESTOSTERONE CYPIONATE AND ESTRADIOL CYPIONATE, UP TO 1 ML	D	N	51	A		2049
J1070	INJECTION, TESTOSTERONE CYPIONATE, UP TO 100 MG	D	N	51	A		2049
J1080	INJECTION, TESTOSTERONE CYPIONATE, 1 CC, 200 MG	D	N	51	A		2049
J1094	INJECTION, DEXAMETHASONE ACETATE, 1 MG	D	N	51	A		2049
J1100	INJECTION, DEXAMETHASONE SODIUM PHOSPHATE, 1MG	D	N	51	A		2049
J1110	INJECTON, DIHYDROERGOTAMINE MESYLATE, PER 1 MG	D	N	51	A		2049
J1120	INJECTION, ACETAZOLAMIDE SODIUM, UP TO 500 MG	D	N	51	A		2049
J1160	INJECTION, DIGOXIN, UP TO 0.5 MG	D	N	51	A		2049
J1162	INJECTION, DIGOXIN IMMUNE FAB (OVINE), PER VIAL	D	N	51	A		2049
J1165	INJECTION, PHENYTOIN SODIUM, PER 50 MG	D	N	51	A		2049
J1170	INJECTION, HYDROMORPHONE, UP TO 4 MG	D	N	51	A		2049
J1180	INJECTION, DYPHYLLINE, UP TO 500 MG	D	N	51	A		2049

HCPCS Code	Statute	Lab Cert	X-Ref	ASC Pay Grp	ASC Pay Group Eff. Date	Proc Notes	BETOS	TOS	Anest	Code Add Date	Code Effective Date	Code Term Date
J0744							O1E	1, P	0	20020101	20020101	
J0745							O1E	1, P	0	19860101	19970101	
J0760							O1E	1, P	0	19820101	19970101	
J0770							O1E	1, P	0	19820101	19970101	
J0780							O1E	1, P	0	19840101	19970101	
J0795				YY	20080101	0095	O1E	1, P	0	20060101	20060101	
J0800				YY	20080101		O1E	1, P	0	19820101	19970101	
J0833				YY	20100101		O1E	1, P	0	20100101	20100101	
J0834				YY	20100101		O1E	1, P	0	20100101	20100101	
J0835							O1E	1, P	0	19950101	20100101	20091231
J0850				YY	20080101		O1E	1, P	0	19820101	19970101	
J0878				YY	20080101		O1E	1, P	0	20050101	20050101	
J0881				YY	20080101	0132	O1E	1, L	0	20060101	20060101	
J0882							O1E	1, L	0	20060101	20060101	
J0885				YY	20080101		O1E	9	0	20060101	20060101	
J0886							O1E	1, L	0	20060101	20070101	
J0894				YY	20080101		O1E	1, P	0	20070101	20070101	
J0895			Q0087				O1E	1, P	0	19920101	20010101	
J0900							O1E	1, P	0	19820101	19970101	
J0945				YY	20100101		O1E	1, P	0	19820101	19970101	
J0970							O1E	1, P	0	19820101	19970101	
J1000							O1E	1, P	0	19820101	19970101	
J1020							O1E	1, P	0	19820101	19970101	
J1030							O1E	1, P	0	19820101	19970101	
J1040							O1E	1, P	0	19820101	19970101	
J1051							O1E	1, P	0	20030101	20030101	
J1055	1862A1						O1E	1, P	0	19940101	19970101	
J1056							O1E	1, P	0	20020101	20030101	
J1060							O1E	1, P	0	19820101	19970101	
J1070							O1E	1, P	0	19820101	19970101	
J1080							O1E	1, P	0	19820101	19970101	
J1094							O1E	1, P	0	20030101	20030101	
J1100							O1E	1, P	0	19820101	20010101	
J1110							O1E	1, P	0	19820101	19970101	
J1120							O1E	1, P	0	19820101	19970101	
J1160							O1E	1, P	0	19820101	19970101	
J1162				YY	20080101	0095	O1E	1, P	e	20060101	20060101	
J1165							O1E	1, P	s	19820101	19970101	
J1170							O1E	1, P	0	19820101	19970101	
J1180							O1E	1, P	0	19820101	19970101	

HCPCS Code	Long Description	Coverage	Action	PI	MPI	CIM	MCM
J1190	INJECTION, DEXRAZOXANE HYDROCHLORIDE, PER 250 MG	D	N	51	A		2049
J1200	INJECTION, DIPHENHYDRAMINE HCL, UP TO 50 MG	D	N	51	A		2049
J1205	INJECTION, CHLOROTHIAZIDE SODIUM, PER 500 MG	D	N	51	A		2049
J1212	INJECTION, DMSO, DIMETHYL SULFOXIDE, 50%, 50 ML	D	N	51	A	45-23	2049
J1230	INJECTION, METHADONE HCL, UP TO 10 MG	D	N	51	A		2049
J1240	INJECTION, DIMENHYDRINATE, UP TO 50 MG	D	N	51	A		2049
J1245	INJECTION, DIPYRIDAMOLE, PER 10 MG	D	N	51	A		15030, 2049
J1250	INJECTION, DOBUTAMINE HYDROCHLORIDE, PER 250 MG	D	N	51	A		2049
J1260	INJECTION, DOLASETRON MESYLATE, 10 MG	D	N	51	A		2049
J1265	INJECTION, DOPAMINE HCL, 40 MG	C	N	51	A		
J1267	INJECTION, DORIPENEM, 10 MG	C	N	51	A		
J1270	INJECTION, DOXERCALCIFEROL, 1 MCG	C	N	51	A		
J1300	INJECTION, ECULIZUMAB, 10 MG	C	N	51	A		
J1320	INJECTION, AMITRIPTYLINE HCL, UP TO 20 MG	D	N	51	A		2049
J1324	INJECTION, ENFUVIRTIDE, 1 MG	C	N	51	A		
J1325	INJECTION, EPOPROSTENOL, 0.5 MG	D	N	51	A		2049
J1327	INJECTION, EPTIFIBATIDE, 5 MG	D	N	51	A		2049
J1330	INJECTION, ERGONOVINE MALEATE, UP TO 0.2 MG	D	N	51	A		2049
J1335	INJECTION, ERTAPENEM SODIUM, 500 MG	C	N	51	A		
J1364	INJECTION, ERYTHROMYCIN LACTOBIONATE, PER 500 MG	D	N	51	A		2049
J1380	INJECTION, ESTRADIOL VALERATE, UP TO 10 MG	D	N	51	A		2049
J1390	INJECTION, ESTRADIOL VALERATE, UP TO 20 MG	D	N	51	A		2049
J1410	INJECTION, ESTROGEN CONJUGATED, PER 25 MG	D	N	51	A		2049
J1430	INJECTION, ETHANOLAMINE OLEATE, 100 MG	D	N	51	A		2049
J1435	INJECTION, ESTRONE, PER 1 MG	D	N	51	A		2049
J1436	INJECTION, ETIDRONATE DISODIUM, PER 300 MG	D	N	51	A		2049
J1438	INJECTION, ETANERCEPT, 25 MG (CODE MAY BE USED FOR MEDICARE WHEN DRUG ADMINISTERED UNDER THE DIRECT SUPERVISION OF A PHYSICIAN, NOT FOR USE WHEN DRUG IS SELF ADMINISTERED)	D	N	51	A		2049
J1440	INJECTION, FILGRASTIM (G-CSF), 300 MCG	D	N	51	A		2049
J1441	INJECTION, FILGRASTIM (G-CSF), 480 MCG	D	N	51	A		2049
J1450	INJECTION FLUCONAZOLE, 200 MG	D	N	51	A		2049.5
J1451	INJECTION, FOMEPIZOLE, 15 MG	D	N	51	A		2049
J1452	INJECTION, FOMIVIRSEN SODIUM, INTRAOCULAR, 1.65 MG	D	N	51	A		2049.3
J1453	INJECTION, FOSAPREPITANT, 1 MG	C	N	51	A		
J1455	INJECTION, FOSCARNET SODIUM, PER 1000 MG	D	N	51	A		2049
J1457	INJECTION, GALLIUM NITRATE, 1 MG	C	N	51	A		
J1458	INJECTION, GALSULFASE, 1 MG	C	N	51	A		
J1459	INJECTION, IMMUNE GLOBULIN (PRIVIGEN), INTRAVENOUS, NON-LYOPHILIZED (E.G. LIQUID), 500 MG	C	N	51	A		
J1460	INJECTION, GAMMA GLOBULIN, INTRAMUSCULAR, 1 CC	D	N	51	A		2049
J1470	INJECTION, GAMMA GLOBULIN, INTRAMUSCULAR, 2 CC	D	N	51	A		2049
J1480	INJECTION, GAMMA GLOBULIN, INTRAMUSCULAR, 3 CC	D	N	51	A		2049
J1490	INJECTION, GAMMA GLOBULIN, INTRAMUSCULAR, 4 CC	D	N	51	A		2049
J1500	INJECTION, GAMMA GLOBULIN, INTRAMUSCULAR, 5 CC	D	N	51	A		2049
J1510	INJECTION, GAMMA GLOBULIN, INTRAMUSCULAR, 6 CC	D	N	51	A		2049
J1520	INJECTION, GAMMA GLOBULIN, INTRAMUSCULAR, 7 CC	D	N	51	A		2049
J1530	INJECTION, GAMMA GLOBULIN, INTRAMUSCULAR, 8 CC	D	N	51	A		2049

HCPCS Code	Statute	Lab Cert	X-Ref	ASC Pay Grp	ASC Pay Group Eff. Date	Proc Notes	BETOS	TOS	Anest	Code Add Date	Code Effective Date	Code Term Date
J1190				YY	20080101		O1E	1, P	0	19970101	19970101	
J1200							O1E	1, P	0	19820101	19970101	
J1205				YY	20080101		O1E	1, P	0	19820101	19970101	
J1212				YY	20090101		O1E	1, P	0	19860101	19970101	
J1230							O1E	1, P	0	19820101	19970101	
J1240							O1E	1, P	0	19840101	19970101	
J1245							O1E	1, P	0	19930101	19980101	
J1250							O1E	1, P	0	19960101	19970101	
J1260							O1D	1, P	0	19990101	20000101	
J1265							O1E	1, P	0	20060101	20060101	
J1267				YY	20090101		O1E	1, P	0	20090101	20090101	
J1270							O1E	1, P	0	20020101	20020101	
J1300				YY	20080101		O1E	1, P	0	20080101	20080101	
J1320							O1E	1, P	0	19820101	19970101	
J1324				YY	20100101		O1E	1, P	0	20070101	20070101	
J1325							O1E	1, P	0	19980101	19980101	
J1327				YY	20080101		O1E	1, P	0	20000101	20000101	
J1330							O1E	1, P	0	19860101	19970101	
J1335							O1E	1, P	0	20040101	20040101	
J1364							O1E	1, P	0	19950101	19970101	
J1380							O1E	1, P	0	19820101	19970101	
J1390							O1E	1, P	0	19820101	19970101	
J1410				YY	20080101		O1E	1, P	0	19820101	19970101	
J1430				YY	20080101	0095	O1E	1, P	0	20060101	20060101	
J1435							O1E	1, P	0	19820101	19970101	
J1436				YY	20080101		O1E	1, P	0	19900101	19970101	
J1438				YY	20080101		O1E	1, P	0	20000101	20000101	
J1440				YY	20080101		O1E	1, P	0	19940101	19970101	
J1441				YY	20080101		O1E	1, P	0	19940101	19970101	
J1450							O1E	1, P	0	20000101	20000101	
J1451				YY	20080101	0095	O1E	1, P	0	20060101	20060101	
J1452							O1E	1, P	0	20010101	20010101	
J1453				YY	20090101		O1E	1, P	0	20090101	20090101	
J1455							O1E	1, P	0	19930101	19970101	
J1457				YY	20080101		O1E	1, P	0	20050101	20050101	
J1458				YY	20080101		O1E	1, P	0	20070101	20070101	
J1459				YY	20090101		O1E	1, P	0	20090101	20090101	
J1460				YY	20080101		O1E	1, P	0	19840101	19970101	
J1470				YY	20080101		O1E	1, P	0	19840101	19970101	
J1480				YY	20080101		O1E	1, P	0	19850101	19970101	
J1490				YY	20080101		O1E	1, P	0	19840101	19970101	
J1500				YY	20080101		O1E	1, P	0	19840101	19970101	
J1510				YY	20080101		O1E	1, P	0	19840101	19970101	
J1520				YY	20080101		O1E	1, P	0	19840101	19970101	
J1530				YY	20080101		O1E	1, P	0	19840101	19970101	

HCPCS Code	Long Description	Coverage	Action	PI	MPI	CIM	MCM
J1540	INJECTION, GAMMA GLOBULIN, INTRAMUSCULAR, 9 CC	D	N	51	A		2049
J1550	INJECTION, GAMMA GLOBULIN, INTRAMUSCULAR, 10 CC	D	N	51	A		2049
J1560	INJECTION, GAMMA GLOBULIN, INTRAMUSCULAR, OVER 10 CC	D	N	51	A		2049
J1561	INJECTION, IMMUNE GLOBULIN, (GAMUNEX), INTRAVENOUS, NON-LYOPHILIZED (E.G. LIQUID), 500 MG	D	N	51	A		2049
J1562	INJECTION, IMMUNE GLOBULIN (VIVAGLOBIN), 100 MG	C	N	51	A		
J1565	INJECTION, RESPIRATORY SYNCYTIAL VIRUS IMMUNE GLOBULIN, INTRAVENOUS, 50 MG	D	D	51	A		2049
J1566	INJECTION, IMMUNE GLOBULIN, INTRAVENOUS, LYOPHILIZED (E.G. POWDER), NOT OTHERWISE SPECIFIED, 500 MG	D	N	51	A		2049
J1567	INJECTION, IMMUNE GLOBULIN, INTRAVENOUS, NON-LYOPHILIZED (E.G. LIQUID), 500 MG	I	N	00	9		
J1568	INJECTION, IMMUNE GLOBULIN, (OCTAGAM), INTRAVENOUS, NON-LYOPHILIZED (E.G. LIQUID), 500 MG	C	N	51	A		
J1569	INJECTION, IMMUNE GLOBULIN, (GAMMAGARD LIQUID), INTRAVENOUS, NON-LYOPHILIZED, (E.G. LIQUID), 500 MG	D	N	51	A		2049
J1570	INJECTION, GANCICLOVIR SODIUM, 500 MG	D	N	51	A		2049
J1571	INJECTION, HEPATITIS B IMMUNE GLOBULIN (HEPAGAM B), INTRAMUSCULAR, 0.5 ML	D	N	51	A		2049
J1572	INJECTION, IMMUNE GLOBULIN, (FLEBOGAMMA/ FLEBOGAMMA DIF), INTRAVENOUS, NON-LYOPHILIZED (E.G. LIQUID), 500 MG	D	N	51	A		2049
J1573	INJECTION, HEPATITIS B IMMUNE GLOBULIN (HEPAGAM B), INTRAVENOUS, 0.5 ML	C	N	51	A		
J1580	INJECTION, GARAMYCIN, GENTAMICIN, UP TO 80 MG	D	N	51	A		2049
J1590	INJECTION, GATIFLOXACIN, 10MG	C	N	51	A		
J1595	INJECTION, GLATIRAMER ACETATE, 20 MG	D	N	51	A		2049
J1600	INJECTION, GOLD SODIUM THIOMALATE, UP TO 50 MG	D	N	51	A		2049
J1610	INJECTION, GLUCAGON HYDROCHLORIDE, PER 1 MG	D	N	51	A		2049
J1620	INJECTION, GONADORELIN HYDROCHLORIDE, PER 100 MCG	D	N	51	A		2049
J1626	INJECTION, GRANISETRON HYDROCHLORIDE, 100 MCG	D	N	51	A		2049
J1630	INJECTION, HALOPERIDOL, UP TO 5 MG	D	N	51	A		2049
J1631	INJECTION, HALOPERIDOL DECANOATE, PER 50 MG	D	N	51	A		2049
J1640	INJECTION, HEMIN, 1 MG	D	N	51	A		2049
J1642	INJECTION, HEPARIN SODIUM, (HEPARIN LOCK FLUSH), PER 10 UNITS	D	N	51	A		2049
J1644	INJECTION, HEPARIN SODIUM, PER 1000 UNITS	D	N	51	A		2049
J1645	INJECTION, DALTEPARIN SODIUM, PER 2500 IU	D	N	51	A		2049
J1650	INJECTION, ENOXAPARIN SODIUM, 10 MG	C	N	51	A		
J1652	INJECTION, FONDAPARINUX SODIUM, 0.5 MG	D	N	51	A		2049
J1655	INJECTION, TINZAPARIN SODIUM, 1000 IU	C	N	51	A		
J1670	INJECTION, TETANUS IMMUNE GLOBULIN, HUMAN, UP TO 250 UNITS	D	N	51	A		2049
J1675	INJECTION, HISTRELIN ACETATE, 10 MICROGRAMS	D	N	51	A		2049
J1680	INJECTION, HUMAN FIBRINOGEN CONCENTRATE, 100 MG	C	A	51	A		
J1700	INJECTION, HYDROCORTISONE ACETATE, UP TO 25 MG	D	N	51	A		2049
J1710	INJECTION, HYDROCORTISONE SODIUM PHOSPHATE, UP TO 50 MG	D	N	51	A		2049

HCPCS Code	Statute	Lab Cert	X-Ref	ASC Pay Grp	ASC Pay Group Eff. Date	Proc Notes	BETOS	TOS	Anest	Code Add Date	Code Effective Date	Code Term Date
J1540				YY	20080101		O1E	1, P	0	19840101	19970101	
J1550				YY	20080101		O1E	1, P	0	19840101	19970101	
J1560				YY	20080101		O1E	1, P	0	19840101	19970101	
J1561				YY	20080101		O1E	1, P	0	20080101	20080101	
J1562				YY	20080101		O1E	1, P	0	20070101	20080101	
J1565							O1E	1, P	0	19980101	20100101	20091231
J1566				YY	20080101		O1E	1, P	0	20060101	20080101	
J1567							O1E	1, P	0	20060101	20080101	20071231
J1568				YY	20080101		O1E	1, P	0	20080101	20080101	
J1569				YY	20080101		O1E	1, P	0	20080101	20080101	
J1570							O1E	1, P	0	19940101	19970101	
J1571				YY	20080101		O1E	1, P	0	20080101	20090101	
J1572				YY	20080101		O1E	1, P	0	20080101	20090101	
J1573				YY	20080101		O1E	1, P	0	20080101	20090101	
J1580							O1E	1, P	0	19840101	19970101	
J1590							O1E	1, P	0	20020101	20020101	
J1595				YY	20080101		O1E	1, P	0	20040101	20040101	
J1600							O1E	1, P	0	19820101	19970101	
J1610				YY	20080101		O1E	1, P	0	19860101	19970101	
J1620				YY	20080101		O1E	1, P	0	19820101	19970101	
J1626							O1E	1, P	0	19980101	20090101	
J1630							O1E	1, P	0	19860101	19970101	
J1631							O1E	1, P	0	19890101	19970101	
J1640				YY	20080101	0095	O1E	1, P	0	20060101	20060101	
J1642							O1E	1, P	0	19950101	19970101	
J1644							O1E	1,L,P	0	19950101	20030101	
J1645							O1E	1, P	0	19970101	20020701	
J1650							O1E	1, P	0	19960101	20040101	
J1652				YY	20080101		O1E	1, P	0	20030101	20030101	
J1655							O1E	1, P	0	20020101	20020701	
J1670				YY	20080101		O1E	1, P	0	19860101	19970101	
J1675						0095	O1E	1, G	0	20060101	20060101	
J1680				YY	20100101		O1E	1, P	0	20100101	20100101	
J1700							O1E	1, P	0	19820101	19970101	
J1710							O1E	1, P	0	19820101	19970101	

HCPCS Code	Long Description	Coverage	Action	PI	MPI	CIM	MCM
J1720	INJECTION, HYDROCORTISONE SODIUM SUCCINATE, UP TO 100 MG	D	N	51	A		2049
J1730	INJECTION, DIAZOXIDE, UP TO 300 MG	D	N	51	A		2049
J1740	INJECTION, IBANDRONATE SODIUM, 1 MG	C	N	51	A		
J1742	INJECTION, IBUTILIDE FUMARATE, 1 MG	D	N	51	A		2049
J1743	INJECTION, IDURSULFASE, 1 MG	C	N	51	A		
J1745	INJECTION INFLIXIMAB, 10 MG	D	N	51	A		2049
J1750	INJECTION, IRON DEXTRAN, 50 MG	D	N	51	A		2049.5
J1751	INJECTION, IRON DEXTRAN 165, 50 MG	I	N	00	9		
J1752	INJECTION, IRON DEXTRAN 267, 50 MG	I	N	00	9		
J1756	INJECTION, IRON SUCROSE, 1 MG	C	N	51	A		
J1785	INJECTION, IMIGLUCERASE, PER UNIT	D	N	51	A		2049
J1790	INJECTION, DROPERIDOL, UP TO 5 MG	D	N	51	A		2049
J1800	INJECTION, PROPRANOLOL HCL, UP TO 1 MG	D	N	51	A		2049
J1810	INJECTION, DROPERIDOL AND FENTANYL CITRATE, UP TO 2 ML AMPULE	D	N	51	A		2049
J1815	INJECTION, INSULIN, PER 5 UNITS	D	N	51	A	60-14	2049
J1817	INSULIN FOR ADMINISTRATION THROUGH DME (I.E., INSULIN PUMP) PER 50 UNITS	C	N	51	A		
J1825	INJECTION, INTERFERON BETA-1A, 33 MCG	I	N	00	9		
J1830	INJECTION INTERFERON BETA-1B, 0.25 MG (CODE MAY BE USED FOR MEDICARE WHEN DRUG ADMINISTERED UNDER THE DIRECT SUPERVISION OF A PHYSICIAN, NOT FOR USE WHEN DRUG IS SELF ADMINISTERED)	D	N	51	A		2049
J1835	INJECTION, ITRACONAZOLE, 50 MG	C	N	51	A		
J1840	INJECTION, KANAMYCIN SULFATE, UP TO 500 MG	D	N	51	A		2049
J1850	INJECTION, KANAMYCIN SULFATE, UP TO 75 MG	D	N	51	A		2049
J1885	INJECTION, KETOROLAC TROMETHAMINE, PER 15 MG	D	N	51	A		2049
J1890	INJECTION, CEPHALOTHIN SODIUM, UP TO 1 GRAM	D	N	51	A		2049
J1930	INJECTION, LANREOTIDE, 1 MG	C	N	51	A		
J1931	INJECTION, LARONIDASE, 0.1 MG	C	N	51	A		
J1940	INJECTION, FUROSEMIDE, UP TO 20 MG	D	N	51	A		2049
J1945	INJECTION, LEPIRUDIN, 50 MG	D	N	51	A		2049
J1950	INJECTION, LEUPROLIDE ACETATE (FOR DEPOT SUSPENSION), PER 3.75 MG	D	N	51	A		2049
J1953	INJECTION, LEVETIRACETAM, 10 MG	C	N	51	A		
J1955	INJECTION, LEVOCARNITINE, PER 1 GM	D	N	51	A		2049
J1956	INJECTION, LEVOFLOXACIN, 250 MG	D	N	51	A		2049
J1960	INJECTION, LEVORPHANOL TARTRATE, UP TO 2 MG	D	N	51	A		2049
J1980	INJECTION, HYOSCYAMINE SULFATE, UP TO 0.25 MG	D	N	51	A		2049
J1990	INJECTION, CHLORDIAZEPOXIDE HCL, UP TO 100 MG	D	N	51	A		2049
J2001	INJECTION, LIDOCAINE HCL FOR INTRAVENOUS INFUSION, 10 MG	D	N	51	A		2049
J2010	INJECTION, LINCOMYCIN HCL, UP TO 300 MG	D	N	51	A		2049
J2020	INJECTION, LINEZOLID, 200MG	C	N	51	A		
J2060	INJECTION, LORAZEPAM, 2 MG	D	N	51	A		2049
J2150	INJECTION, MANNITOL, 25% IN 50 ML	D	N	51	A		2049
J2170	INJECTION, MECASERMIN, 1 MG	C	N	51	A		
J2175	INJECTION, MEPERIDINE HYDROCHLORIDE, PER 100 MG	D	N	51	A		2049

HCPCS Code	Statute	Lab Cert	X-Ref	ASC Pay Grp	ASC Pay Group Eff. Date	Proc Notes	BETOS	TOS	Anest	Code Add Date	Code Effective Date	Code Term Date
J1720							O1E	1, P	0	19820101	19970101	
J1730				YY	20080101		O1E	1, P	0	19820101	19970101	
J1740				YY	20080101		O1E	1, P	0	20070101	20070101	
J1742				YY	20080101		O1E	1, P	0	19980101	19980101	
J1743				YY	20080101		O1E	1, P	0	20080101	20080101	
J1745				YY	20080101		O1E	1, P	0	20000101	20000101	
J1750				YY	20090101		O1E	1, P	0	20051231	20090101	
J1751							O1E	1, P	0	20060101	20090101	20081231
J1752							O1E	1, P	0	20060101	20090101	20081231
J1756				YY	20080101		O1E	1, P	0	20030101	20030101	
J1785				YY	20080101		O1E	1, P	0	19950101	19970101	
J1790							O1E	1, P	0	19820101	19970101	
J1800							O1E	1, P	0	19820101	19970101	
J1810							O1E	1, P	0	19820101	19970101	
J1815							O1E	1, P	0	20030101	20030101	
J1817				YY	20100101		D1G	1, P	0	20030101	20030101	
J1825							O1E	1	0	19980101	20030101	
J1830				YY	20080101		O1E	1	0	19820101	20000101	
J1835							O1E	1, P	0	20020101	20020101	
J1840							O1E	1, P	0	19820101	19970101	
J1850							O1E	1, P	0	19820101	19970101	
J1885							O1E	1, P	0	19930101	19970101	
J1890							O1E	1, P	0	19820101	19970101	
J1930				YY	20090101		O1E	1, P	0	20090101	20090101	
J1931				YY	20080101		O1E	1, P	0	20050101	20050101	
J1940							O1E	1, P	0	19820101	19970101	
J1945				YY	20080101	0095	O1E	1, P	0	20060101	20060101	
J1950				YY	20080101		O1E	1, P	0	19860101	19970101	
J1953				YY	20090101		O1E	1, P	0	20090101	20090101	
J1955							O1E	1, P	0	19960101	19970101	
J1956							O1E	1, P	0	19990101	19990101	
J1960							O1E	1, P	0	19820101	19970101	
J1980							O1E	1, P	0	19820101	19970101	
J1990							O1E	1, P	0	19820101	19970101	
J2001							O1E	1, P	0	20040101	20040101	
J2010							O1E	1, P	0	19820101	19970101	
J2020				YY	20080101		O1E	1, P	0	20020101	20020101	
J2060							O1E	1, P	0	19820101	19970101	
J2150							O1E	1, P	s	19860101	19970101	
J2170							O1E	1, P	0	20070101	20070101	
J2175							O1E	1, P	0	19860101	19970101	

HCPCS Code	Long Description	Coverage	Action	PI	MPI	CIM	MCM
J2180	INJECTION, MEPERIDINE AND PROMETHAZINE HCL, UP TO 50 MG	D	N	51	A		2049
J2185	INJECTION, MEROPENEM, 100 MG	C	N	51	A		
J2210	INJECTION, METHYLERGONOVINE MALEATE, UP TO 0.2 MG	D	N	51	A		2049
J2248	INJECTION, MICAFUNGIN SODIUM, 1 MG	C	N	51	A		
J2250	INJECTION, MIDAZOLAM HYDROCHLORIDE, PER 1 MG	D	N	51	A		2049
J2260	INJECTION, MILRINONE LACTATE, 5 MG	D	N	51	A		2049
J2270	INJECTION, MORPHINE SULFATE, UP TO 10 MG	D	N	51	A		2049
J2271	INJECTION, MORPHINE SULFATE, 100MG	D	N	51	A	60-14a	2049
J2275	INJECTION, MORPHINE SULFATE (PRESERVATIVE-FREE STERILE SOLUTION), PER 10 MG	D	N	51	A	60-14b	2049
J2278	INJECTION, ZICONOTIDE, 1 MICROGRAM	D	N	51	A		
J2280	INJECTION, MOXIFLOXACIN, 100 MG	C	N	51	A		
J2300	INJECTION, NALBUPHINE HYDROCHLORIDE, PER 10 MG	D	N	51	A		2049
J2310	INJECTION, NALOXONE HYDROCHLORIDE, PER 1 MG	D	N	51	A		2049
J2315	INJECTION, NALTREXONE, DEPOT FORM, 1 MG	C	N	51	A		
J2320	INJECTION, NANDROLONE DECANOATE, UP TO 50 MG	D	N	51	A		2049
J2321	INJECTION, NANDROLONE DECANOATE, UP TO 100 MG	D	N	51	A		2049
J2322	INJECTION, NANDROLONE DECANOATE, UP TO 200 MG	D	N	51	A		2049
J2323	INJECTION, NATALIZUMAB, 1 MG	C	N	51	A		
J2325	INJECTION, NESIRITIDE, 0.1 MG	D	N	51	A		2049
J2353	INJECTION, OCTREOTIDE, DEPOT FORM FOR INTRAMUSCULAR INJECTION, 1 MG	C	N	51	A		
J2354	INJECTION, OCTREOTIDE, NON-DEPOT FORM FOR SUBCUTANEOUS OR INTRAVENOUS INJECTION, 25 MCG	C	N	51	A		
J2355	INJECTION, OPRELVEKIN, 5 MG	D	N	51	A		2049
J2357	INJECTION, OMALIZUMAB, 5 MG	C	N	51	A		
J2360	INJECTION, ORPHENADRINE CITRATE, UP TO 60 MG	D	N	51	A		2049
J2370	INJECTION, PHENYLEPHRINE HCL, UP TO 1 ML	D	N	51	A		2049
J2400	INJECTION, CHLOROPROCAINE HYDROCHLORIDE, PER 30 ML	D	N	51	A		2049
J2405	INJECTION, ONDANSETRON HYDROCHLORIDE, PER 1 MG	D	N	51	A		2049
J2410	INJECTION, OXYMORPHONE HCL, UP TO 1 MG	D	N	51	A		2049
J2425	INJECTION, PALIFERMIN, 50 MICROGRAMS	C	N	51	A		
J2430	INJECTION, PAMIDRONATE DISODIUM, PER 30 MG	D	N	51	A		2049
J2440	INJECTION, PAPAVERINE HCL, UP TO 60 MG	D	N	51	A		2049
J2460	INJECTION, OXYTETRACYCLINE HCL, UP TO 50 MG	D	N	51	A		2049
J2469	INJECTION, PALONOSETRON HCL, 25 MCG	C	N	51	A		
J2501	INJECTION, PARICALCITOL, 1 MCG	D	N	51	A		2049
J2503	INJECTION, PEGAPTANIB SODIUM, 0.3 MG	C	N	51	A		
J2504	INJECTION, PEGADEMASE BOVINE, 25 IU	D	N	51	A		2049
J2505	INJECTION, PEGFILGRASTIM, 6 MG	C	N	53	A		
J2510	INJECTION, PENICILLIN G PROCAINE, AQUEOUS, UP TO 600,000 UNITS	D	N	51	A		2049
J2513	INJECTION, PENTASTARCH, 10% SOLUTION, 100 ML	D	N	51	A		2049
J2515	INJECTION, PENTOBARBITAL SODIUM, PER 50 MG	D	N	51	A		2049
J2540	INJECTION, PENICILLIN G POTASSIUM, UP TO 600,000 UNITS	D	N	51	A		2049
J2543	INJECTION, PIPERACILLIN SODIUM/TAZOBACTAM SODIUM, 1 GRAM/0.125 GRAMS (1.125 GRAMS)	D	N	51	A		2049

HCPCS Code	Statute	Lab Cert	X-Ref	ASC Pay Grp	ASC Pay Group Eff. Date	Proc Notes	BETOS	TOS	Anest	Code Add Date	Code Effective Date	Code Term Date
J2180							O1E	1, P	0	19820101	19970101	
J2185							O1E	1, P	0	20040101	20040101	
J2210							O1E	1, P	0	19820101	19970101	
J2248				YY	20080101		O1E	1, P	0	20070101	20070101	
J2250							O1E	1, P	0	19960101	19970101	
J2260							O1E	1, P	0	19860101	20010101	
J2270							O1E	1, P	0	19820101	19970101	
J2271							O1E	1, P	0	19990101	20010101	
J2275							O1E	1, P	0	19930101	20010101	
J2278				YY	20080101	0123	O1E	1, P	0	20060101	20060101	
J2280							O1E	1, P	0	20040101	20040101	
J2300							O1E	1, P	0	19960101	19970101	
J2310							O1E	1, P	0	19960101	19970101	
J2315				YY	20080101		O1E	1, P	0	20070101	20070101	
J2320				YY	20100101		O1E	1, P	0	19860101	19970101	
J2321				YY	20100101		O1E	1, P	0	19870101	19970101	
J2322				YY	20100101		O1E	1, P	0	19870101	19970101	
J2323				YY	20080101		O1E	1, P	0	20080101	20080101	
J2325				YY	20080101		O1E	1, P	0	20060101	20060101	
J2353				YY	20080101		O1E	1, P	0	20040101	20040101	
J2354							O1E	1, P	0	20040101	20040101	
J2355				YY	20080101		O1E	1, P	0	19990101	19990101	
J2357				YY	20080101		O1E	1, P	0	20050101	20050101	
J2360							O1E	1, P	0	19820101	19970101	
J2370							O1E	1, P	0	19820101	19970101	
J2400							O1E	1, P	0	19860101	19970101	
J2405							O1E	1, P	0	19930101	19970101	
J2410							O1E	1, P	0	19820101	19970101	
J2425				YY	20080101		O1E	1, P	0	20060101	20060101	
J2430				YY	20080101		O1E	1, P	0	19820101	19970101	
J2440							O1E	1, P	0	19860101	19970101	
J2460							O1E	1, P	0	19820101	19970101	
J2469				YY	20080101		O1E	1, P	0	20050101	20090101	
J2501							O1E	1, P	0	20030101	20030101	
J2503				YY	20080101	0095	O1E	1, P	0	20060101	20060101	
J2504				YY	20080101	0095	O1E	1, P	0	20060101	20060101	
J2505				YY	20080101		O1E	1, P	0	20040101	20040101	
J2510							O1E	1, P	0	19820101	19970101	
J2513				YY	20080101	0095	O1E	1, P	0	20060101	20060101	
J2515							O1E	1, P	0	19820101	19970101	
J2540							O1E	1, P	0	19820101	19970101	
J2543							O1E	1, P	0	20000101	20010101	

HCPCS Code	Long Description	Coverage	Action	PI	MPI	CIM	MCM
J2545	PENTAMIDINE ISETHIONATE, INHALATION SOLUTION, FDA-APPROVED FINAL PRODUCT, NON-COMPOUNDED, ADMINISTERED THROUGH DME, UNIT DOSE FORM, PER 300 MG	D	N	51	A		
J2550	INJECTION, PROMETHAZINE HCL, UP TO 50 MG	D	N	51	A		2049
J2560	INJECTION, PHENOBARBITAL SODIUM, UP TO 120 MG	D	N	51	A		2049
J2562	INJECTION, PLERIXAFOR, 1 MG	C	A	51	A		
J2590	INJECTION, OXYTOCIN, UP TO 10 UNITS	D	N	51	A		2049
J2597	INJECTION, DESMOPRESSIN ACETATE, PER 1 MCG	D	N	51	A		2049
J2650	INJECTION, PREDNISOLONE ACETATE, UP TO 1 ML	D	N	51	A		2049
J2670	INJECTION, TOLAZOLINE HCL, UP TO 25 MG	D	N	51	A		2049
J2675	INJECTION, PROGESTERONE, PER 50 MG	D	N	51	A		2049
J2680	INJECTION, FLUPHENAZINE DECANOATE, UP TO 25 MG	D	N	51	A		2049
J2690	INJECTION, PROCAINAMIDE HCL, UP TO 1 GM	D	N	51	A		2049
J2700	INJECTION, OXACILLIN SODIUM, UP TO 250 MG	D	N	51	A		2049
J2710	INJECTION, NEOSTIGMINE METHYLSULFATE, UP TO 0.5 MG	D	N	51	A		2049
J2720	INJECTION, PROTAMINE SULFATE, PER 10 MG	D	N	51	A		2049
J2724	INJECTION, PROTEIN C CONCENTRATE, INTRAVENOUS, HUMAN, 10 IU	C	N	51	A		
J2725	INJECTION, PROTIRELIN, PER 250 MCG	D	N	51	A		2049
J2730	INJECTION, PRALIDOXIME CHLORIDE, UP TO 1 GM	D	N	51	A		2049
J2760	INJECTION, PHENTOLAMINE MESYLATE, UP TO 5 MG	D	N	51	A		2049
J2765	INJECTION, METOCLOPRAMIDE HCL, UP TO 10 MG	D	N	51	A		2049
J2770	INJECTION, QUINUPRISTIN/DALFOPRISTIN, 500 MG (150/350)	D	N	51	A		2049
J2778	INJECTION, RANIBIZUMAB, 0.1 MG	C	N	51	A		
J2780	INJECTION, RANITIDINE HYDROCHLORIDE, 25 MG	D	N	51	A		2049
J2783	INJECTION, RASBURICASE, 0.5 MG	C	N	51	A		
J2785	INJECTION, REGADENOSON, 0.1 MG	C	N	51	A		
J2788	INJECTION, RHO D IMMUNE GLOBULIN, HUMAN, MINIDOSE, 50 MICROGRAMS (250 I.U.)	D	N	51	A		2049
J2790	INJECTION, RHO D IMMUNE GLOBULIN, HUMAN, FULL DOSE, 300 MICROGRAMS (1500 I.U.)	D	N	51	A		2049
J2791	INJECTION, RHO(D) IMMUNE GLOBULIN (HUMAN), (RHOPHYLAC), INTRAMUSCULAR OR INTRAVENOUS, 100 IU	D	N	51	A		2049
J2792	INJECTION, RHO D IMMUNE GLOBULIN, INTRAVENOUS, HUMAN, SOLVENT DETERGENT, 100 IU	D	N	51	A		2049
J2793	INJECTION, RILONACEPT, 1 MG	D	A	51	A		2049
J2794	INJECTION, RISPERIDONE, LONG ACTING, 0.5 MG	C	N	51	A		
J2795	INJECTION, ROPIVACAINE HYDROCHLORIDE, 1 MG	C	N	51	A		
J2796	INJECTION, ROMIPLOSTIM, 10 MICROGRAMS	C	A	51	A		
J2800	INJECTION, METHOCARBAMOL, UP TO 10 ML	D	N	51	A		2049
J2805	INJECTION, SINCALIDE, 5 MICROGRAMS	C	N	51	A		
J2810	INJECTION, THEOPHYLLINE, PER 40 MG	D	N	51	A		2049
J2820	INJECTION, SARGRAMOSTIM (GM-CSF), 50 MCG	D	N	51	A		2049
J2850	INJECTION, SECRETIN, SYNTHETIC, HUMAN, 1 MICROGRAM	D	N	51	A		2049
J2910	INJECTION, AUROTHIOGLUCOSE, UP TO 50 MG	D	N	51	A		2049
J2912	INJECTION, SODIUM CHLORIDE, 0.9%, PER 2 ML	D	N	51	A		2049
J2916	INJECTION, SODIUM FERRIC GLUCONATE COMPLEX IN SUCROSE INJECTION, 12.5 MG	D	N	51	A		2049.2, 2049.4

HCPCS Code	Statute	Lab Cert	X-Ref	ASC Pay Grp	ASC Pay Group Eff. Date	Proc Notes	BETOS	TOS	Anest	Code Add Date	Code Effective Date	Code Term Date
J2545						0127	D1G	1, P	0	19920101	20080101	
J2550							O1E	1, P	0	19820101	19970101	
J2560							O1E	1, P	0	19820101	19970101	
J2562				YY	20100101		O1E	1, P	0	20100101	20100101	
J2590							O1E	1, P	0	19860101	19970101	
J2597							O1E	1, P	0	19960101	19970101	
J2650							O1E	1, P	0	19820101	19970101	
J2670							O1E	1, P	0	19860101	19970101	
J2675							O1E	1, P	0	19860101	20020701	
J2680							O1E	1, P	0	19820101	19970101	
J2690							O1E	1, P	0	19820101	19970101	
J2700							O1E	1, P	0	19820101	19970101	
J2710							O1E	1, P	0	19820101	19970101	
J2720							O1E	1, P	0	19820101	19970101	
J2724				YY	20080101		O1E	1, P	0	20080101	20090101	
J2725							O1E	1, P	0	19950101	19970101	
J2730				YY	20080101		O1E	1, P	0	19860101	19970101	
J2760							O1E	1, P	0	19820101	19970101	
J2765							O1E	1, P	0	19820101	19970101	
J2770				YY	20080101		O1E	1, P	0	20010101	20010101	
J2778				YY	20080101		O1E	1, P	0	20080101	20080101	
J2780							O1E	1, P	0	20000101	20000101	
J2783				YY	20080101		O1E	1, P	0	20040101	20040101	
J2785				YY	20090101		O1E	1, P	0	20090101	20090101	
J2788				YY	20080101		O1E	1, P	0	20030101	20090101	
J2790				YY	20080101		O1E	1, P	0	19860101	20090101	
J2791				YY	20080101		O1E	1, P	0	20080101	20080101	
J2792				YY	20080101		O1E	1, P	0	19990101	19990101	
J2793				YY	20100101		O1E	1, P	0	20100101	20100101	
J2794				YY	20080101		O1E	1, P	0	20050101	20050101	
J2795							O1E	1, P	0	20010101	20010101	
J2796				YY	20100101		O1E	1, P	0	20100101	20100101	
J2800							O1E	1, P	0	19820101	19970101	
J2805							O1E	1, P	0	20060101	20060101	
J2810							O1E	1, P	0	19820101	19970101	
J2820				YY	20080101		O1E	1, P	0	19820101	19980101	
J2850				YY	20080101		O1E	1, P	0	20060101	20060101	
J2910							O1E	1, P	0	19820101	19970101	
J2912							O1E	1, P	0	19860101	20070101	20061231
J2916							O1E	1, P	0	20030101	20030101	

HCPCS Code	Long Description	Coverage	Action	PI	MPI	CIM	MCM
J2920	INJECTION, METHYLPREDNISOLONE SODIUM SUCCINATE, UP TO 40 MG	D	N	51	A		2049
J2930	INJECTION, METHYLPREDNISOLONE SODIUM SUCCINATE, UP TO 125 MG	D	N	51	A		2049
J2940	INJECTION, SOMATREM, 1 MG	D	N	51	A		2049
J2941	INJECTION, SOMATROPIN, 1 MG	D	N	51	A		2049
J2950	INJECTION, PROMAZINE HCL, UP TO 25 MG	D	N	51	A		2049
J2993	INJECTION, RETEPLASE, 18.1 MG	D	N	51	A		2049
J2995	INJECTION, STREPTOKINASE, PER 250,000 IU	D	N	51	A		2049
J2997	INJECTION, ALTEPLASE RECOMBINANT, 1 MG	D	N	51	A		2049
J3000	INJECTION, STREPTOMYCIN, UP TO 1 GM	D	N	51	A		2049
J3010	INJECTION, FENTANYL CITRATE, 0.1 MG	D	N	51	A		2049
J3030	INJECTION, SUMATRIPTAN SUCCINATE, 6 MG (CODE MAY BE USED FOR MEDICARE WHEN DRUG ADMINISTERED UNDER THE DIRECT SUPERVISION OF A PHYSICIAN, NOT FOR USE WHEN DRUG IS SELF ADMINISTERED)	D	N	51	A		2049
J3070	INJECTION, PENTAZOCINE, 30 MG	D	N	51	A		2049
J3100	INJECTION, TENECTEPLASE, 50MG	C	N	51	A		
J3101	INJECTION, TENECTEPLASE, 1 MG	C	N	51	A		
J3105	INJECTION, TERBUTALINE SULFATE, UP TO 1 MG	D	N	51	A		2049
J3110	INJECTION, TERIPARATIDE, 10 MCG	D	N	51	A		
J3120	INJECTION, TESTOSTERONE ENANTHATE, UP TO 100 MG	D	N	51	A		2049
J3130	INJECTION, TESTOSTERONE ENANTHATE, UP TO 200 MG	D	N	51	A		2049
J3140	INJECTION, TESTOSTERONE SUSPENSION, UP TO 50 MG	D	N	51	A		2049
J3150	INJECTION, TESTOSTERONE PROPIONATE, UP TO 100 MG	D	N	51	A		2049
J3230	INJECTION, CHLORPROMAZINE HCL, UP TO 50 MG	D	N	51	A		2049
J3240	INJECTION, THYROTROPIN ALPHA, 0.9 MG, PROVIDED IN 1.1 MG VIAL	D	N	51	A		2049
J3243	INJECTION, TIGECYCLINE, 1 MG	C	N	51	A		
J3246	INJECTION, TIROFIBAN HCL, 0.25MG	C	N	51	A		
J3250	INJECTION, TRIMETHOBENZAMIDE HCL, UP TO 200 MG	D	N	51	A		2049
J3260	INJECTION, TOBRAMYCIN SULFATE, UP TO 80 MG	D	N	51	A		2049
J3265	INJECTION, TORSEMIDE, 10 MG/ML	D	N	51	A		2049
J3280	INJECTION, THIETHYLPERAZINE MALEATE, UP TO 10 MG	D	N	51	A		2049
J3285	INJECTION, TREPROSTINIL, 1 MG	C	N	51	A		
J3300	INJECTION, TRIAMCINOLONE ACETONIDE, PRESERVATIVE FREE, 1 MG	D	N	51	A		
J3301	INJECTION, TRIAMCINOLONE ACETONIDE, NOT OTHERWISE SPECIFIED, 10 MG	D	N	51	A		2049
J3302	INJECTION, TRIAMCINOLONE DIACETATE, PER 5MG	D	N	51	A		2049
J3303	INJECTION, TRIAMCINOLONE HEXACETONIDE, PER 5MG	D	N	51	A		2049
J3305	INJECTION, TRIMETREXATE GLUCURONATE, PER 25 MG	D	N	51	A		2049
J3310	INJECTION, PERPHENAZINE, UP TO 5 MG	D	N	51	A		2049
J3315	INJECTION, TRIPTORELIN PAMOATE, 3.75 MG	D	N	51	A		2049
J3320	INJECTION, SPECTINOMYCIN DIHYDROCHLORIDE, UP TO 2 GM	D	N	51	A		2049
J3350	INJECTION, UREA, UP TO 40 GM	D	N	51	A		2049
J3355	INJECTION, UROFOLLITROPIN, 75 IU	D	N	51	A		2049
J3360	INJECTION, DIAZEPAM, UP TO 5 MG	D	N	51	A		2049
J3364	INJECTION, UROKINASE, 5000 IU VIAL	D	N	51	A		2049

HCPCS Code	Statute	Lab Cert	X-Ref	ASC Pay Grp	ASC Pay Group Eff. Date	Proc Notes	BETOS	TOS	Anest	Code Add Date	Code Effective Date	Code Term Date
J2920							O1E	1, P	0	19820101	19970101	
J2930							O1E	1, P	0	19840101	19970101	
J2940	1861s2b			YY	20080101		O1E	1, P	0	20020101	20020101	
J2941	1861s2b			YY	20080101		O1E	1, P	0	20020101	20020101	
J2950							O1E	1, P	0	19820101	19970101	
J2993				YY	20080101		O1E	1, P	0	20010101	20010101	
J2995				YY	20080101		O1E	1, P	0	19860101	19970101	
J2997				YY	20080101		O1E	1, P	0	20010101	20010101	
J3000							O1E	1, P	0	19820101	19970101	
J3010							O1E	1, P	0	19820101	20010101	
J3030				YY	20080101		O1E	1, P	0	19860101	20000101	
J3070							O1E	1, P	0	19820101	20030101	
J3100							O1E	1, P	0	20020101	20090101	20081231
J3101				YY	20090101		O1E	1, P	0	20090101	20090101	
J3105							O1E	1, P	0	19870101	19970101	
J3110						0120	O1E	1, P	0	20050101	20050101	
J3120							O1E	1, P	0	19820101	19970101	
J3130							O1E	1, P	0	19820101	19970101	
J3140							O1E	1, P	0	19820101	19970101	
J3150							O1E	1, P	0	19820101	19970101	
J3230							O1E	1, P	0	19820101	19970101	
J3240				YY	20080101		O1E	1, P	0	19860101	20030101	
J3243				YY	20080101		O1E	1, P	0	20070101	20070101	
J3246				YY	20080101		O1E	1, P	0	20050101	20050101	
J3250							O1E	1, P	0	19820101	19970101	
J3260							O1E	1, P	0	19820101	19970101	
J3265							O1E	1, P	0	19960101	19970101	
J3280							O1E	1, P	0	19820101	19970101	
J3285				YY	20080101		O1E	1, P	0	20060101	20060101	
J3300				YY	20090101	0127	O1E	1, P	0	20090101	20090101	
J3301							O1E	1, P	0	19910101	20090101	
J3302							O1E	1, P	0	19910101	19970101	
J3303							O1E	1, P	0	19910101	19970101	
J3305				YY	20080101		O1E	1, P	0	19960101	19970101	
J3310							O1E	1, P	0	19820101	19970101	
J3315				YY	20080101		O1E	1, P	0	20030101	20030101	
J3320							O1E	1, P	0	19820101	19970101	
J3350							O1E	1, P	0	19860101	19970101	
J3355				YY	20080101	0095	O1E	1, P	0	20060101	20060101	
J3360							O1E	1, P	0	19820101	19970101	
J3364							O1E	1, P	0	19930101	19970101	

HCPCS Code	Long Description	Coverage	Action	PI	MPI	CIM	MCM
J3365	INJECTION, IV, UROKINASE, 250,000 I.U. VIAL	D	N	51	A		2049
J3370	INJECTION, VANCOMYCIN HCL, 500 MG	D	N	51	A	60-14	2049
J3396	INJECTION, VERTEPORFIN, 0.1 MG	D	N	51	A		35-100, 45-30
J3400	INJECTION, TRIFLUPROMAZINE HCL, UP TO 20 MG	D	N	51	A		2049
J3410	INJECTION, HYDROXYZINE HCL, UP TO 25 MG	D	N	51	A		2049
J3411	INJECTION, THIAMINE HCL, 100 MG	C	N	51	A		
J3415	INJECTION, PYRIDOXINE HCL, 100 MG	C	N	51	A		
J3420	INJECTION, VITAMIN B-12 CYANOCOBALAMIN, UP TO 1000 MCG	D	N	51	A	45-4	2049
J3430	INJECTION, PHYTONADIONE (VITAMIN K), PER 1 MG	D	N	51	A		2049
J3465	INJECTION, VORICONAZOLE, 10 MG	D	N	51	A		2049
J3470	INJECTION, HYALURONIDASE, UP TO 150 UNITS	D	N	51	A		2049
J3471	INJECTION, HYALURONIDASE, OVINE, PRESERVATIVE FREE, PER 1 USP UNIT (UP TO 999 USP UNITS)	D	N	51	A		
J3472	INJECTION, HYALURONIDASE, OVINE, PRESERVATIVE FREE, PER 1000 USP UNITS	D	N	51	A		
J3473	INJECTION, HYALURONIDASE, RECOMBINANT, 1 USP UNIT	D	N	51	A		2049
J3475	INJECTION, MAGNESIUM SULFATE, PER 500 MG	D	N	51	A		2049
J3480	INJECTION, POTASSIUM CHLORIDE, PER 2 MEQ	D	N	51	A		2049
J3485	INJECTION, ZIDOVUDINE, 10 MG	D	N	51	A		2049
J3486	INJECTION, ZIPRASIDONE MESYLATE, 10 MG	C	N	51	A		
J3487	INJECTION, ZOLEDRONIC ACID (ZOMETA), 1 MG	C	N	51	A		
J3488	INJECTION, ZOLEDRONIC ACID (RECLAST), 1 MG	D	N	51	A		
J3490	UNCLASSIFIED DRUGS	D	N	51	A		2049
J3520	EDETATE DISODIUM, PER 150 MG	M	N	00	9	35-64, 45-20	
J3530	NASAL VACCINE INHALATION	D	N	51	A		2049
J3535	DRUG ADMINISTERED THROUGH A METERED DOSE INHALER	M	N	00	9		2050.5
J3570	LAETRILE, AMYGDALIN, VITAMIN B17	M	N	00	9	45-10	
J3590	UNCLASSIFIED BIOLOGICS	C	N	51	A		
J7030	INFUSION, NORMAL SALINE SOLUTION , 1000 CC	D	N	51	A		2049
J7040	INFUSION, NORMAL SALINE SOLUTION, STERILE (500 ML=1 UNIT)	D	N	51	A		2049
J7042	5% DEXTROSE/NORMAL SALINE (500 ML = 1 UNIT)	D	N	51	A		2049
J7050	INFUSION, NORMAL SALINE SOLUTION , 250 CC	D	N	51	A		2049
J7060	5% DEXTROSE/WATER (500 ML = 1 UNIT)	D	N	51	A		2049
J7070	INFUSION, D5W, 1000 CC	D	N	51	A		2049
J7100	INFUSION, DEXTRAN 40, 500 ML	D	N	51	A		2049
J7110	INFUSION, DEXTRAN 75, 500 ML	D	N	51	A		2049
J7120	RINGERS LACTATE INFUSION, UP TO 1000 CC	D	N	51	A		2049
J7130	HYPERTONIC SALINE SOLUTION, 50 OR 100 MEQ, 20 CC VIAL	D	N	51	A		2049
J7185	INJECTION, FACTOR VIII (ANTIHEMOPHILIC FACTOR, RECOMBINANT) (XYNTHA), PER I.U.	C	A	51	A		
J7186	INJECTION, ANTIHEMOPHILIC FACTOR VIII/VON WILLEBRAND FACTOR COMPLEX (HUMAN),PER FACTOR VIII I.U.	D	N	51	A		2049
J7187	INJECTION, VON WILLEBRAND FACTOR COMPLEX (HUMATE-P), PER IU VWF:RCO	D	N	51	A		2049
J7188	INJECTION, VON WILLEBRAND FACTOR COMPLEX, HUMAN, IU	D	N	51	A	35.30	2049.5
J7189	FACTOR VIIA (ANTIHEMOPHILIC FACTOR, RECOMBINANT), PER 1 MICROGRAM	D	N	51	A		2049

HCPCS Code	Statute	Lab Cert	X-Ref	ASC Pay Grp	ASC Pay Group Eff. Date	Proc Notes	BETOS	TOS	Anest	Code Add Date	Code Effective Date	Code Term Date
J3365			Q0089	YY	20080101		O1E	1, P	0	19920101	19970101	
J3370							O1E	1, P	0	19860101	20000101	
J3396				YY	20080101		O1E	9	0	20050101	20050101	
J3400							O1E	1, P	0	19820101	19970101	
J3410							O1E	1, P	0	19820101	19970101	
J3411							O1E	1, P	0	20040101	20040101	
J3415							O1E	1, P	0	20040101	20040101	
J3420							O1E	1, P	0	19860101	19970101	
J3430							O1E	1, P	0	19820101	19970101	
J3465				YY	20080101		O1E	1, P	0	20040101	20040101	
J3470							O1E	1, P	0	19820101	19970101	
J3471						0123	O1E	1, P	0	20060101	20060101	
J3472						0123	O1E	1, P	0	20060101	20060101	
J3473							O1E	1, P	0	20070101	20070101	
J3475							O1E	1, P	0	19960101	19970101	
J3480							O1E	1, P	0	19960101	19970101	
J3485							O1E	1, P	0	20010101	20010101	
J3486							O1E	1, P	0	20040101	20040101	
J3487				YY	20080101		O1E	1, P	0	20030101	20080101	
J3488				YY	20080101	0135	O1E	1, P	0	20080101	20080101	
J3490							O1E	1, P	0	19860101	19970101	
J3520							O1E	1, P	0	19860101	19960101	
J3530							O1E	1, P	0	19860101	19970101	
J3535							O1E	1, P	0	19940101	19970101	
J3570							O1E	1, P	0	19860101	19960101	
J3590							O1E	1, P	0	20030101	20030101	
J7030							O1E	1, P	0	19820101	19970101	
J7040							O1E	1, P	0	19840101	19970101	
J7042							O1E	1, P	0	19840101	19970101	
J7050							O1E	1, P	0	19820101	19970101	
J7060							O1E	1, P	0	19850101	19970101	
J7070							O1E	1, P	0	19820101	19970101	
J7100							O1E	1, P	0	19820101	19970101	
J7110							O1E	1, P	0	19820101	19970101	
J7120							O1E	1, P	0	19820101	19970101	
J7130							O1E	1, P	0	19840101	19970101	
J7185				YY	20100101		O1E	1, P	0	20100101	20100101	
J7186				YY	20090101		O1E	1, P	0	20090101	20090101	
J7187				YY	20080101		O1E	1, P	0	20070101	20080101	
J7188						0095	O1E	1, P	0	20060101	20070101	20061231
J7189				YY	20080101		O1E	1, P	0	20060101	20060101	

HCPCS Code	Long Description	Coverage	Action	PI	MPI	CIM	MCM
J7190	FACTOR VIII (ANTIHEMOPHILIC FACTOR, HUMAN) PER I.U.	D	N	51	A		2049
J7191	FACTOR VIII (ANTIHEMOPHILIC FACTOR (PORCINE)), PER I.U.	D	N	51	A		2049
J7192	FACTOR VIII (ANTIHEMOPHILIC FACTOR, RECOMBINANT) PER I.U., NOT OTHERWISE SPECIFIED	D	C	51	A		2049
J7193	FACTOR IX (ANTIHEMOPHILIC FACTOR, PURIFIED, NON-RECOMBINANT) PER I.U.	D	N	51	A		2049
J7194	FACTOR IX, COMPLEX, PER I.U.	D	N	51	A		2049
J7195	FACTOR IX (ANTIHEMOPHILIC FACTOR, RECOMBINANT) PER I.U.	D	N	51	A		2049
J7197	ANTITHROMBIN III (HUMAN), PER I.U.	D	N	51	A		2049
J7198	ANTI-INHIBITOR, PER I.U.	D	N	51	A	45-24	2049
J7199	HEMOPHILIA CLOTTING FACTOR, NOT OTHERWISE CLASSIFIED	D	N	51	A	45-24	2049
J7300	INTRAUTERINE COPPER CONTRACEPTIVE	S	N	00	9		
J7302	LEVONORGESTREL-RELEASING INTRAUTERINE CONTRACEPTIVE SYSTEM, 52 MG	S	N	00	9		
J7303	CONTRACEPTIVE SUPPLY, HORMONE CONTAINING VAGINAL RING, EACH	S	N	00	9		
J7304	CONTRACEPTIVE SUPPLY, HORMONE CONTAINING PATCH, EA.	S	N	00	9		
J7306	LEVONORGESTREL (CONTRACEPTIVE) IMPLANT SYSTEM, INCLUDING IMPLANTS AND SUPPLIES	I	N	00	9		
J7307	ETONOGESTREL (CONTRACEPTIVE) IMPLANT SYSTEM, INCLUDING IMPLANT AND SUPPLIES	I	N	00	9		
J7308	AMINOLEVULINIC ACID HCL FOR TOPICAL ADMINISTRATION, 20%, SINGLE UNIT DOSAGE FORM (354 MG)	C	N	51	A		
J7310	GANCICLOVIR, 4.5 MG, LONG-ACTING IMPLANT	D	N	51	A		2049
J7311	FLUOCINOLONE ACETONIDE, INTRAVITREAL IMPLANT	C	N	51	A		
J7317	SODIUM HYALURONATE, PER 20 TO 25 MG DOSE FOR INTRA-ARTICULAR INJECTION	C	N	51	A		
J7319	HYALURONAN (SODIUM HYALURONATE) OR DERIVATIVE, INTRA-ARTICULAR INJECTION, PER INJECTION	I	N	00	9		
J7320	HYLAN G-F 20, 16 MG, FOR INTRA-ARTICULAR INJECTION	C	N	51	A		
J7321	HYALURONAN OR DERIVATIVE, HYALGAN OR SUPARTZ, FOR INTRA-ARTICULAR INJECTION, PER DOSE	C	N	51	A		
J7322	HYALURONAN OR DERIVATIVE, SYNVISC, FOR INTRA-ARTICULAR INJECTION, PER DOSE	C	D	51	A		
J7323	HYALURONAN OR DERIVATIVE, EUFLEXXA, FOR INTRA-ARTICULAR INJECTION, PER DOSE	C	N	51	A		
J7324	HYALURONAN OR DERIVATIVE, ORTHOVISC, FOR INTRA-ARTICULAR INJECTION, PER DOSE	C	N	51	A		
J7325	HYALURONAN OR DERIVATIVE, SYNVISC OR SYNVISC-ONE, FOR INTRA-ARTICULAR INJECTION, 1 MG	C	A	51	A		
J7330	AUTOLOGOUS CULTURED CHONDROCYTES, IMPLANT	C	N	57	A		
J7340	DERMAL AND EPIDERMAL, (SUBSTITUTE) TISSUE OF HUMAN ORIGIN, WITH OR WITHOUT BIOENGINEERED OR PROCESSED ELEMENTS, WITH METABOLICALLY ACTIVE ELEMENTS, PER SQUARE CENTIMETER	C	N	51	A		
J7341	DERMAL (SUBSTITUTE) TISSUE OF NON-HUMAN ORIGIN, WITH OR WITHOUT OTHER BIOENGINEERED OR PROCESSED ELEMENTS, WITH METABOLICALLY ACTIVE ELEMENTS, PER SQUARE CENTIMETER	C	N	51	A		

HCPCS Code	Statute	Lab Cert	X-Ref	ASC Pay Grp	ASC Pay Group Eff. Date	Proc Notes	BETOS	TOS	Anest	Code Add Date	Code Effective Date	Code Term Date
J7190				YY	20080101		O1E	1, P	0	19860101	19990101	
J7191				YY	20090101		O1E	1, P	0	19960101	19980101	
J7192				YY	20080101		O1E	1, P	0	19940101	20100101	
J7193				YY	20080101		O1E	1, P	0	20020101	20020101	
J7194				YY	20080101		O1E	1, P	0	19860101	19980101	
J7195				YY	20080101		O1E	1, P	0	20020101	20020101	
J7197				YY	20100101		O1E	1, P	0	19920101	19970101	
J7198				YY	20080101		O1E	1, P	0	20000101	20000101	
J7199							O1E	1, P	0	20000101	20000101	
J7300	1862A1						P6C	9	0	19860101	19950401	
J7302	1862a1						P6C	9	0	20020101	20020101	
J7303	1862.1						Z2	9	0	20040101	20040101	
J7304	1862.1						Z2	9	0	20050101	20050101	
J7306							P6C	9	0	20060101	20060101	
J7307							Z2	9	0	20080101	20080101	
J7308				YY	20080101		O1E	1	0	20020101	20040101	
J7310				YY	20080101		O1E	9	0	19970101	19970101	
J7311				YY	20080101		O1E	Q	0	20070101	20070101	
J7317							O1E	1	0	20030101	20070101	20061231
J7319							O1E	1	0	20070101	20070401	20070331
J7320							O1E	1	0	19990101	20070101	20061231
J7321				YY	20080101		O1E	1	0	20080101	20080101	
J7322							O1E	1	0	20080101	20100101	20091231
J7323				YY	20080101		O1E	1	0	20080101	20080101	
J7324				YY	20080101		O1E	1	0	20080101	20080101	
J7325				YY	20100101		O1E	1, P	0	20100101	20100101	
J7330							O1E	1, P	0	20010101	20020701	
J7340							O1E	1	0	20020101	20090101	20081231
J7341							O1E	1	0	20060101	20090101	20081231

HCPCS Code	Long Description	Coverage	Action	PI	MPI	CIM	MCM
J7342	DERMAL (SUBSTITUTE) TISSUE OF HUMAN ORIGIN, WITH OR WITHOUT OTHER BIOENGINEERED OR PROCESSED ELEMENTS, WITH METABOLICALLY ACTIVE ELEMENTS, PER SQUARE CENTIMETER	C	N	46	A		
J7343	DERMAL AND EPIDERMAL, (SUBSTITUTE) TISSUE OF NON-HUMAN ORIGIN, WITH OR WITHOUT OTHER BIOENGINEERED OR PROCESSED ELEMENTS, WITHOUT METABOLICALLY ACTIVE ELEMENTS, PER SQUARE CENTIMETER	C	N	51	A		
J7344	DERMAL (SUBSTITUTE) TISSUE OF HUMAN ORIGIN, WITH OR WITHOUT OTHER BIOENGINEERED OR PROCESSED ELEMENTS, WITHOUT METABOLICALLY ACTIVE ELEMENTS, PER SQUARE CENTIMETER	C	N	51	A		
J7345	DERMAL (SUBSTITUTE) TISSUE OF NON-HUMAN ORIGIN, WITH OR WITHOUT OTHER BIOENGINEERED OR PROCESSED ELEMENTS, WITHOUT METABOLICALLY ACTIVE ELEMENTS, PER SQUARE CENTIMETER	C	N	51	A		
J7346	DERMAL (SUBSTITUTE) TISSUE OF HUMAN ORIGIN, INJECTABLE, WITH OR WITHOUT OTHER BIOENGINEERED OR PROCESSED ELEMENTS, BUT WITHOUT METABOLICALLY ACTIVE ELEMENTS, 1 CC	C	N	51	A		
J7347	DERMAL (SUBSTITUTE) TISSUE OF NONHUMAN ORIGIN, WITH OR WITHOUT OTHER BIOENGINEERED OR PROCESSED ELEMENTS, WITHOUT METABOLICALLY ACTIVE ELEMENTS (INTEGRA MATRIX), PER SQUARE CENTIMETER	C	N	51	A		
J7348	DERMAL (SUBSTITUTE) TISSUE OF NONHUMAN ORIGIN, WITH OR WITHOUT OTHER BIOENGINEERED OR PROCESSED ELEMENTS, WITHOUT METABOLICALLY ACTIVE ELEMENTS (TISSUEMEND), PER SQUARE CENTIMETER	C	N	51	A		
J7349	DERMAL (SUBSTITUTE) TISSUE OF NONHUMAN ORIGIN, WITH OR WITHOUT OTHER BIOENGINEERED OR PROCESSED ELEMENTS, WITHOUT METABOLICALLY ACTIVE ELEMENTS (PRIMATRIX), PER SQUARE CENTIMETER	C	N	51	A		
J7350	DERMAL (SUBSTITUTE) TISSUE OF HUMAN ORIGIN, INJECTABLE, WITH OR WITHOUT OTHER BIOENGINEERED OR PROCESSED ELEMENTS, BUT WITHOUT METABOLIZED ACTIVE ELEMENTS, PER 10 MG	C	N	51	A		
J7500	AZATHIOPRINE, ORAL, 50 MG	D	N	51	A		2049.5
J7501	AZATHIOPRINE, PARENTERAL, 100 MG	D	N	51	A		2049
J7502	CYCLOSPORINE, ORAL, 100 MG	D	N	57	A		2049.5
J7504	LYMPHOCYTE IMMUNE GLOBULIN, ANTITHYMOCYTE GLOBULIN, EQUINE, PARENTERAL, 250 MG	D	N	51	A	45-22	2049
J7505	MUROMONAB-CD3, PARENTERAL, 5 MG	D	N	51	A		2049
J7506	PREDNISONE, ORAL, PER 5MG	D	N	51	A		2049.5
J7507	TACROLIMUS, ORAL, PER 1 MG	D	N	51	A		2049.5
J7509	METHYLPREDNISOLONE ORAL, PER 4 MG	D	N	51	A		2049.5
J7510	PREDNISOLONE ORAL, PER 5 MG	D	N	51	A		2049.5
J7511	LYMPHOCYTE IMMUNE GLOBULIN, ANTITHYMOCYTE GLOBULIN, RABBIT, PARENTERAL, 25MG	C	N	51	A		

HCPCS Code	Statute	Lab Cert	X-Ref	ASC Pay Grp	ASC Pay Group Eff. Date	Proc Notes	BETOS	TOS	Anest	Code Add Date	Code Effective Date	Code Term Date
J7342							O1E	1	0	20030101	20090101	20081231
J7343							O1E	1	0	20050101	20090101	20081231
J7344							O1E	1	0	20050101	20090101	20081231
J7345							O1E	1	0	20070101	20080101	20071231
J7346							O1E	1	0	20070101	20090101	20081231
J7347							O1E	1	0	20080101	20090101	20081231
J7348							O1E	1	0	20080101	20090101	20081231
J7349							O1E	1	0	20080101	20090101	20081231
J7350							O1E	1, S	0	20030101	20070101	20061231
J7500							O1E	1, G	0	19880101	20000101	
J7501				YY	20080101		O1E	1, G	0	19880101	20000101	
J7502				YY	20080101		O1E	1, G	0	20000101	20000101	
J7504				YY	20080101		O1E	1, G	0	19880101	20020101	
J7505				YY	20080101		O1E	1, G	0	19880101	20010101	
J7506							O1E	1, G	0	19890101	20000101	
J7507				YY	20080101		O1E	1, G	0	19950101	20000101	
J7509							O1E	1, G	0	19960101	20000101	
J7510							O1E	1, G	0	19960101	20000101	
J7511				YY	20080101		O1E	1, G	0	20020101	20020101	

HCPCS Code	Long Description	Coverage	Action	PI	MPI	CIM	MCM
J7513	DACLIZUMAB, PARENTERAL, 25 MG	D	N	51	A		2049.5
J7515	CYCLOSPORINE, ORAL, 25 MG	C	N	51	A		
J7516	CYCLOSPORIN, PARENTERAL, 250 MG	C	N	51	A		
J7517	MYCOPHENOLATE MOFETIL, ORAL, 250 MG	C	N	51	A		
J7518	MYCOPHENOLIC ACID, ORAL, 180 MG	D	N	51	A		2050.5, 4471, 52
J7520	SIROLIMUS, ORAL, 1 MG	D	N	51	A		2049.5
J7525	TACROLIMUS, PARENTERAL, 5 MG	D	N	51	A		2049.5
J7599	IMMUNOSUPPRESSIVE DRUG, NOT OTHERWISE CLASSIFIED	D	N	51	A		2049.5
J7602	ALBUTEROL, ALL FORMULATIONS INCLUDING SEPARATED ISOMERS, INHALATION SOLUTION, FDA-APPROVED FINAL PRODUCT, NON-COMPOUNDED, ADMINISTERED THROUGH DME, CONCENTRATED FORM, PER 1 MG (ALBUTEROL) OR PER 0.5 MG (LEVALBUTEROL)	I	N	00	9		
J7603	ALBUTEROL, ALL FORMULATIONS INCLUDING SEPARATED ISOMERS, INHALATION SOLUTION, FDA-APPROVED FINAL PRODUCT, NON-COMPOUNDED, ADMINISTERED THROUGH DME, UNIT DOSE, PER 1 MG (ALBUTEROL) OR PER 0.5 MG (LEVALBUTEROL)	I	N	00	9		
J7604	ACETYLCYSTEINE, INHALATION SOLUTION, COMPOUNDED PRODUCT, ADMINISTERED THROUGH DME, UNIT DOSE FORM, PER GRAM	C	N	51	A		
J7605	ARFORMOTEROL, INHALATION SOLUTION, FDA APPROVED FINAL PRODUCT, NON-COMPOUNDED, ADMINISTERED THROUGH DME, UNIT DOSE FORM, 15 MICROGRAMS	C	N	51	A		
J7606	FORMOTEROL FUMARATE, INHALATION SOLUTION, FDA APPROVED FINAL PRODUCT, NON-COMPOUNDED, ADMINISTERED THROUGH DME, UNIT DOSE FORM, 20 MICROGRAMS	C	N	51	A		
J7607	LEVALBUTEROL, INHALATION SOLUTION, COMPOUNDED PRODUCT, ADMINISTERED THROUGH DME, CONCENTRATED FORM, 0.5 MG	C	N	51	A		
J7608	ACETYLCYSTEINE, INHALATION SOLUTION, FDA-APPROVED FINAL PRODUCT, NON-COMPOUNDED, ADMINISTERED THROUGH DME, UNIT DOSE FORM, PER GRAM	D	N	51	A		
J7609	ALBUTEROL, INHALATION SOLUTION, COMPOUNDED PRODUCT, ADMINISTERED THROUGH DME, UNIT DOSE, 1 MG	C	N	51	A		
J7610	ALBUTEROL, INHALATION SOLUTION, COMPOUNDED PRODUCT, ADMINISTERED THROUGH DME, CONCENTRATED FORM, 1 MG	C	N	51	A		
J7611	ALBUTEROL, INHALATION SOLUTION, FDA-APPROVED FINAL PRODUCT, NON-COMPOUNDED, ADMINISTERED THROUGH DME, CONCENTRATED FORM, 1 MG	D	F	00	9		2100.5
J7612	LEVALBUTEROL, INHALATION SOLUTION, FDA-APPROVED FINAL PRODUCT, NON-COMPOUNDED, ADMINISTERED THROUGH DME, CONCENTRATED FORM, 0.5 MG	D	F	00	9		2100.5
J7613	ALBUTEROL, INHALATION SOLUTION, FDA-APPROVED FINAL PRODUCT, NON-COMPOUNDED, ADMINISTERED THROUGH DME, UNIT DOSE, 1 MG	D	F	00	9		2100.5

HCPCS Code	Statute	Lab Cert	X-Ref	ASC Pay Grp	ASC Pay Group Eff. Date	Proc Notes	BETOS	TOS	Anest	Code Add Date	Code Effective Date	Code Term Date
J7513				YY	20080101		O1E	1, G	0	19990101	20000101	
J7515				YY	20100101		O1E	1, G	0	20000101	20000101	
J7516				YY	20090101		O1E	1, G	0	20000101	20000101	
J7517				YY	20080101		O1E	1, G	0	20000101	20000101	
J7518							O1E	1, G	0	20050101	20050101	
J7520				YY	20080101		O1E	1, G	0	20010101	20010101	
J7525				YY	20080101		O1E	1, G	0	20010101	20010101	
J7599							O1E	1, G	0	19960101	20000101	
J7602							O1E	1, P	0	20080101	20090101	20081231
J7603							O1E	1, P	0	20080101	20090101	20081231
J7604							D1G	1, P	0	20080101	20080101	
J7605							D1G	1, P	0	20080101	20080101	
J7606							D1G	1, P	0	20090101	20090101	
J7607							D1G	1, P	0	20070101	20070101	
J7608						0135	D1G	1, P	0	20000101	20080101	
J7609							D1G	1, P	0	20070101	20070101	
J7610							D1G	1, P	0	20070101	20070101	
J7611							D1G	1, P	0	20050101	20090701	
J7612							D1G	1, P	0	20050101	20090701	
J7613							D1G	1, P	0	20050101	20090701	

HCPCS Code	Long Description	Coverage	Action	PI	MPI	CIM	MCM
J7614	LEVALBUTEROL, INHALATION SOLUTION, FDA-APPROVED FINAL PRODUCT, NON-COMPOUNDED, ADMINISTERED THROUGH DME, UNIT DOSE, 0.5 MG	D	F	00	9		2100.5
J7615	LEVALBUTEROL, INHALATION SOLUTION, COMPOUNDED PRODUCT, ADMINISTERED THROUGH DME, UNIT DOSE, 0.5 MG	C	N	51	A		
J7620	ALBUTEROL, UP TO 2.5 MG AND IPRATROPIUM BROMIDE, UP TO 0.5 MG, FDA-APPROVED FINAL PRODUCT, NON-COMPOUNDED, ADMINISTERED THROUGH DME	D	N	51	A		
J7622	BECLOMETHASONE, INHALATION SOLUTION, COMPOUNDED PRODUCT, ADMINISTERED THROUGH DME, UNIT DOSE FORM, PER MILLIGRAM	C	N	51	A		
J7624	BETAMETHASONE, INHALATION SOLUTION, COMPOUNDED PRODUCT, ADMINISTERED THROUGH DME, UNIT DOSE FORM, PER MILLIGRAM	C	N	51	A		
J7626	BUDESONIDE, INHALATION SOLUTION, FDA-APPROVED FINAL PRODUCT, NON-COMPOUNDED, ADMINISTERED THROUGH DME, UNIT DOSE FORM, UP TO 0.5 MG	C	N	51	A		
J7627	BUDESONIDE, INHALATION SOLUTION, COMPOUNDED PRODUCT, ADMINISTERED THROUGH DME, UNIT DOSE FORM, UP TO 0.5 MG	C	N	51	A		
J7628	BITOLTEROL MESYLATE, INHALATION SOLUTION, COMPOUNDED PRODUCT, ADMINISTERED THROUGH DME, CONCENTRATED FORM, PER MILLIGRAM	D	N	51	A		
J7629	BITOLTEROL MESYLATE, INHALATION SOLUTION, COMPOUNDED PRODUCT, ADMINISTERED THROUGH DME, UNIT DOSE FORM, PER MILLIGRAM	D	N	51	A		
J7631	CROMOLYN SODIUM, INHALATION SOLUTION, FDA-APPROVED FINAL PRODUCT, NON-COMPOUNDED, ADMINISTERED THROUGH DME, UNIT DOSE FORM, PER 10 MILLIGRAMS	D	N	51	A		
J7632	CROMOLYN SODIUM, INHALATION SOLUTION, COMPOUNDED PRODUCT, ADMINISTERED THROUGH DME, UNIT DOSE FORM, PER 10 MILLIGRAMS	C	N	51	A		
J7633	BUDESONIDE, INHALATION SOLUTION, FDA-APPROVED FINAL PRODUCT, NON-COMPOUNDED, ADMINISTERED THROUGH DME, CONCENTRATED FORM, PER 0.25 MILLIGRAM	C	N	51	A		
J7634	BUDESONIDE, INHALATION SOLUTION, COMPOUNDED PRODUCT, ADMINISTERED THROUGH DME, CONCENTRATED FORM, PER 0.25 MILLIGRAM	C	N	51	A		
J7635	ATROPINE, INHALATION SOLUTION, COMPOUNDED PRODUCT, ADMINISTERED THROUGH DME, CONCENTRATED FORM, PER MILLIGRAM	D	N	51	A		
J7636	ATROPINE, INHALATION SOLUTION, COMPOUNDED PRODUCT, ADMINISTERED THROUGH DME, UNIT DOSE FORM, PER MILLIGRAM	D	N	51	A		
J7637	DEXAMETHASONE, INHALATION SOLUTION, COMPOUNDED PRODUCT, ADMINISTERED THROUGH DME, CONCENTRATED FORM, PER MILLIGRAM	D	N	51	A		

HCPCS Code	Statute	Lab Cert	X-Ref	ASC Pay Grp	ASC Pay Group Eff. Date	Proc Notes	BETOS	TOS	Anest	Code Add Date	Code Effective Date	Code Term Date
J7614							D1G	1, P	0	20050101	20090701	
J7615							D1G	1, P	0	20070101	20070101	
J7620						0135	D1G	1, P	0	20060101	20070101	
J7622							D1G	1, P	0	20020101	20070101	
J7624							D1G	1, P	0	20020101	20070101	
J7626							D1G	1, P	0	20020101	20070101	
J7627							D1G	1, P	0	20060101	20070101	
J7628						0135	D1G	1, P	0	20000101	20070101	
J7629						0135	D1G	1, P	0	20000101	20070101	
J7631						0135	D1G	1, P	0	20000101	20080101	
J7632							D1G	1, P	0	20080101	20080101	
J7633							D1G	1, P	0	20030101	20070101	
J7634							D1G	1, P	0	20070101	20070101	
J7635						0135	D1G	1, P	0	20000101	20070101	
J7636						0135	D1G	1, P	0	20000101	20070101	
J7637						0135	D1G	1, P	0	20000101	20070101	

HCPCS Code	Long Description	Coverage	Action	PI	MPI	CIM	MCM
J7638	DEXAMETHASONE, INHALATION SOLUTION, COMPOUNDED PRODUCT, ADMINISTERED THROUGH DME, UNIT DOSE FORM, PER MILLIGRAM	D	N	51	A		
J7639	DORNASE ALFA, INHALATION SOLUTION, FDA-APPROVED FINAL PRODUCT, NON-COMPOUNDED, ADMINISTERED THROUGH DME, UNIT DOSE FORM, PER MILLIGRAM	D	N	51	A		
J7640	FORMOTEROL, INHALATION SOLUTION, COMPOUNDED PRODUCT, ADMINISTERED THROUGH DME, UNIT DOSE FORM, 12 MICROGRAMS	C	N	00	9		
J7641	FLUNISOLIDE, INHALATION SOLUTION, COMPOUNDED PRODUCT, ADMINISTERED THROUGH DME, UNIT DOSE, PER MILLIGRAM	C	N	51	A		
J7642	GLYCOPYRROLATE, INHALATION SOLUTION, COMPOUNDED PRODUCT, ADMINISTERED THROUGH DME, CONCENTRATED FORM, PER MILLIGRAM	D	N	51	A		
J7643	GLYCOPYRROLATE, INHALATION SOLUTION, COMPOUNDED PRODUCT, ADMINISTERED THROUGH DME, UNIT DOSE FORM, PER MILLIGRAM	D	N	51	A		
J7644	IPRATROPIUM BROMIDE, INHALATION SOLUTION, FDA-APPROVED FINAL PRODUCT, NON-COMPOUNDED, ADMINISTERED THROUGH DME, UNIT DOSE FORM, PER MILLIGRAM	D	N	51	A		
J7645	IPRATROPIUM BROMIDE, INHALATION SOLUTION, COMPOUNDED PRODUCT, ADMINISTERED THROUGH DME, UNIT DOSE FORM, PER MILLIGRAM	C	N	51	A		
J7647	ISOETHARINE HCL, INHALATION SOLUTION, COMPOUNDED PRODUCT, ADMINISTERED THROUGH DME, CONCENTRATED FORM, PER MILLIGRAM	C	N	51	A		
J7648	ISOETHARINE HCL, INHALATION SOLUTION, FDA-APPROVED FINAL PRODUCT, NON-COMPOUNDED, ADMINISTERED THROUGH DME, CONCENTRATED FORM, PER MILLIGRAM	D	N	51	A		
J7649	ISOETHARINE HCL, INHALATION SOLUTION, FDA-APPROVED FINAL PRODUCT, NON-COMPOUNDED, ADMINISTERED THROUGH DME, UNIT DOSE FORM, PER MILLIGRAM	D	N	51	A		
J7650	ISOETHARINE HCL, INHALATION SOLUTION, COMPOUNDED PRODUCT, ADMINISTERED THROUGH DME, UNIT DOSE FORM, PER MILLIGRAM	C	N	51	A		
J7657	ISOPROTERENOL HCL, INHALATION SOLUTION, COMPOUNDED PRODUCT, ADMINISTERED THROUGH DME, CONCENTRATED FORM, PER MILLIGRAM	C	N	51	A		
J7658	ISOPROTERENOL HCL, INHALATION SOLUTION, FDA-APPROVED FINAL PRODUCT, NON-COMPOUNDED, ADMINISTERED THROUGH DME, CONCENTRATED FORM, PER MILLIGRAM	D	N	51	A		
J7659	ISOPROTERENOL HCL, INHALATION SOLUTION, FDA-APPROVED FINAL PRODUCT, NON-COMPOUNDED, ADMINISTERED THROUGH DME, UNIT DOSE FORM, PER MILLIGRAM	D	N	51	A		

HCPCS Code	Statute	Lab Cert	X-Ref	ASC Pay Grp	ASC Pay Group Eff. Date	Proc Notes	BETOS	TOS	Anest	Code Add Date	Code Effective Date	Code Term Date
J7638						0135	D1G	1, P	0	20000101	20070101	
J7639						0135	D1G	1, P	0	20000101	20090101	
J7640							D1G	1, P	0	20060101	20070101	
J7641							D1G	1, P	0	20020101	20070101	
J7642						0135	D1G	1, P	0	20000101	20070101	
J7643						0135	D1G	1, P	0	20000101	20070101	
J7644						0135	D1G	1, P	0	20000101	20070101	
J7645							D1G	1, P	0	20070101	20070101	
J7647							D1G	1, P	0	20070101	20070101	
J7648						0135	D1G	1, P	0	20000101	20070101	
J7649						0135	D1G	1, P	0	20000101	20070101	
J7650							D1G	1, P	0	20070101	20070101	
J7657							D1G	1, P	0	20070101	20070101	
J7658						0135	D1G	1, P	0	20000101	20070101	
J7659						0135	D1G	1, P	0	20000101	20070101	

HCPCS Code	Long Description	Coverage	Action	PI	MPI	CIM	MCM
J7660	ISOPROTERENOL HCL, INHALATION SOLUTION, COMPOUNDED PRODUCT, ADMINISTERED THROUGH DME, UNIT DOSE FORM, PER MILLIGRAM	C	N	51	A		
J7667	METAPROTERENOL SULFATE, INHALATION SOLUTION, COMPOUNDED PRODUCT, CONCENTRATED FORM, PER 10 MILLIGRAMS	C	N	51	A		
J7668	METAPROTERENOL SULFATE, INHALATION SOLUTION, FDA-APPROVED FINAL PRODUCT, NON-COMPOUNDED, ADMINISTERED THROUGH DME, CONCENTRATED FORM, PER 10 MILLIGRAMS	D	N	51	A		
J7669	METAPROTERENOL SULFATE, INHALATION SOLUTION, FDA-APPROVED FINAL PRODUCT, NON-COMPOUNDED, ADMINISTERED THROUGH DME, UNIT DOSE FORM, PER 10 MILLIGRAMS	D	N	51	A		
J7670	METAPROTERENOL SULFATE, INHALATION SOLUTION, COMPOUNDED PRODUCT, ADMINISTERED THROUGH DME, UNIT DOSE FORM, PER 10 MILLIGRAMS	C	N	51	A		
J7674	METHACHOLINE CHLORIDE ADMINISTERED AS INHALATION SOLUTION THROUGH A NEBULIZER, PER 1 MG	C	N	51	A		
J7676	PENTAMIDINE ISETHIONATE, INHALATION SOLUTION, COMPOUNDED PRODUCT, ADMINISTERED THROUGH DME, UNIT DOSE FORM, PER 300 MG	C	N	51	A		
J7680	TERBUTALINE SULFATE, INHALATION SOLUTION, COMPOUNDED PRODUCT, ADMINISTERED THROUGH DME, CONCENTRATED FORM, PER MILLIGRAM	D	N	51	A		
J7681	TERBUTALINE SULFATE, INHALATION SOLUTION, COMPOUNDED PRODUCT, ADMINISTERED THROUGH DME, UNIT DOSE FORM, PER MILLIGRAM	D	N	51	A		
J7682	TOBRAMYCIN, INHALATION SOLUTION, FDA-APPROVED FINAL PRODUCT, NON-COMPOUNDED, UNIT DOSE FORM, ADMINISTERED THROUGH DME, PER 300 MILLIGRAMS	D	N	51	A		
J7683	TRIAMCINOLONE, INHALATION SOLUTION, COMPOUNDED PRODUCT, ADMINISTERED THROUGH DME, CONCENTRATED FORM, PER MILLIGRAM	D	N	51	A		
J7684	TRIAMCINOLONE, INHALATION SOLUTION, COMPOUNDED PRODUCT, ADMINISTERED THROUGH DME, UNIT DOSE FORM, PER MILLIGRAM	D	N	51	A		
J7685	TOBRAMYCIN, INHALATION SOLUTION, COMPOUNDED PRODUCT, ADMINISTERED THROUGH DME, UNIT DOSE FORM, PER 300 MILLIGRAMS	C	N	51	A		
J7699	NOC DRUGS, INHALATION SOLUTION ADMINISTERED THROUGH DME	D	N	51	A		
J7799	NOC DRUGS, OTHER THAN INHALATION DRUGS, ADMINISTERED THROUGH DME	D	N	51	A		2100.5
J8498	ANTIEMETIC DRUG, RECTAL/SUPPOSITORY, NOT OTHERWISE SPECIFIED	D	N	51	A		
J8499	PRESCRIPTION DRUG, ORAL, NON CHEMOTHERAPEUTIC, NOS	M	N	00	9		2049
J8501	APREPITANT, ORAL, 5 MG	D	N	51	A		
J8510	BUSULFAN; ORAL, 2 MG	D	N	51	A		2049.5

HCPCS Code	Statute	Lab Cert	X-Ref	ASC Pay Grp	ASC Pay Group Eff. Date	Proc Notes	BETOS	TOS	Anest	Code Add Date	Code Effective Date	Code Term Date
J7660							D1G	1, P	0	20070101	20070101	
J7667							D1G	1, P	0	20070101	20070101	
J7668						0135	D1G	1, P	0	20000101	20070101	
J7669						0135	D1G	1, P	0	20000101	20070101	
J7670							D1G	1, P	0	20070101	20070101	
J7674							O1E	1, P	0	20050101	20050101	
J7676							D1G	1, P	0	20080101	20080101	
J7680						0135	D1G	1, P	0	20000101	20070101	
J7681						0135	D1G	1, P	0	20000101	20070101	
J7682						0135	D1G	1, P	0	20000101	20070101	
J7683						0135	D1G	1, P	0	20000101	20070101	
J7684						0135	D1G	1, P	0	20000101	20070101	
J7685							D1G	1, P	0	20070101	20070101	
J7699						0135	D1G	1, P	0	19930101	20070101	
J7799							D1G	1, P	0	19930101	20020701	
J8498	1861s2T						O1D	1	0	20060101	20060101	
J8499							O1E	1, P	0	19950101	19970101	
J8501				YY	20080101	0119	O1E	1, G	0	20050101	20050101	
J8510							O1D	1, P	0	20000101	20000101	

HCPCS Code	Long Description	Coverage	Action	PI	MPI	CIM	MCM
J8515	CABERGOLINE, ORAL, 0.25 MG	M	N	00	9		2049.5
J8520	CAPECITABINE, ORAL, 150 MG	D	N	51	A		2049.5
J8521	CAPECITABINE, ORAL, 500 MG	D	N	51	A		2049.5
J8530	CYCLOPHOSPHAMIDE; ORAL, 25 MG	D	N	51	A		2049.5
J8540	DEXAMETHASONE, ORAL, 0.25 MG	D	N	51	A		2049.5
J8560	ETOPOSIDE; ORAL, 50 MG	D	N	51	A		2049.5
J8565	GEFITINIB, ORAL, 250 MG	I	N	00	9		
J8597	ANTIEMETIC DRUG, ORAL, NOT OTHERWISE SPECIFIED	D	N	51	A		
J8600	MELPHALAN; ORAL, 2 MG	D	N	51	A		2049.5
J8610	METHOTREXATE; ORAL, 2.5 MG	D	N	51	A		2049.5
J8650	NABILONE, ORAL, 1 MG	C	N	51	A		
J8700	TEMOZOLOMIDE, ORAL, 5 MG	D	N	51	A		2049.5C
J8705	TOPOTECAN, ORAL, 0.25 MG	C	N	51	A		
J8999	PRESCRIPTION DRUG, ORAL, CHEMOTHERAPEUTIC, NOS	D	N	51	A		2049.5
J9000	INJECTION, DOXORUBICIN HYDROCHLORIDE, 10 MG	D	N	51	A		2049
J9001	INJECTION, DOXORUBICIN HYDROCHLORIDE, ALL LIPID FORMULATIONS, 10 MG	D	N	51	A		2049
J9010	INJECTION, ALEMTUZUMAB, 10 MG	D	N	51	A		
J9015	INJECTION, ALDESLEUKIN, PER SINGLE USE VIAL	D	N	51	A		2049
J9017	INJECTION, ARSENIC TRIOXIDE, 1 MG	C	N	51	A		
J9020	INJECTION, ASPARAGINASE, 10,000 UNITS	D	N	51	A		2049
J9025	INJECTION, AZACITIDINE, 1 MG	C	N	51	A		
J9027	INJECTION, CLOFARABINE, 1 MG	C	N	51	A		
J9031	BCG (INTRAVESICAL) PER INSTILLATION	D	N	51	A		2049
J9033	INJECTION, BENDAMUSTINE HCL, 1 MG	C	N	51	A		
J9035	INJECTION, BEVACIZUMAB, 10 MG	C	N	51	A		
J9040	INJECTION, BLEOMYCIN SULFATE, 15 UNITS	D	N	51	A		2049
J9041	INJECTION, BORTEZOMIB, 0.1 MG	C	N	51	A		
J9045	INJECTION, CARBOPLATIN, 50 MG	D	N	51	A		2049
J9050	INJECTION, CARMUSTINE, 100 MG	D	N	51	A		2049
J9055	INJECTION, CETUXIMAB, 10 MG	C	N	51	A		
J9060	CISPLATIN, POWDER OR S0LUTION, PER 10 MG	D	N	51	A		2049
J9062	CISPLATIN, 50 MG	D	N	51	A		2049
J9065	INJECTION, CLADRIBINE, PER 1 MG	D	N	51	A		2049
J9070	CYCLOPHOSPHAMIDE, 100 MG	D	N	51	A		2049
J9080	CYCLOPHOSPHAMIDE, 200 MG	D	N	51	A		2049
J9090	CYCLOPHOSPHAMIDE, 500 MG	D	N	51	A		2049
J9091	CYCLOPHOSPHAMIDE, 1.0 GRAM	D	N	51	A		2049
J9092	CYCLOPHOSPHAMIDE, 2.0 GRAM	D	N	51	A		2049
J9093	CYCLOPHOSPHAMIDE, LYOPHILIZED, 100 MG	D	N	51	A		2049
J9094	CYCLOPHOSPHAMIDE, LYOPHILIZED, 200 MG	D	N	51	A		2049
J9095	CYCLOPHOSPHAMIDE, LYOPHILIZED, 500 MG	D	N	51	A		2049
J9096	CYCLOPHOSPHAMIDE, LYOPHILIZED, 1.0 GRAM	D	N	51	A		2049
J9097	CYCLOPHOSPHAMIDE, LYOPHILIZED, 2.0 GRAM	D	N	51	A		2049
J9098	INJECTION, CYTARABINE LIPOSOME, 10 MG	C	N	51	A		
J9100	INJECTION, CYTARABINE, 100 MG	D	N	51	A		2049
J9110	INJECTION, CYTARABINE, 500 MG	D	N	51	A		2049
J9120	INJECTION, DACTINOMYCIN, 0.5 MG	D	N	51	A		2049
J9130	DACARBAZINE, 100 MG	D	N	51	A		2049

HCPCS Code	Statute	Lab Cert	X-Ref	ASC Pay Grp	ASC Pay Group Eff. Date	Proc Notes	BETOS	TOS	Anest	Code Add Date	Code Effective Date	Code Term Date
J8515							O1E	1, P	0	20060101	20060101	
J8520				YY	20080101		O1D	1, P	0	20000101	20000101	
J8521				YY	20080101		O1D	1, P	0	20000101	20000101	
J8530							O1D	1,G,P	0	19950101	19970831	
J8540	1861(s)2T						O1E	1	0	20060101	20060101	
J8560				YY	20080101		O1D	1, P	0	19950101	19970101	
J8565							O1E	9	0	20050101	20050101	
J8597	1861s2T						O1D	1	0	20060101	20060101	
J8600							O1D	1, P	0	19950101	19970101	
J8610							O1D	1,G,P	0	19950101	19970831	
J8650							O1E	1, G	0	20070101	20070101	
J8700				YY	20080101		O1D	1, P	0	20010101	20010101	
J8705				YY	20090101		O1D	1, P	0	20090101	20090101	
J8999							O1D	1, P	0	19950101	19970101	
J9000							O1D	1, P	0	19840101	20090101	
J9001				YY	20080101		O1E	1, P	0	20000101	20090101	
J9010	1833T			YY	20080101		O1E	1, P	0	20030101	20090101	
J9015				YY	20080101		O1D	1, P	0	19960101	20090101	
J9017				YY	20080101		O1D	1, P	0	20020101	20090101	
J9020				YY	20080101		O1D	1, P	0	19840101	20090101	
J9025				YY	20080101		O1D	1, P	0	20060101	20060101	
J9027				YY	20080101		O1E	1, P	0	20060101	20060101	
J9031				YY	20080101		O1D	1, P	0	19910101	19970101	
J9033				YY	20090101		O1D	1, P	0	20090101	20090101	
J9035				YY	20080101		O1E	1, P	0	20050101	20050101	
J9040							O1D	1, P	0	19840101	20090101	
J9041				YY	20080101		O1E	1, P	0	20050101	20050101	
J9045							O1D	1, P	0	19900101	20090101	
J9050				YY	20080101		O1D	1, P	0	19840101	20090101	
J9055				YY	20080101		O1E	1, P	0	20050101	20050101	
J9060							O1D	1, P	0	19840101	19970101	
J9062							O1D	1, P	0	19820101	19970101	
J9065				YY	20080101		O1D	1, P	0	19950101	19970101	
J9070							O1D	1, P	0	19840101	19970101	
J9080							O1D	1, P	0	19940101	19970101	
J9090							O1D	1, P	0	19940101	19970101	
J9091							O1D	1, P	0	19940101	19970101	
J9092							O1D	1, P	0	19940101	19970101	
J9093							O1D	1, P	0	19880101	19970101	
J9094							O1D	1, P	0	19940101	19970101	
J9095							O1D	1, P	0	19940101	19970101	
J9096							O1D	1, P	0	19940101	19970101	
J9097							O1D	1, P	0	19940101	19970101	
J9098				YY	20080101		O1E	1, P	0	20040101	20090101	
J9100							O1D	1, P	0	19860101	20090101	
J9110							O1D	1, P	0	19940101	20090101	
J9120				YY	20080101		O1D	1, P	0	19840101	20090101	
J9130							O1D	1, P	0	19860101	20040101	

HCPCS Code	Long Description	Coverage	Action	PI	MPI	CIM	MCM
J9140	DACARBAZINE, 200 MG	D	N	51	A		2049
J9150	INJECTION, DAUNORUBICIN, 10 MG	D	N	51	A		2049
J9151	INJECTION, DAUNORUBICIN CITRATE, LIPOSOMAL FORMULATION, 10 MG	D	N	51	A		2049
J9155	INJECTION, DEGARELIX, 1 MG	C	A	51	A		
J9160	INJECTION, DENILEUKIN DIFTITOX, 300 MICROGRAMS	C	N	51	A		
J9165	INJECTION, DIETHYLSTILBESTROL DIPHOSPHATE, 250 MG	D	N	51	A		2049
J9170	INJECTION, DOCETAXEL, 20 MG	D	D	51	A		2049
J9171	INJECTION, DOCETAXEL, 1 MG	D	A	51	A		2049
J9175	INJECTION, ELLIOTTS' B SOLUTION, 1 ML	D	N	51	A		2049
J9178	INJECTION, EPIRUBICIN HCL, 2 MG	C	N	51	A		
J9181	INJECTION, ETOPOSIDE, 10 MG	D	N	51	A		2049
J9182	ETOPOSIDE, 100 MG	D	N	51	A		2049
J9185	INJECTION, FLUDARABINE PHOSPHATE, 50 MG	D	N	51	A		2049
J9190	INJECTION, FLUOROURACIL, 500 MG	D	N	51	A		2049
J9200	INJECTION, FLOXURIDINE, 500 MG	D	N	51	A		2049
J9201	INJECTION, GEMCITABINE HYDROCHLORIDE, 200 MG	D	N	51	A		2049
J9202	GOSERELIN ACETATE IMPLANT, PER 3.6 MG	D	N	51	A		2049
J9206	INJECTION, IRINOTECAN, 20 MG	D	N	51	A		2049
J9207	INJECTION, IXABEPILONE, 1 MG	C	N	51	A		
J9208	INJECTION, IFOSFAMIDE, 1 GRAM	D	N	51	A		2049
J9209	INJECTION, MESNA, 200 MG	D	N	51	A		2049
J9211	INJECTION, IDARUBICIN HYDROCHLORIDE, 5 MG	D	N	51	A		2049
J9212	INJECTION, INTERFERON ALFACON-1, RECOMBINANT, 1 MICROGRAM	D	N	51	A		2049
J9213	INJECTION, INTERFERON, ALFA-2A, RECOMBINANT, 3 MILLION UNITS	D	N	51	A		2049
J9214	INJECTION, INTERFERON, ALFA-2B, RECOMBINANT, 1 MILLION UNITS	D	N	51	A		2049
J9215	INJECTION, INTERFERON, ALFA-N3, (HUMAN LEUKOCYTE DERIVED), 250,000 IU	D	N	51	A		2049
J9216	INJECTION, INTERFERON, GAMMA 1-B, 3 MILLION UNITS	D	N	51	A		2049
J9217	LEUPROLIDE ACETATE (FOR DEPOT SUSPENSION), 7.5 MG	D	N	51	A		2049
J9218	LEUPROLIDE ACETATE, PER 1 MG	D	N	51	A		2049
J9219	LEUPROLIDE ACETATE IMPLANT, 65 MG	D	N	51	A		2049
J9225	HISTRELIN IMPLANT (VANTAS), 50 MG	D	N	51	A		2049
J9226	HISTRELIN IMPLANT (SUPPRELIN LA), 50 MG	D	N	51	A		2049
J9230	INJECTION, MECHLORETHAMINE HYDROCHLORIDE, (NITROGEN MUSTARD), 10 MG	D	N	51	A		2049
J9245	INJECTION, MELPHALAN HYDROCHLORIDE, 50 MG	D	N	51	A		2049
J9250	METHOTREXATE SODIUM, 5 MG	D	N	51	A		2049
J9260	METHOTREXATE SODIUM, 50 MG	D	N	51	A		2049
J9261	INJECTION, NELARABINE, 50 MG	C	N	51	A		
J9263	INJECTION, OXALIPLATIN, 0.5 MG	C	N	51	A		
J9264	INJECTION, PACLITAXEL PROTEIN-BOUND PARTICLES, 1 MG	C	N	51	A		
J9265	INJECTION, PACLITAXEL, 30 MG	D	N	51	A		2049
J9266	INJECTION, PEGASPARGASE, PER SINGLE DOSE VIAL	D	N	51	A		2049
J9268	INJECTION, PENTOSTATIN, 10 MG	D	N	51	A		2049
J9270	INJECTION, PLICAMYCIN, 2.5 MG	D	N	51	A		2049

HCPCS Code	Statute	Lab Cert	X-Ref	ASC Pay Grp	ASC Pay Group Eff. Date	Proc Notes	BETOS	TOS	Anest	Code Add Date	Code Effective Date	Code Term Date
J9140							O1D	1, P	0	19940101	19970101	
J9150				YY	20080101		O1D	1, P	0	19860101	20090101	
J9151				YY	20080101		O1D	1, P	0	19990101	20090101	
J9155				YY	20100101		O1E	1, P	0	20100101	20100101	
J9160				YY	20080101		O1E	1, P	0	20010101	20090101	
J9165				YY	20090101		O1D	1, P	0	19880101	20090101	
J9170							O1D	1, P	0	19980101	20100101	20091231
J9171				YY	20100101		O1E	1, P	0	20100101	20100101	
J9175						0095	O1E	1, P	0	20060101	20060101	
J9178				YY	20080101		O1E	1, P	0	20040101	20040101	
J9181							O1D	1, P	0	19870101	20090101	
J9182							O1D	1, P	0	19870101	20090101	20081231
J9185				YY	20080101		O1D	1, P	0	19940101	20090101	
J9190							O1D	1, P	0	19840101	20090101	
J9200				YY	20080101		O1D	1, P	0	19840101	20090101	
J9201				YY	20080101		O1D	1, P	0	19980101	20090101	
J9202				YY	20080101		O1D	1, P	0	19910101	19970101	
J9206				YY	20080101		O1D	1, P	0	19980101	20090101	
J9207				YY	20090101		O1D	1, P	0	20090101	20090101	
J9208				YY	20080101		O1D	1, P	0	19900101	20090101	
J9209				YY	20080101		O1D	1, P	0	19900101	20090101	
J9211				YY	20080101		O1D	1, P	0	19930101	20090101	
J9212				YY	20100101		O1E	1, P	0	19990101	20090101	
J9213				YY	20080101		O1D	G	0	19930101	20090101	
J9214				YY	20080101		O1D	G	0	19930101	20090101	
J9215				YY	20080101		O1D	G	0	19930101	20090101	
J9216				YY	20080101		O1D	G	0	19930101	20090101	
J9217				YY	20080101		O1D	1, P	0	19910101	19970101	
J9218				YY	20080101	0014	O1D	1, P	0	19900101	19970101	
J9219				YY	20080101		O1D	1, P	0	20010101	20010101	
J9225				YY	20080101		O1D	1, P	0	20060101	20080101	
J9226				YY	20080101		O1D	1, P	0	20080101	20080101	
J9230				YY	20080101		O1D	1, P	0	19860101	20090101	
J9245				YY	20080101		O1D	1, P	0	19950101	19970101	
J9250							O1D	1, P	0	19940101	19970101	
J9260							O1D	1, P	0	19840101	19970101	
J9261				YY	20080101		O1E	1, P	0	20070101	20070101	
J9263				YY	20080101		O1D	1, P	0	20040101	20040101	
J9264				YY	20080101		O1E	1, P	0	20060101	20070101	
J9265							O1D	1, P	0	19940101	20090101	
J9266				YY	20080101		O1D	1, P	0	19960101	20090101	
J9268				YY	20080101		O1D	1, P	0	19940101	20090101	
J9270							O1D	1, P	0	19840101	20090101	

HCPCS Code	Long Description	Coverage	Action	PI	MPI	CIM	MCM
J9280	MITOMYCIN, 5 MG	D	N	51	A		2049
J9290	MITOMYCIN, 20 MG	D	N	51	A		2049
J9291	MITOMYCIN, 40 MG	D	N	51	A		2049
J9293	INJECTION, MITOXANTRONE HYDROCHLORIDE, PER 5 MG	D	N	51	A		2049
J9300	INJECTION, GEMTUZUMAB OZOGAMICIN, 5 MG	C	N	51	A		
J9303	INJECTION, PANITUMUMAB, 10 MG	C	N	51	A		
J9305	INJECTION, PEMETREXED, 10 MG	C	N	51	A		
J9310	INJECTION, RITUXIMAB, 100 MG	D	N	51	A		2049
J9320	INJECTION, STREPTOZOCIN, 1 GRAM	D	N	51	A		2049
J9328	INJECTION, TEMOZOLOMIDE, 1 MG	C	A	51	A		
J9330	INJECTION, TEMSIROLIMUS, 1 MG	C	N	51	A		
J9340	INJECTION, THIOTEPA, 15 MG	D	N	51	A		2049
J9350	INJECTION, TOPOTECAN, 4 MG	D	N	51	A		2049
J9355	INJECTION, TRASTUZUMAB, 10 MG	C	N	51	A		
J9357	INJECTION, VALRUBICIN, INTRAVESICAL, 200 MG	D	N	51	A		2049
J9360	INJECTION, VINBLASTINE SULFATE, 1 MG	D	N	51	A		2049
J9370	VINCRISTINE SULFATE, 1 MG	D	N	51	A		2049
J9375	VINCRISTINE SULFATE, 2 MG	D	N	51	A		2049
J9380	VINCRISTINE SULFATE, 5 MG	D	N	51	A		2049
J9390	INJECTION, VINORELBINE TARTRATE, 10 MG	D	N	51	A		2049
J9395	INJECTION, FULVESTRANT, 25 MG	C	N	51	A		
J9600	INJECTION, PORFIMER SODIUM, 75 MG	D	N	51	A		2049
J9999	NOT OTHERWISE CLASSIFIED, ANTINEOPLASTIC DRUGS	D	N	51	A	45-16	2049
K0001	STANDARD WHEELCHAIR	C	N	36	A		
K0002	STANDARD HEMI (LOW SEAT) WHEELCHAIR	C	N	36	A		
K0003	LIGHTWEIGHT WHEELCHAIR	C	N	36	A		
K0004	HIGH STRENGTH, LIGHTWEIGHT WHEELCHAIR	C	N	36	A		
K0005	ULTRALIGHTWEIGHT WHEELCHAIR	C	N	32	A		
K0006	HEAVY DUTY WHEELCHAIR	C	N	36	A		
K0007	EXTRA HEAVY DUTY WHEELCHAIR	C	N	36	A		
K0009	OTHER MANUAL WHEELCHAIR/BASE	C	N	46	A		
K0010	STANDARD - WEIGHT FRAME MOTORIZED/POWER WHEELCHAIR	C	N	36	A		
K0011	STANDARD - WEIGHT FRAME MOTORIZED/POWER WHEELCHAIR WITH PROGRAMMABLE CONTROL PARAMETERS FOR SPEED ADJUSTMENT, TREMOR DAMPENING, ACCELERATION CONTROL AND BRAKING	C	N	36	A		
K0012	LIGHTWEIGHT PORTABLE MOTORIZED/POWER WHEELCHAIR	C	N	36	A		
K0014	OTHER MOTORIZED/POWER WHEELCHAIR BASE	C	N	36	A		
K0015	DETACHABLE, NON-ADJUSTABLE HEIGHT ARMREST, EACH	C	N	32	A		
K0017	DETACHABLE, ADJUSTABLE HEIGHT ARMREST, BASE, EACH	C	N	32	A		
K0018	DETACHABLE, ADJUSTABLE HEIGHT ARMREST, UPPER PORTION, EACH	C	N	32	A		
K0019	ARM PAD, EACH	C	N	32	A		
K0020	FIXED, ADJUSTABLE HEIGHT ARMREST, PAIR	C	N	32	A		
K0037	HIGH MOUNT FLIP-UP FOOTREST, EACH	C	N	32	A		
K0038	LEG STRAP, EACH	C	N	32	A		
K0039	LEG STRAP, H STYLE, EACH	C	N	32	A		
K0040	ADJUSTABLE ANGLE FOOTPLATE, EACH	C	N	32	A		

HCPCS Code	Statute	Lab Cert	X-Ref	ASC Pay Grp	ASC Pay Group Eff. Date	Proc Notes	BETOS	TOS	Anest	Code Add Date	Code Effective Date	Code Term Date
J9280				YY	20080101		O1D	1, P	0	19860101	19970101	
J9290				YY	20080101		O1D	1, P	0	19940101	19970101	
J9291				YY	20080101		O1D	1, P	0	19890101	19970101	
J9293				YY	20080101		O1D	1, P	0	19900101	19970101	
J9300				YY	20080101		O1D	1, P	0	20020101	20090101	
J9303				YY	20080101		O1D	1, P	0	20080101	20080101	
J9305				YY	20080101		O1E	1, P	0	20050101	20050101	
J9310				YY	20080101		O1D	1, P	0	19990101	20090101	
J9320				YY	20080101		O1D	1, P	0	19860101	20090101	
J9328				YY	20100101		O1D	1, P	0	20100101	20100101	
J9330				YY	20090101		O1D	1, P	0	20090101	20090101	
J9340				YY	20080101		O1D	1, P	0	19840101	20090101	
J9350				YY	20080101		O1D	1, P	0	19980101	20090101	
J9355				YY	20080101		O1E	1, P	0	20000101	20090101	
J9357				YY	20080101		O1E	1, P	0	20000101	20090101	
J9360							O1D	1, P	0	19860101	20090101	
J9370							O1D	1, P	0	19860101	19970101	
J9375							O1D	1, P	0	19880101	19970101	
J9380							O1D	1, P	0	19940101	19970101	
J9390							O1D	1, P	0	19960101	20090101	
J9395				YY	20080101		O1E	1, P	0	20040101	20040101	
J9600				YY	20080101		O1D	1, P	0	19980101	20090101	
J9999							O1D	1, P	0	19860101	19970101	
K0001							D1D	R	0	19940101	19940101	
K0002							D1D	R	0	19940101	19940101	
K0003							D1D	R	0	19940101	19940101	
K0004							D1D	R	0	19940101	19940101	
K0005							D1D	A,P,R	0	19940101	19940101	
K0006							D1D	R	0	19940101	19940101	
K0007							D1D	R	0	19940101	19940101	
K0009							D1D	A,P,R	0	19940101	19940101	
K0010							D1D	A,P,R	0	19940101	19970505	
K0011							D1D	A,P,R	0	19940101	19970505	
K0012							D1D	A,P,R	0	19940101	19970505	
K0014							D1D	A,P,R	0	19940101	20010101	
K0015							D1D	A,P,R	0	19940101	19940101	
K0017							D1D	A,P,R	0	19940101	19940101	
K0018							D1D	A,P,R	0	19940101	19940101	
K0019							D1D	A,P,R	0	19940101	19940101	
K0020							D1D	A,P,R	0	19940101	19940101	
K0037							D1D	A,P,R	0	19940101	19940101	
K0038							D1D	A,P,R	0	19940101	19940101	
K0039							D1D	A,P,R	0	19940101	19940101	
K0040							D1D	A,P,R	0	19940101	19940101	

HCPCS Code	Long Description	Coverage	Action	PI	MPI	CIM	MCM
K0041	LARGE SIZE FOOTPLATE, EACH	C	N	32	A		
K0042	STANDARD SIZE FOOTPLATE, EACH	C	N	32	A		
K0043	FOOTREST, LOWER EXTENSION TUBE, EACH	C	N	32	A		
K0044	FOOTREST, UPPER HANGER BRACKET, EACH	C	N	32	A		
K0045	FOOTREST, COMPLETE ASSEMBLY	C	N	32	A		
K0046	ELEVATING LEGREST, LOWER EXTENSION TUBE, EACH	C	N	32	A		
K0047	ELEVATING LEGREST, UPPER HANGER BRACKET, EACH	C	N	32	A		
K0050	RATCHET ASSEMBLY	C	N	32	A		
K0051	CAM RELEASE ASSEMBLY, FOOTREST OR LEGREST, EACH	C	N	32	A		
K0052	SWINGAWAY, DETACHABLE FOOTRESTS, EACH	C	N	32	A		
K0053	ELEVATING FOOTRESTS, ARTICULATING (TELESCOPING), EA.	C	N	32	A		
K0056	SEAT HEIGHT LESS THAN 17" OR EQUAL TO OR GREATER THAN 21" FOR A HIGH STRENGTH, LIGHTWEIGHT, OR ULTRALIGHTWEIGHT WHEELCHAIR	C	N	32	A		
K0065	SPOKE PROTECTORS, EACH	C	N	32	A		
K0069	REAR WHEEL ASSEMBLY, COMPLETE, WITH SOLID TIRE, SPOKES OR MOLDED, EACH	C	N	32	A		
K0070	REAR WHEEL ASSEMBLY, COMPLETE, WITH PNEUMATIC TIRE, SPOKES OR MOLDED, EACH	C	N	32	A		
K0071	FRONT CASTER ASSEMBLY, COMPLETE, WITH PNEUMATIC TIRE, EACH	C	N	32	A		
K0072	FRONT CASTER ASSEMBLY, COMPLETE, WITH SEMI-PNEUMATIC TIRE, EACH	C	N	32	A		
K0073	CASTER PIN LOCK,EACH	C	N	32	A		
K0077	FRONT CASTER ASSEMBLY, COMPLETE, WITH SOLID TIRE, EA.	C	N	32	A		
K0090	REAR WHEEL TIRE FOR POWER WHEELCHAIR, ANY SIZE, EA.	C	N	32	A		
K0091	REAR WHEEL TIRE TUBE OTHER THAN ZERO PRESSURE FOR POWER WHEELCHAIR, ANY SIZE, EACH	C	N	32	A		
K0092	REAR WHEEL ASSEMBLY FOR POWER WHEELCHAIR, COMPLETE, EACH	C	N	32	A		
K0093	REAR WHEEL, ZERO PRESSURE TIRE TUBE (FLAT FREE INSERT) FOR POWER WHEELCHAIR, ANY SIZE, EACH	C	N	32	A		
K0094	WHEEL TIRE FOR POWER BASE, ANY SIZE, EACH	C	N	32	A		
K0095	WHEEL TIRE TUBE OTHER THAN ZERO PRESSURE FOR EACH BASE, ANY SIZE, EACH	C	N	32	A		
K0096	WHEEL ASSEMBLY FOR POWER BASE, COMPLETE, EACH	C	N	32	A		
K0097	WHEEL ZERO PRESSURE TIRE TUBE (FLAT FREE INSERT) FOR POWER BASE, ANY SIZE, EACH	C	N	32	A		
K0098	DRIVE BELT FOR POWER WHEELCHAIR	C	N	32	A		
K0099	FRONT CASTER FOR POWER WHEELCHAIR, EACH	C	N	32	A		
K0105	IV HANGER, EACH	C	N	32	A		
K0108	WHEELCHAIR COMPONENT OR ACCESSORY, NOT OTHERWISE SPECIFIED	C	N	46	A		
K0195	ELEVATING LEG RESTS, PAIR (FOR USE WITH CAPPED RENTAL WHEELCHAIR BASE)	D	N	36	A	60-9	
K0455	INFUSION PUMP USED FOR UNINTERRUPTED PARENTERAL ADMINISTRATION OF MEDICATION, (E.G., EPOPROSTENOL OR TREPROSTINOL)	D	N	31	A	60-14	

HCPCS Code	Statute	Lab Cert	X-Ref	ASC Pay Grp	ASC Pay Group Eff. Date	Proc Notes	BETOS	TOS	Anest	Code Add Date	Code Effective Date	Code Term Date
K0041							D1D	A,P,R	0	19940101	19940101	
K0042							D1D	A,P,R	0	19940101	19940101	
K0043							D1D	A,P,R	0	19940101	19940101	
K0044							D1D	A,P,R	0	19940101	19940101	
K0045							D1D	A,P,R	0	19940101	19940101	
K0046							D1D	A,P,R	0	19940101	19940101	
K0047							D1D	A,P,R	0	19940101	19940101	
K0050							D1D	A,P,R	0	19940101	19940101	
K0051							D1D	A,P,R	0	19940101	19940101	
K0052							D1D	A,P,R	0	19940101	19940101	
K0053							D1D	A,P,R	0	19940101	19940101	
K0056							D1D	A,P,R	0	19940101	19990101	
K0065							D1D	A,P,R	0	19940101	20000101	
K0069							D1D	A,P,R	0	19940101	19940101	
K0070							D1D	A,P,R	0	19940101	19940101	
K0071							D1D	A,P,R	0	19940101	19940101	
K0072							D1D	A,P,R	0	19940101	19940101	
K0073							D1D	A,P,R	0	19940101	19940101	
K0077							D1D	A,P,R	0	19940101	19940101	
K0090							D1D	A,P,R	0	19940101	20070101	20061231
K0091							D1D	A,P,R	0	19940101	20070101	20061231
K0092							D1D	A,P,R	0	19940101	20070101	20061231
K0093							D1D	A,P,R	0	19940101	20070101	20061231
K0094							D1D	A,P,R	0	19940101	20070101	20061231
K0095							D1D	A,P,R	0	19940101	20070101	20061231
K0096							D1D	A,P,R	0	19940101	20070101	20061231
K0097							D1D	A,P,R	0	19940101	20070101	20061231
K0098							D1D	A,P,R	0	19940101	19940101	
K0099							D1D	A,P,R	0	19940101	20070101	20061231
K0105							D1D	A,P,R	0	19940101	20000101	
K0108							D1D	A,P,R	0	19940101	19990701	
K0195							D1D	R	0	19930101	19930101	
K0455							D1E	R	0	19980101	20030701	

HCPCS Code	Long Description	Coverage	Action	PI	MPI	CIM	MCM
K0462	TEMPORARY REPLACEMENT FOR PATIENT OWNED EQUIPMENT BEING REPAIRED, ANY TYPE	D	N	32	A		5102.3
K0552	SUPPLIES FOR EXTERNAL DRUG INFUSION PUMP, SYRINGE TYPE CARTRIDGE, STERILE, EACH	D	N	34	A	60-14	
K0553	COMBINATION ORAL/NASAL MASK, USED WITH CONTINUOUS POSITIVE AIRWAY PRESSURE DEVICE, EACH	C	N	32	A		
K0554	ORAL CUSHION FOR COMBINATION ORAL/NASAL MASK, REPLACEMENT ONLY, EACH	C	N	32	A		
K0555	NASAL PILLOWS FOR COMBINATION ORAL/NASAL MASK, REPLACEMENT ONLY, PAIR	C	N	32	A		
K0601	REPLACEMENT BATTERY FOR EXTERNAL INFUSION PUMP OWNED BY PATIENT, SILVER OXIDE, 1.5 VOLT, EACH	C	N	32	A		
K0602	REPLACEMENT BATTERY FOR EXTERNAL INFUSION PUMP OWNED BY PATIENT, SILVER OXIDE, 3 VOLT, EACH	C	N	32	A		
K0603	REPLACEMENT BATTERY FOR EXTERNAL INFUSION PUMP OWNED BY PATIENT, ALKALINE, 1.5 VOLT, EACH	C	N	32	A		
K0604	REPLACEMENT BATTERY FOR EXTERNAL INFUSION PUMP OWNED BY PATIENT, LITHIUM, 3.6 VOLT, EACH	C	N	32	A		
K0605	REPLACEMENT BATTERY FOR EXTERNAL INFUSION PUMP OWNED BY PATIENT, LITHIUM, 4.5 VOLT, EACH	C	N	32	A		
K0606	AUTOMATIC EXTERNAL DEFIBRILLATOR, WITH INTEGRATED ELECTROCARDIOGRAM ANALYSIS, GARMENT TYPE	C	N	36	A		
K0607	REPLACEMENT BATTERY FOR AUTOMATED EXTERNAL DEFIBRILLATOR, GARMENT TYPE ONLY, EACH	C	N	32	A		
K0608	REPLACEMENT GARMENT FOR USE WITH AUTOMATED EXTERNAL DEFIBRILLATOR, EACH	C	N	32	A		
K0609	REPLACEMENT ELECTRODES FOR USE WITH AUTOMATED EXTERNAL DEFIBRILLATOR, GARMENT TYPE ONLY, EACH	C	N	34	A		
K0669	WHEELCHAIR ACCESSORY, WHEELCHAIR SEAT OR BACK CUSHION, DOES NOT MEET SPECIFIC CODE CRITERIA OR NO WRITTEN CODING VERIFICATION FROM DME PDAC	C	N	32	A		
K0672	ADDITION TO LOWER EXTREMITY ORTHOSIS, REMOVABLE SOFT INTERFACE, ALL COMPONENTS, REPLACEMENT ONLY, EA.	C	N	38	A		
K0730	CONTROLLED DOSE INHALATION DRUG DELIVERY SYSTEM	C	N	36	A		
K0733	POWER WHEELCHAIR ACCESSORY, 12 TO 24 AMP HOUR SEALED LEAD ACID BATTERY, EACH (E.G., GEL CELL, ABSORBED GLASSMAT)	C	N	32	A		
K0734	SKIN PROTECTION WHEELCHAIR SEAT CUSHION, ADJUSTABLE, WIDTH LESS THAN 22 INCHES, ANY DEPTH	C	N	32	A		
K0735	SKIN PROTECTION WHEELCHAIR SEAT CUSHION, ADJUSTABLE, WIDTH 22 INCHES OR GREATER, ANY DEPTH	C	N	32	A		
K0736	SKIN PROTECTION AND POSITIONING WHEELCHAIR SEAT CUSHION, ADJUSTABLE, WIDTH LESS THAN 22 INCHES, ANY DEPTH	C	N	32	A		
K0737	SKIN PROTECTION AND POSITIONING WHEELCHAIR SEAT CUSHION, ADJUSTABLE, WIDTH 22 INCHES OR GREATER, ANY DEPTH	C	N	32	A		

HCPCS Code	Statute	Lab Cert	X-Ref	ASC Pay Grp	ASC Pay Group Eff. Date	Proc Notes	BETOS	TOS	Anest	Code Add Date	Code Effective Date	Code Term Date
K0462							D1E	9	0	19980701	19980701	
K0552							D1E	P	0	20030701	20030701	
K0553			A7027				D1E	A,P,R	0	20070701	20080101	20071231
K0553												
K0554			A7028				D1E	A,P,R	0	20070701	20080101	20071231
K0555			A7029				D1E	A,P,R	0	20070701	20080101	20071231
K0601							D1E	A,P,R	0	20030401	20030401	
K0602							D1E	A,P,R	0	20030401	20030401	
K0603							D1E	A,P,R	0	20030401	20030401	
K0604							D1E	A,P,R	0	20030401	20030401	
K0605							D1E	A,P,R	0	20030401	20030401	
K0606							D1E	A,P,R	0	20030701	20030701	
K0607							D1E	A,P,R	0	20030701	20030701	
K0608							D1E	A,P,R	0	20030701	20030701	
K0609							D1E	P	0	20030701	20030701	
K0669							D1D	A,P,R	0	20040701	20090101	
K0672							D1F	P	0	20080401	20080401	
K0730							D1E	R	0	20050701	20050701	
K0733							D1D	A,P,R	0	20060701	20060701	
K0734							D1D	A,P,R	0	20060701	20060701	
K0735							D1D	A,P,R	0	20060701	20060701	
K0736							D1D	A,P,R	0	20060701	20060701	
K0737							D1D	A,P,R	0	20060701	20060701	

HCPCS Code	Long Description	Coverage	Action	PI	MPI	CIM	MCM
K0738	PORTABLE GASEOUS OXYGEN SYSTEM, RENTAL; HOME COMPRESSOR USED TO FILL PORTABLE OXYGEN CYLINDERS; INCLUDES PORTABLE CONTAINERS, REGULATOR, FLOWMETER, HUMIDIFIER, CANNULA OR MASK, AND TUBING	C	N	33	A		
K0739	REPAIR OR NONROUTINE SERVICE FOR DURABLE MEDICAL EQUIPMENT OTHER THAN OXYGEN EQUIPMENT REQUIRING THE SKILL OF A TECHNICIAN, LABOR COMPONENT, PER 15 MINUTES	C	A	46	A		
K0740	REPAIR OR NONROUTINE SERVICE FOR OXYGEN EQUIPMENT REQUIRING THE SKILL OF A TECHNICIAN, LABOR COMPONENT, PER 15 MINUTES	M	A	00	9		
K0800	POWER OPERATED VEHICLE, GROUP 1 STANDARD, PATIENT WEIGHT CAPACITY UP TO AND INCLUDING 300 POUNDS	C	N	32	A		
K0801	POWER OPERATED VEHICLE, GROUP 1 HEAVY DUTY, PATIENT WEIGHT CAPACITY 301 TO 450 POUNDS	C	N	32	A		
K0802	POWER OPERATED VEHICLE, GROUP 1 VERY HEAVY DUTY, PATIENT WEIGHT CAPACITY 451 TO 600 POUNDS	C	N	32	A		
K0806	POWER OPERATED VEHICLE, GROUP 2 STANDARD, PATIENT WEIGHT CAPACITY UP TO AND INCLUDING 300 POUNDS	C	N	32	A		
K0807	POWER OPERATED VEHICLE, GROUP 2 HEAVY DUTY, PATIENT WEIGHT CAPACITY 301 TO 450 POUNDS	C	N	32	A		
K0808	POWER OPERATED VEHICLE, GROUP 2 VERY HEAVY DUTY, PATIENT WEIGHT CAPACITY 451 TO 600 POUNDS	C	N	32	A		
K0812	POWER OPERATED VEHICLE, NOT OTHERWISE CLASSIFIED	C	N	32	A		
K0813	POWER WHEELCHAIR, GROUP 1 STANDARD, PORTABLE, SLING/SOLID SEAT AND BACK, PATIENT WEIGHT CAPACITY UP TO AND INCLUDING 300 POUNDS	C	N	36	A		
K0814	POWER WHEELCHAIR, GROUP 1 STANDARD, PORTABLE, CAPTAINS CHAIR, PATIENT WEIGHT CAPACITY UP TO AND INCLUDING 300 POUNDS	C	N	36	A		
K0815	POWER WHEELCHAIR, GROUP 1 STANDARD, SLING/SOLID SEAT AND BACK, PATIENT WEIGHT CAPACITY UP TO AND INCLUDING 300 POUNDS	C	N	36	A		
K0816	POWER WHEELCHAIR, GROUP 1 STANDARD, CAPTAINS CHAIR, PATIENT WEIGHT CAPACITY UP TO AND INCLUDING 300 POUNDS	C	N	36	A		
K0820	POWER WHEELCHAIR, GROUP 2 STANDARD, PORTABLE, SLING/SOLID SEAT/BACK, PATIENT WEIGHT CAPACITY UP TO AND INCLUDING 300 POUNDS	C	N	36	A		
K0821	POWER WHEELCHAIR, GROUP 2 STANDARD, PORTABLE, CAPTAINS CHAIR, PATIENT WEIGHT CAPACITY UP TO AND INCLUDING 300 POUNDS	C	N	36	A		
K0822	POWER WHEELCHAIR, GROUP 2 STANDARD, SLING/SOLID SEAT/BACK, PATIENT WEIGHT CAPACITY UP TO AND INCLUDING 300 POUNDS	C	N	36	A		
K0823	POWER WHEELCHAIR, GROUP 2 STANDARD, CAPTAINS CHAIR, PATIENT WEIGHT CAPACITY UP TO & INCLUDING 300 POUNDS	C	N	36	A		
K0824	POWER WHEELCHAIR, GROUP 2 HEAVY DUTY, SLING/SOLID SEAT/BACK, PATIENT WEIGHT CAPACITY 301 TO 450 POUNDS	C	N	36	A		

HCPCS Code	Statute	Lab Cert	X-Ref	ASC Pay Grp	ASC Pay Group Eff. Date	Proc Notes	BETOS	TOS	Anest	Code Add Date	Code Effective Date	Code Term Date
K0738							D1C	P, R	0	20061001	20061001	
K0739							D1E	9	0	20090401	20090401	
K0740						0157	D1C	9	0	20090401	20090401	
K0800							D1D	A,P,R	0	20061001	20061001	
K0801							D1D	A,P,R	0	20061001	20061001	
K0802							D1D	A,P,R	0	20061001	20061001	
K0806							D1D	A,P,R	0	20061001	20061001	
K0807							D1D	A,P,R	0	20061001	20061001	
K0808							D1D	A,P,R	0	20061001	20061001	
K0812							D1D	A,P,R	0	20061001	20061001	
K0813							D1D	A,P,R	0	20061001	20061001	
K0814							D1D	A,P,R	0	20061001	20061001	
K0815							D1D	A,P,R	0	20061001	20061001	
K0816							D1D	A,P,R	0	20061001	20061001	
K0820							D1D	A,P,R	0	20061001	20061001	
K0821							D1D	A,P,R	0	20061001	20061001	
K0822							D1D	A,P,R	0	20061001	20061001	
K0823							D1D	A,P,R	0	20061001	20061001	
K0824							D1D	A,P,R	0	20061001	20061001	

HCPCS Code	Long Description	Coverage	Action	PI	MPI	CIM	MCM
K0825	POWER WHEELCHAIR, GROUP 2 HEAVY DUTY, CAPTAINS CHAIR, PATIENT WEIGHT CAPACITY 301 TO 450 POUNDS	C	N	36	A		
K0826	POWER WHEELCHAIR, GROUP 2 VERY HEAVY DUTY, SLING/SOLID SEAT/BACK, PATIENT WEIGHT CAPACITY 451 TO 600 POUNDS	C	N	36	A		
K0827	POWER WHEELCHAIR, GROUP 2 VERY HEAVY DUTY, CAPTAINS CHAIR, PATIENT WEIGHT CAPACITY 451 TO 600 POUNDS	C	N	36	A		
K0828	POWER WHEELCHAIR, GROUP 2 EXTRA HEAVY DUTY, SLING/SOLID SEAT/BACK, PATIENT WEIGHT CAPACITY 601 POUNDS OR MORE	C	N	36	A		
K0829	POWER WHEELCHAIR, GROUP 2 EXTRA HEAVY DUTY, CAPTAINS CHAIR, PATIENT WEIGHT 601 POUNDS OR MORE	C	N	36	A		
K0830	POWER WHEELCHAIR, GROUP 2 STANDARD, SEAT ELEVATOR, SLING/SOLID SEAT/BACK, PATIENT WEIGHT CAPACITY UP TO AND INCLUDING 300 POUNDS	C	N	36	A		
K0831	POWER WHEELCHAIR, GROUP 2 STANDARD, SEAT ELEVATOR, CAPTAINS CHAIR, PATIENT WEIGHT CAPACITY UP TO AND INCLUDING 300 POUNDS	C	N	36	A		
K0835	POWER WHEELCHAIR, GROUP 2 STANDARD, SINGLE POWER OPTION, SLING/SOLID SEAT/BACK, PATIENT WEIGHT CAPACITY UP TO AND INCLUDING 300 POUNDS	C	N	36	A		
K0836	POWER WHEELCHAIR, GROUP 2 STANDARD, SINGLE POWER OPTION, CAPTAINS CHAIR, PATIENT WEIGHT CAPACITY UP TO AND INCLUDING 300 POUNDS	C	N	36	A		
K0837	POWER WHEELCHAIR, GROUP 2 HEAVY DUTY, SINGLE POWER OPTION, SLING/SOLID SEAT/BACK, PATIENT WEIGHT CAPACITY 301 TO 450 POUNDS	C	N	36	A		
K0838	POWER WHEELCHAIR, GROUP 2 HEAVY DUTY, SINGLE POWER OPTION, CAPTAINS CHAIR, PATIENT WEIGHT CAPACITY 301 TO 450 POUNDS	C	N	36	A		
K0839	POWER WHEELCHAIR, GROUP 2 VERY HEAVY DUTY, SINGLE POWER OPTION SLING/SOLID SEAT/BACK, PATIENT WEIGHT CAPACITY 451 TO 600 POUNDS	C	N	36	A		
K0840	POWER WHEELCHAIR, GROUP 2 EXTRA HEAVY DUTY, SINGLE POWER OPTION, SLING/SOLID SEAT/BACK, PATIENT WEIGHT CAPACITY 601 POUNDS OR MORE	C	N	36	A		
K0841	POWER WHEELCHAIR, GROUP 2 STANDARD, MULTIPLE POWER OPTION, SLING/SOLID SEAT/BACK, PATIENT WEIGHT CAPACITY UP TO AND INCLUDING 300 POUNDS	C	N	36	A		
K0842	POWER WHEELCHAIR, GROUP 2 STANDARD, MULTIPLE POWER OPTION, CAPTAINS CHAIR, PATIENT WEIGHT CAPACITY UP TO AND INCLUDING 300 POUNDS	C	N	36	A		
K0843	POWER WHEELCHAIR, GROUP 2 HEAVY DUTY, MULTIPLE POWER OPTION, SLING/SOLID SEAT/BACK, PATIENT WEIGHT CAPACITY 301 TO 450 POUNDS	C	N	36	A		
K0848	POWER WHEELCHAIR, GROUP 3 STANDARD, SLING/SOLID SEAT/BACK, PATIENT WEIGHT CAPACITY UP TO AND INCLUDING 300 POUNDS	C	N	36	A		

HCPCS Code	Statute	Lab Cert	X-Ref	ASC Pay Grp	ASC Pay Group Eff. Date	Proc Notes	BETOS	TOS	Anest	Code Add Date	Code Effective Date	Code Term Date
K0825							D1D	A,P,R	0	20061001	20061001	
K0826							D1D	A,P,R	0	20061001	20061001	
K0827							D1D	A,P,R	0	20061001	20061001	
K0828							D1D	A,P,R	0	20061001	20061001	
K0829							D1D	A,P,R	0	20061001	20061001	
K0830							D1D	A,P,R	0	20061001	20061001	
K0831							D1D	A,P,R	0	20061001	20061001	
K0835							D1D	A,P,R	0	20061001	20061001	
K0836							D1D	A,P,R	0	20061001	20061001	
K0837							D1D	A,P,R	0	20061001	20061001	
K0838							D1D	A,P,R	0	20061001	20061001	
K0839							D1D	A,P,R	0	20061001	20061001	
K0840							D1D	A,P,R	0	20061001	20061001	
K0841							D1D	A,P,R	0	20061001	20061001	
K0842							D1D	A,P,R	0	20061001	20061001	
K0843							D1D	A,P,R	0	20061001	20061001	
K0848							D1D	A,P,R	0	20061001	20061001	
K0848							D1D	A,P,R	0	20061001	20061001	

HCPCS Code	Long Description	Coverage	Action	PI	MPI	CIM	MCM
K0849	POWER WHEELCHAIR, GROUP 3 STANDARD, CAPTAINS CHAIR, PATIENT WEIGHT CAPACITY UP TO & INCLUDING 300 POUNDS	C	N	36	A		
K0850	POWER WHEELCHAIR, GROUP 3 HEAVY DUTY, SLING/SOLID SEAT/BACK, PATIENT WEIGHT CAPACITY 301 TO 450 POUNDS	C	N	36	A		
K0851	POWER WHEELCHAIR, GROUP 3 HEAVY DUTY, CAPTAINS CHAIR, PATIENT WEIGHT CAPACITY 301 TO 450 POUNDS	C	N	36	A		
K0852	POWER WHEELCHAIR, GROUP 3 VERY HEAVY DUTY, SLING/SOLID SEAT/BACK, PATIENT WEIGHT CAPACITY 451 TO 600 POUNDS	C	N	36	A		
K0853	POWER WHEELCHAIR, GROUP 3 VERY HEAVY DUTY, CAPTAINS CHAIR, PATIENT WEIGHT CAPACITY 451 TO 600 POUNDS	C	N	36	A		
K0854	POWER WHEELCHAIR, GROUP 3 EXTRA HEAVY DUTY, SLING/SOLID SEAT/BACK, PATIENT WEIGHT CAPACITY 601 POUNDS OR MORE	C	N	36	A		
K0855	POWER WHEELCHAIR, GROUP 3 EXTRA HEAVY DUTY, CAPTAINS CHAIR, PATIENT WEIGHT CAPACITY 601 POUNDS OR MORE	C	N	36	A		
K0856	POWER WHEELCHAIR, GROUP 3 STANDARD, SINGLE POWER OPTION, SLING/SOLID SEAT/BACK, PATIENT WEIGHT CAPACITY UP TO AND INCLUDING 300 POUNDS	C	N	36	A		
K0857	POWER WHEELCHAIR, GROUP 3 STANDARD, SINGLE POWER OPTION, CAPTAINS CHAIR, PATIENT WEIGHT CAPACITY UP TO AND INCLUDING 300 POUNDS	C	N	36	A		
K0858	POWER WHEELCHAIR, GROUP 3 HEAVY DUTY, SINGLE POWER OPTION, SLING/SOLID SEAT/BACK, PATIENT WEIGHT 301 TO 450 POUNDS	C	N	36	A		
K0859	POWER WHEELCHAIR, GROUP 3 HEAVY DUTY, SINGLE POWER OPTION, CAPTAINS CHAIR, PATIENT WEIGHT CAPACITY 301 TO 450 POUNDS	C	N	36	A		
K0860	POWER WHEELCHAIR, GROUP 3 VERY HEAVY DUTY, SINGLE POWER OPTION, SLING/SOLID SEAT/BACK, PATIENT WEIGHT CAPACITY 451 TO 600 POUNDS	C	N	36	A		
K0861	POWER WHEELCHAIR, GROUP 3 STANDARD, MULTIPLE POWER OPTION, SLING/SOLID SEAT/BACK, PATIENT WEIGHT CAPACITY UP TO AND INCLUDING 300 POUNDS	C	N	36	A		
K0862	POWER WHEELCHAIR, GROUP 3 HEAVY DUTY, MULTIPLE POWER OPTION, SLING/SOLID SEAT/BACK, PATIENT WEIGHT CAPACITY 301 TO 450 POUNDS	C	N	36	A		
K0863	POWER WHEELCHAIR, GROUP 3 VERY HEAVY DUTY, MULTIPLE POWER OPTION, SLING/SOLID SEAT/BACK, PATIENT WEIGHT CAPACITY 451 TO 600 POUNDS	C	N	36	A		
K0864	POWER WHEELCHAIR, GROUP 3 EXTRA HEAVY DUTY, MULTIPLE POWER OPTION, SLING/SOLID SEAT/BACK, PATIENT WEIGHT CAPACITY 601 POUNDS OR MORE	C	N	36	A		
K0868	POWER WHEELCHAIR, GROUP 4 STANDARD, SLING/SOLID SEAT/BACK, PATIENT WEIGHT CAPACITY UP TO AND INCLUDING 300 POUNDS	C	N	36	A		
K0869	POWER WHEELCHAIR, GROUP 4 STANDARD, CAPTAINS CHAIR, PATIENT WEIGHT CAPACITY UP TO & INCLUDING 300 POUNDS	C	N	36	A		

HCPCS Code	Statute	Lab Cert	X-Ref	ASC Pay Grp	ASC Pay Group Eff. Date	Proc Notes	BETOS	TOS	Anest	Code Add Date	Code Effective Date	Code Term Date
K0849							D1D	A,P,R	0	20061001	20061001	
K0850							D1D	A,P,R	0	20061001	20061001	
K0851							D1D	A,P,R	0	20061001	20061001	
K0852							D1D	A,P,R	0	20061001	20061001	
K0853							D1D	A,P,R	0	20061001	20061001	
K0854							D1D	A,P,R	0	20061001	20061001	
K0855							D1D	A,P,R	0	20061001	20061001	
K0856							D1D	A,P,R	0	20061001	20061001	
K0857							D1D	A,P,R	0	20061001	20061001	
K0858							D1D	A,P,R	0	20061001	20061001	
K0859							D1D	A,P,R	00	20061001	20061001	
K0860							D1D	A,P,R	0	20061001	20061001	
K0861							D1D	A,P,R	0	20061001	20061001	
K0862							D1D	A,P,R	0	20061001	20061001	
K0863							D1D	A,P,R	0	20061001	20061001	
K0864							D1D	A,P,R	0	20061001	20061001	
K0868							D1D	A,P,R	0	20061001	20061001	
K0869							D1D	A,P,R	0	20061001	20061001	

HCPCS Code	Long Description	Coverage	Action	PI	MPI	CIM	MCM
K0870	POWER WHEELCHAIR, GROUP 4 HEAVY DUTY, SLING/SOLID SEAT/BACK, PATIENT WEIGHT CAPACITY 301 TO 450 POUNDS	C	N	36	A		
K0871	POWER WHEELCHAIR, GROUP 4 VERY HEAVY DUTY, SLING/SOLID SEAT/BACK, PATIENT WEIGHT CAPACITY 451 TO 600 POUNDS	C	N	36	A		
K0877	POWER WHEELCHAIR, GROUP 4 STANDARD, SINGLE POWER OPTION, SLING/SOLID SEAT/BACK, PATIENT WEIGHT CAPACITY UP TO AND INCLUDING 300 POUNDS	C	N	36	A		
K0878	POWER WHEELCHAIR, GROUP 4 STANDARD, SINGLE POWER OPTION, CAPTAINS CHAIR, PATIENT WEIGHT CAPACITY UP TO AND INCLUDING 300 POUNDS	C	N	36	A		
K0879	POWER WHEELCHAIR, GROUP 4 HEAVY DUTY, SINGLE POWER OPTION, SLING/SOLID SEAT/BACK, PATIENT WEIGHT CAPACITY 301 TO 450 POUNDS	C	N	36	A		
K0880	POWER WHEELCHAIR, GROUP 4 VERY HEAVY DUTY, SINGLE POWER OPTION, SLING/SOLID SEAT/BACK, PATIENT WEIGHT 451 TO 600 POUNDS	C	N	36	A		
K0884	POWER WHEELCHAIR, GROUP 4 STANDARD, MULTIPLE POWER OPTION, SLING/SOLID SEAT/BACK, PATIENT WEIGHT CAPACITY UP TO AND INCLUDING 300 POUNDS	C	N	36	A		
K0885	POWER WHEELCHAIR, GROUP 4 STANDARD, MULTIPLE POWER OPTION, CAPTAINS CHAIR, PATIENT WEIGHT CAPACITY UP TO AND INCLUDING 300 POUNDS	C	N	36	A		
K0886	POWER WHEELCHAIR, GROUP 4 HEAVY DUTY, MULTIPLE POWER OPTION, SLING/SOLID SEAT/BACK, PATIENT WEIGHT CAPACITY 301 TO 450 POUNDS	C	N	36	A		
K0890	POWER WHEELCHAIR, GROUP 5 PEDIATRIC, SINGLE POWER OPTION, SLING/SOLID SEAT/BACK, PATIENT WEIGHT CAPACITY UP TO AND INCLUDING 125 POUNDS	C	N	36	A		
K0891	POWER WHEELCHAIR, GROUP 5 PEDIATRIC, MULTIPLE POWER OPTION, SLING/SOLID SEAT/BACK, PATIENT WEIGHT CAPACITY UP TO AND INCLUDING 125 POUNDS	C	N	36	A		
K0898	POWER WHEELCHAIR, NOT OTHERWISE CLASSIFIED	C	N	36	A		
K0899	POWER MOBILITY DEVICE, NOT CODED BY DME PDAC OR DOES NOT MEET CRITERIA	C	N	36	A		
L0100	CRANIAL ORTHOSIS (HELMET), WITH OR WITHOUT SOFT INTERFACE, MOLDED TO PATIENT MODEL	C	N	38	A		
L0110	CRANIAL ORTHOSIS (HELMET), WITH OR WITHOUT SOFT-INTERFACE, NON-MOLDED	C	N	38	A		
L0112	CRANIAL CERVICAL ORTHOSIS, CONGENITAL TORTICOLLIS TYPE, WITH OR WITHOUT SOFT INTERFACE MATERIAL, ADJUSTABLE RANGE OF MOTION JOINT, CUSTOM FABRICATED	C	N	38	A		
L0113	CRANIAL CERVICAL ORTHOSIS, TORTICOLLIS TYPE, WITH OR WITHOUT JOINT, WITH OR WITHOUT SOFT INTERFACE MATERIAL, PREFABRICATED, INCLUDES FITTING AND ADJUSTMENT	C	N	38	A		
L0120	CERVICAL, FLEXIBLE, NON-ADJUSTABLE (FOAM COLLAR)	C	N	38	A		
L0130	CERVICAL, FLEXIBLE, THERMOPLASTIC COLLAR, MOLDED TO PATIENT	C	N	38	A		

HCPCS Code	Statute	Lab Cert	X-Ref	ASC Pay Grp	ASC Pay Group Eff. Date	Proc Notes	BETOS	TOS	Anest	Code Add Date	Code Effective Date	Code Term Date
K0870							D1D	A,P,R	0	20061001	20061001	
K0871							D1D	A,P,R	0	20061001	20061001	
K0877							D1D	A,P,R	0	20061001	20061001	
K0878							D1D	A,P,R	0	20061001	20061001	
K0879							D1D	A,P,R	0	20061001	20061001	
K0880							D1D	A,P,R	0	20061001	20061001	
K0884							D1D	A,P,R	0	20061001	20061001	
K0885							D1D	A,P,R	0	20061001	20061001	
K0886							D1D	A,P,R	0	20061001	20061001	
K0890							D1D	A,P,R	0	20061001	20061001	
K0890 K0891							D1D	A,P,R	0	20061001	20061001	
K0898							D1D	A,P,R	0	20061001	20061001	
K0899							D1D	A,P,R	0	20061001	20090101	
L0100							D1F	P	0	19820101	20070101	20061231
L0110							D1F	P	0	19820101	20070101	20061231
L0112							D1F	P	0	20040101	20040101	
L0113							D1F	P	0	20090101	20090101	
L0120							D1F	P	0	19820101	19960101	
L0130							D1F	P	0	19840101	19960101	

L Codes

HCPCS Code	Long Description	Coverage	Action	PI	MPI	CIM	MCM
L0140	CERVICAL, SEMI-RIGID, ADJUSTABLE (PLASTIC COLLAR)	C	N	38	A		
L0150	CERVICAL, SEMI-RIGID, ADJUSTABLE MOLDED CHIN CUP (PLASTIC COLLAR WITH MANDIBULAR/OCCIPITAL PIECE)	C	N	38	A		
L0160	CERVICAL, SEMI-RIGID, WIRE FRAME OCCIPITAL/ MANDIBULAR SUPPORT	C	N	38	A		
L0170	CERVICAL, COLLAR, MOLDED TO PATIENT MODEL	C	N	38	A		
L0172	CERVICAL, COLLAR, SEMI-RIGID THERMOPLASTIC FOAM, TWO PIECE	C	N	38	A		
L0174	CERVICAL, COLLAR, SEMI-RIGID, THERMOPLASTIC FOAM, TWO PIECE WITH THORACIC EXTENSION	C	N	38	A		
L0180	CERVICAL, MULTIPLE POST COLLAR, OCCIPITAL/ MANDIBULAR SUPPORTS, ADJUSTABLE	C	N	38	A		
L0190	CERVICAL, MULTIPLE POST COLLAR, OCCIPITAL/ MANDIBULAR SUPPORTS, ADJUSTABLE CERVICAL BARS (SOMI, GUILFORD, TAYLOR TYPES)	C	N	38	A		
L0200	CERVICAL, MULTIPLE POST COLLAR, OCCIPITAL/ MANDIBULAR SUPPORTS, ADJUSTABLE CERVICAL BARS, AND THORACIC EXTENSION	C	N	38	A		
L0210	THORACIC, RIB BELT	C	D	38	A		
L0220	THORACIC, RIB BELT, CUSTOM FABRICATED	C	N	38	A		
L0430	SPINAL ORTHOSIS, ANTERIOR-POSTERIOR-LATERAL CONTROL, WITH INTERFACE MATERIAL, CUSTOM FITTED (DEWALL POSTURE PROTECTOR ONLY)	C	N	38	A		
L0450	TLSO, FLEXIBLE, PROVIDES TRUNK SUPPORT, UPPER THORACIC REGION, PRODUCES INTRACAVITARY PRESSURE TO REDUCE LOAD ON THE INTEVERTEBRAL DISKS WITH RIGID STAYS OR PANEL(S), INCLUDES SHOULDER STRAPS AND CLOSURES, PREFABRICATED, INCLUDES FITTING AND ADJUSTMENT	C	N	38	A		
L0452	TLSO, FLEXIBLE, PROVIDES TRUNK SUPPORT, UPPER THORACIC REGION, PRODUCES INTRACAVITARY PRESSURE TO REDUCE LOAD ON THE INTERVERTEBRAL DISKS WITH RIGID STAYS OR PANEL(S), INCLUDES SHOULDER STRAPS AND CLOSURES, CUSTOM FABRICATED	C	N	38	A		
L0454	TLSO FLEXIBLE, PROVIDES TRUNK SUPPORT, EXTENDS FROM SACROCOCCYGEAL JUNCTION TO ABOVE T-9 VERTEBRA, RESTRICTS GROSS TRUNK MOTION IN THE SAGITTAL PLANE, PRODUCES INTRACAVITARY PRESSURE TO REDUCE LOAD ON THE INTERVERTEBRAL DISKS WITH RIGID STAYS OR PANEL(S), INCLUDES SHOULDER STRAPS AND CLOSURES, PREFABRICATED, INCLUDES FITTING AND ADJUSTMENT	C	N	38	A		
L0456	TLSO, FLEXIBLE, PROVIDES TRUNK SUPPORT, THORACIC REGION, RIGID POSTERIOR PANEL AND SOFT ANTERIOR APRON, EXTENDS FROM THE SACROCOCCYGEAL JUNCTION AND TERMINATES JUST INFERIOR TO THE SCAPULAR SPINE, RESTRICTS GROSS TRUNK MOTION IN THE SAGITTAL PLANE, PRODUCES INTRACAVITARY PRESSURE TO REDUCE LOAD ON THE INTERVERTEBRAL DISKS, INCLUDES STRAPS AND CLOSURES, PREFABRICATED, INCLUDES FITTING & ADJUSTMENT	C	N	38	A		

HCPCS Code	Statute	Lab Cert	X-Ref	ASC Pay Grp	ASC Pay Group Eff. Date	Proc Notes	BETOS	TOS	Anest	Code Add Date	Code Effective Date	Code Term Date
L0140							D1F	P	0	19820101	19960101	
L0150							D1F	P	0	19820101	19960101	
L0160							D1F	P	0	19820101	19960101	
L0170							D1F	P	0	19860101	19960101	
L0172							D1F	P	0	19880101	19960101	
L0174							D1F	P	0	19880101	19960101	
L0180							D1F	P	0	19840101	19960101	
L0190							D1F	P	0	19820101	19960101	
L0200							D1F	P	0	19840101	19960101	
L0210							D1F	P	0	19820101	20100101	20091231
L0220							D1F	P	0	19820101	19960101	
L0430							D1F	P	0	19880101	20050101	
L0450							D1F	P	0	20030101	20030101	
L0452							D1F	P	0	20030101	20030101	
L0454							D1F	P	0	20030101	20030101	
L0456							D1F	P	0	20030101	20030101	
L0456							D1F	P	0			

HCPCS Code	Long Description	Coverage	Action	PI	MPI	CIM	MCM
L0458	TLSO, TRIPLANAR CONTROL, MODULAR SEGMENTED SPINAL SYSTEM, TWO RIGID PLASTIC SHELLS, POSTERIOR EXTENDS FROM THE SACROCOCCYGEAL JUNCTION AND TERMINATES JUST INFERIOR TO THE SCAPULAR SPINE, ANTERIOR EXTENDS FROM THE SYMPHYSIS PUBIS TO THE XIPHOID, SOFT LINER, RESTRICTS GROSS TRUNK MOTION IN THE SAGITTAL, CORONAL, AND TRANVERSE PLANES, LATERAL STRENGTH IS PROVIDED BY OVERLAPPING PLASTIC AND STABILIZING CLOSURES, INCLUDES STRAPS AND CLOSURES, PREFABRICATED, INCLUDES FITTING & ADJUSTMENT	C	N	38	A		
L0460	TLSO, TRIPLANAR CONTROL, MODULAR SEGMENTED SPINAL SYSTEM, TWO RIGID PLASTIC SHELLS, POSTERIOR EXTENDS FROM THE SACROCOCCYGEAL JUNCTION AND TERMINATES JUST INFERIOR TO THE SCAPULAR SPINE, ANTERIOR EXTENDS FROM THE SYMPHYSIS PUBIS TO THE STERNAL NOTCH, SOFT LINER, RESTRICTS GROSS TRUNK MOTION IN THE SAGITTAL, CORONAL, AND TRANVERSE PLANES, LATERAL STRENGTH IS PROVIDED BY OVERLAPPING PLASTIC AND STABILIZING CLOSURES, INCLUDES STRAPS AND CLOSURES, PREFABRICATED, INCLUDES FITTING AND ADJUSTMENT	C	N	38	A		
L0462	TLSO, TRIPLANAR CONTROL, MODULAR SEGMENTED SPINAL SYSTEM, THREE RIGID PLASTIC SHELLS, POSTERIOR EXTENDS FROM THE SACROCOCCYGEAL JUNCTION AND TERMINATES JUST INFERIOR TO THE SCAPULAR SPINE, ANTERIOR EXTENDS FROM THE SYMPHYSIS PUBIS TO THE STERNAL NOTCH, SOFT LINER, RESTRICTS GROSS TRUNK MOTION IN THE SAGITTAL, CORONAL, AND TRANSVERSE PLANES, LATERAL STRENGTH IS PROVIDED BY OVERLAPPING PLASTIC AND STABILIZING CLOSURES, INCLUDES STRAPS AND CLOSURES, PREFABRICATED, INCLUDES FITTING AND ADJUSTMENT	C	N	38	A		
L0464	TLSO, TRIPLANAR CONTROL, MODULAR SEGMENTED SPINAL SYSTEM, FOUR RIGID PLASTIC SHELLS, POSTERIOR EXTENDS FROM SACROCOCCYGEAL JUNCTION AND TERMINATES JUST INFERIOR TO SCAPULAR SPINE, ANTERIOR EXTENDS FROM SYMPHYSIS PUBIS TO THE STERNAL NOTCH, SOFT LINER, RESTRICTS GROSS TRUNK MOTION IN SAGITTAL, CORONAL, AND TRANVERSE PLANES, LATERAL STRENGTH IS PROVIDED BY OVERLAPPING PLASTIC AND STABILIZING CLOSURES, INCLUDES STRAPS AND CLOSURES, PREFABRICATED, INCLUDES FITTING AND ADJUSTMENT	C	N	38	A		
L0466	TLSO, SAGITTAL CONTROL, RIGID POSTERIOR FRAME AND FLEXIBLE SOFT ANTERIOR APRON WITH STRAPS, CLOSURES AND PADDING, RESTRICTS GROSS TRUNK MOTION IN SAGITTAL PLANE, PRODUCES INTRACAVITARY PRESSURE TO REDUCE LOAD ON INTERVERTEBRAL DISKS, INCLUDES FITTING AND SHAPING THE FRAME, PREFABRICATED, INCLUDES FITTING AND ADJUSTMENT	C	N	38	A		

HCPCS Code	Statute	Lab Cert	X-Ref	ASC Pay Grp	ASC Pay Group Eff. Date	Proc Notes	BETOS	TOS	Anest	Code Add Date	Code Effective Date	Code Term Date
L0458							D1F	P	0	20030101	20030101	
L0460							D1F	P	0	20030101	20030101	
L0462							D1F	P	0	20030101	20030101	
L0464							D1F	P	0	20030101	20030101	
L0466							D1F	P	0	20030101	20030101	
L0466							D1F	P	0	20030101	20030101	

HCPCS Code	Long Description	Coverage	Action	PI	MPI	CIM	MCM
L0468	TLSO, SAGITTAL-CORONAL CONTROL, RIGID POSTERIOR FRAME AND FLEXIBLE SOFT ANTERIOR APRON WITH STRAPS, CLOSURES AND PADDING, EXTENDS FROM SACROCOCCYGEAL JUNCTION OVER SCAPULAE, LATERAL STRENGTH PROVIDED BY PELVIC, THORACIC, AND LATERAL FRAME PIECES, RESTRICTS GROSS TRUNK MOTION IN SAGITTAL, AND CORONAL PLANES, PRODUCES INTRACAVITARY PRESSURE TO REDUCE LOAD ON INTERVERTEBRAL DISKS, INCLUDES FITTING AND SHAPING THE FRAME, PREFABRICATED, INCLUDES FITTING AND ADJUSTMENT	C	N	38	A		
L0470	TLSO, TRIPLANAR CONTROL, RIGID POSTERIOR FRAME AND FLEXIBLE SOFT ANTERIOR APRON WITH STRAPS, CLOSURES AND PADDING, EXTENDS FROM SACROCOCCYGEAL JUNCTION TO SCAPULA, LATERAL STRENGTH PROVIDED BY PELVIC, THORACIC, AND LATERAL FRAME PIECES, ROTATIONAL STRENGTH PROVIDED BY SUBCLAVICULAR EXTENSIONS, RESTRICTS GROSS TRUNK MOTION IN SAGITTAL, CORONAL, AND TRANVERSE PLANES, PRODUCES INTRACAVITARY PRESSURE TO REDUCE LOAD ON THE INTERVERTEBRAL DISKS, INCLUDES FITTING AND SHAPING THE FRAME, PREFABRICATED, INCLUDES FITTING AND ADJUSTMENT	C	N	38	A		
L0472	TLSO, TRIPLANAR CONTROL, HYPEREXTENSION, RIGID ANTERIOR AND LATERAL FRAME EXTENDS FROM SYMPHYSIS PUBIS TO STERNAL NOTCH WITH TWO ANTERIOR COMPONENTS (ONE PUBIC AND ONE STERNAL), POSTERIOR AND LATERAL PADS WITH STRAPS AND CLOSURES, LIMITS SPINAL FLEXION, RESTRICTS GROSS TRUNK MOTION IN SAGITTAL, CORONAL, AND TRANSVERSE PLANES, INCLUDES FITTING AND SHAPING THE FRAME, PREFABRICATED, INCLUDES FITTING AND ADJUSTMENT	C	N	38	A		
L0480	TLSO, TRIPLANAR CONTROL, ONE PIECE RIGID PLASTIC SHELL WITHOUT INTERFACE LINER, WITH MULTIPLE STRAPS AND CLOSURES, POSTERIOR EXTENDS FROM SACROCOCCYGEAL JUNCTION AND TERMINATES JUST INFERIOR TO SCAPULAR SPINE, ANTERIOR EXTENDS FROM SYMPHYSIS PUBIS TO STERNAL NOTCH, ANTERIOR OR POSTERIOR OPENING, RESTRICTS GROSS TRUNK MOTION IN SAGITTAL, CORONAL, AND TRANSVERSE PLANES, INCLUDES A CARVED PLASTER OR CAD-CAM MODEL, CUSTOM FABRICATED	C	N	38	A		
L0482	TLSO, TRIPLANAR CONTROL, ONE PIECE RIGID PLASTIC SHELL WITH INTERFACE LINER, MULTIPLE STRAPS AND CLOSURES, POSTERIOR EXTENDS FROM SACROCOCCYGEAL JUNCTION AND TERMINATES JUST INFERIOR TO SCAPULAR SPINE, ANTERIOR EXTENDS FROM SYMPHYSIS PUBIS TO STERNAL NOTCH, ANTERIOR OR POSTERIOR OPENING, RESTRICTS GROSS TRUNK MOTION IN SAGITTAL, CORONAL, AND TRANSVERSE PLANES, INCLUDES A CARVED PLASTER OR CAD-CAM MODEL, CUSTOM FABRICATED	C	N	38	A		

HCPCS Code	Statute	Lab Cert	X-Ref	ASC Pay Grp	ASC Pay Group Eff. Date	Proc Notes	BETOS	TOS	Anest	Code Add Date	Code Effective Date	Code Term Date
L0468							D1F	P	0	20030101	20030101	
L0470							D1F	P	0	20030101	20030101	
L0472							D1F	P	0	20030101	20030101	
L0480							D1F	P	0	20030101	20040101	
L0482							D1F	P	0	20030101	20030101	

HCPCS Code	Long Description	Coverage	Action	PI	MPI	CIM	MCM
L0484	TLSO, TRIPLANAR CONTROL, TWO PIECE RIGID PLASTIC SHELL WITHOUT INTERFACE LINER, WITH MULTIPLE STRAPS AND CLOSURES, POSTERIOR EXTENDS FROM SACROCOCCYGEAL JUNCTION AND TERMINATES JUST INFERIOR TO SCAPULAR SPINE, ANTERIOR EXTENDS FROM SYMPHYSIS PUBIS TO STERNAL NOTCH, LATERAL STRENGTH IS ENHANCED BY OVERLAPPING PLASTIC, RESTRICTS GROSS TRUNK MOTION IN THE SAGITTAL, CORONAL, AND TRANSVERSE PLANES, INCLUDES A CARVED PLASTER OR CAD-CAM MODEL, CUSTOM FABRICATED	C	N	38	A		
L0486	TLSO, TRIPLANAR CONTROL, TWO PIECE RIGID PLASTIC SHELL WITH INTERFACE LINER, MULTIPLE STRAPS AND CLOSURES, POSTERIOR EXTENDS FROM SACROCOCCYGEAL JUNCTION AND TERMINATES JUST INFERIOR TO SCAPULAR SPINE, ANTERIOR EXTENDS FROM SYMPHYSIS PUBIS TO STERNAL NOTCH, LATERAL STRENGTH IS ENHANCED BY OVERLAPPING PLASTIC, RESTRICTS GROSS TRUNK MOTION IN THE SAGITTAL, CORONAL, AND TRANSVERSE PLANES, INCLUDES A CARVED PLASTER OR CAD-CAM MODEL, CUSTOM FABRICATED	C	N	38	A		
L0488	TLSO, TRIPLANAR CONTROL, ONE PIECE RIGID PLASTIC SHELL WITH INTERFACE LINER, MULTIPLE STRAPS AND CLOSURES, POSTERIOR EXTENDS FROM SACROCOCCYGEAL JUNCTION AND TERMINATES JUST INFERIOR TO SCAPULAR SPINE, ANTERIOR EXTENDS FROM SYMPHYSIS PUBIS TO STERNAL NOTCH, ANTERIOR OR POSTERIOR OPENING, RESTRICTS GROSS TRUNK MOTION IN SAGITTAL, CORONAL, AND TRANSVERSE PLANES, PREFABRICATED, INCLUDES FITTING AND ADJUSTMENT	C	N	38	A		
L0490	TLSO, SAGITTAL-CORONAL CONTROL, ONE PIECE RIGID PLASTIC SHELL, WITH OVERLAPPING REINFORCED ANTERIOR, WITH MULTIPLE STRAPS AND CLOSURES, POSTERIOR EXTENDS FROM SACROCOCCYGEAL JUNCTION AND TERMINATES AT OR BEFORE THE T-9 VERTEBRA, ANTERIOR EXTENDS FROM SYMPHYSIS PUBIS TO XIPHOID, ANTERIOR OPENING, RESTRICTS GROSS TRUNK MOTION IN SAGITTAL AND CORONAL PLANES, PREFABRICATED, INCLUDES FITTING AND ADJUSTMENT	C	N	38	A		
L0491	TLSO, SAGITTAL-CORONAL CONTROL, MODULAR SEGMENTED SPINAL SYSTEM, TWO RIGID PLASTIC SHELLS, POSTERIOR EXTENDS FROM THE SACROCOCCYGEAL JUNCTION AND TERMINATES JUST INFERIOR TO THE SCAPULAR SPINE, ANTERIOR EXTENDS FROM THE SYMPHYSIS PUBIS TO THE XIPHOID, SOFT LINER, RESTRICTS GROSS TRUNK MOTION IN THE SAGITTAL AND CORONAL PLANES, LATERAL STRENGTH IS PROVIDED BY OVERLAPPING PLASTIC AND STABILIZING CLOSURES, INCLUDES STRAPS AND CLOSURES, PREFABRICATED, INCLUDES FITTING AND ADJUSTMENT	C	N	38	A		

HCPCS Code	Statute	Lab Cert	X-Ref	ASC Pay Grp	ASC Pay Group Eff. Date	Proc Notes	BETOS	TOS	Anest	Code Add Date	Code Effective Date	Code Term Date
L0484							D1F	P	0	20030101	20030101	
L0486							D1F	P	0	20030101	20030101	
L0488							D1F	P	0	20030101	20030101	
L0490							D1F	P	0	20030101	20030101	
L0491							D1F	P	0	20060101	20060101	

HCPCS Code	Long Description	Coverage	Action	PI	MPI	CIM	MCM
L0492	TLSO, SAGITTAL-CORONAL CONTROL, MODULAR SEGMENTED SPINAL SYSTEM, THREE RIGID PLASTIC SHELLS, POSTERIOR EXTENDS FROM THE SACROCOCCYGEAL JUNCTION AND TERMINATES JUST INFERIOR TO THE SCAPULAR SPINE, ANTERIOR EXTENDS FROM THE SYMPHYSIS PUBIS TO THE XIPHOID, SOFT LINER, RESTRICTS GROSS TRUNK MOTION IN THE SAGITTAL AND CORONAL PLANES, LATERAL STRENGTH IS PROVIDED BY OVERLAPPING PLASTIC AND STABILIZING CLOSURES, INCLUDES STRAPS AND CLOSURES, PREFABRICATED, INCLUDES FITTING AND ADJUSTMENT	C	N	38	A		
L0621	SACROILIAC ORTHOSIS, FLEXIBLE, PROVIDES PELVIC-SACRAL SUPPORT, REDUCES MOTION ABOUT THE SACROILIAC JOINT, INCLUDES STRAPS, CLOSURES, MAY INCLUDE PENDULOUS ABDOMEN DESIGN, PREFABRICATED, INCLUDES FITTING AND ADJUSTMENT	C	N	38	A		
L0622	SACROILIAC ORTHOSIS, FLEXIBLE, PROVIDES PELVIC-SACRAL SUPPORT, REDUCES MOTION ABOUT THE SACROILIAC JOINT, INCLUDES STRAPS, CLOSURES, MAY INCLUDE PENDULOUS ABDOMEN DESIGN, CUSTOM FABRICATED	C	N	38	A		
L0623	SACROILIAC ORTHOSIS, PROVIDES PELVIC-SACRAL SUPPORT, WITH RIGID OR SEMI-RIGID PANELS OVER THE SACRUM AND ABDOMEN, REDUCES MOTION ABOUT THE SACROILIAC JOINT, INCLUDES STRAPS, CLOSURES, MAY INCLUDE PENDULOUS ABDOMEN DESIGN, PREFABRICATED, INCLUDES FITTING AND ADJUSTMENT	C	N	38	A		
L0624	SACROILIAC ORTHOSIS, PROVIDES PELVIC-SACRAL SUPPORT, WITH RIGID OR SEMI-RIGID PANELS PLACED OVER THE SACRUM AND ABDOMEN, REDUCES MOTION ABOUT THE SACROILIAC JOINT, INCLUDES STRAPS, CLOSURES, MAY INCLUDE PENDULOUS ABDOMEN DESIGN, CUSTOM FABRICATED	C	N	38	A		
L0625	LUMBAR ORTHOSIS, FLEXIBLE, PROVIDES LUMBAR SUPPORT, POSTERIOR EXTENDS FROM L-1 TO BELOW L-5 VERTEBRA, PRODUCES INTRACAVITARY PRESSURE TO REDUCE LOAD ON THE INTERVERTEBRAL DISCS, INCLUDES STRAPS, CLOSURES, MAY INCLUDE PENDULOUS ABDOMEN DESIGN, SHOULDER STRAPS, STAYS, PREFABRICATED, INCLUDES FITTING AND ADJUSTMENT	C	N	38	A		
L0626	LUMBAR ORTHOSIS, SAGITTAL CONTROL, WITH RIGID POSTERIOR PANEL(S), POSTERIOR EXTENDS FROM L-1 TO BELOW L-5 VERTEBRA, PRODUCES INTRACAVITARY PRESSURE TO REDUCE LOAD ON THE INTERVERTEBRAL DISCS, INCLUDES STRAPS, CLOSURES, MAY INCLUDE PADDING, STAYS, SHOULDER STRAPS, PENDULOUS ABDOMEN DESIGN, PREFABRICATED, INCLUDES FITTING AND ADJUSTMENT	C	N	38	A		

HCPCS Code	Statute	Lab Cert	X-Ref	ASC Pay Grp	ASC Pay Group Eff. Date	Proc Notes	BETOS	TOS	Anest	Code Add Date	Code Effective Date	Code Term Date
L0492							D1F	P	0	20060101	20060101	
L0621							D1F	P	0	20060101	20060101	
L0622							D1F	P	0	20060101	20060101	
L0623							D1F	P	0	20060101	20060101	
L0624							D1F	P	0	20060101	20060101	
L0625							D1F	P	0	20060101	20060101	
L0626							D1F	P	0	20060101	20060101	

HCPCS Code	Long Description	Coverage	Action	PI	MPI	CIM	MCM
L0627	LUMBAR ORTHOSIS, SAGITTAL CONTROL, WITH RIGID ANTERIOR AND POSTERIOR PANELS, POSTERIOR EXTENDS FROM L-1 TO BELOW L-5 VERTEBRA, PRODUCES INTRACAVITARY PRESSURE TO REDUCE LOAD ON THE INTERVERTEBRAL DISCS, INCLUDES STRAPS, CLOSURES, MAY INCLUDE PADDING, SHOULDER STRAPS, PENDULOUS ABDOMEN DESIGN, PREFABRICATED, INCLUDES FITTING AND ADJUSTMENT	C	N	38	A		
L0628	LUMBAR-SACRAL ORTHOSIS, FLEXIBLE, PROVIDES LUMBO-SACRAL SUPPORT, POSTERIOR EXTENDS FROM SACROCOCCYGEAL JUNCTION TO T-9 VERTEBRA, PRODUCES INTRACAVITARY PRESSURE TO REDUCE LOAD ON THE INTERVERTEBRAL DISCS, INCLUDES STRAPS, CLOSURES, MAY INCLUDE STAYS, SHOULDER STRAPS, PENDULOUS ABDOMEN DESIGN, PREFABRICATED, INCLUDES FITTING AND ADJUSTMENT	C	N	38	A		
L0629	LUMBAR-SACRAL ORTHOSIS, FLEXIBLE, PROVIDES LUMBO-SACRAL SUPPORT, POSTERIOR EXTENDS FROM SACROCOCCYGEAL JUNCTION TO T-9 VERTEBRA, PRODUCES INTRACAVITARY PRESSURE TO REDUCE LOAD ON THE INTERVERTEBRAL DISCS, INCLUDES STRAPS, CLOSURES, MAY INCLUDE STAYS, SHOULDER STRAPS, PENDULOUS ABDOMEN DESIGN, CUSTOM FABRICATED	C	N	38	A		
L0630	LUMBAR-SACRAL ORTHOSIS, SAGITTAL CONTROL, WITH RIGID POSTERIOR PANEL(S),POSTERIOR EXTENDS FROM SACROCOCCYGEAL JUNCTION TO T-9 VERTEBRA, PRODUCES INTRACAVITARY PRESSURE TO REDUCE LOAD ON THE INTERVERTEBRAL DISCS, INCLUDES STRAPS, CLOSURES, MAY INCLUDE PADDING, STAYS, SHOULDER STRAPS, PENDULOUS ABDOMEN DESIGN, PREFABRICATED, INCLUDES FITTING AND ADJUSTMENT	C	N	38	A		
L0631	LUMBAR-SACRAL ORTHOSIS, SAGITTAL CONTROL, WITH RIGID ANTERIOR AND POSTERIOR PANELS, POSTERIOR EXTENDS FROM SACROCOCCYGEAL JUNCTION TO T-9 VERTEBRA, PRODUCES INTRACAVITARY PRESSURE TO REDUCE LOAD ON THE INTERVERTEBRAL DISCS, INCLUDES STRAPS, CLOSURES, MAY INCLUDE PADDING, SHOULDER STRAPS, PENDULOUS ABDOMEN DESIGN, PREFABRICATED, INCLUDES FITTING AND ADJUSTMENT	C	N	38	A		
L0632	LUMBAR-SACRAL ORTHOSIS, SAGITTAL CONTROL, WITH RIGID ANTERIOR AND POSTERIOR PANELS, POSTERIOR EXTENDS FROM SACROCOCCYGEAL JUNCTION TO T-9 VERTEBRA, PRODUCES INTRACAVITARY PRESSURE TO REDUCE LOAD ON THE INTERVERTEBRAL DISCS, INCLUDES STRAPS, CLOSURES, MAY INCLUDE PADDING, SHOULDER STRAPS, PENDULOUS ABDOMEN DESIGN, CUSTOM FABRICATED	C	N	38	A		

HCPCS Code	Statute	Lab Cert	X-Ref	ASC Pay Grp	ASC Pay Group Eff. Date	Proc Notes	BETOS	TOS	Anest	Code Add Date	Code Effective Date	Code Term Date
L0627							D1F	P	0	20060101	20060101	
L0628							D1F	P	0	20060101	20060101	
L0629							D1F	P	0	20060101	20060101	
L0630							D1F	P	0	20060101	20060101	
L0631							D1F	P	0	20060101	20070101	
L0632							D1F	P	0	20060101	20060101	

HCPCS Code	Long Description	Coverage	Action	PI	MPI	CIM	MCM
L0633	LUMBAR-SACRAL ORTHOSIS, SAGITTAL-CORONAL CONTROL, WITH RIGID POSTERIOR FRAME/PANEL(S), POSTERIOR EXTENDS FROM SACROCOCCYGEAL JUNCTION TO T-9 VERTEBRA, LATERAL STRENGTH PROVIDED BY RIGID LATERAL FRAME/PANELS, PRODUCES INTRACAVITARY PRESSURE TO REDUCE LOAD ON INTERVERTEBRAL DISCS, INCLUDES STRAPS, CLOSURES, MAY INCLUDE PADDING, STAYS, SHOULDER STRAPS, PENDULOUS ABDOMEN DESIGN, PREFABRICATED, INCLUDES FITTING AND ADJUSTMENT	C	N	38	A		
L0634	LUMBAR-SACRAL ORTHOSIS, SAGITTAL-CORONAL CONTROL, WITH RIGID POSTERIOR FRAME/PANEL(S), POSTERIOR EXTENDS FROM SACROCOCCYGEAL JUNCTION TO T-9 VERTEBRA, LATERAL STRENGTH PROVIDED BY RIGID LATERAL FRAME/PANEL(S), PRODUCES INTRACAVITARY PRESSURE TO REDUCE LOAD ON INTERVERTEBRAL DISCS, INCLUDES STRAPS, CLOSURES, MAY INCLUDE PADDING, STAYS, SHOULDER STRAPS, PENDULOUS ABDOMEN DESIGN, CUSTOM FABRICATED	C	N	38	A		
L0635	LUMBAR-SACRAL ORTHOSIS, SAGITTAL-CORONAL CONTROL, LUMBAR FLEXION, RIGID POSTERIOR FRAME/PANEL(S), LATERAL ARTICULATING DESIGN TO FLEX THE LUMBAR SPINE, POSTERIOR EXTENDS FROM SACROCOCCYGEAL JUNCTION TO T-9 VERTEBRA, LATERAL STRENGTH PROVIDED BY RIGID LATERAL FRAME/PANEL(S), PRODUCES INTRACAVITARY PRESSURE TO REDUCE LOAD ON INTERVERTEBRAL DISCS, INCLUDES STRAPS, CLOSURES, MAY INCLUDE PADDING, ANTERIOR PANEL, PENDULOUS ABDOMEN DESIGN, PREFABRICATED, INCLUDES FITTING & ADJUSTMENT	C	N	38	A		
L0636	LUMBAR SACRAL ORTHOSIS, SAGITTAL-CORONAL CONTROL, LUMBAR FLEXION, RIGID POSTERIOR FRAME/PANELS, LATERAL ARTICULATING DESIGN TO FLEX THE LUMBAR SPINE, POSTERIOR EXTENDS FROM SACROCOCCYGEAL JUNCTION TO T-9 VERTEBRA, LATERAL STRENGTH PROVIDED BY RIGID LATERAL FRAME/PANELS, PRODUCES INTRACAVITARY PRESSURE TO REDUCE LOAD ON INTERVERTEBRAL DISCS, INCLUDES STRAPS, CLOSURES, MAY INCLUDE PADDING, ANTERIOR PANEL, PENDULOUS ABDOMEN DESIGN, CUSTOM FABRICATED	C	N	38	A		
L0637	LUMBAR-SACRAL ORTHOSIS, SAGITTAL-CORONAL CONTROL, WITH RIGID ANTERIOR AND POSTERIOR FRAME/PANELS, POSTERIOR EXTENDS FROM SACROCOCCYGEAL JUNCTION TO T-9 VERTEBRA, LATERAL STRENGTH PROVIDED BY RIGID LATERAL FRAME/PANELS, PRODUCES INTRACAVITARY PRESSURE TO REDUCE LOAD ON INTERVERTEBRAL DISCS, INCLUDES STRAPS, CLOSURES, MAY INCLUDE PADDING, SHOULDER STRAPS, PENDULOUS ABDOMEN DESIGN, PREFABRICATED, INCLUDES FITTING AND ADJUSTMENT	C	N	38	A		

HCPCS Code	Statute	Lab Cert	X-Ref	ASC Pay Grp	ASC Pay Group Eff. Date	Proc Notes	BETOS	TOS	Anest	Code Add Date	Code Effective Date	Code Term Date
L0633							D1F	P	0	20060101	20060101	
L0634							D1F	P	0	20060101	20060101	
L0635							D1F	P	0	20060101	20060101	
L0636							D1F	P	0	20060101	20060101	
L0637							D1F	P	0	20060101	20060101	

L Codes

HCPCS Code	Long Description	Coverage	Action	PI	MPI	CIM	MCM
L0638	LUMBAR-SACRAL ORTHOSIS, SAGITTAL-CORONAL CONTROL, WITH RIGID ANTERIOR AND POSTERIOR FRAME/PANELS, POSTERIOR EXTENDS FROM SACROCOCCYGEAL JUNCTION TO T-9 VERTEBRA, LATERAL STRENGTH PROVIDED BY RIGID LATERAL FRAME/PANELS, PRODUCES INTRACAVITARY PRESSURE TO REDUCE LOAD ON INTERVERTEBRAL DISCS, INCLUDES STRAPS, CLOSURES, MAY INCLUDE PADDING, SHOULDER STRAPS, PENDULOUS ABDOMEN DESIGN, CUSTOM FABRICATED	C	N	38	A		
L0639	LUMBAR-SACRAL ORTHOSIS, SAGITTAL-CORONAL CONTROL, RIGID SHELL(S)/PANEL(S),POSTERIOR EXTENDS FROM SACROCOCCYGEAL JUNCTION TO T-9 VERTEBRA, ANTERIOR EXTENDS FROM SYMPHYSIS PUBIS TO XYPHOID, PRODUCES INTRACAVITARY PRESSURE TO REDUCE LOAD ON THE INTERVERTEBRAL DISCS, OVERALL STRENGTH IS PROVIDED BY OVERLAPPING RIGID MATERIAL AND STABILIZING CLOSURES, INCLUDES STRAPS, CLOSURES, MAY INCLUDE SOFT INTERFACE, PENDULOUS ABDOMEN DESIGN, PREFABRICATED, INCLUDES FITTING AND ADJUSTMENT	C	N	38	A		
L0640	LUMBAR-SACRAL ORTHOSIS, SAGITTAL-CORONAL CONTROL, RIGID SHELL(S)/PANEL(S),POSTERIOR EXTENDS FROM SACROCOCCYGEAL JUNCTION TO T-9 VERTEBRA, ANTERIOR EXTENDS FROM SYMPHYSIS PUBIS TO XYPHOID, PRODUCES INTRACAVITARY PRESSURE TO REDUCE LOAD ON THE INTERVERTEBRAL DISCS, OVERALL STRENGTH IS PROVIDED BY OVERLAPPING RIGID MATERIAL AND STABILIZING CLOSURES, INCLUDES STRAPS, CLOSURES, MAY INCLUDE SOFT INTERFACE, PENDULOUS ABDOMEN DESIGN, CUSTOM FABRICATED	C	N	38	A		
L0700	CERVICAL-THORACIC-LUMBAR-SACRAL-ORTHOSES (CTLSO), ANTERIOR-POSTERIOR-LATERAL CONTROL, MOLDED TO PATIENT MODEL, (MINERVA TYPE)	C	N	38	A		
L0710	CTLSO, ANTERIOR-POSTERIOR-LATERAL-CONTROL, MOLDED TO PATIENT MODEL, WITH INTERFACE MATERIAL, (MINERVA TYPE)	C	N	38	A		
L0810	HALO PROCEDURE, CERVICAL HALO INCORPORATED INTO JACKET VEST	C	N	38	A		
L0820	HALO PROCEDURE, CERVICAL HALO INCORPORATED INTO PLASTER BODY JACKET	C	N	38	A		
L0830	HALO PROCEDURE, CERVICAL HALO INCORPORATED INTO MILWAUKEE TYPE ORTHOSIS	C	N	38	A		
L0859	ADDITION TO HALO PROCEDURE, MAGNETIC RESONANCE IMAGE COMPATIBLE SYSTEMS, RINGS AND PINS, ANY MATERIAL	C	N	38	A		
L0861	ADDITION TO HALO PROCEDURE, REPLACEMENT LINER/INTERFACE MATERIAL	C	N	38	A		
L0960	TORSO SUPPORT, POST SURGICAL SUPPORT, PADS FOR POST SURGICAL SUPPORT	C	N	38	A		
L0970	TLSO, CORSET FRONT	C	N	38	A		

HCPCS Code	Statute	Lab Cert	X-Ref	ASC Pay Grp	ASC Pay Group Eff. Date	Proc Notes	BETOS	TOS	Anest	Code Add Date	Code Effective Date	Code Term Date
L0638							D1F	P	0	20060101	20060101	
L0639							D1F	P	0	20060101	20060101	
L0640							D1F	P	0	20060101	20060101	
L0700							D1F	P	0	19840101	19960101	
L0710							D1F	P	0	19840101	19960101	
L0810							D1F	P	0	19860101	19960101	
L0820							D1F	P	0	19860101	19960101	
L0830							D1F	P	0	19860101	19960101	
L0859							D1F	P	0	20060101	20060101	
L0859 L0861							D1F	P	0	20040101	20040101	
L0960							D1F	P	0	19860101	20080101	20071231
L0970							D1F	P	0	19820101	19960101	

HCPCS Code	Long Description	Coverage	Action	PI	MPI	CIM	MCM
L0972	LSO, CORSET FRONT	C	N	38	A		
L0974	TLSO, FULL CORSET	C	N	38	A		
L0976	LSO, FULL CORSET	C	N	38	A		
L0978	AXILLARY CRUTCH EXTENSION	C	N	38	A		
L0980	PERONEAL STRAPS, PAIR	C	N	38	A		
L0982	STOCKING SUPPORTER GRIPS, SET OF FOUR (4)	C	N	38	A		
L0984	PROTECTIVE BODY SOCK, EACH	C	N	38	A		
L0999	ADDITION TO SPINAL ORTHOSIS, NOT OTHERWISE SPECIFIED	C	N	46	A		
L1000	CERVICAL-THORACIC-LUMBAR-SACRAL ORTHOSIS (CTLSO) (MILWAUKEE), INCLUSIVE OF FURNISHING INITIAL ORTHOSIS, INCLUDING MODEL	C	N	38	A		
L1001	CERVICAL THORACIC LUMBAR SACRAL ORTHOSIS, IMMOBILIZER, INFANT SIZE, PREFABRICATED, INCLUDES FITTING AND ADJUSTMENT	C	N	38	A		
L1005	TENSION BASED SCOLIOSIS ORTHOSIS AND ACCESSORY PADS, INCLUDES FITTING AND ADJUSTMENT	C	N	38	A		
L1010	ADDITION TO CERVICAL-THORACIC-LUMBAR-SACRAL ORTHOSIS (CTLSO) OR SCOLIOSIS ORTHOSIS, AXILLA SLING	C	N	38	A		
L1020	ADDITION TO CTLSO OR SCOLIOSIS ORTHOSIS, KYPHOSIS PAD	C	N	38	A		
L1025	ADDITION TO CTLSO OR SCOLIOSIS ORTHOSIS, KYPHOSIS PAD, FLOATING	C	N	38	A		
L1030	ADDITION TO CTLSO OR SCOLIOSIS ORTHOSIS, LUMBAR BOLSTER PAD	C	N	38	A		
L1040	ADDITION TO CTLSO OR SCOLIOSIS ORTHOSIS, LUMBAR OR LUMBAR RIB PAD	C	N	38	A		
L1050	ADDITION TO CTLSO OR SCOLIOSIS ORTHOSIS, STERNAL PAD	C	N	38	A		
L1060	ADDITION TO CTLSO OR SCOLIOSIS ORTHOSIS, THORACIC PAD	C	N	38	A		
L1070	ADDITION TO CTLSO OR SCOLIOSIS ORTHOSIS, TRAPEZIUS SLING	C	N	38	A		
L1080	ADDITION TO CTLSO OR SCOLIOSIS ORTHOSIS, OUTRIGGER	C	N	38	A		
L1085	ADDITION TO CTLSO OR SCOLIOSIS ORTHOSIS, OUTRIGGER, BILATERAL WITH VERTICAL EXTENSIONS	C	N	38	A		
L1090	ADDITION TO CTLSO OR SCOLIOSIS ORTHOSIS, LUMBAR SLING	C	N	38	A		
L1100	ADDITION TO CTLSO OR SCOLIOSIS ORTHOSIS, RING FLANGE, PLASTIC OR LEATHER	C	N	38	A		
L1110	ADDITION TO CTLSO OR SCOLIOSIS ORTHOSIS, RING FLANGE, PLASTIC OR LEATHER, MOLDED TO PATIENT MODEL	C	N	38	A		
L1120	ADDITION TO CTLSO, SCOLIOSIS ORTHOSIS, COVER FOR UPRIGHT, EACH	C	N	38	A		
L1200	THORACIC-LUMBAR-SACRAL-ORTHOSIS (TLSO), INCLUSIVE OF FURNISHING INITIAL ORTHOSIS ONLY	C	N	38	A		
L1210	ADDITION TO TLSO, (LOW PROFILE), LATERAL THORACIC EXTENSION	C	N	38	A		
L1220	ADDITION TO TLSO, (LOW PROFILE), ANTERIOR THORACIC EXTENSION	C	N	38	A		
L1230	ADDITION TO TLSO, (LOW PROFILE), MILWAUKEE TYPE SUPERSTRUCTURE	C	N	38	A		
L1240	ADDITION TO TLSO, (LOW PROFILE), LUMBAR DEROTATION PAD	C	N	38	A		
L1250	ADDITION TO TLSO, (LOW PROFILE), ANTERIOR ASIS PAD	C	N	38	A		

HCPCS Code	Statute	Lab Cert	X-Ref	ASC Pay Grp	ASC Pay Group Eff. Date	Proc Notes	BETOS	TOS	Anest	Code Add Date	Code Effective Date	Code Term Date
L0972							D1F	P	0	19820101	19960101	
L0974							D1F	P	0	19820101	19960101	
L0976							D1F	P	0	19820101	19960101	
L0978							D1F	P	0	19820101	19960101	
L0980							D1F	P	0	19860101	19960101	
L0982							D1F	P	0	19820101	19960101	
L0984							D1F	P	0	19940101	19960101	
L0999							D1F	P	0	19980101	19980101	
L1000							D1F	P	0	19860101	19960101	
L1001							D1F	P	0	20070101	20070101	
L1005							D1F	P	0	20020101	20020101	
L1010							D1F	P	0	19860101	19960101	
L1020							D1F	P	0	19860101	19960101	
L1025							D1F	P	0	19880101	19960101	
L1030							D1F	P	0	19860101	19960101	
L1040							D1F	P	0	19860101	19960101	
L1050							D1F	P	0	19860101	19960101	
L1060							D1F	P	0	19860101	19960101	
L1070							D1F	P	0	19860101	19960101	
L1080							D1F	P	0	19860101	19960101	
L1085							D1F	P	0	19880101	19960101	
L1090							D1F	P	0	19860101	19960101	
L1100							D1F	P	0	19860101	19960101	
L1110							D1F	P	0	19860101	19960101	
L1120							D1F	P	0	19860101	19960101	
L1200							D1F	P	0	19860101	19960101	
L1210							D1F	P	0	19860101	19960101	
L1220							D1F	P	0	19860101	19960101	
L1230							D1F	P	0	19860101	19960101	
L1240							D1F	P	0	19880101	19960101	
L1250							D1F	P	0	19880101	19960101	

HCPCS Code	Long Description	Coverage	Action	PI	MPI	CIM	MCM
L1260	ADDITION TO TLSO, (LOW PROFILE), ANTERIOR THORACIC DEROTATION PAD	C	N	38	A		
L1270	ADDITION TO TLSO, (LOW PROFILE), ABDOMINAL PAD	C	N	38	A		
L1280	ADDITION TO TLSO, (LOW PROFILE), RIB GUSSET (ELASTIC), EA.	C	N	38	A		
L1290	ADDITION TO TLSO, (LOW PROFILE), LATERAL TROCHANTERIC PAD	C	N	38	A		
L1300	OTHER SCOLIOSIS PROCEDURE, BODY JACKET MOLDED TO PATIENT MODEL	C	N	38	A		
L1310	OTHER SCOLIOSIS PROCEDURE, POST-OPERATIVE BODY JACKET	C	N	38	A		
L1499	SPINAL ORTHOSIS, NOT OTHERWISE SPECIFIED	C	N	46	A		
L1500	THORACIC-HIP-KNEE-ANKLE ORTHOSIS (THKAO), MOBILITY FRAME (NEWINGTON, PARAPODIUM TYPES)	C	N	38	A		
L1510	THKAO, STANDING FRAME, WITH OR WITHOUT TRAY AND ACCESSORIES	C	N	38	A		
L1520	THKAO, SWIVEL WALKER	C	N	38	A		
L1600	HIP ORTHOSIS, ABDUCTION CONTROL OF HIP JOINTS, FLEXIBLE, FREJKA TYPE WITH COVER, PREFABRICATED, INCLUDES FITTING AND ADJUSTMENT	C	N	38	A		
L1610	HIP ORTHOSIS, ABDUCTION CONTROL OF HIP JOINTS, FLEXIBLE, (FREJKA COVER ONLY),PREFABRICATED, INCLUDES FITTING AND ADJUSTMENT	C	N	38	A		
L1620	HIP ORTHOSIS, ABDUCTION CONTROL OF HIP JOINTS, FLEXIBLE, (PAVLIK HARNESS),PREFABRICATED, INCLUDES FITTING AND ADJUSTMENT	C	N	38	A		
L1630	HIP ORTHOSIS, ABDUCTION CONTROL OF HIP JOINTS, SEMI-FLEXIBLE (VON ROSEN TYPE),CUSTOM-FABRICATED	C	N	38	A		
L1640	HIP ORTHOSIS, ABDUCTION CONTROL OF HIP JOINTS, STATIC, PELVIC BAND OR SPREADER BAR, THIGH CUFFS, CUSTOM-FABRICATED	C	N	38	A		
L1650	HIP ORTHOSIS, ABDUCTION CONTROL OF HIP JOINTS, STATIC, ADJUSTABLE, (ILFLED TYPE), PREFABRICATED, INCLUDES FITTING & ADJUSTMENT	C	N	38	A		
L1652	HIP ORTHOSIS, BILATERAL THIGH CUFFS WITH ADJUSTABLE ABDUCTOR SPREADER BAR, ADULT SIZE, PREFABRICATED, INCLUDES FITTING AND ADJUSTMENT, ANY TYPE	C	N	38	A		
L1660	HIP ORTHOSIS, ABDUCTION CONTROL OF HIP JOINTS, STATIC, PLASTIC, PREFABRICATED, INCLUDES FITTING & ADJUSTMENT	C	N	38	A		
L1680	HIP ORTHOSIS, ABDUCTION CONTROL OF HIP JOINTS, DYNAMIC, PELVIC CONTROL, ADJUSTABLE HIP MOTION CONTROL, THIGH CUFFS (RANCHO HIP ACTION TYPE), CUSTOM FABRICATED	C	N	38	A		
L1685	HIP ORTHOSIS, ABDUCTION CONTROL OF HIP JOINT, POSTOPERATIVE HIP ABDUCTION TYPE, CUSTOM FABRICATED	C	N	38	A		
L1686	HIP ORTHOSIS, ABDUCTION CONTROL OF HIP JOINT, POSTOPERATIVE HIP ABDUCTION TYPE, PREFABRICATED, INCLUDES FITTING AND ADJUSTMENT	C	N	38	A		
L1690	COMBINATION, BILATERAL, LUMBO-SACRAL, HIP, FEMUR ORTHOSIS PROVIDING ADDUCTION & INTERNAL ROTATION CONTROL, PREFABRICATED, INCLUDES FITTING & ADJUSTMENT	C	N	38	A		

HCPCS Code	Statute	Lab Cert	X-Ref	ASC Pay Grp	ASC Pay Group Eff. Date	Proc Notes	BETOS	TOS	Anest	Code Add Date	Code Effective Date	Code Term Date
L1260							D1F	P	0	19880101	19960101	
L1270							D1F	P	0	19880101	19960101	
L1280							D1F	P	0	19880101	19960101	
L1290							D1F	P	0	19880101	19960101	
L1300							D1F	P	0	19860101	19960101	
L1310							D1F	P	0	19860101	19960101	
L1499							D1F	P	0	19820101	19980101	
L1500							D1F	P	0	19860101	19960101	
L1510							D1F	P	0	19820101	20020101	
L1520							D1F	P	0	19820101	19960101	
L1600							D1F	P	0	19860101	20010101	
L1610							D1F	P	0	19820101	20010101	
L1620							D1F	P	0	19820101	20010101	
L1630							D1F	P	0	19820101	20010101	
L1640							D1F	P	0	19820101	20010101	
L1650							D1F	P	0	19820101	20010101	
L1652							D1F	P	0	20030101	20030101	
L1660							D1F	P	0	19820101	20010101	
L1680							D1F	P	0	19820101	20010101	
L1685							D1F	P	0	19880101	20010101	
L1686							D1F	P	0	19890101	20010101	
L1690							D1F	P	0	19990101	20010101	

HCPCS Code	Long Description	Coverage	Action	PI	MPI	CIM	MCM
L1700	LEGG PERTHES ORTHOSIS, (TORONTO TYPE), CUSTOM-FABRICATED	C	N	38	A		
L1710	LEGG PERTHES ORTHOSIS, (NEWINGTON TYPE), CUSTOM FABRICATED	C	N	38	A		
L1720	LEGG PERTHES ORTHOSIS, TRILATERAL, (TACHDIJAN TYPE), CUSTOM-FABRICATED	C	N	38	A		
L1730	LEGG PERTHES ORTHOSIS, (SCOTTISH RITE TYPE), CUSTOM-FABRICATED	C	N	38	A		
L1755	LEGG PERTHES ORTHOSIS, (PATTEN BOTTOM TYPE), CUSTOM-FABRICATED	C	N	38	A		
L1800	KNEE ORTHOSIS, ELASTIC WITH STAYS, PREFABRICATED, INCLUDES FITTING AND ADJUSTMENT	C	D	38	A		
L1810	KNEE ORTHOSIS, ELASTIC WITH JOINTS, PREFABRICATED, INCLUDES FITTING AND ADJUSTMENT	C	N	38	A		
L1815	KNEE ORTHOSIS, ELASTIC OR OTHER ELASTIC TYPE MATERIAL WITH CONDYLAR PAD(S),PREFABRICATED, INCLUDES FITTING AND ADJUSTMENT	C	D	38	A		
L1820	KNEE ORTHOSIS, ELASTIC WITH CONDYLAR PADS AND JOINTS, WITH OR WITHOUT PATELLAR CONTROL, PREFABRICATED, INCLUDES FITTING AND ADJUSTMENT	C	N	38	A		
L1825	KNEE ORTHOSIS, ELASTIC KNEE CAP, PREFABRICATED, INCLUDES FITTING AND ADJUSTMENT	C	D	38	A		
L1830	KNEE ORTHOSIS, IMMOBILIZER, CANVAS LONGITUDINAL, PREFABRICATED, INCLUDES FITTING AND ADJUSTMENT	C	N	38	A		
L1831	KNEE ORTHOSIS, LOCKING KNEE JOINT(S), POSITIONAL ORTHOSIS, PREFABRICATED, INCLUDES FITTING & ADJUSTMENT	C	N	38	A		
L1832	KNEE ORTHOSIS, ADJUSTABLE KNEE JOINTS (UNICENTRIC OR POLYCENTRIC), POSITIONAL ORTHOSIS, RIGID SUPPORT, PREFABRICATED, INCLUDES FITTING AND ADJUSTMENT	C	N	38	A		
L1834	KNEE ORTHOSIS, WITHOUT KNEE JOINT, RIGID, CUSTOM-FABRICATED	C	N	38	A		
L1836	KNEE ORTHOSIS, RIGID, WITHOUT JOINT(S), INCLUDES SOFT INTERFACE MATERIAL, PREFABRICATED, INCLUDES FITTING AND ADJUSTMENT	C	N	38	A		
L1840	KNEE ORTHOSIS, DEROTATION, MEDIAL-LATERAL, ANTERIOR CRUCIATE LIGAMENT, CUSTOM FABRICATED	C	N	38	A		
L1843	KNEE ORTHOSIS, SINGLE UPRIGHT, THIGH AND CALF, WITH ADJUSTABLE FLEXION AND EXTENSION JOINT (UNICENTRIC OR POLYCENTRIC), MEDIAL-LATERAL AND ROTATION CONTROL, WITH OR WITHOUT VARUS/VALGUS ADJUSTMENT, PREFABRICATED, INCLUDES FITTING AND ADJUSTMENT	C	N	38	A		
L1844	KNEE ORTHOSIS, SINGLE UPRIGHT, THIGH AND CALF, WITH ADJUSTABLE FLEXION AND EXTENSION JOINT (UNICENTRIC OR POLYCENTRIC), MEDIAL-LATERAL AND ROTATION CONTROL, WITH OR WITHOUT VARUS/VALGUS ADJUSTMENT, CUSTOM FABRICATED	C	N	38	A		

HCPCS Code	Statute	Lab Cert	X-Ref	ASC Pay Grp	ASC Pay Group Eff. Date	Proc Notes	BETOS	TOS	Anest	Code Add Date	Code Effective Date	Code Term Date
L1700							D1F	P	0	19820101	20010101	
L1710							D1F	P	0	19820101	20010101	
L1720							D1F	P	0	19850101	20010101	
L1730							D1F	P	0	19820101	20010101	
L1755							D1F	P	0	19880101	20010101	
L1800							D1F	P	0	19860101	20100101	20091231
L1810							D1F	P	0	19820101	20010101	
L1815							D1F	P	0	19880101	20100101	20091231
L1820							D1F	P	0	19860101	20050101	
L1825							D1F	P	0	19850101	20100101	20091231
L1830							D1F	P	0	19860101	20010101	
L1831							D1F	P	0	20040101	20040101	
L1832							D1F	P	0	19890101	20060101	
L1834							D1F	P	0	19890101	20010101	
L1836							D1F	P	0	20030101	20030101	
L1840							D1F	P	0	19860101	20010101	
L1843							D1F	P	0	19980101	20060101	
L1844							D1F	P	0	19930101	20060101	

HCPCS Code	Long Description	Coverage	Action	PI	MPI	CIM	MCM
L1845	KNEE ORTHOSIS, DOUBLE UPRIGHT, THIGH AND CALF, WITH ADJUSTABLE FLEXION AND EXTENSION JOINT (UNICENTRIC OR POLYCENTRIC), MEDIAL-LATERAL AND ROTATION CONTROL, WITH OR WITHOUT VARUS/VALGUS ADJUSTMENT, PREFABRICATED, INCLUDES FITTING AND ADJUSTMENT	C	N	38	A		
L1846	KNEE ORTHOSIS, DOUBLE UPRIGHT, THIGH AND CALF, WITH ADJUSTABLE FLEXION AND EXTENSION JOINT (UNICENTRIC OR POLYCENTRIC), MEDIAL-LATERAL AND ROTATION CONTROL, WITH OR WITHOUT VARUS/VALGUS ADJUSTMENT, CUSTOM FABRICATED	C	N	38	A		
L1847	KNEE ORTHOSIS, DOUBLE UPRIGHT WITH ADJUSTABLE JOINT, WITH INFLATABLE AIR SUPPORT CHAMBER(S), PREFABRICATED, INCLUDES FITTING AND ADJUSTMENT	C	N	38	A		
L1850	KNEE ORTHOSIS, SWEDISH TYPE, PREFABRICATED, INCLUDES FITTING AND ADJUSTMENT	C	N	38	A		
L1855	KNEE ORTHOSIS, MOLDED PLASTIC, THIGH AND CALF SECTIONS, WITH DOUBLE UPRIGHT KNEE JOINTS, CUSTOM-FABRICATED	C	N	38	A		
L1858	KNEE ORTHOSIS, MOLDED PLASTIC, POLYCENTRIC KNEE JOINTS, PNEUMATIC KNEE PADS (CTI), CUSTOM-FABRICATED	C	N	38	A		
L1860	KNEE ORTHOSIS, MODIFICATION OF SUPRACONDYLAR PROSTHETIC SOCKET, CUSTOM-FABRICATED (SK)	C	N	38	A		
L1870	KNEE ORTHOSIS, DOUBLE UPRIGHT, THIGH AND CALF LACERS WITH KNEE JOINTS, CUSTOM-FABRICATED	C	N	38	A		
L1880	KNEE ORTHOSIS, DOUBLE UPRIGHT, NON-MOLDED THIGH & CALF CUFFS/LACERS WITH KNEE JOINTS, CUSTOM-FABRICATED	C	N	38	A		
L1900	ANKLE FOOT ORTHOSIS, SPRING WIRE, DORSIFLEXION ASSIST CALF BAND, CUSTOM-FABRICATED	C	N	38	A		
L1901	ANKLE ORTHOSIS, ELASTIC, PREFABRICATED, INCLUDES FITTING AND ADJUSTMENT (E.G. NEOPRENE, LYCRA)	C	D	38	A		
L1902	ANKLE FOOT ORTHOSIS, ANKLE GAUNTLET, PREFABRICATED, INCLUDES FITTING AND ADJUSTMENT	C	N	38	A		
L1904	ANKLE FOOT ORTHOSIS, MOLDED ANKLE GAUNTLET, CUSTOM-FABRICATED	C	N	38	A		
L1906	ANKLE FOOT ORTHOSIS, MULTILIGAMENTUS ANKLE SUPPORT, PREFABRICATED, INCLUDES FITTING AND ADJUSTMENT	C	N	38	A		
L1907	AFO, SUPRAMALLEOLAR WITH STRAPS, WITH OR WITHOUT INTERFACE/PADS, CUSTOM FABRICATED	C	N	38	A		
L1910	ANKLE FOOT ORTHOSIS, POSTERIOR, SINGLE BAR, CLASP, ATTACHMENT TO SHOE COUNTER PREFABRICATED, INCLUDES FITTING AND ADJUSTMENT	C	N	38	A		
L1920	ANKLE FOOT ORTHOSIS, SINGLE UPRIGHT WITH STATIC OR ADJUSTABLE STOP (PHELPS OR PERLSTEIN TYPE), CUSTOM-FABRICATED	C	N	38	A		
L1930	ANKLE FOOT ORTHOSIS, PLASTIC OR OTHER MATERIAL, PREFABRICATED, INCLUDES FITTING AND ADJUSTMENT	C	N	38	A		
L1932	AFO, RIGID ANTERIOR TIBIAL SECTION, TOTAL CARBON FIBER OR EQUAL MATERIAL, PREFABRICATED, INCLUDES FITTING AND ADJUSTMENT	C	N	38	A		

HCPCS Code	Statute	Lab Cert	X-Ref	ASC Pay Grp	ASC Pay Group Eff. Date	Proc Notes	BETOS	TOS	Anest	Code Add Date	Code Effective Date	Code Term Date
L1845							D1F	P	0	19880101	20060101	
L1846							D1F	P	0	19880101	20060101	
L1847							D1F	P	0	19990101	20010101	
L1850							D1F	P	0	19820101	20010101	
L1855			L1846				D1F	P	0	19880101	20080101	20071231
L1858			L1846				D1F	P	0	19880101	20080101	20071231
L1860							D1F	P	0	19820101	20010101	
L1870			L1846				D1F	P	0	19820101	20080101	20071231
L1880			L1846				D1F	P	0	19820101	20080101	20071231
L1900							D1F	P	0	19860101	20010101	
L1901							D1F	P	0	20030101	20100101	20091231
L1902							D1F	P	0	19880101	20010101	
L1904							D1F	P	0	19880101	20010101	
L1906							D1F	P	0	19880101	20010101	
L1907							D1F	P	0	20040101	20040101	
L1910							D1F	P	0	19820101	20010101	
L1920							D1F	P	0	19820101	20010101	
L1930							D1F	P	0	19820101	20020101	
L1932							D1F	P	0	20050101	20050101	

HCPCS Code	Long Description	Coverage	Action	PI	MPI	CIM	MCM
L1940	ANKLE FOOT ORTHOSIS, PLASTIC OR OTHER MATERIAL, CUSTOM-FABRICATED	C	N	38	A		
L1945	ANKLE FOOT ORTHOSIS, PLASTIC, RIGID ANTERIOR TIBIAL SECTION (FLOOR REACTION),CUSTOM-FABRICATED	C	N	38	A		
L1950	ANKLE FOOT ORTHOSIS, SPIRAL, (INSTITUTE OF REHABILITATIVE MEDICINE TYPE),PLASTIC, CUSTOM-FABRICATED	C	N	38	A		
L1951	ANKLE FOOT ORTHOSIS, SPIRAL, (INSTITUTE OF REHABILITATIVE MEDICINE TYPE),PLASTIC OR OTHER MATERIAL, PREFABRICATED, INCLUDES FITTING AND ADJUSTMENT	C	N	38	A		
L1960	ANKLE FOOT ORTHOSIS, POSTERIOR SOLID ANKLE, PLASTIC, CUSTOM-FABRICATED	C	N	38	A		
L1970	ANKLE FOOT ORTHOSIS, PLASTIC WITH ANKLE JOINT, CUSTOM-FABRICATED	C	N	38	A		
L1971	ANKLE FOOT ORTHOSIS, PLASTIC OR OTHER MATERIAL WITH ANKLE JOINT, PREFABRICATED, INCLUDES FITTING AND ADJUSTMENT	C	N	38	A		
L1980	ANKLE FOOT ORTHOSIS, SINGLE UPRIGHT FREE PLANTAR DORSIFLEXION, SOLID STIRRUP, CALF BAND/CUFF (SINGLE BAR 'BK' ORTHOSIS), CUSTOM-FABRICATED	C	N	38	A		
L1990	ANKLE FOOT ORTHOSIS, DOUBLE UPRIGHT FREE PLANTAR DORSIFLEXION, SOLID STIRRUP, CALF BAND/CUFF (DOUBLE BAR 'BK' ORTHOSIS), CUSTOM-FABRICATED	C	N	38	A		
L2000	KNEE ANKLE FOOT ORTHOSIS, SINGLE UPRIGHT, FREE KNEE, FREE ANKLE, SOLID STIRRUP, THIGH AND CALF BANDS/CUFFS (SINGLE BAR 'AK' ORTHOSIS), CUSTOM-FABRICATED	C	N	38	A		
L2005	KNEE ANKLE FOOT ORTHOSIS, ANY MATERIAL, SINGLE OR DOUBLE UPRIGHT, STANCE CONTROL, AUTOMATIC LOCK AND SWING PHASE RELEASE, MECHANICAL ACTIVATION, INCLUDES ANKLE JOINT, ANY TYPE, CUSTOM FABRICATED	C	N	38	A		
L2010	KNEE ANKLE FOOT ORTHOSIS, SINGLE UPRIGHT, FREE ANKLE, SOLID STIRRUP, THIGH AND CALF BANDS/CUFFS (SINGLE BAR 'AK' ORTHOSIS), WITHOUT KNEE JOINT, CUSTOM-FABRICATED	C	N	38	A		
L2020	KNEE ANKLE FOOT ORTHOSIS, DOUBLE UPRIGHT, FREE ANKLE, SOLID STIRRUP, THIGH AND CALF BANDS/CUFFS (DOUBLE BAR 'AK' ORTHOSIS), CUSTOM-FABRICATED	C	N	38	A		
L2030	KNEE ANKLE FOOT ORTHOSIS, DOUBLE UPRIGHT, FREE ANKLE, SOLID STIRRUP, THIGH AND CALF BANDS/CUFFS, (DOUBLE BAR 'AK' ORTHOSIS), WITHOUT KNEE JOINT, CUSTOM FABRICATED	C	N	38	A		
L2034	KNEE ANKLE FOOT ORTHOSIS, FULL PLASTIC, SINGLE UPRIGHT, WITH OR WITHOUT FREE MOTION KNEE, MEDIAL LATERAL ROTATION CONTROL, WITH OR WITHOUT FREE MOTION ANKLE, CUSTOM FABRICATED	C	N	38	A		
L2035	KNEE ANKLE FOOT ORTHOSIS, FULL PLASTIC, STATIC (PEDIATRIC SIZE), WITHOUT FREEMOTION ANKLE, PREFABRICATED, INCLUDES FITTING AND ADJUSTMENT	C	N	38	A		

HCPCS Code	Statute	Lab Cert	X-Ref	ASC Pay Grp	ASC Pay Group Eff. Date	Proc Notes	BETOS	TOS	Anest	Code Add Date	Code Effective Date	Code Term Date
L1940							D1F	P	0	19820101	20020101	
L1945							D1F	P	0	19890101	20010101	
L1950							D1F	P	0	19820101	20040101	
L1951							D1F	P	0	20040101	20040101	
L1960							D1F	P	0	19820101	20010101	
L1970							D1F	P	0	19820101	20010101	
L1971							D1F	P	0	20040101	20040101	
L1980							D1F	P	0	19820101	20010101	
L1990							D1F	P	0	19820101	20010101	
L2000							D1F	P	0	19850101	20010101	
L2005							D1F	P	0	20050101	20050101	
L2010							D1F	P	0	19860101	20010101	
L2020							D1F	P	0	19850101	20010101	
L2030							D1F	P	0	19860101	20010101	
L2034							D1F	P	0	20060101	20060101	
L2035							D1F	P	0	19980101	20050101	

HCPCS Code	Long Description	Coverage	Action	PI	MPI	CIM	MCM
L2036	KNEE ANKLE FOOT ORTHOSIS, FULL PLASTIC, DOUBLE UPRIGHT, WITH OR WITHOUT FREE MOTION KNEE, WITH OR WITHOUT FREE MOTION ANKLE, CUSTOM FABRICATED	C	N	38	A		
L2037	KNEE ANKLE FOOT ORTHOSIS, FULL PLASTIC, SINGLE UPRIGHT, WITH OR WITHOUT FREE MOTION KNEE, WITH OR WITHOUT FREE MOTION ANKLE, CUSTOM FABRICATED	C	N	38	A		
L2038	KNEE ANKLE FOOT ORTHOSIS, FULL PLASTIC, WITH OR WITHOUT FREE MOTION KNEE, MULTI-AXIS ANKLE, CUSTOM FABRICATED	C	N	38	A		
L2040	HIP KNEE ANKLE FOOT ORTHOSIS, TORSION CONTROL, BILATERAL ROTATION STRAPS, PELVIC BAND/BELT, CUSTOM FABRICATED	C	N	38	A		
L2050	HIP KNEE ANKLE FOOT ORTHOSIS, TORSION CONTROL, BILATERAL TORSION CABLES, HIP JOINT, PELVIC BAND/BELT, CUSTOM-FABRICATED	C	N	38	A		
L2060	HIP KNEE ANKLE FOOT ORTHOSIS, TORSION CONTROL, BILATERAL TORSION CABLES, BALL BEARING HIP JOINT, PELVIC BAND/ BELT, CUSTOM-FABRICATED	C	N	38	A		
L2070	HIP KNEE ANKLE FOOT ORTHOSIS, TORSION CONTROL, UNILATERAL ROTATION STRAPS, PELVIC BAND/BELT, CUSTOM FABRICATED	C	N	38	A		
L2080	HIP KNEE ANKLE FOOT ORTHOSIS, TORSION CONTROL, UNILATERAL TORSION CABLE, HIP JOINT, PELVIC BAND/BELT, CUSTOM-FABRICATED	C	N	38	A		
L2090	HIP KNEE ANKLE FOOT ORTHOSIS, TORSION CONTROL, UNILATERAL TORSION CABLE, BALL BEARING HIP JOINT, PELVIC BAND/ BELT, CUSTOM-FABRICATED	C	N	38	A		
L2106	ANKLE FOOT ORTHOSIS, FRACTURE ORTHOSIS, TIBIAL FRACTURE CAST ORTHOSIS, THERMOPLASTIC TYPE CASTING MATERIAL, CUSTOM-FABRICATED	C	N	38	A		
L2108	ANKLE FOOT ORTHOSIS, FRACTURE ORTHOSIS, TIBIAL FRACTURE CAST ORTHOSIS, CUSTOM-FABRICATED	C	N	38	A		
L2112	ANKLE FOOT ORTHOSIS, FRACTURE ORTHOSIS, TIBIAL FRACTURE ORTHOSIS, SOFT, PREFABRICATED, INCLUDES FITTING AND ADJUSTMENT	C	N	38	A		
L2114	ANKLE FOOT ORTHOSIS, FRACTURE ORTHOSIS, TIBIAL FRACTURE ORTHOSIS, SEMI-RIGID, PREFABRICATED, INCLUDES FITTING AND ADJUSTMENT	C	N	38	A		
L2116	ANKLE FOOT ORTHOSIS, FRACTURE ORTHOSIS, TIBIAL FRACTURE ORTHOSIS, RIGID, PREFABRICATED, INCLUDES FITTING AND ADJUSTMENT	C	N	38	A		
L2126	KNEE ANKLE FOOT ORTHOSIS, FRACTURE ORTHOSIS, FEMORAL FRACTURE CAST ORTHOSIS, THERMOPLASTIC TYPE CASTING MATERIAL, CUSTOM-FABRICATED	C	N	38	A		
L2128	KNEE ANKLE FOOT ORTHOSIS, FRACTURE ORTHOSIS, FEMORAL FRACTURE CAST ORTHOSIS, CUSTOM-FABRICATED	C	N	38	A		
L2132	KAFO, FRACTURE ORTHOSIS, FEMORAL FRACTURE CAST ORTHOSIS, SOFT, PREFABRICATED, INCLUDES FITTING AND ADJUSTMENT	C	N	38	A		

HCPCS Code	Statute	Lab Cert	X-Ref	ASC Pay Grp	ASC Pay Group Eff. Date	Proc Notes	BETOS	TOS	Anest	Code Add Date	Code Effective Date	Code Term Date
L2036							D1F	P	0	19880101	20060101	
L2037							D1F	P	0	19890101	20060101	
L2038							D1F	P	0	19890101	20060101	
L2040							D1F	P	0	19860101	20010101	
L2050							D1F	P	0	19820101	20010101	
L2060							D1F	P	0	19820101	20010101	
L2070							D1F	P	0	19820101	20010101	
L2080							D1F	P	0	19860101	20010101	
L2090							D1F	P	0	19840101	20010101	
L2106							D1F	P	0	19880101	20010101	
L2108							D1F	P	0	19880101	20010101	
L2112							D1F	P	0	19880101	20010101	
L2114							D1F	P	0	19880101	20010101	
L2116							D1F	P	0	19880101	20010101	
L2126							D1F	P	0	19880101	20010101	
L2128							D1F	P	0	19880101	20010101	
L2132							D1F	P	0	19880101	20010101	

HCPCS Code	Long Description	Coverage	Action	PI	MPI	CIM	MCM
L2134	KAFO, FRACTURE ORTHOSIS, FEMORAL FRACTURE CAST ORTHOSIS, SEMI-RIGID, PREFABRICATED, INCLUDES FITTING AND ADJUSTMENT	C	N	38	A		
L2136	KAFO, FRACTURE ORTHOSIS, FEMORAL FRACTURE CAST ORTHOSIS, RIGID, PREFABRICATED, INCLUDES FITTING AND ADJUSTMENT	C	N	38	A		
L2180	ADDITION TO LOWER EXTREMITY FRACTURE ORTHOSIS, PLASTIC SHOE INSERT WITH ANKLE JOINTS	C	N	38	A		
L2182	ADDITION TO LOWER EXTREMITY FRACTURE ORTHOSIS, DROP LOCK KNEE JOINT	C	N	38	A		
L2184	ADDITION TO LOWER EXTREMITY FRACTURE ORTHOSIS, LIMITED MOTION KNEE JOINT	C	N	38	A		
L2186	ADDITION TO LOWER EXTREMITY FRACTURE ORTHOSIS, ADJUSTABLE MOTION KNEE JOINT, LERMAN TYPE	C	N	38	A		
L2188	ADDITION TO LOWER EXTREMITY FRACTURE ORTHOSIS, QUADRILATERAL BRIM	C	N	38	A		
L2190	ADDITION TO LOWER EXTREMITY FRACTURE ORTHOSIS, WAIST BELT	C	N	38	A		
L2192	ADDITION TO LOWER EXTREMITY FRACTURE ORTHOSIS, HIP JOINT, PELVIC BAND, THIGH FLANGE, AND PELVIC BELT	C	N	38	A		
L2200	ADDITION TO LOWER EXTREMITY, LIMITED ANKLE MOTION, EACH JOINT	C	N	38	A		
L2210	ADDITION TO LOWER EXTREMITY, DORSIFLEXION ASSIST (PLANTAR FLEXION RESIST), EACH JOINT	C	N	38	A		
L2220	ADDITION TO LOWER EXTREMITY, DORSIFLEXION AND PLANTAR FLEXION ASSIST/RESIST, EACH JOINT	C	N	38	A		
L2230	ADDITION TO LOWER EXTREMITY, SPLIT FLAT CALIPER STIRRUPS AND PLATE ATTACHMENT	C	N	38	A		
L2232	ADDITION TO LOWER EXTREMITY ORTHOSIS, ROCKER BOTTOM FOR TOTAL CONTACT ANKLE FOOT ORTHOSIS, FOR CUSTOM FABRICATED ORTHOSIS ONLY	C	N	38	A		
L2240	ADDITION TO LOWER EXTREMITY, ROUND CALIPER AND PLATE ATTACHMENT	C	N	38	A		
L2250	ADDITION TO LOWER EXTREMITY, FOOT PLATE, MOLDED TO PATIENT MODEL, STIRRUP ATTACHMENT	C	N	38	A		
L2260	ADDITION TO LOWER EXTREMITY, REINFORCED SOLID STIRRUP (SCOTT-CRAIG TYPE)	C	N	38	A		
L2265	ADDITION TO LOWER EXTREMITY, LONG TONGUE STIRRUP	C	N	38	A		
L2270	ADDITION TO LOWER EXTREMITY, VARUS/VALGUS CORRECTION ('T') STRAP, PADDED/LINED OR MALLEOLUS PAD	C	N	38	A		
L2275	ADDITION TO LOWER EXTREMITY, VARUS/VALGUS CORRECTION, PLASTIC MODIFICATION, PADDED/LINED	C	N	38	A		
L2280	ADDITION TO LOWER EXTREMITY, MOLDED INNER BOOT	C	N	38	A		
L2300	ADDITION TO LOWER EXTREMITY, ABDUCTION BAR (BILATERAL HIP INVOLVEMENT), JOINTED, ADJUSTABLE	C	N	38	A		
L2310	ADDITION TO LOWER EXTREMITY, ABDUCTION BAR-STRAIGHT	C	N	38	A		
L2320	ADDITION TO LOWER EXTREMITY, NON-MOLDED LACER, FOR CUSTOM FABRICATED ORTHOSIS ONLY	C	N	38	A		

HCPCS Code	Statute	Lab Cert	X-Ref	ASC Pay Grp	ASC Pay Group Eff. Date	Proc Notes	BETOS	TOS	Anest	Code Add Date	Code Effective Date	Code Term Date
L2134							D1F	P	0	19880101	20010101	
L2136							D1F	P	0	19880101	20010101	
L2180							D1F	P	0	19880101	19960101	
L2182							D1F	P	0	19880101	19960101	
L2184							D1F	P	0	19880101	19960101	
L2186							D1F	P	0	19880101	19960101	
L2188							D1F	P	0	19880101	19960101	
L2190							D1F	P	0	19880101	19960101	
L2192							D1F	P	0	19880101	19960101	
L2200							D1F	P	0	19860101	19960101	
L2210							D1F	P	0	19860101	19960101	
L2220							D1F	P	0	19860101	19960101	
L2230							D1F	P	0	19860101	19960101	
L2232							D1F	P	0	20050101	20050101	
L2240							D1F	P	0	19860101	19960101	
L2250							D1F	P	0	19860101	19960101	
L2260							D1F	P	0	19860101	19960101	
L2265							D1F	P	0	19890101	19960101	
L2270							D1F	P	0	19860101	19960101	
L2275							D1F	P	0	19940101	19960101	
L2280							D1F	P	0	19860101	19960101	
L2300							D1F	P	0	19860101	19960101	
L2310							D1F	P	0	19860101	19960101	
L2320							D1F	P	0	19860101	20050101	

HCPCS Code	Long Description	Coverage	Action	PI	MPI	CIM	MCM
L2330	ADDITION TO LOWER EXTREMITY, LACER MOLDED TO PATIENT MODEL, FOR CUSTOM FABRICATED ORTHOSIS ONLY	C	N	38	A		
L2335	ADDITION TO LOWER EXTREMITY, ANTERIOR SWING BAND	C	N	38	A		
L2340	ADDITION TO LOWER EXTREMITY, PRE-TIBIAL SHELL, MOLDED TO PATIENT MODEL	C	N	38	A		
L2350	ADDITION TO LOWER EXTREMITY, PROSTHETIC TYPE, (BK) SOCKET, MOLDED TO PATIENT MODEL, (USED FOR 'PTB' 'AFO' ORTHOSES)	C	N	38	A		
L2360	ADDITION TO LOWER EXTREMITY, EXTENDED STEEL SHANK	C	N	38	A		
L2370	ADDITION TO LOWER EXTREMITY, PATTEN BOTTOM	C	N	38	A		
L2375	ADDITION TO LOWER EXTREMITY, TORSION CONTROL, ANKLE JOINT AND HALF SOLID STIRRUP	C	N	38	A		
L2380	ADDITION TO LOWER EXTREMITY, TORSION CONTROL, STRAIGHT KNEE JOINT, EACH JOINT	C	N	38	A		
L2385	ADDITION TO LOWER EXTREMITY, STRAIGHT KNEE JOINT, HEAVY DUTY, EACH JOINT	C	N	38	A		
L2387	ADDITION TO LOWER EXTREMITY, POLYCENTRIC KNEE JOINT, FOR CUSTOM FABRICATED KNEE ANKLE FOOT ORTHOSIS, EACH JOINT	C	N	38	A		
L2390	ADDITION TO LOWER EXTREMITY, OFFSET KNEE JOINT, EACH JOINT	C	N	38	A		
L2395	ADDITION TO LOWER EXTREMITY, OFFSET KNEE JOINT, HEAVY DUTY, EACH JOINT	C	N	38	A		
L2397	ADDITION TO LOWER EXTREMITY ORTHOSIS, SUSPENSION SLEEVE	C	N	38	A		
L2405	ADDITION TO KNEE JOINT, DROP LOCK, EACH	C	N	38	A		
L2415	ADDITION TO KNEE LOCK WITH INTEGRATED RELEASE MECHANISM (BAIL, CABLE, OR EQUAL), ANY MATERIAL, EACH JOINT	C	N	38	A		
L2425	ADDITION TO KNEE JOINT, DISC OR DIAL LOCK FOR ADJUSTABLE KNEE FLEXION, EACH JOINT	C	N	38	A		
L2430	ADDITION TO KNEE JOINT, RATCHET LOCK FOR ACTIVE AND PROGRESSIVE KNEE EXTENSION, EACH JOINT	C	N	38	A		
L2492	ADDITION TO KNEE JOINT, LIFT LOOP FOR DROP LOCK RING	C	N	38	A		
L2500	ADDITION TO LOWER EXTREMITY, THIGH/WEIGHT BEARING, GLUTEAL/ ISCHIAL WEIGHT BEARING, RING	C	N	38	A		
L2510	ADDITION TO LOWER EXTREMITY, THIGH/WEIGHT BEARING, QUADRI- LATERAL BRIM, MOLDED TO PATIENT MODEL	C	N	38	A		
L2520	ADDITION TO LOWER EXTREMITY, THIGH/WEIGHT BEARING, QUADRI- LATERAL BRIM, CUSTOM FITTED	C	N	38	A		
L2525	ADDITION TO LOWER EXTREMITY, THIGH/WEIGHT BEARING, ISCHIAL CONTAINMENT/NARROW M-L BRIM MOLDED TO PATIENT MODEL	C	N	38	A		
L2526	ADDITION TO LOWER EXTREMITY, THIGH/WEIGHT BEARING, ISCHIAL CONTAINMENT/NARROW M-L BRIM, CUSTOM FITTED	C	N	38	A		
L2530	ADDITION TO LOWER EXTREMITY, THIGH-WEIGHT BEARING, LACER, NON-MOLDED	C	N	38	A		
L2540	ADDITION TO LOWER EXTREMITY, THIGH/WEIGHT BEARING, LACER, MOLDED TO PATIENT MODEL	C	N	38	A		

HCPCS Code	Statute	Lab Cert	X-Ref	ASC Pay Grp	ASC Pay Group Eff. Date	Proc Notes	BETOS	TOS	Anest	Code Add Date	Code Effective Date	Code Term Date
L2330							D1F	P	0	19860101	20050101	
L2335							D1F	P	0	19880101	19960101	
L2340							D1F	P	0	19860101	19960101	
L2350							D1F	P	0	19860101	19960101	
L2360							D1F	P	0	19860101	19960101	
L2370							D1F	P	0	19880101	19960101	
L2375							D1F	P	0	19880101	19960101	
L2380							D1F	P	0	19880101	19960101	
L2385							D1F	P	0	19880101	19960101	
L2387							D1F	P	0	20060101	20060101	
L2390							D1F	P	0	19880101	19960101	
L2395							D1F	P	0	19880101	19960101	
L2397							D1F	P	0	19940101	19960101	
L2405							D1F	P	0	19880101	20060101	
L2415							D1F	P	0	19880101	20020101	
L2425							D1F	P	0	19880101	19960101	
L2430							D1F	P	0	19970101	19970101	
L2492							D1F	P	0	19880101	19960101	
L2500							D1F	P	0	19860101	19960101	
L2510							D1F	P	0	19860101	19960101	
L2520							D1F	P	0	19860101	19960101	
L2525							D1F	P	0	19890101	19960101	
L2526							D1F	P	0	19890101	19960101	
L2530							D1F	P	0	19860101	19960101	
L2540							D1F	P	0	19860101	19960101	

HCPCS Code	Long Description	Coverage	Action	PI	MPI	CIM	MCM
L2550	ADDITION TO LOWER EXTREMITY, THIGH/WEIGHT BEARING, HIGH ROLL CUFF	C	N	38	A		
L2570	ADDITION TO LOWER EXTREMITY, PELVIC CONTROL, HIP JOINT, CLEVIS TYPE TWO POSITION JOINT, EACH	C	N	38	A		
L2580	ADDITION TO LOWER EXTREMITY, PELVIC CONTROL, PELVIC SLING	C	N	38	A		
L2600	ADDITION TO LOWER EXTREMITY, PELVIC CONTROL, HIP JOINT, CLEVIS TYPE, OR THRUST BEARING, FREE, EACH	C	N	38	A		
L2610	ADDITION TO LOWER EXTREMITY, PELVIC CONTROL, HIP JOINT, CLEVIS OR THRUST BEARING, LOCK, EACH	C	N	38	A		
L2620	ADDITION TO LOWER EXTREMITY, PELVIC CONTROL, HIP JOINT, HEAVY DUTY, EACH	C	N	38	A		
L2622	ADDITION TO LOWER EXTREMITY, PELVIC CONTROL, HIP JOINT, ADJUSTABLE FLEXION, EACH	C	N	38	A		
L2624	ADDITION TO LOWER EXTREMITY, PELVIC CONTROL, HIP JOINT, ADJUSTABLE FLEXION, EXTENSION, ABDUCTION CONTROL, EACH	C	N	38	A		
L2627	ADDITION TO LOWER EXTREMITY, PELVIC CONTROL, PLASTIC, MOLDED TO PATIENT MODEL, RECIPROCATING HIP JOINT AND CABLES	C	N	38	A		
L2628	ADDITION TO LOWER EXTREMITY, PELVIC CONTROL, METAL FRAME, RECIPROCATING HIP JOINT AND CABLES	C	N	38	A		
L2630	ADDITION TO LOWER EXTREMITY, PELVIC CONTROL, BAND AND BELT, UNILATERAL	C	N	38	A		
L2640	ADDITION TO LOWER EXTREMITY, PELVIC CONTROL, BAND AND BELT, BILATERAL	C	N	38	A		
L2650	ADDITION TO LOWER EXTREMITY, PELVIC AND THORACIC CONTROL, GLUTEAL PAD, EACH	C	N	38	A		
L2660	ADDITION TO LOWER EXTREMITY, THORACIC CONTROL, THORACIC BAND	C	N	38	A		
L2670	ADDITION TO LOWER EXTREMITY, THORACIC CONTROL, PARASPINAL UPRIGHTS	C	N	38	A		
L2680	ADDITION TO LOWER EXTREMITY, THORACIC CONTROL, LATERAL SUPPORT UPRIGHTS	C	N	38	A		
L2750	ADDITION TO LOWER EXTREMITY ORTHOSIS, PLATING CHROME OR NICKEL, PER BAR	C	N	38	A		
L2755	ADDITION TO LOWER EXTREMITY ORTHOSIS, HIGH STRENGTH, LIGHTWEIGHT MATERIAL, ALL HYBRID LAMINATION/PREPREG COMPOSITE, PER SEGMENT, FOR CUSTOM FABRICATED ORTHOSIS ONLY	C	N	38	A		
L2760	ADDITION TO LOWER EXTREMITY ORTHOSIS, EXTENSION, PER EXTENSION, PER BAR (FOR LINEAL ADJUSTMENT FOR GROWTH)	C	N	38	A		
L2768	ORTHOTIC SIDE BAR DISCONNECT DEVICE, PER BAR	C	N	38	A		
L2770	ADDITION TO LOWER EXTREMITY ORTHOSIS, ANY MATERIAL - PER BAR OR JOINT	C	D	38	A		
L2780	ADDITION TO LOWER EXTREMITY ORTHOSIS, NON-CORROSIVE FINISH, PER BAR	C	N	38	A		

HCPCS Code	Statute	Lab Cert	X-Ref	ASC Pay Grp	ASC Pay Group Eff. Date	Proc Notes	BETOS	TOS	Anest	Code Add Date	Code Effective Date	Code Term Date
L2550							D1F	P	0	19860101	19960101	
L2570							D1F	P	0	19860101	19960101	
L2580							D1F	P	0	19860101	19960101	
L2600							D1F	P	0	19860101	19960101	
L2610							D1F	P	0	19860101	19960101	
L2620							D1F	P	0	19860101	19960101	
L2622							D1F	P	0	19880101	19960101	
L2624							D1F	P	0	19880101	19960101	
L2627							D1F	P	0	19890101	19960101	
L2628							D1F	P	0	19890101	19960101	
L2630							D1F	P	0	19860101	19960101	
L2640							D1F	P	0	19860101	19960101	
L2650							D1F	P	0	19860101	19960101	
L2660							D1F	P	0	19860101	19960101	
L2670							D1F	P	0	19860101	19960101	
L2680							D1F	P	0	19860101	19960101	
L2750							D1F	P	0	19860101	19960101	
L2755							D1F	P	0	19970101	20050101	
L2760							D1F	P	0	19860101	19960101	
L2768							D1F	P	0	20020101	20020101	
L2770							D1F	P	0	19860101	20100101	20091231
L2780							D1F	P	0	19860101	19960101	

HCPCS Code	Long Description	Coverage	Action	PI	MPI	CIM	MCM
L2785	ADDITION TO LOWER EXTREMITY ORTHOSIS, DROP LOCK RETAINER, EACH	C	N	38	A		
L2795	ADDITION TO LOWER EXTREMITY ORTHOSIS, KNEE CONTROL, FULL KNEECAP	C	N	38	A		
L2800	ADDITION TO LOWER EXTREMITY ORTHOSIS, KNEE CONTROL, KNEE CAP, MEDIAL OR LATERAL PULL, FOR USE WITH CUSTOM FABRICATED ORTHOSIS ONLY	C	N	38	A		
L2810	ADDITION TO LOWER EXTREMITY ORTHOSIS, KNEE CONTROL, CONDYLAR PAD	C	N	38	A		
L2820	ADDITION TO LOWER EXTREMITY ORTHOSIS, SOFT INTERFACE FOR MOLDED PLASTIC, BELOW KNEE SECTION	C	N	38	A		
L2830	ADDITION TO LOWER EXTREMITY ORTHOSIS, SOFT INTERFACE FOR MOLDED PLASTIC, ABOVE KNEE SECTION	C	N	38	A		
L2840	ADDITION TO LOWER EXTREMITY ORTHOSIS, TIBIAL LENGTH SOCK, FRACTURE OR EQUAL, EACH	C	N	38	A		
L2850	ADDITION TO LOWER EXTREMITY ORTHOSIS, FEMORAL LENGTH SOCK, FRACTURE OR EQUAL, EACH	C	N	38	A		
L2860	ADDITION TO LOWER EXTREMITY JOINT, KNEE OR ANKLE, CONCENTRIC ADJUSTABLE TORSION STYLE MECHANISM, EA.	C	N	00	9		
L2861	ADDITION TO LOWER EXTREMITY JOINT, KNEE OR ANKLE, CONCENTRIC ADJUSTABLE TORSION STYLE MECHANISM FOR CUSTOM FABRICATED ORTHOTICS ONLY, EACH	I	A	00	9		
L2999	LOWER EXTREMITY ORTHOSES, NOT OTHERWISE SPECIFIED	C	N	46	A		
L3000	FOOT, INSERT, REMOVABLE, MOLDED TO PATIENT MODEL, , 'UCB' TYPE, BERKELEY SHELLEACH	D	N	00	9		2323
L3001	FOOT, INSERT, REMOVABLE, MOLDED TO PATIENT MODEL, SPENCO, EACH	D	N	00	9		2323
L3002	FOOT, INSERT, REMOVABLE, MOLDED TO PATIENT MODEL, PLASTAZOTE OR EQUAL, EACH	D	N	00	9		2323
L3003	FOOT, INSERT, REMOVABLE, MOLDED TO PATIENT MODEL, SILICONE GEL, EACH	D	N	00	9		2323
L3010	FOOT, INSERT, REMOVABLE, MOLDED TO PATIENT MODEL, LONGITUDINAL ARCH SUPPORT, EACH	D	N	00	9		2323
L3020	FOOT, INSERT, REMOVABLE, MOLDED TO PATIENT MODEL, LONGITUDINAL/ METATARSAL SUPPORT, EACH	D	N	00	9		2323
L3030	FOOT, INSERT, REMOVABLE, FORMED TO PATIENT FOOT, EA.	D	N	00	9		2323
L3031	FOOT, INSERT/PLATE, REMOVABLE, ADDITION TO LOWER EXTREMITY ORTHOSIS, HIGH STRENGTH, LIGHTWEIGHT MATERIAL, ALL HYBRID LAMINATION/PREPREG COMPOSITE, EACH	C	N	00	9		
L3040	FOOT, ARCH SUPPORT, REMOVABLE, PREMOLDED, LONGITUDINAL, EACH	D	N	00	9		2323
L3050	FOOT, ARCH SUPPORT, REMOVABLE, PREMOLDED, METATARSAL, EACH	D	N	00	9		2323
L3060	FOOT, ARCH SUPPORT, REMOVABLE, PREMOLDED, LONGITUDINAL/ METATARSAL, EACH	D	N	00	9		2323
L3070	FOOT, ARCH SUPPORT, NON-REMOVABLE ATTACHED TO SHOE, LONGITUDINAL, EACH	D	N	00	9		2323

HCPCS Code	Statute	Lab Cert	X-Ref	ASC Pay Grp	ASC Pay Group Eff. Date	Proc Notes	BETOS	TOS	Anest	Code Add Date	Code Effective Date	Code Term Date
L2785							D1F	P	0	19880101	19960101	
L2795							D1F	P	0	19880101	19960101	
L2800							D1F	P	0	19880101	20050101	
L2810							D1F	P	0	19880101	19960101	
L2820							D1F	P	0	19880101	19960101	
L2830							D1F	P	0	19880101	19960101	
L2840							D1F	P	0	19890101	19960101	
L2850							D1F	P	0	19890101	19960101	
L2860							D1F	P	0	19950101	20090101	20081231
L2861							D1F	P	0	20100101	20100101	
L2999							D1F	P	0	19820101	19980101	
L3000							D1F	P	0	19820101	19970101	
L3001							D1F	P	0	19840101	19970101	
L3002							D1F	P	0	19840101	19970101	
L3003							D1F	P	0	19840101	19970101	
L3010							D1F	P	0	19820101	19970101	
L3020							D1F	P	0	19860101	19970101	
L3030							D1F	P	0	19860101	19970101	
L3031							D1F	P	0	20040101	20050101	
L3040							D1F	P	0	19820101	19970101	
L3050							D1F	P	0	19820101	19970101	
L3060							D1F	P	0	19820101	19970101	
L3070							D1F	P	0	19840101	19970101	

HCPCS Code	Long Description	Coverage	Action	PI	MPI	CIM	MCM
L3080	FOOT, ARCH SUPPORT, NON-REMOVABLE ATTACHED TO SHOE, METATARSAL, EACH	D	N	00	9		2323
L3090	FOOT, ARCH SUPPORT, NON-REMOVABLE ATTACHED TO SHOE, LONGITUDINAL/METATARSAL, EACH	D	N	00	9		2323
L3100	HALLUS-VALGUS NIGHT DYNAMIC SPLINT	D	N	00	9		2323
L3140	FOOT, ABDUCTION ROTATION BAR, INCLUDING SHOES	D	N	00	9		2323
L3150	FOOT, ABDUCTION ROTATATION BAR, WITHOUT SHOES	D	N	00	9		2323
L3160	FOOT, ADJUSTABLE SHOE-STYLED POSITIONING DEVICE	C	N	00	9		
L3170	FOOT, PLASTIC, SILICONE OR EQUAL, HEEL STABILIZER, EA.	D	N	00	9		2323
L3201	ORTHOPEDIC SHOE, OXFORD WITH SUPINATOR OR PRONATOR, INFANT	D	N	00	9		2323
L3202	ORTHOPEDIC SHOE, OXFORD WITH SUPINATOR OR PRONATOR, CHILD	D	N	00	9		2323
L3203	ORTHOPEDIC SHOE, OXFORD WITH SUPINATOR OR PRONATOR, JUNIOR	D	N	00	9		2323
L3204	ORTHOPEDIC SHOE, HIGHTOP WITH SUPINATOR OR PRONATOR, INFANT	D	N	00	9		2323
L3206	ORTHOPEDIC SHOE, HIGHTOP WITH SUPINATOR OR PRONATOR, CHILD	D	N	00	9		2323
L3207	ORTHOPEDIC SHOE, HIGHTOP WITH SUPINATOR OR PRONATOR, JUNIOR	D	N	00	9		2323
L3208	SURGICAL BOOT, EACH, INFANT	D	N	00	9		2079
L3209	SURGICAL BOOT, EACH, CHILD	D	N	00	9		2079
L3211	SURGICAL BOOT, EACH, JUNIOR	D	N	00	9		2079
L3212	BENESCH BOOT, PAIR, INFANT	D	N	00	9		2079
L3213	BENESCH BOOT, PAIR, CHILD	D	N	00	9		2079
L3214	BENESCH BOOT, PAIR, JUNIOR	D	N	00	9		2079
L3215	ORTHOPEDIC FOOTWEAR, LADIES SHOE, OXFORD, EACH	S	N	00	9		
L3216	ORTHOPEDIC FOOTWEAR, LADIES SHOE, DEPTH INLAY, EA.	S	N	00	9		
L3217	ORTHOPEDIC FOOTWEAR, LADIES SHOE, HIGHTOP, DEPTH INLAY, EACH	S	N	00	9		
L3219	ORTHOPEDIC FOOTWEAR, MENS SHOE, OXFORD, EACH	S	N	00	9		
L3221	ORTHOPEDIC FOOTWEAR, MENS SHOE, DEPTH INLAY, EACH	S	N	00	9		
L3222	ORTHOPEDIC FOOTWEAR, MENS SHOE, HIGHTOP, DEPTH INLAY, EACH	S	N	00	9		
L3224	ORTHOPEDIC FOOTWEAR, WOMAN'S SHOE, OXFORD, USED AS AN INTEGRAL PART OF A BRACE (ORTHOSIS)	D	N	38	A		2323D
L3225	ORTHOPEDIC FOOTWEAR, MAN'S SHOE, OXFORD, USED AS AN INTEGRAL PART OF A BRACE (ORTHOSIS)	D	N	38	A		2323D
L3230	ORTHOPEDIC FOOTWEAR, CUSTOM SHOE, DEPTH INLAY, EA.	D	N	00	9		2323
L3250	ORTHOPEDIC FOOTWEAR, CUSTOM MOLDED SHOE, REMOVABLE INNER MOLD, PROSTHETIC SHOE, EACH	D	N	00	9		2323
L3251	FOOT, SHOE MOLDED TO PATIENT MODEL, SILICONE SHOE, EACH	D	N	00	9		2323
L3252	FOOT, SHOE MOLDED TO PATIENT MODEL, PLASTAZOTE (OR SIMILAR), CUSTOM FABRICATED, EACH	D	N	00	9		2323
L3253	FOOT, MOLDED SHOE PLASTAZOTE (OR SIMILAR) CUSTOM FITTED, EACH	D	N	00	9		2323
L3254	NON-STANDARD SIZE OR WIDTH	D	N	00	9		2323

HCPCS Code	Statute	Lab Cert	X-Ref	ASC Pay Grp	ASC Pay Group Eff. Date	Proc Notes	BETOS	TOS	Anest	Code Add Date	Code Effective Date	Code Term Date
L3080							D1F	P	0	19840101	19970101	
L3090							D1F	P	0	19840101	19970101	
L3100							D1F	P	0	19850101	19970101	
L3140							D1F	P	0	19820101	19970101	
L3150							D1F	P	0	19840101	19970101	
L3160							D1F	P	0	19860101	19950101	
L3170							D1F	P	0	19840101	20060101	
L3201							D1F	P	0	19840101	19970101	
L3202							D1F	P	0	19840101	19970101	
L3203							D1F	P	0	19840101	19970101	
L3204							D1F	P	0	19840101	19970101	
L3206							D1F	P	0	19840101	19970101	
L3207							D1F	P	0	19840101	19970101	
L3208							D1F	P	0	19840101	19960101	
L3209							D1F	P	0	19840101	19960101	
L3211							D1F	P	0	19840101	19960101	
L3212							D1F	P	0	19840101	19960101	
L3213							D1F	P	0	19840101	19960101	
L3214							D1F	P	0	19840101	19960101	
L3215	1862A8						D1F	P	0	19840101	20060101	
L3216	1862A8						D1F	P	0	19840101	20060101	
L3217	1862A8						D1F	P	0	19840101	20060101	
L3219	1862A8						D1F	P	0	19840101	20060101	
L3221	1862A8						D1F	P	0	19840101	20060101	
L3222	1862A8						D1F	P	0	19840101	20060101	
L3224							D1F	P	0	19950101	19950101	
L3225							D1F	P	0	19950101	19950101	
L3230							D1F	P	0	19840101	20060101	
L3250							D1F	P	0	19840101	19970101	
L3251							D1F	P	0	19840101	19970101	
L3252							D1F	P	0	19840101	19970101	
L3253							D1F	P	0	19840101	19970101	
L3254							D1F	P	0	19840101	19970101	

HCPCS Code	Long Description	Coverage	Action	PI	MPI	CIM	MCM
L3255	NON-STANDARD SIZE OR LENGTH	D	N	00	9		2323
L3257	ORTHOPEDIC FOOTWEAR, ADDITIONAL CHARGE FOR SPLIT SIZE	D	N	00	9		2323
L3260	SURGICAL BOOT/SHOE, EACH	D	N	00	9		2079
L3265	PLASTAZOTE SANDAL, EACH	C	N	00	9		
L3300	LIFT, ELEVATION, HEEL, TAPERED TO METATARSALS, PER INCH	D	N	00	9		2323
L3310	LIFT, ELEVATION, HEEL AND SOLE, NEOPRENE, PER INCH	D	N	00	9		2323
L3320	LIFT, ELEVATION, HEEL AND SOLE, CORK, PER INCH	D	N	00	9		2323
L3330	LIFT, ELEVATION, METAL EXTENSION (SKATE)	D	N	00	9		2323
L3332	LIFT, ELEVATION, INSIDE SHOE, TAPERED, UP TO ONE-HALF INCH	D	N	00	9		2323
L3334	LIFT, ELEVATION, HEEL, PER INCH	D	N	00	9		2323
L3340	HEEL WEDGE, SACH	D	N	00	9		2323
L3350	HEEL WEDGE	D	N	00	9		2323
L3360	SOLE WEDGE, OUTSIDE SOLE	D	N	00	9		2323
L3370	SOLE WEDGE, BETWEEN SOLE	D	N	00	9		2323
L3380	CLUBFOOT WEDGE	D	N	00	9		2323
L3390	OUTFLARE WEDGE	D	N	00	9		2323
L3400	METATARSAL BAR WEDGE, ROCKER	D	N	00	9		2323
L3410	METATARSAL BAR WEDGE, BETWEEN SOLE	D	N	00	9		2323
L3420	FULL SOLE AND HEEL WEDGE, BETWEEN SOLE	D	N	00	9		2323
L3430	HEEL, COUNTER, PLASTIC REINFORCED	D	N	00	9		2323
L3440	HEEL, COUNTER, LEATHER REINFORCED	D	N	00	9		2323
L3450	HEEL, SACH CUSHION TYPE	D	N	00	9		2323
L3455	HEEL, NEW LEATHER, STANDARD	D	N	00	9		2323
L3460	HEEL, NEW RUBBER, STANDARD	D	N	00	9		2323
L3465	HEEL, THOMAS WITH WEDGE	D	N	00	9		2323
L3470	HEEL, THOMAS EXTENDED TO BALL	D	N	00	9		2323
L3480	HEEL, PAD AND DEPRESSION FOR SPUR	D	N	00	9		2323
L3485	HEEL, PAD, REMOVABLE FOR SPUR	D	N	00	9		2323
L3500	ORTHOPEDIC SHOE ADDITION, INSOLE, LEATHER	D	N	00	9		2323
L3510	ORTHOPEDIC SHOE ADDITION, INSOLE, RUBBER	D	N	00	9		2323
L3520	ORTHOPEDIC SHOE ADDITION, INSOLE, FELT COVERED WITH LEATHER	D	N	00	9		2323
L3530	ORTHOPEDIC SHOE ADDITION, SOLE, HALF	D	N	00	9		2323
L3540	ORTHOPEDIC SHOE ADDITION, SOLE, FULL	D	N	00	9		2323
L3550	ORTHOPEDIC SHOE ADDITION, TOE TAP STANDARD	D	N	00	9		2323
L3560	ORTHOPEDIC SHOE ADDITION, TOE TAP, HORSESHOE	D	N	00	9		2323
L3570	ORTHOPEDIC SHOE ADDITION, SPECIAL EXTENSION TO INSTEP (LEATHER WITH EYELETS)	D	N	00	9		2323
L3580	ORTHOPEDIC SHOE ADDITION, CONVERT INSTEP TO VELCRO CLOSURE	D	N	00	9		2323
L3590	ORTHOPEDIC SHOE ADDITION, CONVERT FIRM SHOE COUNTER TO SOFT COUNTER	D	N	00	9		2323
L3595	ORTHOPEDIC SHOE ADDITION, MARCH BAR	D	N	00	9		2323
L3600	TRANSFER OF AN ORTHOSIS FROM ONE SHOE TO ANOTHER, CALIPER PLATE, EXISTING	D	N	00	9		2323

HCPCS Code	Statute	Lab Cert	X-Ref	ASC Pay Grp	ASC Pay Group Eff. Date	Proc Notes	BETOS	TOS	Anest	Code Add Date	Code Effective Date	Code Term Date
L3255							D1F	P	0	19840101	19970101	
L3257							D1F	P	0	19880101	19970101	
L3260							D1F	P	0	19840101	20030101	
L3265							D1F	P	0	19840101	19960101	
L3300							D1F	P	0	19860101	19970101	
L3310							D1F	P	0	19860101	19970101	
L3320							D1F	P	0	19860101	19970101	
L3330							D1F	P	0	19860101	19970101	
L3332							D1F	P	0	19860101	19970101	
L3334							D1F	P	0	19860101	19970101	
L3340							D1F	P	0	19820101	19970101	
L3350							D1F	P	0	19820101	19970101	
L3360							D1F	P	0	19840101	19970101	
L3370							D1F	P	0	19840101	19970101	
L3380							D1F	P	0	19820101	19970101	
L3390							D1F	P	0	19820101	19970101	
L3400							D1F	P	0	19840101	19970101	
L3410							D1F	P	0	19840101	19970101	
L3420							D1F	P	0	19840101	19970101	
L3430							D1F	P	0	19850101	19970101	
L3440							D1F	P	0	19840101	19970101	
L3450							D1F	P	0	19840101	19970101	
L3455							D1F	P	0	19840101	19970101	
L3460							D1F	P	0	19840101	19970101	
L3465							D1F	P	0	19840101	19970101	
L3470							D1F	P	0	19840101	19970101	
L3480							D1F	P	0	19840101	19970101	
L3485							D1F	P	0	19840101	19970101	
L3500							D1F	P	0	19860101	19990101	
L3510							D1F	P	0	19860101	19990101	
L3520							D1F	P	0	19860101	19990101	
L3530							D1F	P	0	19860101	19990101	
L3540							D1F	P	0	19860101	19990101	
L3550							D1F	P	0	19860101	19990101	
L3560							D1F	P	0	19860101	19990101	
L3570							D1F	P	0	19860101	19990101	
L3580							D1F	P	0	19860101	19990101	
L3590							D1F	P	0	19860101	19990101	
L3595							D1F	P	0	19860101	19990101	
L3600							D1F	P	0	19860101	19970101	

HCPCS Code	Long Description	Coverage	Action	PI	MPI	CIM	MCM
L3610	TRANSFER OF AN ORTHOSIS FROM ONE SHOE TO ANOTHER, CALIPER PLATE, NEW	D	N	00	9		2323
L3620	TRANSFER OF AN ORTHOSIS FROM ONE SHOE TO ANOTHER, SOLID STIRRUP, EXISTING	D	N	00	9		2323
L3630	TRANSFER OF AN ORTHOSIS FROM ONE SHOE TO ANOTHER, SOLID STIRRUP, NEW	D	N	00	9		2323
L3640	TRANSFER OF AN ORTHOSIS FROM ONE SHOE TO ANOTHER, DENNIS BROWNE SPLINT (RIVETON), BOTH SHOES	D	N	00	9		2323
L3649	ORTHOPEDIC SHOE, MODIFICATION, ADDITION OR TRANSFER, NOT OTHERWISE SPECIFIED	D	N	00	9		2323
L3650	SHOULDER ORTHOSIS, FIGURE OF EIGHT DESIGN ABDUCTION RESTRAINER, PREFABRICATED, INCLUDES FITTING AND ADJUSTMENT	C	N	38	A		
L3651	SHOULDER ORTHOSIS, SINGLE SHOULDER, ELASTIC, PREFABRICATED, INCLUDES FITTING AND ADJUSTMENT (E.G. NEOPRENE, LYCRA)	C	D	38	A		
L3652	SHOULDER ORTHOSIS, DOUBLE SHOULDER, ELASTIC, PREFABRICATED, INCLUDES FITTING AND ADJUSTMENT (E.G. NEOPRENE, LYCRA)	C	D	38	A		
L3660	SHOULDER ORTHOSIS, FIGURE OF EIGHT DESIGN ABDUCTION RESTRAINER, CANVAS AND WEBBING, PREFABRICATED, INCLUDES FITTING AND ADJUSTMENT	C	N	38	A		
L3670	SHOULDER ORTHOSIS, ACROMIO/CLAVICULAR (CANVAS AND WEBBING TYPE), PREFABRICATED, INCLUDES FITTING AND ADJUSTMENT	C	N	38	A		
L3671	SHOULDER ORTHOSIS, SHOULDER CAP DESIGN, WITHOUT JOINTS, MAY INCLUDE SOFT INTERFACE, STRAPS, CUSTOM FABRICATED, INCLUDES FITTING AND ADJUSTMENT	C	N	38	A		
L3672	SHOULDER ORTHOSIS, ABDUCTION POSITIONING (AIRPLANE DESIGN), THORACIC COMPONENT AND SUPPORT BAR, WITHOUT JOINTS, MAY INLCUDE SOFT INTERFACE, STRAPS, CUSTOM FABRICATED, INCLUDES FITTING & ADJUSTMENT	C	N	38	A		
L3673	SHOULDER ORTHOSIS, ABDUCTION POSITIONING (AIRPLANE DESIGN), THORACIC COMPONENT AND SUPPORT BAR, INCLUDES NONTORSION JOINT/TURNBUCKLE, MAY INCLUDE SOFT INTERFACE, STRAPS, CUSTOM FABRICATED, INCLUDES FITTING AND ADJUSTMENT	C	N	38	A		
L3675	SHOULDER ORTHOSIS, VEST TYPE ABDUCTION RESTRAINER, CANVAS WEBBING TYPE OR EQUAL, PREFABRICATED, INCLUDES FITTING AND ADJUSTMENT	C	N	38	A		
L3677	SHOULDER ORTHOSIS, HARD PLASTIC, SHOULDER STABILIZER, PRE-FABRICATED, INCLUDES FITTING AND ADJUSTMENT	D	N	00	9		2130
L3700	ELBOW HORTHOSIS, ELASTIC WITH STAYS, PREFABRICATED, INCLUDES FITTING AND ADJUSTMENT	C	D	38	A		
L3701	ELBOW ORTHOSIS, ELASTIC, PREFABRICATED, INCLUDES FITTING AND ADJUSTMENT (E.G. NEOPRENE, LYCRA)	C	D	38	A		
L3702	ELBOW ORTHOSIS, WITHOUT JOINTS, MAY INCLUDE SOFT INTERFACE, STRAPS, CUSTOM FABRICATED, INCLUDES FITTING AND ADJUSTMENT	C	N	38	A		

HCPCS Code	Statute	Lab Cert	X-Ref	ASC Pay Grp	ASC Pay Group Eff. Date	Proc Notes	BETOS	TOS	Anest	Code Add Date	Code Effective Date	Code Term Date
L3610							D1F	P	0	19860101	19970101	
L3620							D1F	P	0	19860101	19970101	
L3630							D1F	P	0	19860101	19970101	
L3640							D1F	P	0	19860101	19970101	
L3649							D1F	P	0	19820101	19990101	
L3650							D1F	P	0	19860101	20010101	
L3651							D1F	P	0	20030101	20100101	20091231
L3652							D1F	P	0	20030101	20100101	20091231
L3660							D1F	P	0	19820101	20010101	
L3670							D1F	P	0	19820101	20010101	
L3671							D1F	P	0	20060101	20060101	
L3672							D1F	P	0	20060101	20060101	
L3673							D1F	P	0	20060101	20060101	
L3675							D1F	P	0	19990101	20010101	
L3677							Z2	P	0	20020101	20020101	
L3700							D1F	P	0	19820101	20100101	20091231
L3701							D1F	P	0	20030101	20100101	20091231
L3702							D1F	P	0	20060101	20060101	

L Codes

HCPCS Code	Long Description	Coverage	Action	PI	MPI	CIM	MCM
L3710	ELBOW ORTHOSIS, ELASTIC WITH METAL JOINTS, PREFABRICATED, INCLUDES FITTING AND ADJUSTMENT	C	N	38	A		
L3720	ELBOW ORTHOSIS, DOUBLE UPRIGHT WITH FOREARM/ARM CUFFS, FREE MOTION, CUSTOM-FABRICATED	C	N	38	A		
L3730	ELBOW ORTHOSIS, DOUBLE UPRIGHT WITH FOREARM/ARM CUFFS, EXTENSION/ FLEXION ASSIST, CUSTOM-FABRICATED	C	N	38	A		
L3740	ELBOW ORTHOSIS, DOUBLE UPRIGHT WITH FOREARM/ARM CUFFS, ADJUSTABLE POSITION LOCK WITH ACTIVE CONTROL, CUSTOM-FABRICATED	C	N	38	A		
L3760	ELBOW ORTHOSIS, WITH ADJUSTABLE POSITION LOCKING JOINT(S), PREFABRICATED, INCLUDES FITTING AND ADJUSTMENTS, ANY TYPE	C	N	38	A		
L3762	ELBOW ORTHOSIS, RIGID, WITHOUT JOINTS, INCLUDES SOFT INTERFACE MATERIAL, PREFABRICATED, INCLUDES FITTING AND ADJUSTMENT	C	N	38	A		
L3763	ELBOW WRIST HAND ORTHOSIS, RIGID, WITHOUT JOINTS, MAY INCLUDE SOFT INTERFACE, STRAPS, CUSTOM FABRICATED, INCLUDES FITTING AND ADJUSTMENT	C	N	38	A		
L3764	ELBOW WRIST HAND ORTHOSIS, INCLUDES ONE OR MORE NONTORSION JOINTS, ELASTIC BANDS, TURNBUCKLES, MAY INCLUDE SOFT INTERFACE, STRAPS, CUSTOM FABRICATED, INCLUDES FITTING AND ADJUSTMENT	C	N	38	A		
L3765	ELBOW WRIST HAND FINGER ORTHOSIS, RIGID, WITHOUT JOINTS, MAY INCLUDE SOFT INTERFACE, STRAPS, CUSTOM FABRICATED, INCLUDES FITTING AND ADJUSTMENT	C	N	38	A		
L3766	ELBOW WRIST HAND FINGER ORTHOSIS, INCLUDES ONE OR MORE NONTORSION JOINTS, ELASTIC BANDS, TURNBUCKLES, MAY INCLUDE SOFT INTERFACE, STRAPS, CUSTOM FABRICATED, INCLUDES FITTING AND ADJUSTMENT	C	N	38	A		
L3800	WRIST HAND FINGER ORTHOSIS, SHORT OPPONENS, NO ATTACHMENTS, CUSTOM-FABRICATED	C	N	38	A		
L3805	WRIST HAND FINGER ORTHOSIS, LONG OPPONENS, NO ATTACHMENT, CUSTOM-FABRICATED	C	N	38	A		
L3806	WRIST HAND FINGER ORTHOSIS, INCLUDES ONE OR MORE NONTORSION JOINT(S),TURNBUCKLES, ELASTIC BANDS/ SPRINGS, MAY INCLUDE SOFT INTERFACE MATERIAL, STRAPS, CUSTOM FABRICATED, INCLUDES FITTING AND ADJUSTMENT	C	N	38	A		
L3807	WRIST HAND FINGER ORTHOSIS, WITHOUT JOINT(S), PREFABRICATED, INCLUDES FITTING & ADJUSTMENTS, ANY TYPE	C	N	38	A		
L3808	WRIST HAND FINGER ORTHOSIS, RIGID WITHOUT JOINTS, MAY INCLUDE SOFT INTERFACE MATERIAL; STRAPS, CUSTOM FABRICATED, INCLUDES FITTING & ADJUSTMENT	C	N	38	A		
L3810	WHFO, ADDITION TO SHORT AND LONG OPPONENS, THUMB ABDUCTION ('C') BAR	C	N	38	A		
L3815	WHFO, ADDITION TO SHORT AND LONG OPPONENS, SECOND M.P. ABDUCTION ASSIST	C	N	38	A		

HCPCS Code	Statute	Lab Cert	X-Ref	ASC Pay Grp	ASC Pay Group Eff. Date	Proc Notes	BETOS	TOS	Anest	Code Add Date	Code Effective Date	Code Term Date
L3710							D1F	P	0	19860101	20010101	
L3720							D1F	P	0	19840101	20010101	
L3730							D1F	P	0	19820101	20010101	
L3740							D1F	P	0	19820101	20010101	
L3760							D1F	P	0	20010101	20010101	
L3762							D1F	P	0	20030101	20030101	
L3763							D1F	P	0	20060101	20060101	
L3764							D1F	P	0	20060101	20060101	
L3765							D1F	P	0	20060101	20060101	
L3766							D1F	P	0	20060101	20060101	
L3800			L3808				D1F	P	0	19820101	20080101	20071231
L3805			L3808				D1F	P	0	19820101	20080101	20071231
L3806							D1F	P	0	20070101	20080101	
L3807							D1F	P	0	20000101	20010101	
L3808							D1F	P	0	20070101	20070101	
L3810							D1F	P	0	19860101	20080101	20071231
L3815							D1F	P	0	19860101	20080101	20071231

HCPCS Code	Long Description	Coverage	Action	PI	MPI	CIM	MCM
L3820	WHFO, ADDITION TO SHORT AND LONG OPPONENS, I.P. EXTENSION ASSIST, WITH M.P. EXTENSION STOP	C	N	38	A		
L3825	WHFO, ADDITION TO SHORT AND LONG OPPONENS, M.P. EXTENSION STOP	C	N	38	A		
L3830	WHFO, ADDITION TO SHORT AND LONG OPPONENS, M.P. EXTENSION ASSIST	C	N	38	A		
L3835	WHFO, ADDITION TO SHORT AND LONG OPPONENS, M.P. SPRING EXTENSION ASSIST	C	N	38	A		
L3840	WHFO, ADDITION TO SHORT AND LONG OPPONENS, SPRING SWIVEL THUMB	C	N	38	A		
L3845	WHFO, ADDITION TO SHORT AND LONG OPPONENS, THUMB I.P. EXTENSION ASSIST, WITH M.P. STOP	C	N	38	A		
L3850	WHO, ADDITION TO SHORT AND LONG OPPONENS, ACTION WRIST, WITH DORSIFLEXION ASSIST	C	N	38	A		
L3855	WHFO, ADDITION TO SHORT AND LONG OPPONENS, ADJUSTABLE M.P. FLEXION CONTROL	C	N	38	A		
L3860	WHFO, ADDITION TO SHORT AND LONG OPPONENS, ADJUSTABLE M.P. FLEXION CONTROL AND I.P.	C	N	38	A		
L3890	ADDITION TO UPPER EXTREMITY JOINT, WRIST OR ELBOW, CONCENTRIC ADJUSTABLE TORSION STYLE MECHANISM, EA.	C	N	00	9		
L3891	ADDITION TO UPPER EXTREMITY JOINT, WRIST OR ELBOW, CONCENTRIC ADJUSTABLE TORSION STYLE MECHANISM FOR CUSTOM FABRICATED ORTHOTICS ONLY, EACH	I	A	00	9		
L3900	WRIST HAND FINGER ORTHOSIS, DYNAMIC FLEXOR HINGE, RECIPROCAL WRIST EXTENSION/FLEXION, FINGER FLEXION/EXTENSION, WRIST OR FINGER DRIVEN, CUSTOM-FABRICATED	C	N	38	A		
L3901	WRIST HAND FINGER ORTHOSIS, DYNAMIC FLEXOR HINGE, RECIPROCAL WRIST EXTENSION/FLEXION, FINGER FLEXION/EXTENSION, CABLE DRIVEN, CUSTOM-FABRICATED	C	N	38	A		
L3902	WRIST HAND FINGER ORTHOSIS, EXTERNAL POWERED, COMPRESSED GAS, CUSTOM-FABRICATED	I	N	00	9		
L3904	WRIST HAND FINGER ORTHOSIS, EXTERNAL POWERED, ELECTRIC, CUSTOM-FABRICATED	C	N	38	A		
L3905	WRIST HAND ORTHOSIS, INCLUDES ONE OR MORE NONTORSION JOINTS, ELASTIC BANDS, TURNBUCKLES, MAY INCLUDE SOFT INTERFACE, STRAPS, CUSTOM FABRICATED, INCLUDES FITTING & ADJUSTMENT	C	N	38	A		
L3906	WRIST HAND ORTHOSIS, WITHOUT JOINTS, MAY INCLUDE SOFT INTERFACE, STRAPS, CUSTOM FABRICATED, INCLUDES FITTING AND ADJUSTMENT	C	N	38	A		
L3907	WRIST HAND FINGER ORTHOSIS, WRIST GAUNTLET WITH THUMB SPICA, CUSTOM-FABRICATED	C	N	38	A		
L3908	WRIST HAND ORTHOSIS, WRIST EXTENSION CONTROL COCK-UP, NON MOLDED, PREFABRICATED, INCLUDES FITTING AND ADJUSTMENT	C	N	38	A		
L3909	WRIST ORTHOSIS, ELASTIC, PREFABRICATED, INCLUDES FITTING AND ADJUSTMENT (E.G. NEOPRENE, LYCRA)	C	D	38	A		
L3910	WRIST HAND FINGER ORTHOSIS, SWANSON DESIGN, PREFABRICATED, INCLUDES FITTING AND ADJUSTMENT	C	N	38	A		

HCPCS Code	Statute	Lab Cert	X-Ref	ASC Pay Grp	ASC Pay Group Eff. Date	Proc Notes	BETOS	TOS	Anest	Code Add Date	Code Effective Date	Code Term Date
L3820							D1F	P	0	19860101	20080101	20071231
L3825							D1F	P	0	19860101	20080101	20071231
L3830							D1F	P	0	19860101	20080101	20071231
L3835							D1F	P	0	19860101	20080101	20071231
L3840							D1F	P	0	19860101	20080101	20071231
L3845							D1F	P	0	19860101	20080101	20071231
L3850							D1F	P	0	19860101	20080101	20071231
L3855							D1F	P	0	19860101	20080101	20071231
L3860							D1F	P	0	19860101	20080101	20071231
L3890							D1F	P	0	19950101	20090101	20081231
L3891							D1F	P	0	20100101	20100101	
L3900							D1F	P	0	19860101	20010101	
L3901							D1F	P	0	19840101	20010101	
							D1F	P	0	19850101	20070101	20061231
L3904							D1F	P	0	19820101	20010101	
L3905							D1F	P	0	20060101	20060101	
L3906							D1F	P	0	19860101	20060101	
L3907			L3808				D1F	P	0	19880101	20080101	20071231
L3908							D1F	P	0	19860101	20010101	
L3909							D1F	P	0	20030101	20100101	20091231
L3910			L3931				D1F	P	0	19820101	20080101	20071231

HCPCS Code	Long Description	Coverage	Action	PI	MPI	CIM	MCM
L3911	WRIST HAND FINGER ORTHOSIS, ELASTIC, PREFABRICATED, INCLUDES FITTING & ADJUSTMENT (E.G. NEOPRENE, LYCRA)	C	D	38	A		
L3912	HAND FINGER ORTHOSIS, FLEXION GLOVE WITH ELASTIC FINGER CONTROL, PREFABRICATED, INCLUDES FITTING AND ADJUSTMENT	C	N	38	A		
L3913	HAND FINGER ORTHOSIS, WITHOUT JOINTS, MAY INCLUDE SOFT INTERFACE, STRAPS, CUSTOM FABRICATED, INCLUDES FITTING AND ADJUSTMENT	C	N	38	A		
L3914	WRIST HAND ORTHOSIS, WRIST EXTENSION COCK-UP, PREFABRICATED, INCLUDES FITTING/ADJUSTMENT	C	N	38	A		
L3915	WRIST HAND ORTHOSIS, INCLUDES ONE OR MORE NONTORSION JOINT(S), ELASTIC BANDS, TURNBUCKLES, MAY INCLUDE SOFT INTERFACE, STRAPS, PREFABRICATED INCLUDES FITTING AND ADJUSTMENT	C	N	38	A		
L3916	WRIST HAND FINGER ORTHOSIS, WRIST EXTENSION COCK-UP WITH OUTRIGGER, PREFABRICATED, INCLUDES FITTING AND ADJUSTMENT	C	N	38	A		
L3917	HAND ORTHOSIS, METACARPAL FRACTURE ORTHOSIS, PREFABRICATED, INCLUDES FITTING AND ADJUSTMENT	C	N	38	A		
L3918	HAND FINGER ORTHOSIS, KNUCKLE BENDER, PREFABRICATED, INCLUDES FITTING AND ADJUSTMENT	C	N	38	A		
L3919	HAND ORTHOSIS, WITHOUT JOINTS, MAY INCLUDE SOFT INTERFACE, STRAPS, CUSTOM FABRICATED, INCLUDES FITTING AND ADJUSTMENT	C	N	38	A		
L3920	HAND FINGER ORTHOSIS, KNUCKLE BENDER WITH OUTRIGGER, PREFABRICATED, INCLUDES FITTING AND ADJUSTMENT	C	N	38	A		
L3921	HAND FINGER ORTHOSIS, INCLUDES ONE OR MORE NONTORSION JOINTS, ELASTIC BANDS, TURNBUCKLES, MAY INCLUDE SOFT INTERFACE, STRAPS, CUSTOM FABRICATED, INCLUDES FITTING AND ADJUSTMENT	C	N	38	A		
L3922	HAND FINGER ORTHOSIS, KNUCKLE BENDER, TWO SEGMENT TO FLEX JOINTS, PREFABRICATED, INCLUDES FITTING AND ADJUSTMENT	C	N	38	A		
L3923	HAND FINGER ORTHOSIS, WITHOUT JOINTS, MAY INCLUDE SOFT INTERFACE, STRAPS, PREFABRICATED, INCLUDES FITTING AND ADJUSTMENT	C	N	38	A		
L3924	WRIST HAND FINGER ORTHOSIS, OPPENHEIMER, PREFABRICATED, INCLUDES FITTING AND ADJUSTMENT	C	N	38	A		
L3925	FINGER ORTHOSIS, PROXIMAL INTERPHALANGEAL (PIP)/ DISTAL INTERPHALANGEAL (DIP), NON TORSION JOINT/SPRING, EXTENSION/FLEXION, MAY INCLUDE SOFT INTERFACE MATERIAL, PREFABRICATED, INCLUDES FITTING AND ADJUSTMENT	C	N	38	A		
L3926	WRIST HAND FINGER ORTHOSIS, THOMAS SUSPENSION, PREFABRICATED, INCLUDES FITTING AND ADJUSTMENT	C	N	38	A		
L3927	FINGER ORTHOSIS, PROXIMAL INTERPHALANGEAL (PIP)/ DISTAL INTERPHALANGEAL (DIP), WITHOUT JOINT/SPRING, EXTENSION/FLEXION (E.G. STATIC OR RING TYPE), MAY INCLUDE SOFT INTERFACE MATERIAL, PREFABRICATED, INCLUDES FITTING AND ADJUSTMENT	C	N	38	A		

HCPCS Code	Statute	Lab Cert	X-Ref	ASC Pay Grp	ASC Pay Group Eff. Date	Proc Notes	BETOS	TOS	Anest	Code Add Date	Code Effective Date	Code Term Date
L3911							D1F	P	0	20030101	20100101	20091231
L3912							D1F	P	0	19820101	20010101	
L3913							D1F	P	0	20060101	20060101	
L3914			L3908				D1F	P	0	19860101	20070101	20061231
L3915							D1F	P	0	20070101	20070101	
L3916			L3931				D1F	P	0	19860101	20080101	20071231
L3917							D1F	P	0	20040101	20040101	
L3918			L3929				D1F	P	0	19820101	20080101	20071231
L3919							D1F	P	0	20060101	20060101	
L3920			L3929				D1F	P	0	19820101	20080101	20071231
L3921							D1F	P	0	20060101	20060101	
L3922			L3929				D1F	P	0	19820101	20080101	20071231
L3923							D1F	P	0	20010101	20060101	
L3924			L3931				D1F	P	0	19820101	20080101	20071231
L3925							D1F	P	0	20080101	20080101	
L3926			L3931				D1F	P	0	19820101	20080101	20071231
L3927							D1F	P	0	20080101	20080101	

HCPCS Code	Long Description	Coverage	Action	PI	MPI	CIM	MCM
L3928	HAND FINGER ORTHOSIS, FINGER EXTENSION, WITH CLOCK SPRING, PREFABRICATED, INCLUDES FITTING & ADJUSTMENT	C	N	38	A		
L3929	HAND FINGER ORTHOSIS, INCLUDES ONE OR MORE NONTORSION JOINT(S), TURNBUCKLES, ELASTIC BANDS/SPRINGS, MAY INCLUDE SOFT INTERFACE MATERIAL, STRAPS, PREFABRICATED, INCLUDES FITTING AND ADJUSTMENT	C	N	38	A		
L3930	WRIST HAND FINGER ORTHOSIS, FINGER EXTENSION, WITH WRIST SUPPORT, PREFABRICATED, INCLUDES FITTING AND ADJUSTMENT	C	N	38	A		
L3931	WRIST HAND FINGER ORTHOSIS, INCLUDES ONE OR MORE NONTORSION JOINT(S),TURNBUCKLES, ELASTIC BANDS/SPRINGS, MAY INCLUDE SOFT INTERFACE MATERIAL, STRAPS, PREFABRICATED, INCLUDES FITTING & ADJUSTMENT	C	N	38	A		
L3932	FINGER ORTHOSIS, SAFETY PIN, SPRING WIRE, PREFABRICATED, INCLUDES FITTING AND ADJUSTMENT	C	N	38	A		
L3933	FINGER ORTHOSIS, WITHOUT JOINTS, MAY INCLUDE SOFT INTERFACE, CUSTOM FABRICATED, INCLUDES FITTING AND ADJUSTMENT	C	N	38	A		
L3934	FINGER ORTHOSIS, SAFETY PIN, MODIFIED, PREFABRICATED, INCLUDES FITTING AND ADJUSTMENT	C	N	38	A		
L3935	FINGER ORTHOSIS, NONTORSION JOINT, MAY INCLUDE SOFT INTERFACE, CUSTOM FABRICATED, INCLUDES FITTING AND ADJUSTMENT	C	N	38	A		
L3936	WRIST HAND FINGER ORTHOSIS, PALMER, PREFABRICATED, INCLUDES FITTING AND ADJUSTMENT	C	N	38	A		
L3938	WRIST HAND FINGER ORTHOSIS, DORSAL WRIST, PREFABRICATED, INCLUDES FITTING AND ADJUSTMENT	C	N	38	A		
L3940	WRIST HAND FINGER ORTHOSIS, DORSAL WRIST, WITH OUTRIGGER ATTACHMENT, PREFABRICATED, INCLUDES FITTING AND ADJUSTMENT	C	N	38	A		
L3942	HAND FINGER ORTHOSIS, REVERSE KNUCKLE BENDER, PREFABRICATED, INCLUDES FITTING AND ADJUSTMENT	C	N	38	A		
L3944	HAND FINGER ORTHOSIS, REVERSE KNUCKLE BENDER, WITH OUTRIGGER, PREFABRICATED, INCLUDES FITTING AND ADJUSTMENT	C	N	38	A		
L3946	HAND FINGER ORTHOSIS, COMPOSITE ELASTIC, PREFABRICATED, INCLUDES FITTING AND ADJUSTMENT	C	N	38	A		
L3948	FINGER ORTHOSIS, FINGER KNUCKLE BENDER, PREFABRICATED, INCLUDES FITTING AND ADJUSTMENT	C	N	38	A		
L3950	WRIST HAND FINGER ORTHOSIS, COMBINATION OPPENHEIMER, WITH KNUCKLE BENDER AND TWO ATTACHMENTS, PREFABRICATED, INCLUDES FITTING AND ADJUSTMENT	C	N	38	A		
L3952	WRIST HAND FINGER ORTHOSIS, COMBINATION OPPENHEIMER, WITH REVERSE KNUCKLE AND TWO ATTACHMENTS, PREFABRICATED, INCLUDES FITTING AND ADJUSTMENT	C	N	38	A		
L3954	HAND FINGER ORTHOSIS, SPREADING HAND, PREFABRICATED, INCLUDES FITTING AND ADJUSTMENT	C	N	38	A		
L3956	ADDITION OF JOINT TO UPPER EXTREMITY ORTHOSIS, ANY MATERIAL; PER JOINT	C	N	38	A		

HCPCS Code	Statute	Lab Cert	X-Ref	ASC Pay Grp	ASC Pay Group Eff. Date	Proc Notes	BETOS	TOS	Anest	Code Add Date	Code Effective Date	Code Term Date
L3928			L3929				D1F	P	0	19820101	20080101	20071231
L3929							D1F	P	0	20080101	20080101	
L3930			L3931				D1F	P	0	19820101	20080101	20071231
L3931							D1F	P	0	20080101	20080101	
L3932			L3925				D1F	P	0	19820101	20080101	20071231
L3933							D1F	P	0	20060101	20060101	
L3934			L3925				D1F	P	0	19820101	20080101	20071231
L3935							D1F	P	0	20060101	20060101	
L3936			L3931				D1F	P	0	19820101	20080101	20071231
L3938			L3931				D1F	P	0	19820101	20080101	20071231
L3940			L3931				D1F	P	0	19820101	20080101	20071231
L3942			L3929				D1F	P	0	19820101	20080101	20071231
L3944			L3929				D1F	P	0	19820101	20080101	20071231
L3946			L3929				D1F	P	0	19820101	20080101	20071231
L3948			L3925				D1F	P	0	19820101	20080101	20071231
L3950			L3931				D1F	P	0	19820101	20080101	20071231
L3952			L3931				D1F	P	0	19820101	20080101	20071231
L3954			L3923				D1F	P	0	19820101	20080101	20071231
L3956							D1F	P	0	19970101	19970101	

HCPCS Code	Long Description	Coverage	Action	PI	MPI	CIM	MCM
L3960	SHOULDER ELBOW WRIST HAND ORTHOSIS, ABDUCTION POSITIONING, AIRPLANE DESIGN, PREFABRICATED, INCLUDES FITTING AND ADJUSTMENT	C	N	38	A		
L3961	SHOULDER ELBOW WRIST HAND ORTHOSIS, SHOULDER CAP DESIGN, WITHOUT JOINTS, MAY INCLUDE SOFT INTERFACE, STRAPS, CUSTOM FABRICATED, INCLUDES FITTING AND ADJUSTMENT	C	N	38	A		
L3962	SHOULDER ELBOW WRIST HAND ORTHOSIS, ABDUCTION POSITIONING, ERBS PALSEY DESIGN, PREFABRICATED, INCLUDES FITTING AND ADJUSTMENT	C	N	38	A		
L3964	SHOULDER ELBOW ORTHOSIS, MOBILE ARM SUPPORT ATTACHED TO WHEELCHAIR, BALANCED, ADJUSTABLE, PREFABRICATED, INCLUDES FITTING AND ADJUSTMENT	C	N	32	A		
L3965	SHOULDER ELBOW ORTHOSIS, MOBILE ARM SUPPORT ATTACHED TO WHEELCHAIR, BALANCED, ADJUSTABLE RANCHO TYPE, PREFABRICATED, INCLUDES FITTING AND ADJUSTMENT	C	N	32	A		
L3966	SHOULDER ELBOW ORTHOSIS, MOBILE ARM SUPPORT ATTACHED TO WHEELCHAIR, BALANCED, RECLINING, PREFABRICATED, INCLUDES FITTING AND ADJUSTMENT	C	N	32	A		
L3967	SHOULDER ELBOW WRIST HAND ORTHOSIS, ABDUCTION POSITIONING (AIRPLANE DESIGN),THORACIC COMPONENT AND SUPPORT BAR, WITHOUT JOINTS, MAY INCLUDE SOFT INTERFACE, STRAPS, CUSTOM FABRICATED, INCLUDES FITTING AND ADJUSTMENT	C	N	38	A		
L3968	SHOULDER ELBOW ORTHOSIS, MOBILE ARM SUPPORT ATTACHED TO WHEELCHAIR, BALANCED, FRICTION ARM SUPPORT (FRICTION DAMPENING TO PROXIMAL AND DISTAL JOINTS), PREFABRICATED, INCLUDES FITTING & ADJUSTMENT	C	N	32	A		
L3969	SHOULDER ELBOW ORTHOSIS, MOBILE ARM SUPPORT, MONOSUSPENSION ARM AND HAND SUPPORT, OVERHEAD ELBOW FOREARM HAND SLING SUPPORT, YOKE TYPE SUSPENSION SUPPORT, PREFABRICATED, INCLUDES FITTING AND ADJUSTMENT	C	N	32	A		
L3970	SEO, ADDITION TO MOBILE ARM SUPPORT, ELEVATING PROXIMAL ARM	C	N	32	A		
L3971	SHOULDER ELBOW WRIST HAND ORTHOSIS, SHOULDER CAP DESIGN, INCLUDES ONE OR MORE NONTORSION JOINTS, ELASTIC BANDS, TURNBUCKLES, MAY INCLUDE SOFT INTERFACE, STRAPS, CUSTOM FABRICATED, INCLUDES FITTING AND ADJUSTMENT	C	N	38	A		
L3972	SEO, ADDITION TO MOBILE ARM SUPPORT, OFFSET OR LATERAL ROCKER ARM WITH ELASTIC BALANCE CONTROL	C	N	32	A		
L3973	SHOULDER ELBOW WRIST HAND ORTHOSIS, ABDUCTION POSITIONING (AIRPLANE DESIGN),THORACIC COMPONENT AND SUPPORT BAR, INCLUDES ONE OR MORE NONTORSION JOINTS, ELASTIC BANDS, TURNBUCKLES, MAY INCLUDE SOFT INTERFACE, STRAPS, CUSTOM FABRICATED, INCLUDES FITTING AND ADJUSTMENT	C	N	38	A		

HCPCS Code	Statute	Lab Cert	X-Ref	ASC Pay Grp	ASC Pay Group Eff. Date	Proc Notes	BETOS	TOS	Anest	Code Add Date	Code Effective Date	Code Term Date
L3960							D1F	P	0	19860101	20010101	
L3961							D1F	P	0	20060101	20060101	
L3962							D1F	P	0	19820101	20010101	
L3964							D1D	A,P,R	0	19860101	20010101	
L3965							D1D	A,P,R	0	19840101	20010101	
L3966							D1D	A,P,R	0	19860101	20010101	
L3967							D1F	P	0	20060101	20060101	
L3968							D1D	A,P,R	0	19860101	20010101	
L3969							D1D	A,P,R	0	19880101	20010101	
L3970							D1D	A,P,R	0	19860101	19980101	
L3971							D1F	P	0	20060101	20060101	
L3972							D1D	A,P,R	0	19860101	19980101	
L3973							D1F	P	0	20060101	20060101	

HCPCS Code	Long Description	Coverage	Action	PI	MPI	CIM	MCM
L3974	SEO, ADDITION TO MOBILE ARM SUPPORT, SUPINATOR	C	N	32	A		
L3975	SHOULDER ELBOW WRIST HAND FINGER ORTHOSIS, SHOULDER CAP DESIGN, WITHOUT JOINTS, MAY INCLUDE SOFT INTERFACE, STRAPS, CUSTOM FABRICATED, INCLUDES FITTING AND ADJUSTMENT	C	N	38	A		
L3976	SHOULDER ELBOW WRIST HAND FINGER ORTHOSIS, ABDUCTION POSITIONING (AIRPLANE DESIGN), THORACIC COMPONENT AND SUPPORT BAR, WITHOUT JOINTS, MAY INCLUDE SOFT	C	N	38	A		
L3976	INTERFACE, STRAPS, CUSTOM FABRICATED, INCLUDES FITTING AND ADJUSTMENT						
L3977	SHOULDER ELBOW WRIST HAND FINGER ORTHOSIS, SHOULDER CAP DESIGN, INCLUDES ONE OR MORE NONTORSION JOINTS, ELASTIC BANDS, TURNBUCKLES, MAY INCLUDE SOFT INTERFACE, STRAPS, CUSTOM FABRICATED, INCLUDES FITTING AND ADJUSTMENT	C	N	38	A		
L3978	SHOULDER ELBOW WRIST HAND FINGER ORTHOSIS, ABDUCTION POSITIONING (AIRPLANE DESIGN), THORACIC COMPONENT AND SUPPORT BAR, INCLUDES ONE OR MORE NONTORSION JOINTS, ELASTIC BANDS, TURNBUCKLES, MAY INCLUDE SOFT INTERFACE, STRAPS, CUSTOM FABRICATED, INCLUDES FITTING AND ADJUSTMENT	C	N	38	A		
L3980	UPPER EXTREMITY FRACTURE ORTHOSIS, HUMERAL, PREFABRICATED, INCLUDES FITTING AND ADJUSTMENT	C	N	38	A		
L3982	UPPER EXTREMITY FRACTURE ORTHOSIS, RADIUS/ULNAR, PREFABRICATED, INCLUDES FITTING AND ADJUSTMENT	C	N	38	A		
L3984	UPPER EXTREMITY FRACTURE ORTHOSIS, WRIST, PREFABRICATED, INCLUDES FITTING AND ADJUSTMENT	C	N	38	A		
L3985	UPPER EXTREMITY FRACTURE ORTHOSIS, FOREARM, HAND WITH WRIST HINGE, CUSTOM-FABRICATED	C	N	38	A		
L3986	UPPER EXTREMITY FRACTURE ORTHOSIS, COMBINATION OF HUMERAL, RADIUS/ULNAR, WRIST, (EXAMPLE--COLLES' FRACTURE), CUSTOM FABRICATED	C	N	38	A		
L3995	ADDITION TO UPPER EXTREMITY ORTHOSIS, SOCK, FRACTURE OR EQUAL, EACH	C	N	38	A		
L3999	UPPER LIMB ORTHOSIS, NOT OTHERWISE SPECIFIED	C	N	46	A		
L4000	REPLACE GIRDLE FOR SPINAL ORTHOSIS (CTLSO OR SO)	C	N	38	A		
L4002	REPLACEMENT STRAP, ANY ORTHOSIS, INCLUDES ALL COMPONENTS, ANY LENGTH, ANY TYPE	C	N	38	A		
L4010	REPLACE TRILATERAL SOCKET BRIM	C	N	38	A		
L4020	REPLACE QUADRILATERAL SOCKET BRIM, MOLDED TO PATIENT MODEL	C	N	38	A		
L4030	REPLACE QUADRILATERAL SOCKET BRIM, CUSTOM FITTED	C	N	38	A		
L4040	REPLACE MOLDED THIGH LACER, FOR CUSTOM FABRICATED ORTHOSIS ONLY	C	N	38	A		
L4045	REPLACE NON-MOLDED THIGH LACER, FOR CUSTOM FABRICATED ORTHOSIS ONLY	C	N	38	A		
L4050	REPLACE MOLDED CALF LACER, FOR CUSTOM FABRICATED ORTHOSIS ONLY	C	N	38	A		

HCPCS Code	Statute	Lab Cert	X-Ref	ASC Pay Grp	ASC Pay Group Eff. Date	Proc Notes	BETOS	TOS	Anest	Code Add Date	Code Effective Date	Code Term Date
L3974							D1D	A,P,R	0	19860101	19980101	
L3975							D1F	P	0	20060101	20060101	
L3976							D1F	P	0	20060101	20060101	
					L3976							
L3977							D1F	P	0	20060101	20060101	
L3978							D1F	P	0	20060101	20060101	
L3980							D1F	P	0	19820101	20010101	
L3982							D1F	P	0	19840101	20010101	
L3984							D1F	P	0	19820101	20010101	
L3985			L3764				D1F	P	0	19880101	20080101	20071231
L3986			L3763				D1F	P	0	19840101	20080101	20071231
L3995							D1F	P	0	19890101	19960101	
L3999							D1F	P	0	19820101	19980101	
L4000							D1F	P	0	19850101	20020101	
L4002							D1F	P	0	20050101	20050101	
L4010							D1F	P	0	19850101	19960101	
L4020							D1F	P	0	19850101	19960101	
L4030							D1F	P	0	19850101	19960101	
L4040							D1F	P	0	19850101	20050101	
L4045							D1F	P	0	19880101	20050101	
L4050							D1F	P	0	19850101	20050101	

HCPCS Code	Long Description	Coverage	Action	PI	MPI	CIM	MCM
L4055	REPLACE NON-MOLDED CALF LACER, FOR CUSTOM FABRICATED ORTHOSIS ONLY	C	N	38	A		
L4060	REPLACE HIGH ROLL CUFF	C	N	38	A		
L4070	REPLACE PROXIMAL AND DISTAL UPRIGHT FOR KAFO	C	N	38	A		
L4080	REPLACE METAL BANDS KAFO, PROXIMAL THIGH	C	N	38	A		
L4090	REPLACE METAL BANDS KAFO-AFO, CALF OR DISTAL THIGH	C	N	38	A		
L4100	REPLACE LEATHER CUFF KAFO, PROXIMAL THIGH	C	N	38	A		
L4110	REPLACE LEATHER CUFF KAFO-AFO, CALF OR DISTAL THIGH	C	N	38	A		
L4130	REPLACE PRETIBIAL SHELL	C	N	38	A		
L4205	REPAIR OF ORTHOTIC DEVICE, LABOR COMPONENT, PER 15 MINUTES	D	N	46	A		2100.4
L4210	REPAIR OF ORTHOTIC DEVICE, REPAIR OR REPLACE MINOR PARTS	D	N	46	A		2133, 2100.4, 2130D
L4350	ANKLE CONTROL ORTHOSIS, STIRRUP STYLE, RIGID, INCLUDES ANY TYPE INTERFACE (E.G., PNEUMATIC, GEL), PREFABRICATED, INCLUDES FITTING AND ADJUSTMENT	C	N	38	A		
L4360	WALKING BOOT, PNEUMATIC AND/OR VACUUM, WITH OR WITHOUT JOINTS, WITH OR WITHOUT INTERFACE MATERIAL, PREFABRICATED, INCLUDES FITTING AND ADJUSTMENT	C	N	38	A		
L4370	PNEUMATIC FULL LEG SPLINT, PREFABRICATED, INCLUDES FITTING AND ADJUSTMENT	C	N	38	A		
L4380	PNEUMATIC KNEE SPLINT, PREFABRICATED, INCLUDES FITTING AND ADJUSTMENT	C	N	38	A		
L4386	WALKING BOOT, NON-PNEUMATIC, WITH OR WITHOUT JOINTS, WITH OR WITHOUT INTERFACE MATERIAL, PREFABRICATED, INCLUDES FITTING AND ADJUSTMENT	C	N	38	A		
L4392	REPLACEMENT, SOFT INTERFACE MATERIAL, STATIC AFO	C	N	38	A		
L4394	REPLACE SOFT INTERFACE MATERIAL, FOOT DROP SPLINT	C	N	38	A		
L4396	STATIC OR DYNAMIC ANKLE FOOT ORTHOSIS, INCLUDING SOFT INTERFACE MATERIAL, ADJUSTABLE FOR FIT, FOR POSITIONING, MAY BE USED FOR MINIMAL AMBULATION, PREFABRICATED, INCLUDES FITTING AND ADJUSTMENT	C	C	38	A		
L4398	FOOT DROP SPLINT, RECUMBENT POSITIONING DEVICE, PREFABRICATED, INCLUDES FITTING AND ADJUSTMENT	C	N	38	A		
L5000	PARTIAL FOOT, SHOE INSERT WITH LONGITUDINAL ARCH, TOE FILLER	D	N	38	A		2323
L5010	PARTIAL FOOT, MOLDED SOCKET, ANKLE HEIGHT, WITH TOE FILLER	D	N	38	A		2323
L5020	PARTIAL FOOT, MOLDED SOCKET, TIBIAL TUBERCLE HEIGHT, WITH TOE FILLER	D	N	38	A		2323
L5050	ANKLE, SYMES, MOLDED SOCKET, SACH FOOT	C	N	38	A		
L5060	ANKLE, SYMES, METAL FRAME, MOLDED LEATHER SOCKET, ARTICULATED ANKLE/FOOT	C	N	38	A		
L5100	BELOW KNEE, MOLDED SOCKET, SHIN, SACH FOOT	C	N	38	A		
L5105	BELOW KNEE, PLASTIC SOCKET, JOINTS AND THIGH LACER, SACH FOOT	C	N	38	A		
L5150	KNEE DISARTICULATION (OR THROUGH KNEE), MOLDED SOCKET, EXTERNAL KNEE JOINTS, SHIN, SACH FOOT	C	N	38	A		

HCPCS Code	Statute	Lab Cert	X-Ref	ASC Pay Grp	ASC Pay Group Eff. Date	Proc Notes	BETOS	TOS	Anest	Code Add Date	Code Effective Date	Code Term Date
L4055							D1F	P	0	19880101	20050101	
L4060							D1F	P	0	19850101	19960101	
L4070							D1F	P	0	19860101	19960101	
L4080							D1F	P	0	19860101	19960101	
L4090							D1F	P	0	19850101	19960101	
L4100							D1F	P	0	19860101	19960101	
L4110							D1F	P	0	19850101	19960101	
L4130							D1F	P	0	19840101	19960101	
L4205							D1F	P	0	19970101	19970101	
L4210							D1F	P	0	19850101	19960101	
L4350							D1F	P	0	19890101	20040101	
L4360							D1F	P	0	19890101	20090101	
L4370							D1F	P	0	19890101	20030101	
L4380							D1F	P	0	19890101	20030101	
L4386							D1F	P	0	20030101	20040101	
L4392							D1F	P	0	19970101	20010101	
L4394							D1F	P	0	19970101	19970101	
L4396							D1F	P	0	19970101	20100101	
L4398							D1F	P	0	19970101	20010101	
L5000							D1F	P	0	19820101	19960101	
L5010							D1F	P	0	19820101	19960101	
L5020							D1F	P	0	19820101	19960101	
L5050							D1F	P	0	19850101	19960101	
L5060							D1F	P	0	19850101	19960101	
L5100							D1F	P	0	19820101	19960101	
L5105							D1F	P	0	19890101	19960101	
L5150							D1F	P	0	19820101	19960101	

HCPCS Code	Long Description	Coverage	Action	PI	MPI	CIM	MCM
L5160	KNEE DISARTICULATION (OR THROUGH KNEE), MOLDED SOCKET, BENT KNEE CONFIGURATION, EXTERNAL KNEE JOINTS, SHIN, SACH FOOT	C	N	38	A		
L5200	ABOVE KNEE, MOLDED SOCKET, SINGLE AXIS CONSTANT FRICTION KNEE, SHIN, SACH FOOT	C	N	38	A		
L5210	ABOVE KNEE, SHORT PROSTHESIS, NO KNEE JOINT ('STUBBIES'), WITH FOOT BLOCKS, NO ANKLE JOINTS, EACH	C	N	38	A		
L5220	ABOVE KNEE, SHORT PROSTHESIS, NO KNEE JOINT ('STUBBIES'), WITH ARTICULATED ANKLE/FOOT, DYNAMICALLY ALIGNED, EACH	C	N	38	A		
L5230	ABOVE KNEE, FOR PROXIMAL FEMORAL FOCAL DEFICIENCY, CONSTANT FRICTION KNEE, SHIN, SACH FOOT	C	N	38	A		
L5250	HIP DISARTICULATION, CANADIAN TYPE; MOLDED SOCKET, HIP JOINT, SINGLE AXIS CONSTANT FRICTION KNEE, SHIN, SACH FOOT	C	N	38	A		
L5270	HIP DISARTICULATION, TILT TABLE TYPE; MOLDED SOCKET, LOCKING HIP JOINT, SINGLE AXIS CONSTANT FRICTION KNEE, SHIN, SACH FOOT	C	N	38	A		
L5280	HEMIPELVECTOMY, CANADIAN TYPE; MOLDED SOCKET, HIP JOINT, SINGLE AXIS CONSTANT FRICTION KNEE, SHIN, SACH FOOT	C	N	38	A		
L5301	BELOW KNEE, MOLDED SOCKET, SHIN, SACH FOOT, ENDOSKELETAL SYSTEM	C	N	38	A		
L5311	KNEE DISARTICULATION (OR THROUGH KNEE), MOLDED SOCKET, EXTERNAL KNEE JOINTS, SHIN, SACH FOOT, ENDOSKELETAL SYSTEM	C	N	38	A		
L5321	ABOVE KNEE, MOLDED SOCKET, OPEN END, SACH FOOT, ENDOSKELETAL SYSTEM, SINGLE AXIS KNEE	C	N	38	A		
L5331	HIP DISARTICULATION, CANADIAN TYPE, MOLDED SOCKET, ENDOSKELETAL SYSTEM, HIP JOINT, SINGLE AXIS KNEE, SACH FOOT	C	N	38	A		
L5341	HEMIPELVECTOMY, CANADIAN TYPE, MOLDED SOCKET, ENDOSKELETAL SYSTEM, HIP JOINT, SINGLE AXIS KNEE, SACH FOOT	C	N	38	A		
L5400	IMMEDIATE POST SURGICAL OR EARLY FITTING, APPLICATION OF INITIAL RIGID DRESSING, INCLUDING FITTING, ALIGNMENT, SUSPENSION, AND ONE CAST CHANGE, BELOW KNEE	C	N	38	A		
L5410	IMMEDIATE POST SURGICAL OR EARLY FITTING, APPLICATION OF INITIAL RIGID DRESSING, INCLUDING FITTING, ALIGNMENT AND SUSPENSION, BELOW KNEE, EACH ADDITIONAL CAST CHANGE AND REALIGNMENT	C	N	38	A		
L5420	IMMEDIATE POST SURGICAL OR EARLY FITTING, APPLICATION OF INITIAL RIGID DRESSING, INCLUDING FITTING, ALIGNMENT AND SUSPENSION AND ONE CAST CHANGE 'AK' OR KNEE DISARTICULATION	C	N	38	A		
L5430	IMMEDIATE POST SURGICAL OR EARLY FITTING, APPLICATION OF INITIAL RIGID DRESSING, INCL. FITTING, ALIGNMENT & SUSPENSION, 'AK' OR KNEE DISARTICULATION, EACH ADDITIONAL CAST CHANGE AND REALIGNMENT	C	N	38	A		

HCPCS Code	Statute	Lab Cert	X-Ref	ASC Pay Grp	ASC Pay Group Eff. Date	Proc Notes	BETOS	TOS	Anest	Code Add Date	Code Effective Date	Code Term Date
							D1F	P	0	19820101	19960101	
L5200							D1F	P	0	19820101	19960101	
L5210							D1F	P	0	19820101	19960101	
L5220							D1F	P	0	19820101	19960101	
L5230							D1F	P	0	19820101	19960101	
L5250							D1F	P	0	19820101	19960101	
L5270							D1F	P	0	19820101	19960101	
L5280							D1F	P	0	19820101	19960101	
L5301							D1F	P	0	20020101	20020101	
L5311							D1F	P	0	20020101	20020101	
L5321							D1F	P	0	20020101	20020101	
L5331							D1F	P	0	20020101	20020101	
L5341							D1F	P	0	20020101	20020101	
L5400							D1F	P	0	19820101	19960101	
L5410							D1F	P	0	19860101	19960101	
L5420							D1F	P	0	19820101	19960101	
L5430							D1F	P	0	19860101	19960101	

HCPCS Code	Long Description	Coverage	Action	PI	MPI	CIM	MCM
L5450	IMMEDIATE POST SURGICAL OR EARLY FITTING, APPLICATION OF NON-WEIGHT BEARING RIGID DRESSING, BELOW KNEE	C	N	38	A		
L5460	IMMEDIATE POST SURGICAL OR EARLY FITTING, APPLICATION OF NON-WEIGHT BEARING RIGID DRESSING, ABOVE KNEE	C	N	38	A		
L5500	INITIAL, BELOW KNEE 'PTB' TYPE SOCKET, NON-ALIGNABLE SYSTEM, PYLON, NO COVER, SACH FOOT, PLASTER SOCKET, DIRECT FORMED	C	N	38	A		
L5505	INITIAL, ABOVE KNEE - KNEE DISARTICULATION, ISCHIAL LEVEL SOCKET, NON-ALIGNABLE SYSTEM, PYLON, NO COVER, SACH FOOT, PLASTER SOCKET, DIRECT FORMED	C	N	38	A		
L5510	PREPARATORY, BELOW KNEE 'PTB' TYPE SOCKET, NON-ALIGNABLE SYSTEM, PYLON, NO COVER, SACH FOOT, PLASTER SOCKET, MOLDED TO MODEL	C	N	38	A		
L5520	PREPARATORY, BELOW KNEE 'PTB' TYPE SOCKET, NON-ALIGNABLE SYSTEM, PYLON, NO COVER, SACH FOOT, THERMOPLASTIC OR EQUAL, DIRECT FORMED	C	N	38	A		
L5530	PREPARATORY, BELOW KNEE 'PTB' TYPE SOCKET, NON-ALIGNABLE SYSTEM, PYLON, NO COVER, SACH FOOT, THERMOPLASTIC OR EQUAL, MOLDED TO MODEL	C	N	38	A		
L5535	PREPARATORY, BELOW KNEE 'PTB' TYPE SOCKET, NON-ALIGNABLE SYSTEM, NO COVER, SACH FOOT, PREFABRICATED, ADJUSTABLE OPEN END SOCKET	C	N	38	A		
L5540	PREPARATORY, BELOW KNEE 'PTB' TYPE SOCKET, NON-ALIGNABLE SYSTEM, PYLON, NO COVER, SACH FOOT, LAMINATED SOCKET, MOLDED TO MODEL	C	N	38	A		
L5560	PREPARATORY, ABOVE KNEE- KNEE DISARTICULATION, ISCHIAL LEVEL SOCKET, NON-ALIGNABLE SYSTEM, PYLON, NO COVER, SACH FOOT, PLASTER SOCKET, MOLDED TO MODEL	C	N	38	A		
L5570	PREPARATORY, ABOVE KNEE - KNEE DISARTICULATION, ISCHIAL LEVEL SOCKET, NON-ALIGNABLE SYSTEM, PYLON, NO COVER, SACH FOOT, THERMOPLASTIC OR EQUAL, DIRECT FORMED	C	N	38	A		
L5580	PREPARATORY, ABOVE KNEE - KNEE DISARTICULATION ISCHIAL LEVEL SOCKET, NON-ALIGNABLE SYSTEM, PYLON, NO COVER, SACH FOOT, THERMOPLASTIC OR EQUAL, MOLDED TO MODEL	C	N	38	A		
L5585	PREPARATORY, ABOVE KNEE - KNEE DISARTICULATION, ISCHIAL LEVEL SOCKET, NON-ALIGNABLE SYSTEM, PYLON, NO COVER, SACH FOOT, PREFABRICATED ADJUSTABLE OPEN END SOCKET	C	N	38	A		
L5590	PREPARATORY, ABOVE KNEE - KNEE DISARTICULATION ISCHIAL LEVEL SOCKET, NON-ALIGNABLE SYSTEM, PYLON NO COVER, SACH FOOT, LAMINATED SOCKET, MOLDED TO MODEL	C	N	38	A		
L5595	PREPARATORY, HIP DISARTICULATION-HEMIPELVECTOMY, PYLON, NO COVER, SACH FOOT, THERMOPLASTIC OR EQUAL, MOLDED TO PATIENT MODEL	C	N	38	A		
L5600	PREPARATORY, HIP DISARTICULATION-HEMIPELVECTOMY, PYLON, NO COVER, SACH FOOT, LAMINATED SOCKET, MOLDED TO PATIENT MODEL	C	N	38	A		

HCPCS Code	Statute	Lab Cert	X-Ref	ASC Pay Grp	ASC Pay Group Eff. Date	Proc Notes	BETOS	TOS	Anest	Code Add Date	Code Effective Date	Code Term Date
L5450							D1F	P	0	19820101	19960101	
L5460							D1F	P	0	19820101	19960101	
L5500							D1F	P	0	19860101	19960101	
L5505							D1F	P	0	19860101	19960101	
L5510							D1F	P	0	19860101	19960101	
L5520							D1F	P	0	19860101	19960101	
L5530							D1F	P	0	19860101	19960101	
L5535							D1F	P	0	19890101	19960101	
L5540							D1F	P	0	19860101	19960101	
L5560							D1F	P	0	19860101	19960101	
L5570							D1F	P	0	19860101	19960101	
L5580							D1F	P	0	19860101	19960101	
L5585							D1F	P	0	19880101	19960101	
L5590							D1F	P	0	19860101	19960101	
L5595							D1F	P	0	19890101	19960101	
L5600							D1F	P	0	19890101	19960101	

HCPCS Code	Long Description	Coverage	Action	PI	MPI	CIM	MCM
L5610	ADDITION TO LOWER EXTREMITY, ENDOSKELETAL SYSTEM, ABOVE KNEE, HYDRACADENCE SYSTEM	C	N	38	A		
L5611	ADDITION TO LOWER EXTREMITY, ENDOSKELETAL SYSTEM, ABOVE KNEE - KNEE DISARTICULATION, 4 BAR LINKAGE, WITH FRICTION SWING PHASE CONTROL	C	N	38	A		
L5613	ADDITION TO LOWER EXTREMITY, ENDOSKELETAL SYSTEM, ABOVE KNEE-KNEE DISARTICULATION, 4 BAR LINKAGE, WITH HYDRAULIC SWING PHASE CONTROL	C	N	38	A		
L5614	ADDITION TO LOWER EXTREMITY, EXOSKELETAL SYSTEM, ABOVE KNEE-KNEE DISARTICULATION, 4 BAR LINKAGE, WITH PNEUMATIC SWING PHASE CONTROL	C	N	38	A		
L5616	ADDITION TO LOWER EXTREMITY, ENDOSKELETAL SYSTEM, ABOVE KNEE, UNIVERSAL MULTIPLEX SYSTEM, FRICTION SWING PHASE CONTROL	C	N	38	A		
L5617	ADDITION TO LOWER EXTREMITY, QUICK CHANGE SELF-ALIGNING UNIT, ABOVE KNEE OR BELOW KNEE, EACH	C	N	38	A		
L5618	ADDITION TO LOWER EXTREMITY, TEST SOCKET, SYMES	C	N	38	A		
L5620	ADDITION TO LOWER EXTREMITY, TEST SOCKET, BELOW KNEE	C	N	38	A		
L5622	ADDITION TO LOWER EXTREMITY, TEST SOCKET, KNEE DISARTICULATION	C	N	38	A		
L5624	ADDITION TO LOWER EXTREMITY, TEST SOCKET, ABOVE KNEE	C	N	38	A		
L5626	ADDITION TO LOWER EXTREMITY, TEST SOCKET, HIP DISARTICULATION	C	N	38	A		
L5628	ADDITION TO LOWER EXTREMITY, TEST SOCKET, HEMIPELVECTOMY	C	N	38	A		
L5629	ADDITION TO LOWER EXTREMITY, BELOW KNEE, ACRYLIC SOCKET	C	N	38	A		
L5630	ADDITION TO LOWER EXTREMITY, SYMES TYPE, EXPANDABLE WALL SOCKET	C	N	38	A		
L5631	ADDITION TO LOWER EXTREMITY, ABOVE KNEE OR KNEE DISARTICULATION, ACRYLIC SOCKET	C	N	38	A		
L5632	ADDITION TO LOWER EXTREMITY, SYMES TYPE, 'PTB' BRIM DESIGN SOCKET	C	N	38	A		
L5634	ADDITION TO LOWER EXTREMITY, SYMES TYPE, POSTERIOR OPENING (CANADIAN) SOCKET	C	N	38	A		
L5636	ADDITION TO LOWER EXTREMITY, SYMES TYPE, MEDIAL OPENING SOCKET	C	N	38	A		
L5637	ADDITION TO LOWER EXTREMITY, BELOW KNEE, TOTAL CONTACT	C	N	38	A		
L5638	ADDITION TO LOWER EXTREMITY, BELOW KNEE, LEATHER SOCKET	C	N	38	A		
L5639	ADDITION TO LOWER EXTREMITY, BELOW KNEE, WOOD SOCKET	C	N	38	A		
L5640	ADDITION TO LOWER EXTREMITY, KNEE DISARTICULATION, LEATHER SOCKET	C	N	38	A		
L5642	ADDITION TO LOWER EXTREMITY, ABOVE KNEE, LEATHER SOCKET	C	N	38	A		
L5643	ADDITION TO LOWER EXTREMITY, HIP DISARTICULATION, FLEXIBLE INNER SOCKET, EXTERNAL FRAME	C	N	38	A		

HCPCS Code	Statute	Lab Cert	X-Ref	ASC Pay Grp	ASC Pay Group Eff. Date	Proc Notes	BETOS	TOS	Anest	Code Add Date	Code Effective Date	Code Term Date
L5610							D1F	P	0	19860101	19960101	
L5611							D1F	P	0	19890101	19960101	
L5613							D1F	P	0	19890101	19960101	
L5614							D1F	P	0	19940101	19960101	
L5616							D1F	P	0	19860101	19960101	
L5617							D1F	P	0	19960101	19960101	
L5618							D1F	P	0	19860101	19960101	
L5620							D1F	P	0	19860101	19960101	
L5622							D1F	P	0	19860101	19960101	
L5624							D1F	P	0	19860101	19960101	
L5626							D1F	P	0	19860101	19960101	
L5628							D1F	P	0	19860101	19960101	
L5629							D1F	P	0	19890101	19960101	
L5630							D1F	P	0	19860101	19960101	
L5631							D1F	P	0	19890101	19960101	
L5632							D1F	P	0	19860101	19960101	
L5634							D1F	P	0	19860101	19960101	
L5636							D1F	P	0	19860101	19960101	
L5637							D1F	P	0	19890101	19960101	
L5638							D1F	P	0	19860101	19960101	
L5639							D1F	P	0	19890101	19960101	
L5640							D1F	P	0	19860101	19960101	
L5642							D1F	P	0	19860101	19960101	
L5643							D1F	P	0	19880101	19960101	

HCPCS Code	Long Description	Coverage	Action	PI	MPI	CIM	MCM
L5644	ADDITION TO LOWER EXTREMITY, ABOVE KNEE, WOOD SOCKET	C	N	38	A		
L5645	ADDITION TO LOWER EXTREMITY, BELOW KNEE, FLEXIBLE INNER SOCKET, EXTERNAL FRAME	C	N	38	A		
L5646	ADDITION TO LOWER EXTREMITY, BELOW KNEE, AIR, FLUID, GEL OR EQUAL, CUSHION SOCKET	C	N	38	A		
L5647	ADDITION TO LOWER EXTREMITY, BELOW KNEE SUCTION SOCKET	C	N	38	A		
L5648	ADDITION TO LOWER EXTREMITY, ABOVE KNEE, AIR, FLUID, GEL OR EQUAL, CUSHION SOCKET	C	N	38	A		
L5649	ADDITION TO LOWER EXTREMITY, ISCHIAL CONTAINMENT/NARROW M-L SOCKET	C	N	38	A		
L5650	ADDITIONS TO LOWER EXTREMITY, TOTAL CONTACT, ABOVE KNEE OR KNEE DISARTICULATION SOCKET	C	N	38	A		
L5651	ADDITION TO LOWER EXTREMITY, ABOVE KNEE, FLEXIBLE INNER SOCKET, EXTERNAL FRAME	C	N	38	A		
L5652	ADDITION TO LOWER EXTREMITY, SUCTION SUSPENSION, ABOVE KNEE OR KNEE DISARTICULATION SOCKET	C	N	38	A		
L5653	ADDITION TO LOWER EXTREMITY, KNEE DISARTICULATION, EXPANDABLE WALL SOCKET	C	N	38	A		
L5654	ADDITION TO LOWER EXTREMITY, SOCKET INSERT, SYMES, (KEMBLO, PELITE, ALIPLAST, PLASTAZOTE OR EQUAL)	C	N	38	A		
L5655	ADDITION TO LOWER EXTREMITY, SOCKET INSERT, BELOW KNEE (KEMBLO, PELITE, ALIPLAST, PLASTAZOTE OR EQUAL)	C	N	38	A		
L5656	ADDITION TO LOWER EXTREMITY, SOCKET INSERT, KNEE DISARTICULATION (KEMBLO, PELITE, ALIPLAST, PLASTAZOTE OR EQUAL)	C	N	38	A		
L5658	ADDITION TO LOWER EXTREMITY, SOCKET INSERT, ABOVE KNEE (KEMBLO, PELITE, ALIPLAST, PLASTAZOTE OR EQUAL)	C	N	38	A		
L5661	ADDITION TO LOWER EXTREMITY, SOCKET INSERT, MULTI-DUROMETER SYMES	C	N	38	A		
L5665	ADDITION TO LOWER EXTREMITY, SOCKET INSERT, MULTI-DUROMETER, BELOW KNEE	C	N	38	A		
L5666	ADDITION TO LOWER EXTREMITY, BELOW KNEE, CUFF SUSPENSION	C	N	38	A		
L5668	ADDITION TO LOWER EXTREMITY, BELOW KNEE, MOLDED DISTAL CUSHION	C	N	38	A		
L5670	ADDITION TO LOWER EXTREMITY, BELOW KNEE, MOLDED SUPRACONDYLAR SUSPENSION ('PTS' OR SIMILAR)	C	N	38	A		
L5671	ADDITION TO LOWER EXTREMITY, BELOW KNEE / ABOVE KNEE SUSPENSION LOCKING MECHANISM (SHUTTLE, LANYARD OR EQUAL), EXCLUDES SOCKET INSERT	C	N	38	A		
L5672	ADDITION TO LOWER EXTREMITY, BELOW KNEE, REMOVABLE MEDIAL BRIM SUSPENSION	C	N	38	A		
L5673	ADDITION TO LOWER EXTREMITY, BELOW KNEE/ABOVE KNEE, CUSTOM FABRICATED FROM EXISTING MOLD OR PRE-FABRICATED, SOCKET INSERT, SILICONE GEL, ELASTOMERIC OR EQUAL, FOR USE WITH LOCKING MECHANISM	C	N	38	A		

HCPCS Code	Statute	Lab Cert	X-Ref	ASC Pay Grp	ASC Pay Group Eff. Date	Proc Notes	BETOS	TOS	Anest	Code Add Date	Code Effective Date	Code Term Date
L5644							D1F	P	0	19860101	19960101	
L5645							D1F	P	0	19880101	20001213	
L5646							D1F	P	0	19860101	20040101	
L5647							D1F	P	0	19880101	19960101	
L5648							D1F	P	0	19860101	20040101	
L5649							D1F	P	0	19880101	19960101	
L5650							D1F	P	0	19860101	19960101	
L5651							D1F	P	0	19880101	19960101	
L5652							D1F	P	0	19860101	19960101	
L5653							D1F	P	0	19860101	19960101	
L5654							D1F	P	0	19860101	19960101	
L5655							D1F	P	0	19860101	19960101	
L5656							D1F	P	0	19860101	19960101	
L5658							D1F	P	0	19860101	19960101	
L5661							D1F	P	0	19880101	19960101	
L5665							D1F	P	0	19880101	19960101	
L5666							D1F	P	0	19860101	19960101	
L5668							D1F	P	0	19860101	19960101	
L5670							D1F	P	0	19860101	19960101	
L5671							D1F	P	0	20020101	20020101	
L5672							D1F	P	0	19860101	19960101	
L5673							D1F	P	0	20040101	20040101	

L Codes

HCPCS Code	Long Description	Coverage	Action	PI	MPI	CIM	MCM
L5676	ADDITIONS TO LOWER EXTREMITY, BELOW KNEE, KNEE JOINTS, SINGLE AXIS, PAIR	C	N	38	A		
L5677	ADDITIONS TO LOWER EXTREMITY, BELOW KNEE, KNEE JOINTS, POLYCENTRIC, PAIR	C	N	38	A		
L5678	ADDITIONS TO LOWER EXTREMITY, BELOW KNEE, JOINT COVERS, PAIR	C	N	38	A		
L5679	ADDITION TO LOWER EXTREMITY, BELOW KNEE/ABOVE KNEE, CUSTOM FABRICATED FROM EXISTING MOLD OR PRE-FABRICATED, SOCKET INSERT, SILICONE GEL, ELASTOMERIC OR EQUAL, NOT FOR USE WITH LOCKING MECHANISM	C	N	38	A		
L5680	ADDITION TO LOWER EXTREMITY, BELOW KNEE, THIGH LACER, NONMOLDED	C	N	38	A		
L5681	ADDITION TO LOWER EXTREMITY, BELOW KNEE/ABOVE KNEE, CUSTOM FABRICATED SOCKET INSERT FOR CONGENITAL OR ATYPICAL TRAUMATIC AMPUTEE, SILICONE GEL, ELASTOMERIC OR EQUAL, FOR USE WITH OR WITHOUT LOCKING MECHANISM, INITIAL ONLY (FOR OTHER THAN INITIAL, USE CODE L5673 OR L5679)	C	N	38	A		
L5682	ADDITION TO LOWER EXTREMITY, BELOW KNEE, THIGH LACER, GLUTEAL/ISCHIAL, MOLDED	C	N	38	A		
L5683	ADDITION TO LOWER EXTREMITY, BELOW KNEE/ABOVE KNEE, CUSTOM FABRICATED SOCKET INSERT FOR OTHER THAN CONGENITAL OR ATYPICAL TRAUMATIC AMPUTEE, SILICONE GEL, ELASTOMERIC OR EQUAL, FOR USE WITH OR WITHOUT LOCKING MECHANISM, INITIAL ONLY (FOR OTHER THAN INITIAL, USE CODE L5673 OR L5679)	C	N	38	A		
L5684	ADDITION TO LOWER EXTREMITY, BELOW KNEE, FORK STRAP	C	N	38	A		
L5685	ADDITION TO LOWER EXTREMITY PROSTHESIS, BELOW KNEE, SUSPENSION/SEALING SLEEVE, WITH OR WITHOUT VALVE, ANY MATERIAL, EACH	C	N	38	A		
L5686	ADDITION TO LOWER EXTREMITY, BELOW KNEE, BACK CHECK (EXTENSION CONTROL)	C	N	38	A		
L5688	ADDITION TO LOWER EXTREMITY, BELOW KNEE, WAIST BELT, WEBBING	C	N	38	A		
L5690	ADDITION TO LOWER EXTREMITY, BELOW KNEE, WAIST BELT, PADDED AND LINED	C	N	38	A		
L5692	ADDITION TO LOWER EXTREMITY, ABOVE KNEE, PELVIC CONTROL BELT, LIGHT	C	N	38	A		
L5694	ADDITION TO LOWER EXTREMITY, ABOVE KNEE, PELVIC CONTROL BELT, PADDED AND LINED	C	N	38	A		
L5695	ADDITION TO LOWER EXTREMITY, ABOVE KNEE, PELVIC CONTROL, SLEEVE SUSPENSION, NEOPRENE OR EQUAL, EA.	C	N	38	A		
L5696	ADDITION TO LOWER EXTREMITY, ABOVE KNEE OR KNEE DISARTICULATION, PELVIC JOINT	C	N	38	A		
L5697	ADDITION TO LOWER EXTREMITY, ABOVE KNEE OR KNEE DISARTICULATION, PELVIC BAND	C	N	38	A		
L5698	ADDITION TO LOWER EXTREMITY, ABOVE KNEE OR KNEE DISARTICULATION, SILESIAN BANDAGE	C	N	38	A		
L5699	ALL LOWER EXTREMITY PROSTHESES, SHOULDER HARNESS	C	N	38	A		

HCPCS Code	Statute	Lab Cert	X-Ref	ASC Pay Grp	ASC Pay Group Eff. Date	Proc Notes	BETOS	TOS	Anest	Code Add Date	Code Effective Date	Code Term Date
L5676							D1F	P	0	19860101	19960101	
L5677							D1F	P	0	19880101	19960101	
L5678							D1F	P	0	19840101	19960101	
L5679							D1F	P	0	20040101	20040101	
L5680							D1F	P	0	19860101	19960101	
L5681							D1F	P	0	20040101	20040101	
L5682							D1F	P	0	19860101	19960101	
L5683							D1F	P	0	20040101	20040101	
L5684							D1F	P	0	19860101	19960101	
L5685							D1F	P	0	20050101	20050101	
L5685												
L5686							D1F	P	0	19860101	19960101	
L5688							D1F	P	0	19860101	19960101	
L5690							D1F	P	0	19860101	19960101	
L5692							D1F	P	0	19860101	19960101	
L5694							D1F	P	0	19860101	19960101	
L5695							D1F	P	0	19890101	19960101	
L5696							D1F	P	0	19860101	19960101	
L5697							D1F	P	0	19860101	19960101	
L5698							D1F	P	0	19860101	19960101	
L5699							D1F	P	0	19860101	19960101	

L Codes

HCPCS Code	Long Description	Coverage	Action	PI	MPI	CIM	MCM
L5700	REPLACEMENT, SOCKET, BELOW KNEE, MOLDED TO PATIENT MODEL	C	N	38	A		
L5701	REPLACEMENT, SOCKET, ABOVE KNEE/KNEE DISARTICULATION, INCLUDING ATTACHMENT PLATE, MOLDED TO PATIENT MODEL	C	N	38	A		
L5702	REPLACEMENT, SOCKET, HIP DISARTICULATION, INCLUDING HIP JOINT, MOLDED TO PATIENT MODEL	C	N	38	A		
L5703	ANKLE, SYMES, MOLDED TO PATIENT MODEL, SOCKET WITHOUT SOLID ANKLE CUSHION HEEL (SACH) FOOT, REPLACEMENT ONLY	C	N	38	A		
L5704	CUSTOM SHAPED PROTECTIVE COVER, BELOW KNEE	C	N	38	A		
L5705	CUSTOM SHAPED PROTECTIVE COVER, ABOVE KNEE	C	N	38	A		
L5706	CUSTOM SHAPED PROTECTIVE COVER, KNEE DISARTICULATION	C	N	38	A		
L5707	CUSTOM SHAPED PROTECTIVE COVER, HIP DISARTICULATION	C	N	38	A		
L5710	ADDITION, EXOSKELETAL KNEE-SHIN SYSTEM, SINGLE AXIS, MANUAL LOCK	C	N	38	A		
L5711	ADDITIONS EXOSKELETAL KNEE-SHIN SYSTEM, SINGLE AXIS, MANUAL LOCK, ULTRA-LIGHT MATERIAL	C	N	38	A		
L5712	ADDITION, EXOSKELETAL KNEE-SHIN SYSTEM, SINGLE AXIS, FRICTION SWING AND STANCE PHASE CONTROL (SAFETY KNEE)	C	N	38	A		
L5714	ADDITION, EXOSKELETAL KNEE-SHIN SYSTEM, SINGLE AXIS, VARIABLE FRICTION SWING PHASE CONTROL	C	N	38	A		
L5716	ADDITION, EXOSKELETAL KNEE-SHIN SYSTEM, POLYCENTRIC, MECHANICAL STANCE PHASE LOCK	C	N	38	A		
L5718	ADDITION, EXOSKELETAL KNEE-SHIN SYSTEM, POLYCENTRIC, FRICTION SWING AND STANCE PHASE CONTROL	C	N	38	A		
L5722	ADDITION, EXOSKELETAL KNEE-SHIN SYSTEM, SINGLE AXIS, PNEUMATIC SWING, FRICTION STANCE PHASE CONTROL	C	N	38	A		
L5724	ADDITION, EXOSKELETAL KNEE-SHIN SYSTEM, SINGLE AXIS, FLUID SWING PHASE CONTROL	C	N	38	A		
L5726	ADDITION, EXOSKELETAL KNEE-SHIN SYSTEM, SINGLE AXIS, EXTERNAL JOINTS FLUID SWING PHASE CONTROL	C	N	38	A		
L5728	ADDITION, EXOSKELETAL KNEE-SHIN SYSTEM, SINGLE AXIS, FLUID SWING AND STANCE PHASE CONTROL	C	N	38	A		
L5780	ADDITION, EXOSKELETAL KNEE-SHIN SYSTEM, SINGLE AXIS, PNEUMATIC/HYDRA PNEUMATIC SWING PHASE CONTROL	C	N	38	A		
L5781	ADDITION TO LOWER LIMB PROSTHESIS, VACUUM PUMP, RESIDUAL LIMB VOLUME MANAGEMENT AND MOISTURE EVACUATION SYSTEM	C	N	38	A		
L5782	ADDITION TO LOWER LIMB PROSTHESIS, VACUUM PUMP, RESIDUAL LIMB VOLUME MANAGEMENT AND MOISTURE EVACUATION SYSTEM, HEAVY DUTY	C	N	38	A		
L5785	ADDITION, EXOSKELETAL SYSTEM, BELOW KNEE, ULTRA-LIGHT MATERIAL (TITANIUM, CARBON FIBER OR EQUAL)	C	N	38	A		
L5790	ADDITION, EXOSKELETAL SYSTEM, ABOVE KNEE, ULTRA-LIGHT MATERIAL (TITANIUM, CARBON FIBER OR EQUAL)	C	N	38	A		

HCPCS Code	Statute	Lab Cert	X-Ref	ASC Pay Grp	ASC Pay Group Eff. Date	Proc Notes	BETOS	TOS	Anest	Code Add Date	Code Effective Date	Code Term Date
L5700							D1F	P	0	19940101	19940101	
L5701							D1F	P	0	19940101	19940101	
L5702							D1F	P	0	19940101	19940101	
L5703							D1F	P	0	20060101	20060101	
L5704							D1F	P	0	19940101	20020101	
L5705							D1F	P	0	19940101	20020101	
L5706							D1F	P	0	19940101	20020101	
L5707							D1F	P	0	19940101	20020101	
L5710							D1F	P	0	19860101	19960101	
L5711							D1F	P	0	19880101	19960101	
L5712							D1F	P	0	19860101	19960101	
L5714							D1F	P	0	19860101	19960101	
L5716							D1F	P	0	19860101	19960101	
L5718							D1F	P	0	19860101	19960101	
L5722							D1F	P	0	19860101	19960101	
L5724							D1F	P	0	19860101	19960101	
L5726							D1F	P	0	19860101	19960101	
L5728							D1F	P	0	19860101	19960101	
L5780							D1F	P	0	19860101	19960101	
L5781							D1F	P	0	20030101	20030101	
L5782							D1F	P	0	20030101	20030101	
L5785							D1F	P	0	19880101	19960101	
L5790							D1F	P	0	19880101	19960101	

HCPCS Code	Long Description	Coverage	Action	PI	MPI	CIM	MCM
L5795	ADDITION, EXOSKELETAL SYSTEM, HIP DISARTICULATION, ULTRA-LIGHT MATERIAL (TITANIUM, CARBON FIBER OR EQUAL)	C	N	38	A		
L5810	ADDITION, ENDOSKELETAL KNEE-SHIN SYSTEM, SINGLE AXIS, MANUAL LOCK	C	N	38	A		
L5811	ADDITION, ENDOSKELETAL KNEE-SHIN SYSTEM, SINGLE AXIS, MANUAL LOCK, ULTRA-LIGHT MATERIAL	C	N	38	A		
L5812	ADDITION, ENDOSKELETAL KNEE-SHIN SYSTEM, SINGLE AXIS, FRICTION SWING & STANCE PHASE CONTROL (SAFETY KNEE)	C	N	38	A		
L5814	ADDITION, ENDOSKELETAL KNEE-SHIN SYSTEM, POLYCENTRIC, HYDRAULIC SWING PHASE CONTROL, MECHANICAL STANCE PHASE LOCK	C	N	38	A		
L5816	ADDITION, ENDOSKELETAL KNEE-SHIN SYSTEM, POLYCENTRIC, MECHANICAL STANCE PHASE LOCK	C	N	38	A		
L5818	ADDITION, ENDOSKELETAL KNEE-SHIN SYSTEM, POLYCENTRIC, FRICTION SWING, & STANCE PHASE CONTROL	C	N	38	A		
L5822	ADDITION, ENDOSKELETAL KNEE-SHIN SYSTEM, SINGLE AXIS, PNEUMATIC SWING, FRICTION STANCE PHASE CONTROL	C	N	38	A		
L5824	ADDITION, ENDOSKELETAL KNEE-SHIN SYSTEM, SINGLE AXIS, FLUID SWING PHASE CONTROL	C	N	38	A		
L5826	ADDITION, ENDOSKELETAL KNEE-SHIN SYSTEM, SINGLE AXIS, HYDRAULIC SWING PHASE CONTROL, WITH MINIATURE HIGH ACTIVITY FRAME	C	N	38	A		
L5828	ADDITION, ENDOSKELETAL KNEE-SHIN SYSTEM, SINGLE AXIS, FLUID SWING AND STANCE PHASE CONTROL	C	N	38	A		
L5830	ADDITION, ENDOSKELETAL KNEE-SHIN SYSTEM, SINGLE AXIS, PNEUMATIC/ SWING PHASE CONTROL	C	N	38	A		
L5840	ADDITION, ENDOSKELETAL KNEE/SHIN SYSTEM, 4-BAR LINKAGE OR MULTIAXIAL, PNEUMATIC SWING PHASE CONTROL	C	N	38	A		
L5845	ADDITION, ENDOSKELETAL, KNEE-SHIN SYSTEM, STANCE FLEXION FEATURE, ADJUSTABLE	C	N	38	A		
L5848	ADDITION TO ENDOSKELETAL KNEE-SHIN SYSTEM, FLUID STANCE EXTENSION, DAMPENING FEATURE, WITH OR WITHOUT ADJUSTABILITY	C	N	38	A		
L5850	ADDITION, ENDOSKELETAL SYSTEM, ABOVE KNEE OR HIP DISARTICULATION, KNEE EXTENSION ASSIST	C	N	38	A		
L5855	ADDITION, ENDOSKELETAL SYSTEM, HIP DISARTICULATION, MECHANICAL HIP EXTENSION ASSIST	C	N	38	A		
L5856	ADDITION TO LOWER EXTREMITY PROSTHESIS, ENDOSKELETAL KNEE-SHIN SYSTEM, MICROPROCESSOR CONTROL FEATURE, SWING AND STANCE PHASE, INCLUDES ELECTRONIC SENSOR(S), ANY TYPE	C	N	38	A		
L5857	ADDITION TO LOWER EXTREMITY PROSTHESIS, ENDOSKELETAL KNEE-SHIN SYSTEM, MICROPROCESSOR CONTROL FEATURE, SWING PHASE ONLY, INCLUDES ELECTRONIC SENSOR(S), ANY TYPE	C	N	38	A		

HCPCS Code	Statute	Lab Cert	X-Ref	ASC Pay Grp	ASC Pay Group Eff. Date	Proc Notes	BETOS	TOS	Anest	Code Add Date	Code Effective Date	Code Term Date
L5795							D1F	P	0	19880101	19960101	
L5810							D1F	P	0	19880101	19960101	
L5811							D1F	P	0	19880101	19960101	
L5812							D1F	P	0	19880101	19960101	
L5814							D1F	P	0	19970101	19970101	
L5816							D1F	P	0	19880101	19960101	
L5818							D1F	P	0	19880101	19960101	
L5822							D1F	P	0	19880101	19960101	
L5824							D1F	P	0	19880101	19960101	
L5826							D1F	P	0	19980101	19990101	
L5828							D1F	P	0	19880101	19960101	
L5830							D1F	P	0	19880101	19960101	
L5840							D1F	P	0	19940101	19990101	
L5845							D1F	P	0	19960101	19960101	
L5848							D1F	P	0	20030101	20070101	
L5850							D1F	P	0	19880101	19960101	
L5855							D1F	P	0	19940101	19950101	
L5856							D1F	P	0	20050101	20050101	
L5857							D1F	P	0	20050101	20050101	

L Codes

HCPCS Code	Long Description	Coverage	Action	PI	MPI	CIM	MCM
L5858	ADDITION TO LOWER EXTREMITY PROSTHESIS, ENDOSKELETAL KNEE SHIN SYSTEM, MICROPROCESSOR CONTROL FEATURE, STANCE PHASE ONLY, INCLUDES ELECTRONIC SENSOR(S), ANY TYPE	C	N	38	A		
L5910	ADDITION, ENDOSKELETAL SYSTEM, BELOW KNEE, ALIGNABLE SYSTEM	C	N	38	A		
L5920	ADDITION, ENDOSKELETAL SYSTEM, ABOVE KNEE OR HIP DISARTICULATION, ALIGNABLE SYSTEM	C	N	38	A		
L5925	ADDITION, ENDOSKELETAL SYSTEM, ABOVE KNEE, KNEE DISARTICULATION OR HIP DISARTICULATION, MANUAL LOCK	C	N	38	A		
L5930	ADDITION, ENDOSKELETAL SYSTEM, HIGH ACTIVITY KNEE CONTROL FRAME	C	N	38	A		
L5940	ADDITION, ENDOSKELETAL SYSTEM, BELOW KNEE, ULTRA-LIGHT MATERIAL (TITANIUM, CARBON FIBER OR EQUAL)	C	N	38	A		
L5950	ADDITION, ENDOSKELETAL SYSTEM, ABOVE KNEE, ULTRA-LIGHT MATERIAL (TITANIUM, CARBON FIBER OR EQUAL)	C	N	38	A		
L5960	ADDITION, ENDOSKELETAL SYSTEM, HIP DISARTICULATION, ULTRA-LIGHT MATERIAL (TITANIUM, CARBON FIBER OR EQUAL)	C	N	38	A		
L5962	ADDITION, ENDOSKELETAL SYSTEM, BELOW KNEE, FLEXIBLE PROTECTIVE OUTER SURFACE COVERING SYSTEM	C	N	38	A		
L5964	ADDITION, ENDOSKELETAL SYSTEM, ABOVE KNEE, FLEXIBLE PROTECTIVE OUTER SURFACE COVERING SYSTEM	C	N	38	A		
L5966	ADDITION, ENDOSKELETAL SYSTEM, HIP DISARTICULATION, FLEXIBLE PROTECTIVE OUTER SURFACE COVERING SYSTEM	C	N	38	A		
L5968	ADDITION TO LOWER LIMB PROSTHESIS, MULTIAXIAL ANKLE WITH SWING PHASE ACTIVE DORSIFLEXION FEATURE	C	N	38	A		
L5970	ALL LOWER EXTREMITY PROSTHESES, FOOT, EXTERNAL KEEL, SACH FOOT	C	N	38	A		
L5971	ALL LOWER EXTREMITY PROSTHESIS, SOLID ANKLE CUSHION HEEL (SACH) FOOT, REPLACEMENT ONLY	C	N	38	A		
L5972	ALL LOWER EXTREMITY PROSTHESES, FLEXIBLE KEEL FOOT (SAFE, STEN, BOCK DYNAMIC OR EQUAL)	C	N	38	A		
L5973	ENDOSKELETAL ANKLE FOOT SYSTEM, MICROPROCESSOR CONTROLLED FEATURE, DORSIFLEXION AND/OR PLANTAR FLEXION CONTROL, INCLUDES POWER SOURCE	C	A	38	A		
L5974	ALL LOWER EXTREMITY PROSTHESES, FOOT, SINGLE AXIS ANKLE/FOOT	C	N	38	A		
L5975	ALL LOWER EXTREMITY PROSTHESIS, COMBINATION SINGLE AXIS ANKLE AND FLEXIBLE KEEL FOOT	C	N	38	A		
L5976	ALL LOWER EXTREMITY PROSTHESES, ENERGY STORING FOOT (SEATTLE CARBON COPY II OR EQUAL)	C	N	38	A		
L5978	ALL LOWER EXTREMITY PROSTHESES, FOOT, MULTIAXIAL ANKLE/FOOT	C	N	38	A		
L5979	ALL LOWER EXTREMITY PROSTHESIS, MULTI-AXIAL ANKLE, DYNAMIC RESPONSE FOOT, ONE PIECE SYSTEM	C	N	38	A		
L5980	ALL LOWER EXTREMITY PROSTHESES, FLEX FOOT SYSTEM	C	N	38	A		
L5981	ALL LOWER EXTREMITY PROSTHESES, FLEX-WALK SYSTEM OR EQUAL	C	N	38	A		

HCPCS Code	Statute	Lab Cert	X-Ref	ASC Pay Grp	ASC Pay Group Eff. Date	Proc Notes	BETOS	TOS	Anest	Code Add Date	Code Effective Date	Code Term Date
L5858							D1F	P	0	20060101	20060101	
L5910							D1F	P	0	19880101	19960101	
L5920							D1F	P	0	19880101	19960101	
L5925							D1F	P	0	19940101	20000101	
L5930							D1F	P	0	19960101	19960101	
L5940							D1F	P	0	19880101	19960101	
L5950							D1F	P	0	19880101	19960101	
L5960							D1F	P	0	19880101	19960101	
L5962							D1F	P	0	19940101	19940101	
L5964							D1F	P	0	19940101	19940101	
L5966							D1F	P	0	19940101	19940101	
L5968							D1F	P	0	19990101	20000101	
L5970							D1F	P	0	19890101	19960101	
L5971							D1F	P	0	20060101	20060101	
L5972							D1F	P	0	19890101	19960101	
L5973							D1F	P	0	20100101	20100101	
L5974							D1F	P	0	19890101	19960101	
L5975							D1F	P	0	19990101	19990101	
L5976							D1F	P	0	19890101	19960101	
L5978							D1F	P	0	19890101	19960101	
L5979							D1F	P	0	19940101	20010101	
L5980							D1F	P	0	19890101	19960101	
L5981							D1F	P	0	19940101	19940101	

HCPCS Code	Long Description	Coverage	Action	PI	MPI	CIM	MCM
L5982	ALL EXOSKELETAL LOWER EXTREMITY PROSTHESES, AXIAL ROTATION UNIT	C	N	38	A		
L5984	ALL ENDOSKELETAL LOWER EXTREMITY PROSTHESIS, AXIAL ROTATION UNIT, WITH OR WITHOUT ADJUSTABILITY	C	N	38	A		
L5985	ALL ENDOSKELETAL LOWER EXTREMITY PROSTHESES, DYNAMIC PROSTHETIC PYLON	C	N	38	A		
L5986	ALL LOWER EXTREMITY PROSTHESES, MULTI-AXIAL ROTATION UNIT ('MCP' OR EQUAL)	C	N	38	A		
L5987	ALL LOWER EXTREMITY PROSTHESIS, SHANK FOOT SYSTEM WITH VERTICAL LOADING PYLON	C	N	38	A		
L5988	ADDITION TO LOWER LIMB PROSTHESIS, VERTICAL SHOCK REDUCING PYLON FEATURE	C	N	38	A		
L5990	ADDITION TO LOWER EXTREMITY PROSTHESIS, USER ADJUSTABLE HEEL HEIGHT	C	N	38	A		
L5993	ADDITION TO LOWER EXTREMITY PROSTHESIS, HEAVY DUTY FEATURE, FOOT ONLY, (FOR PATIENT WEIGHT GREATER THAN 300 LBS)	C	N	38	A		
L5994	ADDITION TO LOWER EXTREMITY PROSTHESIS, HEAVY DUTY FEATURE, KNEE ONLY, (FOR PATIENT WEIGHT GREATER THAN 300 LBS)	C	N	38	A		
L5995	ADDITION TO LOWER EXTREMITY PROSTHESIS, HEAVY DUTY FEATURE, OTHER THAN FOOT OR KNEE, (FOR PATIENT WEIGHT GREATER THAN 300 LBS)	C	N	38	A		
L5999	LOWER EXTREMITY PROSTHESIS, NOT OTHERWISE SPECIFIED	C	N	46	A		
L6000	PARTIAL HAND, ROBIN-AIDS, THUMB REMAINING (OR EQUAL)	C	N	38	A		
L6010	PARTIAL HAND, ROBIN-AIDS, LITTLE AND/OR RING FINGER REMAINING (OR EQUAL)	C	N	38	A		
L6020	PARTIAL HAND, ROBIN-AIDS, NO FINGER REMAINING (OR EQUAL)	C	N	38	A		
L6025	TRANSCARPAL/METACARPAL OR PARTIAL HAND DISARTICULATION PROSTHESIS, EXTERNAL POWER, SELF-SUSPENDED, INNER SOCKET WITH REMOVABLE FOREARM SECTION, ELECTRODES AND CABLES, TWO BATTERIES, CHARGER, MYOELECTRIC CONTROL OF TERMINAL DEVICE	C	N	38	A		
L6050	WRIST DISARTICULATION, MOLDED SOCKET, FLEXIBLE ELBOW HINGES, TRICEPS PAD	C	N	38	A		
L6055	WRIST DISARTICULATION, MOLDED SOCKET WITH EXPANDABLE INTERFACE, FLEXIBLE ELBOW HINGES, TRICEPS PAD	C	N	38	A		
L6100	BELOW ELBOW, MOLDED SOCKET, FLEXIBLE ELBOW HINGE, TRICEPS PAD	C	N	38	A		
L6110	BELOW ELBOW, MOLDED SOCKET, (MUENSTER OR NORTHWESTERN SUSPENSION TYPES)	C	N	38	A		
L6120	BELOW ELBOW, MOLDED DOUBLE WALL SPLIT SOCKET, STEP-UP HINGES, HALF CUFF	C	N	38	A		
L6130	BELOW ELBOW, MOLDED DOUBLE WALL SPLIT SOCKET, STUMP ACTIVATED LOCKING HINGE, HALF CUFF	C	N	38	A		
L6200	ELBOW DISARTICULATION, MOLDED SOCKET, OUTSIDE LOCKING HINGE, FOREARM	C	N	38	A		

HCPCS Code	Statute	Lab Cert	X-Ref	ASC Pay Grp	ASC Pay Group Eff. Date	Proc Notes	BETOS	TOS	Anest	Code Add Date	Code Effective Date	Code Term Date
L5982							D1F	P	0	19890101	19960101	
L5984							D1F	P	0	19890101	20040101	
L5985							D1F	P	0	19960101	19960101	
L5986							D1F	P	0	19890101	19960101	
L5987							D1F	P	0	19970101	19970101	
L5988							D1F	P	0	19990101	20000101	
L5990							D1F	P	0	20020101	20020101	
L5993							D1F	P	0	20070101	20090101	20081231
L5994							D1F	P	0	20070101	20090101	20081231
L5995							D1F	P	0	20030101	20090101	20081231
L5999							D1F	P	0	19820101	19980101	
L6000							D1F	P	0	19820101	19960101	
L6010							D1F	P	0	19820101	19960101	
L6020							D1F	P	0	19820101	19960101	
L6025							D1F	P	0	20030101	20030101	
L6050							D1F	P	0	19820101	19960101	
L6055							D1F	P	0	19880101	19960101	
L6100							D1F	P	0	19820101	19960101	
L6110							D1F	P	0	19820101	19960101	
L6120							D1F	P	0	19820101	19960101	
L6130							D1F	P	0	19820101	19960101	
L6200							D1F	P	0	19820101	19960101	

L Codes

L Codes

HCPCS Code	Long Description	Coverage	Action	PI	MPI	CIM	MCM
L6205	ELBOW DISARTICULATION, MOLDED SOCKET WITH EXPANDABLE INTERFACE, OUTSIDE LOCKING HINGES, FOREARM	C	N	38	A		
L6250	ABOVE ELBOW, MOLDED DOUBLE WALL SOCKET, INTERNAL LOCKING ELBOW, FOREARM	C	N	38	A		
L6300	SHOULDER DISARTICULATION, MOLDED SOCKET, SHOULDER BULKHEAD, HUMERAL SECTION, INTERNAL LOCKING ELBOW, FOREARM	C	N	38	A		
L6310	SHOULDER DISARTICULATION, PASSIVE RESTORATION (COMPLETE PROSTHESIS)	C	N	38	A		
L6320	SHOULDER DISARTICULATION, PASSIVE RESTORATION (SHOULDER CAP ONLY)	C	N	38	A		
L6350	INTERSCAPULAR THORACIC, MOLDED SOCKET, SHOULDER BULKHEAD, HUMERAL SECTION, INTERNAL LOCKING ELBOW, FOREARM	C	N	38	A		
L6360	INTERSCAPULAR THORACIC, PASSIVE RESTORATION (COMPLETE PROSTHESIS)	C	N	38	A		
L6370	INTERSCAPULAR THORACIC, PASSIVE RESTORATION (SHOULDER CAP ONLY)	C	N	38	A		
L6380	IMMEDIATE POST SURGICAL OR EARLY FITTING, APPLICATION OF INITIAL RIGID DRESSING, INCLUDING FITTING ALIGNMENT AND SUSPENSION OF COMPONENTS, AND ONE CAST CHANGE, WRIST DISARTICULATION OR BELOW ELBOW	C	N	38	A		
L6382	IMMEDIATE POST SURGICAL OR EARLY FITTING, APPLICATION OF INITIAL RIGID DRESSING INCLUDING FITTING ALIGNMENT AND SUSPENSION OF COMPONENTS, AND ONE CAST CHANGE, ELBOW DISARTICULATION OR ABOVE ELBOW	C	N	38	A		
L6384	IMMEDIATE POST SURGICAL OR EARLY FITTING, APPLICATION OF INITIAL RIGID DRESSING INCLUDING FITTING ALIGNMENT AND SUSPENSION OF COMPONENTS, AND ONE CAST CHANGE, SHOULDER DISARTICULATION OR INTERSCAPULAR THORACIC	C	N	38	A		
L6386	IMMEDIATE POST SURGICAL OR EARLY FITTING, EACH ADDITIONAL CAST CHANGE AND REALIGNMENT	C	N	38	A		
L6388	IMMEDIATE POST SURGICAL OR EARLY FITTING, APPLICATION OF RIGID DRESSING ONLY	C	N	38	A		
L6400	BELOW ELBOW, MOLDED SOCKET, ENDOSKELETAL SYSTEM, INCLUDING SOFT PROSTHETIC TISSUE SHAPING	C	N	38	A		
L6450	ELBOW DISARTICULATION, MOLDED SOCKET, ENDOSKELETAL SYSTEM, INCLUDING SOFT PROSTHETIC TISSUE SHAPING	C	N	38	A		
L6500	ABOVE ELBOW, MOLDED SOCKET, ENDOSKELETAL SYSTEM, INCLUDING SOFT PROSTHETIC TISSUE SHAPING	C	N	38	A		
L6550	SHOULDER DISARTICULATION, MOLDED SOCKET, ENDOSKELETAL SYSTEM, INCLUDING SOFT PROSTHETIC TISSUE SHAPING	C	N	38	A		
L6570	INTERSCAPULAR THORACIC, MOLDED SOCKET, ENDOSKELETAL SYSTEM, INCLUDING SOFT PROSTHETIC TISSUE SHAPING	C	N	38	A		

HCPCS Code	S t a t u t e	Lab Cert	X-Ref	ASC Pay Grp	ASC Pay Group Eff. Date	Proc Notes	BETOS	TOS	A n e s t	Code Add Date	Code Effective Date	Code Term Date
L6205							D1F	P	0	19880101	19960101	
L6250							D1F	P	0	19820101	19960101	
L6300							D1F	P	0	19820101	19960101	
L6310							D1F	P	0	19820101	19960101	
L6320							D1F	P	0	19820101	19960101	
L6350							D1F	P	0	19840101	19960101	
L6360							D1F	P	0	19860101	19960101	
L6370							D1F	P	0	19860101	19960101	
L6380							D1F	P	0	19880101	19960101	
L6382							D1F	P	0	19880101	19960101	
L6384							D1F	P	0	19880101	19960101	
L6386							D1F	P	0	19880101	19960101	
L6388							D1F	P	0	19880101	19960101	
L6400							D1F	P	0	19820101	19960101	
L6450							D1F	P	0	19820101	19960101	
L6500							D1F	P	0	19820101	19960101	
L6550							D1F	P	0	19840101	19960101	
L6570							D1F	P	0	19840101	19960101	

HCPCS Code	Long Description	Coverage	Action	PI	MPI	CIM	MCM
L6580	PREPARATORY, WRIST DISARTICULATION OR BELOW ELBOW, SINGLE WALL PLASTIC SOCKET, FRICTION WRIST, FLEXIBLE ELBOW HINGES, FIGURE OF EIGHT HARNESS, HUMERAL CUFF, BOWDEN CABLE CONTROL, USMC OR EQUAL PYLON, NO COVER, MOLDED TO PATIENT MODEL	C	N	38	A		
L6582	PREPARATORY, WRIST DISARTICULATION OR BELOW ELBOW, SINGLE WALL SOCKET, FRICTION WRIST, FLEXIBLE ELBOW HINGES, FIGURE OF EIGHT HARNESS, HUMERAL CUFF, BOWDEN CABLE CONTROL, USMC OR EQUAL PYLON, NO COVER, DIRECT FORMED	C	N	38	A		
L6584	PREPARATORY, ELBOW DISARTICULATION OR ABOVE ELBOW, SINGLE WALL PLASTIC SOCKET, FRICTION WRIST, LOCKING ELBOW, FIGURE OF EIGHT HARNESS, FAIR LEAD CABLE CONTROL, USMC OR EQUAL PYLON, NO COVER, MOLDED TO PATIENT MODEL	C	N	38	A		
L6586	PREPARATORY, ELBOW DISARTICULATION OR ABOVE ELBOW, SINGLE WALL SOCKET, FRICTION WRIST, LOCKING ELBOW, FIGURE OF EIGHT HARNESS, FAIR LEAD CABLE CONTROL, USMC OR EQUAL PYLON, NO COVER, DIRECT FORMED	C	N	38	A		
L6588	PREPARATORY, SHOULDER DISARTICULATION OR INTERSCAPULAR THORACIC, SINGLE WALL PLASTIC SOCKET, SHOULDER JOINT, LOCKING ELBOW, FRICTION WRIST, CHEST STRAP, FAIR LEAD CABLE CONTROL, USMC OR EQUAL PYLON, NO COVER, MOLDED TO PATIENT MODEL	C	N	38	A		
L6590	PREPARATORY, SHOULDER DISARTICULATION OR INTERSCAPULAR THORACIC, SINGLE WALL SOCKET, SHOULDER JOINT, LOCKING ELBOW, FRICTION WRIST, CHEST STRAP, FAIR LEAD CABLE CONTROL, USMC OR EQUAL PYLON, NO COVER, DIRECT FORMED	C	N	38	A		
L6600	UPPER EXTREMITY ADDITIONS, POLYCENTRIC HINGE, PAIR	C	N	38	A		
L6605	UPPER EXTREMITY ADDITIONS, SINGLE PIVOT HINGE, PAIR	C	N	38	A		
L6610	UPPER EXTREMITY ADDITIONS, FLEXIBLE METAL HINGE, PAIR	C	N	38	A		
L6611	ADDITION TO UPPER EXTREMITY PROSTHESIS, EXTERNAL POWERED, ADDITIONAL SWITCH, ANY TYPE	C	N	38	A		
L6615	UPPER EXTREMITY ADDITION, DISCONNECT LOCKING WRIST UNIT	C	N	38	A		
L6616	UPPER EXTREMITY ADDITION, ADDITIONAL DISCONNECT INSERT FOR LOCKING WRIST UNIT, EACH	C	N	38	A		
L6620	UPPER EXTREMITY ADDITION, FLEXION/EXTENSION WRIST UNIT, WITH OR WITHOUT FRICTION	C	N	38	A		
L6621	UPPER EXTREMITY PROSTHESIS ADDITION, FLEXION/EXTENSION WRIST WITH OR WITHOUT FRICTION, FOR USE WITH EXTERNAL POWERED TERMINAL DEVICE	C	N	38	A		
L6623	UPPER EXTREMITY ADDITION, SPRING ASSISTED ROTATIONAL WRIST UNIT WITH LATCH RELEASE	C	N	38	A		
L6624	UPPER EXTREMITY ADDITION, FLEXION/EXTENSION AND ROTATION WRIST UNIT	C	N	38	A		
L6625	UPPER EXTREMITY ADDITION, ROTATION WRIST UNIT WITH CABLE LOCK	C	N	38	A		

HCPCS Code	Statute	Lab Cert	X-Ref	ASC Pay Grp	ASC Pay Group Eff. Date	Proc Notes	BETOS	TOS	Anest	Code Add Date	Code Effective Date	Code Term Date
L6580							D1F	P	0	19880101	19960101	
L6582							D1F	P	0	19880101	19960101	
L6584							D1F	P	0	19880101	19960101	
L6586							D1F	P	0	19880101	19960101	
L6588							D1F	P	0	19880101	19960101	
L6590							D1F	P	0	19880101	19960101	
							D1F	P	0	19820101	19960101	
L6605							D1F	P	0	19820101	19960101	
L6610							D1F	P	0	19820101	19960101	
L6611							D1F	P	0	20070101	20070101	
L6615							D1F	P	0	19860101	19960101	
L6616							D1F	P	0	19890101	19960101	
L6620							D1F	P	0	19860101	20040101	
L6621							D1F	P	0	20060101	20060101	
L6623							D1F	P	0	19880101	19960101	
L6624							D1F	P	0	20070101	20070101	
L6625							D1F	P	0	19860101	19960101	

HCPCS Code	Long Description	Coverage	Action	PI	MPI	CIM	MCM
L6628	UPPER EXTREMITY ADDITION, QUICK DISCONNECT HOOK ADAPTER, OTTO BOCK OR EQUAL	C	N	38	A		
L6629	UPPER EXTREMITY ADDITION, QUICK DISCONNECT LAMINATION COLLAR WITH COUPLING PIECE, OTTO BOCK OR EQUAL	C	N	38	A		
L6630	UPPER EXTREMITY ADDITION, STAINLESS STEEL, ANY WRIST	C	N	38	A		
L6632	UPPER EXTREMITY ADDITION, LATEX SUSPENSION SLEEVE, EA.	C	N	38	A		
L6635	UPPER EXTREMITY ADDITION, LIFT ASSIST FOR ELBOW	C	N	38	A		
L6637	UPPER EXTREMITY ADDITION, NUDGE CONTROL ELBOW LOCK	C	N	38	A		
L6638	UPPER EXTREMITY ADDITION TO PROSTHESIS, ELECTRIC LOCKING FEATURE, ONLY FOR USE WITH MANUALLY POWERED ELBOW	C	N	38	A		
L6639	UPPER EXTREMITY ADDITION, HEAVY DUTY FEATURE, ANY ELBOW	C	D	38	A		
L6640	UPPER EXTREMITY ADDITIONS, SHOULDER ABDUCTION JOINT, PAIR	C	N	38	A		
L6641	UPPER EXTREMITY ADDITION, EXCURSION AMPLIFIER, PULLEY TYPE	C	N	38	A		
L6642	UPPER EXTREMITY ADDITION, EXCURSION AMPLIFIER, LEVER TYPE	C	N	38	A		
L6645	UPPER EXTREMITY ADDITION, SHOULDER FLEXION-ABDUCTION JOINT, EACH	C	N	38	A		
L6646	UPPER EXTREMITY ADDITION, SHOULDER JOINT, MULTIPOSITIONAL LOCKING, FLEXION, ADJUSTABLE ABDUCTION FRICTION CONTROL, FOR USE WITH BODY POWERED OR EXTERNAL POWERED SYSTEM	C	N	38	A		
L6647	UPPER EXTREMITY ADDITION, SHOULDER LOCK MECHANISM, BODY POWERED ACTUATOR	C	N	38	A		
L6648	UPPER EXTREMITY ADDITION, SHOULDER LOCK MECHANISM, EXTERNAL POWERED ACTUATOR	C	N	38	A		
L6650	UPPER EXTREMITY ADDITION, SHOULDER UNIVERSAL JOINT, EA.	C	N	38	A		
L6655	UPPER EXTREMITY ADDITION, STANDARD CONTROL CABLE, EXTRA	C	N	38	A		
L6660	UPPER EXTREMITY ADDITION, HEAVY DUTY CONTROL CABLE	C	N	38	A		
L6665	UPPER EXTREMITY ADDITION, TEFLON, OR EQUAL, CABLE LINING	C	N	38	A		
L6670	UPPER EXTREMITY ADDITION, HOOK TO HAND, CABLE ADAPTER	C	N	38	A		
L6672	UPPER EXTREMITY ADDITION, HARNESS, CHEST OR SHOULDER, SADDLE TYPE	C	N	38	A		
L6675	UPPER EXTREMITY ADDITION, HARNESS, (E.G. FIGURE OF EIGHT TYPE), SINGLE CABLE DESIGN	C	N	38	A		
L6676	UPPER EXTREMITY ADDITION, HARNESS, (E.G. FIGURE OF EIGHT TYPE), DUAL CABLE DESIGN	C	N	38	A		
L6677	UPPER EXTREMITY ADDITION, HARNESS, TRIPLE CONTROL, SIMULTANEOUS OPERATION OF TERMINAL DEVICE & ELBOW	C	N	38	A		
L6680	UPPER EXTREMITY ADDITION, TEST SOCKET, WRIST DISARTICULATION OR BELOW ELBOW	C	N	38	A		

HCPCS Code	Statute	Lab Cert	X-Ref	ASC Pay Grp	ASC Pay Group Eff. Date	Proc Notes	BETOS	TOS	Anest	Code Add Date	Code Effective Date	Code Term Date
L6628							D1F	P	0	19880101	19960101	
L6629							D1F	P	0	19880101	19960101	
L6630							D1F	P	0	19860101	19960101	
L6632							D1F	P	0	19880101	19960101	
L6635							D1F	P	0	19860101	19960101	
L6637							D1F	P	0	19880101	19960101	
L6638							D1F	P	0	20030101	20030101	
L6639							D1F	P	0	20070101	20100101	20091231
L6640							D1F	P	0	19820101	19960101	
L6641							D1F	P	0	19880101	19960101	
L6642							D1F	P	0	19880101	19960101	
L6645							D1F	P	0	19860101	19960101	
L6646							D1F	P	0	20030101	20030101	
L6647							D1F	P	0	20030101	20030101	
L6648							D1F	P	0	20030101	20030101	
L6650							D1F	P	0	19860101	19960101	
L6655							D1F	P	0	19860101	19960101	
L6660							D1F	P	0	19860101	19960101	
L6665							D1F	P	0	19860101	19960101	
L6670							D1F	P	0	19860101	19960101	
L6672							D1F	P	0	19860101	19960101	
L6675							D1F	P	0	19860101	20040101	
L6676							D1F	P	0	19860101	20040101	
L6677							D1F	P	0	20060101	20060101	
L6680							D1F	P	0	19860101	19960101	

L Codes

HCPCS Code	Long Description	Coverage	Action	PI	MPI	CIM	MCM
L6682	UPPER EXTREMITY ADDITION, TEST SOCKET, ELBOW DISARTICULATION OR ABOVE ELBOW	C	N	38	A		
L6684	UPPER EXTREMITY ADDITION, TEST SOCKET, SHOULDER DISARTICULATION OR INTERSCAPULAR THORACIC	C	N	38	A		
L6686	UPPER EXTREMITY ADDITION, SUCTION SOCKET	C	N	38	A		
L6687	UPPER EXTREMITY ADDITION, FRAME TYPE SOCKET, BELOW ELBOW OR WRIST DISARTICULATION	C	N	38	A		
L6688	UPPER EXTREMITY ADDITION, FRAME TYPE SOCKET, ABOVE ELBOW OR ELBOW DISARTICULATION	C	N	38	A		
L6689	UPPER EXTREMITY ADDITION, FRAME TYPE SOCKET, SHOULDER DISARTICULATION	C	N	38	A		
L6690	UPPER EXTREMITY ADDITION, FRAME TYPE SOCKET, INTERSCAPULAR-THORACIC	C	N	38	A		
L6691	UPPER EXTREMITY ADDITION, REMOVABLE INSERT, EACH	C	N	38	A		
L6692	UPPER EXTREMITY ADDITION, SILICONE GEL INSERT OR EQUAL, EACH	C	N	38	A		
L6693	UPPER EXTREMITY ADDITION, LOCKING ELBOW, FOREARM COUNTERBALANCE	C	N	38	A		
L6694	ADDITION TO UPPER EXTREMITY PROSTHESIS, BELOW ELBOW/ABOVE ELBOW, CUSTOM FABRICATED FROM EXISTING MOLD OR PREFABRICATED, SOCKET INSERT, SILICONE GEL, ELASTOMERIC OR EQUAL, FOR USE WITH LOCKING MECHANISM	C	N	38	A		
L6695	ADDITION TO UPPER EXTREMITY PROSTHESIS, BELOW ELBOW/ABOVE ELBOW, CUSTOM FABRICATED FROM EXISTING MOLD OR PREFABRICATED, SOCKET INSERT, SILICONE GEL, ELASTOMERIC OR EQUAL, NOT FOR USE WITH LOCKING MECHANISM	C	N	38	A		
L6696	ADDITION TO UPPER EXTREMITY PROSTHESIS, BELOW ELBOW/ABOVE ELBOW, CUSTOM FABRICATED SOCKET INSERT FOR CONGENITAL OR ATYPICAL TRAUMATIC AMPUTEE, SILICONE GEL, ELASTOMERIC OR EQUAL, FOR USE WITH OR WITHOUT LOCKING MECHANISM, INITIAL ONLY (FOR OTHER THAN INITIAL, USE CODE L6694 OR L6695)	C	N	38	A		
L6697	ADDITION TO UPPER EXTREMITY PROSTHESIS, BELOW ELBOW/ABOVE ELBOW, CUSTOM FABRICATED SOCKET INSERT FOR OTHER THAN CONGENITAL OR ATYPICAL TRAUMATIC AMPUTEE, SILICONE GEL, ELASTOMERIC OR EQUAL, FOR USE WITH OR WITHOUT LOCKING MECHANISM, INITIAL ONLY (FOR OTHER THAN INITIAL, USE CODE L6694 OR L6695)	C	N	38	A		
L6698	ADDITION TO UPPER EXTREMITY PROSTHESIS, BELOW ELBOW/ABOVE ELBOW, LOCK MECHANISM, EXCLUDES SOCKET INSERT	C	N	38	A		
L6700	TERMINAL DEVICE, HOOK, DORRANCE, OR EQUAL, MODEL #3	D	N	38	A		2133
L6703	TERMINAL DEVICE, PASSIVE HAND/MITT, ANY MATERIAL, ANY SIZE	C	N	38	A		
L6704	TERMINAL DEVICE, SPORT/RECREATIONAL/WORK ATTACHMENT, ANY MATERIAL, ANY SIZE	C	N	38	A		

HCPCS Code	Statute	Lab Cert	X-Ref	ASC Pay Grp	ASC Pay Group Eff. Date	Proc Notes	BETOS	TOS	Anest	Code Add Date	Code Effective Date	Code Term Date
L6682							D1F	P	0	19860101	19960101	
L6684							D1F	P	0	19860101	19960101	
L6686							D1F	P	0	19880101	19960101	
L6687							D1F	P	0	19880101	19960101	
L6688							D1F	P	0	19880101	19960101	
L6689							D1F	P	0	19880101	19960101	
L6690							D1F	P	0	19880101	19960101	
L6691							D1F	P	0	19880101	19960101	
L6692							D1F	P	0	19890101	19960101	
L6693							D1F	P	0	19990101	20000101	
L6694							D1F	P	0	20050101	20050101	
L6695							D1F	P	0	20050101	20050101	
L6696							D1F	P	0	20050101	20050101	
L6697							D1F	P	0	20050101	20050101	
L6698							D1F	P	0	20050101	20050101	
L6700							D1F	P	0	19860101	20070101	20061231
L6703							D1F	P	0	20070101	20070101	
L6704							D1F	P	0	20070101	20070101	

HCPCS Code	Long Description	Coverage	Action	PI	MPI	CIM	MCM
L6705	TERMINAL DEVICE, HOOK, DORRANCE, OR EQUAL, MODEL #5	D	N	38	A		2133
L6706	TERMINAL DEVICE, HOOK, MECHANICAL, VOLUNTARY OPENING, ANY MATERIAL, ANY SIZE, LINED OR UNLINED	C	N	38	A		
L6707	TERMINAL DEVICE, HOOK, MECHANICAL, VOLUNTARY CLOSING, ANY MATERIAL, ANY SIZE, LINED OR UNLINED	C	N	38	A		
L6708	TERMINAL DEVICE, HAND, MECHANICAL, VOLUNTARY OPENING, ANY MATERIAL, ANY SIZE	C	N	38	A		
L6709	TERMINAL DEVICE, HAND, MECHANICAL, VOLUNTARY CLOSING, ANY MATERIAL, ANY SIZE	C	N	38	A		
L6710	TERMINAL DEVICE, HOOK, DORRANCE, OR EQUAL, MODEL #5X	D	N	38	A		2133
L6711	TERMINAL DEVICE, HOOK, MECHANICAL, VOLUNTARY OPENING, ANY MATERIAL, ANY SIZE, LINED OR UNLINED, PEDIATRIC	C	N	38	A		
L6712	TERMINAL DEVICE, HOOK, MECHANICAL, VOLUNTARY CLOSING, ANY MATERIAL, ANY SIZE, LINED OR UNLINED, PEDIATRIC	C	N	38	A		
L6713	TERMINAL DEVICE, HAND, MECHANICAL, VOLUNTARY OPENING, ANY MATERIAL, ANY SIZE, PEDIATRIC	C	N	38	A		
L6714	TERMINAL DEVICE, HAND, MECHANICAL, VOLUNTARY CLOSING, ANY MATERIAL, ANY SIZE, PEDIATRIC	C	N	38	A		
L6715	TERMINAL DEVICE, HOOK, DORRANCE, OR EQUAL, MODEL #5XA	D	N	38	A		2133
L6720	TERMINAL DEVICE, HOOK, DORRANCE, OR EQUAL, MODEL #6	D	N	38	A		2133
L6721	TERMINAL DEVICE, HOOK OR HAND, HEAVY DUTY, MECHANICAL, VOLUNTARY OPENING, ANY MATERIAL, ANY SIZE, LINED OR UNLINED	C	N	38	A		
L6722	TERMINAL DEVICE, HOOK OR HAND, HEAVY DUTY, MECHANICAL, VOLUNTARY CLOSING, ANY MATERIAL, ANY SIZE, LINED OR UNLINED	C	N	38	A		
L6725	TERMINAL DEVICE, HOOK, DORRANCE, OR EQUAL, MODEL #7	D	N	38	A		2133
L6730	TERMINAL DEVICE, HOOK, DORRANCE, OR EQUAL, MODEL #7LO	D	N	38	A		2133
L6735	TERMINAL DEVICE, HOOK, DORRANCE, OR EQUAL, MODEL #8	D	N	38	A		2133
L6740	TERMINAL DEVICE, HOOK, DORRANCE, OR EQUAL, MODEL #8X	D	N	38	A		2133
L6745	TERMINAL DEVICE, HOOK, DORRANCE, OR EQUAL, MODEL #88X	D	N	38	A		2133
L6750	TERMINAL DEVICE, HOOK, DORRANCE, OR EQUAL, MODEL #10P	D	N	38	A		2133
L6755	TERMINAL DEVICE, HOOK, DORRANCE, OR EQUAL, MODEL #10X	D	N	38	A		2133
L6765	TERMINAL DEVICE, HOOK, DORRANCE, OR EQUAL, MODEL #12P	D	N	38	A		2133
L6770	TERMINAL DEVICE, HOOK, DORRANCE, OR EQUAL, MODEL #99X	D	N	38	A		2133
L6775	TERMINAL DEVICE, HOOK, DORRANCE, OR EQUAL, MODEL #555	D	N	38	A		2133
L6780	TERMINAL DEVICE, HOOK, DORRANCE, OR EQUAL, MODEL #SS555	D	N	38	A		2133

HCPCS Code	Statute	Lab Cert	X-Ref	ASC Pay Grp	ASC Pay Group Eff. Date	Proc Notes	BETOS	TOS	Anest	Code Add Date	Code Effective Date	Code Term Date
L6705							D1F	P	0	19860101	20070101	20061231
L6706							D1F	P	0	20070101	20070101	
L6707							D1F	P	0	20070101	20070101	
L6708							D1F	P	0	20070101	20070101	
L6709							D1F	P	0	20070101	20070101	
L6710							D1F	P	0	19860101	20070101	20061231
L6711							D1F	P	0	20090101	20090101	
L6712							D1F	P	0	20090101	20090101	
L6713							D1F	P	0	20090101	20090101	
L6714							D1F	P	0	20090101	20090101	
L6715							D1F	P	0	19860101	20070101	20061231
L6720							D1F	P	0	19860101	20070101	20061231
L6721							D1F	P	0	20090101	20090101	
L6722							D1F	P	0	20090101	20090101	
L6722												
L6725							D1F	P	0	19860101	20070101	20061231
L6730							D1F	P	0	19860101	20070101	20061231
L6735							D1F	P	0	19860101	20070101	20061231
L6740							D1F	P	0	19860101	20070101	20061231
L6745							D1F	P	0	19860101	20070101	20061231
L6750							D1F	P	0	19860101	20070101	20061231
L6755							D1F	P	0	19860101	20070101	20061231
L6765							D1F	P	0	19860101	20070101	20061231
L6770							D1F	P	0	19860101	20070101	20061231
L6775							D1F	P	0	19860101	20070101	20061231
L6780							D1F	P	0	19860101	20070101	20061231

HCPCS Code	Long Description	Coverage	Action	PI	MPI	CIM	MCM
L6790	TERMINAL DEVICE, HOOK-ACCU HOOK, OR EQUAL	D	N	38	A		2133
L6795	TERMINAL DEVICE, HOOK-2 LOAD, OR EQUAL	D	N	38	A		2133
L6800	TERMINAL DEVICE, HOOK-APRL VC, OR EQUAL	D	N	38	A		2133
L6805	ADDITION TO TERMINAL DEVICE, MODIFIER WRIST UNIT	D	N	38	A		2133
L6806	TERMINAL DEVICE, HOOK, TRS GRIP, GRIP III, VC, OR EQUAL	D	N	38	A		2133
L6807	TERMINAL DEVICE, HOOK, GRIP I, GRIP II, VC, OR EQUAL	D	N	38	A		2133
L6808	TERMINAL DEVICE, HOOK, TRS ADEPT, INFANT OR CHILD, VC, OR EQUAL	D	N	38	A		2133
L6809	TERMINAL DEVICE, HOOK, TRS SUPER SPORT, PASSIVE	D	N	38	A		2133
L6810	ADDITION TO TERMINAL DEVICE, PRECISION PINCH DEVICE	D	N	38	A		2133
L6825	TERMINAL DEVICE, HAND, DORRANCE, VO	D	N	38	A		2133
L6830	TERMINAL DEVICE, HAND, APRL, VC	D	N	38	A		2133
L6835	TERMINAL DEVICE, HAND, SIERRA, VO	D	N	38	A		2133
L6840	TERMINAL DEVICE, HAND, BECKER IMPERIAL	D	N	38	A		2133
L6845	TERMINAL DEVICE, HAND, BECKER LOCK GRIP	D	N	38	A		2133
L6850	TERMINAL DEVICE, HAND, BECKER PLYLITE	D	N	38	A		2133
L6855	TERMINAL DEVICE, HAND, ROBIN-AIDS, VO	D	N	38	A		2133
L6860	TERMINAL DEVICE, HAND, ROBIN-AIDS, VO SOFT	D	N	38	A		2133
L6865	TERMINAL DEVICE, HAND, PASSIVE HAND	D	N	38	A		2133
L6867	TERMINAL DEVICE, HAND, DETROIT INFANT HAND (MECHANICAL)	D	N	38	A		2133
L6868	TERMINAL DEVICE, HAND, PASSIVE INFANT HAND, (STEEPER, HOSMER OR EQUAL)	D	N	38	A		2133
L6870	TERMINAL DEVICE, HAND, CHILD MITT	D	N	38	A		2133
L6872	TERMINAL DEVICE, HAND, NYU CHILD HAND	D	N	38	A		2133
L6873	TERMINAL DEVICE, HAND, MECHANICAL INFANT HAND, STEEPER OR EQUAL	D	N	38	A		2133
L6875	TERMINAL DEVICE, HAND, BOCK, VC	D	N	38	A		2133
L6880	TERMINAL DEVICE, HAND, BOCK, VO	D	N	38	A		2133
L6881	AUTOMATIC GRASP FEATURE, ADDITION TO UPPER LIMB ELECTRIC PROSTHETIC TERMINAL DEVICE	C	N	38	A		
L6882	MICROPROCESSOR CONTROL FEATURE, ADDITION TO UPPER LIMB PROSTHETIC TERMINAL DEVICE	D	N	38	A		2133
L6883	REPLACEMENT SOCKET, BELOW ELBOW/WRIST DISARTICULATION, MOLDED TO PATIENT MODEL, FOR USE WITH OR WITHOUT EXTERNAL POWER	C	N	38	A		
L6884	REPLACEMENT SOCKET, ABOVE ELBOW/ELBOW DISARTICULATION, MOLDED TO PATIENT MODEL, FOR USE WITH OR WITHOUT EXTERNAL POWER	C	N	38	A		
L6885	REPLACEMENT SOCKET, SHOULDER DISARTICULATION/ INTERSCAPULAR THORACIC, MOLDED TO PATIENT MODEL, FOR USE WITH OR WITHOUT EXTERNAL POWER	C	N	38	A		
L6890	ADDITION TO UPPER EXTREMITY PROSTHESIS, GLOVE FOR TERMINAL DEVICE, ANY MATERIAL, PREFABRICATED, INCLUDES FITTING AND ADJUSTMENT	C	N	38	A		
L6895	ADDITION TO UPPER EXTREMITY PROSTHESIS, GLOVE FOR TERMINAL DEVICE, ANY MATERIAL, CUSTOM FABRICATED	C	N	38	A		
L6900	HAND RESTORATION (CASTS, SHADING AND MEASUREMENTS INCLUDED), PARTIAL HAND, WITH GLOVE, THUMB OR ONE FINGER REMAINING	C	N	38	A		

HCPCS Code	Statute	Lab Cert	X-Ref	ASC Pay Grp	ASC Pay Group Eff. Date	Proc Notes	BETOS	TOS	Anest	Code Add Date	Code Effective Date	Code Term Date
L6790							D1F	P	0	19860101	20070101	20061231
L6795							D1F	P	0	19860101	20070101	20061231
L6800							D1F	P	0	19860101	20070101	20061231
L6805							D1F	P	0	19850101	20070101	
L6806							D1F	P	0	19880101	20070101	20061231
L6807							D1F	P	0	19880101	20070101	20061231
L6808							D1F	P	0	19880101	20070101	20061231
L6809							D1F	P	0	19880101	20070101	20061231
L6810							D1F	P	0	19880101	20070101	
L6825							D1F	P	0	19820101	20070101	20061231
L6830							D1F	P	0	19860101	20070101	20061231
L6835							D1F	P	0	19860101	20070101	20061231
L6840							D1F	P	0	19860101	20070101	20061231
L6845							D1F	P	0	19860101	20070101	20061231
L6850							D1F	P	0	19860101	20070101	20061231
L6855							D1F	P	0	19860101	20070101	20061231
L6860							D1F	P	0	19860101	20070101	20061231
L6865							D1F	P	0	19860101	20070101	20061231
L6867							D1F	P	0	19880101	20070101	20061231
L6868							D1F	P	0	19880101	20070101	20061231
L6870							D1F	P	0	19860101	20070101	20061231
L6872							D1F	P	0	19880101	20070101	20061231
L6873							D1F	P	0	19880101	20070101	20061231
L6875							D1F	P	0	19860101	20070101	20061231
L6880							D1F	P	0	19860101	20070101	20061231
L6881							D1F	P	0	20020101	20070101	
L6882							D1F	P	0	20020101	20020101	
L6883							D1F	P	0	20060101	20060101	
L6884							D1F	P	0	20060101	20070101	
L6885							D1F	P	0	20060101	20060101	
L6890							D1F	P	0	19860101	20050101	
L6895							D1F	P	0	19860101	20050101	
L6900							D1F	P	0	19820101	19960101	

HCPCS Code	Long Description	Coverage	Action	PI	MPI	CIM	MCM
L6905	HAND RESTORATION (CASTS, SHADING AND MEASUREMENTS INCLUDED), PARTIAL HAND, WITH GLOVE, MULTIPLE FINGERS REMAINING	C	N	38	A		
L6910	HAND RESTORATION (CASTS, SHADING AND MEASUREMENTS INCLUDED), PARTIAL HAND, WITH GLOVE, NO FINGERS REMAINING	C	N	38	A		
L6915	HAND RESTORATION (SHADING, AND MEASUREMENTS INCLUDED), REPLACEMENT GLOVE FOR ABOVE	C	N	38	A		
L6920	WRIST DISARTICULATION, EXTERNAL POWER, SELF-SUSPENDED INNER SOCKET, REMOVABLE FOREARM SHELL, OTTO BOCK OR EQUAL, SWITCH, CABLES, TWO BATTERIES & ONE CHARGER, SWITCH CONTROL OF TERMINAL DEVICE	C	N	38	A		
L6925	WRIST DISARTICULATION, EXTERNAL POWER, SELF-SUSPENDED INNER SOCKET, REMOVABLE FOREARM SHELL, OTTO BOCK OR EQUAL ELECTRODES, CABLES, TWO BATTERIES AND ONE CHARGER, MYOELECTRONIC CONTROL OF TERMINAL DEVICE	C	N	38	A		
L6930	BELOW ELBOW, EXTERNAL POWER, SELF-SUSPENDED INNER SOCKET, REMOVABLE FOREARM SHELL, OTTO BOCK OR EQUAL SWITCH, CABLES, TWO BATTERIES AND ONE CHARGER, SWITCH CONTROL OF TERMINAL DEVICE	C	N	38	A		
L6935	BELOW ELBOW, EXTERNAL POWER, SELF-SUSPENDED INNER SOCKET, REMOVABLE FOREARM SHELL, OTTO BOCK OR EQUAL ELECTRODES, CABLES, TWO BATTERIES AND ONE CHARGER, MYOELECTRONIC CONTROL OF TERMINAL DEVICE	C	N	38	A		
L6940	ELBOW DISARTICULATION, EXTERNAL POWER, MOLDED INNER SOCKET, REMOVABLE HUMERAL SHELL, OUTSIDE LOCKING HINGES, FOREARM, OTTO BOCK OR EQUAL SWITCH, CABLES, TWO BATTERIES AND ONE CHARGER, SWITCH CONTROL OF TERMINAL DEVICE	C	N	38	A		
L6945	ELBOW DISARTICULATION, EXTERNAL POWER, MOLDED INNER SOCKET, REMOVABLE HUMERAL SHELL, OUTSIDE LOCKING HINGES, FOREARM, OTTO BOCK OR EQUAL ELECTRODES, CABLES, TWO BATTERIES AND ONE CHARGER, MYOELECTRONIC CONTROL OF TERMINAL DEVICE	C	N	38	A		
L6950	ABOVE ELBOW, EXTERNAL POWER, MOLDED INNER SOCKET, REMOVABLE HUMERAL SHELL, INTERNAL LOCKING ELBOW, FOREARM, OTTO BOCK OR EQUAL SWITCH, CABLES, TWO BATTERIES AND ONE CHARGER, SWITCH CONTROL OF TERMINAL DEVICE	C	N	38	A		
L6955	ABOVE ELBOW, EXTERNAL POWER, MOLDED INNER SOCKET, REMOVABLE HUMERAL SHELL, INTERNAL LOCKING ELBOW, FOREARM, OTTO BOCK OR EQUAL ELECTRODES, CABLES, TWO BATTERIES AND ONE CHARGER, MYOELECTRONIC CONTROL OF TERMINAL DEVICE	C	N	38	A		

HCPCS Code	Statute	Lab Cert	X-Ref	ASC Pay Grp	ASC Pay Group Eff. Date	Proc Notes	BETOS	TOS	Anest	Code Add Date	Code Effective Date	Code Term Date
L6905							D1F	P	0	19860101	19960101	
L6910							D1F	P	0	19820101	19960101	
L6915							D1F	P	0	19820101	19960101	
L6920							D1F	P	0	19880101	19960101	
L6925							D1F	P	0	19880101	19960101	
L6930							D1F	P	0	19880101	19960101	
L6935							D1F	P	0	19880101	19960101	
L6940							D1F	P	0	19880101	19960101	
L6945							D1F	P	0	19880101	19960101	
L6950							D1F	P	0	19880101	19960101	
L6955							D1F	P	0	19880101	19960101	

HCPCS Code	Long Description	Coverage	Action	PI	MPI	CIM	MCM
L6960	SHOULDER DISARTICULATION, EXTERNAL POWER, MOLDED INNER SOCKET, REMOVABLE SHOULDER SHELL, SHOULDER BULKHEAD, HUMERAL SECTION, MECHANICAL ELBOW, FOREARM, OTTO BOCK OR EQUAL SWITCH, CABLES, TWO BATTERIES AND ONE CHARGER, SWITCH CONTROL OF TERMINAL DEVICE	C	N	38	A		
L6965	SHOULDER DISARTICULATION, EXTERNAL POWER, MOLDED INNER SOCKET, REMOVABLE SHOULDER SHELL, SHOULDER BULKHEAD, HUMERAL SECTION, MECHANICAL ELBOW, FOREARM, OTTO BOCK OR EQUAL ELECTRODES, CABLES, TWO BATTERIES AND ONE CHARGER, MYOELECTRONIC CONTROL OF TERMINAL DEVICE	C	N	38	A		
L6970	INTERSCAPULAR-THORACIC, EXTERNAL POWER, MOLDED INNER SOCKET, REMOVABLE SHOULDER SHELL, SHOULDER BULKHEAD, HUMERAL SECTION, MECHANICAL ELBOW, FOREARM, OTTO BOCK OR EQUAL SWITCH, CABLES, TWO BATTERIES AND ONE CHARGER, SWITCH CONTROL OF TERMINAL DEVICE	C	N	38	A		
L6975	INTERSCAPULAR-THORACIC, EXTERNAL POWER, MOLDED INNER SOCKET, REMOVABLE SHOULDER SHELL, SHOULDER BULKHEAD, HUMERAL SECTION, MECHANICAL ELBOW, FOREARM, OTTO BOCK OR EQUAL ELECTRODES, CABLES, TWO BATTERIES AND ONE CHARGER, MYOELECTRONIC CONTROL OF TERMINAL DEVICE	C	N	38	A		
L7007	ELECTRIC HAND, SWITCH OR MYOELECTRIC CONTROLLED, ADULT	C	N	38	A		
L7008	ELECTRIC HAND, SWITCH OR MYOELECTRIC, CONTROLLED, PEDIATRIC	C	N	38	A		
L7009	ELECTRIC HOOK, SWITCH OR MYOELECTRIC CONTROLLED, ADULT	C	N	38	A		
L7010	ELECTRONIC HAND, OTTO BOCK, STEEPER OR EQUAL, SWITCH CONTROLLED	C	N	38	A		
L7015	ELECTRONIC HAND, SYSTEM TEKNIK, VARIETY VILLAGE OR EQUAL, SWITCH CONTROLLED	C	N	38	A		
L7020	ELECTRONIC GREIFER, OTTO BOCK OR EQUAL, SWITCH CONTROLLED	C	N	38	A		
L7025	ELECTRONIC HAND, OTTO BOCK OR EQUAL, MYOELECTRONICALLY CONTROLLED	C	N	38	A		
L7030	ELECTRONIC HAND, SYSTEM TEKNIK, VARIETY VILLAGE OR EQUAL, MYOELECTRONICALLY CONTROLLED	C	N	38	A		
L7035	ELECTRONIC GREIFER, OTTO BOCK OR EQUAL, MYOELECTRONICALLY CONTROLLED	C	N	38	A		
L7040	PREHENSILE ACTUATOR, SWITCH CONTROLLED	C	N	38	A		
L7045	ELECTRIC HOOK, SWITCH OR MYOELECTRIC CONTROLLED, PEDIATRIC	C	N	38	A		
L7170	ELECTRONIC ELBOW, HOSMER OR EQUAL, SWITCH CONTROLLED	C	N	38	A		
L7180	ELECTRONIC ELBOW, MICROPROCESSOR SEQUENTIAL CONTROL OF ELBOW AND TERMINAL DEVICE	C	N	38	A		

HCPCS Code	Statute	Lab Cert	X-Ref	ASC Pay Grp	ASC Pay Group Eff. Date	Proc Notes	BETOS	TOS	Anest	Code Add Date	Code Effective Date	Code Term Date
L6960							D1F	P	0	19880101	19960101	
L6960 L6965							D1F	P	0	19880101	19960101	
L6970							D1F	P	0	19880101	19960101	
L6975							D1F	P	0	19880101	19960101	
L7007							D1F	P	0	20070101	20070101	
L7008							D1F	P	0	20070101	20070101	
L7009							D1F	P	0	20070101	20070101	
L7010							D1F	P	0	19880101	20070101	20061231
L7015							D1F	P	0	19880101	20070101	20061231
L7020							D1F	P	0	19880101	20070101	20061231
L7025							D1F	P	0	19880101	20070101	20061231
L7030			L7008				D1F	P	0	19880101	20070101	20061231
L7035			L7009				D1F	P	0	19880101	20070101	20061231
L7040							D1F	P	0	19880101	20070101	
L7045							D1F	P	0	19880101	20070101	
L7170							D1F	P	0	19880101	19960101	
L7180							D1F	P	0	19880101	20050101	

HCPCS Code	Long Description	Coverage	Action	PI	MPI	CIM	MCM
L7181	ELECTRONIC ELBOW, MICROPROCESSOR SIMULTANEOUS CONTROL OF ELBOW AND TERMINAL DEVICE	C	N	38	A		
L7185	ELECTRONIC ELBOW, ADOLESCENT, VARIETY VILLAGE OR EQUAL, SWITCH CONTROLLED	C	N	38	A		
L7186	ELECTRONIC ELBOW, CHILD, VARIETY VILLAGE OR EQUAL, SWITCH CONTROLLED	C	N	38	A		
L7190	ELECTRONIC ELBOW, ADOLESCENT, VARIETY VILLAGE OR EQUAL, MYOELECTRONICALLY CONTROLLED	C	N	38	A		
L7191	ELECTRONIC ELBOW, CHILD, VARIETY VILLAGE OR EQUAL, MYOELECTRONICALLY CONTROLLED	C	N	38	A		
L7260	ELECTRONIC WRIST ROTATOR, OTTO BOCK OR EQUAL	C	N	38	A		
L7261	ELECTRONIC WRIST ROTATOR, FOR UTAH ARM	C	N	38	A		
L7266	SERVO CONTROL, STEEPER OR EQUAL	C	N	38	A		
L7272	ANALOGUE CONTROL, UNB OR EQUAL	C	N	38	A		
L7274	PROPORTIONAL CONTROL, 6-12 VOLT, LIBERTY, UTAH OR EQUAL	C	N	38	A		
L7360	SIX VOLT BATTERY, EACH	C	N	38	A		
L7362	BATTERY CHARGER, SIX VOLT, EACH	C	N	38	A		
L7364	TWELVE VOLT BATTERY, EACH	C	N	38	A		
L7366	BATTERY CHARGER, TWELVE VOLT, EACH	C	N	38	A		
L7367	LITHIUM ION BATTERY, REPLACEMENT	C	N	38	A		
L7368	LITHIUM ION BATTERY CHARGER	C	N	38	A		
L7400	ADDITION TO UPPER EXTREMITY PROSTHESIS, BELOW ELBOW/WRIST DISARTICULATION, ULTRALIGHT MATERIAL (TITANIUM, CARBON FIBER OR EQUAL)	C	N	38	A		
L7401	ADDITION TO UPPER EXTREMITY PROSTHESIS, ABOVE ELBOW DISARTICULATION, ULTRALIGHT MATERIAL (TITANIUM, CARBON FIBER OR EQUAL)	C	N	38	A		
L7402	ADDITION TO UPPER EXTREMITY PROSTHESIS, SHOULDER DISARTICULATION/INTERSCAPULAR THORACIC, ULTRALIGHT MATERIAL (TITANIUM, CARBON FIBER OR EQUAL)	C	N	38	A		
L7403	ADDITION TO UPPER EXTREMITY PROSTHESIS, BELOW ELBOW/WRIST DISARTICULATION, ACRYLIC MATERIAL	C	N	38	A		
L7404	ADDITION TO UPPER EXTREMITY PROSTHESIS, ABOVE ELBOW DISARTICULATION, ACRYLIC MATERIAL	C	N	38	A		
L7405	ADDITION TO UPPER EXTREMITY PROSTHESIS, SHOULDER DISARTICULATION/INTERSCAPULAR THORACIC, ACRYLIC MATERIAL	C	N	38	A		
L7499	UPPER EXTREMITY PROSTHESIS, NOT OTHERWISE SPECIFIED	C	N	46	A		
L7500	REPAIR OF PROSTHETIC DEVICE, HOURLY RATE (EXCLUDES V5335 REPAIR OF ORAL OR LARYNGEAL PROSTHESIS OR ARTIFICIAL LARYNX)	D	N	46	A		2100.4, 2130D, 2133
L7510	REPAIR OF PROSTHETIC DEVICE, REPAIR OR REPLACE MINOR PARTS	D	N	46	A		2100.4, 2130D, 2133
L7520	REPAIR PROSTHETIC DEVICE, LABOR COMPONENT, PER 15 MINUTES	C	N	46	A		
L7600	PROSTHETIC DONNING SLEEVE, ANY MATERIAL, EACH	S	N	00	9		
L7611	TERMINAL DEVICE, HOOK, MECHANICAL, VOLUNTARY OPENING, ANY MATERIAL, ANY SIZE, LINED OR UNLINED, PEDIATRIC	C	N	38	A		

HCPCS Code	Statute	Lab Cert	X-Ref	ASC Pay Grp	ASC Pay Group Eff. Date	Proc Notes	BETOS	TOS	Anest	Code Add Date	Code Effective Date	Code Term Date
L7181							D1F	P	0	20050101	20050101	
L7185							D1F	P	0	19880101	19960101	
L7186							D1F	P	0	19890101	19960101	
L7190							D1F	P	0	19880101	19960101	
L7191							D1F	P	0	19890101	19960101	
L7260							D1F	P	0	19880101	19960101	
L7261							D1F	P	0	19880101	19960101	
L7266							D1F	P	0	19880101	19960101	
L7272							D1F	P	0	19880101	19960101	
L7274							D1F	P	0	19880101	19970101	
L7360							D1F	P	0	19880101	20080101	
L7362							D1F	P	0	19880101	20080101	
L7364							D1F	P	0	19880101	20080101	
L7366							D1F	P	0	19880101	20080101	
L7367							D1F	P	0	20030101	20030101	
L7368							D1F	P	0	20030101	20030101	
L7400							D1F	P	0	20060101	20060101	
L7401							D1F	P	0	20060101	20060101	
L7402							D1F	P	0	20060101	20060101	
L7403							D1F	P	0	20060101	20060101	
L7404							D1F	P	0	20060101	20060101	
L7405							D1F	P	0	20060101	20060101	
L7499							D1F	P	0	19850101	19980101	
L7500							D1F	P	0	19820101	19960101	
L7510							D1F	P	0	19850101	20030101	
L7520							D1F	P	0	19970101	20000101	
L7600	1862(1)(a)						D1F	P	0	20060101	20060101	
L7611			L6711				D1F	P	0	20080101	20090101	20081231

L Codes

HCPCS Code	Long Description	Coverage	Action	PI	MPI	CIM	MCM
L7612	TERMINAL DEVICE, HOOK, MECHANICAL, VOLUNTARY CLOSING, ANY MATERIAL, ANY SIZE, LINED OR UNLINED, PEDIATRIC	C	N	38	A		
L7613	TERMINAL DEVICE, HAND, MECHANICAL, VOLUNTARY OPENING, ANY MATERIAL, ANY SIZE, PEDIATRIC	C	N	38	A		
L7614	TERMINAL DEVICE, HAND, MECHANICAL, VOLUNTARY CLOSING, ANY MATERIAL, ANY SIZE, PEDIATRIC	C	N	38	A		
L7621	TERMINAL DEVICE, HOOK OR HAND, HEAVY DUTY, MECHANICAL, VOLUNTARY OPENING, ANY MATERIAL, ANY SIZE, LINED OR UNLINED	C	N	38	A		
L7622	TERMINAL DEVICE, HOOK OR HAND, HEAVY DUTY, MECHANICAL, VOLUNTARY CLOSING, ANY MATERIAL, ANY SIZE, LINED OR UNLINED	C	N	38	A		
L7900	MALE VACUUM ERECTION SYSTEM	C	N	38	A		
L8000	BREAST PROSTHESIS, MASTECTOMY BRA	D	N	38	A		2130 A
L8001	BREAST PROSTHESIS, MASTECTOMY BRA, WITH INTEGRATED BREAST PROSTHESIS FORM, UNILATERAL	D	N	38	A		2130A
L8002	BREAST PROSTHESIS, MASTECTOMY BRA, WITH INTEGRATED BREAST PROSTHESIS FORM, BILATERAL	D	N	38	A		2130A
L8010	BREAST PROSTHESIS, MASTECTOMY SLEEVE	D	N	00	9		2130 A
L8015	EXTERNAL BREAST PROSTHESIS GARMENT, WITH MASTECTOMY FORM, POST MASTECTOMY	D	N	38	A		2130
L8020	BREAST PROSTHESIS, MASTECTOMY FORM	D	N	38	A		2130 A
L8030	BREAST PROSTHESIS, SILICONE OR EQUAL, WITHOUT INTEGRAL ADHESIVE	D	C	38	A		2130 A
L8031	BREAST PROSTHESIS, SILICONE OR EQUAL, WITH INTEGRAL ADHESIVE	D	A	38	A		2130 A
L8032	NIPPLE PROSTHESIS, REUSABLE, ANY TYPE, EACH	C	A	38	A		
L8035	CUSTOM BREAST PROSTHESIS, POST MASTECTOMY, MOLDED TO PATIENT MODEL	D	N	38	A		2130
L8039	BREAST PROSTHESIS, NOT OTHERWISE SPECIFIED	C	N	46	A		
L8040	NASAL PROSTHESIS, PROVIDED BY A NON-PHYSICIAN	C	N	38	A		
L8041	MIDFACIAL PROSTHESIS, PROVIDED BY A NON-PHYSICIAN	C	N	38	A		
L8042	ORBITAL PROSTHESIS, PROVIDED BY A NON-PHYSICIAN	C	N	38	A		
L8043	UPPER FACIAL PROSTHESIS, PROVIDED BY A NON-PHYSICIAN	C	N	38	A		
L8044	HEMI-FACIAL PROSTHESIS, PROVIDED BY A NON-PHYSICIAN	C	N	38	A		
L8045	AURICULAR PROSTHESIS, PROVIDED BY A NON-PHYSICIAN	C	N	38	A		
L8046	PARTIAL FACIAL PROSTHESIS, PROVIDED BY A NON-PHYSICIAN	C	N	38	A		
L8047	NASAL SEPTAL PROSTHESIS, PROVIDED BY A NON-PHYSICIAN	C	N	38	A		
L8048	UNSPECIFIED MAXILLOFACIAL PROSTHESIS, BY REPORT, PROVIDED BY A NON-PHYSICIAN	C	N	46	A		
L8049	REPAIR OR MODIFICATION OF MAXILLOFACIAL PROSTHESIS, LABOR COMPONENT, 15 MINUTE INCREMENTS, PROVIDED BY A NON-PHYSICIAN	C	N	46	A		
L8300	TRUSS, SINGLE WITH STANDARD PAD	D	N	38	A	70-1,0-2	2133
L8310	TRUSS, DOUBLE WITH STANDARD PADS	D	N	38	A	70-1,0-2	2133
L8320	TRUSS, ADDITION TO STANDARD PAD, WATER PAD	D	N	38	A	70-1,0-2	2133
L8330	TRUSS, ADDITION TO STANDARD PAD, SCROTAL PAD	D	N	38	A	70-1,0-2	2133
L8400	PROSTHETIC SHEATH, BELOW KNEE, EACH	D	N	38	A		2133

HCPCS Code	Statute	Lab Cert	X-Ref	ASC Pay Grp	ASC Pay Group Eff. Date	Proc Notes	BETOS	TOS	Anest	Code Add Date	Code Effective Date	Code Term Date
L7612			L6712				D1F	P	0	20080101	20090101	20081231
L7613			L6713				D1F	P	0	20080101	20090101	20081231
L7614			L6714				D1F	P	0	20080101	20090101	20081231
L7621			L6721				D1F	P	0	20080101	20090101	20081231
L7622			L6722				D1F	P	0	20080101	20090101	20081231
L7900							D1F	P	0	19970101	20030101	
L8000							D1F	P	0	19860101	19960101	
L8001							D1F	P	0	20020101	20020101	
L8002							D1F	P	0	20020101	20020101	
L8010							D1F	P	0	19860101	20050401	
L8015							D1F	P	0	19990101	19990101	
L8020							D1F	P	0	19860101	19960101	
L8030							D1F	P	0	19890101	20100101	
L8031							D1F	P	0	20100101	20100101	
L8032							D1F	P	0	20100101	20100101	
L8035							D1F	P	0	19990101	19990101	
L8039							D1F	P	0	19980101	19980101	
L8040							D1F	P	0	20010101	20010101	
L8041							D1F	P	0	20010101	20010101	
L8042							D1F	P	0	20010101	20010101	
L8043							D1F	P	0	20010101	20010101	
L8044							D1F	P	0	20010101	20010101	
L8045							D1F	P	0	20010101	20010101	
L8046							D1F	P	0	20010101	20010101	
L8047							D1F	P	0	20010101	20010101	
L8048							D1F	P	0	20010101	20010101	
L8049							D1F	P	0	20010101	20010101	
L8300							D1F	P	0	19860101	19960101	
L8310							D1F	P	0	19860101	19960101	
L8320							D1F	P	0	19860101	19960101	
L8330							D1F	P	0	19860101	19960101	
L8400							D1F	P	0	19820101	19960101	

HCPCS Code	Long Description	Coverage	Action	PI	MPI	CIM	MCM
L8410	PROSTHETIC SHEATH, ABOVE KNEE, EACH	D	N	38	A		2133
L8415	PROSTHETIC SHEATH, UPPER LIMB, EACH	D	N	38	A		2133
L8417	PROSTHETIC SHEATH/SOCK, INCLUDING A GEL CUSHION LAYER, BELOW KNEE OR ABOVE KNEE, EACH	C	N	38	A		
L8420	PROSTHETIC SOCK, MULTIPLE PLY, BELOW KNEE, EACH	D	N	38	A		2133
L8430	PROSTHETIC SOCK, MULTIPLE PLY, ABOVE KNEE, EACH	D	N	38	A		2133
L8435	PROSTHETIC SOCK, MULTIPLE PLY, UPPER LIMB, EACH	D	N	38	A		2133
L8440	PROSTHETIC SHRINKER, BELOW KNEE, EACH	D	N	38	A		2133
L8460	PROSTHETIC SHRINKER, ABOVE KNEE, EACH	D	N	38	A		2133
L8465	PROSTHETIC SHRINKER, UPPER LIMB, EACH	D	N	38	A		2133
L8470	PROSTHETIC SOCK, SINGLE PLY, FITTING, BELOW KNEE, EA.	D	N	38	A		2133
L8480	PROSTHETIC SOCK, SINGLE PLY, FITTING, ABOVE KNEE, EA.	D	N	38	A		2133
L8485	PROSTHETIC SOCK, SINGLE PLY, FITTING, UPPER LIMB, EA.	D	N	38	A		2133
L8499	UNLISTED PROCEDURE FOR MISCELLANEOUS PROSTHETIC SERVICES	C	N	46	A		
L8500	ARTIFICIAL LARYNX, ANY TYPE	D	N	38	A	65-5	2130
L8501	TRACHEOSTOMY SPEAKING VALVE	D	N	38	A	65-16	
L8505	ARTIFICIAL LARYNX REPLACEMENT BATTERY / ACCESSORY, ANY TYPE	C	N	46	A		
L8507	TRACHEO-ESOPHAGEAL VOICE PROSTHESIS, PATIENT INSERTED, ANY TYPE, EACH	C	N	38	A		
L8509	TRACHEO-ESOPHAGEAL VOICE PROSTHESIS, INSERTED BY A LICENSED HEALTH CARE PROVIDER, ANY TYPE	C	N	38	A		
L8510	VOICE AMPLIFIER	D	N	38	A	65-5	
L8511	INSERT FOR INDWELLING TRACHEOESOPHAGEAL PROSTHESIS, WITH OR WITHOUT VALVE, REPLACEMENT ONLY, EACH	C	N	38	A		
L8512	GELATIN CAPSULES OR EQUIVALENT, FOR USE WITH TRACHEOESOPHAGEAL VOICE PROSTHESIS, REPLACEMENT ONLY, PER 10	C	N	38	A		
L8513	CLEANING DEVICE USED WITH TRACHEOESOPHAGEAL VOICE PROSTHESIS, PIPET, BRUSH, OR EQUAL, REPLACEMENT ONLY, EACH	C	N	38	A		
L8514	TRACHEOESOPHAGEAL PUNCTURE DILATOR, REPLACEMENT ONLY, EACH	C	N	38	A		
L8515	GELATIN CAPSULE, APPLICATION DEVICE FOR USE WITH TRACHEOESOPHAGEAL VOICE PROSTHESIS, EACH	C	N	37	A		
L8600	IMPLANTABLE BREAST PROSTHESIS, SILICONE OR EQUAL	D	N	38	A	35-47	2130
L8603	INJECTABLE BULKING AGENT, COLLAGEN IMPLANT, URINARY TRACT, 2.5 ML SYRINGE, INCLUDES SHIPPING AND NECESSARY SUPPLIES	D	N	38	A	65.9	
L8604	INJECTABLE BULKING AGENT, DEXTRANOMER/HYALURONIC ACID COPOLYMER IMPLANT, URINARY TRACT, 1 ML, INCLUDES SHIPPING AND NECESSARY SUPPLIES	C	N	00	9		
L8606	INJECTABLE BULKING AGENT, SYNTHETIC IMPLANT, URINARY TRACT, 1 ML SYRINGE, INCLUDES SHIPPING AND NECESSARY SUPPLIES	D	N	38	A	65.9	
L8609	ARTIFICIAL CORNEA	C	N	38	A		
L8610	OCULAR IMPLANT	D	N	38	A		2130
L8612	AQUEOUS SHUNT	D	N	38	A		2130

HCPCS Code	Statute	Lab Cert	X-Ref	ASC Pay Grp	ASC Pay Group Eff. Date	Proc Notes	BETOS	TOS	Anest	Code Add Date	Code Effective Date	Code Term Date
L8410							D1F	P	0	19820101	19960101	
L8415							D1F	P	0	19880101	19960101	
L8417							D1F	P	0	19970101	19970101	
L8420							D1F	P	0	19820101	19990101	
L8430							D1F	P	0	19820101	19990101	
L8435							D1F	P	0	19880101	20000101	
L8440							D1F	P	0	19820101	19960101	
L8460							D1F	P	0	19820101	19960101	
L8465							D1F	P	0	19880101	19960101	
L8470							D1F	P	0	19820101	19990101	
L8480							D1F	P	0	19820101	19990101	
L8485							D1F	P	0	19940101	19990101	
L8499							D1F	P	0	19820101	20020101	
L8500							D1F	P	0	19900101	19960101	
L8501							D1F	P	0	19900101	19960101	
L8505							D1F	P	0	20020101	20020101	
L8507							D1F	P	0	20020101	20020101	
L8509							D1F	P	0	20020101	20020101	
L8510							D1F	P	0	20020101	20020101	
L8511							D1F	P	0	20040101	20040101	
L8512							D1F	P	0	20040101	20040101	
L8513							D1F	P	0	20040101	20040101	
L8514							D1F	P	0	20040101	20040101	
L8515							D1F	P	0	20050101	20050101	
L8600							D1F	P	0	19920101	19971001	
L8603							D1F	P	0	19950101	20010101	
L8604							D1F	P	0	20090101	20090101	
L8606							D1F	P	0	20010101	20010101	
L8609							D1F	P	0	20060101	20060101	
L8610							D1F	P	0	19920101	19971001	
L8612			Q0074				D1F	P	0	19920101	19971001	

HCPCS Code	Long Description	Coverage	Action	PI	MPI	CIM	MCM
L8613	OSSICULA IMPLANT	D	N	38	A		2130
L8614	COCHLEAR DEVICE, INCLUDES ALL INTERNAL AND EXTERNAL COMPONENTS	D	N	38	A	65-14	2130
L8615	HEADSET/HEADPIECE FOR USE WITH COCHLEAR IMPLANT DEVICE, REPLACEMENT	D	N	38	A	65-14	
L8616	MICROPHONE FOR USE WITH COCHLEAR IMPLANT DEVICE, REPLACEMENT	D	N	38	A	65-14	
L8617	TRANSMITTING COIL FOR USE WITH COCHLEAR IMPLANT DEVICE, REPLACEMENT	D	N	38	A	65-14	
L8618	TRANSMITTER CABLE FOR USE WITH COCHLEAR IMPLANT DEVICE, REPLACEMENT	D	N	38	A	65-14	
L8619	COCHLEAR IMPLANT, EXTERNAL SPEECH PROCESSOR AND CONTROLLER, INTEGRATED SYSTEM, REPLACEMENT	D	C	38	A	65-14	
L8621	ZINC AIR BATTERY FOR USE WITH COCHLEAR IMPLANT DEVICE, REPLACEMENT, EACH	C	N	38	A		
L8622	ALKALINE BATTERY FOR USE WITH COCHLEAR IMPLANT DEVICE, ANY SIZE, REPLACEMENT, EACH	C	N	38	A		
L8623	LITHIUM ION BATTERY FOR USE WITH COCHLEAR IMPLANT DEVICE SPEECH PROCESSOR, OTHER THAN EAR LEVEL, REPLACEMENT, EACH	C	N	38	A		
L8624	LITHIUM ION BATTERY FOR USE WITH COCHLEAR IMPLANT DEVICE SPEECH PROCESSOR, EAR LEVEL, REPLACEMENT, EA.	C	N	38	A		
L8627	COCHLEAR IMPLANT, EXTERNAL SPEECH PROCESSOR, COMPONENT, REPLACEMENT	D	A	38	A	65-14	
L8628	COCHLEAR IMPLANT, EXTERNAL CONTROLLER COMPONENT, REPLACEMENT	D	A	38	A	65-14	
L8629	TRANSMITTING COIL AND CABLE, INTEGRATED, FOR USE WITH COCHLEAR IMPLANT DEVICE, REPLACEMENT	D	A			65-14	
L8630	METACARPOPHALANGEAL JOINT IMPLANT	D	N	38	A		2130
L8631	METACARPAL PHALANGEAL JOINT REPLACEMENT, TWO OR MORE PIECES, METAL (E.G.,STAINLESS STEEL OR COBALT CHROME), CERAMIC-LIKE MATERIAL (E.G., PYROCARBON), FOR SURGICAL IMPLANTATION (ALL SIZES, INCLUDES ENTIRE SYSTEM)	D	N	38	A		2130
L8641	METATARSAL JOINT IMPLANT	D	N	38	A		2130
L8642	HALLUX IMPLANT	D	N	38	A		2130
L8658	INTERPHALANGEAL JOINT SPACER, SILICONE OR EQUAL, EA.	D	N	38	A		2130
L8659	INTERPHALANGEAL FINGER JOINT REPLACEMENT, 2 OR MORE PIECES, METAL (E.G.,STAINLESS STEEL OR COBALT CHROME), CERAMIC-LIKE MATERIAL (E.G., PYROCARBON) SURGICAL IMPLANTATION, ANY SIZE	D	N	38	A		2130
L8670	VASCULAR GRAFT MATERIAL, SYNTHETIC, IMPLANT	D	N	38	A		2130
L8680	IMPLANTABLE NEUROSTIMULATOR ELECTRODE (WITH ANY NUMBER OF CONTACT POINTS), EACH	D	C	38	A	65-8	
L8681	PATIENT PROGRAMMER (EXTERNAL) FOR USE WITH IMPLANTABLE PROGRAMMABLE NEUROSTIMULATOR PULSE GENERATOR, REPLACEMENT ONLY	D	N	38	A	65-8	
L8682	IMPLANTABLE NEUROSTIMULATOR RADIOFREQUENCY RECEIVER	D	N	38	A	65-8	

HCPCS Code	Statute	Lab Cert	X-Ref	ASC Pay Grp	ASC Pay Group Eff. Date	Proc Notes	BETOS	TOS	Anest	Code Add Date	Code Effective Date	Code Term Date
L8613							D1F	P	0	19920101	19971001	
L8614							D1F	P	0	19920101	20070101	
L8615							D1F	P	0	20050101	20050101	
L8616							D1F	P	0	20050101	20050101	
L8617							D1F	P	0	20050101	20050101	
L8618							D1F	P	0	20050101	20050101	
L8619							D1F	P	0	19960101	20100101	
L8621							D1F	P	0	20050101	20050101	
L8622							D1F	P	0	20050101	20050101	
L8623							D1F	P	0	20060101	20060101	
L8624							D1F	P	0	20060101	20060101	
L8627							D1F	P	0	20100101	20100101	
L8628							D1F	P	0	20100101	20100101	
L8629							D1F	P	0	20100101	20100101	
L8630							D1F	P	0	19920101	19971001	
L8631							D1F	P	0	20040101	20040101	
L8641							D1F	P	0	19920101	19971001	
L8642			Q0073				D1F	P	0	19920101	19971001	
L8658							D1F	P	0	19920101	20040101	
L8659							D1F	P	0	20040101	20040101	
L8670							D1F	P	0	19920101	19971001	
L8680							D1F	P	0	20060101	20100101	
L8681							D1F	P	0	20060101	20090101	
L8681												
L8682							D1F	P	0	20060101	20060101	

HCPCS Code	Long Description	Coverage	Action	PI	MPI	CIM	MCM
L8683	RADIOFREQUENCY TRANSMITTER (EXTERNAL) FOR USE WITH IMPLANTABLE NEUROSTIMULATOR RADIOFREQUENCY RECEIVER	D	N	38	A	65-8	
L8684	RADIOFREQUENCY TRANSMITTER (EXTERNAL) FOR USE WITH IMPLANTABLE SACRAL ROOT NEUROSTIMULATOR RECEIVER FOR BOWEL AND BLADDER MANAGEMENT, REPLACEMENT	D	N	38	A	65-8	
L8685	IMPLANTABLE NEUROSTIMULATOR PULSE GENERATOR, SINGLE ARRAY, RECHARGEABLE, INCLUDES EXTENSION	D	N	38	A	65-8	
L8686	IMPLANTABLE NEUROSTIMULATOR PULSE GENERATOR, SINGLE ARRAY, NON-RECHARGEABLE, INCLUDES EXTENSION	D	N	38	A	65-8	
L8687	IMPLANTABLE NEUROSTIMULATOR PULSE GENERATOR, DUAL ARRAY, RECHARGEABLE, INCLUDES EXTENSION	D	N	38	A	65-8	
L8688	IMPLANTABLE NEUROSTIMULATOR PULSE GENERATOR, DUAL ARRAY, NON-RECHARGEABLE, INCLUDES EXTENSION	D	N	38	A	65-8	
L8689	EXTERNAL RECHARGING SYSTEM FOR BATTERY (INTERNAL) FOR USE WITH IMPLANTABLE NEUROSTIMULATOR, REPLACEMENT ONLY	D	N	38	A	65-8	
L8690	AUDITORY OSSEOINTEGRATED DEVICE, INCLUDES ALL INTERNAL AND EXTERNAL COMPONENTS	C	N	38	A		
L8691	AUDITORY OSSEOINTEGRATED DEVICE, EXTERNAL SOUND PROCESSOR, REPLACEMENT	C	S	38	A		
L8692	AUDITORY OSSEOINTEGRATED DEVICE, EXTERNAL SOUND PROCESSOR, USED WITHOUT OSSEOINTEGRATION, BODY WORN, INCLUDES HEADBAND OR OTHER MEANS OF EXTERNAL ATTACHMENT	S	A	00	9		
L8695	EXTERNAL RECHARGING SYSTEM FOR BATTERY (EXTERNAL) FOR USE WITH IMPLANTABLE NEUROSTIMULATOR, REPLACEMENT ONLY	D	N	38	A	65-8	
L8699	PROSTHETIC IMPLANT, NOT OTHERWISE SPECIFIED	C	N	46	A		
L9900	ORTHOTIC AND PROSTHETIC SUPPLY, ACCESSORY, AND/OR SERVICE COMPONENT OF ANOTHER HCPCS "L" CODE	C	N	46	A		
M0064	BRIEF OFFICE VISIT FOR THE SOLE PURPOSE OF MONITORING OR CHANGING DRUG PRESCRIPTIONS USED IN THE TREATMENT OF MENTAL PSYCHONEUROTIC & PERSONALITY DISORDERS	D	N	11	A		2476.3
M0075	CELLULAR THERAPY	M	N	00	9	35-5	
M0076	PROLOTHERAPY	M	N	00	9	35-13	
M0100	INTRAGASTRIC HYPOTHERMIA USING GASTRIC FREEZING	M	N	00	9	35-65	
M0300	IV CHELATION THERAPY (CHEMICAL ENDARTERECTOMY)	M	N	00	9	35-64	
M0301	FABRIC WRAPPING OF ABDOMINAL ANEURYSM	M	N	00	9	35-34	
P2028	CEPHALIN FLOCULATION, BLOOD	D	N	57	A	50-34	
P2029	CONGO RED, BLOOD	D	N	57	A	50-34	
P2031	HAIR ANALYSIS (EXCLUDING ARSENIC)	M	N	00	9	50-24	
P2033	THYMOL TURBIDITY, BLOOD	D	N	57	A	50-34	
P2038	MUCOPROTEIN, BLOOD (SEROMUCOID) (MEDICAL NECESSITY PROCEDURE)	D	N	21	A	50-34	
P3000	SCREENING PAPANICOLAOU SMEAR, CERVICAL OR VAGINAL, UP TO THREE SMEARS, BY TECHNICIAN UNDER PHYSICIAN SUPERVISION	D	N	21	A	50-20	

HCPCS Code	Statute	Lab Cert	X-Ref	ASC Pay Grp	ASC Pay Group Eff. Date	Proc Notes	BETOS	TOS	Anest	Code Add Date	Code Effective Date	Code Term Date
L8683							D1F	P	0	20060101	20060101	
L8684							D1F	P	0	20060101	20060101	
L8685							D1F	P	0	20060101	20060101	
L8686							D1F	P	0	20060101	20060101	
L8687							D1F	P	0	20060101	20060101	
L8688							D1F	P	0	20060101	20060101	
L8689							D1F	P	0	20060101	20090101	
L8690							D1F	P	0	20070101	20070101	
L8691							D1F	P	0	20070101	20100101	
L8692	1862(a)(7)						D1F	P	0	20100101	20100101	
L8692												
L8695							D1F	P	0	20070101	20090101	
L8699							D1F	P	0	19980101	19980101	
L9900							D1F	P	0	20000101	20000101	
M0064							M5B	1	0	19920101	19960101	
M0075							Y2	1	0	19860101	19960101	
M0076							Y2	1	0	19860101	19960101	
M0100							P1G	1	0	19860101	20040101	
M0300							Y2	1	0	19860101	19960101	
M0301							P1G	2	0	19860101	20040101	
P2028							T1H	5	0	19860101	19900101	
P2029							T1H	5	0	19860101	19900101	
P2031							T1H	5	0	19860101	19890101	
P2033							T1H	5	0	19860101	19900101	
P2038							T1H	5	0	19860101	19930101	
P3000		630				0045	T1H	5	0	19920101	19950101	

HCPCS Code	Long Description	Coverage	Action	PI	MPI	CIM	MCM
P3001	SCREENING PAPANICOLAOU SMEAR, CERVICAL OR VAGINAL, UP TO THREE SMEARS, REQUIRING INTERPRETATION BY PHYSICIAN	D	N	11,21	C	50-20	
P7001	CULTURE, BACTERIAL, URINE; QUANTITATIVE, SENSITIVITY STUDY	I	N	00	9		
P9010	BLOOD (WHOLE), FOR TRANSFUSION, PER UNIT	D	N	52	A		2455A
P9011	BLOOD, SPLIT UNIT	D	N	52	A		2455A
P9012	CRYOPRECIPITATE, EACH UNIT	D	N	52	A		2455 B
P9016	RED BLOOD CELLS, LEUKOCYTES REDUCED, EACH UNIT	D	N	52	A		2455 B
P9017	FRESH FROZEN PLASMA (SINGLE DONOR), FROZEN WITHIN 8 HOURS OF COLLECTION, EACH UNIT	D	N	52	A		2455 B
P9019	PLATELETS, EACH UNIT	D	N	52	A		2455 B
P9020	PLATELET RICH PLASMA, EACH UNIT	D	N	52	A		2455 B
P9021	RED BLOOD CELLS, EACH UNIT	D	N	52	A		2455A
P9022	RED BLOOD CELLS, WASHED, EACH UNIT	D	N	52	A		2455A
P9023	PLASMA, POOLED MULTIPLE DONOR, SOLVENT/DETERGENT TREATED, FROZEN, EACH UNIT	D	N	52	A		2455 B
P9031	PLATELETS, LEUKOCYTES REDUCED, EACH UNIT	D	N	52	A		2455
P9032	PLATELETS, IRRADIATED, EACH UNIT	D	N	52	A		2455
P9033	PLATELETS, LEUKOCYTES REDUCED, IRRADIATED, EA. UNIT	D	N	52	A		2455
P9034	PLATELETS, PHERESIS, EACH UNIT	D	N	52	A		2455
P9035	PLATELETS, PHERESIS, LEUKOCYTES REDUCED, EACH UNIT	D	N	52	A		2455
P9036	PLATELETS, PHERESIS, IRRADIATED, EACH UNIT	D	N	52	A		2455
P9037	PLATELETS, PHERESIS, LEUKOCYTES REDUCED, IRRADIATED, EACH UNIT	D	N	52	A		2455
P9038	RED BLOOD CELLS, IRRADIATED, EACH UNIT	D	N	52	A		2455
P9039	RED BLOOD CELLS, DEGLYCEROLIZED, EACH UNIT	D	N	52	A		2455
P9040	RED BLOOD CELLS, LEUKOCYTES REDUCED, IRRADIATED, EACH UNIT	D	N	52	A		2455
P9041	INFUSION, ALBUMIN (HUMAN), 5%, 50 ML	C	N	52	A		
P9043	INFUSION, PLASMA PROTEIN FRACTION (HUMAN), 5%, 50 ML	D	N	52	A		2455B
P9044	PLASMA, CRYOPRECIPITATE REDUCED, EACH UNIT	D	N	52	A		2455.B
P9045	INFUSION, ALBUMIN (HUMAN), 5%, 250 ML	C	N	52	A		
P9046	INFUSION, ALBUMIN (HUMAN), 25%, 20 ML	C	N	52	A		
P9047	INFUSION, ALBUMIN (HUMAN), 25%, 50 ML	C	N	52	A		
P9048	INFUSION, PLASMA PROTEIN FRACTION (HUMAN), 5%, 250ML	C	N	52	A		
P9050	GRANULOCYTES, PHERESIS, EACH UNIT	C	N	52	A		
P9051	WHOLE BLOOD OR RED BLOOD CELLS, LEUKOCYTES REDUCED, CMV-NEGATIVE, EACH UNIT	D	N	52	A		
P9052	PLATELETS, HLA-MATCHED LEUKOCYTES REDUCED, APHERESIS/PHERESIS, EACH UNIT	D	N	52	A		
P9053	PLATELETS, PHERESIS, LEUKOCYTES REDUCED, CMV-NEGATIVE, IRRADIATED, EACH UNIT	D	N	52	A		
P9054	WHOLE BLOOD OR RED BLOOD CELLS, LEUKOCYTES REDUCED, FROZEN, DEGLYCEROL, WASHED, EACH UNIT	D	N	52	A		
P9055	PLATELETS, LEUKOCYTES REDUCED, CMV-NEGATIVE, APHERESIS/PHERESIS, EACH UNIT	D	N	52	A		
P9056	WHOLE BLOOD, LEUKOCYTES REDUCED, IRRADIATED, EACH UNIT	D	N	52	A		

HCPCS Code	Statute	Lab Cert	X-Ref	ASC Pay Grp	ASC Pay Group Eff. Date	Proc Notes	BETOS	TOS	Anest	Code Add Date	Code Effective Date	Code Term Date
P3001		630				0045	T1G	5	0	19920101	20020101	
P7001		110	CPT				T1H	5	0	19860101	19960101	
P9010							T1H	0	0	19870101	19870101	
P9011							T1H	0	0	19870101	20070101	
P9012							T1H	9	0	19870101	20010101	
P9016							T1H	0	0	19870101	20010101	
P9017							T1H	9	0	19870101	20040101	
P9019							T1H	9	0	19870101	20010101	
P9020							T1H	9	0	19870101	20010101	
P9021							T1H	0	0	19870101	20010101	
P9022							T1H	0	0	19870101	19870101	
P9023							T1H	9	0	20000101	20010101	
P9031							T1H	9	0	20010101	20010101	
P9032							T1H	9	0	20010101	20010101	
P9033							T1H	9	0	20010101	20010101	
P9034							T1H	9	0	20010101	20010101	
P9035							T1H	9	0	20010101	20010101	
P9036							T1H	9	0	20010101	20010101	
P9037							T1H	9	0	20010101	20010101	
P9038							T1H	0	0	20010101	20010101	
P9039							T1H	0	0	20010101	20010101	
P9040							T1H	0	0	20010101	20010101	
P9041				YY	20080101		T1H	9	0	20010101	20010101	
P9043							T1H	9	0	20010101	20010101	
P9044							T1H	9	0	20010101	20010101	
P9045				YY	20080101		Y2	9	0	20020101	20020101	
P9046				YY	20080101		Y2	9	0	20020101	20020101	
P9047				YY	20080101		Y2	9	0	20020101	20020101	
P9048							Y2	9	0	20020101	20020101	
P9050							Z2	9	0	20020101	20020101	
P9051	1833T						T1H	0	0	20040101	20040101	
P9052	1833T						T1H	9	0	20040101	20040101	
P9053	1833T						T1H	9	0	20040101	20040101	
P9054	1833T						T1H	0	0	20040101	20040101	
P9055	1833T						T1H	9	0	20040101	20040101	
P9056	1833T						T1H	0	0	20040101	20040101	

HCPCS Code	Long Description	Coverage	Action	PI	MPI	CIM	MCM
P9057	RED BLOOD CELLS, FROZEN/DEGLYCEROLIZED/WASHED, LEUKOCYTES REDUCED, IRRADIATED, EACH UNIT	D	N	52	A		
P9058	RED BLOOD CELLS, LEUKOCYTES REDUCED, CMV-NEGATIVE, IRRADIATED, EACH UNIT	D	N	52	A		
P9059	FRESH FROZEN PLASMA BETWEEN 8-24 HOURS OF COLLECTION, EACH UNIT	D	N	52	A		
P9060	FRESH FROZEN PLASMA, DONOR RETESTED, EACH UNIT	D	N	52	A		
P9603	TRAVEL ALLOWANCE ONE WAY IN CONNECTION WITH MEDICALLY NECESSARY LABORATORY SPECIMEN COLLECTION DRAWN FROM HOME BOUND OR NURSING HOME BOUND PATIENT; PRORATED MILES ACTUALLY TRAVELLED.	D	N	22	A		51141K
P9604	TRAVEL ALLOWANCE ONE WAY IN CONNECTION WITH MEDICALLY NECESSARY LABORATORY SPECIMEN COLLECTION DRAWN FROM HOME BOUND OR NURSING HOME BOUND PATIENT; PRORATED TRIP CHARGE.	D	N	22	A		51141K
P9612	CATHETERIZATION FOR COLLECTION OF SPECIMEN, SINGLE PATIENT, ALL PLACES OF SERVICE	D	N	57	A		5114.1D
P9615	CATHETERIZATION FOR COLLECTION OF SPECIMEN (S) (MULTIPLE PATIENTS)	D	N	57	A		51141D
Q0035	CARDIOKYMOGRAPHY	D	N	11	A	50-50	
Q0081	INFUSION THERAPY, USING OTHER THAN CHEMOTHERAPEUTIC DRUGS, PER VISIT	D	N	00	9	60-14	
Q0083	CHEMOTHERAPY ADMINISTRATION BY OTHER THAN INFUSION TECHNIQUE ONLY (EG SUBCUTANEOUS, INTRAMUSCULAR, PUSH), PER VISIT	C	N	00	9		
Q0084	CHEMOTHERAPY ADMINISTRATION BY INFUSION TECHNIQUE ONLY, PER VISIT	D	N	00	9	60-14	
Q0085	CHEMOTHERAPY ADMINISTRATION BY BOTH INFUSION TECHNIQUE AND OTHER TECHIQUE(S) (EG SUBCUTANEOUS, INTRAMUSCULAR, PUSH), PER VISIT	C	N	00	9		
Q0091	SCREENING PAPANICOLAOU SMEAR; OBTAINING, PREPARING AND CONVEYANCE OF CERVICAL OR VAGINAL SMEAR TO LABORATORY	D	N	11	A	50-20	
Q0092	SET-UP PORTABLE X-RAY EQUIPMENT	D	N	11	A		2070.4
Q0111	WET MOUNTS, INCLUDING PREPARATIONS OF VAGINAL, CERVICAL OR SKIN SPECIMENS	C	N	21	A		
Q0112	ALL POTASSIUM HYDROXIDE (KOH) PREPARATIONS	C	N	21	A		
Q0113	PINWORM EXAMINATIONS	C	N	21	A		
Q0114	FERN TEST	C	N	21	A		
Q0115	POST-COITAL DIRECT, QUALITATIVE EXAMINATIONS OF VAGINAL OR CERVICAL MUCOUS	C	N	21	A		
Q0138	INJECTION, FERUMOXYTOL, FOR TREATMENT OF IRON DEFICIENCY ANEMIA, 1 MG (NON-ESRD USE)	C	A	51	A		
Q0139	INJECTION, FERUMOXYTOL, FOR TREATMENT OF IRON DEFICIENCY ANEMIA, 1 MG (FOR ESRD ON DIALYSIS)	C	A	51	A		
Q0144	AZITHROMYCIN DIHYDRATE, ORAL, CAPSULES/POWDER, 1 GRAM	M	N	00	9		

HCPCS Code	Statute	Lab Cert	X-Ref	ASC Pay Grp	ASC Pay Group Eff. Date	Proc Notes	BETOS	TOS	Anest	Code Add Date	Code Effective Date	Code Term Date
P9057	1833T						T1H	0	0	20040101	20040101	
P9058	1833T						T1H	0	0	20040101	20040101	
P9059	1833T						T1H	9	0	20040101	20040101	
P9060	1833T						T1H	9	0	20040101	20040101	
P9603						0039	Y2	5	0	19870101	19920101	
P9604						0039	Y2	5	0	19870101	19920101	
P9612							T1H	5	0	19990101	19990101	
P9615						0040	T1H	5	0	19850101	19920101	
Q0035							T2D	5	0	19890101	19910101	
Q0081						0041	P6C	1	0	19920101	19960101	
Q0083						0041	O1D	1	0	19920101	19960101	
Q0084						0041	O1D	1	0	19920101	19960101	
Q0085						0041	O1D	1	0	19920101	19960101	
Q0091							P6C	1	0	19920101	19960701	
Q0092							I1F	4	0	19930101	19960101	
Q0111		110,20,30					T1H	5	0	19940101	19940101	
Q0112		120					T1H	5	0	19940101	19940101	
Q0113		130					T1H	5	0	19940101	19940101	
Q0114		310					T1H	5	0	19940101	19940101	
Q0115		400					T1H	5	0	19940101	19940101	
Q0138				YY	20100101		O1E	1, P	0	20100101	20100101	
Q0139							O1E	1, P	0	20100101	20100101	
Q0144						0054	O1E	1	0	19960701	20020701	

HCPCS Code	Long Description	Coverage	Action	PI	MPI	CIM	MCM
Q0163	DIPHENHYDRAMINE HYDROCHLORIDE, 50 MG, ORAL, FDA APPROVED PRESCRIPTION ANTI-EMETIC, FOR USE AS A COMPLETE THERAPEUTIC SUBSTITUTE FOR AN IV ANTI-EMETIC AT TIME OF CHEMOTHERAPY TREATMENT NOT TO EXCEED A 48 HOUR DOSAGE REGIMEN	D	N	51	A		
Q0164	PROCHLORPERAZINE MALEATE, 5 MG, ORAL, FDA APPROVED PRESCRIPTION ANTI-EMETIC, FOR USE AS A COMPLETE THERAPEUTIC SUBSTITUTE FOR AN IV ANTI-EMETIC AT THE TIME OF CHEMOTHERAPY TREATMENT, NOT TO EXCEED A 48 HOUR DOSAGE REGIMEN	D	N	51	A		
Q0165	PROCHLORPERAZINE MALEATE, 10 MG, ORAL, FDA APPROVED PRESCRIPTION ANTI-EMETIC, FOR USE AS A COMPLETE THERAPEUTIC SUBSTITUTE FOR AN IV ANTI-EMETIC AT THE TIME OF CHEMOTHERAPY TREATMENT, NOT TO EXCEED A 48 HOUR DOSAGE REGIMEN	D	N	51	A		
Q0166	GRANISETRON HYDROCHLORIDE, 1 MG, ORAL, FDA APPROVED PRESCRIPTION ANTI-EMETIC, FOR USE AS A COMPLETE THERAPEUTIC SUBSTITUTE FOR AN IV ANTI-EMETIC AT THE TIME OF CHEMOTHERAPY TREATMENT, NOT TO EXCEED A 24 HOUR DOSAGE REGIMEN	D	N	51	A		
Q0167	DRONABINOL, 2.5 MG, ORAL, FDA APPROVED PRESCRIPTION ANTI-EMETIC, FOR USE AS A COMPLETE THERAPEUTIC SUBSTITUTE FOR AN IV ANTI-EMETIC AT THE TIME OF CHEMOTHERAPY TREATMENT, NOT TO EXCEED A 48 HOUR DOSAGE REGIMEN	D	N	51	A		
Q0168	DRONABINOL, 5 MG, ORAL, FDA APPROVED PRESCRIPTION ANTI-EMETIC, FOR USE AS A COMPLETE THERAPEUTIC SUBSTITUTE FOR AN IV ANTI-EMETIC AT THE TIME OF CHEMOTHERAPY TREATMENT, NOT TO EXCEED A 48 HOUR DOSAGE REGIMEN	D	N	51	A		
Q0169	PROMETHAZINE HYDROCHLORIDE, 12.5 MG, ORAL, FDA APPROVED PRESCRIPTION ANTI-EMETIC, FOR USE AS A COMPLETE THERAPEUTIC SUBSTITUTE FOR AN IV ANTI-EMETIC AT THE TIME OF CHEMOTHERAPY TREATMENT, NOT TO EXCEED A 48 HOUR DOSAGE REGIMEN	D	N	51	A		
Q0170	PROMETHAZINE HYDROCHLORIDE, 25 MG, ORAL, FDA APPROVED PRESCRIPTION ANTI-EMETIC, FOR USE AS A COMPLETE THERAPEUTIC SUBSTITUTE FOR AN IV ANTI-EMETIC AT THE TIME OF CHEMOTHERAPY TREATMENT, NOT TO EXCEED A 48 HOUR DOSAGE REGIMEN	D	N	51	A		
Q0171	CHLORPROMAZINE HYDROCHLORIDE, 10 MG, ORAL, FDA APPROVED PRESCRIPTION ANTI-EMETIC, FOR USE AS A COMPLETE THERAPEUTIC SUBSTITUTE FOR AN IV ANTI-EMETIC AT THE TIME OF CHEMOTHERAPY TREATMENT, NOT TO EXCEED A 48 HOUR DOSAGE REGIMEN	D	N	51	A		
Q0172	CHLORPROMAZINE HYDROCHLORIDE, 25 MG, ORAL, FDA APPROVED PRESCRIPTION ANTI-EMETIC, FOR USE AS A COMPLETE THERAPEUTIC SUBSTITUTE FOR AN IV ANTI-EMETIC AT THE TIME OF CHEMOTHERAPY TREATMENT, NOT TO EXCEED A 48 HOUR DOSAGE REGIMEN	D	N	51	A		

Q - R Codes

HCPCS Code	Statute	Lab Cert	X-Ref	ASC Pay Grp	ASC Pay Group Eff. Date	Proc Notes	BETOS	TOS	Anest	Code Add Date	Code Effective Date	Code Term Date
Q0163	4557						O1D	1	0	19980401	19980401	
Q0164	4557						O1D	1	0	19980401	19980401	
Q0165	4557						O1D	1	0	19980401	19980401	
Q0166	4557						O1D	1	0	19980401	20090101	
Q0167	4557						O1D	1	0	19980401	19980401	
Q0168	4557						O1D	1	0	19980401	19980401	
Q0169	4557						O1D	1	0	19980401	19980401	
Q0170	4557						O1D	1	0	19980401	19980401	
Q0171	4557						O1D	1	0	19980401	19980401	
Q0172	4557						O1D	1	0	19980401	19980401	

HCPCS Code	Long Description	Coverage	Action	PI	MPI	CIM	MCM
Q0173	TRIMETHOBENZAMIDE HYDROCHLORIDE, 250 MG, ORAL, FDA APPROVED PRESCRIPTION ANTI-EMETIC, FOR USE AS A COMPLETE THERAPEUTIC SUBSTITUTE FOR AN IV ANTI-EMETIC AT THE TIME OF CHEMOTHERAPY TREATMENT, NOT TO EXCEED A 48 HOUR DOSAGE REGIMEN	D	N	51	A		
Q0174	THIETHYLPERAZINE MALEATE, 10 MG, ORAL, FDA APPROVED PRESCRIPTION ANTI-EMETIC, FOR USE AS A COMPLETE THERAPEUTIC SUBSTITUTE FOR AN IV ANTI-EMETIC AT THE TIME OF CHEMOTHERAPY TREATMENT, NOT TO EXCEED A 48 HOUR DOSAGE REGIMEN	D	N	51	A		
Q0175	PERPHENAZINE, 4 MG, ORAL, FDA APPROVED PRESCRIPTION ANTI-EMETIC, FOR USE AS A COMPLETE THERAPEUTIC SUBSTITUTE FOR AN IV ANTI-EMETIC AT THE TIME OF CHEMOTHERAPY TREATMENT, NOT TO EXCEED A 48 HOUR DOSAGE REGIMEN	D	N	51	A		
Q0176	PERPHENAZINE, 8MG, ORAL, FDA APPROVED PRESCRIPTION ANTI-EMETIC, FOR USE AS A COMPLETE THERAPEUTIC SUBSTITUTE FOR AN IV ANTI-EMETIC AT THE TIME OF CHEMOTHERAPY TREATMENT, NOT TO EXCEED A 48 HOUR DOSAGE REGIMEN	D	N	51	A		
Q0177	HYDROXYZINE PAMOATE, 25 MG, ORAL, FDA APPROVED PRESCRIPTION ANTI-EMETIC, FOR USE AS A COMPLETE THERAPEUTIC SUBSTITUTE FOR AN IV ANTI-EMETIC AT THE TIME OF CHEMOTHERAPY TREATMENT, NOT TO EXCEED A 48 HOUR DOSAGE REGIMEN	D	N	51	A		
Q0178	HYDROXYZINE PAMOATE, 50 MG, ORAL, FDA APPROVED PRESCRIPTION ANTI-EMETIC, FOR USE AS A COMPLETE THERAPEUTIC SUBSTITUTE FOR AN IV ANTI-EMETIC AT THE TIME OF CHEMOTHERAPY TREATMENT, NOT TO EXCEED A 48 HOUR DOSAGE REGIMEN	D	N	51	A		
Q0179	ONDANSETRON HYDROCHLORIDE 8 MG, ORAL, FDA APPROVED PRESCRIPTION ANTI-EMETIC, FOR USE AS A COMPLETE THERAPEUTIC SUBSTITUTE FOR AN IV ANTI-EMETIC AT THE TIME OF CHEMOTHERAPY TREATMENT, NOT TO EXCEED A 48 HOUR DOSAGE REGIMEN	D	N	51	A		
Q0180	DOLASETRON MESYLATE, 100 MG, ORAL, FDA APPROVED PRESCRIPTION ANTI-EMETIC, FOR USE AS A COMPLETE THERAPEUTIC SUBSTITUTE FOR AN IV ANTI-EMETIC AT THE TIME OF CHEMOTHERAPY TREATMENT, NOT TO EXCEED A 24 HOUR DOSAGE REGIMEN	D	N	51	A		
Q0181	UNSPECIFIED ORAL DOSAGE FORM, FDA APPROVED PRESCRIPTION ANTI-EMETIC, FOR USE AS A COMPLETE THERAPEUTIC SUBSTITUTE FOR A IV ANTI-EMETIC AT THE TIME OF CHEMOTHERAPY TREATMENT, NOT TO EXCEED A 48 HOUR DOSAGE REGIMEN	D	N	51	A		
Q0480	DRIVER FOR USE WITH PNEUMATIC VENTRICULAR ASSIST DEVICE, REPLACEMENT ONLY	D	N	38	A		
Q0481	MICROPROCESSOR CONTROL UNIT FOR USE WITH ELECTRIC VENTRICULAR ASSIST DEVICE, REPLACEMENT ONLY	D	N	38	A		

HCPCS Code	Statute	Lab Cert	X-Ref	ASC Pay Grp	ASC Pay Group Eff. Date	Proc Notes	BETOS	TOS	Anest	Code Add Date	Code Effective Date	Code Term Date
Q0173	4557						O1D	1	0	19980401	19980401	
Q0174	4557						O1D	1	0	19980401	19980401	
Q0175	4557						O1D	1	0	19980401	19980401	
Q0176	4557						O1D	1	0	19980401	19980401	
Q0177	4557						O1D	1	0	19980401	19980401	
Q0178	4557						O1D	1	0	19980401	19980401	
Q0179	4557						O1D	1	0	19980401	20090101	
Q0180	4557						O1D	1	0	19980401	19980401	
Q0181	4557						O1D	1	0	19980401	19980401	
Q0480						0121	D1F	P	0	20051001	20051001	
Q0481						0121	D1F	P	0	20051001	20051001	

HCPCS Code	Long Description	Coverage	Action	PI	MPI	CIM	MCM
Q0482	MICROPROCESSOR CONTROL UNIT FOR USE WITH ELECTRIC/PNEUMATIC COMBINATION VENTRICULAR ASSIST DEVICE, REPLACEMENT ONLY	D	N	38	A		
Q0483	MONITOR/DISPLAY MODULE FOR USE WITH ELECTRIC VENTRICULAR ASSIST DEVICE, REPLACEMENT ONLY	D	N	38	A		
Q0484	MONITOR/DISPLAY MODULE FOR USE WITH ELECTRIC OR ELECTRIC/PNEUMATIC VENTRICULAR ASSIST DEVICE, REPLACEMENT ONLY	D	N	38	A		
Q0485	MONITOR CONTROL CABLE FOR USE WITH ELECTRIC VENTRICULAR ASSIST DEVICE, REPLACEMENT ONLY	D	N	38	A		
Q0486	MONITOR CONTROL CABLE FOR USE WITH ELECTRIC/PNEUMATIC VENTRICULAR ASSIST DEVICE, REPLACEMENT ONLY	D	N	38	A		
Q0487	LEADS (PNEUMATIC/ELECTRICAL) FOR USE WITH ANY TYPE ELECTRIC/PNEUMATIC VENTRICULAR ASSIST DEVICE, REPLACEMENT ONLY	D	N	38	A		
Q0488	POWER PACK BASE FOR USE WITH ELECTRIC VENTRICULAR ASSIST DEVICE, REPLACEMENT ONLY	D	N	38	A		
Q0489	POWER PACK BASE FOR USE WITH ELECTRIC/PNEUMATIC VENTRICULAR ASSIST DEVICE, REPLACEMENT ONLY	D	N	38	A		
Q0490	EMERGENCY POWER SOURCE FOR USE WITH ELECTRIC VENTRICULAR ASSIST DEVICE, REPLACEMENT ONLY	D	N	38	A		
Q0491	EMERGENCY POWER SOURCE FOR USE WITH ELECTRIC/PNEUMATIC VENTRICULAR ASSIST DEVICE, REPLACEMENT ONLY	D	N	38	A		
Q0492	EMERGENCY POWER SUPPLY CABLE FOR USE WITH ELECTRIC VENTRICULAR ASSIST DEVICE, REPLACEMENT ONLY	D	N	38	A		
Q0493	EMERGENCY POWER SUPPLY CABLE FOR USE WITH ELECTRIC/PNEUMATIC VENTRICULAR ASSIST DEVICE, REPLACEMENT ONLY	D	N	38	A		
Q0494	EMERGENCY HAND PUMP FOR USE WITH ELECTRIC OR ELECTRIC/PNEUMATIC VENTRICULAR ASSIST DEVICE, REPLACEMENT ONLY	D	N	38	A		
Q0495	BATTERY/POWER PACK CHARGER FOR USE WITH ELECTRIC OR ELECTRIC/PNEUMATIC VENTRICULAR ASSIST DEVICE, REPLACEMENT ONLY	D	N	38	A		
Q0496	BATTERY, OTHER THAN LITHIUM-ION, FOR USE WITH ELECTRIC OR ELECTRIC/PNEUMATIC VENTRICULAR ASSIST DEVICE, REPLACEMENT ONLY	D	C	38	A		
Q0497	BATTERY CLIPS FOR USE WITH ELECTRIC OR ELECTRIC/PNEUMATIC VENTRICULAR ASSIST DEVICE, REPLACEMENT ONLY	D	N	38	A		
Q0498	HOLSTER FOR USE WITH ELECTRIC OR ELECTRIC/PNEUMATIC VENTRICULAR ASSIST DEVICE, REPLACEMENT ONLY	D	N	38	A		
Q0499	BELT/VEST FOR USE WITH ELECTRIC OR ELECTRIC/PNEUMATIC VENTRICULAR ASSIST DEVICE, REPLACEMENT ONLY	D	N	38	A		
Q0500	FILTERS FOR USE WITH ELECTRIC OR ELECTRIC/PNEUMATIC VENTRICULAR ASSIST DEVICE, REPLACEMENT ONLY	D	N	38	A		

HCPCS Code	Statute	Lab Cert	X-Ref	ASC Pay Grp	ASC Pay Group Eff. Date	Proc Notes	BETOS	TOS	Anest	Code Add Date	Code Effective Date	Code Term Date
Q0482						0121	D1F	P	0	20051001	20051001	
Q0483						0121	D1F	P	0	20051001	20051001	
Q0484						0121	D1F	P	0	20051001	20051001	
Q0485						0121	D1F	P	0	20051001	20051001	
Q0486						0121	D1F	P	0	20051001	20051001	
Q0487						0121	D1F	P	0	20051001	20051001	
Q0488						0121	D1F	P	0	20051001	20051001	
Q0489						0121	D1F	P	0	20051001	20051001	
Q0490						0121	D1F	P	0	20051001	20051001	
Q0491						0121	D1F	P	0	20051001	20051001	
Q0492						0121	D1F	P	0	20051001	20051001	
Q0493						0121	D1F	P	0	20051001	20051001	
Q0494						0121	D1F	P	0	20051001	20051001	
Q0495						0121	D1F	P	0	20051001	20051001	
Q0496						0121	D1F	P	0	20051001	20100101	
Q0497						0121	D1F	P	0	20051001	20051001	
Q0498						0121	D1F	P	0	20051001	20051001	
Q0499						0121	D1F	P	0	20051001	20051001	
Q0500						0121	D1F	P	0	20051001	20051001	

Q - R Codes

HCPCS Code	Long Description	Coverage	Action	PI	MPI	CIM	MCM
Q0501	SHOWER COVER FOR USE WITH ELECTRIC OR ELECTRIC/PNEUMATIC VENTRICULAR ASSIST DEVICE, REPLACEMENT ONLY	D	N	38	A		
Q0502	MOBILITY CART FOR PNEUMATIC VENTRICULAR ASSIST DEVICE, REPLACEMENT ONLY	D	N	38	A		
Q0503	BATTERY FOR PNEUMATIC VENTRICULAR ASSIST DEVICE, REPLACEMENT ONLY, EACH	D	N	38	A		
Q0504	POWER ADAPTER FOR PNEUMATIC VENTRICULAR ASSIST DEVICE, REPLACEMENT ONLY, VEHICLE TYPE	D	N	38	A		
Q0505	MISCELLANEOUS SUPPLY OR ACCESSORY FOR USE WITH E VENTRICULAR ASSIST DEVIC	D	N	38	A		
Q0506	BATTERY, LITHIUM-ION, FOR USE WITH ELECTRIC OR ELECTRIC/PNEUMATIC VENTRICULAR ASSIST DEVICE, REPLACEMENT ONLY	D	A	38	A		
Q0510	PHARMACY SUPPLY FEE FOR INITIAL IMMUNOSUPPRESSIVE DRUG(S), FIRST MONTH FOLLOWING TRANSPLANT	D	N	46	A		
Q0511	PHARMACY SUPPLY FEE FOR ORAL ANTI-CANCER, ORAL ANTI-EMETIC OR IMMUNOSUPPRESSIVE DRUG(S); FOR THE FIRST PRESCRIPTION IN A 30-DAY PERIOD	D	N	46	A		
Q0512	PHARMACY SUPPLY FEE FOR ORAL ANTI-CANCER, ORAL ANTI-EMETIC OR IMMUNOSUPPRESSIVE DRUG(S); FOR A SUBSEQUENT PRESCRIPTION IN A 30-DAY PERIOD	D	N	46	A		
Q0513	PHARMACY DISPENSING FEE FOR INHALATION DRUG(S); PER 30 DAYS	D	N	46	A		
Q0514	PHARMACY DISPENSING FEE FOR INHALATION DRUG(S); PER 90 DAYS	D	N	46	A		
Q0515	INJECTION, SERMORELIN ACETATE, 1 MICROGRAM	D	N	51	A		2049
Q1003	NEW TECHNOLOGY INTRAOCULAR LENS CATEGORY 3 (REDUCED SPHERICAL ABERRATION)	C	N	57	A		
Q1004	NEW TECHNOLOGY INTRAOCULAR LENS CATEGORY 4 AS DEFINED IN FEDERAL REGISTER NOTICE	D	N	57	A		
Q1005	NEW TECHNOLOGY INTRAOCULAR LENS CATEGORY 5 AS DEFINED IN FEDERAL REGISTER NOTICE	D	N	57	A		
Q2004	IRRIGATION SOLUTION FOR TREATMENT OF BLADDER CALCULI, FOR EXAMPLE RENACIDIN, PER 500 ML	D	N	51	A		2049
Q2009	INJECTION, FOSPHENYTOIN, 50 MG PHENYTOIN EQUIVALENT	D	C	51	A		2049
Q2017	INJECTION, TENIPOSIDE, 50 MG	D	N	51	A		2049
Q2023	INJECTION, FACTOR VIII (ANTIHEMOPHILIC FACTOR, RECOMBINANT) (XYNTHA), PER I.U.	C	D	51	A		
Q2024	INJECTION, BEVACIZUMAB, 0.25 MG	C	D	51	A		
Q3001	RADIOELEMENTS FOR BRACHYTHERAPY, ANY TYPE, EACH	D	N	57	A		15022
Q3014	TELEHEALTH ORIGINATING SITE FACILITY FEE	C	N	53	A		
Q3019	ALS VEHICLE USED, EMERGENCY TRANSPORT, NO ALS LEVEL SERVICES FURNISHED	C	N	52	A		
Q3020	ALS VEHICLE USED, NON-EMERGENCY TRANSPORT, NO ALS LEVEL SERVICE FURNISHED	C	N	52	A		
Q3025	INJECTION, INTERFERON BETA-1A, 11 MCG FOR INTRAMUSCULAR USE	D	N	51	A		2049
Q3026	INJECTION, INTERFERON BETA-1A, 11 MCG FOR SUBCUTANEOUS USE	I	N	00	9		

HCPCS Code	Statute	Lab Cert	X-Ref	ASC Pay Grp	ASC Pay Group Eff. Date	Proc Notes	BETOS	TOS	Anest	Code Add Date	Code Effective Date	Code Term Date
Q0501						0121	D1F	P	0	20051001	20051001	
Q0502						0121	D1F	P	0	20051001	20051001	
Q0503						0121	D1F	P	0	20051001	20051001	
Q0504						0121	D1F	P	0	20051001	20051001	
Q0505						0121	D1F	P	0	20051001	20051001	
Q0506						0121	D1F	P	0	20100101	20100101	
Q0510						0129	O1E	9	0	20060101	20060101	
Q0511						0129	O1E	9	0	20060101	20060101	
Q0512						0129	O1E	9	0	20060101	20090101	
Q0513						0129	O1E	9	0	20060101	20060101	
Q0514						0129	O1E	9	0	20060101	20060101	
Q0515				YY	20080101		O1E	1, P	0	20060101	20060101	
Q1003				YY	20080101		D1F	F	0	19990701	20060227	
Q1004						0086	D1F	F	0	19990701	20031001	
Q1005						0086	D1F	F	0	19990701	20031001	
Q2004	1861S2B			YY	20100101		O1E	1, P	0	20000701	20070101	
Q2009	1861S2B						O1E	1, P	0	20000701	20100101	
Q2017	1861S2B			YY	20080101		O1D	1, P	0	20000701	20070101	
Q2023			J7185				O1E	1, P	0	20090701	20100101	20091231
Q2024							O1E	1, P	0	20091001	20100101	20091231
Q3001							P7A	1	0	20000701	20050101	
Q3014							Y2	9	0	20011001	20011001	
Q3019							O1A	D	0	20020401	20060401	20060331
Q3020							O1A	D	0	20020401	20060401	20060331
Q3025				YY	20080101		O1E	1, P	0	20030101	20030101	
Q3026							O1E	1, P	0	20030101	20030101	

HCPCS Code	Long Description	Coverage	Action	PI	MPI	CIM	MCM
Q3031	COLLAGEN SKIN TEST	D	N	11	A	65-9	
Q4001	CASTING SUPPLIES, BODY CAST ADULT, WITH OR WITHOUT HEAD, PLASTER	C	N	52	A		
Q4002	CAST SUPPLIES, BODY CAST ADULT, WITH OR WITHOUT HEAD, FIBERGLASS	C	N	52	A		
Q4003	CAST SUPPLIES, SHOULDER CAST, ADULT (11 YEARS +), PLASTER	C	N	52	A		
Q4004	CAST SUPPLIES, SHOULDER CAST, ADULT (11 YEARS +), FIBERGLASS	C	N	52	A		
Q4005	CAST SUPPLIES, LONG ARM CAST, ADULT (11 YEARS +), PLASTER	C	N	52	A		
Q4006	CAST SUPPLIES, LONG ARM CAST, ADULT (11 YEARS +), FIBERGLASS	C	N	52	A		
Q4007	CAST SUPPLIES, LONG ARM CAST, PEDIATRIC (0-10 YEARS), PLASTER	C	N	52	A		
Q4008	CAST SUPPLIES, LONG ARM CAST, PEDIATRIC (0-10 YEARS), FIBERGLASS	C	N	52	A		
Q4009	CAST SUPPLIES, SHORT ARM CAST, ADULT (11 YEARS +), PLASTER	C	N	52	A		
Q4010	CAST SUPPLIES, SHORT ARM CAST, ADULT (11 YEARS +), FIBERGLASS	C	N	52	A		
Q4011	CAST SUPPLIES, SHORT ARM CAST, PEDIATRIC (0-10 YEARS), PLASTER	C	N	52	A		
Q4012	CAST SUPPLIES, SHORT ARM CAST, PEDIATRIC (0-10 YEARS), FIBERGLASS	C	N	52	A		
Q4013	CAST SUPPLIES, GAUNTLET CAST (INCLUDES LOWER FOREARM AND HAND), ADULT (11 YEARS +), PLASTER	C	N	52	A		
Q4014	CAST SUPPLIES, GAUNTLET CAST (INCLUDES LOWER FOREARM AND HAND), ADULT (11 YEARS +), FIBERGLASS	C	N	52	A		
Q4015	CAST SUPPLIES, GAUNTLET CAST (INCLUDES LOWER FOREARM AND HAND), PEDIATRIC (0-10 YEARS), PLASTER	C	N	52	A		
Q4016	CAST SUPPLIES, GAUNTLET CAST (INCLUDES LOWER FOREARM AND HAND), PEDIATRIC (0-10 YEARS), FIBERGLASS	C	N	52	A		
Q4017	CAST SUPPLIES, LONG ARM SPLINT, ADULT (11 YEARS +), PLASTER	C	N	52	A		
Q4018	CAST SUPPLIES, LONG ARM SPLINT, ADULT (11 YEARS +), FIBERGLASS	C	N	52	A		
Q4019	CAST SUPPLIES, LONG ARM SPLINT, PEDIATRIC (0-10 YEARS), PLASTER	C	N	52	A		
Q4020	CAST SUPPLIES, LONG ARM SPLINT, PEDIATRIC (0-10 YEARS), FIBERGLASS	C	N	52	A		
Q4021	CAST SUPPLIES, SHORT ARM SPLINT, ADULT (11 YEARS +), PLASTER	C	N	52	A		
Q4022	CAST SUPPLIES, SHORT ARM SPLINT, ADULT (11 YEARS +), FIBERGLASS	C	N	52	A		
Q4023	CAST SUPPLIES, SHORT ARM SPLINT, PEDIATRIC (0-10 YEARS), PLASTER	C	N	52	A		
Q4024	CAST SUPPLIES, SHORT ARM SPLINT, PEDIATRIC (0-10 YEARS), FIBERGLASS	C	N	52	A		

HCPCS Code	Statute	Lab Cert	X-Ref	ASC Pay Grp	ASC Pay Group Eff. Date	Proc Notes	BETOS	TOS	Anest	Code Add Date	Code Effective Date	Code Term Date
Q3031							D1A	5	0	20030401	20041001	
Q4001							D1A	S	0	20010701	20010701	
Q4002							D1A	S	0	20010701	20010701	
Q4003							D1A	S	0	20010701	20010701	
Q4004							D1A	S	0	20010701	20010701	
Q4005							D1A	S	0	20010701	20010701	
Q4006							D1A	S	0	20010701	20010701	
Q4007							D1A	S	0	20010701	20010701	
Q4008							D1A	S	0	20010701	20010701	
Q4009							D1A	S	0	20010701	20010701	
Q4010							D1A	S	0	20010701	20010701	
Q4011							D1A	S	0	20010701	20010701	
Q4012							D1A	S	0	20010701	20010701	
Q4013							D1A	S	0	20010701	20010701	
Q4014							D1A	S	0	20010701	20010701	
Q4015							D1A	S	0	20010701	20010701	
Q4016							D1A	S	0	20010701	20010701	
Q4017							D1A	S	0	20010701	20010701	
Q4018							D1A	S	0	20010701	20010701	
Q4019							D1A	S	0	20010701	20010701	
Q4020							D1A	S	0	20010701	20010701	
Q4021							D1A	S	0	20010701	20010701	
Q4022							D1A	S	0	20010701	20010701	
Q4023							D1A	S	0	20010701	20010701	
Q4024							D1A	S	0	20010701	20010701	

HCPCS Code	Long Description	Coverage	Action	PI	MPI	CIM	MCM
Q4025	CAST SUPPLIES, HIP SPICA (ONE OR BOTH LEGS), ADULT (11 YEARS +), PLASTER	C	N	52	A		
Q4026	CAST SUPPLIES, HIP SPICA (ONE OR BOTH LEGS), ADULT (11 YEARS +), FIBERGLASS	C	N	52	A		
Q4027	CAST SUPPLIES, HIP SPICA (ONE OR BOTH LEGS), PEDIATRIC (0-10 YEARS), PLASTER	C	N	52	A		
Q4028	CAST SUPPLIES, HIP SPICA (ONE OR BOTH LEGS), PEDIATRIC (0-10 YEARS), FIBERGLASS	C	N	52	A		
Q4029	CAST SUPPLIES, LONG LEG CAST, ADULT (11 YEARS +), PLASTER	C	N	52	A		
Q4030	CAST SUPPLIES, LONG LEG CAST, ADULT (11 YEARS +), FIBERGLASS	C	N	52	A		
Q4031	CAST SUPPLIES, LONG LEG CAST, PEDIATRIC (0-10 YEARS), PLASTER	C	N	52	A		
Q4032	CAST SUPPLIES, LONG LEG CAST, PEDIATRIC (0-10 YEARS), FIBERGLASS	C	N	52	A		
Q4033	CAST SUPPLIES, LONG LEG CYLINDER CAST, ADULT (11 YEARS +), PLASTER	C	N	52	A		
Q4034	CAST SUPPLIES, LONG LEG CYLINDER CAST, ADULT (11 YEARS +), FIBERGLASS	C	N	52	A		
Q4035	CAST SUPPLIES, LONG LEG CYLINDER CAST, PEDIATRIC (0-10 YEARS), PLASTER	C	N	52	A		
Q4036	CAST SUPPLIES, LONG LEG CYLINDER CAST, PEDIATRIC (0-10 YEARS), FIBERGLASS	C	N	52	A		
Q4037	CAST SUPPLIES, SHORT LEG CAST, ADULT (11 YEARS +), PLASTER	C	N	52	A		
Q4038	CAST SUPPLIES, SHORT LEG CAST, ADULT (11 YEARS +), FIBERGLASS	C	N	52	A		
Q4039	CAST SUPPLIES, SHORT LEG CAST, PEDIATRIC (0-10 YEARS), PLASTER	C	N	52	A		
Q4040	CAST SUPPLIES, SHORT LEG CAST, PEDIATRIC (0-10 YEARS), FIBERGLASS	C	N	52	A		
Q4041	CAST SUPPLIES, LONG LEG SPLINT, ADULT (11 YEARS +), PLASTER	C	N	52	A		
Q4042	CAST SUPPLIES, LONG LEG SPLINT, ADULT (11 YEARS +), FIBERGLASS	C	N	52	A		
Q4043	CAST SUPPLIES, LONG LEG SPLINT, PEDIATRIC (0-10 YEARS), PLASTER	C	N	52	A		
Q4044	CAST SUPPLIES, LONG LEG SPLINT, PEDIATRIC (0-10 YEARS), FIBERGLASS	C	N	52	A		
Q4045	CAST SUPPLIES, SHORT LEG SPLINT, ADULT (11 YEARS +), PLASTER	C	N	52	A		
Q4046	CAST SUPPLIES, SHORT LEG SPLINT, ADULT (11 YEARS +), FIBERGLASS	C	N	52	A		
Q4047	CAST SUPPLIES, SHORT LEG SPLINT, PEDIATRIC (0-10 YEARS), PLASTER	C	N	52	A		
Q4048	CAST SUPPLIES, SHORT LEG SPLINT, PEDIATRIC (0-10 YEARS), FIBERGLASS	C	N	52	A		
Q4049	FINGER SPLINT, STATIC	C	N	52	A		

HCPCS Code	Statute	Lab Cert	X-Ref	ASC Pay Grp	ASC Pay Group Eff. Date	Proc Notes	BETOS	TOS	Anest	Code Add Date	Code Effective Date	Code Term Date
Q4025							D1A	S	0	20010701	20010701	
Q4026							D1A	S	0	20010701	20010701	
Q4027							D1A	S	0	20010701	20010701	
Q4028							D1A	S	0	20010701	20010701	
Q4029							D1A	S	0	20010701	20010701	
Q4030							D1A	S	0	20010701	20010701	
Q4031							D1A	S	0	20010701	20010701	
Q4032							D1A	S	0	20010701	20010701	
Q4033							D1A	S	0	20010701	20010701	
Q4034							D1A	S	0	20010701	20010701	
Q4035							D1A	S	0	20010701	20010701	
Q4036							D1A	S	0	20010701	20010701	
Q4037							D1A	S	0	20010701	20010701	
Q4038							D1A	S	0	20010701	20010701	
Q4039							D1A	S	0	20010701	20010701	
Q4040							D1A	S	0	20010701	20010701	
Q4041							D1A	S	0	20010701	20010701	
Q4042							D1A	S	0	20010701	20010701	
Q4043							D1A	S	0	20010701	20010701	
Q4044							D1A	S	0	20010701	20010701	
Q4045							D1A	S	0	20010701	20010701	
Q4046							D1A	S	0	20010701	20010701	
Q4047							D1A	S	0	20010701	20010701	
Q4048							D1A	S	0	20010701	20010701	
Q4049							D1A	S	0	20010701	20010701	

HCPCS Code	Long Description	Coverage	Action	PI	MPI	CIM	MCM
Q4050	CAST SUPPLIES, FOR UNLISTED TYPES AND MATERIALS OF CASTS	C	N	57	A		
Q4051	SPLINT SUPPLIES, MISCELLANEOUS (INCLUDES THERMOPLASTICS, STRAPPING, FASTENERS, PADDING AND OTHER SUPPLIES)	C	N	57	A		
Q4074	ILOPROST, INHALATION SOLUTION, FDA-APPROVED FINAL PRODUCT, NON-COMPOUNDED, ADMINISTERED THROUGH DME, UNIT DOSE FORM, UP TO 20 MICROGRAMS	C	A	51	A		
Q4079	INJECTION, NATALIZUMAB, 1 MG	C	N	51	A		
Q4080	ILOPROST, INHALATION SOLUTION, FDA-APPROVED FINAL PRODUCT, NON-COMPOUNDED, ADMINISTERED THROUGH DME, UNIT DOSE FORM, 20 MICROGRAMS	C	D	51	A		
Q4081	INJECTION, EPOETIN ALFA, 100 UNITS (FOR ESRD ON DIALYSIS)	D	N	57	A		4273.1
Q4082	DRUG OR BIOLOGICAL, NOT OTHERWISE CLASSIFIED, PART B DRUG COMPETITIVE ACQUISITION PROGRAM (CAP)	C	N	51	A		
Q4083	HYALURONAN OR DERIVATIVE, HYALGAN OR SUPARTZ, FOR INTRA-ARTICULAR INJECTION, PER DOSE	C	N	51	A		
Q4084	HYALURONAN OR DERIVATIVE, SYNVISC, FOR INTRA-ARTICULAR INJECTION, PER DOSE	C	N	51	A		
Q4085	HYALURONAN OR DERIVATIVE, EUFLEXXA, FOR INTRA-ARTICULAR INJECTION, PER DOSE	C	N	51	A		
Q4086	HYALURONAN OR DERIVATIVE, ORTHOVISC, FOR INTRA-ARTICULAR INJECTION, PER DOSE	C	N	51	A		
Q4087	INJECTION, IMMUNE GLOBULIN, (OCTAGAM), INTRAVENOUS, NON-LYOPHILIZED (E.G. LIQUID), 500 MG	C	N	51	A		
Q4088	INJECTION, IMMUNE GLOBULIN, (GAMMAGARD LIQUID), INTRAVENOUS, NON-LYOPHILIZED, (E.G. LIQUID), 500 MG	D	N	51	A		2049
Q4089	INJECTION, RHO(D) IMMUNE GLOBULIN (HUMAN), (RHOPHYLAC), INTRAMUSCULAR OR INTRAVENOUS, 100 IU	D	N	51	A		2049
Q4090	INJECTION, HEPATITIS B IMMUNE GLOBULIN (HEPAGAM B), INTRAMUSCULAR, 0.5 ML	D	N	51	A		2049
Q4091	INJECTION, IMMUNE GLOBULIN, (FLEBOGAMMA), INTRAVENOUS, NON-LYOPHILIZED, (E.G. LIQUID), 500 MG	D	N	51	A		2049
Q4092	INJECTION, IMMUNE GLOBULIN, (GAMUNEX), INTRAVENOUS, NON-LYOPHILIZED (E.G. LIQUID), 500 MG	D	N	51	A		2049
Q4093	ALBUTEROL, ALL FORMULATIONS INCLUDING SEPARATED ISOMERS, INHALATION SOLUTION, FDA-APPROVED FINAL PRODUCT, NON-COMPOUNDED, ADMINISTERED THROUGH DME, CONCENTRATED FORM, PER 1 MG (ALBUTEROL) OR PER 0.5 MG (LEVALBUTEROL)	D	N	51	A		
Q4094	ALBUTEROL, ALL FORMULATIONS INCLUDING SEPARATED ISOMERS, INHALATION SOLUTION, FDA-APPROVED FINAL PRODUCT, NON-COMPOUNDED, ADMINISTERED THROUGH DME, UNIT DOSE, PER 1 MG (ALBUTEROL) OR PER 0.5 MG (LEVALBUTEROL)	D	N	51	A		
Q4095	INJECTION, ZOLEDRONIC ACID (RECLAST), 1 MG	D	N	51	A		
Q4096	INJECTION, VON WILLEBRAND FACTOR COMPLEX, HUMAN, RISTOCETIN COFACTOR (NOT OTHERWISE SPECIFIED), PER I.U. VWF: RCO	D	N	51	A		2049

HCPCS Code	Statute	Lab Cert	X-Ref	ASC Pay Grp	ASC Pay Group Eff. Date	Proc Notes	BETOS	TOS	Anest	Code Add Date	Code Effective Date	Code Term Date
Q4050							D1A	S	0	20010701	20010701	
Q4051							D1A	S	0	20010701	20010701	
Q4074							D1G	1, P	0	20100101	20100101	
Q4079			J2323				O1E	1, P	0	20050101	20080101	20071231
Q4080							D1G	1, P	0	20050701	20100101	20091231
Q4081							O1E	1, L	0	20070101	20070101	
Q4082							D1E	1, L	0	20070101	20070101	
Q4083			J7321				O1E	1	0	20070101	20080101	20071231
Q4084			J7322				O1E	1	0	20070101	20080101	20071231
Q4085			J7323				O1E	1	0	20070101	20080101	20071231
Q4086			J7324				O1E	1	0	20070101	20080101	20071231
Q4087			J1568				O1E	1, P	0	20070701	20080101	20071231
Q4088			J1569				O1E	1, P	0	20070701	20080101	20071231
Q4089			J2791				O1E	1, P	0	20070701	20080101	20071231
Q4090			J1571				O1E	1, P	0	20070701	20080101	20071231
Q4091			J1572				O1E	1, P	0	20070701	20080101	20071231
Q4092			J1561				O1E	1, P	0	20070701	20080101	20071231
Q4093			J7602			0135	O1E	1, P	0	20070701	20080101	20071231
Q4094			J7603			0135	O1E	1, P	0	20070701	20080101	20071231
Q4095			J3488			0135	O1E	1, P	0	20070701	20080101	20071231
Q4096							O1E	1, P	0	20080401	20090101	20081231

HCPCS Code	Long Description	Coverage	Action	PI	MPI	CIM	MCM
Q4097	INJECTION, IMMUNE GLOBULIN (PRIVIGEN), INTRAVENOUS, NON-LYOPHILIZED (E.G. LIQUID), 500 MG	C	N	51	A		
Q4098	INJECTION, IRON DEXTRAN, 50 MG	C	N	51	A		
Q4099	FORMOTEROL FUMARATE, INHALATION SOLUTION, FDA APPROVED FINAL PRODUCT, NON-COMPOUNDED, ADMINISTERED THROUGH DME, UNIT DOSE FORM, 20 MICROGRAMS	C	N	51	A		
Q4100	SKIN SUBSTITUTE, NOT OTHERWISE SPECIFIED	C	N	51	A		
Q4101	SKIN SUBSTITUTE, APLIGRAF, PER SQUARE CENTIMETER	C	N	51	A		
Q4102	SKIN SUBSTITUTE, OASIS WOUND MATRIX, PER SQUARE CENTIMETER	C	N	51	A		
Q4103	SKIN SUBSTITUTE, OASIS BURN MATRIX, PER SQUARE CENTIMETER	C	N	51	A		
Q4104	SKIN SUBSTITUTE, INTEGRA BILAYER MATRIX WOUND DRESSING (BMWD), PER SQUARE CENTIMETER	C	N	51	A		
Q4105	SKIN SUBSTITUTE, INTEGRA DERMAL REGENERATION TEMPLATE (DRT), PER SQUARE CENTIMETER	C	N	51	A		
Q4106	SKIN SUBSTITUTE, DERMAGRAFT, PER SQUARE CENTIMETER	C	N	51	A		
Q4107	SKIN SUBSTITUTE, GRAFTJACKET, PER SQUARE CENTIMETER	C	N	51	A		
Q4108	SKIN SUBSTITUTE, INTEGRA MATRIX, PER SQUARE CENTIMETER	C	N	51	A		
Q4109	SKIN SUBSTITUTE, TISSUEMEND, PER SQUARE CENTIMETER	C	N	51	A		
Q4110	SKIN SUBSTITUTE, PRIMATRIX, PER SQUARE CENTIMETER	C	N	51	A		
Q4111	SKIN SUBSTITUTE, GAMMAGRAFT, PER SQUARE CENTIMETER	C	N	51	A		
Q4112	ALLOGRAFT, CYMETRA, INJECTABLE, 1CC	C	N	51	A		
Q4113	ALLOGRAFT, GRAFTJACKET EXPRESS, INJECTABLE, 1CC	C	N	51	A		
Q4114	INTEGRA FLOWABLE WOUND MATRIX, INJECTABLE, 1CC	C	N	51	A		
Q4115	SKIN SUBSTITUTE, ALLOSKIN, PER SQUARE CENTIMETER	C	A	51	A		
Q4116	SKIN SUBSTITUTE, ALLODERM, PER SQUARE CENTIMETER	C	A	51	A		
Q5001	HOSPICE CARE PROVIDED IN PATIENT'S HOME/RESIDENCE	D	N	00	9		
Q5002	HOSPICE CARE PROVIDED IN ASSISTED LIVING FACILITY	D	N	00	9		
Q5003	HOSPICE CARE PROVIDED IN NURSING LONG TERM CARE FACILITY (LTC) OR NON-SKILLED NURSING FACILITY (NF)	D	N	00	9		
Q5004	HOSPICE CARE PROVIDED IN SKILLED NURSING FACILITY (SNF)	D	N	00	9		
Q5005	HOSPICE CARE PROVIDED IN INPATIENT HOSPITAL	D	N	00	9		
Q5006	HOSPICE CARE PROVIDED IN INPATIENT HOSPICE FACILITY	D	N	00	9		
Q5007	HOSPICE CARE PROVIDED IN LONG TERM CARE FACILITY	D	N	00	9		
Q5008	HOSPICE CARE PROVIDED IN INPATIENT PSYCHIATRIC FACILITY	D	N	00	9		
Q5009	HOSPICE CARE PROVIDED IN PLACE NOT OTHERWISE (NOS) SPECIFIED	D	N	00	9		
Q9945	LOW OSMOLAR CONTRAST MATERIAL, UP TO 149 MG/ML IODINE CONCENTRATION, PER ML	D	N	51	A		15022
Q9946	LOW OSMOLAR CONTRAST MATERIAL, 150-199 MG/ML IODINE CONCENTRATION, PER ML	D	N	51	A		15022
Q9947	LOW OSMOLAR CONTRAST MATERIAL, 200-249 MG/ML IODINE CONCENTRATION, PER ML	D	N	51	A		15022
Q9948	LOW OSMOLAR CONTRAST MATERIAL, 250-299 MG/ML IODINE CONCENTRATION, PER ML	D	N	51	A		15022

Q - R Codes

HCPCS Code	Statute	Lab Cert	X-Ref	ASC Pay Grp	ASC Pay Group Eff. Date	Proc Notes	BETOS	TOS	Anest	Code Add Date	Code Effective Date	Code Term Date
Q4097			J1459				O1E	1, P	0	20080401	20090101	20081231
Q4098			J1750				O1E	1, P	0	20080401	20090101	20081231
Q4099			J7606				D1G	1, P	0	20080401	20090101	20081231
Q4100							O1E	1	0	20090101	20090101	
Q4101				YY	20090101		O1E	1	0	20090101	20090101	
Q4102				YY	20090101		O1E	1	0	20090101	20090101	
Q4103				YY	20090101		O1E	1	0	20090101	20090101	
Q4104				YY	20090101		O1E	1	0	20090101	20090101	
Q4105				YY	20090101		O1E	1	0	20090101	20090101	
Q4106				YY	20090101		O1E	1	0	20090101	20090101	
Q4107				YY	20090101		O1E	1	0	20090101	20090101	
Q4108				YY	20090101		O1E	1	0	20090101	20090101	
Q4109							O1E	1	0	20090101	20090101	
Q4110				YY	20090101		O1E	1	0	20090101	20090101	
Q4111				YY	20090101		O1E	1	0	20090101	20090101	
Q4112				YY	20090101		O1E	1	0	20090101	20090101	
Q4113				YY	20090101		O1E	1	0	20090101	20090101	
Q4114				YY	20090101		O1E	1	0	20090101	20090101	
Q4115				YY	20090701		O1E	1	0	20090701	20090701	
Q4116				YY	20090701		O1E	1	0	20090701	20090701	
Q5001						0133	Y2	1, L	0	20070101	20070101	
Q5002						0133	Y2	1, L	0	20070101	20070101	
Q5003						0133	Y2	1, L	0	20070101	20070101	
Q5004						0133	Y2	1, L	0	20070101	20070101	
Q5005						0133	Y2	1, L	0	20070101	20070101	
Q5006						0133	Y2	1, L	0	20070101	20070101	
Q5007						0133	Y2	1, L	0	20070101	20070101	
Q5008						0133	Y2	1, L	0	20070101	20070101	
Q5009						0133	Y2	1, L	0	20070101	20070101	
Q9945							I1E	4	0	20050401	20080101	20071231
Q9946							I1E	4	0	20050401	20080101	20071231
Q9947							I1E	4	0	20050401	20080101	20071231
Q9948							I1E	4	0	20050401	20080101	20071231

HCPCS Code	Long Description	Coverage	Action	PI	MPI	CIM	MCM
Q9949	LOW OSMOLAR CONTRAST MATERIAL, 300-349 MG/ML IODINE CONCENTRATION, PER ML	D	N	51	A		15022
Q9950	LOW OSMOLAR CONTRAST MATERIAL, 350-399 MG/ML IODINE CONCENTRATION, PER ML	D	N	51	A		15022
Q9951	LOW OSMOLAR CONTRAST MATERIAL, 400 OR GREATER MG/ML IODINE CONCENTRATION, PER ML	D	N	51	A		15022
Q9952	INJECTION, GADOLINIUM-BASED MAGNETIC RESONANCE CONTRAST AGENT, PER ML	D	N	57	A		15022
Q9953	INJECTION, IRON-BASED MAGNETIC RESONANCE CONTRAST AGENT, PER ML	D	N	57	A		15022
Q9954	ORAL MAGNETIC RESONANCE CONTRAST AGENT, PER 100 ML	D	N	57	A		15022
Q9955	INJECTION, PERFLEXANE LIPID MICROSPHERES, PER ML	C	N	57	A		
Q9956	INJECTION, OCTAFLUOROPROPANE MICROSPHERES, PER ML	C	N	57	A		
Q9957	INJECTION, PERFLUTREN LIPID MICROSPHERES, PER ML	C	N	57	A		
Q9958	HIGH OSMOLAR CONTRAST MATERIAL, UP TO 149 MG/ML IODINE CONCENTRATION, PER ML	D	N	51	A		15022
Q9959	HIGH OSMOLAR CONTRAST MATERIAL, 150-199 MG/ML IODINE CONCENTRATION, PER ML	D	N	51	A		15022
Q9960	HIGH OSMOLAR CONTRAST MATERIAL, 200-249 MG/ML IODINE CONCENTRATION, PER ML	D	N	51	A		15022
Q9961	HIGH OSMOLAR CONTRAST MATERIAL, 250-299 MG/ML IODINE CONCENTRATION, PER ML	D	N	51	A		15022
Q9962	HIGH OSMOLAR CONTRAST MATERIAL, 300-349 MG/ML IODINE CONCENTRATION, PER ML	D	N	51	A		15022
Q9963	HIGH OSMOLAR CONTRAST MATERIAL, 350-399 MG/ML IODINE CONCENTRATION, PER ML	D	N	51	A		15022
Q9964	HIGH OSMOLAR CONTRAST MATERIAL, 400 OR GREATER MG/ML IODINE CONCENTRATION, PER ML	D	N	51	A		15022
Q9965	LOW OSMOLAR CONTRAST MATERIAL, 100-199 MG/ML IODINE CONCENTRATION, PER ML	D	N	51	A		15022
Q9966	LOW OSMOLAR CONTRAST MATERIAL, 200-299 MG/ML IODINE CONCENTRATION, PER ML	D	N	51	A		15022
Q9967	LOW OSMOLAR CONTRAST MATERIAL, 300-399 MG/ML IODINE CONCENTRATION, PER ML	D	N	51	A		15022
Q9968	INJECTION, NON-RADIOACTIVE, NON-CONTRAST, VISUALIZATION ADJUNCT (E.G.,METHYLENE BLUE, ISOSULFAN BLUE), 1 MG	C	A	51	A		
R0070	TRANSPORTATION OF PORTABLE X-RAY EQUIPMENT AND PERSONNEL TO HOME OR NURSING HOME, PER TRIP TO FACILITY OR LOCATION, ONE PATIENT SEEN	D	N	13	A		2070.4, 5244.B
R0075	TRANSPORTATION OF PORTABLE X-RAY EQUIPMENT AND PERSONNEL TO HOME OR NURSING HOME, PER TRIP TO FACILITY OR LOCATION, MORE THAN ONE PATIENT SEEN	D	N	13	A		2070.4, 5244.B
R0076	TRANSPORTATION OF PORTABLE EKG TO FACILITY OR LOCATION, PER PATIENT	D	N	13	A	50-15	2070.1, 2070.4
R0075	TRANSPORTATION OF PORTABLE X-RAY EQUIPMENT AND PERSONNEL TO HOME OR NURSING HOME, PER TRIP TO FACILITY OR LOCATION, MORE THAN ONE PATIENT SEEN	D	N	13	A		2070.4, 5244B
R0076	TRANSPORTATION OF PORTABLE EKG TO FACILITY OR LOCATION, PER PATIENT	D	N	13	A	50-15	2070.1, 2070.4

HCPCS Code	Statute	Lab Cert	X-Ref	ASC Pay Grp	ASC Pay Group Eff. Date	Proc Notes	BETOS	TOS	Anest	Code Add Date	Code Effective Date	Code Term Date
Q9949							I1E	4	0	20050401	20080101	20071231
Q9950							I1E	4	0	20050401	20080101	20071231
Q9951							I1E	4	0	20050401	20050401	
Q9952							I1F	4	0	20050401	20080101	20071231
Q9953							I1F	4	0	20050401	20050401	
Q9954							I1F	4	0	20050401	20050401	
Q9955							I1F	4	0	20050401	20050401	
Q9956							I1F	4	0	20050401	20050401	
Q9957							I1F	4	0	20050401	20050401	
Q9958							I1E	4	0	20050701	20050701	
Q9959							I1E	4	0	20050701	20050701	
Q9960							I1E	4	0	20050701	20050701	
Q9961							I1E	4	0	20050701	20050701	
Q9962							I1E	4	0	20050701	20050701	
Q9963							I1E	4	0	20050701	20050701	
Q9964							I1E	4	0	20050701	20050701	
Q9965							I1E	4	0	20080101	20080101	
Q9966							I1E	4	0	20080101	20080101	
Q9967							I1E	4	0	20080101	20080101	
Q9968				YY	20100101		I1E	4	0	20100101	20100101	
R0070							I1F	4	0	19820101	19980101	
R0075							I1F	4	0	19860101	19980101	
R0076						0061	I1F	5	0	19840101	19980101	
R0075							I1F	4	0	19860101	19980101	
R0076						0061	I1F	5	0	19840101	19980101	

HCPCS Code	Long Description	Coverage	Action	PI	MPI	CIM	MCM
S0012	BUTORPHANOL TARTRATE, NASAL SPRAY, 25 MG	I	N	00	9		
S0014	TACRINE HYDROCHLORIDE, 10 MG	I	N	00	9		
S0017	INJECTION, AMINOCAPROIC ACID, 5 GRAMS	I	N	00	9		
S0020	INJECTION, BUPIVICAINE HYDROCHLORIDE, 30 ML	I	N	00	9		
S0021	INJECTION, CEFOPERAZONE SODIUM, 1 GRAM	I	N	00	9		
S0023	INJECTION, CIMETIDINE HYDROCHLORIDE, 300 MG	I	N	00	9		
S0028	INJECTION, FAMOTIDINE, 20 MG	I	N	00	9		
S0030	INJECTION, METRONIDAZOLE, 500 MG	I	N	00	9		
S0032	INJECTION, NAFCILLIN SODIUM, 2 GRAMS	I	N	00	9		
S0034	INJECTION, OFLOXACIN, 400 MG	I	N	00	9		
S0039	INJECTION, SULFAMETHOXAZOLE AND TRIMETHOPRIM, 10 ML	I	N	00	9		
S0040	INJECTION, TICARCILLIN DISODIUM AND CLAVULANATE POTASSIUM, 3.1 GRAMS	I	N	00	9		
S0073	INJECTION, AZTREONAM, 500 MG	I	N	00	9		
S0074	INJECTION, CEFOTETAN DISODIUM, 500 MG	I	N	00	9		
S0077	INJECTION, CLINDAMYCIN PHOSPHATE, 300 MG	I	N	00	9		
S0078	INJECTION, FOSPHENYTOIN SODIUM, 750 MG	I	N	00	9		
S0080	INJECTION, PENTAMIDINE ISETHIONATE, 300 MG	I	N	00	9		
S0081	INJECTION, PIPERACILLIN SODIUM, 500 MG	I	N	00	9		
S0088	IMATINIB, 100 MG	I	N	00	9		
S0090	SILDENAFIL CITRATE, 25 MG	I	N	00	9		
S0091	GRANISETRON HYDROCHLORIDE, 1MG (FOR CIRCUMSTANCES FALLING UNDER THE MEDICARE STATUTE, USE Q0166)	I	N	00	9		
S0092	INJECTION, HYDROMORPHONE HYDROCHLORIDE, 250 MG (LOADING DOSE FOR INFUSION PUMP)	I	N	00	9		
S0093	INJECTION, MORPHINE SULFATE, 500 MG (LOADING DOSE FOR INFUSION PUMP)	I	N	00	9		
S0104	ZIDOVUDINE, ORAL, 100 MG	I	N	00	9		
S0106	BUPROPION HCL SUSTAINED RELEASE TABLET, 150 MG, PER BOTTLE OF 60 TABLETS	I	N	00	9		
S0108	MERCAPTOPURINE, ORAL, 50 MG	I	N	00	9		
S0109	METHADONE, ORAL, 5 MG	I	N	00	9		
S0116	BEVACIZUMAB, 100 MG	I	N	00	9		
S0117	TRETINOIN, TOPICAL, 5 GRAMS	I	N	00	9		
S0122	INJECTION, MENOTROPINS, 75 IU	I	N	00	9		
S0126	INJECTION, FOLLITROPIN ALFA, 75 IU	I	N	00	9		
S0128	INJECTION, FOLLITROPIN BETA, 75 IU	I	N	00	9		
S0132	INJECTION, GANIRELIX ACETATE, 250 MCG	I	N	00	9		
S0133	HISTRELIN, IMPLANT, 50 MG	I	N	00	9		
S0136	CLOZAPINE, 25 MG	I	N	00	9		
S0137	DIDANOSINE (DDI), 25 MG	I	N	00	9		
S0138	FINASTERIDE, 5 MG	I	N	00	9		
S0139	MINOXIDIL, 10 MG	I	N	00	9		
S0140	SAQUINAVIR, 200 MG	I	N	00	9		
S0141	ZALCITABINE (DDC), 0.375 MG	I	N	00	9		
S0142	COLISTIMETHATE SODIUM, INHALATION SOLUTION ADMINISTERED THROUGH DME, CONCENTRATED FORM, PER MG	I	N	00	9		

HCPCS Code	Statute	Lab Cert	X-Ref	ASC Pay Grp	ASC Pay Group Eff. Date	Proc Notes	BETOS	TOS	Anest	Code Add Date	Code Effective Date	Code Term Date
S0012						0088	Z2	1	0	20000101	20000101	
S0014						0088	Z2	1, P	0	20000101	20000101	
S0017						0088	Z2	1, P	0	20000101	20000101	
S0020						0088	Z2	1, P	0	20000101	20000101	
S0021						0088	Z2	1, P	0	20000101	20000101	
S0023						0088	Z2	1, P	0	20000101	20000101	
S0028						0088	Z2	1, P	0	20000101	20000101	
S0030						0088	Z2	1, P	0	20000101	20000101	
S0032						0088	Z2	1, P	0	20000101	20000101	
S0034						0088	Z2	1, P	0	20000101	20000101	
S0039						0088	Z2	1, P	0	20000101	20000101	
S0040						0088	Z2	1, P	0	20000101	20000101	
S0073						0088	Z2	1, P	0	20000101	20000101	
S0074						0088	Z2	1, P	0	20000101	20000101	
S0077						0088	Z2	1, P	0	20000101	20000101	
S0078						0088	Z2	1, P	0	20000101	20000101	
S0080						0088	Z2	1, P	0	20000101	20000101	
S0081						0088	Z2	1, P	0	20000101	20000101	
S0088						0088	Z2	9	0	20020101	20081001	
S0090						0088	Z2	1, P	0	20000101	20000101	
S0091						0088	Z2	9	0	20020101	20010701	
S0092						0088	Z2	9	0	20020101	20010701	
S0093						0088	Z2	9	0	20020101	20010701	
S0104							Z2	1	0	20021001	20021001	
S0106							Z2	9	0	20020401	20020401	
S0108							Z2	9	0	20020401	20020401	
S0109							Z2	9	0	20041001	20041001	
S0116							Z2	9	0	20040701	20060701	20060630
S0117							Z2	9	0	20040701	20040701	
S0122							Z2	1, P	0	20020401	20020401	
S0126							Z2	1, P	0	20020401	20020401	
S0128							Z2	1, P	0	20020401	20020401	
S0132							Z2	1, P	0	20020401	20020401	
S0133							Z2	9	0	20050701	20060401	20060331
S0136							Z2	9	0	20030401	20030401	
S0137							Z2	9	0	20030401	20030401	
S0138							Z2	9	0	20030401	20030401	
S0139							Z2	9	0	20030401	20030401	
S0140							Z2	9	0	20030401	20030401	
S0141							Z2	9	0	20030401	20081001	20080930
S0142							Z2	9	0	20050401	20050401	

HCPCS Code	Long Description	Coverage	Action	PI	MPI	CIM	MCM
S0143	AZTREONAM, INHALATION SOLUTION ADMINISTERED THROUGH DME, CONCENTRATED FORM, PER GRAM	I	N	00	9		
S0145	INJECTION, PEGYLATED INTERFERON ALFA-2A, 180 MCG PER ML	I	N	00	9		
S0146	INJECTION, PEGYLATED INTERFERON ALFA-2B, 10 MCG PER 0.5 ML	I	N	00	9		
S0147	INJECTION, ALGLUCOSIDASE ALFA, 20 MG	I	N	00	9		
S0155	STERILE DILUTANT FOR EPOPROSTENOL, 50ML	I	N	00	9		
S0156	EXEMESTANE, 25 MG	I	N	00	9		
S0157	BECAPLERMIN GEL 0.01%, 0.5 GM	I	N	00	9		
S0160	DEXTROAMPHETAMINE SULFATE, 5 MG	I	N	00	9		
S0161	CALCITROL, 0.25 MG	I	N	00	9		
S0162	INJECTION, EFALIZUMAB, 125 MG	I	D	00	9		
S0164	INJECTION, PANTOPRAZOLE SODIUM, 40 MG	I	N	00	9		
S0166	INJECTION, OLANZAPINE, 2.5 MG	I	N	00	9		
S0167	INJECTION, APOMORPHINE HYDROCHLORIDE, 1 MG	I	N	00	9		
S0170	ANASTROZOLE, ORAL, 1MG	I	N	00	9		
S0171	INJECTION, BUMETANIDE, 0.5MG	I	N	00	9		
S0172	CHLORAMBUCIL, ORAL, 2MG	I	N	00	9		
S0174	DOLASETRON MESYLATE, ORAL 50MG (FOR CIRCUMSTANCES FALLING UNDER THE MEDICARE STATUTE, USE Q0180)	I	N	00	9		
S0175	FLUTAMIDE, ORAL, 125MG	I	N	00	9		
S0176	HYDROXYUREA, ORAL, 500MG	I	N	00	9		
S0177	LEVAMISOLE HYDROCHLORIDE, ORAL, 50MG	I	N	00	9		
S0178	LOMUSTINE, ORAL, 10MG	I	N	00	9		
S0179	MEGESTROL ACETATE, ORAL, 20MG	I	N	00	9		
S0180	ETONOGESTREL (CONTRACEPTIVE) IMPLANT SYSTEM, INCLUDING IMPLANT AND SUPPLIES	I	N	00	9		
S0181	ONDANSETRON HYDROCHLORIDE, ORAL, 4MG (FOR CIRCUMSTANCES FALLING UNDER THE MEDICARE STATUTE, USE Q0179)	I	N	00	9		
S0182	PROCARBAZINE HYDROCHLORIDE, ORAL, 50MG	I	N	00	9		
S0183	PROCHLORPERAZINE MALEATE, ORAL, 5MG (FOR CIRCUMSTANCES FALLING UNDER THE MEDICARE STATUTE, USE Q0164 - Q0165)	I	N	00	9		
S0187	TAMOXIFEN CITRATE, ORAL, 10MG	I	N	00	9		
S0189	TESTOSTERONE PELLET, 75MG	I	N	00	9		
S0190	MIFEPRISTONE, ORAL, 200 MG	I	N	00	9		
S0191	MISOPROSTOL, ORAL, 200 MCG	I	N	00	9		
S0194	DIALYSIS/STRESS VITAMIN SUPPLEMENT, ORAL, 100 CAPSULES	I	N	00	9		
S0195	PNEUMOCOCCAL CONJUGATE VACCINE, POLYVALENT, INTRAMUSCULAR, FOR CHILDREN FROM FIVE YEARS TO NINE YEARS OF AGE WHO HAVE NOT PREVIOUSLY RECEIVED THE VACCINE	I	N	00	9		
S0196	INJECTABLE POLY-L-LACTIC ACID, RESTORATIVE IMPLANT, 1 ML, FACE (DEEP DERMIS, SUBCUTANEOUS LAYERS)	I	N	00	9		
S0197	PRENATAL VITAMINS, 30-DAY SUPPLY	I	N	00	9		
S0198	INJECTION, PEGAPTANIB SODIUM, 0.3 MG	I	N	00	9		

HCPCS Code	Statute	Lab Cert	X-Ref	ASC Pay Grp	ASC Pay Group Eff. Date	Proc Notes	BETOS	TOS	Anest	Code Add Date	Code Effective Date	Code Term Date
S0143							Z2	9	0	20050401	20090101	20081231
S0145							Z2	9	0	20050701	20050701	
S0146							Z2	9	0	20050701	20050701	
S0147							Z2	9	0	20061001	20080101	20071231
S0155						0088	Z2	9	0	20020101	20020101	
S0156						0088	Z2	9	0	20010101	20010101	
S0157						0088	Z2	9	0	20010101	20010101	
S0160							Z2	9	0	20040401	20040401	
S0161							Z2	9	0	20040401	20040401	
S0162							Z2	9	0	20040401	20091001	20090930
S0164							Z2	9	0	20040401	20040401	
S0166							Z2	9	0	20041001	20041001	
S0167							Z2	9	0	20041001	20070401	20070331
S0170						0088	Z2	1, P	0	20020101	20020101	
S0171						0088	Z2	9	0	20020101	20020101	
S0172						0088	Z2	9	0	20020101	20020101	
S0174						0088	Z2	9	0	20020101	20020101	
S0175						0088	Z2	9	0	20020101	20020101	
S0176						0088	Z2	9	0	20020101	20020101	
S0177						0088	Z2	9	0	20020101	20020101	
S0178						0088	Z2	9	0	20020101	20020101	
S0179						0088	Z2	1, P	0	20020101	20020101	
S0180							Z2	9	0	20070101	20080101	20071231
S0181						0088	Z2	9	0	20020101	20020101	
S0182						0088	Z2	9	0	20020101	20020101	
S0183						0088	Z2	9	0	20020101	20020101	
S0187						0088	Z2	9	0	20020101	20020101	
S0189						0088	Z2	1, P	0	20020101	20020101	
S0190						0088	Z2	9	0	20010101	20010101	
S0191						0088	Z2	9	0	20010101	20010101	
S0194							Z2	9	0	20040401	20040401	
S0195							Z2	9	0	20030101	20030101	
S0196							Z2	9	0	20050101	20050101	
S0197							Z2	9	0	20050401	20050401	
S0198							Z2	9	0	20050701	20060701	20060630

HCPCS Code	Long Description	Coverage	Action	PI	MPI	CIM	MCM
S0199	MEDICALLY INDUCED ABORTION BY ORAL INGESTION OF MEDICATION INCLUDING ALL ASSOCIATED SERVICES AND SUPPLIES (E.G., PATIENT COUNSELING, OFFICE VISITS, CONFIRMATION OF PREGNANCY BY HCG, ULTRASOUND TO CONFIRM DURATION OF PREGNANCY, ULTRASOUND TO CONFIRM COMPLETION OF ABORTION) EXCEPT DRUGS	I	N	00	9		
S0201	PARTIAL HOSPITALIZATION SERVICES, LESS THAN 24 HOURS, PER DIEM	I	N	00	9		
S0207	PARAMEDIC INTERCEPT, NON-HOSPITAL-BASED ALS SERVICE (NON-VOLUNTARY), NON-TRANSPORT	I	N	00	9		
S0208	PARAMEDIC INTERCEPT, HOSPITAL-BASED ALS SERVICE (NON-VOLUNTARY), NON-TRANSPORT	I	N	00	9		
S0209	WHEELCHAIR VAN, MILEAGE, PER MILE	I	N	00	9		
S0215	NON-EMERGENCY TRANSPORTATION; MILEAGE, PER MILE	I	N	00	9		
S0220	MEDICAL CONFERENCE BY A PHYSICIAN WITH INTERDISCIPLINARY TEAM OF HEALTH PROFESSIONALS OR REPRESENTATIVES OF COMMUNITY AGENCIES TO COORDINATE ACTIVITIES OF PATIENT CARE (PATIENT IS PRESENT); APPROXIMATELY 30 MINUTES	I	N	00	9		
S0221	MEDICAL CONFERENCE BY A PHYSICIAN WITH INTERDISCIPLINARY TEAM OF HEALTH PROFESSIONALS OR REPRESENTATIVES OF COMMUNITY AGENCIES TO COORDINATE ACTIVITIES OF PATIENT CARE (PATIENT IS PRESENT); APPROXIMATELY 60 MINUTES	I	N	00	9		
S0250	COMPREHENSIVE GERIATRIC ASSESSMENT AND TREATMENT PLANNING PERFORMED BY ASSESSMENT TEAM	I	N	00	9		
S0255	HOSPICE REFERRAL VISIT (ADVISING PATIENT AND FAMILY OF CARE OPTIONS) PERFORMED BY NURSE, SOCIAL WORKER, OR OTHER DESIGNATED STAFF	I	N	00	9		
S0257	COUNSELING AND DISCUSSION REGARDING ADVANCE DIRECTIVES OR END OF LIFE CARE PLANNING AND DECISIONS, WITH PATIENT AND/OR SURROGATE (LIST SEPARATELY IN ADDITION TO CODE FOR APPROPRIATE EVALUATION AND MANAGEMENT SERVICE)	I	N	00	9		
S0260	HISTORY AND PHYSICAL (OUTPATIENT OR OFFICE) RELATED TO SURGICAL PROCEDURE (LIST SEPARATELY IN ADDITION TO CODE FOR APPROPRIATE EVALUATION AND MANAGEMENT SERVICE)	I	N	00	9		
S0265	GENETIC COUNSELING, UNDER PHYSICIAN SUPERVISION, EACH 15 MINUTES	I	N	00	9		
S0270	PHYSICIAN MANAGEMENT OF PATIENT HOME CARE, STANDARD MONTHLY CASE RATE (PER 30 DAYS)	I	N	00	9		
S0271	PHYSICIAN MANAGEMENT OF PATIENT HOME CARE, HOSPICE MONTHLY CASE RATE (PER 30 DAYS)	I	N	00	9		
S0272	PHYSICIAN MANAGEMENT OF PATIENT HOME CARE, EPISODIC CARE MONTHLY CASE RATE (PER 30 DAYS)	I	N	00	9		
S0273	PHYSICIAN VISIT AT MEMBER'S HOME, OUTSIDE OF A CAPITATION ARRANGEMENT	I	N	00	9		

HCPCS Code	Statute	Lab Cert	X-Ref	ASC Pay Grp	ASC Pay Group Eff. Date	Proc Notes	BETOS	TOS	Anest	Code Add Date	Code Effective Date	Code Term Date
S0199						0088	Z2	9	0	20010101	20010101	
S0199												
S0201							Z2	9	0	20021001	20021001	
S0207							Z2	9	0	20021001	20021001	
S0208						0088	Z2	D	0	20020101	20020101	
S0209						0088	Z2	D	0	20020101	20020101	
S0215						0088	Z2	D	0	20020101	20020401	
S0220						0088	Z2	9	0	20010101	20010101	
S0221						0088	Z2	9	0	20010101	20010101	
S0250						0088	Z2	9	0	20020101	20020101	
S0255						0088	Z2	9	0	20020101	20020101	
S0257							Z2	9	0	20050101	20050101	
S0260						0088	Z2	9	0	20020101	20020101	
S0265							Z2	9	0	20050701	20050701	
S0270							Z2	9	0	20070401	20070401	
S0271							Z2	9	0	20070401	20070401	
S0272							Z2	9	0	20070401	20070401	
S0273							Z2	9	0	20070401	20070401	

HCPCS Code	Long Description	Coverage	Action	PI	MPI	CIM	MCM
S0274	NURSE PRACTITIONER VISIT AT MEMBER'S HOME, OUTSIDE OF A CAPITATION ARRANGEMENT	I	N	00	9		
S0280	MEDICAL HOME PROGRAM, COMPREHENSIVE CARE COORDINATION AND PLANNING, INITIAL PLAN	I	A	00	9		
S0281	MEDICAL HOME PROGRAM, COMPREHENSIVE CARE COORDINATION AND PLANNING, MAINTENANCE OF PLAN	I	A	00	9		
S0302	COMPLETED EARLY PERIODIC SCREENING DIAGNOSIS AND TREATMENT (EPSDT) SERVICE (LIST IN ADDITION TO CODE FOR APPROPRIATE EVALUATION & MANAGEMENT SERVICE)	I	N	00	9		
S0310	HOSPITALIST SERVICES (LIST SEPARATELY IN ADDITION TO CODE FOR APPROPRIATE EVALUATION AND MANAGEMENT SERVICE)	I	N	00	9		
S0315	DISEASE MANAGEMENT PROGRAM; INITIAL ASSESSMENT AND INITIATION OF THE PROGRAM	I	N	00	9		
S0316	DISEASE MANAGEMENT PROGRAM, FOLLOW-UP/ REASSESSMENT	I	N	00	9		
S0317	DISEASE MANAGEMENT PROGRAM; PER DIEM	I	N	00	9		
S0320	TELEPHONE CALLS BY A REGISTERED NURSE TO A DISEASE MANAGEMENT PROGRAM MEMBER FOR MONITORING PURPOSES; PER MONTH	I	N	00	9		
S0340	LIFESTYLE MODIFICATION PROGRAM FOR MANAGEMENT OF CORONARY ARTERY DISEASE, INCLUDING ALL SUPPORTIVE SERVICES; FIRST QUARTER / STAGE	I	N	00	9		
S0341	LIFESTYLE MODIFICATION PROGRAM FOR MANAGEMENT OF CORONARY ARTERY DISEASE, INCLUDING ALL SUPPORTIVE SERVICES; SECOND OR THIRD QUARTER / STAGE	I	N	00	9		
S0342	LIFESTYLE MODIFICATION PROGRAM FOR MANAGEMENT OF CORONARY ARTERY DISEASE, INCLUDING ALL SUPPORTIVE SERVICES; FOURTH QUARTER / STAGE	I	N	00	9		
S0345	ELECTROCARDIOGRAPHIC MONITORING UTILIZING A HOME COMPUTERIZED TELEMETRY STATION WITH AUTOMATIC ACTIVATION AND REAL-TIME NOTIFICATION OF MONITORING STATION, 24-HOUR ATTENDED MONITORING, INCLUDING RECORDING, MONITORING, RECEIPT OF TRANSMISSIONS, ANALYSIS, AND PHYSICIAN REVIEW AND INTERPRETATION; PER 24-HOUR PERIOD	I	D	00	9		
S0346	ELECTROCARDIOGRAPHIC MONITORING UTILIZING A HOME COMPUTERIZED TELEMETRY STATION WITH AUTOMATIC ACTIVATION AND REAL-TIME NOTIFICATION OF MONITORING STATION, 24-HOUR ATTENDED MONITORING, INCLUDING RECORDING, MONITORING, RECEIPT OF TRANSMISSIONS, AND ANALYSIS; PER 24-HOUR PERIOD	I	D	00	9		
S0347	ELECTROCARDIOGRAPHIC MONITORING UTILIZING A HOME COMPUTERIZED TELEMETRY STATION WITH AUTOMATIC ACTIVATION AND REAL-TIME NOTIFICATION OF MONITORING STATION, 24-HOUR ATTENDED MONITORING, INCLUDING PHYSICIAN REVIEW AND INTERPRETATION; 24-HOUR PERIOD	I	D	00	9		

HCPCS Code	Statute	Lab Cert	X-Ref	ASC Pay Grp	ASC Pay Group Eff. Date	Proc Notes	BETOS	TOS	Anest	Code Add Date	Code Effective Date	Code Term Date
S0274							Z2	9	0	20070401	20070401	
S0280							Z2	9	0	20100101	20100101	
S0281							Z2	9	0	20100101	20100101	
S0281												
S0302						0088	Z2	9	0	20020101	20020101	
S0310						0088	Z2	9	0	20020101	20020101	
S0315							Z2	9	0	20021001	20021001	
S0316							Z2	9	0	20021001	20061001	
S0317							Z2	9	0	20030701	20030701	
S0320							Z2	9	0	20021001	20021001	
S0340						0088	Z2	9	0	20020101	20020101	
S0341						0088	Z2	9	0	20020101	20020101	
S0341												
S0342						0088	Z2	9	0	20020101	20020101	
S0345							Z2	9	0	20060401	20100101	20091231
S0346							Z2	9	0	20060401	20100101	20091231
S0347							Z2	9	0	20060401	20100101	20091231

HCPCS Code	Long Description	Coverage	Action	PI	MPI	CIM	MCM
S0390	ROUTINE FOOT CARE; REMOVAL AND/OR TRIMMING OF CORNS, CALLUSES AND/OR NAILS AND PREVENTIVE MAINTENANCE IN SPECIFIC MEDICAL CONDITIONS (E.G. DIABETES), PER VISIT	I	N	00	9		
S0395	IMPRESSION CASTING OF A FOOT PERFORMED BY A PRACTITIONER OTHER THAN THE MANUFACTURER OF THE ORTHOTIC	I	N	00	9		
S0400	GLOBAL FEE FOR EXTRACORPOREAL SHOCK WAVE LITHOTRIPSY TREATMENT OF KIDNEY STONE(S)	I	N	00	9		
S0500	DISPOSABLE CONTACT LENS, PER LENS	I	N	00	9		
S0504	SINGLE VISION PRESCRIPTION LENS (SAFETY, ATHLETIC, OR SUNGLASS), PER LENS	I	N	00	9		
S0506	BIFOCAL VISION PRESCRIPTION LENS (SAFETY, ATHLETIC, OR SUNGLASS), PER LENS	I	N	00	9		
S0508	TRIFOCAL VISION PRESCRIPTION LENS (SAFETY, ATHLETIC, OR SUNGLASS), PER LENS	I	N	00	9		
S0510	NON-PRESCRIPTION LENS (SAFETY, ATHLETIC, OR SUNGLASS), PER LENS	I	N	00	9		
S0512	DAILY WEAR SPECIALTY CONTACT LENS, PER LENS	I	N	00	9		
S0514	COLOR CONTACT LENS, PER LENS	I	N	00	9		
S0515	SCLERAL LENS, LIQUID BANDAGE DEVICE, PER LENS	I	N	00	9		
S0516	SAFETY EYEGLASS FRAMES	I	N	00	9		
S0518	SUNGLASSES FRAMES	I	N	00	9		
S0580	POLYCARBONATE LENS (LIST THIS CODE IN ADDITION TO THE BASIC CODE FOR THE LENS)	I	N	00	9		
S0581	NONSTANDARD LENS (LIST THIS CODE IN ADDITION TO THE BASIC CODE FOR THE LENS)	I	N	00	9		
S0590	INTEGRAL LENS SERVICE, MISCELLANEOUS SERVICES REPORTED SEPARATELY	I	N	00	9		
S0592	COMPREHENSIVE CONTACT LENS EVALUATION	I	N	00	9		
S0595	DISPENSING NEW SPECTACLE LENSES FOR PATIENT SUPPLIED FRAME	I	N	00	9		
S0601	SCREENING PROCTOSCOPY	I	N	00	9		
S0605	DIGITAL RECTAL EXAMINATION, MALE, ANNUAL	I	D	00	9		
S0610	ANNUAL GYNECOLOGICAL EXAMINATION, NEW PATIENT	I	N	00	9		
S0612	ANNUAL GYNECOLOGICAL EXAMINATION, ESTABLISHED PATIENT	I	N	00	9		
S0613	ANNUAL GYNECOLOGICAL EXAMINATION; CLINICAL BREAST EXAMINATION WITHOUT PELVIC EVALUATION	I	N	00	9		
S0618	AUDIOMETRY FOR HEARING AID EVALUATION TO DETERMINE THE LEVEL AND DEGREE OF HEARING LOSS	I	N	00	9		
S0620	ROUTINE OPHTHALMOLOGICAL EXAMINATION INCLUDING REFRACTION; NEW PATIENT	I	N	00	9		
S0621	ROUTINE OPHTHALMOLOGICAL EXAMINATION INCLUDING REFRACTION; ESTABLISHED PATIENT	I	N	00	9		
S0622	PHYSICAL EXAM FOR COLLEGE, NEW OR ESTABLISHED PATIENT (LIST SEPARATELY IN ADDITION TO APPROPRIATE EVALUATION AND MANAGEMENT CODE)	I	N	00	9		

HCPCS Code	Statute	Lab Cert	X-Ref	ASC Pay Grp	ASC Pay Group Eff. Date	Proc Notes	BETOS	TOS	Anest	Code Add Date	Code Effective Date	Code Term Date
S0390							Z2	9	0	20020401	20020401	
S0395						0088	Z2	9	0	20020101	20020101	
S0400						0088	Z2	9	0	20020101	20020101	
S0500						0088	Z2	Q	0	20010701	20010701	
S0504						0088	Z2	Q	0	20010701	20010701	
S0506						0088	Z2	Q	0	20010701	20010701	
S0508						0088	Z2	Q	0	20010701	20010701	
S0510						0088	Z2	Q	0	20010701	20010701	
S0512						0088	Z2	Q	0	20010701	20010701	
S0514						0088	Z2	Q	0	20010701	20010701	
S0515							Z2	9	0	20041001	20041001	
S0516						0088	Z2	Q	0	20010701	20010701	
S0518						0088	Z2	Q	0	20010701	20010701	
S0580						0088	Z2	Q	0	20010701	20010701	
S0581						0088	Z2	Q	0	20010701	20010701	
S0590						0088	Z2	Q	0	20010701	20010701	
S0592						0088	Z2	Q	0	20010701	20010701	
S0595							Z2	9	0	20050401	20050401	
S0601						0088	Z2	9	0	20000101	20000101	
S0605						0088	Z2	9	0	20000101	20100101	20091231
S0610						0088	Z2	9	0	20000101	20000101	
S0612						0088	Z2	9	0	20000101	20000101	
S0613							Z2	9	0	20050701	20050701	
S0618							Z2	9	0	20040401	20040401	
S0620						0088	Z2	9	0	20000101	20000101	
S0621						0088	Z2	9	0	20000101	20000101	
S0622						0088	Z2	9	0	20020101	20020101	

HCPCS Code	Long Description	Coverage	Action	PI	MPI	CIM	MCM
S0625	RETINAL TELESCREENING BY DIGITAL IMAGING OF MULTIPLE DIFFERENT FUNDUS AREAS TO SCREEN FOR VISION-THREATENING CONDITIONS, INCLUDING IMAGING, INTERPRETATION AND REPORT	I	N	00	9		
S0630	REMOVAL OF SUTURES; BY A PHYSICIAN OTHER THAN THE PHYSICIAN WHO ORIGINALLY CLOSED THE WOUND	I	N	00	9		
S0800	LASER IN SITU KERATOMILEUSIS (LASIK)	I	N	00	9		
S0810	PHOTOREFRACTIVE KERATECTOMY (PRK)	I	N	00	9		
S0812	PHOTOTHERAPEUTIC KERATECTOMY (PTK)	I	N	00	9		
S0820	COMPUTERIZED CORNEAL TOPOGRAPHY, UNILATERAL	I	N	00	9		
S1001	DELUXE ITEM, PATIENT AWARE (LIST IN ADDITION TO CODE FOR BASIC ITEM)	I	N	00	9		
S1002	CUSTOMIZED ITEM (LIST IN ADDITION TO CODE FOR BASIC ITEM)	I	N	00	9		
S1015	IV TUBING EXTENSION SET	I	N	00	9		
S1016	NON-PVC (POLYVINYL CHLORIDE) INTRAVENOUS ADMINISTRATION SET, FOR USE WITH DRUGS THAT ARE NOT STABLE IN PVC E.G. PACLITAXEL	I	N	00	9		
S1025	INHALED NITRIC OXIDE FOR THE TREATMENT OF HYPOXIC RESPIRATORY FAILURE IN THE NEONATE; PER DIEM	I	N	00	9		
S1030	CONTINUOUS NONINVASIVE GLUCOSE MONITORING DEVICE, PURCHASE (FOR PHYSICIAN INTERPRETATION OF DATA, USE CPT CODE)	I	N	00	9		
S1031	CONTINUOUS NONINVASIVE GLUCOSE MONITORING DEVICE, RENTAL, INCLUDING SENSOR, SENSOR REPLACEMENT, AND DOWNLOAD TO MONITOR (FOR PHYSICIAN INTERPRETATION OF DATA, USE CPT CODE)	I	N	00	9		
S1040	CRANIAL REMOLDING ORTHOSIS, PEDIATRIC, RIGID, WITH SOFT INTERFACE MATERIAL, CUSTOM FABRICATED, INCLUDES FITTING AND ADJUSTMENT(S)	I	N	00	9		
S2053	TRANSPLANTATION OF SMALL INTESTINE AND LIVER ALLOGRAFTS	I	N	00	9		
S2054	TRANSPLANTATION OF MULTIVISCERAL ORGANS	I	N	00	9		
S2055	HARVESTING OF DONOR MULTIVISCERAL ORGANS, WITH PREPARATION AND MAINTENANCE OF ALLOGRAFTS; FROM CADAVER DONOR	I	N	00	9		
S2060	LOBAR LUNG TRANSPLANTATION	I	N	00	9		
S2061	DONOR LOBECTOMY (LUNG) FOR TRANSPLANTATION, LIVING DONOR	I	N	00	9		
S2065	SIMULTANEOUS PANCREAS KIDNEY TRANSPLANTATION	I	N	00	9		
S2066	BREAST RECONSTRUCTION WITH GLUTEAL ARTERY PERFORATOR (GAP) FLAP, INCLUDING HARVESTING OF THE FLAP, MICROVASCULAR TRANSFER, CLOSURE OF DONOR SITE AND SHAPING THE FLAP INTO A BREAST, UNILATERAL	I	N	00	9		
S2067	BREAST RECONSTRUCTION OF A SINGLE BREAST WITH "STACKED" DEEP INFERIOR EPIGASTRIC PERFORATOR (DIEP) FLAP(S) AND/OR GLUTEAL ARTERY PERFORATOR (GAP) FLAP(S), INCLUDING HARVESTING OF THE FLAP(S), MICROVASCULAR TRANSFER, CLOSURE OF DONOR SITE(S) AND SHAPING THE FLAP INTO A BREAST, UNILATERAL	I	N	00	9		

HCPCS Code	Statute	Lab Cert	X-Ref	ASC Pay Grp	ASC Pay Group Eff. Date	Proc Notes	BETOS	TOS	Anest	Code Add Date	Code Effective Date	Code Term Date
S0625							Z2	9	0	20050401	20050401	
S0630						0088	Z2	9	0	20010101	20010101	
S0630												
S0800						0088	Z2	9	0	20000101	20000101	
S0810						0088	Z2	2, 9	0	20000101	20000101	
S0812						0088	Z2	Q	0	20010701	20010701	
S0820						0088	Z2	9	0	20010101	20070401	20070331
S1001						0088	Z2	P	0	20010701	20010701	
S1002						0088	Z2	P	0	20010701	20010701	
S1015						0088	Z2	9	0	20010101	20010101	
S1016						0088	Z2	9	0	20010101	20010101	
S1025						0088	Z2	1	0	20020101	20070401	20070331
S1030						0088	Z2	P, R	0	20020101	20020101	
S1031						0088	Z2	A,P,R	0	20020101	20020101	
S1040							Z2	P	0	20021001	20070101	
S2053						0088	Z2	2, 9	0	20000101	20000101	
S2054						0088	Z2	9	0	20000101	20000101	
S2055						0088	Z2	9	0	20000101	20000101	
S2060						0088	Z2	9	0	20010101	20010101	
S2061						0088	Z2	9	0	20010101	20010101	
S2065						0088	Z2	2	0	20010701	20010701	
S2066							Z2	2	0	20070701	20070701	
S2067							Z2	2	0	20070701	20070701	
S2067												

HCPCS Code	Long Description	Coverage	Action	PI	MPI	CIM	MCM
S2068	BREAST RECONSTRUCTION WITH DEEP INFERIOR EPIGASTRIC PERFORATOR (DIEP) FLAP OR SUPERFICIAL INFERIOR EPIGASTRIC ARTERY (SIEA) FLAP, INCLUDING HARVESTING OF THE FLAP, MICROVASCULAR TRANSFER, CLOSURE OF DONOR SITE AND SHAPING THE FLAP INTO A BREAST, UNILATERA	I	N	00	9		
S2070	CYSTOURETHROSCOPY, WITH URETEROSCOPY AND/OR PYELOSCOPY; WITH ENDOSCOPIC LASER TREATMENT OF URETERAL CALCULI (INCLUDES URETERAL CATHETERIZATION)	I	N	00	9		
S2075	LAPAROSCOPY, SURGICAL; REPAIR INCISIONAL OR VENTRAL HERNIA	I	N	00	9		
S2076	LAPAROSCOPY, SURGICAL; REPAIR UMBILICAL HERNIA	I	N	00	9		
S2077	LAPAROSCOPY, SURGICAL; IMPLANTATION OF MESH OR OTHER PROSTHESIS FOR INCISIONAL OR VENTRAL HERNIA REPAIR (LIST SEPARATELY IN ADDITION TO CODE FOR INCISIONAL OR VENTRAL HERNIA REPAIR)	I	N	00	9		
S2078	LAPAROSCOPIC SUPRACERVICAL HYSTERECTOMY (SUBTOTAL HYSTERECTOMY), WITH OR WITHOUT REMOVAL OF TUBE(S), WITH OR WITHOUT REMOVAL OF OVARY(S)	I	N	00	9		
S2079	LAPAROSCOPIC ESOPHAGOMYOTOMY (HELLER TYPE)	I	N	00	9		
S2080	LASER-ASSISTED UVULOPALATOPLASTY (LAUP)	I	N	00	9		
S2083	ADJUSTMENT OF GASTRIC BAND DIAMETER VIA SUBCUTANEOUS PORT BY INJECTION OR ASPIRATION OF SALINE	I	N	00	9		
S2095	TRANSCATHETER OCCLUSION OR EMBOLIZATION FOR TUMOR DESTRUCTION, PERCUTANEOUS, ANY METHOD, USING YTTRIUM-90 MICROSPHERES	I	N	00	9		
S2102	ISLET CELL TISSUE TRANSPLANT FROM PANCREAS; ALLOGENEIC	I	N	00	9		
S2103	ADRENAL TISSUE TRANSPLANT TO BRAIN	I	N	00	9		
S2107	ADOPTIVE IMMUNOTHERAPY I.E. DEVELOPMENT OF SPECIFIC ANTI-TUMOR REACTIVITY (E.G. TUMOR-INFILTRATING LYMPHOCYTE THERAPY) PER COURSE OF TREATMENT	I	N	00	9		
S2112	ARTHROSCOPY, KNEE, SURGICAL FOR HARVESTING OF CARTILAGE (CHONDROCYTE CELLS)	I	N	00	9		
S2114	ARTHROSCOPY, SHOULDER, SURGICAL; TENODESIS OF BICEPS	I	N	00	9		
S2115	OSTEOTOMY, PERIACETABULAR, WITH INTERNAL FIXATION	I	N	00	9		
S2117	ARTHROEREISIS, SUBTALAR	I	N	00	9		
S2118	METAL-ON-METAL TOTAL HIP RESURFACING, INCLUDING ACETABULAR AND FEMORAL COMPONENTS	D	F	00	9		
S2120	LOW DENSITY LIPOPROTEIN (LDL) APHERESIS USING HEPARIN-INDUCED EXTRACORPOREAL LDL PRECIPITATION	I	N	00	9		
S2135	NEUROLYSIS, BY INJECTION, OF METATARSAL NEUROMA/ INTERDIGITAL NEURITIS, ANY INTERSPACE OF THE FOOT	I	N	00	9		
S2140	CORD BLOOD HARVESTING FOR TRANSPLANTATION, ALLOGENEIC	I	N	00	9		
S2142	CORD BLOOD-DERIVED STEM-CELL TRANSPLANTATION, ALLOGENEIC	I	N	00	9		

HCPCS Code	Statute	Lab Cert	X-Ref	ASC Pay Grp	ASC Pay Group Eff. Date	Proc Notes	BETOS	TOS	Anest	Code Add Date	Code Effective Date	Code Term Date
S2068							Z2	9	0	20060101	20070701	
S2070							Z2	9	0	20031001	20031001	
S2075							Z2	9	0	20051001	20090101	20081231
S2076							Z2	9	0	20051001	20090101	20081231
S2077							Z2	9	0	20051001	20090101	20081231
S2078							Z2	9	0	20060101	20070701	20070630
S2079							Z2	9	0	20060101	20060101	
S2080						0088	Z2	9	0	20020101	20020101	
S2083							Z2	9	0	20040401	20040401	
S2095							Z2	9	0	20040101	20040101	
S2102						0088	Z2	9	0	20010101	20010101	
S2103						0088	Z2	9	0	20010101	20010101	
S2107							Z2	9	0	20020401	20020401	
S2112						0088	Z2	2	0	20010701	20010701	
S2114							Z2	9	0	20051001	20080101	20071231
S2115						0088	Z2	9	0	20020101	20020101	
S2117							Z2	9	0	20051001	20051001	
S2118						0162	Z2	9	0	20081001	20100101	
S2120						0088	Z2	9	0	20010101	20010101	
S2135							Z2	9	0	20040101	20090101	20081231
S2140						0088	Z2	9	0	20010101	20010101	
S2142						0088	Z2	9	0	20010101	20010101	

HCPCS Code	Long Description	Coverage	Action	PI	MPI	CIM	MCM
S2150	BONE MARROW OR BLOOD-DERIVED STEM CELLS (PERIPHERAL OR UMBILICAL), ALLOGENEIC OR AUTOLOGOUS, HARVESTING, TRANSPLANTATION, AND RELATED COMPLICATIONS; INCLUDING: PHERESIS AND CELL PREPARATION/STORAGE; MARROW ABLATIVE THERAPY; DRUGS, SUPPLIES, HOSPITALIZATION WITH OUTPATIENT FOLLOW-UP; MEDICAL/SURGICAL,DIAGNOSTIC, EMERGENCY, AND REHABILITATIVE SERVICES; AND THE NUMBER OF DAYS OF PRE-AND POST-TRANSPLANT CARE IN THE GLOBAL DEFINITION	I	N	00	9		
S2152	SOLID ORGAN(S), COMPLETE OR SEGMENTAL, SINGLE ORGAN OR COMBINATION OF ORGANS; DECEASED OR LIVING DONOR (S), PROCUREMENT, TRANSPLANTATION, AND RELATED COMPLICATIONS; INCLUDING: DRUGS; SUPPLIES; HOSPITALIZATION WITH OUTPATIENT FOLLOW-UP; MEDICAL/SURGICAL, DIAGNOSTIC, EMERGENCY, AND REHABILITATIVE SERVICES, AND THE NUMBER OF DAYS OF PRE- AND POST-TRANSPLANT CARE IN THE GLOBAL DEFINITION	I	N	00	9		
S2202	ECHOSCLEROTHERAPY	I	N	00	9		
S2205	MINIMALLY INVASIVE DIRECT CORONARY ARTERY BYPASS SURGERY INVOLVING MINI-THORACOTOMY OR MINI-STERNOTOMY SURGERY, PERFORMED UNDER DIRECT VISION; USING ARTERIAL GRAFT(S), SINGLE CORONARY ARTERIAL GRAFT	I	N	00	9		
S2206	MINIMALLY INVASIVE DIRECT CORONARY ARTERY BYPASS SURGERY INVOLVING MINI-THORACOTOMY OR MINI-STERNOTOMY SURGERY, PERFORMED UNDER DIRECT VISION; USING ARTERIAL GRAFT(S), TWO CORONARY ARTERIAL GRAFTS	I	N	00	9		
S2207	MINIMALLY INVASIVE DIRECT CORONARY ARTERY BYPASS SURGERY INVOLVING MINI-THORACOTOMY OR MINI-STERNOTOMY SURGERY, PERFORMED UNDER DIRECT VISION; USING VENOUS GRAFT ONLY, SINGLE CORONARY VENOUS GRAFT	I	N	00	9		
S2208	MINIMALLY INVASIVE DIRECT CORONARY ARTERY BYPASS SURGERY INVOLVING MINI-THORACOTOMY OR MINI-STERNOTOMY SURGERY, PERFORMED UNDER DIRECT VISION; USING SINGLE ARTERIAL AND VENOUS GRAFT(S), SINGLE VENOUS GRAFT	I	N	00	9		
S2209	MINIMALLY INVASIVE DIRECT CORONARY ARTERY BYPASS SURGERY INVOLVING MINI-THORACOTOMY OR MINI-STERNOTOMY SURGERY, PERFORMED UNDER DIRECT VISION; USING TWO ARTERIAL GRAFTS AND SINGLE VENOUS GRAFT	I	N	00	9		
S2213	IMPLANTATION OF GASTRIC ELECTRICAL STIMULATION DEVICE	I	N	00	9		
S2225	MYRINGOTOMY, LASER-ASSISTED	I	N	00	9		
S2230	IMPLANTATION OF MAGNETIC COMPONENT OF SEMI-IMPLANTABLE HEARING DEVICE ON OSSICLES IN MIDDLE EAR	I	N	00	9		
S2235	IMPLANTATION OF AUDITORY BRAIN STEM IMPLANT	I	N	00	9		

HCPCS Code	Statute	Lab Cert	X-Ref	ASC Pay Grp	ASC Pay Group Eff. Date	Proc Notes	BETOS	TOS	Anest	Code Add Date	Code Effective Date	Code Term Date
S2150						0088	Z2	9	0	20020101	20040401	
S2152							Z2	9	0	20040401	20040401	
S2202						0088	Z2	9	0	20010101	20010101	
S2205						0088	Z2	9	0	20000101	20000101	
S2206						0088	Z2	9	0	20000101	20000101	
S2207						0088	Z2	9	0	20000101	20000101	
S2208						0088	Z2	9	0	20000101	20000101	
S2209						0088	Z2	9	0	20000101	20000101	
S2213							Z2	9	0	20031001	20070401	20070331
S2225							Z2	9	0	20040101	20040101	
S2230							Z2	9	0	20031001	20031001	
S2235							Z2	9	0	20031001	20031001	

HCPCS Code	Long Description	Coverage	Action	PI	MPI	CIM	MCM
S2250	UTERINE ARTERY EMBOLIZATION FOR UTERINE FIBROIDS	I	N	00	9		
S2260	INDUCED ABORTION, 17 TO 24 WEEKS	I	N	00	9		
S2262	ABORTION FOR MATERNAL INDICATION, 25 WEEKS OR GREATER	I	N	00	9		
S2265	INDUCED ABORTION, 25 TO 28 WEEKS	I	N	00	9		
S2266	INDUCED ABORTION, 29 TO 31 WEEKS	I	N	00	9		
S2267	INDUCED ABORTION, 32 WEEKS OR GREATER	I	N	00	9		
S2270	INSERTION OF VAGINAL CYLINDER FOR APPLICATION OF RADIATION SOURCE OR CLINICAL BRACHYTHERAPY (REPORT SEPARATELY IN ADDITION TO RADIATION SOURCE DELIVERY)	D	F	00	9		
S2300	ARTHROSCOPY, SHOULDER, SURGICAL; WITH THERMALLY-INDUCED CAPSULORRHAPHY	I	N	00	9		
S2325	HIP CORE DECOMPRESSION	I	N	00	9		
S2340	CHEMODENERVATION OF ABDUCTOR MUSCLE(S) OF VOCAL CORD	I	N	00	9		
S2341	CHEMODENERVATION OF ADDUCTOR MUSCLE(S) OF VOCAL CORD	I	N	00	9		
S2342	NASAL ENDOSCOPY FOR POST-OPERATIVE DEBRIDEMENT FOLLOWING FUNCTIONAL ENDOSCOPIC SINUS SURGERY, NASAL AND/OR SINUS CAVITY(S), UNILATERAL OR BILATERAL	I	N	00	9		
S2344	NASAL/SINUS ENDOSCOPY, SURGICAL; WITH ENLARGEMENT OF SINUS OSTIUM OPENING USING INFLATABLE DEVICE (I.E., BALLOON SINUPLASTY)	I	N	00	9		
S2348	DECOMPRESSION PROCEDURE, PERCUTANEOUS, OF NUCLEUS PULPOSUS OF INTERVERTEBRAL DISC, USING RADIOFREQUENCY ENERGY, SINGLE OR MULTIPLE LEVELS, LUMBAR	I	N	00	9		
S2350	DISKECTOMY, ANTERIOR, WITH DECOMPRESSION OF SPINAL CORD AND/OR NERVE ROOT(S), INCLUDING OSTEOPHYTECTOMY; LUMBAR, SINGLE INTERSPACE	I	N	00	9		
S2351	DISKECTOMY, ANTERIOR, WITH DECOMPRESSION OF SPINAL CORD AND/OR NERVE ROOT(S),INCLUDING OSTEOPHYTECTOMY; LUMBAR, EACH ADDITIONAL INTERSPACE (LIST SEPARATELY IN ADDITION TO CODE FOR PRIMARY PROCEDURE)	I	N	00	9		
S2360	PERCUTANEOUS VERTEBROPLASTY, ONE VERTEBRAL BODY, UNILATERAL OR BILATERAL INJECTION; CERVICAL	I	N	00	9		
S2361	EACH ADDITIONAL CERVICAL VERTEBRAL BODY (LIST SEPARATELY IN ADDITION TO CODE FOR PRIMARY PROCEDURE)	I	N	00	9		
S2362	KYPHOPLASTY, ONE VERTEBRAL BODY, UNILATERAL OR BILATERAL INJECTION	I	N	00	9		
S2363	KYPHOPLASTY, ONE VERTEBRAL BODY, UNILATERAL OR BILATERAL INJECTION; EACH ADDITIONAL VERTEBRAL BODY (LIST SEPARATELY IN ADDITION TO CODE FOR PRIMARY PROCEDURE)	I	N	00	9		
S2400	REPAIR, CONGENITAL DIAPHRAGMATIC HERNIA IN THE FETUS USING TEMPORARY TRACHEAL OCCLUSION, PROCEDURE PERFORMED IN UTERO	I	N	00	9		

HCPCS Code	Statute	Lab Cert	X-Ref	ASC Pay Grp	ASC Pay Group Eff. Date	Proc Notes	BETOS	TOS	Anest	Code Add Date	Code Effective Date	Code Term Date
S2250						0088	Z2	9	0	20020101	20070401	20070331
S2260						0088	Z2	9	0	20020101	20070101	
S2262							Z2	9	0	20021001	20070101	20061231
S2265							Z2	9	0	20021001	20070101	
S2266							Z2	9	0	20021001	20070101	
S2267							Z2	9	0	20021001	20070101	
S2270						0162	Z2	9	0	20081001	20100101	
S2300						0088	Z2	9	0	20000101	20000101	
S2325							Z2	9	0	20061001	20061001	
S2340						0088	Z2	9	0	20010101	20010101	
S2341						0088	Z2	9	0	20020101	20020101	
S2342						0088	Z2	9	0	20020101	20020101	
S2342												
S2344							Z2	9	0	20070101	20070101	
S2348							Z2	9	0	20050101	20050101	
S2350						0088	Z2	9	0	20000101	20000101	
S2351						0088	Z2	9	0	20000101	20000101	
S2360						0088	Z2	9	0	20020101	20020101	
S2361						0088	Z2	9	0	20020101	20020101	
S2362							Z2	9	0	20040101	20060401	20060331
S2363							Z2	9	0	20040101	20060401	20060331
S2400						0088	Z2	2	0	20020101	20020401	

HCPCS Code	Long Description	Coverage	Action	PI	MPI	CIM	MCM
S2401	REPAIR, URINARY TRACT OBSTRUCTION IN THE FETUS, PROCEDURE PERFORMED IN UTERO	I	N	00	9		
S2402	REPAIR, CONGENITAL CYSTIC ADENOMATOID MALFORMATION IN THE FETUS, PROCEDURE PERFORMED IN UTERO	I	N	00	9		
S2403	REPAIR, EXTRALOBAR PULMONARY SEQUESTRATION IN THE FETUS, PROCEDURE PERFORMED IN UTERO	I	N	00	9		
S2404	REPAIR, MYELOMENINGOCELE IN THE FETUS, PROCEDURE PERFORMED IN UTERO	I	N	00	9		
S2405	REPAIR OF SACROCOCCYGEAL TERATOMA IN THE FETUS, PROCEDURE PERFORMED IN UTERO	I	N	00	9		
S2409	REPAIR, CONGENITAL MALFORMATION OF FETUS, PROCEDURE PERFORMED IN UTERO, NOT OTHERWISE CLASSIFIED	I	N	00	9		
S2411	FETOSCOPIC LASER THERAPY FOR TREATMENT OF TWIN-TO-TWIN TRANSFUSION SYNDROME	I	N	00	9		
S2900	SURGICAL TECHNIQUES REQUIRING USE OF ROBOTIC SURGICAL SYSTEM (LIST SEPARATELY IN ADDITION TO CODE FOR PRIMARY PROCEDURE)	I	N	00	9		
S3000	DIABETIC INDICATOR; RETINAL EYE EXAM, DILATED, BILATERAL	I	N	00	9		
S3005	PERFORMANCE MEASUREMENT, EVALUATION OF PATIENT SELF ASSESSMENT, DEPRESSION	I	N	00	9		
S3600	STAT LABORATORY REQUEST (SITUATIONS OTHER THAN S3601)	I	N	00	9		
S3601	EMERGENCY STAT LABORATORY CHARGE FOR PATIENT WHO IS HOMEBOUND OR RESIDING IN A NURSING FACILITY	I	N	00	9		
S3618	BLOOD CHEMISTRY FOR FREE BETA HUMAN CHORIONIC GONADOTROPIN (HCG)	I	N	00	9		
S3620	NEWBORN METABOLIC SCREENING PANEL, INCLUDES TEST KIT, POSTAGE AND THE LABORATORY TESTS SPECIFIED BY THE STATE FOR INCLUSION IN THIS PANEL (E.G. GALACTOSE; HEMOGLOBIN, ELECTROPHORESIS; HYDROXYPROGESTERONE, 17-D; PHENYLANINE (PKU); AND THYROXINE, TOTAL)	I	N	00	9		
S3625	MATERNAL SERUM TRIPLE MARKER SCREEN INCLUDING ALPHA-FETOPROTEIN (AFP), ESTRIOL, AND HUMAN CHORIONIC GONADOTROPIN (HCG)	I	N	00	9		
S3626	MATERNAL SERUM QUADRUPLE MARKER SCREEN INCLUDING, ALPHA-FETOPROTEIN (AFP) ESTRIOL, HUMAN CHORIONIC GONADOTROPIN (HCG) AND INHIBIN A	I	N	00	9		
S3628	PLACENTAL ALPHA MICROGLOBULIN-1 RAPID IMMUNOASSAY FOR DETECTION OF RUPTURE OF FETAL MEMBRANES	D	F	00	9		
S3630	EOSINOPHIL COUNT, BLOOD, DIRECT	I	N	00	9		
S3645	HIV-1 ANTIBODY TESTING OF ORAL MUCOSAL TRANSUDATE	I	N	00	9		
S3650	SALIVA TEST, HORMONE LEVEL; DURING MENOPAUSE	I	N	00	9		
S3652	SALIVA TEST, HORMONE LEVEL; TO ASSESS PRETERM LABOR RISK	I	N	00	9		
S3655	ANTISPERM ANTIBODIES TEST (IMMUNOBEAD)	I	N	00	9		
S3701	IMMUNOASSAY FOR NUCLEAR MATRIX PROTEIN 22 (NMP-22), QUANTITATIVE	I	N	00	9		
S3708	GASTROINTESTINAL FAT ABSORPTION STUDY	I	N	00	9		

HCPCS Code	Statute	Lab Cert	X-Ref	ASC Pay Grp	ASC Pay Group Eff. Date	Proc Notes	BETOS	TOS	Anest	Code Add Date	Code Effective Date	Code Term Date
S2401						0088	Z2	2	0	20020101	20020101	
S2402						0088	Z2	2	0	20020101	20020101	
S2403						0088	Z2	2	0	20020101	20020101	
S2404						0088	Z2	2	0	20020101	20020101	
S2405							Z2	9	0	20020401	20020401	
S2409						0088	Z2	2	0	20020101	20020101	
S2411						0088	Z2	9	0	20020101	20020101	
S2900							Z2	9	0	20050701	20050701	
S3000							Z2	9	0	20030401	20030401	
S3005							Z2	9	0	20050401	20050401	
S3600						0088	Z2	9	0	20020101	20020101	
S3601						0088	Z2	9	0	20020101	20020101	
S3601												
S3618							Z2	9	0	20070401	20080101	20071231
S3620						0088	Z2	9	0	20010101	20010101	
S3625							Z2	9	0	20030701	20030701	
S3626							Z2	9	0	20051001	20051001	
S3628						0162	Z2	9	0	20080401	20100101	
S3630						0088	Z2	9	0	20020101	20020101	
S3645						0088	Z2	9	0	20000101	20000101	
S3650						0088	Z2	9	0	20000101	20000101	
S3652						0088	Z2	9	0	20000101	20000101	
S3655							Z2	9	0	20021001	20021001	
S3701						0088	Z2	9	0	20020101	20060401	20060331
S3708						0088	Z2	9	0	20010101	20010101	

HCPCS Code	Long Description	Coverage	Action	PI	MPI	CIM	MCM
S3711	CIRCULATING TUMOR CELL TEST	D	F	00	9		
S3713	KRAS MUTATION ANALYSIS TESTING	I	A	00	9		
S3800	GENETIC TESTING FOR AMYOTROPHIC LATERAL SCLEROSIS (ALS)	I	N	00	9		
S3818	COMPLETE GENE SEQUENCE ANALYSIS; BRCA1 GENE	I	N	00	9		
S3819	COMPLETE GENE SEQUENCE ANALYSIS; BRCA2 GENE	I	N	00	9		
S3820	COMPLETE BRCA1 AND BRCA2 GENE SEQUENCE ANALYSIS FOR SUSCEPTIBILITY TO BREAST AND OVARIAN CANCER	I	N	00	9		
S3822	SINGLE MUTATION ANALYSIS (IN INDIVIDUAL WITH A KNOWN BRCA1 OR BRCA2 MUTATION IN THE FAMILY) FOR SUSCEPTIBILITY TO BREAST AND OVARIAN CANCER	I	N	00	9		
S3823	THREE-MUTATION BRCA1 AND BRCA2 ANALYSIS FOR SUSCEPTIBILITY TO BREAST AND OVARIAN CANCER IN ASHKENAZI INDIVIDUALS	I	N	00	9		
S3828	COMPLETE GENE SEQUENCE ANALYSIS; MLH1 GENE	I	N	00	9		
S3829	COMPLETE GENE SEQUENCE ANALYSIS; MLH2 GENE	I	N	00	9		
S3830	COMPLETE MLH1 AND MLH2 GENE SEQUENCE ANALYSIS FOR HEREDITARY NONPOLYPOSIS COLORECTAL CANCER (HNPCC) GENETIC TESTING	I	N	00	9		
S3831	SINGLE-MUTATION ANALYSIS (IN INDIVIDUAL WITH A KNOWN MLH1 AND MLH2 MUTATION IN THE FAMILY) FOR HEREDITARY NONPOLYPOSIS COLORECTAL CANCER (HNPCC) GENETIC TESTING	I	N	00	9		
S3833	COMPLETE APC GENE SEQUENCE ANALYSIS FOR SUSCEPTIBILITY TO FAMILIAL ADENOMATOUS POLYPOSIS (FAP) AND ATTENUATED FAP	I	N	00	9		
S3834	SINGLE-MUTATION ANALYSIS (IN INDIVIDUAL WITH A KNOWN APC MUTATION IN THE FAMILY) FOR SUSCEPTIBILITY TO FAMILIAL ADENOMATOUS POLYPOSIS (FAP) AND ATTENUATED FAP	I	N	00	9		
S3835	COMPLETE GENE SEQUENCE ANALYSIS FOR CYSTIC FIBROSIS GENETIC TESTING	I	N	00	9		
S3837	COMPLETE GENE SEQUENCE ANALYSIS FOR HEMOCHROMATOSIS GENETIC TESTING	I	N	00	9		
S3840	DNA ANALYSIS FOR GERMLINE MUTATIONS OF THE RET PROTO-ONCOGENE FOR SUSCEPTIBILITY TO MULTIPLE ENDOCRINE NEOPLASIA TYPE 2	I	N	00	9		
S3841	GENETIC TESTING FOR RETINOBLASTOMA	I	N	00	9		
S3842	GENETIC TESTING FOR VON HIPPEL-LINDAU DISEASE	I	N	00	9		
S3843	DNA ANALYSIS OF THE F5 GENE FOR SUSCEPTIBILITY TO FACTOR V LEIDEN THROMBOPHILIA	I	N	00	9		
S3844	DNA ANALYSIS OF THE CONNEXIN 26 GENE (GJB2) FOR SUSCEPTIBILITY TO CONGENITAL, PROFOUND DEAFNESS	I	N	00	9		
S3845	GENETIC TESTING FOR ALPHA-THALASSEMIA	I	N	00	9		
S3846	GENETIC TESTING FOR HEMOGLOBIN E BETA-THALASSEMIA	I	N	00	9		
S3847	GENETIC TESTING FOR TAY-SACHS DISEASE	I	N	00	9		
S3848	GENETIC TESTING FOR GAUCHER DISEASE	I	N	00	9		
S3849	GENETIC TESTING FOR NIEMANN-PICK DISEASE	I	N	00	9		
S3850	GENETIC TESTING FOR SICKLE CELL ANEMIA	I	N	00	9		

HCPCS Code	Statute	Lab Cert	X-Ref	ASC Pay Grp	ASC Pay Group Eff. Date	Proc Notes	BETOS	TOS	Anest	Code Add Date	Code Effective Date	Code Term Date
S3711						0162	Z2	9	0	20090101	20100101	
S3713							Z2	9	0	20091001	20091001	
S3800							Z2	9	0	20070701	20070701	
S3818						0088	Z2	5	0	20010701	20010701	
S3819						0088	Z2	5	0	20010701	20010701	
S3820							Z2	9	0	20030401	20030401	
S3822							Z2	9	0	20030401	20030401	
S3823							Z2	9	0	20030401	20030401	
S3823												
S3828							Z2	9	0	20030401	20030401	
S3829							Z2	9	0	20030401	20030401	
S3830						0088	Z2	9	0	20020101	20020101	
S3831						0088	Z2	9	0	20020101	20020101	
S3833							Z2	9	0	20030401	20030401	
S3834							Z2	9	0	20030401	20030401	
S3835						0088	Z2	9	0	20020101	20020101	
S3837						0088	Z2	9	0	20020101	20020101	
S3840							Z2	9	0	20030701	20030701	
S3841							Z2	9	0	20030701	20030701	
S3842							Z2	9	0	20030701	20030701	
S3843							Z2	9	0	20030701	20030701	
S3844							Z2	9	0	20030701	20030701	
S3845							Z2	9	0	20030701	20030701	
S3846							Z2	9	0	20030701	20030701	
S3847							Z2	9	0	20030701	20030701	
S3848							Z2	9	0	20030701	20030701	
S3849							Z2	9	0	20030701	20030701	
S3850							Z2	9	0	20030701	20030701	

HCPCS Code	Long Description	Coverage	Action	PI	MPI	CIM	MCM
S3851	GENETIC TESTING FOR CANAVAN DISEASE	I	N	00	9		
S3852	DNA ANALYSIS FOR APOE EPSILON 4 ALLELE FOR SUSCEPTIBILITY TO ALZHEIMER'S DISEASE	I	N	00	9		
S3853	GENETIC TESTING FOR MYOTONIC MUSCULAR DYSTROPHY	I	N	00	9		
S3854	GENE EXPRESSION PROFILING PANEL FOR USE IN THE MANAGEMENT OF BREAST CANCER TREATMENT	I	N	00	9		
S3855	GENETIC TESTING FOR DETECTION OF MUTATIONS IN THE PRESENILIN - 1 GENE	I	N	00	9		
S3860	GENETIC TESTING, COMPREHENSIVE CARDIAC ION CHANNEL ANALYSIS, FOR VARIANTS IN 5 MAJOR CARDIAC ION CHANNEL GENES FOR INDIVIDUALS WITH HIGH INDEX OF SUSPICION FOR FAMILIAL LONG QT SYNDROME (LQTS) OR RELATED SYNDROMES	D	F	00	9		
S3861	GENETIC TESTING, SODIUM CHANNEL, VOLTAGE-GATED, TYPE V, ALPHA SUBUNIT (SCN5A) AND VARIANTS FOR SUSPECTED BRUGADA SYNDROME	D	F	00	9		
S3862	GENETIC TESTING, FAMILY-SPECIFIC ION CHANNEL ANALYSIS, FOR BLOOD-RELATIVES OF INDIVIDUALS (INDEX CASE) WHO HAVE PREVIOUSLY TESTED POSITIVE FOR A GENETIC VARIANT OF A CARDIAC ION CHANNEL SYNDROME USING EITHER ONE OF THE ABOVE TEST CONFIGURATIONS OR CONFIRMED RESULTS FROM ANOTHER LABORATORY	D	F	00	9		
S3865	COMPREHENSIVE GENE SEQUENCE ANALYSIS FOR HYPERTROPHIC CARDIOMYOPATHY	I	A	00	9		
S3866	GENETIC ANALYSIS FOR A SPECIFIC GENE MUTATION FOR HYPERTROPHIC CARDIOMYOPATHY (HCM) IN AN INDIVIDUAL WITH A KNOWN HCM MUTATION IN THE FAMILY	I	A	00	9		
S3870	COMPARATIVE GENOMIC HYBRIZATION (CGH) MICROARRAY TESTING FOR DEVELOPMENTAL DELAY, AUTISM SPECTRUM DISORDER AND/OR MENTAL RETARDATION	I	A	00	9		
S3890	DNA ANALYSIS, FECAL, FOR COLORECTAL CANCER SCREENING	I	N	00	9		
S3900	SURFACE ELECTROMYOGRAPHY (EMG)	I	N	00	9		
S3902	BALLISTOCARDIOGRAM	I	N	00	9		
S3904	MASTERS TWO STEP	I	N	00	9		
S3905	NON-INVASIVE ELECTRODIAGNOSTIC TESTING WITH AUTOMATIC COMPUTERIZED HAND-HELD DEVICE TO STIMULATE AND MEASURE NEUROMUSCULAR SIGNALS IN DIAGNOSING AND EVALUATING SYSTEMIC AND ENTRAPMENT NEUROPATHIES	I	N	00	9		
S4005	INTERIM LABOR FACILITY GLOBAL (LABOR OCCURRING BUT NOT RESULTING IN DELIVERY)	I	N	00	9		
S4011	IN VITRO FERTILIZATION; INCLUDING BUT NOT LIMITED TO IDENTIFICATION AND INCUBATION OF MATURE OOCYTES, FERTILIZATION WITH SPERM, INCUBATION OF EMBRYO(S), AND SUBSEQUENT VISUALIZATION FOR DETERMINATION OF DEVELOPMENT	I	N	00	9		
S4013	COMPLETE CYCLE, GAMETE INTRAFALLOPIAN TRANSFER (GIFT), CASE RATE	I	N	00	9		
S4014	COMPLETE CYCLE, ZYGOTE INTRAFALLOPIAN TRANSFER (ZIFT), CASE RATE	I	N	00	9		

HCPCS Code	Statute	Lab Cert	X-Ref	ASC Pay Grp	ASC Pay Group Eff. Date	Proc Notes	BETOS	TOS	Anest	Code Add Date	Code Effective Date	Code Term Date
S3851							Z2	9	0	20030701	20030701	
S3852							Z2	9	0	20030701	20030701	
S3853							Z2	9	0	20040101	20040101	
S3854							Z2	9	0	20060101	20060101	
S3855							Z2	9	0	20070101	20070101	
S3860						0162	Z2	9	0	20081001	20100101	
S3861						0162	Z2	9	0	20081001	20100101	
S3862						0162	Z2	9	0	20081001	20100101	
S3865							Z2	9	0	20090401	20090401	
S3866							Z2	9	0	20090401	20090401	
S3870							Z2	9	0	20090401	20090401	
S3890							Z2	9	0	20040401	20040401	
S3900						0088	Z2	9	0	20010701	20010701	
S3902						0088	Z2	9	0	20010101	20010101	
S3904						0088	Z2	9	0	20010101	20010101	
S3905							Z2	9	0	20070701	20070701	
S4005							Z2	9	0	20020401	20020401	
S4011						0088	Z2	9	0	20020101	20020101	
S4013							Z2	9	0	20020401	20020401	
S4014							Z2	9	0	20020401	20020401	

HCPCS Code	Long Description	Coverage	Action	PI	MPI	CIM	MCM
S4015	COMPLETE IN VITRO FERTILIZATION CYCLE, NOT OTHERWISE SPECIFIED, CASE RATE	I	N	00	9		
S4016	FROZEN IN VITRO FERTILIZATION CYCLE, CASE RATE	I	N	00	9		
S4017	INCOMPLETE CYCLE, TREATMENT CANCELLED PRIOR TO STIMULATION, CASE RATE	I	N	00	9		
S4018	FROZEN EMBRYO TRANSFER PROCEDURE CANCELLED	I	N	00	9		
S4020	IN VITRO FERTILIZATION PROCEDURE CANCELLED BEFORE ASPIRATION, CASE RATE	I	N	00	9		
S4021	IN VITRO FERTILIZATION PROCEDURE CANCELLED AFTER ASPIRATION, CASE RATE	I	N	00	9		
S4022	ASSISTED OOCYTE FERTILIZATION, CASE RATE	I	N	00	9		
S4023	DONOR EGG CYCLE, INCOMPLETE, CASE RATE	I	N	00	9		
S4025	DONOR SERVICES FOR IN VITRO FERTILIZATION (SPERM OR EMBRYO), CASE RATE	I	N	00	9		
S4026	PROCUREMENT OF DONOR SPERM FROM SPERM BANK	I	N	00	9		
S4027	STORAGE OF PREVIOUSLY FROZEN EMBRYOS	I	N	00	9		
S4028	MICROSURGICAL EPIDIDYMAL SPERM ASPIRATION (MESA)	I	N	00	9		
S4030	SPERM PROCUREMENT AND CRYOPRESERVATION SERVICES; INITIAL VISIT	I	N	00	9		
S4031	SPERM PROCUREMENT AND CRYOPRESERVATION SERVICES; SUBSEQUENT VISIT	I	N	00	9		
S4035	STIMULATED INTRAUTERINE INSEMINATION (IUI), CASE RATE	I	N	00	9		
S4036	INTRAVAGINAL CULTURE (IVC), CASE RATE	I	N	00	9		
S4037	CRYOPRESERVED EMBRYO TRANSFER, CASE RATE	I	N	00	9		
S4040	MONITORING AND STORAGE OF CRYOPRESERVED EMBRYOS, PER 30 DAYS	I	N	00	9		
S4042	MANAGEMENT OF OVULATION INDUCTION (INTERPRETATION OF DIAGNOSTIC TESTS AND STUDIES, NON-FACE-TO-FACE MEDICAL MANAGEMENT OF THE PATIENT), PER CYCLE	I	A	00	9		
S4981	INSERTION OF LEVONORGESTREL-RELEASING INTRAUTERINE SYSTEM	I	N	00	9		
S4989	CONTRACEPTIVE INTRAUTERINE DEVICE (E.G. PROGESTACERT IUD), INCLUDING IMPLANTS AND SUPPLIES	I	N	00	9		
S4990	NICOTINE PATCHES, LEGEND	I	N	00	9		
S4991	NICOTINE PATCHES, NON-LEGEND	I	N	00	9		
S4993	CONTRACEPTIVE PILLS FOR BIRTH CONTROL	I	N	00	9		
S4995	SMOKING CESSATION GUM	I	N	00	9		
S5000	PRESCRIPTION DRUG, GENERIC	I	N	00	9		
S5001	PRESCRIPTION DRUG, BRAND NAME	I	N	00	9		
S5010	5% DEXTROSE AND 0.45% NORMAL SALINE, 1000 ML	I	N	00	9		
S5011	5% DEXTROSE IN LACTATED RINGER'S, 1000 ML	I	N	00	9		
S5012	5% DEXTROSE WITH POTASSIUM CHLORIDE, 1000 ML	I	N	00	9		
S5013	5% DEXTROSE/0.45% NORMAL SALINE WITH POTASSIUM CHLORIDE AND MAGNESIUM SULFATE, 1000 ML	I	N	00	9		
S5014	5% DEXTROSE/0.45% NORMAL SALINE WITH POTASSIUM CHLORIDE AND MAGNESIUM SULFATE, 1500 ML	I	N	00	9		
S5035	HOME INFUSION THERAPY, ROUTINE SERVICE OF INFUSION DEVICE (E.G. PUMP MAINTENANCE)	I	N	00	9		
S5036	HOME INFUSION THERAPY, REPAIR OF INFUSION DEVICE (E.G. PUMP REPAIR)	I	N	00	9		

HCPCS Code	Statute	Lab Cert	X-Ref	ASC Pay Grp	ASC Pay Group Eff. Date	Proc Notes	BETOS	TOS	Anest	Code Add Date	Code Effective Date	Code Term Date
S4015						0088	Z2	9	0	20020101	20020401	
S4016						0088	Z2	9	0	20020101	20020101	
S4017							Z2	9	0	20020401	20020401	
S4018						0088	Z2	9	0	20020101	20020101	
S4020						0088	Z2	9	0	20020101	20020101	
S4021						0088	Z2	9	0	20020101	20020101	
S4022						0088	Z2	9	0	20020101	20020101	
S4023							Z2	9	0	20020401	20020401	
S4025						0088	Z2	9	0	20020101	20020101	
S4026						0088	Z2	9	0	20020101	20020101	
S4027						0088	Z2	9	0	20020101	20020101	
S4028						0088	Z2	9	0	20020101	20020101	
S4030						0088	Z2	9	0	20020101	20020101	
S4031						0088	Z2	9	0	20020101	20020101	
S4035							Z2	9	0	20020401	20020401	
S4036							Z2	9	0	20020401	20070101	20061231
S4037							Z2	9	0	20020401	20020401	
S4040							Z2	9	0	20020401	20020401	
S4042							Z2	9	0	20050101	20050101	
S4981						0088	Z2	2	0	20010701	20010701	
S4989						0088	Z2	9	0	20020101	20020101	
S4990						0088	Z2	9	0	20020101	20020101	
S4991						0088	Z2	9	0	20020101	20020101	
S4993							Z2	9	0	20020401	20020401	
S4995							Z2	9	0	20020401	20020401	
S5000						0088	Z2	9	0	20010101	20010101	
S5001						0088	Z2	9	0	20010101	20010101	
S5010						0088	Z2	9	0	20010101	20010101	
S5011						0088	Z2	9	0	20010101	20010101	
S5012						0088	Z2	9	0	20010101	20010101	
S5013						0088	Z2	9	0	20010101	20010101	
S5014						0088	Z2	9	0	20010101	20010101	
S5035						0088	Z2	9	0	20020101	20020101	
S5036						0088	Z2	9	0	20020101	20020101	

HCPCS Code	Long Description	Coverage	Action	PI	MPI	CIM	MCM
S5100	DAY CARE SERVICES, ADULT; PER 15 MINUTES	I	N	00	9		
S5101	DAY CARE SERVICES, ADULT; PER HALF DAY	I	N	00	9		
S5102	DAY CARE SERVICES, ADULT; PER DIEM	I	N	00	9		
S5105	DAY CARE SERVICES, CENTER-BASED; SERVICES NOT INCLUDED IN PROGRAM FEE, PER DIEM	I	N	00	9		
S5108	HOME CARE TRAINING TO HOME CARE CLIENT, PER 15 MINUTES	I	N	00	9		
S5109	HOME CARE TRAINING TO HOME CARE CLIENT, PER SESSION	I	N	00	9		
S5110	HOME CARE TRAINING, FAMILY; PER 15 MINUTES	I	N	00	9		
S5111	HOME CARE TRAINING, FAMILY; PER SESSION	I	N	00	9		
S5115	HOME CARE TRAINING, NON-FAMILY; PER 15 MINUTES	I	N	00	9		
S5116	HOME CARE TRAINING, NON-FAMILY; PER SESSION	I	N	00	9		
S5120	CHORE SERVICES; PER 15 MINUTES	I	N	00	9		
S5121	CHORE SERVICES; PER DIEM	I	N	00	9		
S5125	ATTENDANT CARE SERVICES; PER 15 MINUTES	I	N	00	9		
S5126	ATTENDANT CARE SERVICES; PER DIEM	I	N	00	9		
S5130	HOMEMAKER SERVICE, NOS; PER 15 MINUTES	I	N	00	9		
S5131	HOMEMAKER SERVICE, NOS; PER DIEM	I	N	00	9		
S5135	COMPANION CARE, ADULT (E.G. IADL/ADL); PER 15 MINUTES	I	N	00	9		
S5136	COMPANION CARE, ADULT (E.G. IADL/ADL); PER DIEM	I	N	00	9		
S5140	FOSTER CARE, ADULT; PER DIEM	I	N	00	9		
S5141	FOSTER CARE, ADULT; PER MONTH	I	N	00	9		
S5145	FOSTER CARE, THERAPEUTIC, CHILD; PER DIEM	I	N	00	9		
S5146	FOSTER CARE, THERAPEUTIC, CHILD; PER MONTH	I	N	00	9		
S5150	UNSKILLED RESPITE CARE, NOT HOSPICE; PER 15 MINUTES	I	N	00	9		
S5151	UNSKILLED RESPITE CARE, NOT HOSPICE; PER DIEM	I	N	00	9		
S5160	EMERGENCY RESPONSE SYSTEM; INSTALLATION AND TESTING	I	N	00	9		
S5161	EMERGENCY RESPONSE SYSTEM; SERVICE FEE, PER MONTH (EXCLUDES INSTALLATION AND TESTING)	I	N	00	9		
S5162	EMERGENCY RESPONSE SYSTEM; PURCHASE ONLY	I	N	00	9		
S5165	HOME MODIFICATIONS; PER SERVICE	I	N	00	9		
S5170	HOME DELIVERED MEALS, INCLUDING PREPARATION; PER MEAL	I	N	00	9		
S5175	LAUNDRY SERVICE, EXTERNAL, PROFESSIONAL; PER ORDER	I	N	00	9		
S5180	HOME HEALTH RESPIRATORY THERAPY, INITIAL EVALUATION	I	N	00	9		
S5181	HOME HEALTH RESPIRATORY THERAPY, NOS, PER DIEM	I	N	00	9		
S5185	MEDICATION REMINDER SERVICE, NON-FACE-TO-FACE; PER MONTH	I	N	00	9		
S5190	WELLNESS ASSESSMENT, PERFORMED BY NON-PHYSICIAN	I	N	00	9		
S5199	PERSONAL CARE ITEM, NOS, EACH	I	N	00	9		
S5497	HOME INFUSION THERAPY, CATHETER CARE / MAINTENANCE, NOT OTHERWISE CLASSIFIED; INCLUDES ADMINISTRATIVE SERVICES, PROFESSIONAL PHARMACY SERVICES, CARE COORDINATION, AND ALL NECESSARY SUPPLIES AND EQUIPMENT (DRUGS AND NURSING VISITS CODED SEPARATELY), PER DIEM	I	N	00	9		

HCPCS Code	Statute	Lab Cert	X-Ref	ASC Pay Grp	ASC Pay Group Eff. Date	Proc Notes	BETOS	TOS	Anest	Code Add Date	Code Effective Date	Code Term Date
S5100							Z2	9	0	20030101	20030101	
S5101							Z2	9	0	20030101	20030101	
S5102							Z2	9	0	20030101	20030101	
S5105							Z2	9	0	20030101	20030101	
S5108							Z2	9	0	20030401	20030401	
S5109							Z2	9	0	20030401	20030401	
S5110							Z2	9	0	20030101	20030101	
S5111							Z2	9	0	20030101	20030101	
S5115							Z2	9	0	20030101	20030101	
S5116							Z2	9	0	20030101	20030101	
S5120							Z2	9	0	20030101	20030101	
S5121							Z2	9	0	20030101	20030101	
S5125							Z2	9	0	20030101	20030101	
S5126							Z2	9	0	20030101	20030101	
S5130							Z2	9	0	20030101	20030101	
S5131							Z2	9	0	20030101	20030101	
S5135							Z2	9	0	20030101	20030101	
S5136							Z2	9	0	20030101	20030101	
S5140							Z2	9	0	20030101	20030101	
S5141							Z2	9	0	20030101	20030101	
S5145							Z2	9	0	20030101	20030101	
S5146							Z2	9	0	20030101	20030101	
S5150							Z2	9	0	20030101	20030101	
S5151							Z2	9	0	20030101	20030101	
S5160							Z2	9	0	20030101	20030101	
S5161							Z2	9	0	20030101	20030101	
S5162							Z2	9	0	20030101	20030101	
S5165							Z2	9	0	20030101	20030101	
S5170							Z2	9	0	20030101	20030101	
S5175							Z2	9	0	20030101	20030101	
S5180							Z2	9	0	20030101	20030101	
S5181							Z2	9	0	20030101	20030101	
S5185							Z2	9	0	20030101	20030101	
S5190							Z2	9	0	20030101	20030101	
S5199							Z2	9	0	20030101	20030101	
S5497						0088	Z2	9	0	20020101	20020101	

HCPCS Code	Long Description	Coverage	Action	PI	MPI	CIM	MCM
S5498	HOME INFUSION THERAPY, CATHETER CARE / MAINTENANCE, SIMPLE (SINGLE LUMEN),INCLUDES ADMINISTRATIVE SERVICES, PROFESSIONAL PHARMACY SERVICES, CARE COORDINATION AND ALL NECESSARY SUPPLIES AND EQUIPMENT, (DRUGS AND NURSING VISITS CODED SEPARATELY), PER DIEM	I	N	00	9		
S5501	HOME INFUSION THERAPY, CATHETER CARE / MAINTENANCE, COMPLEX (MORE THAN ONE LUMEN), INCLUDES ADMINISTRATIVE SERVICES, PROFESSIONAL PHARMACY SERVICES, CARE COORDINATION, AND ALL NECESSARY SUPPLIES AND EQUIPMENT (DRUGS AND NURSING VISITS CODED SEPARATELY), PER DIEM	I	N	00	9		
S5502	HOME INFUSION THERAPY, CATHETER CARE / MAINTENANCE, IMPLANTED ACCESS DEVICE, INCLUDES ADMINISTRATIVE SERVICES, PROFESSIONAL PHARMACY SERVICES, CARE COORDINATION AND ALL NECESSARY SUPPLIES AND EQUIPMENT, (DRUGS & NURSING VISITS CODED SEPARATELY), PER DIEM (USE THIS CODE FOR INTERIM MAINTENANCE OF VASCULAR ACCESS NOT CURRENTLY IN USE)	I	N	00	9		
S5517	HOME INFUSION THERAPY, ALL SUPPLIES NECESSARY FOR RESTORATION OF CATHETER PATENCY OR DECLOTTING	I	N	00	9		
S5518	HOME INFUSION THERAPY, ALL SUPPLIES NECESSARY FOR CATHETER REPAIR	I	N	00	9		
S5520	HOME INFUSION THERAPY, ALL SUPPLIES (INCLUDING CATHETER) NECESSARY FOR A PERIPHERALLY INSERTED CENTRAL VENOUS CATHETER (PICC) LINE INSERTION	I	N	00	9		
S5521	HOME INFUSION THERAPY, ALL SUPPLIES (INCLUDING CATHETER) NECESSARY FOR A MIDLINE CATHETER INSERTION	I	N	00	9		
S5522	HOME INFUSION THERAPY, INSERTION OF PERIPHERALLY INSERTED CENTRAL VENOUS CATHETER (PICC), NURSING SERVICES ONLY (NO SUPPLIES OR CATHETER INCLUDED)	I	N	00	9		
S5523	HOME INFUSION THERAPY, INSERTION OF MIDLINE VENOUS CATHETER, NURSING SERVICES ONLY (NO SUPPLIES OR CATHETER INCLUDED)	I	N	00	9		
S5550	INSULIN, RAPID ONSET, 5 UNITS	I	N	00	9		
S5551	INSULIN, MOST RAPID ONSET (LISPRO OR ASPART); 5 UNITS	I	N	00	9		
S5552	INSULIN, INTERMEDIATE ACTING (NPH OR LENTE); 5 UNITS	I	N	00	9		
S5553	INSULIN, LONG ACTING; 5 UNITS	I	N	00	9		
S5560	INSULIN DELIVERY DEVICE, REUSABLE PEN; 1.5 ML SIZE	I	N	00	9		
S5561	INSULIN DELIVERY DEVICE, REUSABLE PEN; 3 ML SIZE	I	N	00	9		
S5565	INSULIN CARTRIDGE FOR USE IN INSULIN DELIVERY DEVICE OTHER THAN PUMP; 150 UNITS	I	N	00	9		
S5566	INSULIN CARTRIDGE FOR USE IN INSULIN DELIVERY DEVICE OTHER THAN PUMP; 300 UNITS	I	N	00	9		
S5570	INSULIN DELIVERY DEVICE, DISPOSABLE PEN (INCLUDING INSULIN); 1.5 ML SIZE	I	N	00	9		
S5571	INSULIN DELIVERY DEVICE, DISPOSABLE PEN (INCLUDING INSULIN); 3 ML SIZE	I	N	00	9		
S8030	SCLERAL APPLICATION OF TANTALUM RING(S) FOR LOCALIZATION OF LESIONS FOR PROTON BEAM THERAPY	I	N	00	9		

HCPCS Code	Statute	Lab Cert	X-Ref	ASC Pay Grp	ASC Pay Group Eff. Date	Proc Notes	BETOS	TOS	Anest	Code Add Date	Code Effective Date	Code Term Date
S5498						0088	Z2	9	0	20020101	20020101	
S5501						0088	Z2	9	0	20020101	20020101	
S5502						0088	Z2	9	0	20020101	20020101	
S5517						0088	Z2	9	0	20020101	20020101	
S5518						0088	Z2	9	0	20020101	20020101	
S5520						0088	Z2	9	0	20020101	20020101	
S5521						0088	Z2	9	0	20020101	20020101	
S5522						0088	Z2	9	0	20020101	20020101	
S5523						0088	Z2	9	0	20020101	20060701	
S5550							Z2	9	0	20031001	20031001	
S5551							Z2	9	0	20031001	20031001	
S5552							Z2	9	0	20031001	20031001	
S5553							Z2	9	0	20031001	20031001	
S5560							Z2	9	0	20031001	20031001	
S5561							Z2	9	0	20031001	20031001	
S5565							Z2	9	0	20031001	20031001	
S5566							Z2	9	0	20031001	20031001	
S5570							Z2	9	0	20031001	20031001	
S5571							Z2	9	0	20031001	20031001	
S8030						0088	Z2	9	0	20020101	20020101	

HCPCS Code	Long Description	Coverage	Action	PI	MPI	CIM	MCM
S8035	MAGNETIC SOURCE IMAGING	I	N	00	9		
S8037	MAGNETIC RESONANCE CHOLANGIOPANCREATOGRAPHY (MRCP)	I	N	00	9		
S8040	TOPOGRAPHIC BRAIN MAPPING	I	N	00	9		
S8042	MAGNETIC RESONANCE IMAGING (MRI), LOW-FIELD	I	N	00	9		
S8049	INTRAOPERATIVE RADIATION THERAPY (SINGLE ADMINISTRATION)	I	N	00	9		
S8055	ULTRASOUND GUIDANCE FOR MULTIFETAL PREGNANCY REDUCTION(S), TECHNICAL COMPONENT (ONLY TO BE USED WHEN THE PHYSICIAN DOING THE REDUCTION PROCEDURE DOES NOT PERFORM THE ULTRASOUND, GUIDANCE IS INCLUDED IN THE CPT CODE FOR MULTIFETAL PREGNANCY REDUCTION - 59866)	I	N	00	9		
S8075	COMPUTER ANALYSIS OF FULL-FIELD DIGITAL MAMMOGRAM AND FURTHER PHYSICIAN REVIEW FOR INTERPRETATION, MAMMOGRAPHY (LIST SEPARATELY IN ADDITION TO CODE FOR PRIMARY PROCEDURE)	I	N	00	9		
S8080	SCINTIMAMMOGRAPHY (RADIOIMMUNOSCINTIGRAPHY OF THE BREAST), UNILATERAL, INCLUDING SUPPLY OF RADIOPHARMACEUTICAL	I	N	00	9		
S8085	FLUORINE-18 FLUORODEOXYGLUCOSE (F-18 FDG) IMAGING USING DUAL-HEAD COINCIDENCE DETECTION SYSTEM (NON-DEDICATED PET SCAN)	I	N	00	9		
S8092	ELECTRON BEAM COMPUTED TOMOGRAPHY (ALSO KNOWN AS ULTRAFAST CT, CINE CT)	I	N	00	9		
S8093	COMPUTED TOMOGRAPHIC ANGIOGRAPHY, CORONARY ARTERIES, WITH CONTRAST MATERIAL(S)	I	N	00	9		
S8096	PORTABLE PEAK FLOW METER	I	N	00	9		
S8097	ASTHMA KIT (INCLUDING BUT NOT LIMITED TO PORTABLE PEAK EXPIRATORY FLOW METER, INSTRUCTIONAL VIDEO, BROCHURE, AND/OR SPACER)	I	N	00	9		
S8100	HOLDING CHAMBER OR SPACER FOR USE WITH AN INHALER OR NEBULIZER; WITHOUT MASK	I	N	00	9		
S8101	HOLDING CHAMBER OR SPACER FOR USE WITH AN INHALER OR NEBULIZER; WITH MASK	I	N	00	9		
S8110	PEAK EXPIRATORY FLOW RATE (PHYSICIAN SERVICES)	I	N	00	9		
S8120	OXYGEN CONTENTS, GASEOUS, 1 UNIT EQUALS 1 CUBIC FOOT	I	N	00	9		
S8121	OXYGEN CONTENTS, LIQUID, 1 UNIT EQUALS 1 POUND	I	N	00	9		
S8185	FLUTTER DEVICE	I	N	00	9		
S8186	SWIVEL ADAPTOR	I	N	00	9		
S8189	TRACHEOSTOMY SUPPLY, NOT OTHERWISE CLASSIFIED	I	N	00	9		
S8190	ELECTRONIC SPIROMETER (OR MICROSPIROMETER)	I	D	00	9		
S8210	MUCUS TRAP	I	N	00	9		
S8260	ORAL ORTHOTIC FOR TREATMENT OF SLEEP APNEA, INCLUDES FITTING, FABRICATION, AND MATERIALS	I	N	00	9		
S8262	MANDIBULAR ORTHOPEDIC REPOSITIONING DEVICE, EACH	I	N	00	9		
S8265	HABERMAN FEEDER FOR CLEFT LIP/PALATE	I	N	00	9		
S8270	ENURESIS ALARM, USING AUDITORY BUZZER AND/OR VIBRATION DEVICE	I	N	00	9		

HCPCS Code	Statute	Lab Cert	X-Ref	ASC Pay Grp	ASC Pay Group Eff. Date	Proc Notes	BETOS	TOS	Anest	Code Add Date	Code Effective Date	Code Term Date
S8035						0088	Z2	9	0	20000101	20000101	
S8037						0088	Z2	4	0	20010701	20010701	
S8040						0088	Z2	9	0	20000101	20000101	
S8042							Z2	9	0	20020401	20020401	
S8049						0088	Z2	9	0	20000101	20000101	
S8055						0088	Z2	9	0	20020101	20020101	
S8075							Z2	9	0	20040101	20060701	20060630
S8080						0088	Z2	9	0	20010101	20010101	
S8085						0088	Z2	9	0	20010101	20010101	
S8092						0088	Z2	9	0	20000101	20000101	
S8093							Z2	9	0	20041001	20060401	20060331
S8096						0088	Z2	9	0	20000101	20000101	
S8097						0088	Z2	9	0	20020101	20020101	
S8100						0088	Z2	9	0	20020101	20020101	
S8101						0088	Z2	9	0	20020101	20020101	
S8110						0088	Z2	9	0	20000101	20000101	
S8120							Z2	9	0	20031001	20031001	
S8121							Z2	9	0	20031001	20031001	
S8185						0088	Z2	9	0	20020101	20020101	
S8186						0088	Z2	9	0	20020101	20020101	
S8189						0088	Z2	9	0	20020101	20020101	
S8190						0088	Z2	9	0	20020101	20090401	20090331
S8210						0088	Z2	9	0	20010101	20010101	
S8260						0088	Z2	P	0	20000101	20060401	20060331
S8262							Z2	9	0	20020401	20020401	
S8265							Z2	9	0	20020401	20020401	
S8270							Z2	9	0	20050701	20050701	

HCPCS Code	Long Description	Coverage	Action	PI	MPI	CIM	MCM
S8301	INFECTION CONTROL SUPPLIES, NOT OTHERWISE SPECIFIED	I	N	00	9		
S8415	SUPPLIES FOR HOME DELIVERY OF INFANT	I	N	00	9		
S8420	GRADIENT PRESSURE AID (SLEEVE AND GLOVE COMBINATION), CUSTOM MADE	I	N	00	9		
S8421	GRADIENT PRESSURE AID (SLEEVE AND GLOVE COMBINATION), READY MADE	I	N	00	9		
S8422	GRADIENT PRESSURE AID (SLEEVE), CUSTOM MADE, MEDIUM WEIGHT	I	N	00	9		
S8423	GRADIENT PRESSURE AID (SLEEVE), CUSTOM MADE, HEAVY WEIGHT	I	N	00	9		
S8424	GRADIENT PRESSURE AID (SLEEVE), READY MADE	I	N	00	9		
S8425	GRADIENT PRESSURE AID (GLOVE), CUSTOM MADE, MEDIUM WEIGHT	I	N	00	9		
S8426	GRADIENT PRESSURE AID (GLOVE), CUSTOM MADE, HEAVY WEIGHT	I	N	00	9		
S8427	GRADIENT PRESSURE AID (GLOVE), READY MADE	I	N	00	9		
S8428	GRADIENT PRESSURE AID (GAUNTLET), READY MADE	I	N	00	9		
S8429	GRADIENT PRESSURE EXTERIOR WRAP	I	N	00	9		
S8430	PADDING FOR COMPRESSION BANDAGE, ROLL	I	N	00	9		
S8431	COMPRESSION BANDAGE, ROLL	I	N	00	9		
S8450	SPLINT, PREFABRICATED, DIGIT (SPECIFY DIGIT BY USE OF MODIFIER)	I	N	00	9		
S8451	SPLINT, PREFABRICATED, WRIST OR ANKLE	I	N	00	9		
S8452	SPLINT, PREFABRICATED, ELBOW	I	N	00	9		
S8460	CAMISOLE, POST-MASTECTOMY	I	N	00	9		
S8490	INSULIN SYRINGES (100 SYRINGES, ANY SIZE)	I	N	00	9		
S8940	EQUESTRIAN/HIPPOTHERAPY, PER SESSION	I	N	00	9		
S8948	APPLICATION OF A MODALITY (REQUIRING CONSTANT PROVIDER ATTENDANCE) TO ONE OR MORE AREAS; LOW-LEVEL LASER; EACH 15 MINUTES	I	N	00	9		
S8950	COMPLEX LYMPHEDEMA THERAPY, EACH 15 MINUTES	I	N	00	9		
S8990	PHYSICAL OR MANIPULATIVE THERAPY PERFORMED FOR MAINTENANCE RATHER THAN RESTORATION	I	N	00	9		
S8999	RESUSCITATION BAG (FOR USE BY PATIENT ON ARTIFICIAL RESPIRATION DURING POWER FAILURE OR OTHER CATASTROPHIC EVENT)	I	N	00	9		
S9001	HOME UTERINE MONITOR WITH OR WITHOUT ASSOCIATED NURSING SERVICES	I	N	00	9		
S9007	ULTRAFILTRATION MONITOR	I	N	00	9		
S9015	AUTOMATED EEG MONITORING	I	N	00	9		
S9022	DIGITAL SUBTRACTION ANGIOGRAPHY (USE IN ADDITION TO CPT CODE FOR THE PROCEDURE FOR FURTHER IDENTIFICATION)	I	N	00	9		
S9024	PARANASAL SINUS ULTRASOUND	I	N	00	9		
S9025	OMNICARDIOGRAM/CARDIOINTEGRAM	I	N	00	9		
S9034	EXTRACORPOREAL SHOCKWAVE LITHOTRIPSY FOR GALL STONES (IF PERFORMED WITH ERCP, USE 43265)	I	N	00	9		
S9055	PROCUREN OR OTHER GROWTH FACTOR PREPARATION TO PROMOTE WOUND HEALING	I	N	00	9		

HCPCS Code	Statute	Lab Cert	X-Ref	ASC Pay Grp	ASC Pay Group Eff. Date	Proc Notes	BETOS	TOS	Anest	Code Add Date	Code Effective Date	Code Term Date
S8301							Z2	9	0	20040701	20040701	
S8415						0088	Z2	9	0	20020101	20020101	
S8420						0088	Z2	9	0	20020101	20020101	
S8421						0088	Z2	9	0	20020101	20020101	
S8422						0088	Z2	9	0	20020101	20020101	
S8423						0088	Z2	9	0	20020101	20020101	
S8424						0088	Z2	9	0	20020101	20020101	
S8425						0088	Z2	9	0	20020101	20020101	
S8426						0088	Z2	9	0	20020101	20020101	
S8427						0088	Z2	9	0	20020101	20020101	
S8428						0088	Z2	9	0	20020101	20020101	
S8429						0088	Z2	9	0	20020101	20020101	
S8430						0088	Z2	9	0	20020101	20020101	
S8431						0088	Z2	9	0	20020101	20020101	
S8450						0088	Z2	P	0	20020101	20020101	
S8451						0088	Z2	P	0	20020101	20020101	
S8452						0088	Z2	P	0	20020101	20020101	
S8460							Z2	9	0	20030401	20030401	
S8490						0088	Z2	S	0	20020101	20020101	
S8940							Z2	9	0	20050401	20050401	
S8948							Z2	9	0	20040101	20040101	
S8950						0088	Z2	9	0	20000101	20000101	
S8990							Z2	9	0	20030401	20030401	
S8999						0088	Z2	9	0	20010101	20010101	
S9001						0088	Z2	9	0	20000101	20000101	
S9007						0088	Z2	9	0	20010101	20010101	
S9015						0088	Z2	9	0	20010101	20010101	
S9022						0088	Z2	9	0	20000101	20060701	20060630
S9024						0088	Z2	9	0	20000101	20000101	
S9025						0088	Z2	9	0	20010101	20010101	
S9034							Z2	9	0	20020401	20020401	
S9055						0088	Z2	9	0	20000101	20000101	

HCPCS Code	Long Description	Coverage	Action	PI	MPI	CIM	MCM
S9056	COMA STIMULATION PER DIEM	I	N	00	9		
S9061	HOME ADMINISTRATION OF AEROSOLIZED DRUG THERAPY (E.G., PENTAMIDINE);ADMINISTRATIVE SERVICES, PROFESSIONAL PHARMACY SERVICES, CARE COORDINATION, ALL NECESSARY SUPPLIES AND EQUIPMENT (DRUGS AND NURSING VISITS CODED SEPARATELY), PER DIEM	I	N	00	9		
S9075	SMOKING CESSATION TREATMENT	I	N	00	9		
S9083	GLOBAL FEE URGENT CARE CENTERS	I	N	00	9		
S9088	SERVICES PROVIDED IN AN URGENT CARE CENTER (LIST IN ADDITION TO CODE FOR SERVICE)	I	N	00	9		
S9090	VERTEBRAL AXIAL DECOMPRESSION, PER SESSION	I	N	00	9		
S9092	CANOLITH REPOSITIONING, PER VISIT	I	N	00	9		
S9097	HOME VISIT FOR WOUND CARE	I	N	00	9		
S9098	HOME VISIT, PHOTOTHERAPY SERVICES (E.G. BILI-LITE), INCLUDING EQUIPMENT RENTAL, NURSING SERVICES, BLOOD DRAW, SUPPLIES, AND OTHER SERVICES, PER DIEM	I	N	00	9		
S9109	CONGESTIVE HEART FAILURE TELEMONITORING, EQUIPMENT RENTAL, INCLUDING TELESCALE, COMPUTER SYSTEM AND SOFTWARE, TELEPHONE CONNECTIONS, AND MAINTENANCE, PER MONTH	I	N	00	9		
S9117	BACK SCHOOL, PER VISIT	I	N	00	9		
S9122	HOME HEALTH AIDE OR CERTIFIED NURSE ASSISTANT, PROVIDING CARE IN THE HOME; PER HOUR	I	N	00	9		
S9123	NURSING CARE, IN THE HOME; BY REGISTERED NURSE, PER HOUR (USE FOR GENERAL NURSING CARE ONLY, NOT TO BE USED WHEN CPT CODES 99500-99602 CAN BE USED)	I	N	00	9		
S9124	NURSING CARE, IN THE HOME; BY LICENSED PRACTICAL NURSE, PER HOUR	I	N	00	9		
S9125	RESPITE CARE, IN THE HOME, PER DIEM	I	N	00	9		
S9126	HOSPICE CARE, IN THE HOME, PER DIEM	I	N	00	9		
S9127	SOCIAL WORK VISIT, IN THE HOME, PER DIEM	I	N	00	9		
S9128	SPEECH THERAPY, IN THE HOME, PER DIEM	I	N	00	9		
S9129	OCCUPATIONAL THERAPY, IN THE HOME, PER DIEM	I	N	00	9		
S9131	PHYSICAL THERAPY; IN THE HOME, PER DIEM	I	N	00	9		
S9140	DIABETIC MANAGEMENT PROGRAM, FOLLOW-UP VISIT TO NON-MD PROVIDER	I	N	00	9		
S9141	DIABETIC MANAGEMENT PROGRAM, FOLLOW-UP VISIT TO R MD PROVIDE	I	N	00	9		
S9145	INSULIN PUMP INITIATION, INSTRUCTION IN INITIAL USE OF PUMP (PUMP NOT INCLUDED)	I	N	00	9		
S9150	EVALUATION BY OCULARIST	I	N	00	9		
S9152	SPEECH THERAPY, RE-EVALUATION	I	N	00	9		
S9208	HOME MANAGEMENT OF PRETERM LABOR, INCLUDING ADMINISTRATIVE SERVICES, PROFESSIONAL PHARMACY SERVICES, CARE COORDINATION, AND ALL NECESSARY SUPPLIES OR EQUIPMENT (DRUGS AND NURSING VISITS CODED SEPARATELY), PER DIEM (DO NOT USE THIS CODE WITH ANY HOME INFUSION PER DIEM CODE)	I	N	00	9		

HCPCS Code	Statute	Lab Cert	X-Ref	ASC Pay Grp	ASC Pay Group Eff. Date	Proc Notes	BETOS	TOS	Anest	Code Add Date	Code Effective Date	Code Term Date
S9056						0088	Z2	9	0	20000101	20000101	
S9061						0088	Z2	9	0	20010101	20020101	
S9075						0088	Z2	9	0	20000101	20000101	
S9083						0088	Z2	9	0	20020101	20020101	
S9088						0088	Z2	9	0	20010101	20020101	
S9090						0088	Z2	9	0	20000101	20000101	
S9092							Z2	9	0	20020401	20090101	20081231
S9097							Z2	9	0	20041001	20041001	
S9098						0088	Z2	9	0	20020101	20020101	
S9109						0088	Z2	9	0	20020101	20020101	
S9117						0088	Z2	9	0	20020101	20020101	
S9122						0088	Z2	9	0	20000101	20000101	
S9123						0088	Z2	9	0	20000101	20040101	
S9124						0088	Z2	9	0	20000101	20000101	
S9125						0088	Z2	9	0	20000101	20000101	
S9126						0088	Z2	9	0	20000101	20000101	
S9127						0088	Z2	9	0	20000101	20000101	
S9128						0088	Z2	9	0	20000101	20000101	
S9129						0088	Z2	9	0	20000101	20000101	
S9131						0088	Z2	9	0	20020101	20020101	
S9140						0088	Z2	9	0	20000101	20000101	
S9141						0088	Z2	9	0	20000101	20000101	
S9145							Z2	9	0	20020401	20020401	
S9150							Z2	9	0	20020401	20020401	
S9152							Z2	9	0	20070701	20070701	
S9208						0088	Z2	9	0	20020101	20020101	

HCPCS Code	Long Description	Coverage	Action	PI	MPI	CIM	MCM
S9209	HOME MANAGEMENT OF PRETERM PREMATURE RUPTURE OF MEMBRANES (PPROM), INCLUDING ADMINISTRATIVE SERVICES, PROFESSIONAL PHARMACY SERVICES, CARE COORDINATION, & ALL NECESSARY SUPPLIES OR EQUIPMENT (DRUGS AND NURSING VISITS CODED SEPARATELY), PER DIEM (DO NOT USE THIS CODE WITH ANY HOME INFUSION PER DIEM CODE)	I	N	00	9		
S9211	HOME MANAGEMENT OF GESTATIONAL HYPERTENSION, INCLUDES ADMINISTRATIVE SERVICES, PROFESSIONAL PHARMACY SERVICES, CARE COORDINATION AND ALL NECESSARY SUPPLIES AND EQUIPMENT (DRUGS AND NURSING VISITS CODED SEPARATELY); PER DIEM (DO NOT USE THIS CODE WITH ANY HOME INFUSION PER DIEM CODE)	I	N	00	9		
S9212	HOME MANAGEMENT OF POSTPARTUM HYPERTENSION, INCLUDES ADMINISTRATIVE SERVICES, PROFESSIONAL PHARMACY SERVICES, CARE COORDINATION, AND ALL NECESSARY SUPPLIES AND EQUIPMENT (DRUGS AND NURSING VISITS CODED SEPARATELY), PER DIEM (DO NOT USE THIS CODE WITH ANY HOME INFUSION PER DIEM CODE)	I	N	00	9		
S9213	HOME MANAGEMENT OF PREECLAMPSIA, INCLUDES ADMINISTRATIVE SERVICES, PROFESSIONAL PHARMACY SERVICES, CARE COORDINATION, AND ALL NECESSARY SUPPLIES AND EQUIPMENT (DRUGS AND NURSING SERVICES CODED SEPARATELY); PER DIEM (DO NOT USE THIS CODE WITH ANY HOME INFUSION PER DIEM CODE)	I	N	00	9		
S9214	HOME MANAGEMENT OF GESTATIONAL DIABETES, INCLUDES ADMINISTRATIVE SERVICES, PROFESSIONAL PHARMACY SERVICES, CARE COORDINATION, AND ALL NECESSARY SUPPLIES AND EQUIPMENT (DRUGS AND NURSING VISITS CODED SEPARATELY); PER DIEM (DO NOT USE THIS CODE WITH ANY HOME INFUSION PER DIEM CODE)	I	N	00	9		
S9325	HOME INFUSION THERAPY, PAIN MANAGEMENT INFUSION; ADMINISTRATIVE SERVICES, PROFESSIONAL PHARMACY SERVICES, CARE COORDINATION, AND ALL NECESSARY SUPPLIES AND EQUIPMENT, (DRUGS AND NURSING VISITS CODED SEPARATELY), PER DIEM (DO NOT USE THIS CODE WITH S9326, S9327 OR S9328)	I	N	00	9		
S9326	HOME INFUSION THERAPY, CONTINUOUS (TWENTY-FOUR HOURS OR MORE) PAIN MANAGEMENT INFUSION; ADMINISTRATIVE SERVICES, PROFESSIONAL PHARMACY SERVICES, CARE COORDINATION AND ALL NECESSARY SUPPLIES AND EQUIPMENT (DRUGS AND NURSING VISITS CODED SEPARATELY), PER DIEM	I	N	00	9		
S9327	HOME INFUSION THERAPY, INTERMITTENT (LESS THAN TWENTY-FOUR HOURS) PAIN MANAGEMENT INFUSION; ADMINISTRATIVE SERVICES, PROFESSIONAL PHARMACY SERVICES, CARE COORDINATION, AND ALL NECESSARY SUPPLIES AND EQUIPMENT (DRUGS AND NURSING VISITS CODED SEPARATELY), PER DIEM	I	N	00	9		

HCPCS Code	Statute	Lab Cert	X-Ref	ASC Pay Grp	ASC Pay Group Eff. Date	Proc Notes	BETOS	TOS	Anest	Code Add Date	Code Effective Date	Code Term Date
S9209						0088	Z2	9	0	20020101	20020101	
S9211						0088	Z2	9	0	20020101	20020101	
S9212						0088	Z2	9	0	20020101	20020101	
S9213						0088	Z2	9	0	20020101	20020101	
S9214						0088	Z2	9	0	20020101	20020101	
S9325						0088	Z2	9	0	20020101	20020101	
S9326						0088	Z2	9	0	20020101	20020101	
S9327						0088	Z2	9	0	20020101	20020101	

HCPCS Code	Long Description	Coverage	Action	PI	MPI	CIM	MCM
S9328	HOME INFUSION THERAPY, IMPLANTED PUMP PAIN MANAGEMENT INFUSION; ADMINISTRATIVE SERVICES, PROFESSIONAL PHARMACY SERVICES, CARE COORDINATION, AND ALL NECESSARY SUPPLIES AND EQUIPMENT (DRUGS AND NURSING VISITS CODED SEPARATELY), PER DIEM	I	N	00	9		
S9329	HOME INFUSION THERAPY, CHEMOTHERAPY INFUSION; ADMINISTRATIVE SERVICES, PROFESSIONAL PHARMACY SERVICES, CARE COORDINATION, AND ALL NECESSARY SUPPLIES AND EQUIPMENT (DRUGS AND NURSING VISITS CODED SEPARATELY), PER DIEM (DO NOT USE THIS CODE WITH S9330 OR S9331)	I	N	00	9		
S9330	HOME INFUSION THERAPY, CONTINUOUS (TWENTY-FOUR HOURS OR MORE) CHEMOTHERAPY INFUSION; ADMINISTRATIVE SERVICES, PROFESSIONAL PHARMACY SERVICES, CARE COORDINATION, AND ALL NECESSARY SUPPLIES AND EQUIPMENT (DRUGS AND NURSING VISITS CODED SEPARATELY), PER DIEM	I	N	00	9		
S9331	HOME INFUSION THERAPY, INTERMITTENT (LESS THAN TWENTY-FOUR HOURS) CHEMOTHERAPY INFUSION; ADMINISTRATIVE SERVICES, PROFESSIONAL PHARMACY SERVICES, CARE COORDINATION, AND ALL NECESSARY SUPPLIES AND EQUIPMENT (DRUGS AND NURSING VISITS CODED SEPARATELY), PER DIEM	I	N	00	9		
S9335	HOME THERAPY, HEMODIALYSIS; ADMINISTRATIVE SERVICES, PROFESSIONAL PHARMACY SERVICES, CARE COORDINATION, AND ALL NECESSARY SUPPLIES AND EQUIPMENT (DRUGS AND NURSING SERVICES CODED SEPARATELY), PER DIEM	I	N	00	9		
S9336	HOME INFUSION THERAPY, CONTINUOUS ANTICOAGULANT INFUSION THERAPY (E.G. HEPARIN), ADMINISTRATIVE SERVICES, PROFESSIONAL PHARMACY SERVICES, CARE COORDINATION AND ALL NECESSARY SUPPLIES AND EQUIPMENT (DRUGS AND NURSING VISITS CODED SEPARATELY), PER DIEM	I	N	00	9		
S9338	HOME INFUSION THERAPY, IMMUNOTHERAPY, ADMINISTRATIVE SERVICES, PROFESSIONAL PHARMACY SERVICES, CARE COORDINATION, AND ALL NECESSARY SUPPLIES AND EQUIPMENT (DRUGS AND NURSING VISITS CODED SEPARATELY), PER DIEM	I	N	00	9		
S9339	HOME THERAPY; PERITONEAL DIALYSIS, ADMINISTRATIVE SERVICES, PROFESSIONAL PHARMACY SERVICES, CARE COORDINATION AND ALL NECESSARY SUPPLIES & EQUIPMENT (DRUGS AND NURSING VISITS CODED SEPARATELY), PER DIEM	I	N	00	9		
S9340	HOME THERAPY; ENTERAL NUTRITION; ADMINISTRATIVE SERVICES, PROFESSIONAL PHARMACY SERVICES, CARE COORDINATION, AND ALL NECESSARY SUPPLIES AND EQUIPMENT (ENTERAL FORMULA AND NURSING VISITS CODED SEPARATELY), PER DIEM	I	N	00	9		

HCPCS Code	Statute	Lab Cert	X-Ref	ASC Pay Grp	ASC Pay Group Eff. Date	Proc Notes	BETOS	TOS	Anest	Code Add Date	Code Effective Date	Code Term Date
S9328						0088	Z2	9	0	20020101	20020101	
S9329						0088	Z2	9	0	20020101	20020101	
S9330							Z2	9	0	20020101	20020101	
S9331						0088	Z2	9	0	20020101	20020101	
S9335							Z2	9	0	20030701	20030701	
S9336						0088	Z2	9	0	20020101	20020101	
S9338						0088	Z2	9	0	20020101	20020101	
S9339						0088	Z2	9	0	20020101	20020101	
S9340						0088	Z2	9	0	20020101	20020101	

HCPCS Code	Long Description	Coverage	Action	PI	MPI	CIM	MCM
S9341	HOME THERAPY; ENTERAL NUTRITION VIA GRAVITY; ADMINISTRATIVE SERVICES, PROFESSIONAL PHARMACY SERVICES, CARE COORDINATION, AND ALL NECESSARY SUPPLIES AND EQUIPMENT (ENTERAL FORMULA AND NURSING VISITS CODED SEPARATELY), PER DIEM	I	N	00	9		
S9342	HOME THERAPY; ENTERAL NUTRITION VIA PUMP; ADMINISTRATIVE SERVICES, PROFESSIONAL PHARMACY SERVICES, CARE COORDINATION, AND ALL NECESSARY SUPPLIES AND EQUIPMENT (ENTERAL FORMULA AND NURSING VISITS CODED SEPARATELY), PER DIEM	I	N	00	9		
S9343	HOME THERAPY; ENTERAL NUTRITION VIA BOLUS; ADMINISTRATIVE SERVICES, PROFESSIONAL PHARMACY SERVICES, CARE COORDINATION, & ALL NECESSARY SUPPLIES AND EQUIPMENT (ENTERAL FORMULA & NURSING VISITS CODED SEPARATELY), PER DIEM	I	N	00	9		
S9345	HOME INFUSION THERAPY, ANTI-HEMOPHILIC AGENT INFUSION THERAPY (E.G. FACTOR VIII); ADMINISTRATIVE SERVICES, PROFESSIONAL PHARMACY SERVICES, CARE COORDINATION, AND ALL NECESSARY SUPPLIES AND EQUIPMENT (DRUGS AND NURSING VISITS CODED SEPARATELY), PER DIEM	I	N	00	9		
S9346	HOME INFUSION THERAPY, ALPHA-1-PROTEINASE INHIBITOR (E.G., PROLASTIN);ADMINISTRATIVE SERVICES, PROFESSIONAL PHARMACY SERVICES, CARE COORDINATION, AND ALL NECESSARY SUPPLIES AND EQUIPMENT (DRUGS AND NURSING VISITS CODED SEPARATELY), PER DIEM	I	N	00	9		
S9347	HOME INFUSION THERAPY, UNINTERRUPTED, LONG-TERM, CONTROLLED RATE INTRAVENOUS OR SUBCUTANEOUS INFUSION THERAPY (E.G. EPOPROSTENOL); ADMINISTRATIVE SERVICES, PROFESSIONAL PHARMACY SERVICES, CARE COORDINATION, AND ALL NECESSARY SUPPLIES & EQUIPMENT (DRUGS AND NURSING VISITS CODED SEPARATELY), PER DIEM	I	N	00	9		
S9348	HOME INFUSION THERAPY, SYMPATHOMIMETIC/INOTROPIC AGENT INFUSION THERAPY (E.G.,DOBUTAMINE); ADMINISTRATIVE SERVICES, PROFESSIONAL PHARMACY SERVICES, CARE COORDINATION, ALL NECESSARY SUPPLIES AND EQUIPMENT (DRUGS AND NURSING VISITS CODED SEPARATELY), PER DIEM	I	N	00	9		
S9349	HOME INFUSION THERAPY, TOCOLYTIC INFUSION THERAPY; ADMINISTRATIVE SERVICES, PROFESSIONAL PHARMACY SERVICES, CARE COORDINATION, AND ALL NECESSARY SUPPLIES AND EQUIPMENT (DRUGS AND NURSING VISITS CODED SEPARATELY), PER DIEM	I	N	00	9		
S9351	HOME INFUSION THERAPY, CONTINUOUS OR INTERMITTENT ANTI-EMETIC INFUSION THERAPY; ADMINISTRATIVE SERVICES, PROFESSIONAL PHARMACY SERVICES, CARE COORDINATION, AND ALL NECESSARY SUPPLIES AND EQUIPMENT (DRUGS & VISITS CODED SEPARATELY), PER DIEM	I	N	00	9		

HCPCS Code	Statute	Lab Cert	X-Ref	ASC Pay Grp	ASC Pay Group Eff. Date	Proc Notes	BETOS	TOS	Anest	Code Add Date	Code Effective Date	Code Term Date
S9341						0088	Z2	9	0	20020101	20020101	
S9342						0088	Z2	9	0	20020101	20020101	
S9343						0088	Z2	9	0	20020101	20020101	
S9345						0088	Z2	9	0	20020101	20020101	
S9346						0088	Z2	9	0	20020101	20020101	
S9347						0088	Z2	9	0	20020101	20030101	
S9348						0088	Z2	9	0	20020101	20020101	
S9349						0088	Z2	9	0	20020101	20020101	
S9351						0088	Z2	9	0	20020101	20070401	

HCPCS Code	Long Description	Coverage	Action	PI	MPI	CIM	MCM
S9353	HOME INFUSION THERAPY, CONTINUOUS INSULIN INFUSION THERAPY; ADMINISTRATIVE SERVICES, PROFESSIONAL PHARMACY SERVICES, CARE COORDINATION, AND ALL NECESSARY SUPPLIES AND EQUIPMENT (DRUGS AND NURSING VISITS CODED SEPARATELY), PER DIEM	I	N	00	9		
S9355	HOME INFUSION THERAPY, CHELATION THERAPY; ADMINISTRATIVE SERVICES, PROFESSIONAL PHARMACY SERVICES, CARE COORDINATION, AND ALL NECESSARY SUPPLIES AND EQUIPMENT (DRUGS AND NURSING VISITS CODED SEPARATELY), PER DIEM	I	N	00	9		
S9357	HOME INFUSION THERAPY, ENZYME REPLACEMENT INTRAVENOUS THERAPY; (E.G. IMIGLUCERASE); ADMINISTRATIVE SERVICES, PROFESSIONAL PHARMACY SERVICES, CARE COORDINATION, AND ALL NECESSARY SUPPLIES AND EQUIPMENT (DRUGS AND NURSING VISITS CODED SEPARATELY), PER DIEM	I	N	00	9		
S9359	HOME INFUSION THERAPY, ANTI-TUMOR NECROSIS FACTOR INTRAVENOUS THERAPY; (E.G. INFLIXIMAB); ADMINISTRATIVE SERVICES, PROFESSIONAL PHARMACY SERVICES, CARE COORDINATION, AND ALL NECESSARY SUPPLIES AND EQUIPMENT (DRUGS AND NURSING VISITS CODED SEPARATELY), PER DIEM	I	N	00	9		
S9361	HOME INFUSION THERAPY, DIURETIC INTRAVENOUS THERAPY; ADMINISTRATIVE SERVICES, PROFESSIONAL PHARMACY SERVICES, CARE COORDINATION, AND ALL NECESSARY SUPPLIES AND EQUIPMENT (DRUGS AND NURSING VISITS CODED SEPARATELY), PER DIEM	I	N	00	9		
S9363	HOME INFUSION THERAPY, ANTI-SPASMOTIC THERAPY; ADMINISTRATIVE SERVICES, PROFESSIONAL PHARMACY SERVICES, CARE COORDINATION, AND ALL NECESSARY SUPPLIES AND EQUIPMENT (DRUGS AND NURSING VISITS CODED SEPARATELY), PER DIEM	I	N	00	9		
S9364	HOME INFUSION THERAPY, TOTAL PARENTERAL NUTRITION (TPN); ADMINISTRATIVE SERVICES, PROFESSIONAL PHARMACY SERVICES, CARE COORDINATION, AND ALL NECESSARY SUPPLIES AND EQUIPMENT INCLUDING STANDARD TPN FORMULA (LIPIDS, SPECIALTY AMINO ACID FORMULAS, DRUGS OTHER THAN IN STANDARD FORMULA AND NURSING VISITS CODED SEPARATELY), PER DIEM (DO NOT USE WITH HOME INFUSION CODES S9365-S9368 USING DAILY VOLUME SCALES)	I	N	00	9		
S9365	HOME INFUSION THERAPY, TOTAL PARENTERAL NUTRITION (TPN); ONE LITER PER DAY, ADMINISTRATIVE SERVICES, PROFESSIONAL PHARMACY SERVICES, CARE COORDINATION, AND ALL NECESSARY SUPPLIES AND EQUIPMENT INCLUDING STANDARD TPN FORMULA (LIPIDS, SPECIALTY AMINO ACID FORMULAS, DRUGS OTHER THAN IN STANDARD FORMULA AND NURSING VISITS CODED SEPARATELY), PER DIEM	I	N	00	9		

HCPCS Code	Statute	Lab Cert	X-Ref	ASC Pay Grp	ASC Pay Group Eff. Date	Proc Notes	BETOS	TOS	Anest	Code Add Date	Code Effective Date	Code Term Date
S9353						0088	Z2	9	0	20020101	20020101	
S9355						0088	Z2	9	0	20020101	20020101	
S9357						0088	Z2	9	0	20020101	20020101	
S9359						0088	Z2	9	0	20020101	20020101	
S9361						0088	Z2	9	0	20020101	20020101	
S9363						0088	Z2	9	0	20020101	20041001	
S9364						0088	Z2	9	0	20020101	20020101	
S9365						0088	Z2	9	0	20020101	20020101	

HCPCS Code	Long Description	Coverage	Action	PI	MPI	CIM	MCM
S9366	HOME INFUSION THERAPY, TOTAL PARENTERAL NUTRITION (TPN); MORE THAN ONE LITER BUT NO MORE THAN TWO LITERS PER DAY, ADMINISTRATIVE SERVICES, PROFESSIONAL PHARMACY SERVICES, CARE COORDINATION, AND ALL NECESSARY SUPPLIES AND EQUIPMENT INCLUDING STANDARD TPN FORMULA (LIPIDS, SPECIALTY AMINO ACID FORMULAS, DRUGS OTHER THAN IN STANDARD FORMULA AND NURSING VISITS CODED SEPARATELY), PER DIEM	I	N	00	9		
S9367	HOME INFUSION THERAPY, TOTAL PARENTERAL NUTRITION (TPN); MORE THAN TWO LITERS BUT NO MORE THAN THREE LITERS PER DAY, ADMINISTRATIVE SERVICES, PROFESSIONAL PHARMACY SERVICES, CARE COORDINATION, AND ALL NECESSARY SUPPLIES AND EQUIPMENT INCLUDING STANDARD TPN FORMULA (LIPIDS, SPECIALTY AMINO ACID FORMULAS, DRUGS OTHER THAN IN STANDARD FORMULA AND NURSING VISITS CODED SEPARATELY), PER DIEM	I	N	00	9		
S9368	HOME INFUSION THERAPY, TOTAL PARENTERAL NUTRITION (TPN); MORE THAN THREE LITERS PER DAY, ADMINISTRATIVE SERVICES, PROFESSIONAL PHARMACY SERVICES, CARE COORDINATION, AND ALL NECESSARY SUPPLIES AND EQUIPMENT INCLUDING STANDARD TPN FORMULA (LIPIDS, SPECIALTY AMINO ACID FORMULAS, DRUGS OTHER THAN IN STANDARD FORMULA AND NURSING VISITS CODED SEPARATELY), PER DIEM	I	N	00	9		
S9370	HOME THERAPY, INTERMITTENT ANTI-EMETIC INJECTION THERAPY; ADMINISTRATIVE SERVICES, PROFESSIONAL PHARMACY SERVICES, CARE COORDINATION, AND ALL NECESSARY SUPPLIES AND EQUIPMENT (DRUGS AND NURSING VISITS CODED SEPARATELY), PER DIEM	I	N	00	9		
S9372	HOME THERAPY; INTERMITTENT ANTICOAGULANT INJECTION THERAPY (E.G. HEPARIN);ADMINISTRATIVE SERVICES, PROFESSIONAL PHARMACY SERVICES, CARE COORDINATION, AND ALL NECESSARY SUPPLIES AND EQUIPMENT (DRUGS AND NURSING VISITS CODED SEPARATELY), PER DIEM (DO NOT USE THIS CODE FOR FLUSHING OF INFUSION DEVICES WITH HEPARIN TO MAINTAIN PATENCY)	I	N	00	9		
S9373	HOME INFUSION THERAPY, HYDRATION THERAPY; ADMINISTRATIVE SERVICES, PROFESSIONAL PHARMACY SERVICES, CARE COORDINATION, AND ALL NECESSARY SUPPLIES AND EQUIPMENT (DRUGS AND NURSING VISITS CODED SEPARATELY), PER DIEM (DO NOT USE WITH HYDRATION THERAPY CODES S9374-S9377 USING DAILY VOLUME SCALES)	I	N	00	9		
S9374	HOME INFUSION THERAPY, HYDRATION THERAPY; ONE LITER PER DAY, ADMINISTRATIVE SERVICES, PROFESSIONAL PHARMACY SERVICES, CARE COORDINATION, AND ALL NECESSARY SUPPLIES AND EQUIPMENT (DRUGS AND NURSING VISITS CODED SEPARATELY), PER DIEM	I	N	00	9		

HCPCS Code	Statute	Lab Cert	X-Ref	ASC Pay Grp	ASC Pay Group Eff. Date	Proc Notes	BETOS	TOS	Anest	Code Add Date	Code Effective Date	Code Term Date
S9366						0088	Z2	9	0	20020101	20020101	
S9367						0088	Z2	9	0	20020101	20020101	
S9368						0088	Z2	9	0	20020101	20020101	
S9370						0088	Z2	9	0	20020101	20020101	
S9372						0088	Z2	9	0	20020101	20020101	
S9373						0088	Z2	9	0	20020101	20020101	
S9374						0088	Z2	9	0	20020101	20020101	

S Codes

HCPCS Code	Long Description	Coverage	Action	PI	MPI	CIM	MCM
S9375	HOME INFUSION THERAPY, HYDRATION THERAPY; MORE THAN ONE LITER BUT NO MORE THAN TWO LITERS PER DAY, ADMINISTRATIVE SERVICES, PROFESSIONAL PHARMACY SERVICES, CARE COORDINATION, AND ALL NECESSARY SUPPLIES AND EQUIPMENT (DRUGS AND NURSING VISITS CODED SEPARATELY), PER DIEM	I	N	00	9		
S9376	HOME INFUSION THERAPY, HYDRATION THERAPY; MORE THAN TWO LITERS BUT NO MORE THAN THREE LITERS PER DAY, ADMINISTRATIVE SERVICES, PROFESSIONAL PHARMACY SERVICES, CARE COORDINATION, AND ALL NECESSARY SUPPLIES AND EQUIPMENT (DRUGS AND NURSING VISITS CODED SEPARATELY), PER DIEM	I	N	00	9		
S9377	HOME INFUSION THERAPY, HYDRATION THERAPY; MORE THAN THREE LITERS PER DAY, ADMINISTRATIVE SERVICES, PROFESSIONAL PHARMACY SERVICES, CARE COORDINATION, AND ALL NECESSARY SUPPLIES (DRUGS AND NURSING VISITS CODED SEPARATELY), PER DIEM	I	N	00	9		
S9379	HOME INFUSION THERAPY, INFUSION THERAPY, NOT OTHERWISE CLASSIFIED; ADMINISTRATIVE SERVICES, PROFESSIONAL PHARMACY SERVICES, CARE COORDINATION, AND ALL NECESSARY SUPPLIES AND EQUIPMENT (DRUGS AND NURSING VISITS CODED SEPARATELY), PER DIEM	I	N	00	9		
S9381	DELIVERY OR SERVICE TO HIGH RISK AREAS REQUIRING ESCORT OR EXTRA PROTECTION, PER VISIT	I	N	00	9		
S9401	ANTICOAGULATION CLINIC, INCLUSIVE OF ALL SERVICES EXCEPT LABORATORY TESTS, PER SESSION	I	N	00	9		
S9430	PHARMACY COMPOUNDING AND DISPENSING SERVICES	I	N	00	9		
S9433	MEDICAL FOOD NUTRITIONALLY COMPLETE, ADMINISTERED ORALLY, PROVIDING 100% OF NUTRITIONAL INTAKE	D	F	00	9		
S9434	MODIFIED SOLID FOOD SUPPLEMENTS FOR INBORN ERRORS OF METABOLISM	I	N	00	9		
S9435	MEDICAL FOODS FOR INBORN ERRORS OF METABOLISM	I	N	00	9		
S9436	CHILDBIRTH PREPARATION/LAMAZE CLASSES, NON-PHYSICIAN PROVIDER, PER SESSION	I	N	00	9		
S9437	CHILDBIRTH REFRESHER CLASSES, NON-PHYSICIAN PROVIDER, PER SESSION	I	N	00	9		
S9438	CESAREAN BIRTH CLASSES, NON-PHYSICIAN PROVIDER, PER SESSION	I	N	00	9		
S9439	VBAC (VAGINAL BIRTH AFTER CESAREAN) CLASSES, NON-PHYSICIAN PROVIDER, PER SESSION	I	N	00	9		
S9441	ASTHMA EDUCATION, NON-PHYSICIAN PROVIDER, PER SESSION	I	N	00	9		
S9442	BIRTHING CLASSES, NON-PHYSICIAN PROVIDER, PER SESSION	I	N	00	9		
S9443	LACTATION CLASSES, NON-PHYSICIAN PROVIDER, PER SESSION	I	N	00	9		
S9444	PARENTING CLASSES, NON-PHYSICIAN PROVIDER, PER SESSION	I	N	00	9		
S9445	PATIENT EDUCATION, NOT OTHERWISE CLASSIFIED, NON-PHYSICIAN PROVIDER, INDIVIDUAL, PER SESSION	I	N	00	9		
S9446	PATIENT EDUCATION, NOT OTHERWISE CLASSIFIED, NON-PHYSICIAN PROVIDER, GROUP, PER SESSION	I	N	00	9		

HCPCS Code	Statute	Lab Cert	X-Ref	ASC Pay Grp	ASC Pay Group Eff. Date	Proc Notes	BETOS	TOS	Anest	Code Add Date	Code Effective Date	Code Term Date
S9375						0088	Z2	9	0	20020101	20020101	
S9376						0088	Z2	9	0	20020101	20020101	
S9377						0088	Z2	9	0	20020101	20020101	
S9379						0088	Z2	9	0	20020101	20020101	
S9381						0088	Z2	9	0	20020101	20020101	
S9401							Z2	9	0	20020401	20020401	
S9430							Z2	9	0	20020401	20020401	
S9433						0162	Z2	9	0	20090101	20100101	
S9434							Z2	9	0	20030401	20030401	
S9435						0088	Z2	9	0	20010101	20010101	
S9436							Z2	9	0	20020401	20020401	
S9437							Z2	9	0	20020401	20020401	
S9438							Z2	9	0	20020401	20020401	
S9439							Z2	9	0	20020401	20020401	
S9441						0088	Z2	9	0	20020101	20020101	
S9442						0088	Z2	9	0	20020101	20020101	
S9443						0088	Z2	9	0	20020101	20020101	
S9444							Z2	9	0	20020401	20020401	
S9445						0088	Z2	9	0	20020101	20020101	
S9446						0088	Z2	9	0	20020101	20020101	

HCPCS Code	Long Description	Coverage	Action	PI	MPI	CIM	MCM
S9447	INFANT SAFETY (INCLUDING CPR) CLASSES, NON-PHYSICIAN	I	N	00	9		
S9449	WEIGHT MANAGEMENT CLASSES, NON-PHYSICIAN PROVIDER, PER SESSION	I	N	00	9		
S9451	EXERCISE CLASSES, NON-PHYSICIAN PROVIDER, PER SESSION	I	N	00	9		
S9452	NUTRITION CLASSES, NON-PHYSICIAN PROVIDER, PER SESSION	I	N	00	9		
S9453	SMOKING CESSATION CLASSES, NON-PHYSICIAN PROVIDER, PER SESSION	I	N	00	9		
S9454	STRESS MANAGEMENT CLASSES, NON-PHYSICIAN PROVIDER, PER SESSION	I	N	00	9		
S9455	DIABETIC MANAGEMENT PROGRAM, GROUP SESSION	I	N	00	9		
S9460	DIABETIC MANAGEMENT PROGRAM, NURSE VISIT	I	N	00	9		
S9465	DIABETIC MANAGEMENT PROGRAM, DIETITIAN VISIT	I	N	00	9		
S9470	NUTRITIONAL COUNSELING, DIETITIAN VISIT	I	N	00	9		
S9472	CARDIAC REHABILITATION PROGRAM, NON-PHYSICIAN PROVIDER, PER DIEM	I	N	00	9		
S9473	PULMONARY REHABILITATION PROGRAM, NON-PHYSICIAN PROVIDER, PER DIEM	I	N	00	9		
S9474	ENTEROSTOMAL THERAPY BY A REGISTERED NURSE CERTIFIED IN ENTEROSTOMAL THERAPY, PER DIEM	I	N	00	9		
S9475	AMBULATORY SETTING SUBSTANCE ABUSE TREATMENT OR DETOXIFICATION SERVICES, PER DIEM	I	N	00	9		
S9476	VESTIBULAR REHABILITATION PROGRAM, NON-PHYSICIAN PROVIDER, PER DIEM	I	N	00	9		
S9480	INTENSIVE OUTPATIENT PSYCHIATRIC SERVICES, PER DIEM	I	N	00	9		
S9482	FAMILY STABILIZATION SERVICES, PER 15 MINUTES	I	N	00	9		
S9484	CRISIS INTERVENTION MENTAL HEALTH SERVICES, PER HOUR	I	N	00	9		
S9485	CRISIS INTERVENTION MENTAL HEALTH SERVICES, PER DIEM	I	N	00	9		
S9490	HOME INFUSION THERAPY, CORTICOSTEROID INFUSION; ADMINISTRATIVE SERVICES, PROFESSIONAL PHARMACY SERVICES, CARE COORDINATION, AND ALL NECESSARY SUPPLIES AND EQUIPMENT (DRUGS AND NURSING VISITS CODED SEPARATELY), PER DIEM	I	N	00	9		
S9494	HOME INFUSION THERAPY, ANTIBIOTIC, ANTIVIRAL, OR ANTIFUNGAL THERAPY; ADMINISTRATIVE SERVICES, PROFESSIONAL PHARMACY SERVICES, CARE COORDINATION, AND ALL NECESSARY SUPPLIES AND EQUIPMENT (DRUGS & NURSING VISITS CODED SEPARATELY, PER DIEM) (DO NOT USE THIS CODE WITH HOME INFUSION CODES FOR HOURLY DOSING SCHEDULES S9497-S9504)	I	N	00	9		
S9497	HOME INFUSION THERAPY, ANTIBIOTIC, ANTIVIRAL, OR ANTIFUNGAL THERAPY; ONCE EVERY 3 HOURS; ADMINISTRATIVE SERVICES, PROFESSIONAL PHARMACY SERVICES, CARE COORDINATION, AND ALL NECESSARY SUPPLIES AND EQUIPMENT (DRUGS AND NURSING VISITS CODED SEPARATELY), PER DIEM	I	N	00	9		

HCPCS Code	Statute	Lab Cert	X-Ref	ASC Pay Grp	ASC Pay Group Eff. Date	Proc Notes	BETOS	TOS	Anest	Code Add Date	Code Effective Date	Code Term Date
S9447							Z2	9	0	20020401	20020401	
S9449							Z2	9	0	20020401	20020401	
S9451							Z2	9	0	20020401	20020401	
S9452							Z2	9	0	20020401	20020401	
S9453							Z2	9	0	20020401	20020401	
S9454							Z2	9	0	20020401	20020401	
S9455						0088	Z2	9	0	20000101	20000101	
S9460						0088	Z2	9	0	20000101	20000101	
S9465						0088	Z2	9	0	20000101	20000101	
S9470						0088	Z2	9	0	20000101	20000101	
S9472						0088	Z2	9	0	20000101	20000101	
S9473						0088	Z2	9	0	20000101	20000101	
S9474						0088	Z2	9	0	20000101	20000101	
S9475						0088	Z2	9	0	20000101	20000101	
S9476							Z2	9	0	20031001	20031001	
S9480						0088	Z2	9	0	20000101	20000101	
S9482							Z2	9	0	20050101	20050101	
S9484							Z2	9	0	20020701	20020701	
S9485						0088	Z2	9	0	20000101	20000101	
S9490							Z2	9	0	20020701	20020701	
S9494						0088	Z2	9	0	20020101	20020101	
S9497						0088	Z2	9	0	20020101	20020101	

HCPCS Code	Long Description	Coverage	Action	PI	MPI	CIM	MCM
S9500	HOME INFUSION THERAPY, ANTIBIOTIC, ANTIVIRAL, OR ANTIFUNGAL THERAPY; ONCE EVERY 24 HOURS; ADMINISTRATIVE SERVICES, PROFESSIONAL PHARMACY SERVICES, CARE COORDINATION, AND ALL NECESSARY SUPPLIES AND EQUIPMENT (DRUGS AND NURSING VISITS CODED SEPARATELY), PER DIEM	I	N	00	9		
S9501	HOME INFUSION THERAPY, ANTIBIOTIC, ANTIVIRAL, OR ANTIFUNGAL THERAPY; ONCE EVERY 12 HOURS; ADMINISTRATIVE SERVICES, PROFESSIONAL PHARMACY SERVICES, CARE COORDINATION, AND ALL NECESSARY SUPPLIES AND EQUIPMENT (DRUGS AND NURSING VISITS CODED SEPARATELY), PER DIEM	I	N	00	9		
S9502	HOME INFUSION THERAPY, ANTIBIOTIC, ANTIVIRAL, OR ANTIFUNGAL THERAPY; ONCE EVERY 8 HOURS, ADMINISTRATIVE SERVICES, PROFESSIONAL PHARMACY SERVICES, CARE COORDINATION, AND ALL NECESSARY SUPPLIES AND EQUIPMENT (DRUGS AND NURSING VISITS CODED SEPARATELY), PER DIEM	I	N	00	9		
S9503	HOME INFUSION THERAPY, ANTIBIOTIC, ANTIVIRAL, OR ANTIFUNGAL; ONCE EVERY 6 HOURS; ADMINISTRATIVE SERVICES, PROFESSIONAL PHARMACY SERVICES, CARE COORDINATION, AND ALL NECESSARY SUPPLIES AND EQUIPMENT (DRUGS AND NURSING VISITS CODED SEPARATELY), PER DIEM	I	N	00	9		
S9504	HOME INFUSION THERAPY, ANTIBIOTIC, ANTIVIRAL, OR ANTIFUNGAL; ONCE EVERY 4 HOURS; ADMINISTRATIVE SERVICES, PROFESSIONAL PHARMACY SERVICES, CARE COORDINATION, AND ALL NECESSARY SUPPLIES AND EQUIPMENT (DRUGS AND NURSING VISITS CODED SEPARATELY), PER DIEM	I	N	00	9		
S9529	ROUTINE VENIPUNCTURE FOR COLLECTION OF SPECIMEN(S), SINGLE HOME BOUND, NURSING HOME, OR SKILLED NURSING FACILITY PATIENT	I	N	00	9		
S9537	HOME THERAPY; HEMATOPOIETIC HORMONE INJECTION THERAPY (E.G.ERYTHROPOIETIN, G-CSF, GM-CSF); ADMINISTRATIVE SERVICES, PROFESSIONAL PHARMACY SERVICES, CARE COORDINATION, AND ALL NECESSARY SUPPLIES AND EQUIPMENT (DRUGS AND NURSING VISITS CODED SEPARATELY), PER DIEM	I	N	00	9		
S9538	HOME TRANSFUSION OF BLOOD PRODUCT(S); ADMINISTRATIVE SERVICES, PROFESSIONAL PHARMACY SERVICES, CARE COORDINATION AND ALL NECESSARY SUPPLIES AND EQUIPMENT (BLOOD PRODUCTS, DRUGS, AND NURSING VISITS CODED SEPARATELY), PER DIEM	I	N	00	9		
S9542	HOME INJECTABLE THERAPY, NOT OTHERWISE CLASSIFIED, INCLUDING ADMINISTRATIVE SERVICES, PROFESSIONAL PHARMACY SERVICES, CARE COORDINATION, AND ALL NECESSARY SUPPLIES AND EQUIPMENT (DRUGS AND NURSING VISITS CODED SEPARATELY), PER DIEM	I	N	00	9		

HCPCS Code	Statute	Lab Cert	X-Ref	ASC Pay Grp	ASC Pay Group Eff. Date	Proc Notes	BETOS	TOS	Anest	Code Add Date	Code Effective Date	Code Term Date
S9500						0088	Z2	9	0	20020101	20020101	
S9501						0088	Z2	9	0	20020101	20020101	
S9502						0088	Z2	9	0	20020101	20020101	
S9503						0088	Z2	9	0	20020101	20020101	
S9504						0088	Z2	9	0	20020101	20020101	
S9529						0088	Z2	5	0	20020101	20020101	
S9537						0088	Z2	9	0	20020101	20020101	
S9538						0088	Z2	9	0	20020101	20020101	
S9542						0088	Z2	9	0	20020101	20020101	

HCPCS Code	Long Description	Coverage	Action	PI	MPI	CIM	MCM
S9558	HOME INJECTABLE THERAPY; GROWTH HORMONE, INCLUDING ADMINISTRATIVE SERVICES, PROFESSIONAL PHARMACY SERVICES, CARE COORDINATION, AND ALL NECESSARY SUPPLIES AND EQUIPMENT (DRUGS AND NURSING VISITS CODED SEPARATELY), PER DIEM	I	N	00	9		
S9559	HOME INJECTABLE THERAPY, INTERFERON, INCLUDING ADMINISTRATIVE SERVICES, PROFESSIONAL PHARMACY SERVICES, CARE COORDINATION, AND ALL NECESSARY SUPPLIES AND EQUIPMENT (DRUGS AND NURSING VISITS CODED SEPARATELY), PER DIEM	I	N	00	9		
S9560	HOME INJECTABLE THERAPY; HORMONAL THERAPY (E.G.; LEUPROLIDE, GOSERELIN),INCLUDING ADMINISTRATIVE SERVICES, PROFESSIONAL PHARMACY SERVICES, CARE COORDINATION, AND ALL NECESSARY SUPPLIES AND EQUIPMENT (DRUGS AND NURSING VISITS CODED SEPARATELY), PER DIEM	I	N	00	9		
S9562	HOME INJECTABLE THERAPY, PALIVIZUMAB, INCLUDING ADMINISTRATIVE SERVICES, PROFESSIONAL PHARMACY SERVICES, CARE COORDINATION, AND ALL NECESSARY SUPPLIES AND EQUIPMENT (DRUGS AND NURSING VISITS CODED SEPARATELY), PER DIEM	I	N	00	9		
S9590	HOME THERAPY, IRRIGATION THERAPY (E.G. STERILE IRRIGATION OF AN ORGAN OR ANATOMICAL CAVITY); INCLUDING ADMINISTRATIVE SERVICES, PROFESSIONAL PHARMACY SERVICES, CARE COORDINATION, AND ALL NECESSARY SUPPLIES AND EQUIPMENT (DRUGS & NURSING VISITS CODED SEPARATELY), PER DIEM	I	N	00	9		
S9810	HOME THERAPY; PROFESSIONAL PHARMACY SERVICES FOR PROVISION OF INFUSION, SPECIALTY DRUG ADMINISTRATION, AND/OR DISEASE STATE MANAGEMENT, NOT OTHERWISE CLASSIFIED, PER HOUR (DO NOT USE THIS CODE WITH ANY PER DIEM CODE)	I	N	00	9		
S9900	SERVICES BY AUTHORIZED CHRISTIAN SCIENCE PRACTITIONER FOR THE PROCESS OF HEALING, PER DIEM; NOT TO BE USED FOR REST OR STUDY; EXCLUDES IN-PATIENT SERVICES	I	N	00	9		
S9970	HEALTH CLUB MEMBERSHIP, ANNUAL	I	N	00	9		
S9975	TRANSPLANT RELATED LODGING, MEALS AND TRANSPORTATION, PER DIEM	I	N	00	9		
S9976	LODGING, PER DIEM, NOT OTHERWISE CLASSIFIED	I	N	00	9		
S9977	MEALS, PER DIEM, NOT OTHERWISE SPECIFIED	I	N	00	9		
S9981	MEDICAL RECORDS COPYING FEE, ADMINISTRATIVE	I	N	00	9		
S9982	MEDICAL RECORDS COPYING FEE, PER PAGE	I	N	00	9		
S9986	NOT MEDICALLY NECESSARY SERVICE (PATIENT IS AWARE THAT SERVICE NOT MEDICALLY NECESSARY)	I	N	00	9		
S9988	SERVICES PROVIDED AS PART OF A PHASE I CLINICAL TRIAL	I	N	00	9		
S9989	SERVICES PROVIDED OUTSIDE OF THE UNITED STATES OF AMERICA (LIST IN ADDITION TO CODE(S) FOR SERVICES(S))	I	N	00	9		
S9990	SERVICES PROVIDED AS PART OF A PHASE II CLINICAL TRIAL	I	N	00	9		

HCPCS Code	Statute	Lab Cert	X-Ref	ASC Pay Grp	ASC Pay Group Eff. Date	Proc Notes	BETOS	TOS	Anest	Code Add Date	Code Effective Date	Code Term Date
S9558						0088	Z2	9	0	20020101	20020101	
S9559						0088	Z2	9	0	20020101	20020101	
S9560						0088	Z2	9	0	20020101	20020101	
S9562							Z2	9	0	20030101	20030101	
S9590							Z2	9	0	20030101	20030101	
S9810						0088	Z2	9	0	20020101	20020101	
S9900							Z2	9	0	20020701	20020701	
S9970							Z2	9	0	20020401	20020401	
S9975							Z2	9	0	20020401	20020401	
S9976							Z2	9	0	20040401	20040401	
S9977							Z2	9	0	20040401	20040401	
S9981						0088	Z2	9	0	20020101	20020101	
S9982						0088	Z2	9	0	20020101	20020101	
S9986						0088	Z2	9	0	20020101	20020101	
S9988							Z2	9	0	20040401	20040401	
S9989						0088	Z2	9	0	20020101	20020101	
S9989												
S9990						0088	Z2	9	0	20000101	20000101	

HCPCS Code	Long Description	Coverage	Action	PI	MPI	CIM	MCM
S9991	SERVICES PROVIDED AS PART OF A PHASE III CLINICAL TRIAL	I	N	00	9		
S9992	TRANSPORTATION COSTS TO AND FROM TRIAL LOCATION AND LOCAL TRANSPORTATION COSTS (E.G., FARES FOR TAXICAB OR BUS) FOR CLINICAL TRIAL PARTICIPANT AND ONE CAREGIVER/COMPANION	I	N	00	9		
S9994	LODGING COSTS (E.G., HOTEL CHARGES) FOR CLINICAL TRIAL PARTICIPANT AND ONE CAREGIVER/COMPANION	I	N	00	9		
S9996	MEALS FOR CLINICAL TRIAL PARTICIPANT AND ONE CAREGIVER/COMPANION	I	N	00	9		
S9999	SALES TAX	I	N	00	9		
T1000	PRIVATE DUTY / INDEPENDENT NURSING SERVICE(S) - LICENSED, UP TO 15 MINUTES	I	N	00	9		
T1001	NURSING ASSESSMENT / EVALUATION	I	N	00	9		
T1002	RN SERVICES, UP TO 15 MINUTES	I	N	00	9		
T1003	LPN/LVN SERVICES, UP TO 15 MINUTES	I	N	00	9		
T1004	SERVICES OF A QUALIFIED NURSING AIDE, UP TO 15 MINUTES	I	N	00	9		
T1005	RESPITE CARE SERVICES, UP TO 15 MINUTES	I	N	00	9		
T1006	ALCOHOL AND/OR SUBSTANCE ABUSE SERVICES, FAMILY/COUPLE COUNSELING	I	N	00	9		
T1007	ALCOHOL AND/OR SUBSTANCE ABUSE SERVICES, TREATMENT PLAN DEVELOPMENT AND/OR MODIFICATION	I	N	00	9		
T1009	CHILD SITTING SERVICES FOR CHILDREN OF THE INDIVIDUAL RECEIVING ALCOHOL AND/OR SUBSTANCE ABUSE SERVICES	I	N	00	9		
T1010	MEALS FOR INDIVIDUALS RECEIVING ALCOHOL AND/OR SUBSTANCE ABUSE SERVICES (WHEN MEALS NOT INCLUDED IN THE PROGRAM)	I	N	00	9		
T1012	ALCOHOL AND/OR SUBSTANCE ABUSE SERVICES, SKILLS DEVELOPMENT	I	N	00	9		
T1013	SIGN LANGUAGE OR ORAL INTERPRETIVE SERVICES, PER 15 MINUTES	I	N	00	9		
T1014	TELEHEALTH TRANSMISSION, PER MINUTE, PROFESSIONAL SERVICES BILL SEPARATELY	I	N	00	9		
T1015	CLINIC VISIT/ENCOUNTER, ALL-INCLUSIVE	I	N	00	9		
T1016	CASE MANAGEMENT, EACH 15 MINUTES	I	N	00	9		
T1017	TARGETED CASE MANAGEMENT, EACH 15 MINUTES	I	N	00	9		
T1018	SCHOOL-BASED INDIVIDUALIZED EDUCATION PROGRAM (IEP) SERVICES, BUNDLED	I	N	00	9		
T1019	PERSONAL CARE SERVICES, PER 15 MINUTES, NOT FOR AN INPATIENT OR RESIDENT OF A HOSPITAL, NURSING FACILITY, ICF/MR OR IMD, PART OF THE INDIVIDUALIZED PLAN OF TREATMENT (CODE MAY NOT BE USED TO IDENTIFY SERVICES PROVIDED BY HOME HEALTH AIDE OR CERTIFIED NURSE ASSISTANT)	I	N	00	9		
T1020	PERSONAL CARE SERVICES, PER DIEM, NOT FOR AN INPATIENT OR RESIDENT OF A HOSPITAL, NURSING FACILITY, ICF/MR OR IMD, PART OF THE INDIVIDUALIZED PLAN OF TREATMENT (CODE MAY NOT BE USED TO IDENTIFY SERVICES PROVIDED BY HOME HEALTH AIDE OR CERTIFIED NURSE ASSISTANT)	I	N	00	9		
T1021	HOME HEALTH AIDE OR CERTIFIED NURSE ASSISTANT, PER VISIT	I	N	00	9		

HCPCS Code	Statute	Lab Cert	X-Ref	ASC Pay Grp	ASC Pay Group Eff. Date	Proc Notes	BETOS	TOS	Anest	Code Add Date	Code Effective Date	Code Term Date
S9991						0088	Z2	9	0	20000101	20000101	
S9992						0088	Z2	9	0	20000101	20000101	
S9994						0088	Z2	9	0	20000101	20000101	
S9996						0088	Z2	9	0	20000101	20000101	
S9999						0088	Z2	9	0	20000101	20000101	
T1000							Z2	9	0	20010701	20010701	
T1001							Z2	9	0	20010701	20010701	
T1002							Z2	9	0	20010701	20010701	
T1003							Z2	9	0	20010701	20010701	
T1004							Z2	9	0	20010701	20010701	
T1005							Z2	9	0	20010701	20010701	
T1006							Z2	9	0	20010701	20010701	
T1007							Z2	9	0	20010701	20010701	
T1009							Z2	9	0	20010701	20010701	
T1010							Z2	9	0	20010701	20010701	
T1012							Z2	9	0	20010701	20010701	
T1013							Z2	9	0	20010701	20030101	
T1014							Z2	9	0	20010701	20010701	
T1015							Z2	1	0	20020101	20020101	
T1016							Z2	9	0	20020701	20020701	
T1017							Z2	9	0	20020701	20020701	
T1018							Z2	9	0	20020701	20020701	
T1019							Z2	9	0	20020701	20020701	
T1020							Z2	9	0	20020701	20020701	
T1021							Z2	9	0	20020701	20020701	

HCPCS Code	Long Description	Coverage	Action	PI	MPI	CIM	MCM
T1022	CONTRACTED HOME HEALTH AGENCY SERVICES, ALL SERVICES PROVIDED UNDER CONTRACT, PER DAY	I	N	00	9		
T1023	SCREENING TO DETERMINE THE APPROPRIATENESS OF CONSIDERATION OF AN INDIVIDUAL FOR PARTICIPATION IN A SPECIFIED PROGRAM, PROJECT OR TREATMENT PROTOCOL, PER ENCOUNTER	I	N	00	9		
T1024	EVALUATION AND TREATMENT BY AN INTEGRATED, SPECIALTY TEAM CONTRACTED TO PROVIDE COORDINATED CARE TO MULTIPLE OR SEVERELY HANDICAPPED CHILDREN, PER ENCOUNTER	I	N	00	9		
T1025	INTENSIVE, EXTENDED MULTIDISCIPLINARY SERVICES PROVIDED IN A CLINIC SETTING TO CHILDREN WITH COMPLEX MEDICAL, PHYSICAL, MENTAL AND PSYCHOSOCIAL IMPAIRMENTS, PER DIEM	I	N	00	9		
T1026	INTENSIVE, EXTENDED MULTIDISCIPLINARY SERVICES PROVIDED IN A CLINIC SETTING TO CHILDREN WITH COMPLEX MEDICAL, PHYSICAL, MEDICAL AND PSYCHOSOCIAL IMPAIRMENTS, PER HOUR	I	N	00	9		
T1027	FAMILY TRAINING AND COUNSELING FOR CHILD DEVELOPMENT, PER 15 MINUTES	I	N	00	9		
T1028	ASSESSMENT OF HOME, PHYSICAL AND FAMILY ENVIRONMENT, TO DETERMINE SUITABILITY TO MEET PATIENT'S MEDICAL NEEDS	I	N	00	9		
T1029	COMPREHENSIVE ENVIRONMENTAL LEAD INVESTIGATION, NOT INCLUDING LABORATORY ANALYSIS, PER DWELLING	I	N	00	9		
T1030	NURSING CARE, IN THE HOME, BY REGISTERED NURSE, PER DIEM	I	N	00	9		
T1031	NURSING CARE, IN THE HOME, BY LICENSED PRACTICAL NURSE, PER DIEM	I	N	00	9		
T1502	ADMINISTRATION OF ORAL, INTRAMUSCULAR AND/OR SUBCUTANEOUS MEDICATION BY HEALTH CARE AGENCY/PROFESSIONAL, PER VISIT	I	N	00	9		
T1503	ADMINISTRATION OF MEDICATION, OTHER THAN ORAL AND/OR INJECTABLE, BY A HEALTH CARE AGENCY/PROFESSIONAL, PER VISIT	I	N	00	9		
T1999	MISCELLANEOUS THERAPEUTIC ITEMS AND SUPPLIES, RETAIL PURCHASES, NOT OTHERWISE CLASSIFIED; IDENTIFY PRODUCT IN "REMARKS"	I	N	00	9		
T2001	NON-EMERGENCY TRANSPORTATION; PATIENT ATTENDANT/ESCORT	I	N	00	9		
T2002	NON-EMERGENCY TRANSPORTATION; PER DIEM	I	N	00	9		
T2003	NON-EMERGENCY TRANSPORTATION; ENCOUNTER/TRIP	I	N	00	9		
T2004	NON-EMERGENCY TRANSPORT; COMMERCIAL CARRIER, MULTI-PASS	I	N	00	9		
T2005	NON-EMERGENCY TRANSPORTATION; STRETCHER VAN	I	N	00	9		
T2007	TRANSPORTATION WAITING TIME, AIR AMBULANCE & NON-EMERGENCY VEHICLE, ONE-HALF (1/2) HOUR INCREMENTS	I	N	00	9		
T2010	PREADMISSION SCREENING AND RESIDENT REVIEW (PASRR) LEVEL I IDENTIFICATION SCREENING, PER SCREEN	I	N	00	9		

HCPCS Code	Statute	Lab Cert	X-Ref	ASC Pay Grp	ASC Pay Group Eff. Date	Proc Notes	BETOS	TOS	Anest	Code Add Date	Code Effective Date	Code Term Date
T1022							Z2	9	0	20030101	20030101	
T1023							Z2	9	0	20030101	20030101	
T1024							Z2	9	0	20030101	20030101	
T1025							Z2	9	0	20030101	20030101	
T1026							Z2	9	0	20030101	20030101	
T1027							Z2	9	0	20030101	20030101	
T1028							Z2	9	0	20030101	20030101	
T1029							Z2	9	0	20030101	20030101	
T1030							Z2	9	0	20030101	20030101	
T1031							Z2	9	0	20030101	20030101	
T1502							Z2	9	0	20030101	20030101	
T1503							Z2	9	0	20070401	20070401	
T1999							Z2	9	0	20030101	20030101	
T2001							Z2	9	0	20020401	20020401	
T2002							Z2	9	0	20020401	20020401	
T2003							Z2	9	0	20020401	20020401	
T2004							Z2	9	0	20020401	20020401	
T2005							Z2	9	0	20020401	20040701	
T2007							Z2	9	0	20030101	20030101	
T2010						0112	Z2	9	0	20030401	20030401	

HCPCS Code	Long Description	Coverage	Action	PI	MPI	CIM	MCM
T2011	PREADMISSION SCREENING AND RESIDENT REVIEW (PASRR) LEVEL II EVALUATION, PER EVALUATION	I	N	00	9		
T2012	HABILITATION, EDUCATIONAL; WAIVER, PER DIEM	I	N	00	9		
T2013	HABILITATION, EDUCATIONAL, WAIVER; PER HOUR	I	N	00	9		
T2014	HABILITATION, PREVOCATIONAL, WAIVER; PER DIEM	I	N	00	9		
T2015	HABILITATION, PREVOCATIONAL, WAIVER; PER HOUR	I	N	00	9		
T2016	HABILITATION, RESIDENTIAL, WAIVER; PER DIEM	I	N	00	9		
T2017	HABILITATION, RESIDENTIAL, WAIVER; 15 MINUTES	I	N	00	9		
T2018	HABILITATION, SUPPORTED EMPLOYMENT, WAIVER; PER DIEM	I	N	00	9		
T2019	HABILITATION, SUPPORTED EMPLOYMENT, WAIVER; PER 15 MINUTES	I	N	00	9		
T2020	DAY HABILITATION, WAIVER; PER DIEM	I	N	00	9		
T2021	DAY HABILITATION, WAIVER; PER 15 MINUTES	I	N	00	9		
T2022	CASE MANAGEMENT, PER MONTH	I	N	00	9		
T2023	TARGETED CASE MANAGEMENT; PER MONTH	I	N	00	9		
T2024	SERVICE ASSESSMENT/PLAN OF CARE DEVELOPMENT, WAIVER	I	N	00	9		
T2025	WAIVER SERVICES; NOT OTHERWISE SPECIFIED (NOS)	I	N	00	9		
T2026	SPECIALIZED CHILDCARE, WAIVER; PER DIEM	I	N	00	9		
T2027	SPECIALIZED CHILDCARE, WAIVER; PER 15 MINUTES	I	N	00	9		
T2028	SPECIALIZED SUPPLY, NOT OTHERWISE SPECIFIED, WAIVER	I	N	00	9		
T2029	SPECIALIZED MEDICAL EQUIPMENT, NOT OTHERWISE SPECIFIED, WAIVER	I	N	00	9		
T2030	ASSISTED LIVING, WAIVER; PER MONTH	I	N	00	9		
T2031	ASSISTED LIVING; WAIVER, PER DIEM	I	N	00	9		
T2032	RESIDENTIAL CARE, NOT OTHERWISE SPECIFIED (NOS), WAIVER; PER MONTH	I	N	00	9		
T2033	RESIDENTIAL CARE, NOT OTHERWISE SPECIFIED (NOS), WAIVER; PER DIEM	I	N	00	9		
T2034	CRISIS INTERVENTION, WAIVER; PER DIEM	I	N	00	9		
T2035	UTILITY SERVICES TO SUPPORT MEDICAL EQUIPMENT AND ASSISTIVE TECHNOLOGY/DEVICES, WAIVER	I	N	00	9		
T2036	THERAPEUTIC CAMPING, OVERNIGHT, WAIVER; EACH SESSION	I	N	00	9		
T2037	THERAPEUTIC CAMPING, DAY, WAIVER; EACH SESSION	I	N	00	9		
T2038	COMMUNITY TRANSITION, WAIVER; PER SERVICE	I	N	00	9		
T2039	VEHICLE MODIFICATIONS, WAIVER; PER SERVICE	I	N	00	9		
T2040	FINANCIAL MANAGEMENT, SELF-DIRECTED, WAIVER; PER 15 MINUTES	I	N	00	9		
T2041	SUPPORTS BROKERAGE, SELF-DIRECTED, WAIVER; PER 15 MINUTES	I	N	00	9		
T2042	HOSPICE ROUTINE HOME CARE; PER DIEM	I	N	00	9		
T2043	HOSPICE CONTINUOUS HOME CARE; PER HOUR	I	N	00	9		
T2044	HOSPICE INPATIENT RESPITE CARE; PER DIEM	I	N	00	9		
T2045	HOSPICE GENERAL INPATIENT CARE; PER DIEM	I	N	00	9		
T2046	HOSPICE LONG TERM CARE, ROOM AND BOARD ONLY; PER DIEM	I	N	00	9		
T2048	BEHAVIORAL HEALTH; LONG-TERM CARE RESIDENTIAL (NON-ACUTE CARE IN A RESIDENTIAL TREATMENT PROGRAM WHERE STAY IS TYPICALLY LONGER THAN 30 DAYS), WITH ROOM AND BOARD, PER DIEM	I	N	00	9		

HCPCS Code	Statute	Lab Cert	X-Ref	ASC Pay Grp	ASC Pay Group Eff. Date	Proc Notes	BETOS	TOS	Anest	Code Add Date	Code Effective Date	Code Term Date
T2011						0113	Z2	9	0	20030401	20030401	
T2012							Z2	9	0	20031001	20031001	
T2013							Z2	9	0	20031001	20031001	
T2014							Z2	9	0	20031001	20031001	
T2015							Z2	9	0	20031001	20031001	
T2016							Z2	9	0	20031001	20031001	
T2017							Z2	9	0	20031001	20031001	
T2018							Z2	9	0	20031001	20031001	
T2019							Z2	9	0	20031001	20031001	
T2020							Z2	9	0	20031001	20031001	
T2021							Z2	9	0	20031001	20031001	
T2022							Z2	9	0	20031001	20031001	
T2023							Z2	9	0	20031001	20031001	
T2024							Z2	9	0	20031001	20031001	
T2025							Z2	9	0	20031001	20031001	
T2026							Z2	9	0	20031001	20031001	
T2027							Z2	9	0	20031001	20031001	
T2028							Z2	9	0	20031001	20031001	
T2029							Z2	9	0	20031001	20031001	
T2030							Z2	9	0	20031001	20031001	
T2031							Z2	9	0	20031001	20031001	
T2032							Z2	9	0	20031001	20031001	
T2033							Z2	9	0	20031001	20031001	
T2034							Z2	9	0	20031001	20031001	
T2035							Z2	9	0	20031001	20031001	
T2036							Z2	9	0	20031001	20031001	
T2037							Z2	9	0	20031001	20031001	
T2038							Z2	9	0	20031001	20031001	
T2039							Z2	9	0	20031001	20031001	
T2040							Z2	9	0	20031001	20031001	
T2041							Z2	9	0	20031001	20031001	
T2042							Z2	9	0	20031001	20031001	
T2043							Z2	9	0	20031001	20031001	
T2044							Z2	9	0	20031001	20031001	
T2045							Z2	9	0	20031001	20031001	
T2046							Z2	9	0	20031001	20031001	
T2048							Z2	9	0	20031001	20031001	

HCPCS Code	Long Description	Coverage	Action	PI	MPI	CIM	MCM
T2049	NON-EMERGENCY TRANSPORTATION; STRETCHER VAN, MILEAGE; PER MILE	I	N	00	9		
T2101	HUMAN BREAST MILK PROCESSING, STORAGE AND DISTRIBUTION ONLY	I	N	00	9		
T4521	ADULT SIZED DISPOSABLE INCONTINENCE PRODUCT, BRIEF/DIAPER, SMALL, EACH	M	N	00	9	60-9	
T4522	ADULT SIZED DISPOSABLE INCONTINENCE PRODUCT, BRIEF/DIAPER, MEDIUM, EACH	M	N	00	9	60-9	
T4523	ADULT SIZED DISPOSABLE INCONTINENCE PRODUCT, BRIEF/DIAPER, LARGE, EACH	M	N	00	9	60-9	
T4524	ADULT SIZED DISPOSABLE INCONTINENCE PRODUCT, BRIEF/DIAPER, EXTRA LARGE, EACH	M	N	00	9	60-9	
T4525	ADULT SIZED DISPOSABLE INCONTINENCE PRODUCT, PROTECTIVE UNDERWEAR/PULL-ON, SMALL SIZE, EACH	M	N	00	9	60-9	
T4526	ADULT SIZED DISPOSABLE INCONTINENCE PRODUCT, PROTECTIVE UNDERWEAR/PULL-ON, MEDIUM SIZE, EACH	M	N	00	9	60-9	
T4527	ADULT SIZED DISPOSABLE INCONTINENCE PRODUCT, PROTECTIVE UNDERWEAR/PULL-ON, LARGE SIZE, EACH	M	N	00	9	60-9	
T4528	ADULT SIZED DISPOSABLE INCONTINENCE PRODUCT, PROTECTIVE UNDERWEAR/PULL-ON, EXTRA LARGE SIZE, EA.	M	N	00	9	60-9	
T4529	PEDIATRIC SIZED DISPOSABLE INCONTINENCE PRODUCT, BRIEF/DIAPER, SMALL/MEDIUM SIZE, EACH	M	N	00	9	60-9	
T4530	PEDIATRIC SIZED DISPOSABLE INCONTINENCE PRODUCT, BRIEF/DIAPER, LARGE SIZE, EACH	M	N	00	9	60-9	
T4531	PEDIATRIC SIZED DISPOSABLE INCONTINENCE PRODUCT, PROTECTIVE UNDERWEAR/PULL-ON, SMALL/MEDIUM SIZE, EA.	M	N	00	9	60-9	
T4532	PEDIATRIC SIZED DISPOSABLE INCONTINENCE PRODUCT, PROTECTIVE UNDERWEAR/PULL-ON, LARGE SIZE, EACH	M	N	00	9	60-9	
T4533	YOUTH SIZED DISPOSABLE INCONTINENCE PRODUCT, BRIEF/DIAPER, EACH	M	N	00	9	60-9	
T4534	YOUTH SIZED DISPOSABLE INCONTINENCE PRODUCT, PROTECTIVE UNDERWEAR/PULL-ON, EACH	M	N	00	9	60-9	
T4535	DISPOSABLE LINER/SHIELD/GUARD/PAD/UNDERGARMENT, FOR INCONTINENCE, EACH	M	N	00	9	60-9	
T4536	INCONTINENCE PRODUCT, PROTECTIVE UNDERWEAR/PULL-ON, REUSABLE, ANY SIZE, EACH	M	N	00	9	60-9	
T4537	INCONTINENCE PRODUCT, PROTECTIVE UNDERPAD, REUSABLE, BED SIZE, EACH	M	N	00	9	60-9	
T4538	DIAPER SERVICE, REUSABLE DIAPER, EACH DIAPER	M	N	00	9	60-9	
T4539	INCONTINENCE PRODUCT, DIAPER/BRIEF, REUSABLE, ANY SIZE, EACH	M	N	00	9	60-9	
T4540	INCONTINENCE PRODUCT, PROTECTIVE UNDERPAD, REUSABLE, CHAIR SIZE, EACH	M	N	00	9	60-9	
T4541	INCONTINENCE PRODUCT, DISPOSABLE UNDERPAD, LARGE, EA.	I	N	00	9		
T4542	INCONTINENCE PRODUCT, DISPOSABLE UNDERPAD, SMALL SIZE, EACH	I	N	00	9		
T4543	DISPOSABLE INCONTINENCE PRODUCT, BRIEF/DIAPER, BARIATRIC, EACH	M	N	00	9	60-9	
T5001	POSITIONING SEAT FOR PERSONS WITH SPECIAL ORTHOPEDIC NEEDS	I	N	00	9		

HCPCS Code	Statute	Lab Cert	X-Ref	ASC Pay Grp	ASC Pay Group Eff. Date	Proc Notes	BETOS	TOS	Anest	Code Add Date	Code Effective Date	Code Term Date
T2049							Z2	9	0	20040701	20040701	
T2101							Z2	9	0	20040101	20040101	
T4521							D1A	9	0	20050101	20050101	
T4522							D1A	9	0	20050101	20050101	
T4523							D1A	9	0	20050101	20050101	
T4524							D1A	9	0	20050101	20050101	
T4525							D1A	9	0	20050101	20050101	
T4526							D1A	9	0	20050101	20050101	
T4527							D1A	9	0	20050101	20050101	
T4528							D1A	9	0	20050101	20050101	
T4529							D1A	9	0	20050101	20050101	
T4530							D1A	9	0	20050101	20050101	
T4531							D1A	9	0	20050101	20050101	
T4532							D1A	9	0	20050101	20050101	
T4533							D1A	9	0	20050101	20050101	
T4534							D1A	9	0	20050101	20050101	
T4535							D1A	9	0	20050101	20050101	
T4536							D1A	9	0	20050101	20050101	
T4537							D1A	9	0	20050101	20050101	
T4538							D1A	9	0	20050101	20050101	
T4539							D1A	9	0	20050101	20050101	
T4540							D1A	9	0	20050101	20050101	
T4541							Z2	9	0	20050101	20050101	
T4542							Z2	9	0	20050101	20050101	
T4543							D1A	9	0	20070101	20070101	
T5001							Z2	P	0	20040101	20070101	

HCPCS Code	Long Description	Coverage	Action	PI	MPI	CIM	MCM
T5999	SUPPLY, NOT OTHERWISE SPECIFIED	I	N	00	9		
V2020	FRAMES, PURCHASES	D	N	38	A		2130
V2025	DELUXE FRAME	M	N	00	9		3045.4
V2100	SPHERE, SINGLE VISION, PLANO TO PLUS OR MINUS 4.00, PER LENS	C	N	38	A		
V2101	SPHERE, SINGLE VISION, PLUS OR MINUS 4.12 TO PLUS OR MINUS 7.00D, PER LENS	C	N	38	A		
V2102	SPHERE, SINGLE VISION, PLUS OR MINUS 7.12 TO PLUS OR MINUS 20.00D, PER LENS	C	N	38	A		
V2103	SPHEROCYLINDER, SINGLE VISION, PLANO TO PLUS OR MINUS 4.00D SPHERE, .12 TO 2.00D CYLINDER, PER LENS	C	N	38	A		
V2104	SPHEROCYLINDER, SINGLE VISION, PLANO TO PLUS OR MINUS 4.00D SPHERE, 2.12 TO 4.00D CYLINDER, PER LENS	C	N	38	A		
V2105	SPHEROCYLINDER, SINGLE VISION, PLANO TO PLUS OR MINUS 4.00D SPHERE, 4.25 TO 6.00D CYLINDER, PER LENS	C	N	38	A		
V2106	SPHEROCYLINDER, SINGLE VISION, PLANO TO PLUS OR MINUS 4.00D SPHERE, OVER 6.00D CYLINDER, PER LENS	C	N	38	A		
V2107	SPHEROCYLINDER, SINGLE VISION, PLUS OR MINUS 4.25 TO PLUS OR MINUS 7.00 SPHERE,.12 TO 2.00D CYLINDER, PER LENS	C	N	38	A		
V2108	SPHEROCYLINDER, SINGLE VISION, PLUS OR MINUS 4.25D TO PLUS OR MINUS 7.00D SPHERE, 2.12 TO 4.00D CYLINDER, PER LENS	C	N	38	A		
V2109	SPHEROCYLINDER, SINGLE VISION, PLUS OR MINUS 4.25 TO PLUS OR MINUS 7.00D SPHERE, 4.25 TO 6.00D CYLINDER, PER LENS	C	N	38	A		
V2110	SPHEROCYLINDER, SINGLE VISION, PLUS OR MINUS 4.25 TO 7.00D SPHERE, OVER 6.00D CYLINDER, PER LENS	C	N	38	A		
V2111	SPHEROCYLINDER, SINGLE VISION, PLUS OR MINUS 7.25 TO PLUS OR MINUS 12.00D SPHERE, .25 TO 2.25D CYLINDER, PER LENS	C	N	38	A		
V2112	SPHEROCYLINDER, SINGLE VISION, PLUS OR MINUS 7.25 TO PLUS OR MINUS 12.00D SPHERE, 2.25D TO 4.00D CYLINDER, PER LENS	C	N	38	A		
V2113	SPHEROCYLINDER, SINGLE VISION, PLUS OR MINUS 7.25 TO PLUS OR MINUS 12.00D SPHERE, 4.25 TO 6.00D CYLINDER, PER LENS	C	N	38	A		
V2114	SPHEROCYLINDER, SINGLE VISION, SPHERE OVER PLUS OR MINUS 12.00D, PER LENS	C	N	38	A		
V2115	LENTICULAR, (MYODISC), PER LENS, SINGLE VISION	C	N	38	A		
V2118	ANISEIKONIC LENS, SINGLE VISION	C	N	38	A		
V2121	LENTICULAR LENS, PER LENS, SINGLE	D	N	38	A		2130.B
V2199	NOT OTHERWISE CLASSIFIED, SINGLE VISION LENS	C	N	46	A		
V2200	SPHERE, BIFOCAL, PLANO TO PLUS OR MINUS 4.00D, PER LENS	C	N	38	A		
V2201	SPHERE, BIFOCAL, PLUS OR MINUS 4.12 TO PLUS OR MINUS 7.00D, PER LENS	C	N	38	A		
V2202	SPHERE, BIFOCAL, PLUS OR MINUS 7.12 TO PLUS OR MINUS 20.00D, PER LENS	C	N	38	A		

HCPCS Code	Statute	Lab Cert	X-Ref	ASC Pay Grp	ASC Pay Group Eff. Date	Proc Notes	BETOS	TOS	Anest	Code Add Date	Code Effective Date	Code Term Date
T5999							Z2	9	0	20040101	20040101	
V2020							D1F	Q	0	19850101	20031001	
V2025							D1F	Q	0	19920101	20031001	
V2100							D1F	Q	0	19850101	20031001	
V2101							D1F	Q	0	19850101	20031001	
V2102							D1F	Q	0	19850101	20031001	
V2103							D1F	Q	0	19850101	20031001	
V2104							D1F	Q	0	19850101	20031001	
V2105							D1F	Q	0	19850101	20031001	
V2106							D1F	Q	0	19850101	20031001	
V2107							D1F	Q	0	19850101	20031001	
V2108							D1F	Q	0	19850101	20031001	
V2109							D1F	Q	0	19850101	20031001	
V2110							D1F	Q	0	19850101	20031001	
V2111							D1F	Q	0	19850101	20031001	
V2112							D1F	Q	0	19850101	20031001	
V2113							D1F	Q	0	19850101	20031001	
V2114							D1F	Q	0	19850101	20031001	
V2115							D1F	Q	0	19850101	20031001	
V2118							D1F	Q	0	19850101	20031001	
V2121							D1F	Q	0	20040101	20040101	
V2199							D1F	Q	0	19850101	20031001	
V2200							D1F	Q	0	19850101	20031001	
V2201							D1F	Q	0	19850101	20031001	
V2202							D1F	Q	0	19850101	20031001	

HCPCS Code	Long Description	Coverage	Action	PI	MPI	CIM	MCM
V2203	SPHEROCYLINDER, BIFOCAL, PLANO TO PLUS OR MINUS 4.00D SPHERE, .12 TO 2.00D CYLINDER, PER LENS	C	N	38	A		
V2204	SPHEROCYLINDER, BIFOCAL, PLANO TO PLUS OR MINUS 4.00D SPHERE, 2.12 TO 4.00D CYLINDER, PER LENS	C	N	38	A		
V2205	SPHEROCYLINDER, BIFOCAL, PLANO TO PLUS OR MINUS 4.00D SPHERE, 4.25 TO 6.00D CYLINDER, PER LENS	C	N	38	A		
V2206	SPHEROCYLINDER, BIFOCAL, PLANO TO PLUS OR MINUS 4.00D SPHERE, OVER 6.00D CYLINDER, PER LENS	C	N	38	A		
V2207	SPHEROCYLINDER, BIFOCAL, PLUS OR MINUS 4.25 TO PLUS OR MINUS 7.00D SPHERE,.12 TO 2.00D CYLINDER, PER LENS	C	N	38	A		
V2208	SPHEROCYLINDER, BIFOCAL, PLUS OR MINUS 4.25 TO PLUS OR MINUS 7.00D SPHERE, 2.12 TO 4.00D CYLINDER, PER LENS	C	N	38	A		
V2209	SPHEROCYLINDER, BIFOCAL, PLUS OR MINUS 4.25 TO PLUS OR MINUS 7.00D SPHERE, 4.25 TO 6.00D CYLINDER, PER LENS	C	N	38	A		
V2210	SPHEROCYLINDER, BIFOCAL, PLUS OR MINUS 4.25 TO PLUS OR MINUS 7.00D SPHERE, OVER 6.00D CYLINDER,PER LENS	C	N	38	A		
V2211	SPHEROCYLINDER, BIFOCAL, PLUS OR MINUS 7.25 TO PLUS OR MINUS 12.00D SPHERE, .25 TO 2.25D CYLINDER, PER LENS	C	N	38	A		
V2212	SPHEROCYLINDER, BIFOCAL, PLUS OR MINUS 7.25 TO PLUS OR MINUS 12.00D SPHERE, 2.25 TO 4.00D CYLINDER, PER LENS	C	N	38	A		
V2213	SPHEROCYLINDER, BIFOCAL, PLUS OR MINUS 7.25 TO PLUS OR MINUS 12.00D SPHERE, 4.25 TO 6.00D CYLINDER, PER LENS	C	N	38	A		
V2214	SPHEROCYLINDER, BIFOCAL, SPHERE OVER PLUS OR MINUS 12.00D, PER LENS	C	N	38	A		
V2215	LENTICULAR (MYODISC), PER LENS, BIFOCAL	C	N	38	A		
V2218	ANISEIKONIC, PER LENS, BIFOCAL	C	N	38	A		
V2219	BIFOCAL SEG WIDTH OVER 28MM	C	N	38	A		
V2220	BIFOCAL ADD OVER 3.25D	C	N	38	A		
V2221	LENTICULAR LENS, PER LENS, BIFOCAL	D	N	38	A		2130.B
V2299	SPECIALTY BIFOCAL (BY REPORT)	C	N	46	A		
V2300	SPHERE, TRIFOCAL, PLANO TO PLUS OR MINUS 4.00D, PER LENS	C	N	38	A		
V2301	SPHERE, TRIFOCAL, PLUS OR MINUS 4.12 TO PLUS OR MINUS 7.00D, PER LENS	C	N	38	A		
V2302	SPHERE, TRIFOCAL, PLUS OR MINUS 7.12 TO PLUS OR MINUS 20.00, PER LENS	C	N	38	A		
V2303	SPHEROCYLINDER, TRIFOCAL, PLANO TO PLUS OR MINUS 4.00D SPHERE, .12-2.00D CYLINDER, PER LENS	C	N	38	A		
V2304	SPHEROCYLINDER, TRIFOCAL, PLANO TO PLUS OR MINUS 4.00D SPHERE, 2.25-4.00D CYLINDER, PER LENS	C	N	38	A		
V2305	SPHEROCYLINDER, TRIFOCAL, PLANO TO PLUS OR MINUS 4.00D SPHERE, 4.25 TO 6.00 CYLINDER, PER LENS	C	N	38	A		
V2306	SPHEROCYLINDER, TRIFOCAL, PLANO TO PLUS OR MINUS 4.00D SPHERE, OVER 6.00D CYLINDER, PER LENS	C	N	38	A		
V2307	SPHEROCYLINDER, TRIFOCAL, PLUS OR MINUS 4.25 TO PLUS OR MINUS 7.00D SPHERE, .12 TO 2.00D CYLINDER, PER LENS	C	N	38	A		
V2308	SPHEROCYLINDER, TRIFOCAL, PLUS OR MINUS 4.25 TO PLUS OR MINUS 7.00D SPHERE, 2.12 TO 4.00D CYLINDER, PER LENS	C	N	38	A		
V2309	SPHEROCYLINDER, TRIFOCAL, PLUS OR MINUS 4.25 TO PLUS OR MINUS 7.00D SPHERE, 4.25 TO 6.00D CYLINDER, PER LENS	C	N	38	A		

HCPCS Code	Statute	Lab Cert	X-Ref	ASC Pay Grp	ASC Pay Group Eff. Date	Proc Notes	BETOS	TOS	Anest	Code Add Date	Code Effective Date	Code Term Date
V2203							D1F	Q	0	19850101	20031001	
V2204							D1F	Q	0	19850101	20031001	
V2205							D1F	Q	0	19850101	20031001	
V2206							D1F	Q	0	19850101	20031001	
V2207							D1F	Q	0	19850101	20031001	
V2208							D1F	Q	0	19850101	20031001	
V2209							D1F	Q	0	19850101	20031001	
V2210							D1F	Q	0	19850101	20031001	
V2211							D1F	Q	0	19850101	20031001	
V2212							D1F	Q	0	19850101	20031001	
V2213							D1F	Q	0	19850101	20031001	
V2214							D1F	Q	0	19850101	20031001	
V2215							D1F	Q	0	19850101	20031001	
V2218							D1F	Q	0	19850101	20031001	
V2219							D1F	Q	0	19850101	20031001	
V2220							D1F	Q	0	19850101	20031001	
V2221							BETOS	Q	0	20040101	20040101	
V2299							D1F	Q	0	19850101	20031001	
V2300							D1F	Q	0	19850101	20031001	
V2301							D1F	Q	0	19850101	20031001	
V2302							D1F	Q	0	19850101	20031001	
V2303							D1F	Q	0	19850101	20031001	
V2304							D1F	Q	0	19850101	20031001	
V2305							D1F	Q	0	19850101	20031001	
V2306							D1F	Q	0	19850101	20031001	
V2307							D1F	Q	0	19850101	20031001	
V2308							D1F	Q	0	19850101	20031001	
V2309							D1F	Q	0	19850101	20031001	

HCPCS Code	Long Description	Coverage	Action	PI	MPI	CIM	MCM
V2310	SPHEROCYLINDER, TRIFOCAL, PLUS OR MINUS 4.25 TO PLUS OR MINUS 7.00D SPHERE, OVER 6.00D CYLINDER, PER LENS	C	N	38	A		
V2311	SPHEROCYLINDER, TRIFOCAL, PLUS OR MINUS 7.25 TO PLUS OR MINUS 12.00D SPHERE,.25 TO 2.25D CYLINDER, PER LENS	C	N	38	A		
V2312	SPHEROCYLINDER, TRIFOCAL, PLUS OR MINUS 7.25 TO PLUS OR MINUS 12.00D SPHERE, 2.25 TO 4.00D CYLINDER, PER LENS	C	N	38	A		
V2313	SPHEROCYLINDER, TRIFOCAL, PLUS OR MINUS 7.25 TO PLUS OR MINUS 12.00D SPHERE, 4.25 TO 6.00D CYLINDER, PER LENS	C	N	38	A		
V2314	SPHEROCYLINDER, TRIFOCAL, SPHERE OVER PLUS OR MINUS 12 .00D, PER LENS	C	N	38	A		
V2315	LENTICULAR, (MYODISC), PER LENS, TRIFOCAL	C	N	38	A		
V2318	ANISEIKONIC LENS, TRIFOCAL	C	N	38	A		
V2319	TRIFOCAL SEG WIDTH OVER 28 MM	C	N	38	A		
V2320	TRIFOCAL ADD OVER 3.25D	C	N	38	A		
V2321	LENTICULAR LENS, PER LENS, TRIFOCAL	D	N	38	A		2130.B
V2399	SPECIALTY TRIFOCAL (BY REPORT)	C	N	46	A		
V2410	VARIABLE ASPHERICITY LENS, SINGLE VISION, FULL FIELD, GLASS OR PLASTIC, PER LENS	C	N	38	A		
V2430	VARIABLE ASPHERICITY LENS, BIFOCAL, FULL FIELD, GLASS OR PLASTIC, PER LENS	C	N	38	A		
V2499	VARIABLE SPHERICITY LENS, OTHER TYPE	C	N	46	A		
V2500	CONTACT LENS, PMMA, SPHERICAL, PER LENS	C	N	38	A		
V2501	CONTACT LENS, PMMA, TORIC OR PRISM BALLAST, PER LENS	C	N	38	A		
V2502	CONTACT LENS PMMA, BIFOCAL, PER LENS	C	N	38	A		
V2503	CONTACT LENS, PMMA, COLOR VISION DEFICIENCY, PER LENS	C	N	38	A		
V2510	CONTACT LENS, GAS PERMEABLE, SPHERICAL, PER LENS	C	N	38	A		
V2511	CONTACT LENS, GAS PERMEABLE, TORIC, PRISM BALLAST, PER LENS	C	N	38	A		
V2512	CONTACT LENS, GAS PERMEABLE, BIFOCAL, PER LENS	C	N	38	A		
V2513	CONTACT LENS, GAS PERMEABLE, EXTENDED WEAR, PER LENS	C	N	38	A		
V2520	CONTACT LENS, HYDROPHILIC, SPHERICAL, PER LENS	D	N	38	A	45-7, 65-1	
V2521	CONTACT LENS, HYDROPHILIC, TORIC, OR PRISM BALLAST, PER LENS	D	N	38	A	45-7, 65-1	
V2522	CONTACT LENS, HYDROPHILLIC, BIFOCAL, PER LENS	D	N	38	A	45-7, 65-1	
V2523	CONTACT LENS, HYDROPHILIC, EXTENDED WEAR, PER LENS	D	N	38	A	45-7, 65-1	
V2530	CONTACT LENS, SCLERAL, GAS IMPERMEABLE, PER LENS (FOR CONTACT LENS MODIFICATION, SEE 92325)	C	N	38	A		
V2531	CONTACT LENS, SCLERAL, GAS PERMEABLE, PER LENS (FOR CONTACT LENS MODIFICATION, SEE 92325)	D	N	38	A	65-3	
V2599	CONTACT LENS, OTHER TYPE	C	N	46	A		
V2600	HAND HELD LOW VISION AIDS AND OTHER NONSPECTACLE MOUNTED AIDS	C	N	46	A		
V2610	SINGLE LENS SPECTACLE MOUNTED LOW VISION AIDS	C	N	46	A		
V2615	TELESCOPIC AND OTHER COMPOUND LENS SYSTEM, INCLUDING DISTANCE VISION TELESCOPIC, NEAR VISION TELESCOPES AND COMPOUND MICROSCOPIC LENS SYSTEM	C	N	46	A		
V2623	PROSTHETIC EYE, PLASTIC, CUSTOM	D	N	38	A		2133
V2624	POLISHING/RESURFACING OF OCULAR PROSTHESIS	C	N	38	A		

HCPCS Code	Statute	Lab Cert	X-Ref	ASC Pay Grp	ASC Pay Group Eff. Date	Proc Notes	BETOS	TOS	Anest	Code Add Date	Code Effective Date	Code Term Date
V2310							D1F	Q	0	19850101	20031001	
V2311							D1F	Q	0	19850101	20031001	
V2312							D1F	Q	0	19850101	20031001	
V2313							D1F	Q	0	19850101	20031001	
V2314							D1F	Q	0	19850101	20031001	
V2315							D1F	Q	0	19850101	20031001	
V2318							D1F	Q	0	19850101	20031001	
V2319							D1F	Q	0	19850101	20031001	
V2320							D1F	Q	0	19850101	20031001	
V2321							D1F	Q	0	20040101	20040101	
V2399							D1F	Q	0	19850101	20031001	
V2410							D1F	Q	0	19840101	20031001	
V2430							D1F	Q	0	19840101	20031001	
V2499							D1F	Q	0	19840101	20031001	
V2500							D1F	Q	0	19850101	20031001	
V2501							D1F	Q	0	19850101	20031001	
V2502							D1F	Q	0	19850101	20031001	
V2503							D1F	Q	0	19850101	20031001	
V2510							D1F	Q	0	19850101	20031001	
V2511							D1F	Q	0	19850101	20031001	
V2512							D1F	Q	0	19850101	20031001	
V2513							D1F	Q	0	19850101	20031001	
V2520							D1F	Q	0	19840101	20031001	
V2521							D1F	Q	0	19850101	20031001	
V2522							D1F	Q	0	19850101	20031001	
V2523							D1F	Q	0	19850101	20031001	
V2530							D1F	Q	0	19850101	20031001	
V2531							D1F	Q	0	19960101	20031001	
V2599							D1F	Q	0	19850101	20031001	
V2600							D1F	Q	0	19850101	20031001	
V2610							D1F	Q	0	19850101	20031001	
V2615							D1F	Q	0	19850101	20031001	
V2623							D1F	P	0	19850101	20031001	
V2624							D1F	P	0	19930101	20031001	

HCPCS Code	Long Description	Coverage	Action	PI	MPI	CIM	MCM
V2625	ENLARGEMENT OF OCULAR PROSTHESIS	C	N	38	A		
V2626	REDUCTION OF OCULAR PROSTHESIS	C	N	38	A		
V2627	SCLERAL COVER SHELL	D	N	38	A	65-3	
V2628	FABRICATION AND FITTING OF OCULAR CONFORMER	C	N	38	A		
V2629	PROSTHETIC EYE, OTHER TYPE	C	N	46	A		
V2630	ANTERIOR CHAMBER INTRAOCULAR LENS	D	N	52	A		2130
V2631	IRIS SUPPORTED INTRAOCULAR LENS	D	N	52	A		2130
V2632	POSTERIOR CHAMBER INTRAOCULAR LENS	D	N	52	A		2130
V2700	BALANCE LENS, PER LENS	C	N	38	A		
V2702	DELUXE LENS FEATURE	M	N	00	9		2130B
V2710	SLAB OFF PRISM, GLASS OR PLASTIC, PER LENS	C	N	38	A		
V2715	PRISM, PER LENS	C	N	38	A		
V2718	PRESS-ON LENS, FRESNELL PRISM, PER LENS	C	N	38	A		
V2730	SPECIAL BASE CURVE, GLASS OR PLASTIC, PER LENS	C	N	38	A		
V2744	TINT, PHOTOCHROMATIC, PER LENS	D	N	38	A		2130B
V2745	ADDITION TO LENS; TINT, ANY COLOR, SOLID, GRADIENT OR EQUAL, EXCLUDES PHOTOCHROMATIC, ANY LENS MATERIAL, PER LENS	D	N	38	A		2130.B
V2750	ANTI-REFLECTIVE COATING, PER LENS	D	N	38	A		2130B
V2755	U-V LENS, PER LENS	D	N	38	A		2130B
V2756	EYE GLASS CASE	C	N	00	9		
V2760	SCRATCH RESISTANT COATING, PER LENS	C	N	38	A		
V2761	MIRROR COATING, ANY TYPE, SOLID, GRADIENT OR EQUAL, ANY LENS MATERIAL, PER LENS	D	N	38	A		2130.B
V2762	POLARIZATION, ANY LENS MATERIAL, PER LENS	D	N	38	A		2130.B
V2770	OCCLUDER LENS, PER LENS	C	N	38	A		
V2780	OVERSIZE LENS, PER LENS	C	N	38	A		
V2781	PROGRESSIVE LENS, PER LENS	C	N	00	9		
V2782	LENS, INDEX 1.54 TO 1.65 PLASTIC OR 1.60 TO 1.79 GLASS, EXCLUDES POLYCARBONATE, PER LENS	D	N	38	A		2130.B
V2783	LENS, INDEX GREATER THAN OR EQUAL TO 1.66 PLASTIC OR GREATER THAN OR EQUAL TO 1.80 GLASS, EXCLUDES POLYCARBONATE, PER LENS	D	N	38	A		2130.B
V2784	LENS, POLYCARBONATE OR EQUAL, ANY INDEX, PER LENS	D	N	38	A		2130.B
V2785	PROCESSING, PRESERVING AND TRANSPORTING CORNEAL TISSUE	C	N	46	A		
V2786	SPECIALTY OCCUPATIONAL MULTIFOCAL LENS, PER LENS	D	N	38	A		2130.B
V2787	ASTIGMATISM CORRECTING FUNCTION OF INTRAOCULAR LENS	S	N	00	9		
V2788	PRESBYOPIA CORRECTING FUNCTION OF INTRAOCULAR LENS	S	N	00	9		
V2790	AMNIOTIC MEMBRANE FOR SURGICAL RECONSTRUCTION, PER PROCEDURE	C	N	57	A		
V2797	VISION SUPPLY, ACCESSORY AND/OR SERVICE COMPONENT OF ANOTHER HCPCS VISION CODE	C	N	00	9		
V2799	VISION SERVICE, MISCELLANEOUS	C	N	46	A		
V5008	HEARING SCREENING	M	N	00	9		2320
V5010	ASSESSMENT FOR HEARING AID	S	N	00	9		
V5011	FITTING/ORIENTATION/CHECKING OF HEARING AID	S	N	00	9		
V5014	REPAIR/MODIFICATION OF A HEARING AID	S	N	00	9		

HCPCS Code	Statute	Lab Cert	X-Ref	ASC Pay Grp	ASC Pay Group Eff. Date	Proc Notes	BETOS	TOS	Anest	Code Add Date	Code Effective Date	Code Term Date
V2625							D1F	P	0	19930101	20031001	
V2626							D1F	P	0	19930101	20031001	
V2627							D1F	P	0	19930101	20031001	
V2628							D1F	P	0	19930101	20031001	
V2629							D1F	P	0	19850101	20031001	
V2630							D1F	Q	0	19850101	20031001	
V2631							D1F	Q	0	19850101	20031001	
V2632							D1F	Q	0	19850101	20031001	
V2700							D1F	Q	0	19850101	20031001	
V2702							D1F	Q	0	20050101	20050101	
V2710							D1F	Q	0	19850101	20031001	
V2715							D1F	Q	0	19850101	20031001	
V2718							D1F	Q	0	19850101	20031001	
V2730							D1F	Q	0	19850101	20031001	
V2744							D1F	Q	0	19850101	20031001	
V2745							D1F	Q	0	20040101	20050101	
V2750							D1F	Q	0	19850101	20031001	
V2755							D1F	Q	0	19850101	20031001	
V2756							Z2	Q	0	20040101	20070101	
V2760							D1F	Q	0	19850101	20031001	
V2761							D1F	Q	0	20040101	20040101	
V2762							D1F	Q	0	20040101	20040101	
V2770							D1F	Q	0	19850101	20031001	
V2780							D1F	Q	0	19850101	20031001	
V2781							D1F	Q	0	19960101	20031001	
V2782							D1F	Q	0	20040101	20040101	
V2783							D1F	Q	0	20040101	20040101	
V2784							D1F	Q	0	20040101	20040101	
V2785				YY	20080101		D1F	Q	0	19900101	20031001	
V2786							D1F	Q	0	20040101	20040101	
V2787	1862(a)(7)						Z2	Q	0	20080101	20080101	
V2788	1862(a)(7)						Z2	Q	0	20060101	20060101	
V2790							Z2	Q	0	20010101	20031001	
V2797							D1F	Q	0	20040101	20040101	
V2799							D1F	Q	0	19850101	20031001	
V5008							O1F	K	0	19900101	19950101	
V5010	1862A7						O1F	K	0	19840101	19950101	
V5011	1862A7						O1F	K	0	19900101	19950101	
V5014	1862A7						O1F	K	0	19900101	19950101	

HCPCS Code	Long Description	Coverage	Action	PI	MPI	CIM	MCM
V5020	CONFORMITY EVALUATION	S	N	00	9		
V5030	HEARING AID, MONAURAL, BODY WORN, AIR CONDUCTION	S	N	00	9		
V5040	HEARING AID, MONAURAL, BODY WORN, BONE CONDUCTION	S	N	00	9		
V5050	HEARING AID, MONAURAL, IN THE EAR	S	N	00	9		
V5060	HEARING AID, MONAURAL, BEHIND THE EAR	S	N	00	9		
V5070	GLASSES, AIR CONDUCTION	S	N	00	9		
V5080	GLASSES, BONE CONDUCTION	S	N	00	9		
V5090	DISPENSING FEE, UNSPECIFIED HEARING AID	S	N	00	9		
V5095	SEMI-IMPLANTABLE MIDDLE EAR HEARING PROSTHESIS	S	N	00	9		
V5100	HEARING AID, BILATERAL, BODY WORN	S	N	00	9		
V5110	DISPENSING FEE, BILATERAL	S	N	00	9		
V5120	BINAURAL, BODY	S	N	00	9		
V5130	BINAURAL, IN THE EAR	S	N	00	9		
V5140	BINAURAL, BEHIND THE EAR	S	N	00	9		
V5150	BINAURAL, GLASSES	S	N	00	9		
V5160	DISPENSING FEE, BINAURAL	S	N	00	9		
V5170	HEARING AID, CROS, IN THE EAR	S	N	00	9		
V5180	HEARING AID, CROS, BEHIND THE EAR	S	N	00	9		
V5190	HEARING AID, CROS, GLASSES	S	N	00	9		
V5200	DISPENSING FEE, CROS	S	N	00	9		
V5210	HEARING AID, BICROS, IN THE EAR	S	N	00	9		
V5220	HEARING AID, BICROS, BEHIND THE EAR	S	N	00	9		
V5230	HEARING AID, BICROS, GLASSES	S	N	00	9		
V5240	DISPENSING FEE, BICROS	S	N	00	9		
V5241	DISPENSING FEE, MONAURAL HEARING AID, ANY TYPE	S	N	00	9		
V5242	HEARING AID, ANALOG, MONAURAL, CIC (COMPLETELY IN THE EAR CANAL)	S	N	00	9		
V5243	HEARING AID, ANALOG, MONAURAL, ITC (IN THE CANAL)	S	N	00	9		
V5244	HEARING AID, DIGITALLY PROGRAMMABLE ANALOG, MONAURAL, CIC	S	N	00	9		
V5245	HEARING AID, DIGITALLY PROGRAMMABLE, ANALOG, MONAURAL, ITC	S	N	00	9		
V5246	HEARING AID, DIGITALLY PROGRAMMABLE ANALOG, MONAURAL, ITE (IN THE EAR)	S	N	00	9		
V5247	HEARING AID, DIGITALLY PROGRAMMABLE ANALOG, MONAURAL, BTE (BEHIND THE EAR)	S	N	00	9		
V5248	HEARING AID, ANALOG, BINAURAL, CIC	S	N	00	9		
V5249	HEARING AID, ANALOG, BINAURAL, ITC	S	N	00	9		
V5250	HEARING AID, DIGITALLY PROGRAMMABLE ANALOG, BINAURAL, CIC	S	N	00	9		
V5251	HEARING AID, DIGITALLY PROGRAMMABLE ANALOG, BINAURAL, ITC	S	N	00	9		
V5252	HEARING AID, DIGITALLY PROGRAMMABLE, BINAURAL, ITE	S	N	00	9		
V5253	HEARING AID, DIGITALLY PROGRAMMABLE, BINAURAL, BTE	S	N	00	9		
V5254	HEARING AID, DIGITAL, MONAURAL, CIC	S	N	00	9		
V5255	HEARING AID, DIGITAL, MONAURAL, ITC	S	N	00	9		
V5256	HEARING AID, DIGITAL, MONAURAL, ITE	S	N	00	9		
V5257	HEARING AID, DIGITAL, MONAURAL, BTE	S	N	00	9		
V5258	HEARING AID, DIGITAL, BINAURAL, CIC	S	N	00	9		

HCPCS Code	Statute	Lab Cert	X-Ref	ASC Pay Grp	ASC Pay Group Eff. Date	Proc Notes	BETOS	TOS	Anest	Code Add Date	Code Effective Date	Code Term Date
V5020	1862A7						O1F	K	0	19840101	19950101	
V5030	1862A7						O1F	K	0	19860101	19950101	
V5040	1862A7						O1F	K	0	19860101	19950101	
V5050	1862A7						O1F	K	0	19820101	20010101	
V5060	1862A7						O1F	K	0	19820101	19950101	
V5070	1862A7						O1F	K	0	19820101	19950101	
V5080	1862A7						O1F	K	0	19820101	19950101	
V5090	1862A7						O1F	K	0	19820101	19950101	
V5095	1862A7						O1F	K	0	20030101	20030101	
V5100	1862A7						O1F	K	0	19820101	19950101	
V5110	1862A7						O1F	K	0	19820101	19950101	
V5120	1862A7						O1F	K	0	19820101	19950101	
V5130	1862A7						O1F	K	0	19820101	19950101	
V5140	1862A7						O1F	K	0	19820101	19950101	
V5150	1862A7						O1F	K	0	19820101	19950101	
V5160	1862A7						O1F	K	0	19820101	19950101	
V5170	1862A7						O1F	K	0	19820101	19950101	
V5180	1862A7						O1F	K	0	19820101	19950101	
V5190	1862A7						O1F	K	0	19820101	19950101	
V5200	1862A7						O1F	K	0	19820101	19950101	
V5210	1862A7						O1F	K	0	19820101	19950101	
V5220	1862A7						O1F	K	0	19820101	19950101	
V5230	1862A7						O1F	K	0	19820101	19950101	
V5240	1862A7						O1F	K	0	19820101	19950101	
V5241	1862A7						O1F	K	0	20020101	20020101	
V5242	1862A7						O1F	K	0	20020101	20020101	
V5243	1862A7						O1F	K	0	20020101	20020101	
V5244	1862A7						O1F	K	0	20020101	20020101	
V5245	1862A7						O1F	K	0	20020101	20020101	
V5246	1862A7						O1F	K	0	20020101	20020101	
V5247	1862A7						O1F	K	0	20020101	20020101	
V5248	1862A7						O1F	K	0	20020101	20020101	
V5249	1862A7						O1F	K	0	20020101	20020101	
V5250	1862A7						O1F	K	0	20020101	20020101	
V5251	1862A7						O1F	K	0	20020101	20020101	
V5252	1862A7						O1F	K	0	20020101	20020101	
V5253	1862A7						O1F	K	0	20020101	20020101	
V5254	1862A7						O1F	K	0	20020101	20020101	
V5255	1862A7						O1F	K	0	20020101	20020101	
V5256	1862A7						O1F	K	0	20020101	20020101	
V5257	1862A7						O1F	K	0	20020101	20020101	
V5258	1862A7						O1F	K	0	20020101	20020101	

HCPCS Code	Long Description	Coverage	Action	PI	MPI	CIM	MCM
V5259	HEARING AID, DIGITAL, BINAURAL, ITC	S	N	00	9		
V5260	HEARING AID, DIGITAL, BINAURAL, ITE	S	N	00	9		
V5261	HEARING AID, DIGITAL, BINAURAL, BTE	S	N	00	9		
V5262	HEARING AID, DISPOSABLE, ANY TYPE, MONAURAL	S	N	00	9		
V5263	HEARING AID, DISPOSABLE, ANY TYPE, BINAURAL	S	N	00	9		
V5264	EAR MOLD/INSERT, NOT DISPOSABLE, ANY TYPE	S	N	00	9		
V5265	EAR MOLD/INSERT, DISPOSABLE, ANY TYPE	S	N	00	9		
V5266	BATTERY FOR USE IN HEARING DEVICE	S	N	00	9		
V5267	HEARING AID SUPPLIES / ACCESSORIES	S	N	00	9		
V5268	ASSISTIVE LISTENING DEVICE, TELEPHONE AMPLIFIER, ANY TYPE	S	N	00	9		
V5269	ASSISTIVE LISTENING DEVICE, ALERTING, ANY TYPE	S	N	00	9		
V5270	ASSISTIVE LISTENING DEVICE, TELEVISION AMPLIFIER, ANY TYPE	S	N	00	9		
V5271	ASSISTIVE LISTENING DEVICE, TELEVISION CAPTION DECODER						
V5272	ASSISTIVE LISTENING DEVICE, TDD	S	N	00	9		
V5273	ASSISTIVE LISTENING DEVICE, FOR USE WITH COCHLEAR IMPLANT	S	N	00	9		
V5274	ASSISTIVE LISTENING DEVICE, NOT OTHERWISE SPECIFIED	S	N	00	9		
V5275	EAR IMPRESSION, EACH	S	N	00	9		
V5298	HEARING AID, NOT OTHERWISE CLASSIFIED	S	N	00	9		
V5299	HEARING SERVICE, MISCELLANEOUS	D	N	13	A		2320
V5336	REPAIR/MODIFICATION OF AUGMENTATIVE COMMUNICATIVE SYSTEM OR DEVICE (EXCLUDES ADAPTIVE HEARING AID)	S	N	00	9		
V5362	SPEECH SCREENING	S	N	00	9		
V5363	LANGUAGE SCREENING	S	N	00	9		
V5364	DYSPHAGIA SCREENING	S	N	00	9		

HCPCS Code	Statute	Lab Cert	X-Ref	ASC Pay Grp	ASC Pay Group Eff. Date	Proc Notes	BETOS	TOS	Anest	Code Add Date	Code Effective Date	Code Term Date
V5259	1862A7						O1F	K	0	20020101	20020101	
V5260	1862A7						O1F	K	0	20020101	20020101	
V5261	1862A7						O1F	K	0	20020101	20020101	
V5262	1862A7						O1F	K	0	20020101	20020101	
V5263	1862A7						O1F	K	0	20020101	20020101	
V5264	1862A7						O1F	K	0	20020101	20020101	
V5265	1862A7						O1F	K	0	20020101	20020101	
V5266	1862A7						O1F	K	0	20020101	20020101	
V5267	1862A7						O1F	K	0	20020101	20020101	
V5268	1862A7						O1F	K	0	20020101	20020101	
V5269	1862A7						O1F	K	0	20020101	20020101	
V5270	1862A7						O1F	K	0	20020101	20020101	
V5272	1862A7						O1F	K	0	20020101	20020101	
V5273	1862A7						O1F	K	0	20020101	20020101	
V5274	1862A7						O1F	K	0	20020101	20020101	
V5275	1862A7						O1F	K	0	20020101	20020101	
V5298	1862A7						O1F	K	0	20030101	20030101	
V5299							O1F	K	0	19820101	19950101	
V5336	1862A7						O1F	1	0	19900101	19910101	
V5362	1862(a)(7)						O1F	1,W	0	19900101	20040101	
V5363	1862(a)(7)						O1F	1,W	0	19900101	20040101	
V5364	1862(a)(7)						O1F	1,W	0	19900101	20040101	

HCPCS Code	Long Description	Coverage	Action	PI	MPI	CIM	MCM

2010 Table of Drugs

IA - Intra-arterial administration

IM - Intramuscular administration

INH - Administration by inhaled solution

IT - Intrathecal

IV - Intravenous administration

SC - Subcutaneous administration

VAR - Various routes of administration

OTH - Other routes of administration

ORAL - Administered orally

Intravenous administration includes all methods, such as gravity infusion, injections, and timed pushes. The 'VAR' posting denotes various routes of administration and is used for drugs that are commonly administered into joints, cavities, tissues, or topical applications, in addition to other parenteral administrations. Listings posted with 'OTH' indicate other administration methods, such as suppositories or catheter injections.

A

Drug	Dosage	Route	Code
Abarelix	10 mg		J0128
Abatacept	10 mg		J0129
Abbokinase, see Urokinase			
Abbokinase, Open Cath, see Urokinase			
Abciximab	10 mg	IV	J0130
Abelcet, see Amphotericin B Lipid Complex			
ABLC, see Amphotericin B			
AbobotulinumtoxintypeA	5 units		J0586
Acetazolamide sodium	up to 500 mg	IM, IV	J1120
Acetylcysteine, injection	100 mg		J0132
Acetylcysteine, unit dose form	per gram	INH	J7604,J7608
Achromycin, see Tetracycline			
ACTH, see Corticotropin			
Acthar, see Corticotropin			
Actimmune, see Interferon gamma 1-B			
Activase, see Alteplase recombinant			
Acyclovir	5 mg		J0133
Adalimumab	20 mg		J0135
Adenocard, see Adenosine			
Adenoscan, see Adenosine			
Adenosine	6 mg	IV	J0150
Adenosine	30 mg	IV	J0152
Adrenalin Chloride, see Adrenalin, epinephrine			
Adrenalin, epinephrine	up to 1 ml ampule	SC, IM	J0170

Adriamycin PFS, see Doxorubicin HCl			
Adriamycin RDF, see Doxorubicin HCl			
Adrucil, see Fluorouracil			
Agalsidase beta	1 mg		J0180
Aggrastat, see Tirofiban hydrochloride			
A-hydroCort, see Hydrocortisone sodium phosphate			
Akineton, see Biperiden			
Alatrofloxacin mesylate, injection	100 mg	IV	J0200
Albuterol	0.5 mg	INH	J7620
Albuterol, concentrated form	1 mg	INH	J7610, J7611
Albuterol, unit dose form	1 mg	INH	J7609, J7613
Aldesleukin	per single use vial	IM, IV	J9015
Aldomet, see Methyldopate HCl			
Alefacept	0.5 mg		J0215
Alemtuzumab	10 mg		J9010
Alferon N, see Interferon alfa-n3			
Alglucerase	per 10 units	IV	J0205
Alglucosidase	10 mg		J0220
Alkaban-AQ, see Vinblastine sulfate			
Alkeran, see Melphalan, oral			
Alpha 1-proteinase inhibitor, human	10 mg	IV	J0256
Alphanate			J7186
Alprostadil, injection injection	1.25 mcg	OTH	J0270
Alprostadil, urethral suppository		OTH	J0275
Alteplase recombinant	1 mg	IV	J2997
Alupent, see Metaproterenol sulfate or Metaproterenol, compounded			
Amcort, see Triamcinolone diacetate			
A-methaPred, see Methylprednisolone sodium succinate			
Amgen, see Interferon alphacon-1			
Amifostine	500 mg	IV	J0207
Amikacin sulfate	100 mg		J0278
Aminolevalinic acid Hcl	unit dose (354 mg)	OTH	J7308
Aminophylline/Aminophyllin	up to 250 mg	IV	J0280
Amiodarone HCl	30 mg	IV	J0282
Amitriptyline HCl	up to 20 mg	IM	J1320
Amobarbital	up to 125 mg	IM, IV	J0300
Amphocin, see Amphotericin B			
Amphotericin B	50 mg	IV	J0285
Amphotericin B, lipid complex	10 mg	IV	J0287-J0289
Ampicillin sodium	up to 500 mg	IM, IV	J0290
Ampicillin sodium/sulbactam sodium	per 1.5 gm	IM, IV	J0295
Amygdalin, see Laetrile, Amygdalin, vitamin B-17			
Amytal, see Amobarbital			
Anabolin LA 100, see Nandrolone decanoate			
Anadulafungin	1 mg		J0348
Ancef, see Cefazolin sodium			
Andrest 90-4, see Testosterone enanthate and estradiol valerate			

Andro-Cyp, see Testosterone cypionate
Andro-Cyp 200, see Testosterone cypionate
Andro L.A. 200, see Testosterone enanthate
Andro-Estro 90-4, see Testosterone enanthate and estradiol valerate
Andro/Fem, see Testosterone cypionate and estradiol cypionate
Androgyn L.A., see Testosterone enanthate and estradiol valerate
Androlone-50, see Nandrolone phenpropionate
Androlone-D 100, see Nandrolone decanoate
Andronaq-50, see Testosterone suspension
Andronaq-LA, see Testosterone cypionate
Andronate-200, see Testosterone cypionate
Andronate-100, see Testosterone cypionate
Andropository 100, see Testosterone enanthate
Andryl 200, see Testosterone enanthate
Anectine, see Succinylcholine chloride
Anergan 25, see Promethazine HCl
Anergan 50, see Promethazine HCl

Anistreplase	30 units	IV	J0350
Anti-Inhibitor	per IU	IV	J7198
Antispas, see Dicyclomine HCl			
Antithrombin III (human)	per IU	IV	J7197
Anzemet, see Dolasetron mesylate injection			
A.P.L., see Chorionic gonadotropin			
Apomorphine Hydrochloride	1 mg		J0364
Apresoline, see Hydralazine HCl			
Aprotinin	10,000 kiu		J0365
AquaMEPHYTON, see Vitamin K			
Aralen, see Chloroquine HCl			
Aramine, see Metaraminol			
Aranesp, see Darbepoetin Alfa			
Arbutamine	1 mg	IV	J0395
Arcalyst, see Rilanocept			
Aredia, see Pamidronate disodium			
Arfonad, see Trimethaphan camsylate			
Arformoterol tartrate	15 mcg		J7605
Aripiprazole	0.25 mg		J0400
Aristocort Forte, see Triamcinolone diacetate			
Aristocort Intralesional, see Triamcinolone diacetate			
Aristospan Intra-Articular, see Triamcinolone hexacetonide			
Aristospan Intralesional, see Triamcinolone hexacetonide			
Arrestin, see Trimethobenzamide HCl			
Arsenic trioxide	1 mg	IV	J9017
Asparaginase	10,000 units	IV, IM	J9020
Astramorph PF, see Morphine sulfate			
Atgam, see Lymphocyte immune globulin			
Ativan, see Lorazepam			
Atropine, concentrated form	per mg	INH	J7635
Atropine, unit dose form	per mg	INH	J7636

Atropine sulfate	0.01 mg	IV, IM, SC	J0461
Atrovent, see Ipratropium bromide			
Aurothioglucose	up to 50 mg	IM	J2910
Autologous cultured chondrocytes implant			J7330
Autoplex T, see Hemophilia clotting factors			
Avonex, see Interferon beta-1a			
Azacitidine	1 mg		J9025
Azathioprine	50 mg	ORAL	J7500
Azathioprine, parenteral	100 mg	IV	J7501
Azithromycin, dihydrate	1 gm	ORAL	Q0144
Azithromycin, injection	500 mg	IV	J0456

B

Baclofen	10 mg	IT	J0475
Baclofen for intrathecal trial	50 mcg	OTH	J0476
Bactocill, see Oxacillin sodium			
BAL in oil, see Dimercaprol			
Banflex, see Orphenadrine citrate			
Basiliximab	20 mg		J0480
BCG (Bacillus Calmette and Guérin), live	per vial instillation	IV	J9031
Beclomethasone inhalation solution, unit dose form	per mg	INH	J7622
Bena-D 10, see Diphenhydramine HCl			
Bena-D 50, see Diphenhydramine HCl			
Benadryl, see Diphenhydramine HCl			
Benahist 10, see Diphenhydramine HCl			
Benahist 50, see Diphenhydramine HCl			
Ben-Allergin-50, see Diphenhydramine HCl			
Bendamustine HCl	1 mg		J9033
Benefix, see Factor IX, recombinant			
Benoject-10, see Diphenhydramine HCl			
Benoject-50, see Diphenhydramine HCl			
Bentyl, see Dicyclomine			
Benztropine mesylate	per 1 mg	IM, IV	J0515
Berubigen, see Vitamin B-12 cyanocobalamin			
Betalin 12, see Vitamin B-12 cyanocobalamin			
Betameth, see Betamethasone sodium phosphate			
Betamethasone acetate			
& betamethasone sodium phosphate	per 3 mg	IM	J0702
Betamethasone inhalation solution, unit dose form	per mg	INH	J7624
Betamethasone sodium phosphate	per 4 mg	IM, IV	J0704
Betaseron, see Interferon beta-1b			
Bethanechol chloride	up to 5 mg	SC	J0520
Bevacizumab	0.25 mg		Q2024
	10 mg		J9035
Bicillin L-A, see Penicillin G benzathine			
Bicillin C-R 900/300, see Penicillin G procaine and penicillin G benzathine			

Bicillin C-R, see Penicillin G benzathine and penicillin G procaine
BiCNU, see Carmustine

Biperiden lactate	per 5 mg	IM, IV	J0190
Bitolterol mesylate,concentrated form	per mg	INH	J7628
Bitolterol mesylate,unit dose form	per mg	INH	J7629
Bivalirudin	1 mg		J0583

Blenoxane, see Bleomycin sulfate

Bleomycin sulfate	15 units	IM, IV, SC	J9040
Bortezomib	0.1 mg		J9041

Botox, see OnabotulinumtoxinA
Brethine, see Terbutaline sulfate or Terbutaline, compounded
Bricanyl Subcutaneous, see Terbutaline sulfate

Brompheniramine maleate	per 10 mg	IM, SC, IV	J0945

Bronkephrine, see Ethylnorepinephrine HCl
Bronkosol, see Isoetharine HCl

Budesonide inhalation solution, concentrated form	0.25 mg	INH	J7633, J7634
Budesonide inhalation solution, unit dose form	0.5 mg	INH	J7626, J7627
Buprenorphine Hydrochloride	0.1 mg		J0592
Busulfan	1 mg		J0594
Busulfan	2 mg	ORAL	J8510
Butorphanol tartrate	1 mg		J0595

C

C1 Esterase Inhibitor	10 units		J0598
Cabergoline	.25 mg	ORAL	J8515

Cafcit, see Caffeine citrate

Caffeine citrate	5 mg	IV	J0706

Caine-1, see Lidocaine Hcl
Caine-2, see Lidocaine HCl
Calcijex, see Calcitriol
Calcimar, see Calcitonin-salmon

Calcitonin-salmon	up to 400 units	SC, IM	J0630
Calcitriol	0.1 mcg	IM	J0636

Calcium Disodium Versenate, see Edetate calcium disodium

Calcium gluconate	per 10 ml	IV	J0610
Calcium glycerophosphate & calcium lactate	per 10 ml	IM, SC	J0620

Calphosan, see Calcium glycerophosphate and calcium lactate
Camptosar, see Irinotecan

Capecitabine	150 mg	ORAL	J8520
Capecitabine	500 mg	ORAL	J8521

Carbocaine with Neo-Cobefrin, see Mepivacaine
Carbocaine, see Mepivacaine

Carboplatin	50 mg	IV	J9045
Carmustine	100 mg	IV	J9050

Carnitor, see Levocarnitine
Carticel, see Autologous cultured chondrocytes

Caspofungin acetate	5 mg	IV	J0637

Cefadyl, see Cephapirin Sodium

Cefazolin sodium	500 mg	IV, IM	J0690
Cefepime hydrochloride	500 mg	IV	J0692
Cefizox, see Ceftizoxime sodium			
Cefotaxime sodium	per 1 g	IV, IM	J0698
Cefoxitin sodium	1 g	IV, IM	J0694
Ceftazidime	per 500 mg	IM, IV	J0713
Ceftizoxime sodium	per 500 mg	IV, IM	J0715
Ceftriaxone sodium	per 250 mg	IV, IM	J0696
Cefuroxime sodium, sterile	per 750 mg	IM, IV	J0697
Celestone Phosphate, see Betamethasone sodium phosphate			
Celestone Soluspan, see Betamethasone acetate			
and betamethasone sodium phosphate			
CellCept, see Mycophenolate mofetil			
Cel-U-Jec, see Betamethasone sodium phosphate			
Cenacort Forte, see Triamcinolone diacetate			
Cenacort A-40, see Triamcinolone acetonide			
Cephalothin sodium	up to 1 g	IM, IV	J1890
Cephapirin sodium	up to 1 g	IV, IM	J0710
Ceredase, see Alglucerase			
Cerezyme, see Imiglucerase			
Certolizumab pegol	1 mg		J0718
Cerubidine, see Daunorubicin HCl			
Cetuximab	10 mg		J9055
Chealamide, see Endrate ethylenediamine-tetra-acetic acid			
Chloramphenicol sodium succinate	up to 1 g	IV	J0720
Chlordiazepoxide HCl	up to 100 mg	IM, IV	J1990
Chloromycetin Sodium Succinate, see Chloramphenicol sodium succinate			
Chloroprocaine HCl	per 30 ml	VAR	J2400
Chlorpromazine HCl,	oral 10 mg	ORAL	Q0171
	25 mg	ORAL	Q0172
Chloroquine HCl	up to 250 mg	IM	J0390
Chlorothiazide sodium	per 500 mg	IV	J1205
Chlorpromazine HCl	up to 50 mg	IM, IV	J3230
Chorex-5, see Chorionic gonadotropin			
Chorex-10, see Chorionic gonadotropin			
Chorignon, see Chorionic gonadotropin			
Chorionic gonadotropin	per 1,000 USP units	IM	J0725
Choron 10, see Chorionic gonadotropin			
Cidofovir	375 mg	IV	J0740
Cilastatin sodium, imipenem	per 250 mg	IV, IM	J0743
Cimzia, see Certolizumab pegol			
Cinryze, see C1 Esterase Inhibitor			
Cipro IV, see Ciprofloxacin			
Ciprofloxacin	200 mg	IV	J0706
Cisplatin, powder or solution	per 10 mg	IV	J9060
Cisplatin	50 mg	IV	J9062
Cladribine	per mg	IV	J9065
Claforan, see Cefotaxime sodium			

Clofarabine	1 mg		J9027
Clonidine Hydrochloride	1 mg	epidural	J0735
Cobex, see Vitamin B-12 cyanocobalamin			
Codeine phosphate	per 30 mg	IM, IV, SC	J0745
Codimal-A, see Brompheniramine maleate			
Cogentin, see Benztropine mesylate			
Colchicine per	1 mg	IV	J0760
Colistimethate sodium	up to 150 mg	IM, IV	J0770
Coly-Mycin M, see Colistimethate sodium			
Compa-Z, see Prochlorperazine			
Compazine, see Prochlorperazine			
Cophene-B, see Brompheniramine maleate			
Copper contraceptive, intrauterine		OTH	J7300
Cordarone, see Amiodarone HCl			
Corgonject-5, see Chorionic gonadotropin			
Corticorelin ovine triflutate	1 mcg		J0795
Corticotropin	up to 40 units	IV, IM, SC	J0800
Cortrosyn, see Cosyntropin			
Cosmegen, see Dactinomycin			
Cosyntropin	per 0.25 mg	IM, IV	J0833, J0834
Cotranzine, see Prochlorperazine			
Cromolyn sodium, unit dose form	per 10 mg	INH	J7631, J7632
Crysticillin 300 A.S., see Penicillin G procaine			
Crysticillin 600 A.S., see Penicillin G procaine			
Cyclophosphamide	100 mg	IV	J9070
	200 mg	IV	J9080
	500 mg	IV	J9090
	1 g	IV	J9091
	2 g	IV	J9092
Cyclophosphamide, lyophilized	100 mg	IV	J9093
	200 mg	IV	J9094
	500 mg	IV	J9095
	1 g	IV	J9096
	2 g	IV	J9097
Cyclophosphamide, oral	25 mg	ORAL	J8530
Cyclosporine, oral	25 mg	ORAL	J7515
	100 mg	ORAL	J7502
Cyclosporine, parenteral	250 mg	IV	J7516
Cytarabine	100 mg	SC, IV	J9100
Cytarabine	500 mg	SC, IV	J9110
Cytarabine liposome	10 mg		J9098
Cytomegalovirus immune globulin intravenous(human)	per vial	IV	J0850
Cytosar-U, see Cytarabine			
Cytovene, see Ganciclovir sodium			
Cytoxan, see Cyclophosphamide; cyclophosphamide, lyophilized; and cyclophosphamide, oral			

D

D-5-W, infusion	1000 cc	IV	J7070
Dacarbazine	100 mg	IV	J9130
	200 mg	IV	J9140
Daclizumab	25 mg	IV	J7513
Dactinomycin	0.5 mg	IV	J9120
Dalalone, see Dexamethasone sodium phosphate			
Dalalone L.A., see Dexamethasone acetate			
Dalteparin sodium	per 2500 IU	SC	J1645
Daptomycin	1 mg		J0878
Darbepoetin Alfa	1 mcg		J0881, J0882
Daunorubicin citrate, liposomal formulation	10 mg	IV	J9151
Daunorubicin HCl	10 mg	IV	J9150
Daunoxome, see Daunorubicin citrate			
DDAVP, see Desmopressin acetate			
Decadron Phosphate, see Dexamethasone sodium phosphate			
Decadron, see Dexamethasone sodium phosphate			
Decadron-LA, see Dexamethasone acetate			
Deca-Durabolin, see Nandrolone decanoate			
Decaject, see Dexamethasone sodium phosphate			
Decaject-L.A., see Dexamethasone acetate			
Decitabine	1 mg		J0894
Decolone-50, see Nandrolone decanoate			
Decolone-100, see Nandrolone decanoate			
De-Comberol, see Testosterone cypionate and estradiol cypionate			
Deferoxamine mesylate	500 mg	IM, SC, IV	J0895
Degarelix	1 mg		J9155
Dehist, see Brompheniramine maleate			
Deladumone OB, see Testosterone enanthate and estradiol valerate			
Deladumone, see Testosterone enanthate and estradiol valerate			
Delatest, see Testosterone enanthate			
Delatestadiol, see Testosterone enanthate and estradiol valerate			
Delatestryl, see Testosterone enanthate			
Delta-Cortef, see Prednisolone, oral			
Delestrogen, see Estradiol valerate			
Demadex, see Torsemide			
Demerol HCl, see Meperidine HCl			
Denileukin diftitox	300 mcg		J9160
DepAndro 100, see Testosterone cypionate			
DepAndro 200, see Testosterone cypionate			
DepAndrogyn, see Testosterone cypionate and estradiol cypionate			
DepGynogen, see Depo-estradiol cypionate			
DepMedalone 40, see Methylprednisolone acetate			
DepMedalone 80, see Methylprednisolone acetate			
Depo-estradiol cypionate	up to 5 mg	IM	J1000
Depogen, see Depo-estradiol cypionate			
Depoject, see Methyprednisolone acetate			

Drug	Dose	Route	Code
Depo-Medrol, see Methylprednisolone acetate			
Depopred-40, see Methylprednisolone acetate			
Depopred-80, see Methylprednisolone acetate			
Depo-Provera, see Medroxyprogesterone acetate			
Depotest, see Testosterone cypionate			
Depo-Testadiol, see Testosterone cypionate and estradiol cypionate			
Depotestogen, see Testosterone cypionate and estradiol cypionate			
Depo-Testosterone, see Testosterone cypionate			
Desferal Mesylate, see Deferoxamine mesylate			
Desmopressin acetate	1 mcg	IV, SC	J2597
Dexacen LA-8, see Dexamethasone acetate			
Dexacen-4, see Dexamethasone sodium phosphate			
Dexamethasone, concentrated form	per mg	INH	J7637
Dexamethasone,unit form	per mg	INH	J7638
Dexamethasone, oral	0.25 mg		J8540
Dexamethasone acetate	1 mg	IM	J1094
Dexamethasone sodium phosphate	1 mg	IM, IV, OTH	J1100
Dexasone, see Dexamethasone sodium phosphate			
Dexasone L.A., see Dexamethasone acetate			
Dexferrum, see Iron Dextran			
Dexone, see Dexamethasone sodium phosphate			
Dexone LA, see Dexamethasone acetate			
Dexrazoxane hydrochloride	250 mg	IV	J1190
Dextran 40	500 ml	IV	J7100
Dextran 75	500 ml	IV	J7110
Dextrose 5%/normal saline solution,	500 ml = 1 unit	IV	J7042
Dextrose/water (5%)	500 ml = 1 unit	IV	J7060
D.H.E. 45, see Dihydroergotamine			
Diamox, see Acetazolamide sodium			
Diazepam up to 5 mg IM, IV J3360			
Diazoxide up to 300 mg IV J1730			
Dibent, see Dicyclomine HCl			
Dicyclomine HCl	up to 20 mg	IM	J0500
Didronel, see Etidronate disodium			
Diethylstilbestrol diphosphate	250 mg	IV	J9165
Diflucan, see Fluconazole			
Digoxin	up to 0.5 mg	IM, IV	J1160
Digoxin immune fab (ovine)	per vial		J1162
Dihydrex, see Diphenhydramine Hcl			
Dihydroergotamine mesylate	per 1 mg	IM, IV	J1110
Dilantin, see Phenytoin sodium			
Dilaudid, see Hydromorphone HCl			
Dilocaine, see Lidocaine HCl			
Dilomine, see Dicyclomine HCl			
Dilor, see Dyphylline			
Dimenhydrinate	up to 50 mg	IM, IV	J1240
Dimercaprol	per 100 mg	IM	J0470
Dimethyl sulfoxide, see DMSO, Dimethylsulfoxide			

Dinate, see Dimenhydrinate
Dioval, see Estradiol valerate
Dioval 40, see Estradiol valerate
Dioval XX, see Estradiol valerate
Diphenacen-50, see Diphenhydramine HCl

Diphenhydramine HCl, injection	up to 50 mg	IV, IM	J1200
Diphenhydramine HCl, oral	50 mg	ORAL	Q0163
Dipyridamole	per 10 mg	IV	J1245

Disotate, see Endrate ethylenediamine-tetra-acetic acid
Di-Spaz, see Dicyclomine HCl
Ditate-DS, see Testosterone enanthate and estradiol valerate
Diuril Sodium, see Chlorothiazide sodium
D-Med 80, see Methylprednisolone acetate

DMSO, Dimethyl sulfoxide 50%,	50 ml	OTH	J1212
Dobutamine HCl	per 250 mg	IV	J1250

Dobutrex, see Dobutamine Hcl

Docetaxel	20 mg	IV	J9170
Dolasetron mesylate, injection	10 mg	IV	J1260
Dolasetron mesylate, tablets	100 mg	ORAL	Q0180

Dolophine HCl, see Methadone Hcl
Dommanate, see Dimenhydrinate
Donbax, see Doripenem

Dopamine HCl	40 mg		J1265

Doribax, see Doripenem

Doripenem	10 mg		J1267
Dornase alpha, unit dose form	per mg	INH	J7639
Doxercalciferol	1 mcg	IV	J1270

Doxil, see Doxorubicin HCL, lipid

Doxorubicin HCL	10 mg	IV	J9000
Doxorubicin HCL, all lipid	10 mg	IV	J9001

Dramamine, see Dimenhydrinate
Dramanate, see Dimenhydrinate
Dramilin, see Dimenhydrinate
Dramocen, see Dimenhydrinate
Dramoject, see Dimenhydrinate

Dronabinol, oral	2.5 mg	ORAL	Q0167
Dronabinol, oral	5 mg	ORAL	Q0168
Droperidol	up to 5 mg	IM, IV	J1790
Drug administered through a metered dose inhaler		INH	J3535
Droperidol and fentanyl citrate	up to 2 ml ampule	IM, IV	J1810

DTIC-Dome, see Dacarbazine
Dua-Gen L.A., see Testosterone enanthate and estradiol valerate cypionate
Duoval P.A., see Testosterone enanthate and estradiol valerate
Durabolin, see Nandrolone phenpropionate
Duraclon, see Clonidine Hydrochloride
Dura-Estrin, see Depo-estradiol cypionate
Duracillin A.S., see Penicillin G procaine
Duragen-10, see Estradiol valerate

Duragen-20, see Estradiol valerate
Duragen-40, see Estradiol valerate
Duralone-40, see Methylprednisolone acetate
Duralone-80, see Methylprednisolone acetate
Duralutin, see Hydroxyprogesterone Caproate
Duramorph, see Morphine sulfate
Duratest-100, see Testosterone cypionate
Duratest-200, see Testosterone cypionate
Duratestrin, see Testosterone cypionate and estradiol cypionate
Durathate-200, see Testosterone enanthate
Dymenate, see Dimenhydrinate

Dyphylline	up to 500 mg	IM	J1180

Dysport, see AbobotulinumtoxintypeA

E

Eculizumab	10 mg		J1300
Edetate calcium disodium	up to 1000 mg	IV, SC, IM	J0600
Edetate disodium	per 150 mg	IV	J3520

Elavil, see Amitriptyline HCl
Ellence, see Epirubicin HCl

Elliotts b solution	1 ml	OTH	J9175

Elspar, see Asparaginase
Emend, see Fosaprepitant
Emete-Con, see Benzquinamide
Eminase, see Anistreplase
Enbrel, see Etanercept
Endrate ethylenediamine-tetra-acetic acid, see Edetate disodium

Enfuvirtide	1 mg		J1324

Enovil, see Amitriptyline HCl

Enoxaparin sodium	10 mg	SC	J1650

Eovist, see Gadoxetate disodium

Epinephrine, adrenalin	up to 1 ml amp	SC, IM	J0170
Epirubicin hydrochloride	2 mg		J9178
Epoetin alfa	1000 units		Q4055
Epoprostenol	0.5 mg	IV	J1325
Eptifibatide, injection	5 mg	IM, IV	J1327
Ergonovine maleate	up to 0.2 mg	IM, IV	J1330
Ertapenem sodium	500 mg		J1335
Erythromycin lactobionate	500 mg	IV	J1364

Estra-D, see Depo-estradiol cypionate
Estra-L 20, see Estradiol valerate
Estra-L 40, see Estradiol valerate
Estra-Testrin, see Testosterone enanthate and estradiol valerate
Estradiol Cypionate, see Depo-estradiol cypionate
Estradiol L.A., see Estradiol valerate
Estradiol L.A. 20, see Estradiol valerate
Estradiol L.A. 40, see Estradiol valerate

Estradiol valerate	up to 10 mg	IM	J1380
	up to 20 mg	IM	J1390
	up to 40 mg	IM	J0970
Estro-Cyp, see Depo-estradiol cypionate			
Estrogen, conjugated	per 25 mg	IV, IM	J1410
Estroject L.A., see Depo-estradiol cypionate			
Estrone per	1 mg	IM	J1435
Estrone 5, see Estrone			
Estrone Aqueous, see Estrone			
Estronol, see Estrone			
Estronol-L.A., see Depo-estradiol cypionate			
Etanercept, injection	25 mg	IM, IV	J1438
Ethanolamine	100 mg		J1430
Ethyol, see Amifostine			
Etidronate disodium	per 300 mg	IV	J1436
Etonogestrel implant			J7307
Etopophos, see Etoposide			
Etoposide	10 mg	IV	J9181
Etoposide, oral	50 mg	ORAL	J8560
Euflexxa			J7323
Everone, see Testosterone Enanthate			

F

Factor VIIa (coagulation factor, recombinant)	1 mcg	IV	J7189
Factor VIII (anti-hemophilic factor, human)	per IU	IV	J7190
Factor VIII (anti-hemophilic factor, porcine)	per IU	IV	J7191
Factor VIII (anti-hemophilic factor, recombinant)	per IU	IV	J7185, J7192
Factor IX (anti-hemophilic factor, purified, non-recombinant)	per IU	IV	J7193
Factor IX (anti-hemophilic factor, recombinant)	per IU	IV	J7195
Factor IX, complex	per IU	IV	J7194
Factors, other hemophilia clotting	per IU	IV	J7196
Factrel, see Gonadorelin HCl			
Faraheme, see Ferumoxytol			
Feiba VH Immuno, see Factors, other hemophilia clotting			
Fentanyl citrate	0.1 mg	IM, IV	J3010
Ferrlecit, see Sodium ferricgluconate complex in sucrose injection			
Ferumoxytol	1 mg		Q0138, Q0139
Filgrastim (G-CSF)	300 mcg	SC, IV	J1440
	480 mcg	SC, IV	J1441
Firmagon, see Degarelix			
Flebogamma	500 mg	IV	J1572
Flexoject, see Orphenadrine citrate			
Flexon, see Orphenadrine citrate			
Flolan, see Epoprostenol			
Floxuridine	500 mg	IV	J9200
Fluconazole	200 mg	IV	J1450

Drug	Amount	Route	Code
Fludara, see Fludarabine phosphate			
Fludarabine phosphate	50 mg	IV	J9185
Flunisolide inhalation solution, unit dose form	per mg	INH	J7641
Fluocinolone			J7311
Fluorouracil	500 mg	IV	J9190
Folex, see Methotrexate sodium			
Folex PFS, see Methotrexate sodium			
Follutein, see Chorionic gonadotropin			
Fomepizole	15 mg		J1451
Fomivirsen sodium	1.65 mg	Intraocular	J1452
Fondaparinux sodium	0.5 mg		J1652
Formoterol	12 mcg	INH J	7640
Formoterol fumarate	20 mcg		J7606
Fortaz, see Ceftazidime			
Fosaprepitant	1 mg		J1453
Foscarnet sodium	per 1,000 mg	IV	J1455
Foscavir, see Foscarnet sodium			
Fosphenytoin	50 mg		Q2009
FUDR, see Floxuridine			
Fulvestrant	25 mg		J9395
Fungizone Intravenous, see Amphotericin B			
Furomide M.D., see Furosemide			
Furosemide	up to 20 mg	IM, IV	J1940

G

Drug	Amount	Route	Code
Gadoxetate disodium	1 ml		A9581
Gallium nitrate	1 mg		J1457
Galsulfase	1 mg		J1458
Gamastan, see Gamma globulin and Immune globulin			
Gammagard Liquid	500 mg		J1569
Gamma globulin	1 cc	IM	J1460
	2 cc	IM	J1470
	3 cc	IM	J1480
	4 cc	IM	J1490
	5 cc	IM	J1500
	6 cc	IM	J1510
	7 cc	IM	J1520
	8 cc	IM	J1530
	9 cc	IM	J1540
	10 cc	IM	J1550
	over 10 cc	IM	J1560
Gammar, see Gamma globulin and Immune globulin			
Gammar-IV, see Immune globulin intravenous (human)			
Gamulin RH, see Rho(D) immune globulin			
Gamunex	500 mg		J1561
Ganciclovir, implant	4.5 mg	OTH	J7310
Ganciclovir sodium	500 mg	IV	J1570
Garamycin, gentamicin	up to 80 mg	IM, IV	J1580

Gatifloxacin	10 mg	IV	J1590
Gefitinib	250 mg		J8565
Gemcitabine HCl	200 mg	IV	J9201
Gemsar, see Gemcitabine Hcl			
Gemtuzumab ozogamicin	5 mg	IV	J9300
Gentamicin Sulfate, see Garamycin, gentamicin			
Gentran, see Dextran 40			
Gentran 75, see Dextran 75			
Gesterol 50, see Progesterone			
Glatiramer Acetate	20 mg		J1595
Glucagon Hcl	per 1 mg	SC, IM, IV	J1610
Glukor, see Chorionic gonadotropin			
Glycopyrrolate, concentrated form	per 1 mg	INH	J7642
Glycopyrrolate, unit dose form	per 1 mg	INH	J7643
Gold sodium thiomalate	up to 50 mg	IM	J1600
Gonadorelin HCl	per 100 mcg	SC, IV	J1620
Gonic, see Chorionic gonadotropin			
Goserelin acetate implant	per 3.6 mg	SC	J9202
Granisetron HCl, injection	100 mcg	IV	J1626
Granisetron HCl, oral	1 mg	ORAL	Q0166
Gynogen L.A. A10,@ see Estradiol valerate			
Gynogen L.A. A20,@ see Estradiol valerate			
Gynogen L.A. A40,@ see Estradiol valerate			

H

Haldol, see Haloperidol			
Haloperidol	up to 5 mg	IM, IV	J1630
Haloperidol decanoate	per 50 mg	IM	J1631
Hectoral, see Doxercalciferol			
Hemin	1 mg		J1640
Hemofil M, see Factor VIII			
Hemophilia clotting factors(e.g., anti-inhibitors)	per IU	IV	J7198
Hemophilia clotting factors, NOC	per IU	IV	J7199
Hepagam B	0.5 ml	IM	J1571
	0.5 ml	IV	J1573
Hep-Lock, see Heparin sodium (heparin lock flush)			
Hep-Lock U/P, see Heparin sodium (heparin lock flush)			
Heparin sodium	1,000 units	IV, SC	J1644
Heparin sodium (heparin lock flush)	10 units	IV	J1642
Herceptin, see Trastuzumab			
Hexadrol Phosphate, see Dexamethasone sodium phosphate			
Histaject, see Brompheniramine maleate			
Histerone 50, see Testosterone suspension			
Histerone 100, see Testosterone suspension			
Histrelin acetate	10 mcg		J1675
Histrelin implant	50 mg		J9225
Human fibrinogen concentrate	100 mg		J1680
Hyalgan			J7321

Drug	Dosage	Route	Code
Hyaluronidase	up to 150 units	SC, IV	J3470
Hyaluronidase, ovine	up to 999 units		J3471
Hyaluronidase, ovine	per 1000 units		J3472
Hyaluronidase recombinant	1 usp		J3473
Hyate:C, see Factor VIII (anti-hemophilic factor (porcine))			
Hybolin Improved, see Nandrolone phenpropionate			
Hybolin Decanoate, see Nandrolone decanoate			
Hycamtin, see Topotecan			
Hydralazine HCl	up to 20 mg	IV, IM	J0360
Hydrate, see Dimenhydrinate			
Hydrocortisone acetate	up to 25 mg	IV, IM, SC	J1700
Hydrocortisone sodium phosphate	up to 50 mg	IV, IM, SC	J1710
Hydrocortisone succinate sodium	up to 100 mg	IV, IM, SC	J1720
Hydrocortone Acetate, see Hydrocortisone acetate			
Hydrocortone Phosphate, see Hydrocortisone sodium phosphate			
Hydromorphone HCl	up to 4 mg	SC, IM, IV	J1170
Hydroxyzine HCl up to	25 mg	IM	J3410
Hydroxyzine Pamoate	25 mg	ORAL	Q0177
	50 mg	ORAL	Q0178
Hylan G-F 20			J7322
Hyoscyamine sulfate	up to 0.25 mg	SC, IM, IV	J1980
Hyperstat IV, see Diazoxide			
Hyper-Tet, see Tetanus immune globulin, human			
HypRho-D, see Rho(D) immune globulin			
Hyrexin-50, see Diphenhydramine HCl			
Hyzine-50, see Hydroxyzine HCl			

I

Drug	Dosage	Route	Code
Ibandronate sodium	1 mg		J1740
Ibutilide fumarate	1 mg	IV	J1742
Idamycin, see Idarubicin HCl			
Idarubicin HCl	5 mg	IV	J9211
Idursulfase	1 mg		J1743
Ifex, see Ifosfamide			
Ifosfamide	1 g	IV	J9208
Iloprost	20 mcg		Q4074
Ilotycin, see Erythromycin glucoptate			
Imferon, see Iron dextran			
Imiglucerase	per unit	IV	J1785
Imitrex, see Sumatriptan succinate			
Immune globulin			
Flebogamma	500 mg	IV	J1572
Gammagard Liquid	500 mg	IV	J1569
Gamunex	500 mg	IV	J1561
HepaGam B	0.5 ml	IM	J1571
HepaGam B	0.5 ml	IV	J1573
NOS	500 mg	IV	J1566
Octagam	500 mg	IV	J1568

Privigen	500 mg	IV	J1459
Rhophylac	100 IU	IM	J2791
Subcutaneous	100 mg		J1562
Immunosuppressive drug, not otherwise classified			J7599
Imuran, see Azathioprine			
Inapsine, see Droperidol			
Inderal, see Propranolol HCl			
Infed, see Iron Dextran			
Infergen, see Interferon alfa-1			
Infliximab, injection	10 mg	IM, IV	J1745
Innohep, see Tinzarparin			
Innovar, see Droperidol with fentanyl citrate			
Insulin	5 units	SC	J1815
Insulin lispro	50 units	SC	J1817
Intal, see Cromolyn sodium or Cromolyn sodium, compounded			
Integrilin, injection, see Eptifibatide			
Interferon alphacon-1, recombinant	1 mcg	SC	J9212
Interferon alfa-2a, recombinant	3 million units	SC, IM	J9213
Interferon alfa-2b, recombinant	1 million units	SC, IM	J9214
Interferon alfa-n3 (human leukocyte derived)	250,000 IU	IM	J9215
Interferon beta-1a	33 mcg	IM	J1825
Interferon beta-1a	11 mcg	IM	Q3025
Interferon beta-1a	11 mcg	SC	Q3026
Interferon beta-1b	0.25 mg	SC	J1830
Interferon gamma-1b	3 million units	SC	J9216
Intrauterine copper contraceptive, see Copper contraceptive, intrauterine			
Ipratropium bromide, unit dose form	per mg	INH	J7644, J7645
Irinotecan	20 mg	IV	J9206
Iron dextran	50 mg		J1750
Iron sucrose	1 mg	IV	J1756
Irrigation solution for Tx of bladder calculi	per 50 ml	OTH	Q2004
Isocaine HCl, see Mepivacaine			
Isoetharine HCl, concentrated form	per mg	INH	J7647, J7648
Isoetharine Hcl, unit dose form	per mg	INH	J7649, J7650
Isoproterenol HCl, concentrated form	per mg	INH	J7657, J7658
Isoproterenol Hcl, unit dose form	per mg	INH	J7659, J7660
Isuprel, see Isoproterenol HCl			
Itraconazole	50 mg	IV	J1835
Ixabepilone	1 mg		J9207
Ixempra, see Ixabepilone			

J

Jenamicin, see Garamycin, gentamicin

K

Kabikinase, see Streptokinase
Kaleinate, see Calcium gluconate

Drug	Dose	Route	Code
Kanamycin sulfate	up to 75 mg	IM, IV	J1850
Kanamycin sulfate	up to 500 mg	IM, IV	J1840
Kantrex, see Kanamycin sulfate			
Keflin, see Cephalothin sodium			
Kefurox, see Cufuroxime sodium			
Kefzol, see Cefazolin sodium			
Kenaject-40, see Triamcinolone acetonide			
Kenalog-10, see Triamcinolone acetonide			
Kenalog-40, see Triamcinolone acetonide			
Keppra, see Levetiracetam			
Kestrone 5, see Estrone			
Ketorolac tromethamine	per 15 mg	IM, IV	J1885
Key-Pred 25, see Prednisolone acetate			
Key-Pred 50, see Prednisolone acetate			
Key-Pred-SP, see Prednisolone sodium phosphate			
K-Flex, see Orphenadrine citrate			
Klebcil, see Kanamycin sulfate			
Koate-HP, see Factor VIII			
Kogenate, see Factor VIII			
Konakion, see Vitamin K, phytonadione, etc.			
Konyne-80, see Factor IX, complex			
Kytril, see Granisetron HCl			

L

Drug	Dose	Route	Code
L.A.E. 20, see Estradiol valerate			
Laetrile, Amygdalin, vitamin B-17			J3570
Lanoxin, see Digoxin			
Lanreotide	1 mg		J1930
Largon, see Propiomazine HCl			
Laronidase	0.1 mg		J1931
Lasix, see Furosemide			
L-Caine, see Lidocaine HCl			
Lepirudin	50 mg		J1945
Leucovorin calcium	per 50 mg	IM, IV	J0640
Leukine, see Sargramostim (GM-CSF)			
Leuprolide acetate (for depot suspension)	per 3.75 mg	IM	J1950
	7.5 mg	IM	J9217
Leuprolide acetate	per 1 mg	IM	J9218
Leuprolide acetate implant	65 mg		J9219
Leustatin, see Cladribine			
Levalbuterol HCl, concentrated form	0.5 mg	INH	J7607, J7612
Levalbuterol HCl, unit dose form	0.5 mg	INH	J7614, J7615
Levaquin I.U., see Levofloxacin			
Levetiracetam	10 mg		J1953
Levocarnitine	per 1 gm	IV	J1955
Levo-Dromoran, see Levorphanol tartrate			
Levofloxacin	250 mg	IV	J1956
Levoleucovorin calcium	0.5 mg		J0641

Levonorgestrel implant			J7306
Levonorgestrel releasing intrauterin contraceptive	52 mg	OTH	J7302
Levorphanol tartrate	up to 2 mg	SC, IV	J1960
Levsin, see Hyoscyamine sulfate			
Levulan Kerastick, see Aminolevulinic acid HCl			
Lexiscan, see Regadenoson			
Librium, see Chlordiazepoxide HCl			
Lidocaine HCl	10 mg	IV	J2001
Lidoject-1, see Lidocaine HCl			
Lidoject-2, see Lidocaine HCl			
Lincocin, see Lincomycin HCl			
Lincomycin HCl	up to 300 mg	IV	J2010
Linezolid	200 mg	IV	J2020
Liquaemin Sodium, see Heparin sodium			
Lioresal, see Baclofen			
LMD (10%), see Dextran 40			
Lovenox, see Enoxaparin sodium			
Lorazepam	2 mg	IM, IV	J2060
Lufyllin, see Dyphylline			
Luminal Sodium, see Phenobarbitol sodium			
Lunelle, see Medroxyprogesterone acetate/estradiol cypionate			
Lupron, see Leuprolide acetate			
Lymphocyte immune globulin,			
anti-thymocyte globulin, equine	250 mg	IV	J7504
anti-thymocyte globulin, rabbit	25 mg	IV	J7511
Lyophilized, see Cyclophosphamide, lyophilized			

M

Magnesium sulfate	500 mg		J3475
Mannitol 25% in	50 ml	IV	J2150
Marmine, see Dimenhydrinate			
Maxipime, see Cefepime hydrochloride			
Mecasermin	1 mg		J2170
Mechlorethamine HCl (nitrogen mustard), HN2	10 mg	IV	J9230
Medralone 40, see Methylprednisolone acetate			
Medralone 80, see Methylprednisolone acetate			
Medrol, see Methylprednisolone			
Medroxyprogesterone acetate	50 mg	IM	J1051
	150 mg	IM	J1055
Medroxyprogesterone acetate/estradiol cypionate	5 mg/25 mg	IM	J1056
Mefoxin, see Cefoxitin sodium			
Melphalan HCl	50 mg	IV	J9245
Melphalan, oral	2 mg	ORAL	J8600
Menoject LA, see Testosterone cypionate and estradiol cypionate			
Mepergan Injection, see Meperdine and promethazine HCl			
Meperidine HCl	per 100 mg	IM, IV, SC	J2175
Meperidine and promethazine HCl	up to 50 mg	IM, IV	J2180
Mepivacaine HCL	per 10 ml	VAR	J0670

Drug	Dose	Route	Code
Meropenem	100 mg		J2185
Mesna	200 mg	IV	J9209
Mesnex, see Mesna			
Metaprel, see Metaproterenol sulfate			
Metaproterenol sulfate, concentrated form	per 10 mg	INH	J7667, J7668
Metaproterenol sulfate, unit dose form	per 10 mg	INH	J7669, J7670
Metaraminol bitartrate	per 10 mg	IV, IM, SC	J0380
Metastron, see Strontium-89 chloride			
Methacholine chloride	1 mg		J7674
Methadone HCl	up to 10 mg	IM, SC	J1230
Methergine, see Methylergonovine maleate			
Methocarbamol	up to 10 ml	IV, IM	J2800
Methotrexate, oral	2.5 mg	ORAL	J8610
Methotrexate sodium	5 mg	IV, IM, IT, IA	J9250
	50 mg	IV, IM, IT, IA	J9260
Methotrexate LPF, see Methotrexate sodium			
Methyldopate HCl	up to 250 mg	IV	J0210
Methylprednisolone, oral	per 4 mg	ORAL	J7509
Methylprednisolone acetate	20 mg	IM	J1020
	40 mg	IM	J1030
	80 mg	IM	J1040
Methylprednisolone sodium succinate	up to 40 mg	IM, IV	J2920
	up to 125 mg	IM, IV	J2930
Metoclopramide HCl	up to 10 mg	IV	J2765
Miacalcin, see Calcitonin-salmon			
Micafungin sodium	1 mg		J2248
Midazolam HCl	per 1 mg	IM, IV	J2250
Milrinone lactate	5 mg	IV	J2260
Mirena, see Levonorgestrel releasing intrauterine contraceptive			
Mithracin, see Plicamycin			
Mitomycin	5 mg	IV	J9280
	20 mg	IV	J9290
	40 mg	IV	J9291
Mitoxantrone HCl	per 5 mg	IV	J9293
Monocid, see Cefonicic sodium			
Monoclate-P, see Factor VIII			
Monoclonal antibodies, parenteral	5 mg	IV	J7505
Mononine, see Factor IX, purified, non-recombinant			
Morphine sulfate	up to 10 mg	IM, IV, SC	J2270
	100 mg	IM, IV, SC	J2271
Morphine sulfate, preservative-free	per 10 mg	SC, IM, IV	J2275
Moxifloxacin	100 mg		J2280
Mozobil, see Plerixafor			
M-Prednisol-40, see Methylprednisolone acetate			
M-Prednisol-80, see Methylprednisolone acetate			
Mucomyst, see Acetylcysteine or Acetylcysteine, compounded			
Mucosol, see Acetylcysteine			
Muromonab-CD3	5 mg	IV	J7505

Muse, see Alprostadil
Mustargen, see Mechlorethamine HCl
Mutamycin, see Mitomycin

Mycophenolic acid	180 mg		J7518
Mycophenolate Mofetil	250 mg	ORAL	J7517

Myleran, see Busulfan
Mylotarg, see Gemtuzumab ozogamicin
Myobloc, see RimabotulinumtoxinB
Myochrysine, see Gold sodium thiomalate
Myolin, see Orphenadrine citrate

N

Nabilone	1 mg	ORAL	J8650
Nalbuphine HCl	per 10 mg	IM, IV, SC	J2300
Naloxone HCl	per 1 mg	IM, IV, SC	J2310
Naltrexone, depot form	1 mg		J2315

Nandrobolic L.A., see Nandrolone decanoate

Nandrolone decanoate	up to 50 mg	IM	J2320
	up to 100 mg	IM	J2321
	up to 200 mg	IM	J2322

Narcan, see Naloxone HCl
Naropin, see Ropivacaine HCl
Nasahist B, see Brompheniramine maleate

Nasal vaccine inhalation		INH	J3530
Natalizumab	1 mg		J2323

Navane, see Thiothixene
Navelbine, see Vinorelbine tartrate
ND Stat, see Brompheniramine maleate
Nebcin, see Tobramycin sulfate
NebuPent, see Pentamidine isethionate

Nelarabine	50 mg		J9261

Nembutal Sodium Solution, see Pentobarbital sodium
Neocyten, see Orphenadrine citrate
Neo-Durabolic, see Nandrolone decanoate
Neoquess, see Dicyclomine HCl
Neosar, see Cyclophosphamide

Neostigmine methylsulfate	up to 0.5 mg I	M, IV, SC	J2710

Neo-Synephrine, see Phenylephrine HCl
Nervocaine 1%, see Lidocaine HCl
Nervocaine 2%, see Lidocaine HCl
Nesacaine, see Chloroprocaine HCL
Nesacaine-MPF, see Chloroprocaine HCl

Nesiritide	0.1 mg		J2325

Neumega, see Oprelvekin
Neupogen, see Filgrastim (G-CSF)
Neutrexin, see Trimetrexate glucuronate
Nipent, see Pentostatin
Nordryl, see Diphenhydramine HCl

Norflex, see Orphenadrine citrate
Norzine, see Thiethylperazine maleate

Not otherwise classified drugs			J3490
Not otherwise classified drugs	other than INH administered thru DME		J7799
Not otherwise classified drugs	INH administered thru DME		J7699
Not otherwise classified drugs, anti-neoplastic			J9999
Not otherwise classified drugs, chemotherapeutic	ORAL		J8999
Not otherwise classified drugs, immunosuppressive			J7599
Not otherwise classified drugs, nonchemotherapeutic	ORAL		J8499

Novantrone, see Mitoxantrone HCl
Novo Seven, see Factor VIIa
NPH, see Insulin
Nplate, see Romiplostim
Nubain, see Nalbuphine HCl
Nulicaine, see Lidocaine HCl
Numorphan, see Oxymorphone HCl
Numorphan H.P., see Oxymorphone HCl

O

Octagam	500 mg			J1568
Octreotide Acetate, injection	1 mg	IM		J2353
	25 mcg	IV, SQ		J2354
Oculinum, see Botulinum toxin type A				
O-Flex, see Orphenadrine citrate				
Omalizumab	5 mg			J2357
Omnipen-N, see Ampicillin				
OnabotulinumtoxinA	1 unit			J0585
Oncaspar, see Pegaspargase				
Oncovin, see Vincristine sulfate				
Ondansetron HCl	1 mg	IV		J2405
Ondansetron HCl, oral	8 mg	ORAL		Q0179
Oprelvekin	5 mg	SC		J2355
Oraminic II, see Brompheniramine maleate				
Ormazine, see Chlorpromazine HCl				
Orphenadrine citrate	up to 60 mg	IV, IM		J2360
Orphenate, see Orphenadrine citrate				
Orthovisc				J7324
Or-Tyl, see Dicyclomine				
Oxacillin sodium	up to 250 mg	IM, IV		J2700
Oxaliplatin	0.5 mg			J9263
Oxymorphone HCl	up to 1 mg	IV, SC, IM		J2410
Oxytetracycline HCl	up to 50 mg	IM		J2460
Oxytocin	up to 10 units	IV, IM		J2590

P

Drug	Dose	Route	Code
Paclitaxel	30 mg	IV	J9265
Paclitaxel protein-bound particles	1 mg		J9264
Palifermin	50 mcg		J2425
Palonosetron HCl	25 mcg		J2469
Pamidronate disodium	per 30 mg	IV	J2430
Panitumumab	10 mg		J9303
Papaverine HCl	up to 60 mg	IV, IM	J2440
Paragard T 380 A, see Copper contraceptive, intrauterine			
Paraplatin, see Carboplatin			
Paricalcitol, injection	1 mcg	IV, IM	J2501
Pegademase bovine	25 iu		J2504
Pegaptinib	0.3 mg		J2503
Pegaspargase	per single dose vial	IM, IV	J9266
Pegfilgrastim	6 mg		J2505
Pemetrexed	10 mg		J9305
Penicillin G benzathine	up to 600,000 units	IM	J0560
	up to 1,200,000 units	IM	J0570
	up to 2,400,000 units	IM	J0580
Penicillin G benzathine and penicillin G procaine			
	2500 units	IM	J0559
Penicillin G potassium	up to 600,000 units	IM, IV	J2540
Penicillin G procaine, aqueous	up to 600,000 units	IM, IV	J2510
Pentamidine isethionate	per 300 mg	INH	J2545, J7676
Pentastarch, 10%	100 ml		J2513
Pentazocine HCl	30 mg	IM, SC, IV	J3070
Pentobarbital sodium	per 50 mg	IM, IV, OTH	J2515
Pentostatin	per 10 mg	IV	J9268
Peforomist, see Formoterol fumarate			
Permapen, see Penicillin G benzathine			
Perphenazine, injection	up to 5 mg	IM, IV	J3310
Perphenazine, tablets	4 mg	ORAL	Q0175
	8 mg	ORAL	Q0176
Persantine IV, see Dipyridamole			
Pfizerpen, see Penicillin G potassium			
Pfizerpen A.S., see Penicillin G procaine			
Phenazine 25, see Promethazine HCl			
Phenazine 50, see Promethazine HCl			
Phenergan, see Promethazine HCl			
Phenobarbital sodium	up to 120 mg	IM, IV	J2560
Phentolamine mesylate	up to 5 mg	IM, IV	J2760
Phenylephrine HCl	up to 1 ml	SC, IM, IV	J2370
Phenytoin sodium	per 50 mg	IM, IV	J1165
Photofrin, see Porfimer sodium			
Phytonadione (Vitamin K)	per 1 mg	IM, SC, IV	J3430
Piperacillin/Tazobactam Sodium, injection	1.125 g	IV	J2543
Pitocin, see Oxytocin			
Plantinol AQ, see Cisplatin			

Drug	Dose	Route	Code
Plas+SD, see Plasma, pooled multiple donor			
Plasma, cryoprecipitate reduced	each unit		P9044
Plasma, pooled multiple donor, frozen,	each unit	IV	P9023
Platinol, see Cisplatin			
Plerixafor	1 mg		J2562
Plicamycin	2,500 mcg	IV	J9270
Polocaine, see Mepivacaine			
Polycillin-N, see Ampicillin			
Porfimer Sodium	75 mg	IV	J9600
Potassium chloride	per 2 mEq	IV	J3480
Pralidoxime chloride	up to 1 g	IV, IM, SC	J2730
Predalone-50, see Prednisolone acetate			
Predcor-25, see Prednisolone acetate			
Predcor-50, see Prednisolone acetate			
Predicort-50, see Prednisolone acetate			
Prednisone	per 5 mg	ORAL	J7506
Prednisolone, oral	5 mg	ORAL	J7510
Prednisolone acetate	up to 1 ml	IM	J2650
Predoject-50, see Prednisolone acetate			
Pregnyl, see Chorionic gonadotropin			
Premarin Intravenous, see Estrogen, conjugated			
Prescription,chemotherapeutic,not otherwise specified		ORAL	J8999
Prescription,nonchemotherapeutic,not otherwise specified		ORAL	J8499
Primacor, see Milrinone lactate			
Primaxin I.M., see Cilastatin sodium, imipenem			
Primaxin I.V., see Cilastatin sodium, imipenem			
Priscoline HCl, see Tolazoline HCl			
Privigen	500 mg		J1459
Pro-Depo, see Hydroxyprogesterone Caproate			
Procainamide HCl	up to 1 g	IM, IV	J2690
Prochlorperazine	up to 10 mg	IM, IV	J0780
Prochlorperazine maleate, oral	5 mg	ORAL	Q0164
	10 mg	ORAL	Q0165
Profasi HP, see Chorionic gonadotropin			
Profilnine Heat-Treated, see Factor IX			
Progestaject, see Progesterone			
Progesterone	per 50 mg		J2675
Prograf, see Tacrolimus, oral or parenteral			
Prokine, see Sargramostim (GM-CSF)			
Prolastin, see Alpha 1-proteinase inhibitor, human			
Proleukin, see Aldesleukin			
Prolixin Decanoate, see Fluphenazine decanoate			
Promazine HCl	up to 25 mg	IM	J2950
Promethazine HCl, injection	up to 50 mg	IM, IV	J2550
Promethazine HCl, oral	12.5 mg	ORAL	Q0169
	25 mg	ORAL	Q0170
Pronestyl, see Procainamide HCl			
Proplex T, see Factor IX			

Proplex SX-T, see Factor IX			
Propranolol HCl	up to 1 mg	IV	J1800
Prorex-25, see Promethazine HCl			
Prorex-50, see Promethazine HCl			
Prostaphlin, see Procainamide HCl			
Prostigmin, see Neostigmine methylsulfate			
Protamine sulfate	per 10 mg	IV	J2720
Protein C Concentrate 10		IU	J2724
Protirelin	per 250 mcg	IV	J2725
Prothazine, see Promethazine HCl			
Protopam Chloride, see Pralidoxime chloride			
Proventil, see Albuterol sulfate, compounded			
Prozine-50, see Promazine HCl			
Pulmicort Respules, see Budesonide			
Pyridoxine HCl	100 mg		J3415

Q

Quelicin, see Succinylcholine chloride			
Quinupristin/dalfopristin	500 mg(150/350)	IV	J2770

R

Ranibizumab	0.1 mg		J2778
Ranitidine HCL, injection	25 mg	IV, IM	J2780
Rapamune, see Sirolimus			
Rasburicase	0.5 mg		J2783
Reclast	1 mg		J3488
Recombinate, see Factor VIII			
Redisol, see Vitamin B-12 cyanocobalamin			
Regadenoson	0.1 mg		J2785
Regitine, see Phentolamine mesylate			
Reglan, see Metoclopramide HCl			
Regular, see Insulin			
Relefact TRH, see Protirelin			
Remicade, see Infliximab, injection			
Reo Pro, see Abciximab			
Rep-Pred 40, see Methylprednisolone acetate			
Rep-Pred 80, see Methylprednisolone acetate			
RespiGam, see Respiratory Syncytial Virus			
Retavase, see Reteplase			
Reteplase	18.8 mg	IV	J2993
Retrovir, see Zidovudine			
Rheomacrodex, see Dextran 40			
Rhesonativ, see Rho(D) immune globulin, human			
Rheumatrex Dose Pack, see Methotrexate, oral			
Rho(D) immune globulin			J2791
Rho(D) immune globulin, human	1 dose package, 300 mcg	IM	J2790
	50 mg	J2788	

Rho(D)immune globulin, human,solvent detergent	100 IU	IV	J2792
RhoGAM, see Rho(D) immune globulin, human			
Rhophylac	100 IU		J2791
Riastap, see Human Fibrinogen concentrate			
Rilonacept	1 mg		J2793
RimabotulinumtoxinB	100 units		J0587
Ringers lactate infusion	up to 1,000 cc	IV	J7120
Risperidone	0.5 mg		J2794
Rituxan, see Rituximab			
Rituximab	100 mg	IV	J9310
Robaxin, see Methocarbamol			
Rocephin, see Ceftriaxone sodium			
Roferon-A, see Interferon alfa-2A, recombinant			
Romiplostim	10 mcg		J2796
Ropivacaine Hydrochloride	1 mg		J2795
Rubex, see Doxorubicin HCl			
Rubramin PC, see Vitamin B-12 cyanocobalamin			

S

Saline solution 5% dextrose,	500 ml	IV	J7042
	infusion, 250 cc	IV	J7050
	infusion, 1,000 cc	IV	J7030
Saline solution, sterile	500 ml = 1 unit	IV, OTH	J7040
Sandimmune, see Cyclosporine			
Sandoglobulin, see Immune globulin intravenous (human)			
Sandostatin Lar Depot, see Octreotide			
Sargramostim (GM-CSF)	50 mcg	IV	J2820
Selestoject, see Betamethasone sodium phosphate			
Sermorelin acetate	1 mcg		Q0515
Sincalide	5 mcg		J2805
Sinusol-B, see Brompheniramine maleate			
Sirolimus	1 mg	Oral	J7520
Sodium ferricgluconate in sucrose	12.5 mg		J2916
Sodium Hyaluronate			
Euflexxa			J7323
Hyalgan			J7321
Orthovisc			J7324
Supartz			J7321
Solganal, see Aurothioglucose			
Solu-Cortef, see Hydrocortisone sodium phosphate (J1710)			
Solu-Medrol, see Methylprednisolone sodium succinate			
Solurex, see Dexamethasone sodium phosphate			
Solurex LA, see Dexamethasone acetate			
Somatrem	1 mg		J2940
Somatropin	1 mg		J2941
Somatulin Depot, see Lanreotide			
Sparine, see Promazine HCl			
Spasmoject, see Dicyclomine HCl			

Spectinomycin HCl	up to 2 g	IM	J3320
Sporanox, see Itraconazole			
Staphcillin, see Methicillin sodium			
Stilphostrol, see Diethylstilbestrol diphosphate			
Streptase, see Streptokinase			
Streptokinase	per 250,000 IU	IV	J2995
Streptomycin Sulfate, see Streptomycin			
Streptomycin	up to 1 g	IM	J3000
Streptozocin	1 gm	IV	J9320
Strontium-89 chloride per millicurie			A9600
Sublimaze, see Fentanyl citrate			
Succinylcholine chloride	up to 20 mg	IV, IM	J0330
Sumatriptan succinate	6 mg	SC J	3030
Supartz			J7321
Surostrin, see Succinycholine chloride			
Sus-Phrine, see Adrenalin, epinephrine			
Synercid, see Quinupristin/dalfopristin			
Synkavite, see Vitamin K, phytonadione, etc.			
Syntocionon, see Oxytocin			
Synvisc and Synvisc-One	1 mg		J7325
Sytobex, see Vitamin B-12 cyanocobalamin			

T

Tacrolimus, oral	per 1 mg	ORAL	J7507
Tacrolimus, parenteral	5 mg		J7525
Talwin, see Pentazocine Hcl			
Taractan, see Chlorprothixene			
Taxol, see Paclitaxel			
Taxotere, see Docetaxel			
Tazidime, see Ceftazidime Technetium TC Sestambi	per dose		A9500
TEEV, see Testosterone enanthate and estradiol valerate			
Temozolomide 1	mg		J9328
	5 mg	ORAL	J8700
Temsirolimus	1 mg		J9330
Tenecteplase	1 mg		J3101
Teniposide	50 mg		Q2017
Tequin, see Gatifloxacin			
Terbutaline sulfate	up to 1 mg	SC, IV	J3105
Terbutaline sulfate, concentrated form	per 1 mg	INH	J7680
Terbutaline sulfate, unit dose form	per 1 mg	INH	J7681
Teriparatide	10 mcg		J3110
Terramycin IM, see Oxytetracycline HCl			
Testa-C, see Testosterone cypionate			
Testadiate, see Testosterone enanthate and estradiol valerate			
Testadiate-Depo, see Testosterone cypionate			
Testaject-LA, see Testosterone cypionate			
Testaqua, see Testosterone suspension			
Test-Estro Cypionates, see Testosterone cypionate and estradiol cypionate			

Test-Estro-C, see Testosterone cypionate and estradiol cypionate
Testex, see Testosterone propionate
Testoject-50, see Testosterone suspension
Testoject-LA, see Testosterone cypionate
Testone LA 200, see Testosterone enanthate
Testone LA 100, see Testosterone enanthate
Testosterone Aqueous, see Testosterone suspension

Testosterone enanthate and estradiol valerate	up to 1 cc	IM	J0900
Testosterone enanthate	up to 100 mg	IM	J3120
	up to 200 mg	IM	J3130
Testosterone cypionate	up to 100 mg	IM	J1070
	1 cc, 200 mg	IM	J1080
Testosterone cypionate and estradiol cypionate	up to 1 ml	IM	J1060
Testosterone propionate	up to 100 mg	IM	J3150
Testosterone suspension	up to 50 mg	IM	J3140

Testradiol 90/4, see Testosterone enanthate and estradiol valerate
Testrin PA, see Testosterone enanthate

Tetanus immune globulin, human	up to 250 units	IM	J1670
Tetracycline	up to 250 mg	IM, IV	J0120
Thallous Chloride TL 201	per MCI		A9505

Theelin Aqueous, see Estrone

Theophylline	per 40 mg	IV	J2810

TheraCys, see BCG live

Thiamine HCl	100 mg		J3411
Thiethylperazine maleate, injection	up to 10 mg	IM	J3280
Thiethylperazine maleate, oral	10 mg	ORAL	Q0174
Thiotepa	15 mg	IV	J9340

Thorazine, see Chlorpromazine HCl
Thymoglobulin, see Immune globulin, anti-thymocyte
Thypinone, see Protirelin
Thyrogen, see Thyrotropin Alfa

Thyrotropin Alfa, injection	0.9 mg	IM, SC	J3240

Tice BCG, see BCG live
Ticon, see Trimethobenzamide HCl
Tigan, see Trimethobenzamide HCl

Tigecycline	1 mg		J3243

Tiject-20, see Trimethobenzamide HCl

Tinzaparin	1000 IU	SC	J1655
Tirofiban Hydrochloride, injection	0.25 mg	IM, IV	J3246

TNKase, see Tenecteplase
Tobi, see Tobramycin, inhalation solution

Tobramycin, inhalation solution	300 mg	INH	J7682, J7685
Tobramycin sulfate	up to 80 mg	IM, IV	J3260

Tofranil, see Imipramine HCl

Tolazoline HCl	up to 25 mg	IV	J2670
Topotecan	0.25 mg	Oral	J8705
	4 mg	IV	J9350

Toradol, see Ketorolac tromethamine

Torecan, see Thiethylperazine maleate
Torisel, see Temsirolimus
Tornalate, see Bitolterol mesylate

| Torsemide | 10 mg/ml | IV | J3265 |

Totacillin-N, see Ampicillin

| Trastuzumab | 10 mg | IV J | 9355 |

Treanda, see Bendamustine HCl

| Treprostinil | 1 mg | | J3285 |

Tri-Kort, see Triamcinolone acetonide
Triam-A, see Triamcinolone acetonide

Triamcinolone, concentrated form	per 1 mg	INH	J7683
Triamcinolone, unit dose	per 1 mg	INH	J7684
Triamcinolone acetonide	1 mg		J3300
	per 10 mg	IM	J3301
Triamcinolone diacetate	per 5 mg	IM	J3302
Triamcinolone hexacetonide	per 5 mg	VAR	J3303

Triesence, see Triamcinolone acetonide

| Triflupromazine HCl | up to 20 mg | IM, IV | J3400 |

Trilafon, see Perphenazine
Trilog, see Triamcinolone acetonide
Trilone, see Triamcinolone diacetate

Trimethobenzamide HCl, injection	up to 200 mg	IM	J3250
Trimethobenzamide HCl, oral	250 mg	ORAL	Q0173
Trimetrexate glucuronate	per 25 mg	IV	J3305
Triptorelin Pamoate	3.75 mg		J3315

Trisenox, see Arsenic trioxide
Trobicin, see Spectinomycin HCl
Trovan, see Alatrofloxacin mesylate
Tysabri, see Natalizumab

U

Ultrazine-10, see Prochlorperazine
Unasyn, see Ampicillin sodium/sulbactam sodium

Unclassified drugs (see also Not elsewhere classified)			J3490
Unspecified oral antiemetic			Q0181
Urea	up to 40 g	IV	J3350

Ureaphil, see Urea
Urecholine, see Bethanechol chloride

Urofollitropin	75 iu		J3355
Urokinase	5,000 IU vial	IV	J3364
	250,000 IU vial	IV	J3365

V

V-Gan 25, see Promethazine HCl
V-Gan 50, see Promethazine HCl
Valergen 10, see Estradiol valerate

Valergen 20, see Estradiol valerate
Valergen 40, see Estradiol valerate
Valertest No. 1, see Testosterone enanthate and estradiol valerate
Valertest No. 2, see Testosterone enanthate and estradiol valerate
Valium, see Diazepam

Valrubicin, intravesical	200 mg	OTH	J9357

Valstar, see Valrubicin
Vancocin, see Vancomycin HCl
Vancoled, see Vancomycin HCl

Vancomycin HCl	500 mg	IV, IM	J3370

Vasoxyl, see Methoxamine HCl
Velban, see Vinblastine sulfate
Velsar, see Vinblastine sulfate
Venofer, see Iron sucrose
Ventolin, see Albuterol sulfate
VePesid, see Etoposide and Etoposide, oral
Versed, see Midazolam HCl

Verteporfin	0.1 mg	IV	J3396

Vesprin, see Triflupromazine HCl
Viadur, see Leuprolide acetate implant

Vinblastine sulfate	1 mg	IV	J9360

Vincasar PFS, see Vincristine sulfate

Vincristine sulfate	1 mg	IV	J9370
	2 mg	IV	J9375
	5 mg	IV	J9380
Vinorelbine tartrate	per 10 mg	IV	J9390

Vistaject-25, see Hydroxyzine HCl
Vistaril, see Hydroxyzine HCl
Vistide, see cidofovir
Visudyne, see Verteporfin

Vitamin K, phytonadione, menadione, menadiol sodium diphosphate	per 1 mg	IM, SC, IV	J3430
Vitamin B-12 cyanocobalamin	up to 1,000 mcg	IM, SC	J3420
Von Willebrand Factor Complex, human	per IU VWF:RCo	IV	J7187
Voriconazole	10 mg		J3465

W

Wehamine, see Dimenhydrinate
Wehdryl, see Diphenhydramine HCL
Wellcovorin, see Leucovorin calcium
Win Rho SD, see Rho(D)immuglobulin, human, solvent detergent
Wyamine Sulfate, see Mephentermine sulfate
Wycillin, see Penicillin G procaine
Wydase, see Hyaluronidase

X

Xeloda, see Capecitabine
Xopenex, see Albuterol

Xylocaine HCL, see Lidocaine HCL

Z

Zanosar, see Streptozocin
Zantac, see Ranitidine HCL
Zemplar, see Paricalcitol
Zenapax, see Daclizumab
Zetran, see Diazepam

Ziconotide	1 mcg		J2278
Zidovudine	10 mg	IV	J3485

Zinacef, see Cefuroxime sodium

Ziprasidone Mesylate	10 mg	J3486

Zithromax, see Azithromycin dihydrate
Zithromax I.V., see Azithromycin, injection
Zofran, see Ondansetron HCl
Zoladex, see Goserelin acetate implant

Zoledronic Acid	1 mg	J3487

Zolicef, see Cefazolin sodium

Zometa	1 mg	J3487

Zosyn, see Piperacillin
Zyvox, see Linezolid

Addendum AA

Addendum AA -- Final ASC Covered Surgical Procedures for CY 2010
(Including Surgical Procedures for Which Payment is Packaged)

NOTE 1: *The Medicare program payment is 80 percent of the total payment amount and beneficiary coinsurance is 20 percent of the total payment amount, except for screening flexible sigmoidoscopies and screening colonoscopies for which the program payment is 75 percent and the beneficiary coinsurance is 25 percent.*

NOTE 2: *Payment indicators for "office-based" procedures (P2, P3) are based on a comparison of the final rates according to the ASC standard ratesetting methodology and the MPFS. Under current law, the MPFS payment rates will have a negative update for CY 2010. For a discussion of those rates, we refer readers to the CY 2010 MPFS final rule.*

**:* *Asterisked codes(*) indicate that the procedure's "office-based," designation is temporary because we have insufficient claims data. We will reconsider this designation when new claims data become available.*

HCPCS Code	HCPCS Short Descriptor	Subject To Multiple Procedure Discounts	CY 2010 Comment Indicator	CY 2010 Payment Indicator	CY 2010 Third Year Transition. Pymt. Weight	CY 2010 Third Year Transition Payment
0016T	Thermotx choroid vasc lesion	Y		R2	5.5965	$234.34
0017T	Photocoagulat macular drusen	Y		R2	5.5965	$234.34
0084T	Temp prostate urethral stent	N	CH	D5		
0086T	L ventricle fill pressure	N	CH	D5		
0099T*	Implant corneal ring	Y		R2	15.5449	$650.91
0100T	Prosth retina receive&gen	Y		G2	38.2338	$1,600.96
0101T	Extracorp shockwv tx,hi enrg	Y		G2	30.396	$1,272.77
0102T	Extracorp shockwv tx,anesth	Y		G2	30.396	$1,272.77
0123T	Scleral fistulization	Y		G2	23.3455	$977.55
0124T*	Conjunctival drug placement	Y		R2	4.3122	$180.56
0170T	Anorectal fistula plug rpr	N	CH	D5		
0176T	Aqu canal dilat w/o retent	Y		A2	37.7011	$1,578.66
0177T	Aqu canal dilat w retent	Y		A2	37.7011	$1,578.66
0186T	Suprachoroidal drug delivery	Y		G2	19.8176	$829.82
0190T	Place intraoc radiation src	Y		G2	19.8176	$829.82
0191T	Insert ant segment drain int	Y		G2	23.3455	$977.55
0192T	Insert ant segment drain ext	Y		G2	40.0704	$1,677.87
0193T	Rf bladder neck microremodel	Y	CH	G2	19.1572	$802.17
0200T	Perq sacral augmt unilat inj	Y		G2	21.0617	$881.92
0201T	Perq sacral augmt bilat inj	Y		G2	30.396	$1,272.77
0213T	Us facet jt inj cerv/t 1 lev	Y	NI	G2	6.8884	$288.44
0214T	Us facet jt inj cerv/t 2 lev	Y	NI	G2	2.4451	$102.38
0215T	Us facet jt inj cerv/t 3 lev	Y	NI	G2	2.4451	$102.38
0216T	Us facet jt inj ls 1 level	Y	NI	G2	6.8884	$288.44
0217T	Us facet jt inj ls 2 level	Y	NI	G2	2.4451	$102.38
0218T	Us facet jt inj ls 3 level	Y	NI	G2	2.4451	$102.38
10021	Fna w/o image	Y		P2	1.4457	$60.54
10022	Fna w/image	Y		G2	4.4	$184.24
10040	Acne surgery	Y		P2	0.8408	$35.21
10060	Drainage of skin abscess	Y		P3		$42.61
10061	Drainage of skin abscess	Y		P2	1.3927	$58.32
10080	Drainage of pilonidal cyst	Y		P2	1.3927	$58.32
10081	Drainage of pilonidal cyst	Y		P3		$108.51
10120	Remove foreign body	Y		P3		$59.08
10121	Remove foreign body	Y		A2	15.1023	$632.38
10140	Drainage of hematoma/fluid	Y		P3		$63.35

HCPCS Code	HCPCS Short Descriptor	Subject To Multiple Procedure Discounts	CY 2010 Comment Indicator	CY 2010 Payment Indicator	CY 2010 Third Year Transition. Pymt. Weight	CY 2010 Third Year Transition Payment
10160	Puncture drainage of lesion	Y	CH	P3		$52.55
10180	Complex drainage, wound	Y		A2	16.472	$689.73
11000	Debride infected skin	Y		P3		$20.17
11001	Debride infected skin add-on	Y		P3		$6.82
11010	Debride skin, fx	Y		A2	4.5669	$191.23
11011	Debride skin/muscle, fx	Y		A2	4.5669	$191.23
11012	Debride skin/muscle/bone, fx	Y		A2	4.5669	$191.23
11040	Debride skin, partial	Y		P3		$18.75
11041	Debride skin, full	Y		P3		$20.45
11042	Debride skin/tissue	Y		A2	2.947	$123.40
11043	Debride tissue/muscle	Y		A2	2.947	$123.40
11044	Debride tissue/muscle/bone	Y		A2	8.3025	$347.65
11055	Trim skin lesion	Y		P3		$21.87
11056	Trim skin lesions, 2 to 4	Y		P3		$23.86
11057	Trim skin lesions, over 4	Y	CH	P3		$26.99
11100	Biopsy, skin lesion	Y	CH	P3		$49.71
11101	Biopsy, skin add-on	Y		P3		$11.65
11200	Removal of skin tags	Y		P2	0.8408	$35.21
11201	Remove skin tags add-on	Y		P3		$4.83
11300	Shave skin lesion	Y	CH	P3		$33.24
11301	Shave skin lesion	Y		P2	0.8408	$35.21
11302	Shave skin lesion	Y		P2	0.8408	$35.21
11303	Shave skin lesion	Y	CH	P3		$55.96
11305	Shave skin lesion	Y	CH	P3		$29.54
11306	Shave skin lesion	Y		P2	0.8408	$35.21
11307	Shave skin lesion	Y		P2	0.8408	$35.21
11308	Shave skin lesion	Y		P2	0.8408	$35.21
11310	Shave skin lesion	Y		P2	0.8408	$35.21
11311	Shave skin lesion	Y		P2	0.8408	$35.21
11312	Shave skin lesion	Y		P2	0.8408	$35.21
11313	Shave skin lesion	Y		P2	0.8408	$35.21
11400	Exc tr-ext b9+marg 0.5 < cm	Y		P3		$56.53
11401	Exc tr-ext b9+marg 0.6-1 cm	Y		P3		$63.63
11402	Exc tr-ext b9+marg 1.1-2 cm	Y		P3		$69.88
11403	Exc tr-ext b9+marg 2.1-3 cm	Y		P3		$74.99
11404	Exc tr-ext b9+marg 3.1-4 cm	Y		A2	14.457	$605.36
11406	Exc tr-ext b9+marg > 4.0 cm	Y		A2	15.1023	$632.38
11420	Exc h-f-nk-sp b9+marg 0.5 <	Y		P3		$53.12
11421	Exc h-f-nk-sp b9+marg 0.6-1	Y		P3		$64.20
11422	Exc h-f-nk-sp b9+marg 1.1-2	Y		P3		$70.16
11423	Exc h-f-nk-sp b9+marg 2.1-3	Y		P3		$78.40
11424	Exc h-f-nk-sp b9+marg 3.1-4	Y		A2	15.1023	$632.38
11426	Exc h-f-nk-sp b9+marg > 4 cm	Y		A2	19.3292	$809.37
11440	Exc face-mm b9+marg 0.5 < cm	Y		P3		$60.50
11441	Exc face-mm b9+marg 0.6-1 cm	Y		P3		$70.16
11442	Exc face-mm b9+marg 1.1-2 cm	Y		P3		$77.26
11443	Exc face-mm b9+marg 2.1-3 cm	Y		P3		$85.50
11444	Exc face-mm b9+marg 3.1-4 cm	Y		A2	7.7878	$326.10
11446	Exc face-mm b9+marg > 4 cm	Y		A2	19.3292	$809.37
11450	Removal, sweat gland lesion	Y		A2	19.3292	$809.37
11451	Removal, sweat gland lesion	Y		A2	19.3292	$809.37

HCPCS Code	HCPCS Short Descriptor	Subject To Multiple Procedure Discounts	CY 2010 Comment Indicator	CY 2010 Payment Indicator	CY 2010 Third Year Transition. Pymt. Weight	CY 2010 Third Year Transition Payment
11462	Removal, sweat gland lesion	Y		A2	19.3292	$809.37
11463	Removal, sweat gland lesion	Y		A2	19.3292	$809.37
11470	Removal, sweat gland lesion	Y		A2	19.3292	$809.37
11471	Removal, sweat gland lesion	Y		A2	19.3292	$809.37
11600	Exc tr-ext mlg+marg 0.5 < cm	Y		P3		$80.39
11601	Exc tr-ext mlg+marg 0.6-1 cm	Y		P3		$96.30
11602	Exc tr-ext mlg+marg 1.1-2 cm	Y		P3		$105.39
11603	Exc tr-ext mlg+marg 2.1-3 cm	Y		P3		$112.77
11604	Exc tr-ext mlg+marg 3.1-4 cm	Y		A2	8.2762	$346.55
11606	Exc tr-ext mlg+marg > 4 cm	Y		A2	15.1023	$632.38
11620	Exc h-f-nk-sp mlg+marg 0.5 <	Y		P3		$82.66
11621	Exc h-f-nk-sp mlg+marg 0.6-1	Y		P3		$97.43
11622	Exc h-f-nk-sp mlg+marg 1.1-2	Y		P3		$107.94
11623	Exc h-f-nk-sp mlg+marg 2.1-3	Y		P3		$117.03
11624	Exc h-f-nk-sp mlg+marg 3.1-4	Y		A2	15.1023	$632.38
11626	Exc h-f-nk-sp mlg+mar > 4 cm	Y		A2	19.3292	$809.37
11640	Exc face-mm malig+marg 0.5 <	Y		P3		$86.92
11641	Exc face-mm malig+marg 0.6-1	Y		P3		$101.98
11642	Exc face-mm malig+marg 1.1-2	Y		P3		$113.62
11643	Exc face-mm malig+marg 2.1-3	Y		P3		$123.28
11644	Exc face-mm malig+marg 3.1-4	Y		A2	15.1023	$632.38
11646	Exc face-mm mlg+marg > 4 cm	Y		A2	19.3292	$809.37
11719	Trim nail(s)	Y		P3		$10.23
11720	Debride nail, 1-5	Y		P3		$12.50
11721	Debride nail, 6 or more	Y		P3		$15.06
11730	Removal of nail plate	Y		P2	0.8408	$35.21
11732	Remove nail plate, add-on	Y		P3		$15.06
11740	Drain blood from under nail	Y		P2	0.4244	$17.77
11750	Removal of nail bed	Y		P3		$81.24
11752	Remove nail bed/finger tip	Y		P3		$113.34
11755	Biopsy, nail unit	Y		P3		$55.68
11760	Repair of nail bed	Y		G2	1.2956	$54.25
11762	Reconstruction of nail bed	Y		P3		$104.25
11765	Excision of nail fold, toe	Y		P2	0.8408	$35.21
11770	Removal of pilonidal lesion	Y		A2	19.6948	$824.68
11771	Removal of pilonidal lesion	Y		A2	19.6948	$824.68
11772	Removal of pilonidal lesion	Y		A2	19.6948	$824.68
11900	Injection into skin lesions	Y		P3		$24.71
11901	Added skin lesions injection	Y	CH	P3		$27.27
11920	Correct skin color defects	Y		P3		$77.26
11921	Correct skin color defects	Y		P3		$85.79
11922	Correct skin color defects	Y		P3		$28.12
11950	Therapy for contour defects	Y		P3		$28.69
11951	Therapy for contour defects	Y		P3		$36.93
11952	Therapy for contour defects	Y	CH	P3		$47.15
11954	Therapy for contour defects	Y		P2	1.2956	$54.25
11960	Insert tissue expander(s)	Y		A2	19.7192	$825.70
11970	Replace tissue expander	Y		A2	36.3344	$1,521.43
11971	Remove tissue expander(s)	Y		A2	18.6836	$782.34
11976	Removal of contraceptive cap	Y		P3		$51.70
11980	Implant hormone pellet(s)	N		P2	0.6403	$26.81

HCPCS Code	HCPCS Short Descriptor	Subject To Multiple Procedure Discounts	CY 2010 Comment Indicator	CY 2010 Payment Indicator	CY 2010 Third Year Transition. Pymt. Weight	CY 2010 Third Year Transition Payment
11981	Insert drug implant device	N		P2	0.6403	$26.81
11982	Remove drug implant device	N		P2	0.6403	$26.81
11983	Remove/insert drug implant	N		P2	0.6403	$26.81
12001	Repair superficial wound(s)	Y		P2	1.2956	$54.25
12002	Repair superficial wound(s)	Y		P2	1.2956	$54.25
12004	Repair superficial wound(s)	Y		P2	1.2956	$54.25
12005	Repair superficial wound(s)	Y		A2	1.4926	$62.50
12006	Repair superficial wound(s)	Y		A2	1.4926	$62.50
12007	Repair superficial wound(s)	Y		A2	1.4926	$62.50
12011	Repair superficial wound(s)	Y		P2	1.2956	$54.25
12013	Repair superficial wound(s)	Y		P2	1.2956	$54.25
12014	Repair superficial wound(s)	Y		P2	1.2956	$54.25
12015	Repair superficial wound(s)	Y		G2	1.2956	$54.25
12016	Repair superficial wound(s)	Y		A2	1.4926	$62.50
12017	Repair superficial wound(s)	Y		A2	1.4926	$62.50
12018	Repair superficial wound(s)	Y		A2	1.4926	$62.50
12020	Closure of split wound	Y		A2	3.706	$155.18
12021	Closure of split wound	Y		A2	2.782	$116.49
12031	Intmd wnd repair s/tr/ext	Y		P2	1.2956	$54.25
12032	Intmd wnd repair s/tr/ext	Y		P2	3.0144	$126.22
12034	Intmd wnd repair s/tr/ext	Y		A2	1.4926	$62.50
12035	Intmd wnd repair s/tr/ext	Y		A2	1.4926	$62.50
12036	Intmd wnd repair s/tr/ext	Y		A2	2.782	$116.49
12037	Intmd wnd repair s/tr/ext	Y		A2	4.1074	$171.99
12041	Intmd wnd repair n-hf/genit	Y		P2	1.2956	$54.25
12042	Intmd wnd repair n-hg/genit	Y		P2	1.2956	$54.25
12044	Intmd wnd repair n-hg/genit	Y		A2	1.4926	$62.50
12045	Intmd wnd repair n-hg/genit	Y		A2	2.782	$116.49
12046	Intmd wnd repair n-hg/genit	Y		A2	2.782	$116.49
12047	Intmd wnd repair n-hg/genit	Y		A2	4.1074	$171.99
12051	Intmd wnd repair face/mm	Y		P2	1.2956	$54.25
12052	Intmd wnd repair face/mm	Y		P2	1.2956	$54.25
12053	Intmd wnd repair face/mm	Y		P2	1.2956	$54.25
12054	Intmd wnd repair, face/mm	Y		A2	1.4926	$62.50
12055	Intmd wnd repair face/mm	Y		A2	2.782	$116.49
12056	Intmd wnd repair face/mm	Y		A2	2.782	$116.49
12057	Intmd wnd repair face/mm	Y		A2	4.1074	$171.99
13100	Repair of wound or lesion	Y		A2	5.0314	$210.68
13101	Repair of wound or lesion	Y		A2	5.0314	$210.68
13102	Repair wound/lesion add-on	Y		A2	3.706	$155.18
13120	Repair of wound or lesion	Y		A2	2.782	$116.49
13121	Repair of wound or lesion	Y		A2	2.782	$116.49
13122	Repair wound/lesion add-on	Y		A2	1.4926	$62.50
13131	Repair of wound or lesion	Y		A2	2.782	$116.49
13132	Repair of wound or lesion	Y		A2	3.706	$155.18
13133	Repair wound/lesion add-on	Y		A2	2.782	$116.49
13150	Repair of wound or lesion	Y		A2	5.0314	$210.68
13151	Repair of wound or lesion	Y		A2	5.0314	$210.68
13152	Repair of wound or lesion	Y		A2	5.0314	$210.68
13153	Repair wound/lesion add-on	Y		A2	2.782	$116.49
13160	Late closure of wound	Y		A2	19.7192	$825.70

HCPCS Code	HCPCS Short Descriptor	Subject To Multiple Procedure Discounts	CY 2010 Comment Indicator	CY 2010 Payment Indicator	CY 2010 Third Year Transition. Pymt. Weight	CY 2010 Third Year Transition Payment
14000	Skin tissue rearrangement	Y		A2	14.0668	$589.02
14001	Skin tissue rearrangement	Y		A2	14.4325	$604.33
14020	Skin tissue rearrangement	Y		A2	14.4325	$604.33
14021	Skin tissue rearrangement	Y		A2	14.4325	$604.33
14040	Skin tissue rearrangement	Y		A2	14.0668	$589.02
14041	Skin tissue rearrangement	Y		A2	14.4325	$604.33
14060	Skin tissue rearrangement	Y		A2	14.4325	$604.33
14061	Skin tissue rearrangement	Y		A2	14.4325	$604.33
14300	Skin tissue rearrangement	N	CH	D5		
14301	Skin tissue rearrangement	Y	NI	G2	22.8955	$958.70
14302	Skin tissue rearrange add-on	Y	NI	G2	22.8955	$958.70
14350	Skin tissue rearrangement	Y		A2	20.0845	$841.00
15002	Wound prep, trk/arm/leg	Y		A2	5.0314	$210.68
15003	Wound prep, addl 100 cm	Y		A2	5.0314	$210.68
15004	Wound prep, f/n/hf/g	Y		A2	5.0314	$210.68
15005	Wnd prep, f/n/hf/g, addl cm	Y		A2	5.0314	$210.68
15040	Harvest cultured skin graft	Y		A2	2.782	$116.49
15050	Skin pinch graft	Y		A2	5.0314	$210.68
15100	Skin splt grft, trnk/arm/leg	Y		A2	19.7192	$825.70
15101	Skin splt grft t/a/l, add-on	Y		A2	20.0845	$841.00
15110	Epidrm autogrft trnk/arm/leg	Y		A2	5.7323	$240.03
15111	Epidrm autogrft t/a/l add-on	Y		A2	5.0868	$213.00
15115	Epidrm a-grft face/nck/hf/g	Y		A2	5.7323	$240.03
15116	Epidrm a-grft f/n/hf/g addl	Y		A2	5.0868	$213.00
15120	Skn splt a-grft fac/nck/hf/g	Y		A2	19.7192	$825.70
15121	Skn splt a-grft f/n/hf/g add	Y		A2	20.0845	$841.00
15130	Derm autograft, trnk/arm/leg	Y		A2	14.0668	$589.02
15131	Derm autograft t/a/l add-on	Y		A2	13.4213	$561.99
15135	Derm autograft face/nck/hf/g	Y		A2	14.0668	$589.02
15136	Derm autograft, f/n/hf/g add	Y		A2	13.4213	$561.99
15150	Cult epiderm grft t/arm/leg	Y		A2	5.7323	$240.03
15151	Cult epiderm grft t/a/l addl	Y		A2	5.0868	$213.00
15152	Cult epiderm graft t/a/l +%	Y		A2	5.0868	$213.00
15155	Cult epiderm graft, f/n/hf/g	Y		A2	5.7323	$240.03
15156	Cult epidrm grft f/n/hfg add	Y		A2	5.0868	$213.00
15157	Cult epiderm grft f/n/hfg +%	Y		A2	5.0868	$213.00
15170	Acell graft trunk/arms/legs	Y		G2	4.2464	$177.81
15171	Acell graft t/arm/leg add-on	Y		G2	3.0144	$126.22
15175	Acellular graft, f/n/hf/g	Y		G2	4.2464	$177.81
15176	Acell graft, f/n/hf/g add-on	Y		G2	4.2464	$177.81
15200	Skin full graft, trunk	Y		A2	14.4325	$604.33
15201	Skin full graft trunk add-on	Y		A2	13.3659	$559.67
15220	Skin full graft sclp/arm/leg	Y		A2	14.0668	$589.02
15221	Skin full graft add-on	Y		A2	5.0314	$210.68
15240	Skin full grft face/genit/hf	Y		A2	14.4325	$604.33
15241	Skin full graft add-on	Y		A2	5.0314	$210.68
15260	Skin full graft een & lips	Y		A2	14.0668	$589.02
15261	Skin full graft add-on	Y		A2	13.3659	$559.67
15300	Apply skinallogrft, t/arm/lg	Y		A2	5.0314	$210.68
15301	Apply sknallogrft t/a/l addl	Y		A2	5.0314	$210.68
15320	Apply skin allogrft f/n/hf/g	Y		A2	5.0314	$210.68

HCPCS Code	HCPCS Short Descriptor	Subject To Multiple Procedure Discounts	CY 2010 Comment Indicator	CY 2010 Payment Indicator	CY 2010 Third Year Transition. Pymt. Weight	CY 2010 Third Year Transition Payment
15321	Aply sknallogrft f/n/hfg add	Y		A2	5.0314	$210.68
15330	Aply acell alogrft t/arm/leg	Y		A2	5.0314	$210.68
15331	Aply acell grft t/a/l add-on	Y		A2	5.0314	$210.68
15335	Apply acell graft, f/n/hf/g	Y		A2	5.0314	$210.68
15336	Aply acell grft f/n/hf/g add	Y		A2	5.0314	$210.68
15340	Apply cult skin substitute	Y		G2	3.0144	$126.22
15341	Apply cult skin sub add-on	Y		G2	3.0144	$126.22
15360	Apply cult derm sub, t/a/l	Y		G2	3.0144	$126.22
15361	Aply cult derm sub t/a/l add	Y		G2	3.0144	$126.22
15365	Apply cult derm sub f/n/hf/g	Y		G2	3.0144	$126.22
15366	Apply cult derm f/hf/g add	Y		G2	3.0144	$126.22
15400	Apply skin xenograft, t/a/l	Y		A2	5.0314	$210.68
15401	Apply skn xenogrft t/a/l add	Y		A2	5.0314	$210.68
15420	Apply skin xgraft, f/n/hf/g	Y		A2	5.0314	$210.68
15421	Apply skn xgrft f/n/hf/g add	Y		A2	5.0314	$210.68
15430	Apply acellular xenograft	Y		A2	5.0314	$210.68
15431	Apply acellular xgraft add	Y		A2	5.0314	$210.68
15570	Form skin pedicle flap	Y		A2	20.0845	$841.00
15572	Form skin pedicle flap	Y		A2	20.0845	$841.00
15574	Form skin pedicle flap	Y		A2	20.0845	$841.00
15576	Form skin pedicle flap	Y		A2	20.0845	$841.00
15600	Skin graft	Y		A2	20.0845	$841.00
15610	Skin graft	Y		A2	20.0845	$841.00
15620	Skin graft	Y		A2	20.7702	$869.71
15630	Skin graft	Y		A2	20.0845	$841.00
15650	Transfer skin pedicle flap	Y		A2	21.2669	$890.51
15731	Forehead flap w/vasc pedicle	Y		A2	20.0845	$841.00
15732	Muscle-skin graft, head/neck	Y		A2	20.0845	$841.00
15734	Muscle-skin graft, trunk	Y		A2	20.0845	$841.00
15736	Muscle-skin graft, arm	Y		A2	20.0845	$841.00
15738	Muscle-skin graft, leg	Y		A2	20.0845	$841.00
15740	Island pedicle flap graft	Y		A2	14.0668	$589.02
15750	Neurovascular pedicle graft	Y		A2	19.7192	$825.70
15760	Composite skin graft	Y		A2	19.7192	$825.70
15770	Derma-fat-fascia graft	Y		A2	20.0845	$841.00
15775	Hair transplant punch grafts	Y		A2	2.818	$118.00
15776	Hair transplant punch grafts	Y		A2	2.818	$118.00
15780	Abrasion treatment of skin	Y		P3		$331.50
15781	Abrasion treatment of skin	Y		P2	4.1736	$174.76
15782	Abrasion treatment of skin	Y		P2	4.1736	$174.76
15783	Abrasion treatment of skin	Y		P2	2.677	$112.09
15786	Abrasion, lesion, single	Y		P2	0.8408	$35.21
15787	Abrasion, lesions, add-on	Y		P3		$25.00
15788	Chemical peel, face, epiderm	Y		P2	0.8408	$35.21
15789	Chemical peel, face, dermal	Y		P2	1.4745	$61.74
15792	Chemical peel, nonfacial	Y		P2	1.4745	$61.74
15793	Chemical peel, nonfacial	Y		P2	0.8408	$35.21
15819	Plastic surgery, neck	Y		G2	3.0144	$126.22
15820	Revision of lower eyelid	Y		A2	20.0845	$841.00
15821	Revision of lower eyelid	Y		A2	20.0845	$841.00
15822	Revision of upper eyelid	Y		A2	20.0845	$841.00

HCPCS Code	HCPCS Short Descriptor	Subject To Multiple Procedure Discounts	CY 2010 Comment Indicator	CY 2010 Payment Indicator	CY 2010 Third Year Transition. Pymt. Weight	CY 2010 Third Year Transition Payment
15823	Revision of upper eyelid	Y		A2	21.2669	$890.51
15824	Removal of forehead wrinkles	Y		A2	20.0845	$841.00
15825	Removal of neck wrinkles	Y		A2	20.0845	$841.00
15826	Removal of brow wrinkles	Y		A2	20.0845	$841.00
15828	Removal of face wrinkles	Y		A2	20.0845	$841.00
15829	Removal of skin wrinkles	Y		A2	21.2669	$890.51
15830	Exc skin abd	Y		A2	19.6948	$824.68
15832	Excise excessive skin tissue	Y		A2	19.6948	$824.68
15833	Excise excessive skin tissue	Y		A2	19.6948	$824.68
15834	Excise excessive skin tissue	Y		A2	19.6948	$824.68
15835	Excise excessive skin tissue	Y		A2	18.6282	$780.02
15836	Excise excessive skin tissue	Y		A2	15.468	$647.69
15837	Excise excessive skin tissue	Y		G2	16.7399	$700.95
15838	Excise excessive skin tissue	Y		G2	16.7399	$700.95
15839	Excise excessive skin tissue	Y		A2	15.468	$647.69
15840	Graft for face nerve palsy	Y		A2	20.7702	$869.71
15841	Graft for face nerve palsy	Y		A2	20.7702	$869.71
15842	Flap for face nerve palsy	Y		G2	22.8955	$958.70
15845	Skin and muscle repair, face	Y		A2	20.7702	$869.71
15847	Exc skin abd add-on	Y		A2	19.6948	$824.68
15850	Removal of sutures	Y		G2	2.677	$112.09
15851	Removal of sutures	Y		P3		$41.19
15852	Dressing change not for burn	N	CH	R2	0.6403	$26.81
15860	Test for blood flow in graft	N		G2	0.6403	$26.81
15876	Suction assisted lipectomy	Y		A2	20.0845	$841.00
15877	Suction assisted lipectomy	Y		A2	20.0845	$841.00
15878	Suction assisted lipectomy	Y		A2	20.0845	$841.00
15879	Suction assisted lipectomy	Y		A2	20.0845	$841.00
15920	Removal of tail bone ulcer	Y		A2	4.5669	$191.23
15922	Removal of tail bone ulcer	Y		A2	20.7702	$869.71
15931	Remove sacrum pressure sore	Y		A2	19.6948	$824.68
15933	Remove sacrum pressure sore	Y		A2	19.6948	$824.68
15934	Remove sacrum pressure sore	Y		A2	20.0845	$841.00
15935	Remove sacrum pressure sore	Y		A2	20.7702	$869.71
15936	Remove sacrum pressure sore	Y		A2	15.1179	$633.03
15937	Remove sacrum pressure sore	Y		A2	20.7702	$869.71
15940	Remove hip pressure sore	Y		A2	19.6948	$824.68
15941	Remove hip pressure sore	Y		A2	19.6948	$824.68
15944	Remove hip pressure sore	Y		A2	20.0845	$841.00
15945	Remove hip pressure sore	Y		A2	20.7702	$869.71
15946	Remove hip pressure sore	Y		A2	20.7702	$869.71
15950	Remove thigh pressure sore	Y		A2	19.6948	$824.68
15951	Remove thigh pressure sore	Y		A2	20.3802	$853.38
15952	Remove thigh pressure sore	Y		A2	14.4325	$604.33
15953	Remove thigh pressure sore	Y		A2	15.1179	$633.03
15956	Remove thigh pressure sore	Y		A2	14.4325	$604.33
15958	Remove thigh pressure sore	Y		A2	15.1179	$633.03
16000	Initial treatment of burn(s)	Y		P3		$22.72
16020	Dress/debrid p-thick burn, s	Y		P3		$34.37
16025	Dress/debrid p-thick burn, m	Y		A2	1.4893	$62.36
16030	Dress/debrid p-thick burn, l	Y		A2	1.676	$70.18

HCPCS Code	HCPCS Short Descriptor	Subject To Multiple Procedure Discounts	CY 2010 Comment Indicator	CY 2010 Payment Indicator	CY 2010 Third Year Transition. Pymt. Weight	CY 2010 Third Year Transition Payment
16035	Incision of burn scab, initi	Y		G2	1.4745	$61.74
17000	Destruct premalg lesion	Y		P2	0.8408	$35.21
17003	Destruct premalg les, 2-14	Y		P3		$3.12
17004	Destroy premlg lesions 15+	Y		P3		$69.88
17106	Destruction of skin lesions	Y		P2	2.677	$112.09
17107	Destruction of skin lesions	Y		P2	2.677	$112.09
17108	Destruction of skin lesions	Y		P2	2.677	$112.09
17110	Destruct b9 lesion, 1-14	Y		P2	0.8408	$35.21
17111	Destruct lesion, 15 or more	Y		P2	1.4745	$61.74
17250	Chemical cautery, tissue	Y		P3		$38.06
17260	Destruction of skin lesions	Y		P3		$39.77
17261	Destruction of skin lesions	Y		P2	1.4745	$61.74
17262	Destruction of skin lesions	Y		P2	1.4745	$61.74
17263	Destruction of skin lesions	Y		P2	1.4745	$61.74
17264	Destruction of skin lesions	Y		P2	1.4745	$61.74
17266	Destruction of skin lesions	Y	CH	P3		$94.88
17270	Destruction of skin lesions	Y		P2	1.4745	$61.74
17271	Destruction of skin lesions	Y		P2	1.4745	$61.74
17272	Destruction of skin lesions	Y		P2	1.4745	$61.74
17273	Destruction of skin lesions	Y	CH	P3		$86.35
17274	Destruction of skin lesions	Y	CH	P3		$97.72
17276	Destruction of skin lesions	Y	CH	P3		$107.09
17280	Destruction of skin lesions	Y		P2	1.4745	$61.74
17281	Destruction of skin lesions	Y		P3		$73.86
17282	Destruction of skin lesions	Y		P3		$84.37
17283	Destruction of skin lesions	Y	CH	P3		$96.86
17284	Destruction of skin lesions	Y	CH	P3		$108.80
17286	Destruction of skin lesions	Y		P2	2.677	$112.09
17311	Mohs, 1 stage, h/n/hf/g	Y		P2	4.7201	$197.64
17312	Mohs addl stage	Y	CH	P3		$192.88
17313	Mohs, 1 stage, t/a/l	Y		P2	4.7201	$197.64
17314	Mohs, addl stage, t/a/l	Y	CH	P3		$178.96
17315	Mohs surg, addl block	Y		P3		$32.67
17340	Cryotherapy of skin	Y		P3		$12.78
17360	Skin peel therapy	Y		P2	0.8408	$35.21
17380	Hair removal by electrolysis	Y		R2	0.8408	$35.21
19000	Drainage of breast lesion	Y		P3		$54.82
19001	Drain breast lesion add-on	Y		P3		$7.39
19020	Incision of breast lesion	Y		A2	16.472	$689.73
19030	Injection for breast x-ray	N		N1		
19100	Bx breast percut w/o image	Y		A2	4.6708	$195.58
19101	Biopsy of breast, open	Y		A2	20.3074	$850.33
19102	Bx breast percut w/image	Y		A2	6.978	$292.19
19103	Bx breast percut w/device	Y		A2	13.3824	$560.36
19105	Cryosurg ablate fa, each	Y	CH	P2	32.686	$1,368.66
19110	Nipple exploration	Y		A2	20.3074	$850.33
19112	Excise breast duct fistula	Y		A2	20.6727	$865.63
19120	Removal of breast lesion	Y		A2	20.6727	$865.63
19125	Excision, breast lesion	Y		A2	20.6727	$865.63
19126	Excision, addl breast lesion	Y		A2	20.6727	$865.63
19290	Place needle wire, breast	N		N1		

HCPCS Code	HCPCS Short Descriptor	Subject To Multiple Procedure Discounts	CY 2010 Comment Indicator	CY 2010 Payment Indicator	CY 2010 Third Year Transition. Pymt. Weight	CY 2010 Third Year Transition Payment
19291	Place needle wire, breast	N		N1		
19295	Place breast clip, percut	N		N1		
19296	Place po breast cath for rad	Y		A2	49.4283	$2,069.71
19297	Place breast cath for rad	Y		A2	49.4283	$2,069.71
19298	Place breast rad tube/caths	Y		A2	49.4283	$2,069.71
19300	Removal of breast tissue	Y		A2	21.3584	$894.34
19301	Partical mastectomy	Y		A2	20.6727	$865.63
19302	P-mastectomy w/ln removal	Y		A2	35.819	$1,499.85
19303	Mast, simple, complete	Y		A2	28.1131	$1,177.18
19304	Mast, subq	Y		A2	28.1131	$1,177.18
19316	Suspension of breast	Y		A2	28.1131	$1,177.18
19318	Reduction of large breast	Y		A2	33.7344	$1,412.56
19324	Enlarge breast	Y		A2	33.7344	$1,412.56
19325	Enlarge breast with implant	Y		A2	49.4283	$2,069.71
19328	Removal of breast implant	Y		A2	26.4165	$1,106.14
19330	Removal of implant material	Y		A2	26.4165	$1,106.14
19340	Immediate breast prosthesis	Y		A2	32.6834	$1,368.55
19342	Delayed breast prosthesis	Y		A2	44.693	$1,871.43
19350	Breast reconstruction	Y		A2	21.3584	$894.34
19355	Correct inverted nipple(s)	Y		A2	28.1131	$1,177.18
19357	Breast reconstruction	Y		A2	45.8754	$1,920.94
19366	Breast reconstruction	Y		A2	28.6098	$1,197.98
19370	Surgery of breast capsule	Y		A2	28.1131	$1,177.18
19371	Removal of breast capsule	Y		A2	28.1131	$1,177.18
19380	Revise breast reconstruction	Y		A2	34.2311	$1,433.36
19396	Design custom breast implant	Y		G2	32.686	$1,368.66
20000	Incision of abscess	Y		P2	1.3927	$58.32
20005	Incision of deep abscess	Y		A2	18.3436	$768.10
20103	Explore wound, extremity	Y		G2	12.0752	$505.62
20150	Excise epiphyseal bar	Y		G2	44.5617	$1,865.93
20200	Muscle biopsy	Y		A2	15.1023	$632.38
20205	Deep muscle biopsy	Y		A2	15.468	$647.69
20206	Needle biopsy, muscle	Y		A2	6.978	$292.19
20220	Bone biopsy, trocar/needle	Y		A2	7.3224	$306.61
20225	Bone biopsy, trocar/needle	Y		A2	14.9452	$625.80
20240	Bone biopsy, excisional	Y		A2	19.3292	$809.37
20245	Bone biopsy, excisional	Y		A2	19.6948	$824.68
20250	Open bone biopsy	Y		A2	18.7092	$783.41
20251	Open bone biopsy	Y		A2	18.7092	$783.41
20500	Injection of sinus tract	Y		P3		$44.03
20501	Inject sinus tract for x-ray	N		N1		
20520	Removal of foreign body	Y		P3		$79.82
20525	Removal of foreign body	Y		A2	19.6948	$824.68
20526	Ther injection, carp tunnel	Y		P3		$25.28
20550	Inj tendon sheath/ligament	Y		P3		$19.32
20551	Inj tendon origin/insertion	Y		P3		$19.60
20552	Inj trigger point, 1/2 muscl	Y		P3		$18.46
20553	Inject trigger points, =/> 3	Y		P3		$21.02
20555	Place ndl musc/tis for rt	Y	CH	R2	30.396	$1,272.77
20600	Drain/inject, joint/bursa	Y		P3		$19.60
20605	Drain/inject, joint/bursa	Y		P3		$21.87

HCPCS Code	HCPCS Short Descriptor	Subject To Multiple Procedure Discounts	CY 2010 Comment Indicator	CY 2010 Payment Indicator	CY 2010 Third Year Transition. Pymt. Weight	CY 2010 Third Year Transition Payment
20610	Drain/inject, joint/bursa	Y		P3		$31.25
20612	Aspirate/inj ganglion cyst	Y		P3		$21.02
20615	Treatment of bone cyst	Y		P3		$85.50
20650	Insert and remove bone pin	Y		A2	18.7092	$783.41
20662	Application of pelvis brace	Y		R2	21.0617	$881.92
20663	Application of thigh brace	Y		R2	21.0617	$881.92
20665	Removal of fixation device	N		G2	0.6403	$26.81
20670	Removal of support implant	Y		A2	14.457	$605.36
20680	Removal of support implant	Y		A2	19.6948	$824.68
20690	Apply bone fixation device	Y		A2	25.3445	$1,061.25
20692	Apply bone fixation device	Y		A2	25.7101	$1,076.56
20693	Adjust bone fixation device	Y		A2	18.7092	$783.41
20694	Remove bone fixation device	Y		A2	17.6983	$741.08
20696	Comp multiplane ext fixation	Y		G2	30.396	$1,272.77
20697	Comp ext fixate strut change	Y		G2	17.5996	$736.95
20822	Replantation digit, complete	Y		G2	27.0149	$1,131.19
20900	Removal of bone for graft	Y		A2	25.7101	$1,076.56
20902	Removal of bone for graft	Y		A2	26.3955	$1,105.26
20910	Remove cartilage for graft	Y		A2	20.0845	$841.00
20912	Remove cartilage for graft	Y		A2	20.0845	$841.00
20920	Removal of fascia for graft	Y		A2	15.1179	$633.03
20922	Removal of fascia for graft	Y		A2	14.4325	$604.33
20924	Removal of tendon for graft	Y		A2	26.3955	$1,105.26
20926	Removal of tissue for graft	Y		A2	6.7834	$284.04
20950	Fluid pressure, muscle	Y		G2	1.3927	$58.32
20972	Bone/skin graft, metatarsal	Y		G2	50.2514	$2,104.18
20973	Bone/skin graft, great toe	Y		R2	50.2514	$2,104.18
20975	Electrical bone stimulation	N		N1		
20979	Us bone stimulation	N		P3		$19.03
20982	Ablate, bone tumor(s) perq	Y		G2	44.5617	$1,865.93
20985	Cptr-asst dir ms px	N		N1		
21010	Incision of jaw joint	Y		A2	20.4597	$856.71
21011	Exc face les sc < 2 cm	Y	NI	P3		$147.14
21012	Exc face les sc = 2 cm	Y	NI	R2	7.8476	$328.60
21013	Exc face tum deep < 2 cm	Y	NI	P3		$203.96
21014	Exc face tum deep = 2 cm	Y	NI	R2	7.8476	$328.60
21015*	Resect face tum < 2 cm	Y	NI	R2	16.7399	$700.95
21016	Resect face tum = 2 cm	Y	NI	G2	22.3753	$936.92
21025	Excision of bone, lower jaw	Y		A2	33.3886	$1,398.08
21026	Excision of facial bone(s)	Y		A2	33.3886	$1,398.08
21029	Contour of face bone lesion	Y		A2	33.3886	$1,398.08
21030	Excise max/zygoma b9 tumor	Y		P3		$208.78
21031	Remove exostosis, mandible	Y		P3		$171.86
21032	Remove exostosis, maxilla	Y		P3		$174.98
21034	Excise max/zygoma mlg tumor	Y		A2	33.7542	$1,413.39
21040	Excise mandible lesion	Y		A2	20.4597	$856.71
21044	Removal of jaw bone lesion	Y		A2	33.3886	$1,398.08
21046	Remove mandible cyst complex	Y		A2	33.3886	$1,398.08
21047	Excise lwr jaw cyst w/repair	Y		A2	33.3886	$1,398.08
21048	Remove maxilla cyst complex	Y		R2	41.1215	$1,721.88
21050	Removal of jaw joint	Y		A2	33.7542	$1,413.39

HCPCS Code	HCPCS Short Descriptor	Subject To Multiple Procedure Discounts	CY 2010 Comment Indicator	CY 2010 Payment Indicator	CY 2010 Third Year Transition. Pymt. Weight	CY 2010 Third Year Transition Payment
21060	Remove jaw joint cartilage	Y		A2	33.3886	$1,398.08
21070	Remove coronoid process	Y		A2	33.7542	$1,413.39
21073	Mnpj of tmj w/anesth	Y		P3		$160.21
21076	Prepare face/oral prosthesis	Y		P3		$287.19
21077	Prepare face/oral prosthesis	Y		P3		$691.12
21079	Prepare face/oral prosthesis	Y		P3		$495.40
21080	Prepare face/oral prosthesis	Y		P3		$566.42
21081	Prepare face/oral prosthesis	Y		P3		$522.10
21082	Prepare face/oral prosthesis	Y		P3		$500.80
21083	Prepare face/oral prosthesis	Y		P3		$491.99
21084	Prepare face/oral prosthesis	Y		P3		$563.01
21085	Prepare face/oral prosthesis	Y		P3		$224.98
21086	Prepare face/oral prosthesis	Y		P3		$490.29
21087	Prepare face/oral prosthesis	Y		P3		$489.44
21088	Prepare face/oral prosthesis	Y		R2	41.1215	$1,721.88
21100	Maxillofacial fixation	Y		A2	33.3886	$1,398.08
21110	Interdental fixation	Y		P2	7.2897	$305.24
21116	Injection, jaw joint x-ray	N		N1		
21120	Reconstruction of chin	Y		A2	23.5956	$988.02
21121	Reconstruction of chin	Y		A2	23.5956	$988.02
21122	Reconstruction of chin	Y		A2	23.5956	$988.02
21123	Reconstruction of chin	Y		A2	23.5956	$988.02
21125	Augmentation, lower jaw bone	Y		A2	23.5956	$988.02
21127	Augmentation, lower jaw bone	Y		A2	38.4895	$1,611.67
21137	Reduction of forehead	Y		G2	23.8828	$1,000.04
21138	Reduction of forehead	Y		G2	41.1215	$1,721.88
21139	Reduction of forehead	Y		G2	41.1215	$1,721.88
21150	Reconstruct midface, lefort	Y		G2	41.1215	$1,721.88
21181	Contour cranial bone lesion	Y		A2	23.5956	$988.02
21198	Reconstr lwr jaw segment	Y		G2	41.1215	$1,721.88
21199	Reconstr lwr jaw w/advance	Y		G2	41.1215	$1,721.88
21206	Reconstruct upper jaw bone	Y		A2	34.9366	$1,462.90
21208	Augmentation of facial bones	Y		A2	36.5245	$1,529.39
21209	Reduction of facial bones	Y		A2	34.9366	$1,462.90
21210	Face bone graft	Y		A2	36.5245	$1,529.39
21215	Lower jaw bone graft	Y		A2	36.5245	$1,529.39
21230	Rib cartilage graft	Y		A2	36.5245	$1,529.39
21235	Ear cartilage graft	Y		A2	23.5956	$988.02
21240	Reconstruction of jaw joint	Y		A2	34.4396	$1,442.09
21242	Reconstruction of jaw joint	Y		A2	34.9366	$1,462.90
21243	Reconstruction of jaw joint	Y		A2	34.9366	$1,462.90
21244	Reconstruction of lower jaw	Y		A2	36.5245	$1,529.39
21245	Reconstruction of jaw	Y		A2	36.5245	$1,529.39
21246	Reconstruction of jaw	Y		A2	36.5245	$1,529.39
21248	Reconstruction of jaw	Y		A2	36.5245	$1,529.39
21249	Reconstruction of jaw	Y		A2	36.5245	$1,529.39
21260	Revise eye sockets	Y		G2	41.1215	$1,721.88
21267	Revise eye sockets	Y		A2	36.5245	$1,529.39
21270	Augmentation, cheek bone	Y		A2	34.9366	$1,462.90
21275	Revision, orbitofacial bones	Y		A2	36.5245	$1,529.39
21280	Revision of eyelid	Y		A2	34.9366	$1,462.90

HCPCS Code	HCPCS Short Descriptor	Subject To Multiple Procedure Discounts	CY 2010 Comment Indicator	CY 2010 Payment Indicator	CY 2010 Third Year Transition. Pymt. Weight	CY 2010 Third Year Transition Payment
21282	Revision of eyelid	Y		A2	16.4282	$687.90
21295	Revision of jaw muscle/bone	Y		A2	7.3694	$308.58
21296	Revision of jaw muscle/bone	Y		A2	19.8142	$829.68
21310	Treatment of nose fracture	Y		A2	1.6877	$70.67
21315	Treatment of nose fracture	Y		A2	13.1937	$552.46
21320	Treatment of nose fracture	Y		A2	14.8802	$623.08
21325	Treatment of nose fracture	Y		A2	21.5108	$900.72
21330	Treatment of nose fracture	Y		A2	22.0077	$921.53
21335	Treatment of nose fracture	Y		A2	23.5956	$988.02
21336	Treat nasal septal fracture	Y		A2	22.1427	$927.18
21337	Treat nasal septal fracture	Y		A2	14.8802	$623.08
21338	Treat nasoethmoid fracture	Y		A2	21.5108	$900.72
21339	Treat nasoethmoid fracture	Y		A2	22.0077	$921.53
21340	Treatment of nose fracture	Y		A2	34.4396	$1,442.09
21345	Treat nose/jaw fracture	Y		A2	23.5956	$988.02
21355	Treat cheek bone fracture	Y		A2	33.7542	$1,413.39
21356	Treat cheek bone fracture	Y		A2	20.8254	$872.02
21360	Treat cheek bone fracture	Y		G2	23.8828	$1,000.04
21390	Treat eye socket fracture	Y		G2	41.1215	$1,721.88
21400	Treat eye socket fracture	Y		A2	8.0147	$335.60
21401	Treat eye socket fracture	Y		A2	15.2459	$638.39
21406	Treat eye socket fracture	Y		G2	41.1215	$1,721.88
21407	Treat eye socket fracture	Y		G2	41.1215	$1,721.88
21421	Treat mouth roof fracture	Y		A2	21.5108	$900.72
21440	Treat dental ridge fracture	Y		P3		$281.22
21445	Treat dental ridge fracture	Y		A2	21.5108	$900.72
21450	Treat lower jaw fracture	Y		A2	3.3186	$138.96
21451	Treat lower jaw fracture	Y		A2	8.1184	$339.94
21452	Treat lower jaw fracture	Y		A2	14.8802	$623.08
21453	Treat lower jaw fracture	Y		A2	33.7542	$1,413.39
21454	Treat lower jaw fracture	Y		A2	22.0077	$921.53
21461	Treat lower jaw fracture	Y		A2	34.4396	$1,442.09
21462	Treat lower jaw fracture	Y		A2	34.9366	$1,462.90
21465	Treat lower jaw fracture	Y		A2	34.4396	$1,442.09
21480	Reset dislocated jaw	Y		A2	1.6877	$70.67
21485	Reset dislocated jaw	Y		A2	14.8802	$623.08
21490	Repair dislocated jaw	Y		A2	33.7542	$1,413.39
21495	Treat hyoid bone fracture	Y		G2	16.4437	$688.55
21497	Interdental wiring	Y		A2	14.8802	$623.08
21501	Drain neck/chest lesion	Y		A2	16.472	$689.73
21502	Drain chest lesion	Y		A2	18.3436	$768.10
21550	Biopsy of neck/chest	Y		G2	16.7399	$700.95
21552	Exc neck les sc = 3 cm	Y	NI	G2	22.3753	$936.92
21554	Exc neck tum deep = 5 cm	Y	NI	G2	22.3753	$936.92
21555*	Exc neck les sc < 3 cm	Y	NI	P3		$169.58
21556	Exc neck tum deep < 5 cm	Y	NI	G2	22.3753	$936.92
21557	Resect neck tum < 5 cm	Y	NI	G2	16.7399	$700.95
21558	Resect neck tum = 5 cm	Y	NI	G2	22.3753	$936.92
21600	Partial removal of rib	Y		A2	25.3445	$1,061.25
21610	Partial removal of rib	Y		A2	25.3445	$1,061.25
21685	Hyoid myotomy & suspension	Y		G2	7.2897	$305.24

HCPCS Code	HCPCS Short Descriptor	Subject To Multiple Procedure Discounts	CY 2010 Comment Indicator	CY 2010 Payment Indicator	CY 2010 Third Year Transition. Pymt. Weight	CY 2010 Third Year Transition Payment
21700	Revision of neck muscle	Y		A2	18.3436	$768.10
21720	Revision of neck muscle	Y		A2	18.7092	$783.41
21725	Revision of neck muscle	Y		A2	1.5497	$64.89
21800	Treatment of rib fracture	Y		A2	1.7811	$74.58
21805	Treatment of rib fracture	Y		A2	21.0916	$883.17
21820	Treat sternum fracture	Y		A2	1.7811	$74.58
21920	Biopsy soft tissue of back	Y		P3		$119.59
21925	Biopsy soft tissue of back	Y		A2	19.3292	$809.37
21930*	Exc back les sc < 3 cm	Y	NI	P3		$176.97
21931	Exc back les sc = 3 cm	Y	NI	G2	22.3753	$936.92
21932	Exc back tum deep < 5 cm	Y	NI	G2	16.7399	$700.95
21933	Exc back tum deep = 5 cm	Y	NI	G2	22.3753	$936.92
21935	Resect back tum < 5 cm	Y	NI	G2	16.7399	$700.95
21936	Resect back tum = 5 cm	Y	NI	G2	22.3753	$936.92
22102	Remove part, lumbar vertebra	Y		G2	47.0941	$1,971.97
22103	Remove extra spine segment	Y		G2	47.0941	$1,971.97
22305	Treat spine process fracture	Y		A2	1.7811	$74.58
22310	Treat spine fracture	Y		A2	4.0322	$168.84
22315	Treat spine fracture	Y		A2	13.7917	$577.50
22505	Manipulation of spine	Y		A2	13.5199	$566.12
22520	Percut vertebroplasty thor	Y		A2	30.4452	$1,274.83
22521	Percut vertebroplasty lumb	Y		A2	30.4452	$1,274.83
22522	Percut vertebroplasty addl	Y		A2	30.4452	$1,274.83
22523	Percut kyphoplasty, thor	Y		G2	84.8135	$3,551.40
22524	Percut kyphoplasty, lumbar	Y		G2	84.8135	$3,551.40
22525	Percut kyphoplasty, add-on	Y		G2	84.8135	$3,551.40
22900	Exc back tum deep < 5 cm	Y	NI	G2	22.3753	$936.92
22901	Exc back tum deep = 5 cm	Y	NI	G2	22.3753	$936.92
22902	Exc abd les sc < 3 cm	Y	NI	G2	16.7399	$700.95
22903	Exc abd les sc > 3 cm	Y	NI	G2	22.3753	$936.92
22904	Resect abd tum < 5 cm	Y	NI	G2	16.7399	$700.95
22905	Resect abd tum > 5 cm	Y	NI	G2	22.3753	$936.92
23000	Removal of calcium deposits	Y		A2	15.1023	$632.38
23020	Release shoulder joint	Y		A2	35.969	$1,506.13
23030	Drain shoulder lesion	Y		A2	15.8264	$662.70
23031	Drain shoulder bursa	Y		A2	16.8376	$705.04
23035	Drain shoulder bone lesion	Y		A2	18.7092	$783.41
23040	Exploratory shoulder surgery	Y		A2	25.7101	$1,076.56
23044	Exploratory shoulder surgery	Y		A2	26.3955	$1,105.26
23065	Biopsy shoulder tissues	Y		P3		$83.51
23066	Biopsy shoulder tissues	Y		A2	19.3292	$809.37
23071	Exc shoulder les sc > 3 cm	Y	NI	G2	22.3753	$936.92
23073	Exc shoulder tum deep > 5 cm	Y	NI	G2	22.3753	$936.92
23075*	Exc shoulder les sc < 3 cm	Y	NI	P3		$130.38
23076	Exc shoulder tum deep < 5 cm	Y	NI	G2	16.7399	$700.95
23077	Resect shoulder tum < 5 cm	Y	NI	G2	16.7399	$700.95
23078	Resect shoulder tum > 5 cm	Y	NI	G2	22.3753	$936.92
23100	Biopsy of shoulder joint	Y		A2	18.3436	$768.10
23101	Shoulder joint surgery	Y		A2	28.4804	$1,192.56
23105	Remove shoulder joint lining	Y		A2	26.3955	$1,105.26
23106	Incision of collarbone joint	Y		A2	26.3955	$1,105.26

HCPCS Code	HCPCS Short Descriptor	Subject To Multiple Procedure Discounts	CY 2010 Comment Indicator	CY 2010 Payment Indicator	CY 2010 Third Year Transition. Pymt. Weight	CY 2010 Third Year Transition Payment
23107	Explore treat shoulder joint	Y		A2	26.3955	$1,105.26
23120	Partial removal, collar bone	Y		A2	26.8925	$1,126.07
23125	Removal of collar bone	Y		A2	26.8925	$1,126.07
23130	Remove shoulder bone, part	Y		A2	37.5168	$1,570.94
23140	Removal of bone lesion	Y		A2	19.3946	$812.11
23145	Removal of bone lesion	Y		A2	26.8925	$1,126.07
23146	Removal of bone lesion	Y		A2	26.8925	$1,126.07
23150	Removal of humerus lesion	Y		A2	26.3955	$1,105.26
23155	Removal of humerus lesion	Y		A2	26.8925	$1,126.07
23156	Removal of humerus lesion	Y		A2	26.8925	$1,126.07
23170	Remove collar bone lesion	Y		A2	25.3445	$1,061.25
23172	Remove shoulder blade lesion	Y		A2	25.3445	$1,061.25
23174	Remove humerus lesion	Y		A2	25.3445	$1,061.25
23180	Remove collar bone lesion	Y		A2	26.3955	$1,105.26
23182	Remove shoulder blade lesion	Y		A2	26.3955	$1,105.26
23184	Remove humerus lesion	Y		A2	26.3955	$1,105.26
23190	Partial removal of scapula	Y		A2	26.3955	$1,105.26
23195	Removal of head of humerus	Y		A2	26.8925	$1,126.07
23330	Remove shoulder foreign body	Y		A2	7.7878	$326.10
23331	Remove shoulder foreign body	Y		A2	18.6836	$782.34
23350	Injection for shoulder x-ray	N		N1		
23395	Muscle transfer,shoulder/arm	Y		A2	37.5168	$1,570.94
23397	Muscle transfers	Y		A2	69.2933	$2,901.52
23400	Fixation of shoulder blade	Y		A2	28.4804	$1,192.56
23405	Incision of tendon & muscle	Y		A2	25.3445	$1,061.25
23406	Incise tendon(s) & muscle(s)	Y		A2	25.3445	$1,061.25
23410	Repair rotator cuff, acute	Y		A2	37.5168	$1,570.94
23412	Repair rotator cuff, chronic	Y		A2	39.1047	$1,637.43
23415	Release of shoulder ligament	Y		A2	37.5168	$1,570.94
23420	Repair of shoulder	Y		A2	39.1047	$1,637.43
23430	Repair biceps tendon	Y		A2	37.02	$1,550.14
23440	Remove/transplant tendon	Y		A2	37.02	$1,550.14
23450	Repair shoulder capsule	Y		A2	67.7054	$2,835.03
23455	Repair shoulder capsule	Y		A2	69.2933	$2,901.52
23460	Repair shoulder capsule	Y		A2	67.7054	$2,835.03
23462	Repair shoulder capsule	Y		A2	39.1047	$1,637.43
23465	Repair shoulder capsule	Y		A2	67.7054	$2,835.03
23466	Repair shoulder capsule	Y		A2	39.1047	$1,637.43
23480	Revision of collar bone	Y		A2	37.02	$1,550.14
23485	Revision of collar bone	Y		A2	69.2933	$2,901.52
23490	Reinforce clavicle	Y		A2	36.3344	$1,521.43
23491	Reinforce shoulder bones	Y		A2	66.5231	$2,785.52
23500	Treat clavicle fracture	Y		A2	1.7811	$74.58
23505	Treat clavicle fracture	Y		A2	13.7917	$577.50
23515	Treat clavicle fracture	Y		A2	49.8932	$2,089.18
23520	Treat clavicle dislocation	Y		A2	4.0322	$168.84
23525	Treat clavicle dislocation	Y		A2	4.0322	$168.84
23530	Treat clavicle dislocation	Y		A2	35.5372	$1,488.05
23532	Treat clavicle dislocation	Y		A2	22.1427	$927.18
23540	Treat clavicle dislocation	Y		A2	1.7811	$74.58
23545	Treat clavicle dislocation	Y		A2	4.0322	$168.84

HCPCS Code	HCPCS Short Descriptor	Subject To Multiple Procedure Discounts	CY 2010 Comment Indicator	CY 2010 Payment Indicator	CY 2010 Third Year Transition. Pymt. Weight	CY 2010 Third Year Transition Payment
23550	Treat clavicle dislocation	Y		A2	35.5372	$1,488.05
23552	Treat clavicle dislocation	Y		A2	36.2226	$1,516.75
23570	Treat shoulder blade fx	Y		A2	1.7811	$74.58
23575	Treat shoulder blade fx	Y		A2	4.0322	$168.84
23585	Treat scapula fracture	Y		A2	49.8932	$2,089.18
23600	Treat humerus fracture	Y		P2	1.5858	$66.40
23605	Treat humerus fracture	Y		A2	13.7917	$577.50
23615	Treat humerus fracture	Y		A2	50.5787	$2,117.88
23616	Treat humerus fracture	Y		A2	50.5787	$2,117.88
23620	Treat humerus fracture	Y		P2	1.5858	$66.40
23625	Treat humerus fracture	Y		A2	13.7917	$577.50
23630	Treat humerus fracture	Y		A2	51.0756	$2,138.69
23650	Treat shoulder dislocation	Y		A2	1.7811	$74.58
23655	Treat shoulder dislocation	Y		A2	12.8746	$539.10
23660	Treat shoulder dislocation	Y		A2	35.5372	$1,488.05
23665	Treat dislocation/fracture	Y		A2	4.0322	$168.84
23670	Treat dislocation/fracture	Y		A2	49.8932	$2,089.18
23675	Treat dislocation/fracture	Y		A2	1.7811	$74.58
23680	Treat dislocation/fracture	Y		A2	35.5372	$1,488.05
23700	Fixation of shoulder	Y		A2	12.8746	$539.10
23800	Fusion of shoulder joint	Y		A2	67.2085	$2,814.22
23802	Fusion of shoulder joint	Y		A2	39.1047	$1,637.43
23921	Amputation follow-up surgery	Y		A2	13.3659	$559.67
23930	Drainage of arm lesion	Y		A2	15.8264	$662.70
23931	Drainage of arm bursa	Y		A2	16.472	$689.73
23935	Drain arm/elbow bone lesion	Y		A2	18.3436	$768.10
24000	Exploratory elbow surgery	Y		A2	26.3955	$1,105.26
24006	Release elbow joint	Y		A2	26.3955	$1,105.26
24065	Biopsy arm/elbow soft tissue	Y		P3		$115.04
24066	Biopsy arm/elbow soft tissue	Y		A2	15.1023	$632.38
24071	Exc arm/elbow les sc = 3 cm	Y	NI	G2	22.3753	$936.92
24073	Ex arm/elbow tum deep > 5 cm	Y	NI	G2	22.3753	$936.92
24075*	Exc arm/elbow les sc < 3 cm	Y	NI	P3		$210.21
24076	Ex arm/elbow tum deep < 5 cm	Y	NI	G2	16.7399	$700.95
24077	Resect arm/elbow tum < 5 cm	Y	NI	G2	16.7399	$700.95
24079	Resect arm/elbow tum > 5 cm	Y	NI	G2	22.3753	$936.92
24100	Biopsy elbow joint lining	Y		A2	17.6983	$741.08
24101	Explore/treat elbow joint	Y		A2	26.3955	$1,105.26
24102	Remove elbow joint lining	Y		A2	26.3955	$1,105.26
24105	Removal of elbow bursa	Y		A2	18.7092	$783.41
24110	Remove humerus lesion	Y		A2	18.3436	$768.10
24115	Remove/graft bone lesion	Y		A2	25.7101	$1,076.56
24116	Remove/graft bone lesion	Y		A2	25.7101	$1,076.56
24120	Remove elbow lesion	Y		A2	18.7092	$783.41
24125	Remove/graft bone lesion	Y		A2	25.7101	$1,076.56
24126	Remove/graft bone lesion	Y		A2	25.7101	$1,076.56
24130	Removal of head of radius	Y		A2	25.7101	$1,076.56
24134	Removal of arm bone lesion	Y		A2	25.3445	$1,061.25
24136	Remove radius bone lesion	Y		A2	25.3445	$1,061.25
24138	Remove elbow bone lesion	Y		A2	25.3445	$1,061.25
24140	Partial removal of arm bone	Y		A2	25.7101	$1,076.56

HCPCS Code	HCPCS Short Descriptor	Subject To Multiple Procedure Discounts	CY 2010 Comment Indicator	CY 2010 Payment Indicator	CY 2010 Third Year Transition. Pymt. Weight	CY 2010 Third Year Transition Payment
24145	Partial removal of radius	Y		A2	25.7101	$1,076.56
24147	Partial removal of elbow	Y		A2	25.3445	$1,061.25
24149	Radical resection of elbow	Y		G2	30.396	$1,272.77
24152	Resect radius tumor	Y		G2	44.5617	$1,865.93
24153	Extensive radius surgery	N	CH	D5		
24155	Removal of elbow joint	Y		A2	36.3344	$1,521.43
24160	Remove elbow joint implant	Y		A2	25.3445	$1,061.25
24164	Remove radius head implant	Y		A2	25.7101	$1,076.56
24200	Removal of arm foreign body	Y		P3		$85.22
24201	Removal of arm foreign body	Y		A2	15.1023	$632.38
24220	Injection for elbow x-ray	N		N1		
24300	Manipulate elbow w/anesth	Y		G2	14.63	$612.60
24301	Muscle/tendon transfer	Y		A2	26.3955	$1,105.26
24305	Arm tendon lengthening	Y		A2	26.3955	$1,105.26
24310	Revision of arm tendon	Y		A2	18.7092	$783.41
24320	Repair of arm tendon	Y		A2	36.3344	$1,521.43
24330	Revision of arm muscles	Y		A2	66.5231	$2,785.52
24331	Revision of arm muscles	Y		A2	36.3344	$1,521.43
24332	Tenolysis, triceps	Y		G2	21.0617	$881.92
24340	Repair of biceps tendon	Y		A2	36.3344	$1,521.43
24341	Repair arm tendon/muscle	Y		A2	36.3344	$1,521.43
24342	Repair of ruptured tendon	Y		A2	36.3344	$1,521.43
24343	Repr elbow lat ligmnt w/tiss	Y		G2	30.396	$1,272.77
24344	Reconstruct elbow lat ligmnt	Y		G2	84.8135	$3,551.40
24345	Repr elbw med ligmnt w/tissu	Y		A2	25.3445	$1,061.25
24346	Reconstruct elbow med ligmnt	Y		G2	44.5617	$1,865.93
24357	Repair elbow, perc	Y		G2	30.396	$1,272.77
24358	Repair elbow w/deb, open	Y		G2	30.396	$1,272.77
24359	Repair elbow deb/attch open	Y		G2	30.396	$1,272.77
24360	Reconstruct elbow joint	Y		A2	32.7158	$1,369.91
24361	Reconstruct elbow joint	Y		H8	150.2992	$6,293.48
24362	Reconstruct elbow joint	Y		A2	45.772	$1,916.61
24363	Replace elbow joint	Y		H8	151.8871	$6,359.97
24365	Reconstruct head of radius	Y		A2	32.7158	$1,369.91
24366	Reconstruct head of radius	Y		H8	150.2992	$6,293.48
24400	Revision of humerus	Y		A2	37.02	$1,550.14
24410	Revision of humerus	Y		A2	37.02	$1,550.14
24420	Revision of humerus	Y		A2	36.3344	$1,521.43
24430	Repair of humerus	Y		A2	66.5231	$2,785.52
24435	Repair humerus with graft	Y		A2	67.2085	$2,814.22
24470	Revision of elbow joint	Y		A2	36.3344	$1,521.43
24495	Decompression of forearm	Y		A2	25.3445	$1,061.25
24498	Reinforce humerus	Y		A2	66.5231	$2,785.52
24500	Treat humerus fracture	Y		A2	1.7811	$74.58
24505	Treat humerus fracture	Y		A2	1.7811	$74.58
24515	Treat humerus fracture	Y		A2	50.5787	$2,117.88
24516	Treat humerus fracture	Y		A2	50.5787	$2,117.88
24530	Treat humerus fracture	Y		A2	1.7811	$74.58
24535	Treat humerus fracture	Y		A2	4.0322	$168.84
24538	Treat humerus fracture	Y		A2	21.0916	$883.17
24545	Treat humerus fracture	Y		A2	50.5787	$2,117.88

HCPCS Code	HCPCS Short Descriptor	Subject To Multiple Procedure Discounts	CY 2010 Comment Indicator	CY 2010 Payment Indicator	CY 2010 Third Year Transition. Pymt. Weight	CY 2010 Third Year Transition Payment
24546	Treat humerus fracture	Y		A2	51.0756	$2,138.69
24560	Treat humerus fracture	Y		A2	1.7811	$74.58
24565	Treat humerus fracture	Y		A2	1.7811	$74.58
24566	Treat humerus fracture	Y		A2	21.0916	$883.17
24575	Treat humerus fracture	Y		A2	49.8932	$2,089.18
24576	Treat humerus fracture	Y		A2	1.7811	$74.58
24577	Treat humerus fracture	Y		A2	4.0322	$168.84
24579	Treat humerus fracture	Y		A2	49.8932	$2,089.18
24582	Treat humerus fracture	Y		A2	21.0916	$883.17
24586	Treat elbow fracture	Y		A2	50.5787	$2,117.88
24587	Treat elbow fracture	Y		A2	51.0756	$2,138.69
24600	Treat elbow dislocation	Y		A2	1.7811	$74.58
24605	Treat elbow dislocation	Y		A2	13.5199	$566.12
24615	Treat elbow dislocation	Y		A2	49.8932	$2,089.18
24620	Treat elbow fracture	Y		A2	13.7917	$577.50
24635	Treat elbow fracture	Y		A2	49.8932	$2,089.18
24640	Treat elbow dislocation	Y		P3		$47.72
24650	Treat radius fracture	Y		P2	1.5858	$66.40
24655	Treat radius fracture	Y		A2	4.0322	$168.84
24665	Treat radius fracture	Y		A2	36.2226	$1,516.75
24666	Treat radius fracture	Y		A2	50.5787	$2,117.88
24670	Treat ulnar fracture	Y		A2	1.7811	$74.58
24675	Treat ulnar fracture	Y		A2	1.7811	$74.58
24685	Treat ulnar fracture	Y		A2	35.5372	$1,488.05
24800	Fusion of elbow joint	Y		A2	37.02	$1,550.14
24802	Fusion/graft of elbow joint	Y		A2	37.5168	$1,570.94
24925	Amputation follow-up surgery	Y		A2	18.7092	$783.41
25000	Incision of tendon sheath	Y		A2	18.7092	$783.41
25001	Incise flexor carpi radialis	Y		G2	21.0617	$881.92
25020	Decompress forearm 1 space	Y		A2	25.7101	$1,076.56
25023	Decompress forearm 1 space	Y		A2	25.7101	$1,076.56
25024	Decompress forearm 2 spaces	Y		A2	25.7101	$1,076.56
25025	Decompress forearm 2 spaces	Y		A2	25.7101	$1,076.56
25028	Drainage of forearm lesion	Y		A2	17.6983	$741.08
25031	Drainage of forearm bursa	Y		A2	18.3436	$768.10
25035	Treat forearm bone lesion	Y		A2	18.3436	$768.10
25040	Explore/treat wrist joint	Y		A2	26.8925	$1,126.07
25065	Biopsy forearm soft tissues	Y		P3		$116.75
25066	Biopsy forearm soft tissues	Y		A2	19.3292	$809.37
25071	Exc forearm les sc > 3 cm	Y	NI	G2	22.3753	$936.92
25073	Exc forearm tum deep = 3 cm	Y	NI	G2	22.3753	$936.92
25075*	Exc forearm les sc < 3 cm	Y	NI	P3		$140.89
25076	Exc forearm tum deep < 3 cm	Y	NI	G2	16.7399	$700.95
25077	Resect forearm/wrist tum<3cm	Y	NI	G2	16.7399	$700.95
25078	Resect forearm/wrist tum=3cm	Y	NI	G2	22.3753	$936.92
25085	Incision of wrist capsule	Y		A2	18.7092	$783.41
25100	Biopsy of wrist joint	Y		A2	18.3436	$768.10
25101	Explore/treat wrist joint	Y		A2	25.7101	$1,076.56
25105	Remove wrist joint lining	Y		A2	26.3955	$1,105.26
25107	Remove wrist joint cartilage	Y		A2	25.7101	$1,076.56
25109	Excise tendon forearm/wrist	Y		G2	21.0617	$881.92

HCPCS Code	HCPCS Short Descriptor	Subject To Multiple Procedure Discounts	CY 2010 Comment Indicator	CY 2010 Payment Indicator	CY 2010 Third Year Transition. Pymt. Weight	CY 2010 Third Year Transition Payment
25110	Remove wrist tendon lesion	Y		A2	18.7092	$783.41
25111	Remove wrist tendon lesion	Y		A2	18.7092	$783.41
25112	Reremove wrist tendon lesion	Y		A2	19.3946	$812.11
25115	Remove wrist/forearm lesion	Y		A2	19.3946	$812.11
25116	Remove wrist/forearm lesion	Y		A2	19.3946	$812.11
25118	Excise wrist tendon sheath	Y		A2	25.3445	$1,061.25
25119	Partial removal of ulna	Y		A2	25.7101	$1,076.56
25120	Removal of forearm lesion	Y		A2	25.7101	$1,076.56
25125	Remove/graft forearm lesion	Y		A2	25.7101	$1,076.56
25126	Remove/graft forearm lesion	Y		A2	25.7101	$1,076.56
25130	Removal of wrist lesion	Y		A2	25.7101	$1,076.56
25135	Remove & graft wrist lesion	Y		A2	25.7101	$1,076.56
25136	Remove & graft wrist lesion	Y		A2	25.7101	$1,076.56
25145	Remove forearm bone lesion	Y		A2	25.3445	$1,061.25
25150	Partial removal of ulna	Y		A2	25.3445	$1,061.25
25151	Partial removal of radius	Y		A2	25.3445	$1,061.25
25210	Removal of wrist bone	Y		A2	25.7101	$1,076.56
25215	Removal of wrist bones	Y		A2	26.3955	$1,105.26
25230	Partial removal of radius	Y		A2	26.3955	$1,105.26
25240	Partial removal of ulna	Y		A2	26.3955	$1,105.26
25246	Injection for wrist x-ray	N		N1		
25248	Remove forearm foreign body	Y		A2	18.3436	$768.10
25250	Removal of wrist prosthesis	Y		A2	24.699	$1,034.22
25251	Removal of wrist prosthesis	Y		A2	24.699	$1,034.22
25259	Manipulate wrist w/anesthes	Y		G2	17.5996	$736.95
25260	Repair forearm tendon/muscle	Y		A2	26.3955	$1,105.26
25263	Repair forearm tendon/muscle	Y		A2	25.3445	$1,061.25
25265	Repair forearm tendon/muscle	Y		A2	25.7101	$1,076.56
25270	Repair forearm tendon/muscle	Y		A2	26.3955	$1,105.26
25272	Repair forearm tendon/muscle	Y		A2	25.7101	$1,076.56
25274	Repair forearm tendon/muscle	Y		A2	26.3955	$1,105.26
25275	Repair forearm tendon sheath	Y		A2	26.3955	$1,105.26
25280	Revise wrist/forearm tendon	Y		A2	26.3955	$1,105.26
25290	Incise wrist/forearm tendon	Y		A2	25.7101	$1,076.56
25295	Release wrist/forearm tendon	Y		A2	18.7092	$783.41
25300	Fusion of tendons at wrist	Y		A2	25.7101	$1,076.56
25301	Fusion of tendons at wrist	Y		A2	25.7101	$1,076.56
25310	Transplant forearm tendon	Y		A2	36.3344	$1,521.43
25312	Transplant forearm tendon	Y		A2	37.02	$1,550.14
25315	Revise palsy hand tendon(s)	Y		A2	36.3344	$1,521.43
25316	Revise palsy hand tendon(s)	Y		A2	66.5231	$2,785.52
25320	Repair/revise wrist joint	Y		A2	36.3344	$1,521.43
25332	Revise wrist joint	Y		A2	32.7158	$1,369.91
25335	Realignment of hand	Y		A2	36.3344	$1,521.43
25337	Reconstruct ulna/radioulnar	Y		A2	37.5168	$1,570.94
25350	Revision of radius	Y		A2	36.3344	$1,521.43
25355	Revision of radius	Y		A2	36.3344	$1,521.43
25360	Revision of ulna	Y		A2	36.3344	$1,521.43
25365	Revise radius & ulna	Y		A2	36.3344	$1,521.43
25370	Revise radius or ulna	Y		A2	36.3344	$1,521.43
25375	Revise radius & ulna	Y		A2	37.02	$1,550.14

HCPCS Code	HCPCS Short Descriptor	Subject To Multiple Procedure Discounts	CY 2010 Comment Indicator	CY 2010 Payment Indicator	CY 2010 Third Year Transition. Pymt. Weight	CY 2010 Third Year Transition Payment
25390	Shorten radius or ulna	Y		A2	36.3344	$1,521.43
25391	Lengthen radius or ulna	Y		A2	37.02	$1,550.14
25392	Shorten radius & ulna	Y		A2	25.7101	$1,076.56
25393	Lengthen radius & ulna	Y		A2	37.02	$1,550.14
25394	Repair carpal bone, shorten	Y		G2	44.5617	$1,865.93
25400	Repair radius or ulna	Y		A2	36.3344	$1,521.43
25405	Repair/graft radius or ulna	Y		A2	67.2085	$2,814.22
25415	Repair radius & ulna	Y		A2	66.5231	$2,785.52
25420	Repair/graft radius & ulna	Y		A2	67.2085	$2,814.22
25425	Repair/graft radius or ulna	Y		A2	36.3344	$1,521.43
25426	Repair/graft radius & ulna	Y		A2	37.02	$1,550.14
25430	Vasc graft into carpal bone	Y		G2	44.5617	$1,865.93
25431	Repair nonunion carpal bone	Y		G2	44.5617	$1,865.93
25440	Repair/graft wrist bone	Y		A2	67.2085	$2,814.22
25441	Reconstruct wrist joint	Y		H8	150.2992	$6,293.48
25442	Reconstruct wrist joint	Y		H8	150.2992	$6,293.48
25443	Reconstruct wrist joint	Y		A2	45.772	$1,916.61
25444	Reconstruct wrist joint	Y		A2	45.772	$1,916.61
25445	Reconstruct wrist joint	Y		A2	45.772	$1,916.61
25446	Wrist replacement	Y		H8	151.8871	$6,359.97
25447	Repair wrist joint(s)	Y		A2	32.7158	$1,369.91
25449	Remove wrist joint implant	Y		A2	32.7158	$1,369.91
25450	Revision of wrist joint	Y		A2	36.3344	$1,521.43
25455	Revision of wrist joint	Y		A2	36.3344	$1,521.43
25490	Reinforce radius	Y		A2	36.3344	$1,521.43
25491	Reinforce ulna	Y		A2	36.3344	$1,521.43
25492	Reinforce radius and ulna	Y		A2	36.3344	$1,521.43
25500	Treat fracture of radius	Y		P2	1.5858	$66.40
25505	Treat fracture of radius	Y		A2	4.0322	$168.84
25515	Treat fracture of radius	Y		A2	35.5372	$1,488.05
25520	Treat fracture of radius	Y		A2	4.0322	$168.84
25525	Treat fracture of radius	Y		A2	36.2226	$1,516.75
25526	Treat fracture of radius	Y		A2	36.7196	$1,537.56
25530	Treat fracture of ulna	Y		P2	1.5858	$66.40
25535	Treat fracture of ulna	Y		A2	1.7811	$74.58
25545	Treat fracture of ulna	Y		A2	35.5372	$1,488.05
25560	Treat fracture radius & ulna	Y		P2	1.5858	$66.40
25565	Treat fracture radius & ulna	Y		A2	4.0322	$168.84
25574	Treat fracture radius & ulna	Y		A2	49.8932	$2,089.18
25575	Treat fracture radius/ulna	Y		A2	49.8932	$2,089.18
25600	Treat fracture radius/ulna	Y		P2	1.5858	$66.40
25605	Treat fracture radius/ulna	Y		A2	4.0322	$168.84
25606	Treat fx distal radial	Y		A2	21.4573	$898.48
25607	Treat fx rad extra-articul	Y		A2	51.0756	$2,138.69
25608	Treat fx rad intra-articul	Y		A2	51.0756	$2,138.69
25609	Treat fx radial 3+ frag	Y		A2	51.0756	$2,138.69
25622	Treat wrist bone fracture	Y		P2	1.5858	$66.40
25624	Treat wrist bone fracture	Y		A2	4.0322	$168.84
25628	Treat wrist bone fracture	Y		A2	35.5372	$1,488.05
25630	Treat wrist bone fracture	Y		P2	1.5858	$66.40
25635	Treat wrist bone fracture	Y		A2	4.0322	$168.84

HCPCS Code	HCPCS Short Descriptor	Subject To Multiple Procedure Discounts	CY 2010 Comment Indicator	CY 2010 Payment Indicator	CY 2010 Third Year Transition. Pymt. Weight	CY 2010 Third Year Transition Payment
25645	Treat wrist bone fracture	Y		A2	35.5372	$1,488.05
25650	Treat wrist bone fracture	Y		P2	1.5858	$66.40
25651	Pin ulnar styloid fracture	Y		G2	24.7255	$1,035.33
25652	Treat fracture ulnar styloid	Y		G2	43.499	$1,821.43
25660	Treat wrist dislocation	Y		A2	1.7811	$74.58
25670	Treat wrist dislocation	Y		A2	21.4573	$898.48
25671	Pin radioulnar dislocation	Y		A2	20.4461	$856.14
25675	Treat wrist dislocation	Y		A2	1.7811	$74.58
25676	Treat wrist dislocation	Y		A2	21.0916	$883.17
25680	Treat wrist fracture	Y		A2	1.7811	$74.58
25685	Treat wrist fracture	Y		A2	21.4573	$898.48
25690	Treat wrist dislocation	Y		A2	13.7917	$577.50
25695	Treat wrist dislocation	Y		A2	21.0916	$883.17
25800	Fusion of wrist joint	Y		A2	67.2085	$2,814.22
25805	Fusion/graft of wrist joint	Y		A2	37.5168	$1,570.94
25810	Fusion/graft of wrist joint	Y		A2	67.7054	$2,835.03
25820	Fusion of hand bones	Y		A2	37.02	$1,550.14
25825	Fuse hand bones with graft	Y		A2	67.7054	$2,835.03
25830	Fusion, radioulnar jnt/ulna	Y		A2	67.7054	$2,835.03
25907	Amputation follow-up surgery	Y		A2	18.7092	$783.41
25922	Amputate hand at wrist	Y		A2	18.7092	$783.41
25929	Amputation follow-up surgery	Y		A2	14.4325	$604.33
25931	Amputation follow-up surgery	Y		G2	21.0617	$881.92
26010	Drainage of finger abscess	Y		P2	1.3927	$58.32
26011	Drainage of finger abscess	Y		A2	10.9586	$458.87
26020	Drain hand tendon sheath	Y		A2	14.7756	$618.70
26025	Drainage of palm bursa	Y		A2	14.1301	$591.67
26030	Drainage of palm bursa(s)	Y		A2	14.7756	$618.70
26034	Treat hand bone lesion	Y		A2	14.7756	$618.70
26035	Decompress fingers/hand	Y		G2	16.3041	$682.70
26037	Decompress fingers/hand	Y	CH	G2	16.3041	$682.70
26040	Release palm contracture	Y		A2	23.8595	$999.07
26045	Release palm contracture	Y		A2	23.1741	$970.37
26055	Incise finger tendon sheath	Y		A2	14.7756	$618.70
26060	Incision of finger tendon	Y		A2	14.7756	$618.70
26070	Explore/treat hand joint	Y		A2	14.7756	$618.70
26075	Explore/treat finger joint	Y		A2	15.8267	$662.71
26080	Explore/treat finger joint	Y		A2	15.8267	$662.71
26100	Biopsy hand joint lining	Y		A2	14.7756	$618.70
26105	Biopsy finger joint lining	Y		A2	14.1301	$591.67
26110	Biopsy finger joint lining	Y		A2	14.1301	$591.67
26111	Exc hand les sc > 1.5 cm	Y	NI	G2	22.3753	$936.92
26113	Exc hand tum deep > 1.5 cm	Y	NI	G2	22.3753	$936.92
26115*	Exc hand les sc < 1.5 cm	Y	NI	P3		$287.19
26116	Exc hand tum deep < 1.5 cm	Y	NI	G2	16.7399	$700.95
26117	Exc hand tum ra < 3 cm	Y	NI	G2	16.7399	$700.95
26118	Exc hand tum ra > 3 cm	Y	NI	G2	22.3753	$936.92
26121	Release palm contracture	Y		A2	23.8595	$999.07
26123	Release palm contracture	Y		A2	23.8595	$999.07
26125	Release palm contracture	Y		A2	15.8267	$662.71
26130	Remove wrist joint lining	Y		A2	15.141	$634.00

HCPCS Code	HCPCS Short Descriptor	Subject To Multiple Procedure Discounts	CY 2010 Comment Indicator	CY 2010 Payment Indicator	CY 2010 Third Year Transition. Pymt. Weight	CY 2010 Third Year Transition Payment
26135	Revise finger joint, each	Y		A2	23.8595	$999.07
26140	Revise finger joint, each	Y		A2	14.7756	$618.70
26145	Tendon excision, palm/finger	Y		A2	15.141	$634.00
26160	Remove tendon sheath lesion	Y		A2	15.141	$634.00
26170	Removal of palm tendon, each	Y		A2	15.141	$634.00
26180	Removal of finger tendon	Y		A2	15.141	$634.00
26185	Remove finger bone	Y		A2	15.8267	$662.71
26200	Remove hand bone lesion	Y		A2	14.7756	$618.70
26205	Remove/graft bone lesion	Y		A2	23.1741	$970.37
26210	Removal of finger lesion	Y		A2	14.7756	$618.70
26215	Remove/graft finger lesion	Y		A2	15.141	$634.00
26230	Partial removal of hand bone	Y		A2	17.8996	$749.51
26235	Partial removal, finger bone	Y		A2	15.141	$634.00
26236	Partial removal, finger bone	Y		A2	15.141	$634.00
26250	Extensive hand surgery	Y		A2	15.141	$634.00
26255	Extensive hand surgery	N	CH	D5		
26260	Resect prox finger tumor	Y		A2	15.141	$634.00
26261	Extensive finger surgery	N	CH	D5		
26262	Resect distal finger tumor	Y		A2	14.7756	$618.70
26320	Removal of implant from hand	Y		A2	15.1023	$632.38
26340	Manipulate finger w/anesth	Y		G2	4.587	$192.07
26350	Repair finger/hand tendon	Y		A2	22.1632	$928.04
26352	Repair/graft hand tendon	Y		A2	23.8595	$999.07
26356	Repair finger/hand tendon	Y		A2	23.8595	$999.07
26357	Repair finger/hand tendon	Y		A2	23.8595	$999.07
26358	Repair/graft hand tendon	Y		A2	23.8595	$999.07
26370	Repair finger/hand tendon	Y		A2	23.8595	$999.07
26372	Repair/graft hand tendon	Y		A2	23.8595	$999.07
26373	Repair finger/hand tendon	Y		A2	23.1741	$970.37
26390	Revise hand/finger tendon	Y		A2	23.8595	$999.07
26392	Repair/graft hand tendon	Y		A2	23.1741	$970.37
26410	Repair hand tendon	Y		A2	15.141	$634.00
26412	Repair/graft hand tendon	Y		A2	23.1741	$970.37
26415	Excision, hand/finger tendon	Y		A2	23.8595	$999.07
26416	Graft hand or finger tendon	Y		A2	23.1741	$970.37
26418	Repair finger tendon	Y		A2	15.8267	$662.71
26420	Repair/graft finger tendon	Y		A2	23.8595	$999.07
26426	Repair finger/hand tendon	Y		A2	23.1741	$970.37
26428	Repair/graft finger tendon	Y		A2	23.1741	$970.37
26432	Repair finger tendon	Y		A2	15.141	$634.00
26433	Repair finger tendon	Y		A2	15.141	$634.00
26434	Repair/graft finger tendon	Y		A2	23.1741	$970.37
26437	Realignment of tendons	Y		A2	15.141	$634.00
26440	Release palm/finger tendon	Y		A2	15.141	$634.00
26442	Release palm & finger tendon	Y		A2	23.1741	$970.37
26445	Release hand/finger tendon	Y		A2	15.141	$634.00
26449	Release forearm/hand tendon	Y		A2	23.1741	$970.37
26450	Incision of palm tendon	Y		A2	15.141	$634.00
26455	Incision of finger tendon	Y		A2	15.141	$634.00
26460	Incise hand/finger tendon	Y		A2	15.141	$634.00
26471	Fusion of finger tendons	Y		A2	14.7756	$618.70

HCPCS Code	HCPCS Short Descriptor	Subject To Multiple Procedure Discounts	CY 2010 Comment Indicator	CY 2010 Payment Indicator	CY 2010 Third Year Transition. Pymt. Weight	CY 2010 Third Year Transition Payment
26474	Fusion of finger tendons	Y		A2	14.7756	$618.70
26476	Tendon lengthening	Y		A2	14.1301	$591.67
26477	Tendon shortening	Y		A2	14.1301	$591.67
26478	Lengthening of hand tendon	Y		A2	14.1301	$591.67
26479	Shortening of hand tendon	Y		A2	14.1301	$591.67
26480	Transplant hand tendon	Y		A2	23.1741	$970.37
26483	Transplant/graft hand tendon	Y		A2	23.1741	$970.37
26485	Transplant palm tendon	Y		A2	22.8085	$955.06
26489	Transplant/graft palm tendon	Y		A2	23.1741	$970.37
26490	Revise thumb tendon	Y		A2	23.1741	$970.37
26492	Tendon transfer with graft	Y		A2	23.1741	$970.37
26494	Hand tendon/muscle transfer	Y		A2	23.1741	$970.37
26496	Revise thumb tendon	Y		A2	23.1741	$970.37
26497	Finger tendon transfer	Y		A2	23.1741	$970.37
26498	Finger tendon transfer	Y		A2	23.8595	$999.07
26499	Revision of finger	Y		A2	23.1741	$970.37
26500	Hand tendon reconstruction	Y		A2	15.8267	$662.71
26502	Hand tendon reconstruction	Y		A2	23.8595	$999.07
26508	Release thumb contracture	Y		A2	15.141	$634.00
26510	Thumb tendon transfer	Y		A2	23.1741	$970.37
26516	Fusion of knuckle joint	Y		A2	22.1632	$928.04
26517	Fusion of knuckle joints	Y		A2	23.1741	$970.37
26518	Fusion of knuckle joints	Y		A2	23.1741	$970.37
26520	Release knuckle contracture	Y		A2	15.141	$634.00
26525	Release finger contracture	Y		A2	15.141	$634.00
26530	Revise knuckle joint	Y		A2	31.5334	$1,320.40
26531	Revise knuckle with implant	Y		A2	47.3599	$1,983.10
26535	Revise finger joint	Y		A2	32.7158	$1,369.91
26536	Revise/implant finger joint	Y		A2	45.772	$1,916.61
26540	Repair hand joint	Y		A2	15.8267	$662.71
26541	Repair hand joint with graft	Y		A2	25.9444	$1,086.37
26542	Repair hand joint with graft	Y		A2	15.8267	$662.71
26545	Reconstruct finger joint	Y		A2	23.8595	$999.07
26546	Repair nonunion hand	Y		A2	23.8595	$999.07
26548	Reconstruct finger joint	Y		A2	23.8595	$999.07
26550	Construct thumb replacement	Y		A2	22.8085	$955.06
26555	Positional change of finger	Y		A2	23.1741	$970.37
26560	Repair of web finger	Y		A2	14.7756	$618.70
26561	Repair of web finger	Y		A2	23.1741	$970.37
26562	Repair of web finger	Y		A2	23.8595	$999.07
26565	Correct metacarpal flaw	Y		A2	24.3565	$1,019.88
26567	Correct finger deformity	Y		A2	24.3565	$1,019.88
26568	Lengthen metacarpal/finger	Y		A2	23.1741	$970.37
26580	Repair hand deformity	Y		A2	16.3234	$683.51
26587	Reconstruct extra finger	Y		A2	16.3234	$683.51
26590	Repair finger deformity	Y		A2	16.3234	$683.51
26591	Repair muscles of hand	Y		A2	23.1741	$970.37
26593	Release muscles of hand	Y		A2	15.141	$634.00
26596	Excision constricting tissue	Y		A2	14.7756	$618.70
26600	Treat metacarpal fracture	Y		P2	1.5858	$66.40
26605	Treat metacarpal fracture	Y		A2	1.7811	$74.58

HCPCS Code	HCPCS Short Descriptor	Subject To Multiple Procedure Discounts	CY 2010 Comment Indicator	CY 2010 Payment Indicator	CY 2010 Third Year Transition. Pymt. Weight	CY 2010 Third Year Transition Payment
26607	Treat metacarpal fracture	Y		A2	13.7917	$577.50
26608	Treat metacarpal fracture	Y		A2	22.1427	$927.18
26615	Treat metacarpal fracture	Y		A2	36.2226	$1,516.75
26641	Treat thumb dislocation	Y		P2	1.5858	$66.40
26645	Treat thumb fracture	Y		A2	4.0322	$168.84
26650	Treat thumb fracture	Y		A2	21.0916	$883.17
26665	Treat thumb fracture	Y		A2	36.2226	$1,516.75
26670	Treat hand dislocation	Y		P2	1.5858	$66.40
26675	Treat hand dislocation	Y		A2	4.0322	$168.84
26676	Pin hand dislocation	Y		A2	21.0916	$883.17
26685	Treat hand dislocation	Y		A2	21.4573	$898.48
26686	Treat hand dislocation	Y		A2	49.8932	$2,089.18
26700	Treat knuckle dislocation	Y		P2	1.5858	$66.40
26705	Treat knuckle dislocation	Y		A2	1.7811	$74.58
26706	Pin knuckle dislocation	Y		A2	13.7917	$577.50
26715	Treat knuckle dislocation	Y		A2	22.1427	$927.18
26720	Treat finger fracture, each	Y		P2	1.5858	$66.40
26725	Treat finger fracture, each	Y		P2	1.5858	$66.40
26727	Treat finger fracture, each	Y		A2	24.2275	$1,014.48
26735	Treat finger fracture, each	Y		A2	22.1427	$927.18
26740	Treat finger fracture, each	Y		P2	1.5858	$66.40
26742	Treat finger fracture, each	Y		A2	1.7811	$74.58
26746	Treat finger fracture, each	Y		A2	22.6396	$947.99
26750	Treat finger fracture, each	Y		P2	1.5858	$66.40
26755	Treat finger fracture, each	Y		G2	1.5858	$66.40
26756	Pin finger fracture, each	Y		A2	21.0916	$883.17
26765	Treat finger fracture, each	Y		A2	22.1427	$927.18
26770	Treat finger dislocation	Y		G2	1.5858	$66.40
26775	Treat finger dislocation	Y		P3		$143.17
26776	Pin finger dislocation	Y		A2	21.0916	$883.17
26785	Treat finger dislocation	Y		A2	21.0916	$883.17
26820	Thumb fusion with graft	Y		A2	24.3565	$1,019.88
26841	Fusion of thumb	Y		A2	23.8595	$999.07
26842	Thumb fusion with graft	Y		A2	23.8595	$999.07
26843	Fusion of hand joint	Y		A2	23.1741	$970.37
26844	Fusion/graft of hand joint	Y		A2	23.1741	$970.37
26850	Fusion of knuckle	Y		A2	23.8595	$999.07
26852	Fusion of knuckle with graft	Y		A2	23.8595	$999.07
26860	Fusion of finger joint	Y		A2	23.1741	$970.37
26861	Fusion of finger jnt, add-on	Y		A2	22.8085	$955.06
26862	Fusion/graft of finger joint	Y		A2	23.8595	$999.07
26863	Fuse/graft added joint	Y		A2	23.1741	$970.37
26910	Amputate metacarpal bone	Y		A2	23.1741	$970.37
26951	Amputation of finger/thumb	Y		A2	14.7756	$618.70
26952	Amputation of finger/thumb	Y		A2	15.8267	$662.71
26990	Drainage of pelvis lesion	Y		A2	17.6983	$741.08
26991	Drainage of pelvis bursa	Y		A2	17.6983	$741.08
27000	Incision of hip tendon	Y		A2	18.3436	$768.10
27001	Incision of hip tendon	Y		A2	25.7101	$1,076.56
27003	Incision of hip tendon	Y		A2	25.7101	$1,076.56
27033	Exploration of hip joint	Y		A2	36.3344	$1,521.43

HCPCS Code	HCPCS Short Descriptor	Subject To Multiple Procedure Discounts	CY 2010 Comment Indicator	CY 2010 Payment Indicator	CY 2010 Third Year Transition. Pymt. Weight	CY 2010 Third Year Transition Payment
27035	Denervation of hip joint	Y		A2	37.02	$1,550.14
27040	Biopsy of soft tissues	Y		A2	7.7878	$326.10
27041	Biopsy of soft tissues	Y		A2	8.2762	$346.55
27043	Exc hip pelvis les sc > 3 cm	Y	NI	G2	22.3753	$936.92
27045	Exc hip/pelv tum deep > 5 cm	Y	NI	G2	22.3753	$936.92
27047*	Exc hip/pelvis les sc < 3 cm	Y	NI	P3		$200.26
27048	Exc hip/pelv tum deep < 5 cm	Y	NI	G2	16.7399	$700.95
27049	Resect hip/pelv tum < 5 cm	Y	NI	G2	16.7399	$700.95
27050	Biopsy of sacroiliac joint	Y		A2	18.7092	$783.41
27052	Biopsy of hip joint	Y		A2	18.7092	$783.41
27059	Resect hip/pelv tum > 5 cm	Y	NI	G2	22.3753	$936.92
27060	Removal of ischial bursa	Y		A2	19.8916	$832.92
27062	Remove femur lesion/bursa	Y		A2	19.8916	$832.92
27065	Removal of hip bone lesion	Y		A2	19.8916	$832.92
27066	Removal of hip bone lesion	Y		A2	26.8925	$1,126.07
27067	Remove/graft hip bone lesion	Y		A2	26.8925	$1,126.07
27080	Removal of tail bone	Y		A2	25.3445	$1,061.25
27086	Remove hip foreign body	Y		A2	7.7878	$326.10
27087	Remove hip foreign body	Y		A2	18.7092	$783.41
27093	Injection for hip x-ray	N		N1		
27095	Injection for hip x-ray	N		N1		
27097	Revision of hip tendon	Y		A2	25.7101	$1,076.56
27098	Transfer tendon to pelvis	Y		A2	25.7101	$1,076.56
27100	Transfer of abdominal muscle	Y		A2	37.02	$1,550.14
27105	Transfer of spinal muscle	Y		A2	37.02	$1,550.14
27110	Transfer of iliopsoas muscle	Y		A2	37.02	$1,550.14
27111	Transfer of iliopsoas muscle	Y		A2	37.02	$1,550.14
27193	Treat pelvic ring fracture	Y		A2	1.7811	$74.58
27194	Treat pelvic ring fracture	Y		A2	13.5199	$566.12
27200	Treat tail bone fracture	Y	CH	P3		$63.63
27202	Treat tail bone fracture	Y		A2	35.1716	$1,472.74
27220	Treat hip socket fracture	Y		G2	1.5858	$66.40
27230	Treat thigh fracture	Y		A2	1.7811	$74.58
27238	Treat thigh fracture	Y		A2	4.0322	$168.84
27246	Treat thigh fracture	Y		A2	4.0322	$168.84
27250	Treat hip dislocation	Y		A2	1.7811	$74.58
27252	Treat hip dislocation	Y		A2	13.5199	$566.12
27256	Treat hip dislocation	Y		G2	1.5858	$66.40
27257	Treat hip dislocation	Y		A2	13.8856	$581.43
27265	Treat hip dislocation	Y		A2	1.7811	$74.58
27266	Treat hip dislocation	Y		A2	13.5199	$566.12
27267	Cltx thigh fx	Y		G2	1.5858	$66.40
27275	Manipulation of hip joint	Y		A2	13.5199	$566.12
27301	Drain thigh/knee lesion	Y		A2	16.8376	$705.04
27305	Incise thigh tendon & fascia	Y		A2	18.3436	$768.10
27306	Incision of thigh tendon	Y		A2	18.7092	$783.41
27307	Incision of thigh tendons	Y		A2	18.7092	$783.41
27310	Exploration of knee joint	Y		A2	26.3955	$1,105.26
27323	Biopsy, thigh soft tissues	Y		A2	7.7878	$326.10
27324	Biopsy, thigh soft tissues	Y		A2	18.6836	$782.34
27325	Neurectomy, hamstring	Y		A2	15.9795	$669.11

HCPCS Code	HCPCS Short Descriptor	Subject To Multiple Procedure Discounts	CY 2010 Comment Indicator	CY 2010 Payment Indicator	CY 2010 Third Year Transition. Pymt. Weight	CY 2010 Third Year Transition Payment
27326	Neurectomy, popliteal	Y		A2	15.9795	$669.11
27327*	Exc thigh/knee les sc < 3 cm	Y	NI	P3		$182.37
27328	Exc thigh/knee tum deep <5cm	Y	NI	G2	16.7399	$700.95
27329	Resect thigh/knee tum < 5 cm	Y	NI	G2	16.7399	$700.95
27330	Biopsy, knee joint lining	Y		A2	26.3955	$1,105.26
27331	Explore/treat knee joint	Y		A2	26.3955	$1,105.26
27332	Removal of knee cartilage	Y		A2	26.3955	$1,105.26
27333	Removal of knee cartilage	Y		A2	26.3955	$1,105.26
27334	Remove knee joint lining	Y		A2	26.3955	$1,105.26
27335	Remove knee joint lining	Y		A2	26.3955	$1,105.26
27337	Exc thigh/knee les sc > 3 cm	Y	NI	G2	22.3753	$936.92
27339	Exc thigh/knee tum deep >5cm	Y	NI	G2	22.3753	$936.92
27340	Removal of kneecap bursa	Y		A2	18.7092	$783.41
27345	Removal of knee cyst	Y		A2	19.3946	$812.11
27347	Remove knee cyst	Y		A2	19.3946	$812.11
27350	Removal of kneecap	Y		A2	26.3955	$1,105.26
27355	Remove femur lesion	Y		A2	25.7101	$1,076.56
27356	Remove femur lesion/graft	Y		A2	26.3955	$1,105.26
27357	Remove femur lesion/graft	Y		A2	26.8925	$1,126.07
27358	Remove femur lesion/fixation	Y		A2	26.8925	$1,126.07
27360	Partial removal, leg bone(s)	Y		A2	26.8925	$1,126.07
27364	Resect thigh/knee tum >5 cm	Y	NI	G2	22.3753	$936.92
27370	Injection for knee x-ray	N		N1		
27372	Removal of foreign body	Y		A2	22.4651	$940.68
27380	Repair of kneecap tendon	Y		A2	17.6983	$741.08
27381	Repair/graft kneecap tendon	Y		A2	18.7092	$783.41
27385	Repair of thigh muscle	Y		A2	18.7092	$783.41
27386	Repair/graft of thigh muscle	Y		A2	18.7092	$783.41
27390	Incision of thigh tendon	Y		A2	17.6983	$741.08
27391	Incision of thigh tendons	Y		A2	18.3436	$768.10
27392	Incision of thigh tendons	Y		A2	18.7092	$783.41
27393	Lengthening of thigh tendon	Y		A2	25.3445	$1,061.25
27394	Lengthening of thigh tendons	Y		A2	25.7101	$1,076.56
27395	Lengthening of thigh tendons	Y		A2	36.3344	$1,521.43
27396	Transplant of thigh tendon	Y		A2	25.7101	$1,076.56
27397	Transplants of thigh tendons	Y		A2	36.3344	$1,521.43
27400	Revise thigh muscles/tendons	Y		A2	36.3344	$1,521.43
27403	Repair of knee cartilage	Y		A2	26.3955	$1,105.26
27405	Repair of knee ligament	Y		A2	37.02	$1,550.14
27407	Repair of knee ligament	Y		A2	67.2085	$2,814.22
27409	Repair of knee ligaments	Y		A2	37.02	$1,550.14
27416	Osteochondral knee autograft	Y		G2	44.5617	$1,865.93
27418	Repair degenerated kneecap	Y		A2	36.3344	$1,521.43
27420	Revision of unstable kneecap	Y		A2	36.3344	$1,521.43
27422	Revision of unstable kneecap	Y		A2	39.1047	$1,637.43
27424	Revision/removal of kneecap	Y		A2	36.3344	$1,521.43
27425	Lat retinacular release open	Y		A2	28.4804	$1,192.56
27427	Reconstruction, knee	Y		A2	36.3344	$1,521.43
27428	Reconstruction, knee	Y		A2	67.2085	$2,814.22
27429	Reconstruction, knee	Y		A2	67.2085	$2,814.22
27430	Revision of thigh muscles	Y		A2	37.02	$1,550.14

HCPCS Code	HCPCS Short Descriptor	Subject To Multiple Procedure Discounts	CY 2010 Comment Indicator	CY 2010 Payment Indicator	CY 2010 Third Year Transition. Pymt. Weight	CY 2010 Third Year Transition Payment
27435	Incision of knee joint	Y		A2	37.02	$1,550.14
27437	Revise kneecap	Y		A2	32.2191	$1,349.11
27438	Revise kneecap with implant	Y		A2	45.772	$1,916.61
27440	Revision of knee joint	Y		G2	38.1606	$1,597.90
27441	Revision of knee joint	Y		A2	32.7158	$1,369.91
27442	Revision of knee joint	Y		A2	32.7158	$1,369.91
27443	Revision of knee joint	Y		A2	32.7158	$1,369.91
27446	Revision of knee joint	Y		J8	158.2621	$6,626.91
27475	Surgery to stop leg growth	Y	CH	G2	30.396	$1,272.77
27479	Surgery to stop leg growth	Y	CH	G2	30.396	$1,272.77
27496	Decompression of thigh/knee	Y		A2	26.8925	$1,126.07
27497	Decompression of thigh/knee	Y		A2	18.7092	$783.41
27498	Decompression of thigh/knee	Y		A2	25.7101	$1,076.56
27499	Decompression of thigh/knee	Y		A2	25.7101	$1,076.56
27500	Treatment of thigh fracture	Y		A2	4.0322	$168.84
27501	Treatment of thigh fracture	Y		A2	1.7811	$74.58
27502	Treatment of thigh fracture	Y		A2	13.7917	$577.50
27503	Treatment of thigh fracture	Y		A2	1.7811	$74.58
27508	Treatment of thigh fracture	Y		A2	1.7811	$74.58
27509	Treatment of thigh fracture	Y		A2	21.4573	$898.48
27510	Treatment of thigh fracture	Y		A2	4.0322	$168.84
27516	Treat thigh fx growth plate	Y		A2	1.7811	$74.58
27517	Treat thigh fx growth plate	Y		A2	1.7811	$74.58
27520	Treat kneecap fracture	Y		A2	1.7811	$74.58
27530	Treat knee fracture	Y		A2	1.7811	$74.58
27532	Treat knee fracture	Y		A2	13.7917	$577.50
27538	Treat knee fracture(s)	Y		A2	1.7811	$74.58
27550	Treat knee dislocation	Y		A2	1.7811	$74.58
27552	Treat knee dislocation	Y		A2	12.8746	$539.10
27560	Treat kneecap dislocation	Y		A2	1.7811	$74.58
27562	Treat kneecap dislocation	Y		A2	12.8746	$539.10
27566	Treat kneecap dislocation	Y		A2	35.1716	$1,472.74
27570	Fixation of knee joint	Y		A2	12.8746	$539.10
27594	Amputation follow-up surgery	Y		A2	18.7092	$783.41
27600	Decompression of lower leg	Y		A2	18.7092	$783.41
27601	Decompression of lower leg	Y		A2	18.7092	$783.41
27602	Decompression of lower leg	Y		A2	18.7092	$783.41
27603	Drain lower leg lesion	Y		A2	16.472	$689.73
27604	Drain lower leg bursa	Y		A2	18.3436	$768.10
27605	Incision of achilles tendon	Y		A2	17.5755	$735.94
27606	Incision of achilles tendon	Y		A2	17.6983	$741.08
27607	Treat lower leg bone lesion	Y		A2	18.3436	$768.10
27610	Explore/treat ankle joint	Y		A2	25.3445	$1,061.25
27612	Exploration of ankle joint	Y		A2	25.7101	$1,076.56
27613	Biopsy lower leg soft tissue	Y		P3		$110.78
27614	Biopsy lower leg soft tissue	Y		A2	19.3292	$809.37
27615	Resect leg/ankle tum < 5 cm	Y	NI	G2	16.7399	$700.95
27616	Resect leg/ankle tum > 5 cm	Y	NI	G2	22.3753	$936.92
27618*	Exc leg/ankle tum < 3 cm	Y	NI	P3		$188.05
27619	Exc leg/ankle tum deep <5 cm	Y	NI	G2	16.7399	$700.95
27620	Explore/treat ankle joint	Y		A2	26.3955	$1,105.26

HCPCS Code	HCPCS Short Descriptor	Subject To Multiple Procedure Discounts	CY 2010 Comment Indicator	CY 2010 Payment Indicator	CY 2010 Third Year Transition. Pymt. Weight	CY 2010 Third Year Transition Payment
27625	Remove ankle joint lining	Y		A2	26.3955	$1,105.26
27626	Remove ankle joint lining	Y		A2	26.3955	$1,105.26
27630	Removal of tendon lesion	Y		A2	18.7092	$783.41
27632	Exc leg/ankle les sc > 3 cm	Y	NI	G2	22.3753	$936.92
27634	Exc leg/ankle tum deep >5 cm	Y	NI	G2	22.3753	$936.92
27635	Remove lower leg bone lesion	Y		A2	25.7101	$1,076.56
27637	Remove/graft leg bone lesion	Y		A2	25.7101	$1,076.56
27638	Remove/graft leg bone lesion	Y		A2	25.7101	$1,076.56
27640	Partial removal of tibia	Y		A2	35.969	$1,506.13
27641	Partial removal of fibula	Y		A2	25.3445	$1,061.25
27647	Resect talus/calcaneus tum	Y		A2	36.3344	$1,521.43
27648	Injection for ankle x-ray	N		N1		
27650	Repair achilles tendon	Y		A2	36.3344	$1,521.43
27652	Repair/graft achilles tendon	Y		A2	66.5231	$2,785.52
27654	Repair of achilles tendon	Y		A2	36.3344	$1,521.43
27656	Repair leg fascia defect	Y		A2	18.3436	$768.10
27658	Repair of leg tendon, each	Y		A2	17.6983	$741.08
27659	Repair of leg tendon, each	Y		A2	18.3436	$768.10
27664	Repair of leg tendon, each	Y		A2	25.3445	$1,061.25
27665	Repair of leg tendon, each	Y		A2	25.3445	$1,061.25
27675	Repair lower leg tendons	Y		A2	18.3436	$768.10
27676	Repair lower leg tendons	Y		A2	25.7101	$1,076.56
27680	Release of lower leg tendon	Y		A2	25.7101	$1,076.56
27681	Release of lower leg tendons	Y		A2	25.3445	$1,061.25
27685	Revision of lower leg tendon	Y		A2	25.7101	$1,076.56
27686	Revise lower leg tendons	Y		A2	25.7101	$1,076.56
27687	Revision of calf tendon	Y		A2	25.7101	$1,076.56
27690	Revise lower leg tendon	Y		A2	37.02	$1,550.14
27691	Revise lower leg tendon	Y		A2	37.02	$1,550.14
27692	Revise additional leg tendon	Y		A2	36.3344	$1,521.43
27695	Repair of ankle ligament	Y		A2	25.3445	$1,061.25
27696	Repair of ankle ligaments	Y		A2	25.3445	$1,061.25
27698	Repair of ankle ligament	Y		A2	25.3445	$1,061.25
27700	Revision of ankle joint	Y		A2	32.7158	$1,369.91
27704	Removal of ankle implant	Y		A2	18.3436	$768.10
27705	Incision of tibia	Y		A2	35.969	$1,506.13
27707	Incision of fibula	Y		A2	18.3436	$768.10
27709	Incision of tibia & fibula	Y		A2	25.3445	$1,061.25
27720	Repair of tibia	Y	CH	G2	43.499	$1,821.43
27726	Repair fibula nonunion	Y		G2	43.499	$1,821.43
27730	Repair of tibia epiphysis	Y		A2	25.3445	$1,061.25
27732	Repair of fibula epiphysis	Y		A2	25.3445	$1,061.25
27734	Repair lower leg epiphyses	Y		A2	25.3445	$1,061.25
27740	Repair of leg epiphyses	Y		A2	25.3445	$1,061.25
27742	Repair of leg epiphyses	Y		A2	35.969	$1,506.13
27745	Reinforce tibia	Y		A2	66.5231	$2,785.52
27750	Treatment of tibia fracture	Y		A2	1.7811	$74.58
27752	Treatment of tibia fracture	Y		A2	13.7917	$577.50
27756	Treatment of tibia fracture	Y		A2	21.4573	$898.48
27758	Treatment of tibia fracture	Y		A2	36.2226	$1,516.75
27759	Treatment of tibia fracture	Y		A2	50.5787	$2,117.88

HCPCS Code	HCPCS Short Descriptor	Subject To Multiple Procedure Discounts	CY 2010 Comment Indicator	CY 2010 Payment Indicator	CY 2010 Third Year Transition. Pymt. Weight	CY 2010 Third Year Transition Payment
27760	Cltx medial ankle fx	Y		A2	1.7811	$74.58
27762	Cltx med ankle fx w/mnpj	Y		A2	13.7917	$577.50
27766	Optx medial ankle fx	Y		A2	35.5372	$1,488.05
27767	Cltx post ankle fx	Y		G2	1.5858	$66.40
27768	Cltx post ankle fx w/mnpj	Y		G2	1.5858	$66.40
27769	Optx post ankle fx	Y		G2	43.499	$1,821.43
27780	Treatment of fibula fracture	Y		A2	1.7811	$74.58
27781	Treatment of fibula fracture	Y		A2	13.7917	$577.50
27784	Treatment of fibula fracture	Y		A2	35.5372	$1,488.05
27786	Treatment of ankle fracture	Y		A2	1.7811	$74.58
27788	Treatment of ankle fracture	Y		A2	1.7811	$74.58
27792	Treatment of ankle fracture	Y		A2	35.5372	$1,488.05
27808	Treatment of ankle fracture	Y		A2	1.7811	$74.58
27810	Treatment of ankle fracture	Y		A2	4.0322	$168.84
27814	Treatment of ankle fracture	Y		A2	35.5372	$1,488.05
27816	Treatment of ankle fracture	Y		A2	1.7811	$74.58
27818	Treatment of ankle fracture	Y		A2	4.0322	$168.84
27822	Treatment of ankle fracture	Y		A2	35.5372	$1,488.05
27823	Treatment of ankle fracture	Y		A2	49.8932	$2,089.18
27824	Treat lower leg fracture	Y		A2	1.7811	$74.58
27825	Treat lower leg fracture	Y		A2	13.7917	$577.50
27826	Treat lower leg fracture	Y		A2	35.5372	$1,488.05
27827	Treat lower leg fracture	Y		A2	49.8932	$2,089.18
27828	Treat lower leg fracture	Y		A2	50.5787	$2,117.88
27829	Treat lower leg joint	Y		A2	35.1716	$1,472.74
27830	Treat lower leg dislocation	Y		A2	1.7811	$74.58
27831	Treat lower leg dislocation	Y		A2	13.7917	$577.50
27832	Treat lower leg dislocation	Y		A2	35.1716	$1,472.74
27840	Treat ankle dislocation	Y		A2	4.0322	$168.84
27842	Treat ankle dislocation	Y		A2	12.8746	$539.10
27846	Treat ankle dislocation	Y		A2	35.5372	$1,488.05
27848	Treat ankle dislocation	Y		A2	35.5372	$1,488.05
27860	Fixation of ankle joint	Y		A2	12.8746	$539.10
27870	Fusion of ankle joint, open	Y		A2	67.2085	$2,814.22
27871	Fusion of tibiofibular joint	Y		A2	67.2085	$2,814.22
27884	Amputation follow-up surgery	Y		A2	18.7092	$783.41
27889	Amputation of foot at ankle	Y		A2	25.7101	$1,076.56
27892	Decompression of leg	Y		A2	25.7101	$1,076.56
27893	Decompression of leg	Y		A2	25.7101	$1,076.56
27894	Decompression of leg	Y		A2	25.7101	$1,076.56
28001	Drainage of bursa of foot	Y		P3		$109.65
28002	Treatment of foot infection	Y		A2	18.7092	$783.41
28003	Treatment of foot infection	Y		A2	18.7092	$783.41
28005	Treat foot bone lesion	Y		A2	18.5864	$778.27
28008	Incision of foot fascia	Y		A2	18.5864	$778.27
28010	Incision of toe tendon	Y		P3		$80.11
28011	Incision of toe tendons	Y		A2	18.5864	$778.27
28020	Exploration of foot joint	Y		A2	18.221	$762.97
28022	Exploration of foot joint	Y		A2	18.221	$762.97
28024	Exploration of toe joint	Y		A2	18.221	$762.97
28035	Decompression of tibia nerve	Y		A2	17.0305	$713.12

HCPCS Code	HCPCS Short Descriptor	Subject To Multiple Procedure Discounts	CY 2010 Comment Indicator	CY 2010 Payment Indicator	CY 2010 Third Year Transition. Pymt. Weight	CY 2010 Third Year Transition Payment
28039*	Exc foot/toe tum sc > 1.5 cm	Y	NI	P3		$199.69
28041*	Exc foot/toe tum deep >1.5cm	Y	NI	R2	22.3753	$936.92
28043*	Exc foot/toe tum sc < 1.5 cm	Y	NI	P3		$142.03
28045*	Exc foot/toe tum deep <1.5cm	Y	NI	P3		$194.87
28046*	Resect foot/toe tumor < 3 cm	Y	NI	R2	16.7399	$700.95
28047	Resect foot/toe tumor > 3 cm	Y	NI	G2	22.3753	$936.92
28050	Biopsy of foot joint lining	Y		A2	18.221	$762.97
28052	Biopsy of foot joint lining	Y		A2	18.221	$762.97
28054	Biopsy of toe joint lining	Y		A2	18.221	$762.97
28055	Neurectomy, foot	Y		A2	17.0305	$713.12
28060	Partial removal, foot fascia	Y		A2	18.221	$762.97
28062	Removal of foot fascia	Y		A2	18.5864	$778.27
28070	Removal of foot joint lining	Y		A2	18.5864	$778.27
28072	Removal of foot joint lining	Y		A2	18.5864	$778.27
28080	Removal of foot lesion	Y		A2	18.5864	$778.27
28086	Excise foot tendon sheath	Y		A2	18.221	$762.97
28088	Excise foot tendon sheath	Y		A2	18.221	$762.97
28090	Removal of foot lesion	Y		A2	18.5864	$778.27
28092	Removal of toe lesions	Y		A2	18.5864	$778.27
28100	Removal of ankle/heel lesion	Y		A2	18.221	$762.97
28102	Remove/graft foot lesion	Y		A2	40.6016	$1,700.11
28103	Remove/graft foot lesion	Y		A2	40.6016	$1,700.11
28104	Removal of foot lesion	Y		A2	18.221	$762.97
28106	Remove/graft foot lesion	Y		A2	40.6016	$1,700.11
28107	Remove/graft foot lesion	Y		A2	40.6016	$1,700.11
28108	Removal of toe lesions	Y		A2	18.221	$762.97
28110	Part removal of metatarsal	Y		A2	18.5864	$778.27
28111	Part removal of metatarsal	Y		A2	18.5864	$778.27
28112	Part removal of metatarsal	Y		A2	18.5864	$778.27
28113	Part removal of metatarsal	Y		A2	18.5864	$778.27
28114	Removal of metatarsal heads	Y		A2	18.5864	$778.27
28116	Revision of foot	Y		A2	18.5864	$778.27
28118	Removal of heel bone	Y		A2	19.2721	$806.98
28119	Removal of heel spur	Y		A2	19.2721	$806.98
28120	Part removal of ankle/heel	Y		A2	21.3567	$894.27
28122	Partial removal of foot bone	Y		A2	18.5864	$778.27
28124	Partial removal of toe	Y		P3		$185.78
28126	Partial removal of toe	Y		A2	18.5864	$778.27
28130	Removal of ankle bone	Y		A2	18.5864	$778.27
28140	Removal of metatarsal	Y		A2	18.5864	$778.27
28150	Removal of toe	Y		A2	18.5864	$778.27
28153	Partial removal of toe	Y		A2	18.5864	$778.27
28160	Partial removal of toe	Y		A2	18.5864	$778.27
28171	Resect tarsal tumor	Y		A2	18.5864	$778.27
28173	Resect metatarsal tumor	Y		A2	18.5864	$778.27
28175	Resect phalanx of toe tumor	Y		A2	18.5864	$778.27
28190	Removal of foot foreign body	Y		P3		$113.62
28192	Removal of foot foreign body	Y		A2	15.1023	$632.38
28193	Removal of foot foreign body	Y		A2	8.2762	$346.55
28200	Repair of foot tendon	Y		A2	18.5864	$778.27
28202	Repair/graft of foot tendon	Y		A2	18.5864	$778.27

HCPCS Code	HCPCS Short Descriptor	Subject To Multiple Procedure Discounts	CY 2010 Comment Indicator	CY 2010 Payment Indicator	CY 2010 Third Year Transition. Pymt. Weight	CY 2010 Third Year Transition Payment
28208	Repair of foot tendon	Y		A2	18.5864	$778.27
28210	Repair/graft of foot tendon	Y		A2	40.6016	$1,700.11
28220	Release of foot tendon	Y		P3		$175.55
28222	Release of foot tendons	Y		A2	17.5755	$735.94
28225	Release of foot tendon	Y		A2	17.5755	$735.94
28226	Release of foot tendons	Y		A2	17.5755	$735.94
28230	Incision of foot tendon(s)	Y		P3		$171.57
28232	Incision of toe tendon	Y		P3		$164.47
28234	Incision of foot tendon	Y		A2	18.221	$762.97
28238	Revision of foot tendon	Y		A2	40.6016	$1,700.11
28240	Release of big toe	Y		A2	18.221	$762.97
28250	Revision of foot fascia	Y		A2	18.5864	$778.27
28260	Release of midfoot joint	Y		A2	18.5864	$778.27
28261	Revision of foot tendon	Y		A2	18.5864	$778.27
28262	Revision of foot and ankle	Y		A2	19.2721	$806.98
28264	Release of midfoot joint	Y		A2	39.5907	$1,657.78
28270	Release of foot contracture	Y		A2	18.5864	$778.27
28272	Release of toe joint, each	Y		P3		$158.51
28280	Fusion of toes	Y		A2	18.221	$762.97
28285	Repair of hammertoe	Y		A2	18.5864	$778.27
28286	Repair of hammertoe	Y		A2	19.2721	$806.98
28288	Partial removal of foot bone	Y		A2	18.5864	$778.27
28289	Repair hallux rigidus	Y		A2	18.5864	$778.27
28290	Correction of bunion	Y		A2	25.1878	$1,054.69
28292	Correction of bunion	Y		A2	25.1878	$1,054.69
28293	Correction of bunion	Y		A2	25.5535	$1,070.00
28294	Correction of bunion	Y		A2	25.5535	$1,070.00
28296	Correction of bunion	Y		A2	25.5535	$1,070.00
28297	Correction of bunion	Y		A2	25.5535	$1,070.00
28298	Correction of bunion	Y		A2	25.5535	$1,070.00
28299	Correction of bunion	Y		A2	26.7358	$1,119.51
28300	Incision of heel bone	Y		A2	40.2362	$1,684.81
28302	Incision of ankle bone	Y		A2	18.221	$762.97
28304	Incision of midfoot bones	Y		A2	40.2362	$1,684.81
28305	Incise/graft midfoot bones	Y		A2	40.6016	$1,700.11
28306	Incision of metatarsal	Y		A2	19.2721	$806.98
28307	Incision of metatarsal	Y		A2	19.2721	$806.98
28308	Incision of metatarsal	Y		A2	18.221	$762.97
28309	Incision of metatarsals	Y		A2	41.2872	$1,728.82
28310	Revision of big toe	Y		A2	18.5864	$778.27
28312	Revision of toe	Y		A2	18.5864	$778.27
28313	Repair deformity of toe	Y		A2	18.221	$762.97
28315	Removal of sesamoid bone	Y		A2	19.2721	$806.98
28320	Repair of foot bones	Y		A2	41.2872	$1,728.82
28322	Repair of metatarsals	Y		A2	41.2872	$1,728.82
28340	Resect enlarged toe tissue	Y		A2	19.2721	$806.98
28341	Resect enlarged toe	Y		A2	19.2721	$806.98
28344	Repair extra toe(s)	Y		A2	19.2721	$806.98
28345	Repair webbed toe(s)	Y		A2	19.2721	$806.98
28400	Treatment of heel fracture	Y		A2	1.7811	$74.58
28405	Treatment of heel fracture	Y		A2	13.7917	$577.50

HCPCS Code	HCPCS Short Descriptor	Subject To Multiple Procedure Discounts	CY 2010 Comment Indicator	CY 2010 Payment Indicator	CY 2010 Third Year Transition. Pymt. Weight	CY 2010 Third Year Transition Payment
28406	Treatment of heel fracture	Y		A2	21.0916	$883.17
28415	Treat heel fracture	Y		A2	49.8932	$2,089.18
28420	Treat/graft heel fracture	Y		A2	36.2226	$1,516.75
28430	Treatment of ankle fracture	Y		P2	1.5858	$66.40
28435	Treatment of ankle fracture	Y		A2	1.7811	$74.58
28436	Treatment of ankle fracture	Y		A2	21.0916	$883.17
28445	Treat ankle fracture	Y		A2	35.5372	$1,488.05
28446	Osteochondral talus autogrft	Y		G2	50.2514	$2,104.18
28450	Treat midfoot fracture, each	Y		P2	1.5858	$66.40
28455	Treat midfoot fracture, each	Y		P2	1.5858	$66.40
28456	Treat midfoot fracture	Y		A2	21.0916	$883.17
28465	Treat midfoot fracture, each	Y		A2	35.5372	$1,488.05
28470	Treat metatarsal fracture	Y		P2	1.5858	$66.40
28475	Treat metatarsal fracture	Y		P2	1.5858	$66.40
28476	Treat metatarsal fracture	Y		A2	21.0916	$883.17
28485	Treat metatarsal fracture	Y		A2	36.2226	$1,516.75
28490	Treat big toe fracture	Y	CH	P3		$61.64
28495	Treat big toe fracture	Y		P2	1.5858	$66.40
28496	Treat big toe fracture	Y		A2	21.0916	$883.17
28505	Treat big toe fracture	Y		A2	21.4573	$898.48
28510	Treatment of toe fracture	Y		P3		$48.86
28515	Treatment of toe fracture	Y	CH	P3		$63.35
28525	Treat toe fracture	Y		A2	21.4573	$898.48
28530	Treat sesamoid bone fracture	Y		P3		$46.87
28531	Treat sesamoid bone fracture	Y		A2	21.4573	$898.48
28540	Treat foot dislocation	Y		P2	1.5858	$66.40
28545	Treat foot dislocation	Y		A2	20.4461	$856.14
28546	Treat foot dislocation	Y		A2	21.0916	$883.17
28555	Repair foot dislocation	Y		A2	35.1716	$1,472.74
28570	Treat foot dislocation	Y		P3		$67.61
28575	Treat foot dislocation	Y		A2	13.7917	$577.50
28576	Treat foot dislocation	Y		A2	21.4573	$898.48
28585	Repair foot dislocation	Y		A2	21.4573	$898.48
28600	Treat foot dislocation	Y		P2	1.5858	$66.40
28605	Treat foot dislocation	Y		A2	1.7811	$74.58
28606	Treat foot dislocation	Y		A2	21.0916	$883.17
28615	Repair foot dislocation	Y		A2	35.5372	$1,488.05
28630	Treat toe dislocation	Y	CH	P3		$53.12
28635	Treat toe dislocation	Y		A2	12.8746	$539.10
28636	Treat toe dislocation	Y		A2	21.4573	$898.48
28645	Repair toe dislocation	Y		A2	21.4573	$898.48
28660	Treat toe dislocation	Y		P3		$38.92
28665	Treat toe dislocation	Y		A2	12.8746	$539.10
28666	Treat toe dislocation	Y		A2	21.4573	$898.48
28675	Repair of toe dislocation	Y		A2	21.4573	$898.48
28705	Fusion of foot bones	Y		A2	41.2872	$1,728.82
28715	Fusion of foot bones	Y		A2	67.2085	$2,814.22
28725	Fusion of foot bones	Y		A2	41.2872	$1,728.82
28730	Fusion of foot bones	Y		A2	41.2872	$1,728.82
28735	Fusion of foot bones	Y		A2	41.2872	$1,728.82
28737	Revision of foot bones	Y		A2	41.784	$1,749.62

HCPCS Code	HCPCS Short Descriptor	Subject To Multiple Procedure Discounts	CY 2010 Comment Indicator	CY 2010 Payment Indicator	CY 2010 Third Year Transition. Pymt. Weight	CY 2010 Third Year Transition Payment
28740	Fusion of foot bones	Y		A2	41.2872	$1,728.82
28750	Fusion of big toe joint	Y		A2	41.2872	$1,728.82
28755	Fusion of big toe joint	Y		A2	19.2721	$806.98
28760	Fusion of big toe joint	Y		A2	41.2872	$1,728.82
28810	Amputation toe & metatarsal	Y		A2	18.221	$762.97
28820	Amputation of toe	Y		A2	18.221	$762.97
28825	Partial amputation of toe	Y		A2	18.221	$762.97
28890	High energy eswt, plantar f	Y		P3		$141.46
29000	Application of body cast	N		G2	1.0081	$42.21
29010	Application of body cast	N		P2	2.2441	$93.97
29015	Application of body cast	N		P2	2.2441	$93.97
29020	Application of body cast	N		G2	1.0081	$42.21
29025	Application of body cast	N		P2	1.0081	$42.21
29035	Application of body cast	N		P2	2.2441	$93.97
29040	Application of body cast	N		G2	1.0081	$42.21
29044	Application of body cast	N		P2	2.2441	$93.97
29046	Application of body cast	N		G2	2.2441	$93.97
29049	Application of figure eight	N		P3		$34.66
29055	Application of shoulder cast	N	CH	P3		$90.90
29058	Application of shoulder cast	N	CH	P3		$38.06
29065	Application of long arm cast	N		P3		$38.63
29075	Application of forearm cast	N		P3		$37.21
29085	Apply hand/wrist cast	N	CH	P3		$38.06
29086	Apply finger cast	N		P3		$32.10
29105	Apply long arm splint	N		P3		$33.52
29125	Apply forearm splint	N		P3		$29.26
29126	Apply forearm splint	N		P3		$30.96
29130	Application of finger splint	N		P3		$13.35
29131	Application of finger splint	N		P3		$19.03
29200	Strapping of chest	N		P3		$18.75
29220	Strapping of low back	N	CH	D5		
29240	Strapping of shoulder	N		P3		$20.45
29260	Strapping of elbow or wrist	N		P3		$19.88
29280	Strapping of hand or finger	N		P3		$20.17
29305	Application of hip cast	N		P2	2.2441	$93.97
29325	Application of hip casts	N		P2	2.2441	$93.97
29345	Application of long leg cast	N		P3		$50.56
29355	Application of long leg cast	N		P3		$49.99
29358	Apply long leg cast brace	N		P3		$62.49
29365	Application of long leg cast	N		P3		$47.72
29405	Apply short leg cast	N		P3		$35.79
29425	Apply short leg cast	N		P3		$36.08
29435	Apply short leg cast	N		P3		$45.73
29440	Addition of walker to cast	N		P3		$19.60
29445	Apply rigid leg cast	N		P3		$47.72
29450	Application of leg cast	N		P2	1.0081	$42.21
29505	Application, long leg splint	N		P3		$32.67
29515	Application lower leg splint	N		P3		$28.12
29520	Strapping of hip	N		P3		$19.32
29530	Strapping of knee	N		P3		$19.88
29540	Strapping of ankle and/or ft	N		P3		$15.06

HCPCS Code	HCPCS Short Descriptor	Subject To Multiple Procedure Discounts	CY 2010 Comment Indicator	CY 2010 Payment Indicator	CY 2010 Third Year Transition. Pymt. Weight	CY 2010 Third Year Transition Payment
29550	Strapping of toes	N		P3		$15.34
29580	Application of paste boot	N		P3		$20.74
29581	Apply multlay comprs lwr leg	N	NI	P2	1.0081	$42.21
29590	Application of foot splint	N		P3		$16.76
29700	Removal/revision of cast	N		P3		$27.55
29705	Removal/revision of cast	N		P3		$23.58
29710	Removal/revision of cast	N		P3		$42.33
29715	Removal/revision of cast	N	CH	P3		$33.24
29720	Repair of body cast	N		P3		$34.94
29730	Windowing of cast	N		P3		$22.72
29740	Wedging of cast	N		P3		$30.68
29750	Wedging of clubfoot cast	N		P3		$33.52
29800	Jaw arthroscopy/surgery	Y		A2	24.3811	$1,020.91
29804	Jaw arthroscopy/surgery	Y		A2	24.3811	$1,020.91
29805	Shoulder arthroscopy, dx	Y		A2	24.3811	$1,020.91
29806	Shoulder arthroscopy/surgery	Y		A2	37.9409	$1,588.70
29807	Shoulder arthroscopy/surgery	Y		A2	37.9409	$1,588.70
29819	Shoulder arthroscopy/surgery	Y		A2	37.9409	$1,588.70
29820	Shoulder arthroscopy/surgery	Y		A2	37.9409	$1,588.70
29821	Shoulder arthroscopy/surgery	Y		A2	37.9409	$1,588.70
29822	Shoulder arthroscopy/surgery	Y		A2	24.3811	$1,020.91
29823	Shoulder arthroscopy/surgery	Y		A2	37.9409	$1,588.70
29824	Shoulder arthroscopy/surgery	Y		A2	25.5635	$1,070.42
29825	Shoulder arthroscopy/surgery	Y		A2	37.9409	$1,588.70
29826	Shoulder arthroscopy/surgery	Y		A2	37.9409	$1,588.70
29827	Arthroscop rotator cuff repr	Y		A2	39.1233	$1,638.21
29828	Arthroscopy biceps tenodesis	Y		G2	46.7038	$1,955.63
29830	Elbow arthroscopy	Y		A2	24.3811	$1,020.91
29834	Elbow arthroscopy/surgery	Y		A2	24.3811	$1,020.91
29835	Elbow arthroscopy/surgery	Y		A2	24.3811	$1,020.91
29836	Elbow arthroscopy/surgery	Y		A2	24.3811	$1,020.91
29837	Elbow arthroscopy/surgery	Y		A2	24.3811	$1,020.91
29838	Elbow arthroscopy/surgery	Y		A2	24.3811	$1,020.91
29840	Wrist arthroscopy	Y		A2	24.3811	$1,020.91
29843	Wrist arthroscopy/surgery	Y		A2	24.3811	$1,020.91
29844	Wrist arthroscopy/surgery	Y		A2	24.3811	$1,020.91
29845	Wrist arthroscopy/surgery	Y		A2	24.3811	$1,020.91
29846	Wrist arthroscopy/surgery	Y		A2	24.3811	$1,020.91
29847	Wrist arthroscopy/surgery	Y		A2	37.9409	$1,588.70
29848	Wrist endoscopy/surgery	Y		A2	29.1164	$1,219.19
29850	Knee arthroscopy/surgery	Y		A2	25.0667	$1,049.62
29851	Knee arthroscopy/surgery	Y		A2	38.6263	$1,617.40
29855	Tibial arthroscopy/surgery	Y		A2	38.6263	$1,617.40
29856	Tibial arthroscopy/surgery	Y		A2	38.6263	$1,617.40
29860	Hip arthroscopy, dx	Y		A2	38.6263	$1,617.40
29861	Hip arthroscopy/surgery	Y		A2	38.6263	$1,617.40
29862	Hip arthroscopy/surgery	Y		A2	42.6762	$1,786.98
29863	Hip arthroscopy/surgery	Y		A2	38.6263	$1,617.40
29866	Autgrft implnt, knee w/scope	Y		G2	46.7038	$1,955.63
29870	Knee arthroscopy, dx	Y		A2	24.3811	$1,020.91
29871	Knee arthroscopy/drainage	Y		A2	24.3811	$1,020.91

HCPCS Code	HCPCS Short Descriptor	Subject To Multiple Procedure Discounts	CY 2010 Comment Indicator	CY 2010 Payment Indicator	CY 2010 Third Year Transition. Pymt. Weight	CY 2010 Third Year Transition Payment
29873	Knee arthroscopy/surgery	Y		A2	24.3811	$1,020.91
29874	Knee arthroscopy/surgery	Y		A2	24.3811	$1,020.91
29875	Knee arthroscopy/surgery	Y		A2	25.0667	$1,049.62
29876	Knee arthroscopy/surgery	Y		A2	25.0667	$1,049.62
29877	Knee arthroscopy/surgery	Y		A2	25.0667	$1,049.62
29879	Knee arthroscopy/surgery	Y		A2	24.3811	$1,020.91
29880	Knee arthroscopy/surgery	Y		A2	25.0667	$1,049.62
29881	Knee arthroscopy/surgery	Y		A2	25.0667	$1,049.62
29882	Knee arthroscopy/surgery	Y		A2	24.3811	$1,020.91
29883	Knee arthroscopy/surgery	Y		A2	24.3811	$1,020.91
29884	Knee arthroscopy/surgery	Y		A2	24.3811	$1,020.91
29885	Knee arthroscopy/surgery	Y		A2	37.9409	$1,588.70
29886	Knee arthroscopy/surgery	Y		A2	24.3811	$1,020.91
29887	Knee arthroscopy/surgery	Y		A2	24.3811	$1,020.91
29888	Knee arthroscopy/surgery	Y		A2	66.5231	$2,785.52
29889	Knee arthroscopy/surgery	Y		A2	66.5231	$2,785.52
29891	Ankle arthroscopy/surgery	Y		A2	37.9409	$1,588.70
29892	Ankle arthroscopy/surgery	Y		A2	66.5231	$2,785.52
29893	Scope, plantar fasciotomy	Y		A2	22.845	$956.59
29894	Ankle arthroscopy/surgery	Y		A2	24.3811	$1,020.91
29895	Ankle arthroscopy/surgery	Y		A2	24.3811	$1,020.91
29897	Ankle arthroscopy/surgery	Y		A2	24.3811	$1,020.91
29898	Ankle arthroscopy/surgery	Y		A2	24.3811	$1,020.91
29899	Ankle arthroscopy/surgery	Y		A2	37.9409	$1,588.70
29900	Mcp joint arthroscopy, dx	Y		A2	24.3811	$1,020.91
29901	Mcp joint arthroscopy, surg	Y		A2	24.3811	$1,020.91
29902	Mcp joint arthroscopy, surg	Y		A2	24.3811	$1,020.91
29904	Subtalar arthro w/fb rmvl	Y		G2	28.6243	$1,198.59
29905	Subtalar arthro w/exc	Y		G2	28.6243	$1,198.59
29906	Subtalar arthro w/deb	Y		G2	28.6243	$1,198.59
29907	Subtalar arthro w/fusion	Y		G2	46.7038	$1,955.63
30000	Drainage of nose lesion	Y	CH	P3		$119.02
30020	Drainage of nose lesion	Y	CH	P3		$115.33
30100	Intranasal biopsy	Y		P3		$71.30
30110	Removal of nose polyp(s)	Y		P3		$110.50
30115	Removal of nose polyp(s)	Y		A2	14.8802	$623.08
30117	Removal of intranasal lesion	Y		A2	15.2459	$638.39
30118	Removal of intranasal lesion	Y		A2	20.8254	$872.02
30120	Revision of nose	Y		A2	19.8142	$829.68
30124	Removal of nose lesion	Y		R2	7.2897	$305.24
30125	Removal of nose lesion	Y		A2	33.3886	$1,398.08
30130	Excise inferior turbinate	Y		A2	15.2459	$638.39
30140	Resect inferior turbinate	Y		A2	20.4597	$856.71
30150	Partial removal of nose	Y		A2	33.7542	$1,413.39
30160	Removal of nose	Y		A2	34.4396	$1,442.09
30200	Injection treatment of nose	Y		P3		$56.24
30210	Nasal sinus therapy	Y		P3		$71.58
30220	Insert nasal septal button	Y		A2	8.1184	$339.94
30300	Remove nasal foreign body	N		P2	0.6403	$26.81
30310	Remove nasal foreign body	Y		A2	14.2349	$596.06
30320	Remove nasal foreign body	Y		A2	14.8802	$623.08

HCPCS Code	HCPCS Short Descriptor	Subject To Multiple Procedure Discounts	CY 2010 Comment Indicator	CY 2010 Payment Indicator	CY 2010 Third Year Transition. Pymt. Weight	CY 2010 Third Year Transition Payment
30400	Reconstruction of nose	Y		A2	34.4396	$1,442.09
30410	Reconstruction of nose	Y		A2	34.9366	$1,462.90
30420	Reconstruction of nose	Y		A2	34.9366	$1,462.90
30430	Revision of nose	Y		A2	20.8254	$872.02
30435	Revision of nose	Y		A2	34.9366	$1,462.90
30450	Revision of nose	Y		A2	36.5245	$1,529.39
30460	Revision of nose	Y		A2	36.5245	$1,529.39
30462	Revision of nose	Y		A2	38.4895	$1,611.67
30465	Repair nasal stenosis	Y		A2	38.4895	$1,611.67
30520	Repair of nasal septum	Y		A2	21.5108	$900.72
30540	Repair nasal defect	Y		A2	34.9366	$1,462.90
30545	Repair nasal defect	Y		A2	34.9366	$1,462.90
30560	Release of nasal adhesions	Y		A2	3.3186	$138.96
30580	Repair upper jaw fistula	Y		A2	34.4396	$1,442.09
30600	Repair mouth/nose fistula	Y		A2	34.4396	$1,442.09
30620	Intranasal reconstruction	Y		A2	36.5245	$1,529.39
30630	Repair nasal septum defect	Y		A2	23.5956	$988.02
30801	Ablate inf turbinate, superf	Y		A2	7.3694	$308.58
30802	Ablate inf turbinate submuc	Y		A2	14.2349	$596.06
30901	Control of nosebleed	Y	CH	P3		$38.63
30903	Control of nosebleed	Y		A2	1.2409	$51.96
30905	Control of nosebleed	Y		A2	1.2409	$51.96
30906	Repeat control of nosebleed	Y		A2	1.2409	$51.96
30915	Ligation, nasal sinus artery	Y		A2	21.613	$905.00
30920	Ligation, upper jaw artery	Y		A2	21.9786	$920.31
30930	Ther fx, nasal inf turbinate	Y		A2	15.9313	$667.09
31000	Irrigation, maxillary sinus	Y		P3		$91.18
31002	Irrigation, sphenoid sinus	Y		R2	7.2897	$305.24
31020	Exploration, maxillary sinus	Y		A2	20.4597	$856.71
31030	Exploration, maxillary sinus	Y		A2	33.7542	$1,413.39
31032	Explore sinus, remove polyps	Y		A2	34.4396	$1,442.09
31040	Exploration behind upper jaw	Y		R2	23.8828	$1,000.04
31050	Exploration, sphenoid sinus	Y		A2	33.3886	$1,398.08
31051	Sphenoid sinus surgery	Y		A2	34.4396	$1,442.09
31070	Exploration of frontal sinus	Y		A2	20.4597	$856.71
31075	Exploration of frontal sinus	Y		A2	34.4396	$1,442.09
31080	Removal of frontal sinus	Y		A2	34.4396	$1,442.09
31081	Removal of frontal sinus	Y		A2	34.4396	$1,442.09
31084	Removal of frontal sinus	Y		A2	34.4396	$1,442.09
31085	Removal of frontal sinus	Y		A2	34.4396	$1,442.09
31086	Removal of frontal sinus	Y		A2	34.4396	$1,442.09
31087	Removal of frontal sinus	Y		A2	34.4396	$1,442.09
31090	Exploration of sinuses	Y		A2	34.9366	$1,462.90
31200	Removal of ethmoid sinus	Y		A2	33.3886	$1,398.08
31201	Removal of ethmoid sinus	Y		A2	34.9366	$1,462.90
31205	Removal of ethmoid sinus	Y		A2	33.7542	$1,413.39
31231	Nasal endoscopy, dx	Y		P2	1.7627	$73.81
31233	Nasal/sinus endoscopy, dx	Y		A2	1.8155	$76.02
31235	Nasal/sinus endoscopy, dx	Y		A2	17.4415	$730.33
31237	Nasal/sinus endoscopy, surg	Y		A2	18.0871	$757.36
31238	Nasal/sinus endoscopy, surg	Y		A2	17.4415	$730.33

HCPCS Code	HCPCS Short Descriptor	Subject To Multiple Procedure Discounts	CY 2010 Comment Indicator	CY 2010 Payment Indicator	CY 2010 Third Year Transition. Pymt. Weight	CY 2010 Third Year Transition Payment
31239	Nasal/sinus endoscopy, surg	Y		A2	24.6018	$1,030.15
31240	Nasal/sinus endoscopy, surg	Y		A2	18.0871	$757.36
31254	Revision of ethmoid sinus	Y		A2	23.9164	$1,001.45
31255	Removal of ethmoid sinus	Y		A2	25.0988	$1,050.96
31256	Exploration maxillary sinus	Y		A2	23.9164	$1,001.45
31267	Endoscopy, maxillary sinus	Y		A2	23.9164	$1,001.45
31276	Sinus endoscopy, surgical	Y		A2	23.9164	$1,001.45
31287	Nasal/sinus endoscopy, surg	Y		A2	23.9164	$1,001.45
31288	Nasal/sinus endoscopy, surg	Y		A2	23.9164	$1,001.45
31300	Removal of larynx lesion	Y		A2	22.0077	$921.53
31320	Diagnostic incision, larynx	Y		A2	33.3886	$1,398.08
31400	Revision of larynx	Y		A2	33.3886	$1,398.08
31420	Removal of epiglottis	Y		A2	33.3886	$1,398.08
31500	Insert emergency airway	N		G2	2.349	$98.36
31502	Change of windpipe airway	N		G2	1.353	$56.65
31505	Diagnostic laryngoscopy	Y		P2	0.766	$32.07
31510	Laryngoscopy with biopsy	Y		A2	18.0871	$757.36
31511	Remove foreign body, larynx	Y		A2	1.8155	$76.02
31512	Removal of larynx lesion	Y		A2	18.0871	$757.36
31513	Injection into vocal cord	Y		A2	1.8155	$76.02
31515	Laryngoscopy for aspiration	Y		A2	17.4415	$730.33
31520	Dx laryngoscopy, newborn	Y		G2	1.7627	$73.81
31525	Dx laryngoscopy excl nb	Y		A2	17.4415	$730.33
31526	Dx laryngoscopy w/oper scope	Y		A2	18.0871	$757.36
31527	Laryngoscopy for treatment	Y		A2	22.9055	$959.12
31528	Laryngoscopy and dilation	Y		A2	18.0871	$757.36
31529	Laryngoscopy and dilation	Y		A2	18.0871	$757.36
31530	Laryngoscopy w/fb removal	Y		A2	18.0871	$757.36
31531	Laryngoscopy w/fb & op scope	Y		A2	18.4525	$772.66
31535	Laryngoscopy w/biopsy	Y		A2	18.0871	$757.36
31536	Laryngoscopy w/bx & op scope	Y		A2	18.4525	$772.66
31540	Laryngoscopy w/exc of tumor	Y		A2	18.4525	$772.66
31541	Larynscop w/tumr exc + scope	Y		A2	19.1381	$801.37
31545	Remove vc lesion w/scope	Y		A2	24.6018	$1,030.15
31546	Remove vc lesion scope/graft	Y		A2	24.6018	$1,030.15
31560	Laryngoscop w/arytenoidectom	Y		A2	25.0988	$1,050.96
31561	Larynscop, remve cart + scop	Y		A2	25.0988	$1,050.96
31570	Laryngoscope w/vc inj	Y		A2	18.0871	$757.36
31571	Laryngoscop w/vc inj + scope	Y		A2	23.5507	$986.14
31575	Diagnostic laryngoscopy	Y		P3		$51.13
31576	Laryngoscopy with biopsy	Y		A2	18.0871	$757.36
31577	Remove foreign body, larynx	Y		A2	4.516	$189.10
31578	Removal of larynx lesion	Y		A2	23.5507	$986.14
31579	Diagnostic laryngoscopy	Y		P3		$90.33
31580	Revision of larynx	Y		A2	34.9366	$1,462.90
31582	Revision of larynx	Y		A2	34.9366	$1,462.90
31588	Revision of larynx	Y		A2	34.9366	$1,462.90
31590	Reinnervate larynx	Y		A2	34.9366	$1,462.90
31595	Larynx nerve surgery	Y		A2	33.3886	$1,398.08
31603	Incision of windpipe	Y		A2	7.3694	$308.58
31605	Incision of windpipe	Y		G2	7.2897	$305.24

HCPCS Code	HCPCS Short Descriptor	Subject To Multiple Procedure Discounts	CY 2010 Comment Indicator	CY 2010 Payment Indicator	CY 2010 Third Year Transition. Pymt. Weight	CY 2010 Third Year Transition Payment
31611	Surgery/speech prosthesis	Y		A2	20.8254	$872.02
31612	Puncture/clear windpipe	Y		A2	19.8142	$829.68
31613	Repair windpipe opening	Y		A2	20.4597	$856.71
31614	Repair windpipe opening	Y		A2	33.3886	$1,398.08
31615	Visualization of windpipe	Y		A2	7.3694	$308.58
31620	Endobronchial us add-on	N		N1		
31622	Dx bronchoscope/wash	Y		A2	9.3433	$391.23
31623	Dx bronchoscope/brush	Y		A2	9.9888	$418.26
31624	Dx bronchoscope/lavage	Y		A2	9.9888	$418.26
31625	Bronchoscopy w/biopsy(s)	Y		A2	9.9888	$418.26
31626	Bronchoscopy w/markers	Y	NI	G2	9.9216	$415.45
31627	Navigational bronchoscopy	N	NI	N1		
31628	Bronchoscopy/lung bx, each	Y		A2	9.9888	$418.26
31629	Bronchoscopy/needle bx, each	Y		A2	9.9888	$418.26
31630	Bronchoscopy dilate/fx repr	Y		A2	21.1332	$884.91
31631	Bronchoscopy, dilate w/stent	Y		A2	21.1332	$884.91
31632	Bronchoscopy/lung bx, addl	Y		G2	9.9216	$415.45
31633	Bronchoscopy/needle bx addl	Y		G2	9.9216	$415.45
31635	Bronchoscopy w/fb removal	Y		A2	9.9888	$418.26
31636	Bronchoscopy, bronch stents	Y		A2	21.1332	$884.91
31637	Bronchoscopy, stent add-on	Y		A2	9.3433	$391.23
31638	Bronchoscopy, revise stent	Y		A2	21.1332	$884.91
31640	Bronchoscopy w/tumor excise	Y		A2	21.1332	$884.91
31641	Bronchoscopy, treat blockage	Y		A2	21.1332	$884.91
31643	Diag bronchoscope/catheter	Y		A2	9.9888	$418.26
31645	Bronchoscopy, clear airways	Y		A2	9.3433	$391.23
31646	Bronchoscopy, reclear airway	Y		A2	9.3433	$391.23
31656	Bronchoscopy, inj for x-ray	Y		A2	9.3433	$391.23
31715	Injection for bronchus x-ray	N		N1		
31717	Bronchial brush biopsy	Y		A2	4.516	$189.10
31720	Clearance of airways	N		A2	0.5615	$23.51
31730	Intro, windpipe wire/tube	Y		A2	4.516	$189.10
31750	Repair of windpipe	Y		A2	34.9366	$1,462.90
31755	Repair of windpipe	Y		A2	33.3886	$1,398.08
31820	Closure of windpipe lesion	Y		A2	19.8142	$829.68
31825	Repair of windpipe defect	Y		A2	20.4597	$856.71
31830	Revise windpipe scar	Y		A2	20.4597	$856.71
32400	Needle biopsy chest lining	Y		A2	8.8382	$370.08
32405	Biopsy, lung or mediastinum	Y		A2	8.8382	$370.08
32420	Puncture/clear lung	Y		A2	5.2561	$220.09
32421	Thoracentesis for aspiration	Y		A2	5.2561	$220.09
32422	Thoracentesis w/tube insert	Y		G2	5.3117	$222.42
32550	Insert pleural cath	Y		G2	29.1413	$1,220.23
32552	Remove lung catheter	N	NI	G2	1.353	$56.65
32553	Ins mark thor for rt perq	N	NI	G2	13.1619	$551.13
32960	Therapeutic pneumothorax	Y		G2	5.3117	$222.42
32998	Perq rf ablate tx, pul tumor	Y		G2	49.1378	$2,057.55
33010	Drainage of heart sac	Y		A2	5.2561	$220.09
33011	Repeat drainage of heart sac	Y		A2	5.2561	$220.09
33206	Insertion of heart pacemaker	Y		J8	169.4488	$7,095.33
33207	Insertion of heart pacemaker	Y		J8	169.4488	$7,095.33

HCPCS Code	HCPCS Short Descriptor	Subject To Multiple Procedure Discounts	CY 2010 Comment Indicator	CY 2010 Payment Indicator	CY 2010 Third Year Transition. Pymt. Weight	CY 2010 Third Year Transition Payment
33208	Insertion of heart pacemaker	Y		J8	205.4713	$8,603.70
33210	Insertion of heart electrode	Y		G2	46.8172	$1,960.38
33211	Insertion of heart electrode	Y		G2	46.8172	$1,960.38
33212	Insertion of pulse generator	Y		H8	138.5387	$5,801.03
33213	Insertion of pulse generator	Y		H8	152.6905	$6,393.61
33214	Upgrade of pacemaker system	Y		J8	205.4713	$8,603.70
33215	Reposition pacing-defib lead	Y		G2	21.9478	$919.02
33216	Insert 1 electrode pm-defib	Y		G2	46.8172	$1,960.38
33217	Insert 2 electrode pm-defib	Y		G2	46.8172	$1,960.38
33218	Repair lead pace-defib, one	Y		G2	21.9478	$919.02
33220	Repair lead pace-defib, dual	Y		G2	21.9478	$919.02
33222	Revise pocket, pacemaker	Y		A2	14.0668	$589.02
33223	Revise pocket for defib	Y		A2	14.0668	$589.02
33224	Insert pacing lead & connect	Y		J8	303.507	$12,708.75
33225	L ventric pacing lead add-on	Y		J8	303.507	$12,708.75
33226	Reposition l ventric lead	Y		G2	21.9478	$919.02
33233	Removal of pacemaker system	Y		A2	19.0084	$795.94
33234	Removal of pacemaker system	Y		G2	21.9478	$919.02
33235	Removal pacemaker electrode	Y		G2	21.9478	$919.02
33240	Insert pulse generator	Y		J8	500.9758	$20,977.36
33241	Remove pulse generator	Y		G2	21.9478	$919.02
33249	Eltrd/insert pace-defib	Y		J8	632.2356	$26,473.60
33282	Implant pat-active ht record	N		J8	111.8317	$4,682.73
33284	Remove pat-active ht record	Y		G2	7.8476	$328.60
33508	Endoscopic vein harvest	N		N1		
34490	Removal of vein clot	Y		G2	39.1293	$1,638.46
35188	Repair blood vessel lesion	Y		A2	32.9456	$1,379.53
35207	Repair blood vessel lesion	Y		A2	32.9456	$1,379.53
35460	Repair venous blockage	Y	CH	G2	48.4864	$2,030.27
35473	Repair arterial blockage	Y		G2	48.4864	$2,030.27
35475	Repair arterial blockage	Y	CH	G2	48.4864	$2,030.27
35476	Repair venous blockage	Y		G2	48.4864	$2,030.27
35492	Atherectomy, percutaneous	Y		G2	89.2835	$3,738.57
35572	Harvest femoropopliteal vein	N		N1		
35761	Exploration of artery/vein	Y		G2	34.0556	$1,426.01
35875	Removal of clot in graft	Y		A2	36.9952	$1,549.10
35876	Removal of clot in graft	Y		A2	36.9952	$1,549.10
36000	Place needle in vein	N		N1		
36002	Pseudoaneurysm injection trt	N		G2	2.2009	$92.16
36005	Injection ext venography	N		N1		
36010	Place catheter in vein	N		N1		
36011	Place catheter in vein	N		N1		
36012	Place catheter in vein	N		N1		
36013	Place catheter in artery	N		N1		
36014	Place catheter in artery	N		N1		
36015	Place catheter in artery	N		N1		
36100	Establish access to artery	N		N1		
36120	Establish access to artery	N		N1		
36140	Establish access to artery	N		N1		
36145	Artery to vein shunt	N	CH	D5		
36147	Access av dial grft for eval	Y	NI	P2	2.2917	$95.96

HCPCS Code	HCPCS Short Descriptor	Subject To Multiple Procedure Discounts	CY 2010 Comment Indicator	CY 2010 Payment Indicator	CY 2010 Third Year Transition. Pymt. Weight	CY 2010 Third Year Transition Payment
36148	Access av dial grft for proc	N	NI	N1		
36160	Establish access to aorta	N		N1		
36200	Place catheter in aorta	N		N1		
36215	Place catheter in artery	N		N1		
36216	Place catheter in artery	N		N1		
36217	Place catheter in artery	N		N1		
36218	Place catheter in artery	N		N1		
36245	Place catheter in artery	N		N1		
36246	Place catheter in artery	N		N1		
36247	Place catheter in artery	N		N1		
36248	Place catheter in artery	N		N1		
36260	Insertion of infusion pump	Y		A2	24.7544	$1,036.54
36261	Revision of infusion pump	Y		A2	19.0084	$795.94
36262	Removal of infusion pump	Y		A2	18.3631	$768.92
36400	Bl draw < 3 yrs fem/jugular	N		N1		
36405	Bl draw < 3 yrs scalp vein	N		N1		
36406	Bl draw < 3 yrs other vein	N		N1		
36410	Non-routine bl draw > 3 yrs	N		N1		
36416	Capillary blood draw	N		N1		
36420	Vein access cutdown < 1 yr	N	CH	R2	0.222	$9.30
36425	Vein access cutdown > 1 yr	N		R2	0.222	$9.30
36430	Blood transfusion service	N		P3		$25.85
36440	Bl push transfuse, 2 yr or <	N		R2	3.2345	$135.44
36450	Bl exchange/transfuse, nb	N		R2	3.2345	$135.44
36455	Bl exchange/transfuse non-nb	N		G2	3.2345	$135.44
36468	Injection(s), spider veins	Y		R2	0.8408	$35.21
36469	Injection(s), spider veins	Y		R2	0.8408	$35.21
36470	Injection therapy of vein	Y		P2	0.8408	$35.21
36471	Injection therapy of veins	Y		P2	0.8408	$35.21
36475	Endovenous rf, 1st vein	Y		A2	39.958	$1,673.16
36476	Endovenous rf, vein add-on	Y		A2	26.7139	$1,118.59
36478	Endovenous laser, 1st vein	Y		A2	26.7139	$1,118.59
36479	Endovenous laser vein addon	Y		A2	26.7139	$1,118.59
36481	Insertion of catheter, vein	N		N1		
36500	Insertion of catheter, vein	N		N1		
36510	Insertion of catheter, vein	N		N1		
36511	Apheresis wbc	N		G2	11.4253	$478.41
36512	Apheresis rbc	N		G2	11.4253	$478.41
36513	Apheresis platelets	N		G2	11.4253	$478.41
36514	Apheresis plasma	N		G2	11.4253	$478.41
36515	Apheresis, adsorp/reinfuse	N		P2	31.8778	$1,334.82
36516	Apheresis, selective	N		P2	31.8778	$1,334.82
36522	Photopheresis	N		G2	31.8778	$1,334.82
36555	Insert non-tunnel cv cath	Y		A2	9.914	$415.13
36556	Insert non-tunnel cv cath	Y		A2	9.914	$415.13
36557	Insert tunneled cv cath	Y		A2	20.7258	$867.85
36558	Insert tunneled cv cath	Y		A2	20.7258	$867.85
36560	Insert tunneled cv cath	Y		A2	24.7544	$1,036.54
36561	Insert tunneled cv cath	Y		A2	24.7544	$1,036.54
36563	Insert tunneled cv cath	Y		A2	24.7544	$1,036.54
36565	Insert tunneled cv cath	Y		A2	24.7544	$1,036.54

HCPCS Code	HCPCS Short Descriptor	Subject To Multiple Procedure Discounts	CY 2010 Comment Indicator	CY 2010 Payment Indicator	CY 2010 Third Year Transition. Pymt. Weight	CY 2010 Third Year Transition Payment
36566	Insert tunneled cv cath	Y		A2	24.7544	$1,036.54
36568	Insert picc cath	Y		A2	9.914	$415.13
36569	Insert picc cath	Y		A2	9.914	$415.13
36570	Insert picvad cath	Y		A2	21.0912	$883.15
36571	Insert picvad cath	Y		A2	21.0912	$883.15
36575	Repair tunneled cv cath	Y		A2	7.1211	$298.18
36576	Repair tunneled cv cath	Y		A2	10.5593	$442.15
36578	Replace tunneled cv cath	Y		A2	20.7258	$867.85
36580	Replace cvad cath	Y		A2	9.914	$415.13
36581	Replace tunneled cv cath	Y		A2	20.7258	$867.85
36582	Replace tunneled cv cath	Y		A2	24.7544	$1,036.54
36583	Replace tunneled cv cath	Y		A2	24.7544	$1,036.54
36584	Replace picc cath	Y		A2	9.914	$415.13
36585	Replace picvad cath	Y		A2	21.0912	$883.15
36589	Removal tunneled cv cath	Y		A2	6.4758	$271.16
36590	Removal tunneled cv cath	Y		A2	9.914	$415.13
36591	Draw blood off venous device	N		N1		
36592	Collect blood from picc	N		N1		
36593	Declot vascular device	Y		P3		$20.45
36595	Mech remov tunneled cv cath	Y		G2	24.2374	$1,014.89
36596	Mech remov tunneled cv cath	Y		G2	10.6825	$447.31
36597	Reposition venous catheter	Y		G2	10.6825	$447.31
36598	Inj w/fluor, eval cv device	Y		P3		$63.63
36600	Withdrawal of arterial blood	N		N1		
36620	Insertion catheter, artery	N		N1		
36625	Insertion catheter, artery	N		N1		
36640	Insertion catheter, artery	Y		A2	23.7432	$994.20
36680	Insert needle, bone cavity	Y		G2	1.4457	$60.54
36800	Insertion of cannula	Y		A2	25.1408	$1,052.72
36810	Insertion of cannula	Y		A2	25.1408	$1,052.72
36815	Insertion of cannula	Y		A2	25.1408	$1,052.72
36818	Av fuse, uppr arm, cephalic	Y		A2	32.2599	$1,350.82
36819	Av fuse, uppr arm, basilic	Y		A2	32.2599	$1,350.82
36820	Av fusion/forearm vein	Y		A2	32.2599	$1,350.82
36821	Av fusion direct any site	Y		A2	32.2599	$1,350.82
36825	Artery-vein autograft	Y		A2	32.9456	$1,379.53
36830	Artery-vein nonautograft	Y		A2	32.9456	$1,379.53
36831	Open thrombect av fistula	Y		A2	36.9952	$1,549.10
36832	Av fistula revision, open	Y		A2	32.9456	$1,379.53
36833	Av fistula revision	Y		A2	32.9456	$1,379.53
36834	Repair A-V aneurysm	N	CH	D5		
36835	Artery to vein shunt	Y		A2	25.8262	$1,081.42
36860	External cannula declotting	Y		A2	2.4464	$102.44
36861	Cannula declotting	Y		A2	25.1408	$1,052.72
36870	Percut thrombect av fistula	Y		A2	41.1482	$1,723.00
37184	Prim art mech thrombectomy	Y		G2	39.1293	$1,638.46
37185	Prim art m-thrombect add-on	Y		G2	39.1293	$1,638.46
37186	Sec art m-thrombect add-on	Y		G2	39.1293	$1,638.46
37187	Venous mech thrombectomy	Y		G2	39.1293	$1,638.46
37188	Venous m-thrombectomy add-on	Y		G2	39.1293	$1,638.46
37200	Transcatheter biopsy	Y		G2	29.1216	$1,219.41

HCPCS Code	HCPCS Short Descriptor	Subject To Multiple Procedure Discounts	CY 2010 Comment Indicator	CY 2010 Payment Indicator	CY 2010 Third Year Transition. Pymt. Weight	CY 2010 Third Year Transition Payment
37203	Transcatheter retrieval	Y		G2	29.1216	$1,219.41
37250	Iv us first vessel add-on	N		N1		
37251	Iv us each add vessel add-on	N		N1		
37500	Endoscopy ligate perf veins	Y		A2	35.2227	$1,474.88
37607	Ligation of a-v fistula	Y		A2	21.9786	$920.31
37609	Temporal artery procedure	Y		A2	15.1023	$632.38
37650	Revision of major vein	Y		A2	21.613	$905.00
37700	Revise leg vein	Y		A2	21.613	$905.00
37718	Ligate/strip short leg vein	Y		A2	21.9786	$920.31
37722	Ligate/strip long leg vein	Y		A2	35.2227	$1,474.88
37735	Removal of leg veins/lesion	Y		A2	35.2227	$1,474.88
37760	Ligate leg veins radical	Y		A2	21.9786	$920.31
37761*	Ligate leg veins open	Y	NI	R2	25.4208	$1,064.45
37765	Phleb veins - extrem - to 20	Y		R2	25.4208	$1,064.45
37766	Phleb veins - extrem 20+	Y		R2	25.4208	$1,064.45
37780	Revision of leg vein	Y		A2	21.9786	$920.31
37785	Ligate/divide/excise vein	Y		A2	21.9786	$920.31
37790	Penile venous occlusion	Y		A2	27.9431	$1,170.06
38200	Injection for spleen x-ray	N		N1		
38204	Bl donor search management	N		N1		
38206	Harvest auto stem cells	N		G2	11.4253	$478.41
38220	Bone marrow aspiration	Y		P3		$81.24
38221	Bone marrow biopsy	Y		P3		$84.65
38230	Bone marrow collection	N		G2	31.8778	$1,334.82
38241	Bone marrow/stem transplant	N		G2	31.8778	$1,334.82
38242	Lymphocyte infuse transplant	N		R2	11.4253	$478.41
38300	Drainage, lymph node lesion	Y		A2	10.9586	$458.87
38305	Drainage, lymph node lesion	Y		A2	16.472	$689.73
38308	Incision of lymph channels	Y		A2	20.2092	$846.22
38500	Biopsy/removal, lymph nodes	Y		A2	20.2092	$846.22
38505	Needle biopsy, lymph nodes	Y		A2	6.978	$292.19
38510	Biopsy/removal, lymph nodes	Y		A2	20.2092	$846.22
38520	Biopsy/removal, lymph nodes	Y		A2	20.2092	$846.22
38525	Biopsy/removal, lymph nodes	Y		A2	20.2092	$846.22
38530	Biopsy/removal, lymph nodes	Y		A2	20.2092	$846.22
38542	Explore deep node(s), neck	Y		A2	37.5311	$1,571.54
38550	Removal, neck/armpit lesion	Y		A2	20.5746	$861.52
38555	Removal, neck/armpit lesion	Y		A2	21.2602	$890.23
38570	Laparoscopy, lymph node biop	Y		A2	41.2571	$1,727.56
38571	Laparoscopy, lymphadenectomy	Y		A2	59.9976	$2,512.28
38572	Laparoscopy, lymphadenectomy	Y		A2	41.2571	$1,727.56
38700	Removal of lymph nodes, neck	Y		G2	23.5488	$986.06
38740	Remove armpit lymph nodes	Y		A2	37.5311	$1,571.54
38745	Remove armpit lymph nodes	Y		A2	38.5821	$1,615.55
38760	Remove groin lymph nodes	Y		A2	20.2092	$846.22
38790	Inject for lymphatic x-ray	N		N1		
38792	Identify sentinel node	N		N1		
38794	Access thoracic lymph duct	N		N1		
40490	Biopsy of lip	Y		P3		$57.10
40500	Partial excision of lip	Y		A2	14.8802	$623.08
40510	Partial excision of lip	Y		A2	20.4597	$856.71

HCPCS Code	HCPCS Short Descriptor	Subject To Multiple Procedure Discounts	CY 2010 Comment Indicator	CY 2010 Payment Indicator	CY 2010 Third Year Transition. Pymt. Weight	CY 2010 Third Year Transition Payment
40520	Partial excision of lip	Y		A2	14.8802	$623.08
40525	Reconstruct lip with flap	Y		A2	20.4597	$856.71
40527	Reconstruct lip with flap	Y		A2	20.4597	$856.71
40530	Partial removal of lip	Y		A2	20.4597	$856.71
40650	Repair lip	Y		A2	8.1184	$339.94
40652	Repair lip	Y		A2	8.1184	$339.94
40654	Repair lip	Y		A2	8.1184	$339.94
40700	Repair cleft lip/nasal	Y		A2	36.5245	$1,529.39
40701	Repair cleft lip/nasal	Y		A2	36.5245	$1,529.39
40702	Repair cleft lip/nasal	Y		R2	41.1215	$1,721.88
40720	Repair cleft lip/nasal	Y		A2	36.5245	$1,529.39
40761	Repair cleft lip/nasal	Y		A2	33.7542	$1,413.39
40800	Drainage of mouth lesion	Y		P2	1.3927	$58.32
40801	Drainage of mouth lesion	Y		A2	8.0147	$335.60
40804	Removal, foreign body, mouth	N		P2	0.6403	$26.81
40805	Removal, foreign body, mouth	Y		P3		$144.59
40806	Incision of lip fold	Y		P3		$64.48
40808	Biopsy of mouth lesion	Y		P3		$99.14
40810	Excision of mouth lesion	Y		P3		$102.83
40812	Excise/repair mouth lesion	Y		P3		$129.82
40814	Excise/repair mouth lesion	Y		A2	14.8802	$623.08
40816	Excision of mouth lesion	Y		A2	20.4597	$856.71
40818	Excise oral mucosa for graft	Y		A2	3.3186	$138.96
40819	Excise lip or cheek fold	Y		A2	7.3694	$308.58
40820	Treatment of mouth lesion	Y		P3		$146.29
40830	Repair mouth laceration	Y		G2	3.2767	$137.21
40831	Repair mouth laceration	Y		A2	7.3694	$308.58
40840	Reconstruction of mouth	Y		A2	20.4597	$856.71
40842	Reconstruction of mouth	Y		A2	20.8254	$872.02
40843	Reconstruction of mouth	Y		A2	20.8254	$872.02
40844	Reconstruction of mouth	Y		A2	34.9366	$1,462.90
40845	Reconstruction of mouth	Y		A2	34.9366	$1,462.90
41000	Drainage of mouth lesion	Y		P3		$73.86
41005	Drainage of mouth lesion	Y		A2	3.3186	$138.96
41006	Drainage of mouth lesion	Y		A2	19.8142	$829.68
41007	Drainage of mouth lesion	Y		A2	14.2349	$596.06
41008	Drainage of mouth lesion	Y		A2	14.2349	$596.06
41009	Drainage of mouth lesion	Y		A2	3.3186	$138.96
41010	Incision of tongue fold	Y		A2	7.3694	$308.58
41015	Drainage of mouth lesion	Y		A2	3.3186	$138.96
41016	Drainage of mouth lesion	Y		A2	7.3694	$308.58
41017	Drainage of mouth lesion	Y		A2	7.3694	$308.58
41018	Drainage of mouth lesion	Y		A2	7.3694	$308.58
41019	Place needles h&n for rt	Y		G2	23.8828	$1,000.04
41100	Biopsy of tongue	Y		P3		$77.55
41105	Biopsy of tongue	Y		P3		$76.98
41108	Biopsy of floor of mouth	Y		P3		$71.30
41110	Excision of tongue lesion	Y		P3		$103.11
41112	Excision of tongue lesion	Y		A2	14.8802	$623.08
41113	Excision of tongue lesion	Y		A2	14.8802	$623.08
41114	Excision of tongue lesion	Y		A2	20.4597	$856.71

HCPCS Code	HCPCS Short Descriptor	Subject To Multiple Procedure Discounts	CY 2010 Comment Indicator	CY 2010 Payment Indicator	CY 2010 Third Year Transition. Pymt. Weight	CY 2010 Third Year Transition Payment
41115	Excision of tongue fold	Y		P3		$119.31
41116	Excision of mouth lesion	Y		A2	14.2349	$596.06
41120	Partial removal of tongue	Y		A2	22.0077	$921.53
41250	Repair tongue laceration	Y		A2	1.6877	$70.67
41251	Repair tongue laceration	Y		A2	3.3186	$138.96
41252	Repair tongue laceration	Y		A2	8.0147	$335.60
41500	Fixation of tongue	Y		A2	19.8142	$829.68
41510	Tongue to lip surgery	Y		A2	14.2349	$596.06
41512	Tongue suspension	Y	CH	G2	7.2897	$305.24
41520	Reconstruction, tongue fold	Y		A2	8.0147	$335.60
41530	Tongue base vol reduction	Y		G2	23.8828	$1,000.04
41800	Drainage of gum lesion	Y		A2	1.5497	$64.89
41805	Removal foreign body, gum	Y		P3		$132.37
41806	Removal foreign body,jawbone	Y		P3		$159.07
41820	Excision, gum, each quadrant	Y		R2	7.2897	$305.24
41821	Excision of gum flap	Y		G2	7.2897	$305.24
41822	Excision of gum lesion	Y		P3		$130.95
41823	Excision of gum lesion	Y		P3		$190.04
41825	Excision of gum lesion	Y		P3		$104.53
41826	Excision of gum lesion	Y		P3		$135.78
41827	Excision of gum lesion	Y		A2	20.4597	$856.71
41828	Excision of gum lesion	Y		P3		$120.73
41830	Removal of gum tissue	Y		P3		$170.15
41850	Treatment of gum lesion	Y		R2	16.4437	$688.55
41870	Gum graft	Y		G2	23.8828	$1,000.04
41872	Repair gum	Y		P3		$168.16
41874	Repair tooth socket	Y		P3		$163.90
42000	Drainage mouth roof lesion	Y		A2	3.3186	$138.96
42100	Biopsy roof of mouth	Y		P3		$66.19
42104	Excision lesion, mouth roof	Y		P3		$99.14
42106	Excision lesion, mouth roof	Y		P3		$124.13
42107	Excision lesion, mouth roof	Y		A2	20.4597	$856.71
42120	Remove palate/lesion	Y		A2	34.4396	$1,442.09
42140	Excision of uvula	Y		A2	8.0147	$335.60
42145	Repair palate, pharynx/uvula	Y		A2	22.0077	$921.53
42160	Treatment mouth roof lesion	Y		P3		$114.76
42180	Repair palate	Y		A2	3.3186	$138.96
42182	Repair palate	Y		A2	33.3886	$1,398.08
42200	Reconstruct cleft palate	Y		A2	34.9366	$1,462.90
42205	Reconstruct cleft palate	Y		A2	34.9366	$1,462.90
42210	Reconstruct cleft palate	Y		A2	34.9366	$1,462.90
42215	Reconstruct cleft palate	Y		A2	36.5245	$1,529.39
42220	Reconstruct cleft palate	Y		A2	34.9366	$1,462.90
42225	Reconstruct cleft palate	Y	CH	G2	41.1215	$1,721.88
42226	Lengthening of palate	Y		A2	34.9366	$1,462.90
42227	Lengthening of palate	Y	CH	G2	41.1215	$1,721.88
42235	Repair palate	Y		A2	16.4282	$687.90
42260	Repair nose to lip fistula	Y		A2	21.5108	$900.72
42280	Preparation, palate mold	Y		P3		$65.33
42281	Insertion, palate prosthesis	Y		G2	16.4437	$688.55
42300	Drainage of salivary gland	Y		A2	14.2349	$596.06

HCPCS Code	HCPCS Short Descriptor	Subject To Multiple Procedure Discounts	CY 2010 Comment Indicator	CY 2010 Payment Indicator	CY 2010 Third Year Transition. Pymt. Weight	CY 2010 Third Year Transition Payment
42305	Drainage of salivary gland	Y		A2	14.8802	$623.08
42310	Drainage of salivary gland	Y		A2	3.3186	$138.96
42320	Drainage of salivary gland	Y		A2	3.3186	$138.96
42330	Removal of salivary stone	Y		P3		$99.71
42335	Removal of salivary stone	Y		P3		$165.61
42340	Removal of salivary stone	Y		A2	14.8802	$623.08
42400	Biopsy of salivary gland	Y		P3		$55.11
42405	Biopsy of salivary gland	Y		A2	20.4597	$856.71
42408	Excision of salivary cyst	Y		A2	15.2459	$638.39
42409	Drainage of salivary cyst	Y		A2	15.2459	$638.39
42410	Excise parotid gland/lesion	Y		A2	33.7542	$1,413.39
42415	Excise parotid gland/lesion	Y		A2	36.5245	$1,529.39
42420	Excise parotid gland/lesion	Y		A2	36.5245	$1,529.39
42425	Excise parotid gland/lesion	Y		A2	36.5245	$1,529.39
42440	Excise submaxillary gland	Y		A2	33.7542	$1,413.39
42450	Excise sublingual gland	Y		A2	20.4597	$856.71
42500	Repair salivary duct	Y		A2	20.8254	$872.02
42505	Repair salivary duct	Y		A2	34.4396	$1,442.09
42507	Parotid duct diversion	Y		A2	33.7542	$1,413.39
42508	Parotid duct diversion	Y		A2	34.4396	$1,442.09
42509	Parotid duct diversion	Y		A2	34.4396	$1,442.09
42510	Parotid duct diversion	Y		A2	34.4396	$1,442.09
42550	Injection for salivary x-ray	N		N1		
42600	Closure of salivary fistula	Y		A2	14.2349	$596.06
42650	Dilation of salivary duct	Y		P3		$36.64
42660	Dilation of salivary duct	Y		P3		$43.18
42665	Ligation of salivary duct	Y		A2	23.5956	$988.02
42700	Drainage of tonsil abscess	Y		A2	3.3186	$138.96
42720	Drainage of throat abscess	Y		A2	14.2349	$596.06
42725	Drainage of throat abscess	Y		A2	33.3886	$1,398.08
42800	Biopsy of throat	Y		P3		$71.02
42802	Biopsy of throat	Y		A2	14.2349	$596.06
42804	Biopsy of upper nose/throat	Y		A2	14.2349	$596.06
42806	Biopsy of upper nose/throat	Y		A2	20.4597	$856.71
42808	Excise pharynx lesion	Y		A2	20.4597	$856.71
42809	Remove pharynx foreign body	N		G2	0.6403	$26.81
42810	Excision of neck cyst	Y		A2	20.8254	$872.02
42815	Excision of neck cyst	Y		A2	34.9366	$1,462.90
42820	Remove tonsils and adenoids	Y		A2	20.8254	$872.02
42821	Remove tonsils and adenoids	Y		A2	22.0077	$921.53
42825	Removal of tonsils	Y		A2	21.5108	$900.72
42826	Removal of tonsils	Y		A2	21.5108	$900.72
42830	Removal of adenoids	Y		A2	21.5108	$900.72
42831	Removal of adenoids	Y		A2	21.5108	$900.72
42835	Removal of adenoids	Y		A2	21.5108	$900.72
42836	Removal of adenoids	Y		A2	21.5108	$900.72
42860	Excision of tonsil tags	Y		A2	20.8254	$872.02
42870	Excision of lingual tonsil	Y		A2	20.8254	$872.02
42890	Partial removal of pharynx	Y		A2	36.5245	$1,529.39
42892	Revision of pharyngeal walls	Y		A2	36.5245	$1,529.39
42900	Repair throat wound	Y		A2	7.3694	$308.58

HCPCS Code	HCPCS Short Descriptor	Subject To Multiple Procedure Discounts	CY 2010 Comment Indicator	CY 2010 Payment Indicator	CY 2010 Third Year Transition. Pymt. Weight	CY 2010 Third Year Transition Payment
42950	Reconstruction of throat	Y		A2	20.4597	$856.71
42955	Surgical opening of throat	Y		A2	20.4597	$856.71
42960	Control throat bleeding	Y		A2	1.2409	$51.96
42962	Control throat bleeding	Y		A2	33.3886	$1,398.08
42970	Control nose/throat bleeding	Y		R2	1.1023	$46.16
42972	Control nose/throat bleeding	Y		A2	15.2459	$638.39
43030	Throat muscle surgery	Y		G2	16.4437	$688.55
43130	Removal of esophagus pouch	Y	CH	G2	41.1215	$1,721.88
43200	Esophagus endoscopy	Y		A2	8.1776	$342.42
43201	Esoph scope w/submucous inj	Y		A2	8.1776	$342.42
43202	Esophagus endoscopy, biopsy	Y		A2	8.1776	$342.42
43204	Esoph scope w/sclerosis inj	Y		A2	8.1776	$342.42
43205	Esophagus endoscopy/ligation	Y		A2	8.1776	$342.42
43215	Esophagus endoscopy	Y		A2	8.1776	$342.42
43216	Esophagus endoscopy/lesion	Y		A2	8.1776	$342.42
43217	Esophagus endoscopy	Y		A2	8.1776	$342.42
43219	Esophagus endoscopy	Y		A2	20.9104	$875.58
43220	Esoph endoscopy, dilation	Y		A2	8.1776	$342.42
43226	Esoph endoscopy, dilation	Y		A2	8.1776	$342.42
43227	Esoph endoscopy, repair	Y		A2	8.8231	$369.45
43228	Esoph endoscopy, ablation	Y		A2	19.962	$835.87
43231	Esoph endoscopy w/us exam	Y		A2	8.8231	$369.45
43232	Esoph endoscopy w/us fn bx	Y		A2	8.8231	$369.45
43234	Upper GI endoscopy, exam	Y		A2	8.1776	$342.42
43235	Uppr gi endoscopy, diagnosis	Y		A2	8.1776	$342.42
43236	Uppr gi scope w/submuc inj	Y		A2	8.8231	$369.45
43237	Endoscopic us exam, esoph	Y		A2	8.8231	$369.45
43238	Uppr gi endoscopy w/us fn bx	Y		A2	8.8231	$369.45
43239	Upper GI endoscopy, biopsy	Y		A2	8.8231	$369.45
43240	Esoph endoscope w/drain cyst	Y		A2	8.8231	$369.45
43241	Upper GI endoscopy with tube	Y		A2	8.8231	$369.45
43242	Uppr gi endoscopy w/us fn bx	Y		A2	8.8231	$369.45
43243	Upper gi endoscopy & inject	Y		A2	8.8231	$369.45
43244	Upper GI endoscopy/ligation	Y		A2	8.8231	$369.45
43245	Uppr gi scope dilate strictr	Y		A2	8.8231	$369.45
43246	Place gastrostomy tube	Y		A2	8.8231	$369.45
43247	Operative upper GI endoscopy	Y		A2	8.8231	$369.45
43248	Uppr gi endoscopy/guide wire	Y		A2	8.8231	$369.45
43249	Esoph endoscopy, dilation	Y		A2	8.8231	$369.45
43250	Upper GI endoscopy/tumor	Y		A2	8.8231	$369.45
43251	Operative upper GI endoscopy	Y		A2	8.8231	$369.45
43255	Operative upper GI endoscopy	Y		A2	8.8231	$369.45
43256	Uppr gi endoscopy w/stent	Y		A2	21.9213	$917.91
43257	Uppr gi scope w/thrml txmnt	Y		A2	20.3277	$851.18
43258	Operative upper GI endoscopy	Y		A2	9.1887	$384.76
43259	Endoscopic ultrasound exam	Y		A2	9.1887	$384.76
43260	Endo cholangiopancreatograph	Y		A2	18.7713	$786.01
43261	Endo cholangiopancreatograph	Y		A2	18.7713	$786.01
43262	Endo cholangiopancreatograph	Y		A2	18.7713	$786.01
43263	Endo cholangiopancreatograph	Y		A2	18.7713	$786.01
43264	Endo cholangiopancreatograph	Y		A2	18.7713	$786.01

HCPCS Code	HCPCS Short Descriptor	Subject To Multiple Procedure Discounts	CY 2010 Comment Indicator	CY 2010 Payment Indicator	CY 2010 Third Year Transition. Pymt. Weight	CY 2010 Third Year Transition Payment
43265	Endo cholangiopancreatograph	Y		A2	18.7713	$786.01
43267	Endo cholangiopancreatograph	Y		A2	18.7713	$786.01
43268	Endo cholangiopancreatograph	Y		A2	21.5557	$902.60
43269	Endo cholangiopancreatograph	Y		A2	21.5557	$902.60
43271	Endo cholangiopancreatograph	Y		A2	18.7713	$786.01
43272	Endo cholangiopancreatograph	Y		A2	18.7713	$786.01
43273	Endoscopic pancreatoscopy	Y		G2	21.632	$905.80
43450	Dilate esophagus	Y		A2	6.1801	$258.78
43453	Dilate esophagus	Y		A2	6.1801	$258.78
43456	Dilate esophagus	Y		A2	6.194	$259.36
43458	Dilate esophagus	Y		A2	8.1914	$343.00
43600	Biopsy of stomach	Y		A2	8.1776	$342.42
43653	Laparoscopy, gastrostomy	Y		A2	41.2571	$1,727.56
43752	Nasal/orogastric w/stent	N	CH	G2	1.2143	$50.85
43760	Change gastrostomy tube	Y		A2	2.547	$106.65
43761	Reposition gastrostomy tube	Y		A2	8.1776	$342.42
43870	Repair stomach opening	Y		A2	8.1776	$342.42
43886	Revise gastric port, open	Y		G2	22.8955	$958.70
43887	Remove gastric port, open	Y		G2	4.2464	$177.81
43888	Change gastric port, open	Y		G2	22.8955	$958.70
44100	Biopsy of bowel	Y		A2	8.1776	$342.42
44312	Revision of ileostomy	Y		A2	19.0736	$798.67
44340	Revision of colostomy	Y		A2	20.0845	$841.00
44360	Small bowel endoscopy	Y		A2	9.6153	$402.62
44361	Small bowel endoscopy/biopsy	Y		A2	9.6153	$402.62
44363	Small bowel endoscopy	Y		A2	9.6153	$402.62
44364	Small bowel endoscopy	Y		A2	9.6153	$402.62
44365	Small bowel endoscopy	Y		A2	9.6153	$402.62
44366	Small bowel endoscopy	Y		A2	9.6153	$402.62
44369	Small bowel endoscopy	Y		A2	9.6153	$402.62
44370	Small bowel endoscopy/stent	Y		A2	26.6566	$1,116.19
44372	Small bowel endoscopy	Y		A2	9.6153	$402.62
44373	Small bowel endoscopy	Y		A2	9.6153	$402.62
44376	Small bowel endoscopy	Y		A2	9.6153	$402.62
44377	Small bowel endoscopy/biopsy	Y		A2	9.6153	$402.62
44378	Small bowel endoscopy	Y		A2	9.6153	$402.62
44379	S bowel endoscope w/stent	Y		A2	26.6566	$1,116.19
44380	Small bowel endoscopy	Y		A2	8.97	$375.60
44382	Small bowel endoscopy	Y		A2	8.97	$375.60
44383	Ileoscopy w/stent	Y		A2	26.6566	$1,116.19
44385	Endoscopy of bowel pouch	Y		A2	8.4353	$353.21
44386	Endoscopy, bowel pouch/biop	Y		A2	8.4353	$353.21
44388	Colonoscopy	Y		A2	8.4353	$353.21
44389	Colonoscopy with biopsy	Y		A2	8.4353	$353.21
44390	Colonoscopy for foreign body	Y		A2	8.4353	$353.21
44391	Colonoscopy for bleeding	Y		A2	8.4353	$353.21
44392	Colonoscopy & polypectomy	Y		A2	8.4353	$353.21
44393	Colonoscopy, lesion removal	Y		A2	8.4353	$353.21
44394	Colonoscopy w/snare	Y		A2	8.4353	$353.21
44397	Colonoscopy w/stent	Y		A2	20.9104	$875.58
44500	Intro, gastrointestinal tube	Y		G2	6.0982	$255.35

HCPCS Code	HCPCS Short Descriptor	Subject To Multiple Procedure Discounts	CY 2010 Comment Indicator	CY 2010 Payment Indicator	CY 2010 Third Year Transition. Pymt. Weight	CY 2010 Third Year Transition Payment
44701	Intraop colon lavage add-on	N		N1		
45000	Drainage of pelvic abscess	Y		A2	11.9098	$498.70
45005	Drainage of rectal abscess	Y		A2	12.6748	$530.73
45020	Drainage of rectal abscess	Y		A2	12.6748	$530.73
45100	Biopsy of rectum	Y		A2	19.1013	$799.83
45108	Removal of anorectal lesion	Y		A2	19.7469	$826.86
45150	Excision of rectal stricture	Y		A2	19.7469	$826.86
45160	Excision of rectal lesion	Y		A2	19.7469	$826.86
45170	Excision of rectal lesion	N	CH	D5		
45171	Exc rect tum transanal part	Y	NI	G2	13.5029	$565.41
45172	Exc rect tum transanal full	Y	NI	G2	22.9324	$960.25
45190	Destruction, rectal tumor	Y		A2	24.8475	$1,040.44
45300	Proctosigmoidoscopy dx	Y		P3		$55.96
45303	Proctosigmoidoscopy dilate	Y		P2	8.8447	$370.35
45305	Proctosigmoidoscopy w/bx	Y		A2	8.5358	$357.42
45307	Proctosigmoidoscopy fb	Y		A2	18.2767	$765.30
45308	Proctosigmoidoscopy removal	Y		A2	8.5358	$357.42
45309	Proctosigmoidoscopy removal	Y		A2	8.5358	$357.42
45315	Proctosigmoidoscopy removal	Y		A2	8.5358	$357.42
45317	Proctosigmoidoscopy bleed	Y		A2	8.5358	$357.42
45320	Proctosigmoidoscopy ablate	Y		A2	18.2767	$765.30
45321	Proctosigmoidoscopy volvul	Y		A2	18.2767	$765.30
45327	Proctosigmoidoscopy w/stent	Y		A2	20.9104	$875.58
45330	Diagnostic sigmoidoscopy	Y		P3		$70.16
45331	Sigmoidoscopy and biopsy	Y		A2	5.8527	$245.07
45332	Sigmoidoscopy w/fb removal	Y		A2	5.8527	$245.07
45333	Sigmoidoscopy & polypectomy	Y		A2	8.5358	$357.42
45334	Sigmoidoscopy for bleeding	Y		A2	8.5358	$357.42
45335	Sigmoidoscopy w/submuc inj	Y		A2	5.8527	$245.07
45337	Sigmoidoscopy & decompress	Y		A2	5.8527	$245.07
45338	Sigmoidoscopy w/tumr remove	Y		A2	8.5358	$357.42
45339	Sigmoidoscopy w/ablate tumr	Y		A2	8.5358	$357.42
45340	Sig w/balloon dilation	Y		A2	8.5358	$357.42
45341	Sigmoidoscopy w/ultrasound	Y		A2	8.5358	$357.42
45342	Sigmoidoscopy w/us guide bx	Y		A2	8.5358	$357.42
45345	Sigmoidoscopy w/stent	Y		A2	20.9104	$875.58
45355	Surgical colonoscopy	Y		A2	8.4353	$353.21
45378	Diagnostic colonoscopy	Y		A2	9.0806	$380.23
45379	Colonoscopy w/fb removal	Y		A2	9.0806	$380.23
45380	Colonoscopy and biopsy	Y		A2	9.0806	$380.23
45381	Colonoscopy, submucous inj	Y		A2	9.0806	$380.23
45382	Colonoscopy/control bleeding	Y		A2	9.0806	$380.23
45383	Lesion removal colonoscopy	Y		A2	9.0806	$380.23
45384	Lesion remove colonoscopy	Y		A2	9.0806	$380.23
45385	Lesion removal colonoscopy	Y		A2	9.0806	$380.23
45386	Colonoscopy dilate stricture	Y		A2	9.0806	$380.23
45387	Colonoscopy w/stent	Y		A2	20.9104	$875.58
45391	Colonoscopy w/endoscope us	Y		A2	9.0806	$380.23
45392	Colonoscopy w/endoscopic fnb	Y		A2	9.0806	$380.23
45500	Repair of rectum	Y		A2	19.7469	$826.86
45505	Repair of rectum	Y		A2	25.6382	$1,073.55

HCPCS Code	HCPCS Short Descriptor	Subject To Multiple Procedure Discounts	CY 2010 Comment Indicator	CY 2010 Payment Indicator	CY 2010 Third Year Transition. Pymt. Weight	CY 2010 Third Year Transition Payment
45520	Treatment of rectal prolapse	Y		P2	0.8408	$35.21
45541	Correct rectal prolapse	Y	CH	G2	30.7878	$1,289.18
45560	Repair of rectocele	Y		A2	25.6382	$1,073.55
45900	Reduction of rectal prolapse	Y		A2	5.632	$235.83
45905	Dilation of anal sphincter	Y		A2	19.1013	$799.83
45910	Dilation of rectal narrowing	Y		A2	19.1013	$799.83
45915	Remove rectal obstruction	Y		A2	11.9098	$498.70
45990	Surg dx exam, anorectal	Y		A2	18.9819	$794.83
46020	Placement of seton	Y		A2	20.1125	$842.17
46030	Removal of rectal marker	Y		A2	5.632	$235.83
46040	Incision of rectal abscess	Y		A2	20.1125	$842.17
46045	Incision of rectal abscess	Y		A2	19.7469	$826.86
46050	Incision of anal abscess	Y		A2	11.9098	$498.70
46060	Incision of rectal abscess	Y		A2	19.7469	$826.86
46070	Incision of anal septum	Y		G2	13.5029	$565.41
46080	Incision of anal sphincter	Y		A2	20.1125	$842.17
46083	Incise external hemorrhoid	Y		P2	1.932	$80.90
46200	Removal of anal fissure	Y		A2	19.7469	$826.86
46210	Removal of anal crypt	N	CH	D5		
46211	Removal of anal crypts	N	CH	D5		
46220	Excise anal ext tag/papilla	Y		A2	12.0292	$503.70
46221	Ligation of hemorrhoid(s)	Y		P3		$105.39
46230	Removal of anal tags	Y		A2	19.1013	$799.83
46250	Remove ext hem groups = 2	Y		A2	20.1125	$842.17
46255	Remove int/ext hem 1 group	Y		A2	20.1125	$842.17
46257	Remove in/ex hem grp & fiss	Y		A2	20.1125	$842.17
46258	Remove in/ex hem grp w/fistu	Y		A2	20.1125	$842.17
46260	Remove in/ex hem groups = 2	Y		A2	20.1125	$842.17
46261	Remove in/ex hem grps & fiss	Y		A2	20.7979	$870.87
46262	Remove in/ex hem grps w/fist	Y		A2	20.7979	$870.87
46270	Remove anal fist subq	Y		A2	20.1125	$842.17
46275	Remove anal fist inter	Y		A2	20.1125	$842.17
46280	Remove anal fist complex	Y		A2	20.7979	$870.87
46285	Remove anal fist 2 stage	Y		A2	19.1013	$799.83
46288	Repair anal fistula	Y		A2	20.7979	$870.87
46320	Removal of hemorrhoid clot	Y		P3		$71.02
46500	Injection into hemorrhoid(s)	Y		P3		$99.42
46505	Chemodenervation anal musc	Y		G2	22.9324	$960.25
46600	Diagnostic anoscopy	N		P2	0.6403	$26.81
46604	Anoscopy and dilation	Y	CH	P3		$343.71
46606	Anoscopy and biopsy	Y		P3		$113.91
46608	Anoscopy, remove for body	Y		A2	8.5358	$357.42
46610	Anoscopy, remove lesion	Y		A2	18.2767	$765.30
46611	Anoscopy	Y		A2	8.5358	$357.42
46612	Anoscopy, remove lesions	Y		A2	18.2767	$765.30
46614	Anoscopy, control bleeding	Y		P3		$59.08
46615	Anoscopy	Y		A2	18.922	$792.32
46700	Repair of anal stricture	Y		A2	20.1125	$842.17
46706	Repr of anal fistula w/glue	Y		A2	24.9927	$1,046.52
46707	Repair anorectal fist w/plug	Y	NI	G2	30.7878	$1,289.18
46750	Repair of anal sphincter	Y		A2	26.0039	$1,088.86

HCPCS Code	HCPCS Short Descriptor	Subject To Multiple Procedure Discounts	CY 2010 Comment Indicator	CY 2010 Payment Indicator	CY 2010 Third Year Transition. Pymt. Weight	CY 2010 Third Year Transition Payment
46753	Reconstruction of anus	Y		A2	20.1125	$842.17
46754	Removal of suture from anus	Y		A2	19.7469	$826.86
46760	Repair of anal sphincter	Y		A2	25.6382	$1,073.55
46761	Repair of anal sphincter	Y		A2	26.0039	$1,088.86
46762	Implant artificial sphincter	Y		A2	28.7742	$1,204.86
46900	Destruction, anal lesion(s)	Y	CH	P3		$102.83
46910	Destruction, anal lesion(s)	Y		P3		$110.50
46916	Cryosurgery, anal lesion(s)	Y		P2	1.4745	$61.74
46917	Laser surgery, anal lesions	Y		A2	17.1605	$718.56
46922	Excision of anal lesion(s)	Y		A2	17.1605	$718.56
46924	Destruction, anal lesion(s)	Y		A2	17.1605	$718.56
46930*	Destroy internal hemorrhoids	Y		P3		$100.56
46937	Cryotherapy of rectal lesion	N	CH	D5		
46938	Cryotherapy of rectal lesion	N	CH	D5		
46940	Treatment of anal fissure	Y		P3		$80.96
46942	Treatment of anal fissure	Y		P3		$79.25
46945	Remove by ligat int hem grp	Y		P3		$132.09
46946	Remove by ligat int hem grps	Y		A2	12.0292	$503.70
46947	Hemorrhoidopexy by stapling	Y		A2	28.7742	$1,204.86
47000	Needle biopsy of liver	Y		A2	8.8382	$370.08
47001	Needle biopsy, liver add-on	N		N1		
47382	Percut ablate liver rf	Y		G2	49.1378	$2,057.55
47500	Injection for liver x-rays	N		N1		
47505	Injection for liver x-rays	N		N1		
47510	Insert catheter, bile duct	Y		A2	24.6063	$1,030.34
47511	Insert bile duct drain	Y		A2	29.1751	$1,221.65
47525	Change bile duct catheter	Y		A2	12.8875	$539.64
47530	Revise/reinsert bile tube	Y		A2	12.8875	$539.64
47552	Biliary endoscopy thru skin	Y		A2	24.6063	$1,030.34
47553	Biliary endoscopy thru skin	Y		A2	24.9719	$1,045.65
47554	Biliary endoscopy thru skin	Y		A2	24.9719	$1,045.65
47555	Biliary endoscopy thru skin	Y		A2	24.9719	$1,045.65
47556	Biliary endoscopy thru skin	Y		A2	29.1751	$1,221.65
47560	Laparoscopy w/cholangio	Y		A2	30.2178	$1,265.31
47561	Laparo w/cholangio/biopsy	Y		A2	30.2178	$1,265.31
47562	Laparoscopic cholecystectomy	Y		G2	44.8118	$1,876.40
47563	Laparo cholecystectomy/graph	Y		G2	44.8118	$1,876.40
47564	Laparo cholecystectomy/explr	Y		G2	44.8118	$1,876.40
47630	Remove bile duct stone	Y		A2	24.9719	$1,045.65
48102	Needle biopsy, pancreas	Y		A2	8.8382	$370.08
49080	Puncture, peritoneal cavity	Y		A2	5.2561	$220.09
49081	Removal of abdominal fluid	Y		A2	5.2561	$220.09
49180	Biopsy, abdominal mass	Y		A2	8.8382	$370.08
49250	Excision of umbilicus	Y		A2	23.1049	$967.47
49320	Diag laparo separate proc	Y		A2	30.2178	$1,265.31
49321	Laparoscopy, biopsy	Y		A2	30.9032	$1,294.01
49322	Laparoscopy, aspiration	Y		A2	30.9032	$1,294.01
49324	Lap insertion perm ip cath	Y		G2	36.4063	$1,524.44
49325	Lap revision perm ip cath	Y		G2	36.4063	$1,524.44
49326	Lap w/omentopexy add-on	Y		G2	36.4063	$1,524.44
49400	Air injection into abdomen	N		N1		

HCPCS Code	HCPCS Short Descriptor	Subject To Multiple Procedure Discounts	CY 2010 Comment Indicator	CY 2010 Payment Indicator	CY 2010 Third Year Transition. Pymt. Weight	CY 2010 Third Year Transition Payment
49402	Remove foreign body, adbomen	Y		A2	22.0538	$923.46
49411	Ins mark abd/pel for rt perq	N	NI	P3		$281.50
49419	Insrt abdom cath for chemotx	Y		A2	24.1299	$1,010.39
49420	Insert abdom drain, temp	Y		A2	23.758	$994.82
49421	Insert abdom drain, perm	Y		A2	23.758	$994.82
49422	Remove perm cannula/catheter	Y		A2	18.3631	$768.92
49423	Exchange drainage catheter	Y		G2	14.6474	$613.33
49424	Assess cyst, contrast inject	N		N1		
49426	Revise abdomen-venous shunt	Y		A2	22.0538	$923.46
49427	Injection, abdominal shunt	N		N1		
49429	Removal of shunt	Y		G2	21.9478	$919.02
49435	Insert subq exten to ip cath	Y	CH	G2	14.6474	$613.33
49436	Embedded ip cath exit-site	Y	CH	G2	14.6474	$613.33
49440	Place gastrostomy tube perc	Y		G2	8.3675	$350.37
49441	Place duod/jej tube perc	Y		G2	8.3675	$350.37
49442	Place cecostomy tube perc	Y	CH	G2	13.5029	$565.41
49446	Change g-tube to g-j perc	Y		G2	8.3675	$350.37
49450	Replace g/c tube perc	Y		G2	6.0982	$255.35
49451	Replace duod/jej tube perc	Y		G2	6.0982	$255.35
49452	Replace g-j tube perc	Y		G2	6.0982	$255.35
49460	Fix g/colon tube w/device	Y		G2	6.0982	$255.35
49465	Fluoro exam of g/colon tube	N		N1		
49495	Rpr ing hernia baby, reduc	Y		A2	26.5364	$1,111.16
49496	Rpr ing hernia baby, blocked	Y		A2	26.5364	$1,111.16
49500	Rpr ing hernia, init, reduce	Y		A2	26.5364	$1,111.16
49501	Rpr ing hernia, init blocked	Y		A2	30.5863	$1,280.74
49505	Prp i/hern init reduc >5 yr	Y		A2	26.5364	$1,111.16
49507	Prp i/hern init block >5 yr	Y		A2	30.5863	$1,280.74
49520	Rerepair ing hernia, reduce	Y		A2	28.6213	$1,198.46
49521	Rerepair ing hernia, blocked	Y		A2	30.5863	$1,280.74
49525	Repair ing hernia, sliding	Y		A2	26.5364	$1,111.16
49540	Repair lumbar hernia	Y		A2	25.4854	$1,067.15
49550	Rpr rem hernia, init, reduce	Y		A2	27.0334	$1,131.97
49553	Rpr fem hernia, init blocked	Y		A2	30.5863	$1,280.74
49555	Rerepair fem hernia, reduce	Y		A2	27.0334	$1,131.97
49557	Rerepair fem hernia, blocked	Y		A2	30.5863	$1,280.74
49560	Rpr ventral hern init, reduc	Y		A2	26.5364	$1,111.16
49561	Rpr ventral hern init, block	Y		A2	30.5863	$1,280.74
49565	Rerepair ventrl hern, reduce	Y		A2	26.5364	$1,111.16
49566	Rerepair ventrl hern, block	Y		A2	30.5863	$1,280.74
49568	Hernia repair w/mesh	Y		A2	28.6213	$1,198.46
49570	Rpr epigastric hern, reduce	Y		A2	26.5364	$1,111.16
49572	Rpr epigastric hern, blocked	Y		A2	30.5863	$1,280.74
49580	Rpr umbil hern, reduc < 5 yr	Y		A2	26.5364	$1,111.16
49582	Rpr umbil hern, block < 5 yr	Y		A2	30.5863	$1,280.74
49585	Rpr umbil hern, reduc > 5 yr	Y		A2	26.5364	$1,111.16
49587	Rpr umbil hern, block > 5 yr	Y		A2	30.5863	$1,280.74
49590	Repair spigelian hernia	Y		A2	25.851	$1,082.46
49600	Repair umbilical lesion	Y		A2	26.5364	$1,111.16
49650	Lap ing hernia repair init	Y		A2	37.2073	$1,557.98
49651	Lap ing hernia repair recur	Y		A2	39.2921	$1,645.28

HCPCS Code	HCPCS Short Descriptor	Subject To Multiple Procedure Discounts	CY 2010 Comment Indicator	CY 2010 Payment Indicator	CY 2010 Third Year Transition. Pymt. Weight	CY 2010 Third Year Transition Payment
49652	Lap vent/abd hernia repair	Y		G2	69.7991	$2,922.70
49653	Lap vent/abd hern proc comp	Y		G2	69.7991	$2,922.70
49654	Lap inc hernia repair	Y		G2	69.7991	$2,922.70
49655	Lap inc hern repair comp	Y		G2	69.7991	$2,922.70
49656	Lap inc hernia repair recur	Y		G2	69.7991	$2,922.70
49657	Lap inc hern recur comp	Y		G2	69.7991	$2,922.70
50080	Removal of kidney stone	Y	CH	G2	44.6588	$1,870.00
50081	Removal of kidney stone	Y	CH	G2	44.6588	$1,870.00
50200	Renal biopsy perq	Y		A2	8.8382	$370.08
50382	Change ureter stent, percut	Y		G2	24.4172	$1,022.42
50384	Remove ureter stent, percut	Y		G2	16.2968	$682.40
50385	Change stent via transureth	Y		G2	24.4172	$1,022.42
50386	Remove stent via transureth	Y	CH	P2	6.8253	$285.80
50387	Change ext/int ureter stent	Y		G2	14.6474	$613.33
50389	Remove renal tube w/fluoro	Y		G2	6.8253	$285.80
50390	Drainage of kidney lesion	Y		A2	8.8382	$370.08
50391	Instll rx agnt into rnal tub	Y	CH	P3		$42.33
50392	Insert kidney drain	Y		A2	14.1246	$591.44
50393	Insert ureteral tube	Y		A2	20.2152	$846.47
50394	Injection for kidney x-ray	N		N1		
50395	Create passage to kidney	Y		A2	20.2152	$846.47
50396	Measure kidney pressure	Y		A2	2.2002	$92.13
50398	Change kidney tube	Y		A2	12.8875	$539.64
50551	Kidney endoscopy	Y		A2	7.021	$293.99
50553	Kidney endoscopy	Y		A2	20.2152	$846.47
50555	Kidney endoscopy & biopsy	Y		A2	7.021	$293.99
50557	Kidney endoscopy & treatment	Y		A2	20.2152	$846.47
50561	Kidney endoscopy & treatment	Y		A2	20.2152	$846.47
50562	Renal scope w/tumor resect	Y		G2	6.8253	$285.80
50570	Kidney endoscopy	Y		G2	6.8253	$285.80
50572	Kidney endoscopy	Y		G2	6.8253	$285.80
50574	Kidney endoscopy & biopsy	Y		G2	6.8253	$285.80
50575	Kidney endoscopy	Y		G2	34.6334	$1,450.20
50576	Kidney endoscopy & treatment	Y		G2	16.2968	$682.40
50580	Kidney endoscopy & treatment	Y		G2	16.2968	$682.40
50590	Fragmenting of kidney stone	Y		G2	39.5716	$1,656.98
50592	Perc rf ablate renal tumor	Y		G2	49.1378	$2,057.55
50684	Injection for ureter x-ray	N		N1		
50686	Measure ureter pressure	Y	CH	P3		$37.78
50688	Change of ureter tube/stent	Y		A2	12.8875	$539.64
50690	Injection for ureter x-ray	N		N1		
50727	Revise ureter	Y	CH	G2	19.1572	$802.17
50947	Laparo new ureter/bladder	Y		A2	41.2571	$1,727.56
50948	Laparo new ureter/bladder	Y		A2	41.2571	$1,727.56
50951	Endoscopy of ureter	Y		A2	7.021	$293.99
50953	Endoscopy of ureter	Y		A2	7.021	$293.99
50955	Ureter endoscopy & biopsy	Y		A2	20.2152	$846.47
50957	Ureter endoscopy & treatment	Y		A2	20.2152	$846.47
50961	Ureter endoscopy & treatment	Y		A2	20.2152	$846.47
50970	Ureter endoscopy	Y		A2	7.021	$293.99
50972	Ureter endoscopy & catheter	Y		A2	7.021	$293.99

HCPCS Code	HCPCS Short Descriptor	Subject To Multiple Procedure Discounts	CY 2010 Comment Indicator	CY 2010 Payment Indicator	CY 2010 Third Year Transition. Pymt. Weight	CY 2010 Third Year Transition Payment
50974	Ureter endoscopy & biopsy	Y		A2	14.1246	$591.44
50976	Ureter endoscopy & treatment	Y		A2	14.1246	$591.44
50980	Ureter endoscopy & treatment	Y		A2	20.2152	$846.47
51020	Incise & treat bladder	Y		A2	21.9115	$917.50
51030	Incise & treat bladder	Y		A2	21.9115	$917.50
51040	Incise & drain bladder	Y		A2	21.9115	$917.50
51045	Incise bladder/drain ureter	Y		A2	7.3993	$309.83
51050	Removal of bladder stone	Y		A2	21.9115	$917.50
51065	Remove ureter calculus	Y		A2	21.9115	$917.50
51080	Drainage of bladder abscess	Y		A2	15.8264	$662.70
51100	Drain bladder by needle	Y		P3		$25.00
51101	Drain bladder by trocar/cath	Y		P2	1.0484	$43.90
51102	Drain bl w/cath insertion	Y		A2	16.2699	$681.27
51500	Removal of bladder cyst	Y		A2	26.5364	$1,111.16
51520	Removal of bladder lesion	Y		A2	21.9115	$917.50
51535	Repair of ureter lesion	Y	CH	G2	24.4172	$1,022.42
51600	Injection for bladder x-ray	N		N1		
51605	Preparation for bladder xray	N		N1		
51610	Injection for bladder x-ray	N		N1		
51700	Irrigation of bladder	Y		P3		$41.47
51701	Insert bladder catheter	N		P2	0.6403	$26.81
51702	Insert temp bladder cath	N		P2	0.6403	$26.81
51703	Insert bladder cath, complex	Y		P2	1.0484	$43.90
51705	Change of bladder tube	Y	CH	P3		$56.81
51710	Change of bladder tube	Y		A2	6.4758	$271.16
51715	Endoscopic injection/implant	Y		A2	25.4269	$1,064.70
51720	Treatment of bladder lesion	Y		P3		$45.45
51725	Simple cystometrogram	Y	CH	P3		$106.52
51726	Complex cystometrogram	Y		A2	3.3645	$140.88
51727	Cystometrogram w/up	Y	NI	P2	2.8906	$121.04
51728	Cystometrogram w/vp	Y	NI	P2	2.8906	$121.04
51729	Cystometrogram w/vp&up	Y	NI	P2	2.8906	$121.04
51736	Urine flow measurement	Y		P3		$17.04
51741	Electro-uroflowmetry, first	Y		P3		$19.88
51772	Urethra pressure profile	N	CH	D5		
51784	Anal/urinary muscle study	Y		P2	1.0484	$43.90
51785	Anal/urinary muscle study	Y		A2	1.8313	$76.68
51792	Urinary reflex study	Y		P2	1.0484	$43.90
51795	Urine voiding pressure study	N	CH	D5		
51797	Intraabdominal pressure test	Y	CH	P3		$74.71
51798	Us urine capacity measure	N		P3		$14.49
51880	Repair of bladder opening	Y		A2	20.2152	$846.47
51992	Laparo sling operation	Y		A2	37.7042	$1,578.79
52000	Cystoscopy	Y		A2	7.021	$293.99
52001	Cystoscopy, removal of clots	Y		A2	14.5029	$607.28
52005	Cystoscopy & ureter catheter	Y		A2	20.8605	$873.49
52007	Cystoscopy and biopsy	Y		A2	20.8605	$873.49
52010	Cystoscopy & duct catheter	Y		A2	7.3993	$309.83
52204	Cystoscopy w/biopsy(s)	Y		A2	20.8605	$873.49
52214	Cystoscopy and treatment	Y		A2	20.8605	$873.49
52224	Cystoscopy and treatment	Y		A2	20.8605	$873.49

HCPCS Code	HCPCS Short Descriptor	Subject To Multiple Procedure Discounts	CY 2010 Comment Indicator	CY 2010 Payment Indicator	CY 2010 Third Year Transition. Pymt. Weight	CY 2010 Third Year Transition Payment
52234	Cystoscopy and treatment	Y		A2	20.8605	$873.49
52235	Cystoscopy and treatment	Y		A2	21.2261	$888.80
52240	Cystoscopy and treatment	Y		A2	21.2261	$888.80
52250	Cystoscopy and radiotracer	Y		A2	21.9115	$917.50
52260	Cystoscopy and treatment	Y		A2	14.7699	$618.46
52265	Cystoscopy and treatment	Y	CH	P3		$235.77
52270	Cystoscopy & revise urethra	Y		A2	14.7699	$618.46
52275	Cystoscopy & revise urethra	Y		A2	20.8605	$873.49
52276	Cystoscopy and treatment	Y		A2	21.2261	$888.80
52277	Cystoscopy and treatment	Y		A2	20.8605	$873.49
52281	Cystoscopy and treatment	Y		A2	14.7699	$618.46
52282	Cystoscopy, implant stent	Y		A2	33.6233	$1,407.91
52283	Cystoscopy and treatment	Y		A2	20.8605	$873.49
52285	Cystoscopy and treatment	Y		A2	14.7699	$618.46
52290	Cystoscopy and treatment	Y		A2	20.8605	$873.49
52300	Cystoscopy and treatment	Y		A2	20.8605	$873.49
52301	Cystoscopy and treatment	Y		A2	21.2261	$888.80
52305	Cystoscopy and treatment	Y		A2	20.8605	$873.49
52310	Cystoscopy and treatment	Y		A2	14.5029	$607.28
52315	Cystoscopy and treatment	Y		A2	20.8605	$873.49
52317	Remove bladder stone	Y		A2	20.2152	$846.47
52318	Remove bladder stone	Y		A2	20.8605	$873.49
52320	Cystoscopy and treatment	Y		A2	22.4085	$938.31
52325	Cystoscopy, stone removal	Y		A2	21.9115	$917.50
52327	Cystoscopy, inject material	Y		A2	28.5224	$1,194.32
52330	Cystoscopy and treatment	Y		A2	20.8605	$873.49
52332	Cystoscopy and treatment	Y		A2	20.8605	$873.49
52334	Create passage to kidney	Y		A2	21.2261	$888.80
52341	Cysto w/ureter stricture tx	Y		A2	21.2261	$888.80
52342	Cysto w/up stricture tx	Y		A2	21.2261	$888.80
52343	Cysto w/renal stricture tx	Y		A2	21.2261	$888.80
52344	Cysto/uretero, stricture tx	Y		A2	21.2261	$888.80
52345	Cysto/uretero w/up stricture	Y		A2	21.2261	$888.80
52346	Cystouretero w/renal strict	Y		A2	21.2261	$888.80
52351	Cystouretero & or pyeloscope	Y		A2	21.2261	$888.80
52352	Cystouretero w/stone remove	Y		A2	21.9115	$917.50
52353	Cystouretero w/lithotripsy	Y		A2	29.5735	$1,238.33
52354	Cystouretero w/biopsy	Y		A2	21.9115	$917.50
52355	Cystouretero w/excise tumor	Y		A2	21.9115	$917.50
52400	Cystouretero w/congen repr	Y		A2	21.2261	$888.80
52402	Cystourethro cut ejacul duct	Y		A2	21.2261	$888.80
52450	Incision of prostate	Y		A2	21.2261	$888.80
52500	Revision of bladder neck	Y		A2	21.2261	$888.80
52601	Prostatectomy (TURP)	Y		A2	29.5735	$1,238.33
52630	Remove prostate regrowth	Y		A2	28.5224	$1,194.32
52640	Relieve bladder contracture	Y		A2	20.8605	$873.49
52647	Laser surgery of prostate	Y		A2	41.1423	$1,722.75
52648	Laser surgery of prostate	Y		A2	41.1423	$1,722.75
52700	Drainage of prostate abscess	Y		A2	20.8605	$873.49
53000	Incision of urethra	Y		A2	16.4949	$690.69
53010	Incision of urethra	Y		A2	16.4949	$690.69

HCPCS Code	HCPCS Short Descriptor	Subject To Multiple Procedure Discounts	CY 2010 Comment Indicator	CY 2010 Payment Indicator	CY 2010 Third Year Transition. Pymt. Weight	CY 2010 Third Year Transition Payment
53020	Incision of urethra	Y		A2	16.4949	$690.69
53025	Incision of urethra	Y		R2	19.4568	$814.71
53040	Drainage of urethra abscess	Y		A2	17.1402	$717.71
53060	Drainage of urethra abscess	Y		P3		$58.52
53080	Drainage of urinary leakage	Y		A2	17.5058	$733.02
53085	Drainage of urinary leakage	Y		G2	19.4568	$814.71
53200	Biopsy of urethra	Y		A2	16.4949	$690.69
53210	Removal of urethra	Y		A2	26.6093	$1,114.21
53215	Removal of urethra	Y		A2	18.6882	$782.53
53220	Treatment of urethra lesion	Y		A2	25.0613	$1,049.39
53230	Removal of urethra lesion	Y		A2	25.0613	$1,049.39
53235	Removal of urethra lesion	Y		A2	17.5058	$733.02
53240	Surgery for urethra pouch	Y		A2	25.0613	$1,049.39
53250	Removal of urethra gland	Y		A2	17.1402	$717.71
53260	Treatment of urethra lesion	Y		A2	17.1402	$717.71
53265	Treatment of urethra lesion	Y		A2	17.1402	$717.71
53270	Removal of urethra gland	Y		A2	17.1402	$717.71
53275	Repair of urethra defect	Y		A2	17.1402	$717.71
53400	Revise urethra, stage 1	Y		A2	25.4269	$1,064.70
53405	Revise urethra, stage 2	Y		A2	25.0613	$1,049.39
53410	Reconstruction of urethra	Y		A2	25.0613	$1,049.39
53420	Reconstruct urethra, stage 1	Y		A2	25.4269	$1,064.70
53425	Reconstruct urethra, stage 2	Y		A2	25.0613	$1,049.39
53430	Reconstruction of urethra	Y		A2	25.0613	$1,049.39
53431	Reconstruct urethra/bladder	Y		A2	25.0613	$1,049.39
53440	Male sling procedure	N		H8	124.7551	$5,223.87
53442	Remove/revise male sling	Y		A2	24.416	$1,022.37
53444	Insert tandem cuff	N		H8	124.7551	$5,223.87
53445	Insert uro/ves nck sphincter	N		H8	223.2126	$9,346.58
53446	Remove uro sphincter	Y		A2	24.416	$1,022.37
53447	Remove/replace ur sphincter	N		H8	223.2126	$9,346.58
53449	Repair uro sphincter	Y		A2	24.416	$1,022.37
53450	Revision of urethra	Y		A2	24.416	$1,022.37
53460	Revision of urethra	Y		A2	16.4949	$690.69
53502	Repair of urethra injury	Y		A2	17.1402	$717.71
53505	Repair of urethra injury	Y		A2	25.0613	$1,049.39
53510	Repair of urethra injury	Y		A2	17.1402	$717.71
53515	Repair of urethra injury	Y		A2	25.0613	$1,049.39
53520	Repair of urethra defect	Y		A2	25.0613	$1,049.39
53600	Dilate urethra stricture	Y		P3		$31.81
53601	Dilate urethra stricture	Y	CH	P3		$36.93
53605	Dilate urethra stricture	Y		A2	14.7699	$618.46
53620	Dilate urethra stricture	Y		P3		$48.57
53621	Dilate urethra stricture	Y		P3		$51.13
53660	Dilation of urethra	Y	CH	P3		$36.08
53661	Dilation of urethra	Y	CH	P3		$35.22
53665	Dilation of urethra	Y		A2	16.4949	$690.69
53850	Prostatic microwave thermotx	Y	CH	P3		$1,568.87
53852	Prostatic rf thermotx	Y	CH	P3		$1,479.96
53855	Insert prost urethral stent	Y	NI	P2	1.932	$80.90
54000	Slitting of prepuce	Y		A2	17.1402	$717.71

HCPCS Code	HCPCS Short Descriptor	Subject To Multiple Procedure Discounts	CY 2010 Comment Indicator	CY 2010 Payment Indicator	CY 2010 Third Year Transition. Pymt. Weight	CY 2010 Third Year Transition Payment
54001	Slitting of prepuce	Y		A2	17.1402	$717.71
54015	Drain penis lesion	Y		A2	17.523	$733.74
54050	Destruction, penis lesion(s)	Y		P2	0.8408	$35.21
54055	Destruction, penis lesion(s)	Y		P3		$53.40
54056	Cryosurgery, penis lesion(s)	Y		P2	0.8408	$35.21
54057	Laser surg, penis lesion(s)	Y		A2	17.1605	$718.56
54060	Excision of penis lesion(s)	Y		A2	17.1605	$718.56
54065	Destruction, penis lesion(s)	Y		A2	17.1605	$718.56
54100	Biopsy of penis	Y		A2	14.457	$605.36
54105	Biopsy of penis	Y		A2	18.6836	$782.34
54110	Treatment of penis lesion	Y		A2	27.5774	$1,154.75
54111	Treat penis lesion, graft	Y		A2	27.5774	$1,154.75
54112	Treat penis lesion, graft	Y		A2	27.5774	$1,154.75
54115	Treatment of penis lesion	Y		A2	15.8264	$662.70
54120	Partial removal of penis	Y		A2	27.5774	$1,154.75
54150	Circumcision w/regionl block	Y		A2	18.6086	$779.20
54160	Circumcision, neonate	Y		A2	19.2542	$806.23
54161	Circum 28 days or older	Y		A2	19.2542	$806.23
54162	Lysis penil circumic lesion	Y		A2	19.2542	$806.23
54163	Repair of circumcision	Y		A2	19.2542	$806.23
54164	Frenulotomy of penis	Y		A2	19.2542	$806.23
54200	Treatment of penis lesion	Y		P3		$53.97
54205	Treatment of penis lesion	Y		A2	28.6285	$1,198.76
54220	Treatment of penis lesion	Y		A2	2.2002	$92.13
54230	Prepare penis study	N		N1		
54231	Dynamic cavernosometry	Y		P3		$51.13
54235	Penile injection	Y		P3		$36.36
54240	Penis study	Y		P3		$25.85
54250	Penis study	Y		P3		$9.09
54300	Revision of penis	Y		A2	27.9431	$1,170.06
54304	Revision of penis	Y		A2	27.9431	$1,170.06
54308	Reconstruction of urethra	Y		A2	27.9431	$1,170.06
54312	Reconstruction of urethra	Y		A2	27.9431	$1,170.06
54316	Reconstruction of urethra	Y		A2	27.9431	$1,170.06
54318	Reconstruction of urethra	Y		A2	27.9431	$1,170.06
54322	Reconstruction of urethra	Y		A2	27.9431	$1,170.06
54324	Reconstruction of urethra	Y		A2	27.9431	$1,170.06
54326	Reconstruction of urethra	Y		A2	27.9431	$1,170.06
54328	Revise penis/urethra	Y		A2	27.9431	$1,170.06
54340	Secondary urethral surgery	Y		A2	27.9431	$1,170.06
54344	Secondary urethral surgery	Y		A2	27.9431	$1,170.06
54348	Secondary urethral surgery	Y		A2	27.9431	$1,170.06
54352	Reconstruct urethra/penis	Y		A2	27.9431	$1,170.06
54360	Penis plastic surgery	Y		A2	27.9431	$1,170.06
54380	Repair penis	Y		A2	27.9431	$1,170.06
54385	Repair penis	Y		A2	27.9431	$1,170.06
54400	Insert semi-rigid prosthesis	N		H8	125.1205	$5,239.17
54401	Insert self-contd prosthesis	N		H8	224.2235	$9,388.91
54405	Insert multi-comp penis pros	N		H8	224.2235	$9,388.91
54406	Remove muti-comp penis pros	Y		A2	27.9431	$1,170.06
54408	Repair multi-comp penis pros	Y		A2	27.9431	$1,170.06

HCPCS Code	HCPCS Short Descriptor	Subject To Multiple Procedure Discounts	CY 2010 Comment Indicator	CY 2010 Payment Indicator	CY 2010 Third Year Transition. Pymt. Weight	CY 2010 Third Year Transition Payment
54410	Remove/replace penis prosth	N		H8	224.2235	$9,388.91
54415	Remove self-contd penis pros	Y		A2	27.9431	$1,170.06
54416	Remv/repl penis contain pros	N		H8	224.2235	$9,388.91
54420	Revision of penis	Y		A2	28.6285	$1,198.76
54435	Revision of penis	Y		A2	28.6285	$1,198.76
54440	Repair of penis	Y		A2	28.6285	$1,198.76
54450	Preputial stretching	Y		A2	3.3645	$140.88
54500	Biopsy of testis	Y		A2	13.0239	$545.35
54505	Biopsy of testis	Y		A2	18.6086	$779.20
54512	Excise lesion testis	Y		A2	19.2542	$806.23
54520	Removal of testis	Y		A2	19.6196	$821.53
54522	Orchiectomy, partial	Y		A2	19.6196	$821.53
54530	Removal of testis	Y		A2	26.5364	$1,111.16
54550	Exploration for testis	Y		A2	26.5364	$1,111.16
54560	Exploration for testis	Y		G2	22.2756	$932.75
54600	Reduce testis torsion	Y		A2	20.3052	$850.24
54620	Suspension of testis	Y		A2	19.6196	$821.53
54640	Suspension of testis	Y		A2	26.5364	$1,111.16
54660	Revision of testis	Y		A2	19.2542	$806.23
54670	Repair testis injury	Y		A2	19.6196	$821.53
54680	Relocation of testis(es)	Y		A2	19.6196	$821.53
54690	Laparoscopy, orchiectomy	Y		A2	41.2571	$1,727.56
54692	Laparoscopy, orchiopexy	Y		G2	69.7991	$2,922.70
54700	Drainage of scrotum	Y		A2	19.2542	$806.23
54800	Biopsy of epididymis	Y		A2	4.0262	$168.59
54830	Remove epididymis lesion	Y		A2	19.6196	$821.53
54840	Remove epididymis lesion	Y		A2	20.3052	$850.24
54860	Removal of epididymis	Y		A2	19.6196	$821.53
54861	Removal of epididymis	Y		A2	20.3052	$850.24
54865	Explore epididymis	Y		A2	18.6086	$779.20
54900	Fusion of spermatic ducts	Y		A2	20.3052	$850.24
54901	Fusion of spermatic ducts	Y		A2	20.3052	$850.24
55000	Drainage of hydrocele	Y		P3		$52.55
55040	Removal of hydrocele	Y		A2	25.851	$1,082.46
55041	Removal of hydroceles	Y		A2	27.0334	$1,131.97
55060	Repair of hydrocele	Y		A2	20.3052	$850.24
55100	Drainage of scrotum abscess	Y		A2	10.9586	$458.87
55110	Explore scrotum	Y		A2	19.2542	$806.23
55120	Removal of scrotum lesion	Y		A2	19.2542	$806.23
55150	Removal of scrotum	Y		A2	18.6086	$779.20
55175	Revision of scrotum	Y		A2	18.6086	$779.20
55180	Revision of scrotum	Y		A2	19.2542	$806.23
55200	Incision of sperm duct	Y		A2	19.2542	$806.23
55250	Removal of sperm duct(s)	Y		A2	19.2542	$806.23
55300	Prepare, sperm duct x-ray	N		N1		
55400	Repair of sperm duct	Y		A2	18.6086	$779.20
55450	Ligation of sperm duct	Y		P3		$166.74
55500	Removal of hydrocele	Y		A2	19.6196	$821.53
55520	Removal of sperm cord lesion	Y		A2	20.3052	$850.24
55530	Revise spermatic cord veins	Y		A2	20.3052	$850.24
55535	Revise spermatic cord veins	Y		A2	26.5364	$1,111.16

HCPCS Code	HCPCS Short Descriptor	Subject To Multiple Procedure Discounts	CY 2010 Comment Indicator	CY 2010 Payment Indicator	CY 2010 Third Year Transition. Pymt. Weight	CY 2010 Third Year Transition Payment
55540	Revise hernia & sperm veins	Y		A2	27.0334	$1,131.97
55550	Laparo ligate spermatic vein	Y		A2	41.2571	$1,727.56
55600	Incise sperm duct pouch	Y		R2	22.2756	$932.75
55680	Remove sperm pouch lesion	Y		A2	18.6086	$779.20
55700	Biopsy of prostate	Y		A2	10.8951	$456.21
55705	Biopsy of prostate	Y		A2	10.8951	$456.21
55706	Prostate saturation sampling	Y		G2	11.893	$498.00
55720	Drainage of prostate abscess	Y		A2	20.2152	$846.47
55725	Drainage of prostate abscess	Y		A2	20.8605	$873.49
55860	Surgical exposure, prostate	Y		G2	19.1572	$802.17
55870	Electroejaculation	Y		P3		$63.06
55873	Cryoablate prostate	Y		H8	146.626	$6,139.67
55875	Transperi needle place, pros	N		A2	33.6233	$1,407.91
55876	Place rt device/marker, pros	N		P3		$57.66
55920	Place needles pelvic for rt	Y		G2	26.0084	$1,089.05
56405	I & D of vulva/perineum	Y		P3		$35.51
56420	Drainage of gland abscess	Y	CH	P3		$48.57
56440	Surgery for vulva lesion	Y		A2	16.9305	$708.93
56441	Lysis of labial lesion(s)	Y		A2	16.285	$681.90
56442	Hymenotomy	Y		A2	16.285	$681.90
56501	Destroy, vulva lesions, sim	Y		P3		$48.57
56515	Destroy vulva lesion/s compl	Y		A2	18.1714	$760.89
56605	Biopsy of vulva/perineum	Y		P3		$28.12
56606	Biopsy of vulva/perineum	Y		P3		$11.65
56620	Partial removal of vulva	Y		A2	18.4785	$773.75
56625	Complete removal of vulva	Y		A2	20.0664	$840.24
56700	Partial removal of hymen	Y		A2	16.285	$681.90
56740	Remove vagina gland lesion	Y		A2	17.2961	$724.24
56800	Repair of vagina	Y		A2	17.2961	$724.24
56805	Repair clitoris	Y		G2	19.1772	$803.01
56810	Repair of perineum	Y		A2	18.4785	$773.75
56820	Exam of vulva w/scope	Y		P3		$36.08
56821	Exam/biopsy of vulva w/scope	Y	CH	P3		$46.59
57000	Exploration of vagina	Y		A2	16.285	$681.90
57010	Drainage of pelvic abscess	Y		A2	16.9305	$708.93
57020	Drainage of pelvic fluid	Y		A2	7.2135	$302.05
57022	I & d vaginal hematoma, pp	Y	CH	R2	12.0752	$505.62
57023	I & d vag hematoma, non-ob	Y		A2	15.8264	$662.70
57061	Destroy vag lesions, simple	Y		P3		$44.60
57065	Destroy vag lesions, complex	Y		A2	16.285	$681.90
57100	Biopsy of vagina	Y		P3		$28.69
57105	Biopsy of vagina	Y		A2	16.9305	$708.93
57130	Remove vagina lesion	Y		A2	16.9305	$708.93
57135	Remove vagina lesion	Y		A2	16.9305	$708.93
57150	Treat vagina infection	Y		P3		$19.88
57155	Insert uteri tandems/ovoids	Y		A2	7.2135	$302.05
57160	Insert pessary/other device	Y		P3		$29.83
57170	Fitting of diaphragm/cap	Y		P2	0.1263	$5.29
57180	Treat vaginal bleeding	Y		A2	2.1133	$88.49
57200	Repair of vagina	Y		A2	16.285	$681.90
57210	Repair vagina/perineum	Y		A2	16.9305	$708.93

HCPCS Code	HCPCS Short Descriptor	Subject To Multiple Procedure Discounts	CY 2010 Comment Indicator	CY 2010 Payment Indicator	CY 2010 Third Year Transition. Pymt. Weight	CY 2010 Third Year Transition Payment
57220	Revision of urethra	Y		A2	35.194	$1,473.68
57230	Repair of urethral lesion	Y		A2	28.2177	$1,181.56
57240	Repair bladder & vagina	Y		A2	29.4001	$1,231.07
57250	Repair rectum & vagina	Y		A2	29.4001	$1,231.07
57260	Repair of vagina	Y		A2	29.4001	$1,231.07
57265	Extensive repair of vagina	Y		A2	37.9643	$1,589.68
57267	Insert mesh/pelvic flr addon	Y		A2	30.988	$1,297.56
57268	Repair of bowel bulge	Y		A2	28.2177	$1,181.56
57287	Revise/remove sling repair	Y		G2	33.7396	$1,412.78
57288	Repair bladder defect	Y		A2	36.3764	$1,523.19
57289	Repair bladder & vagina	Y		A2	29.4001	$1,231.07
57291	Construction of vagina	Y		A2	29.4001	$1,231.07
57295	Revise vag graft via vagina	Y	CH	G2	19.1772	$803.01
57300	Repair rectum-vagina fistula	Y		A2	28.2177	$1,181.56
57320	Repair bladder-vagina lesion	Y		G2	33.7396	$1,412.78
57400	Dilation of vagina	Y		A2	16.9305	$708.93
57410	Pelvic examination	Y		A2	16.9305	$708.93
57415	Remove vaginal foreign body	Y		A2	16.9305	$708.93
57420	Exam of vagina w/scope	Y		P3		$37.21
57421	Exam/biopsy of vag w/scope	Y		P3		$48.57
57426	Revise prosth vag graft lap	Y	NI	G2	19.1772	$803.01
57452	Exam of cervix w/scope	Y		P3		$35.22
57454	Bx/curett of cervix w/scope	Y		P3		$43.46
57455	Biopsy of cervix w/scope	Y		P3		$45.45
57456	Endocerv curettage w/scope	Y		P3		$44.03
57460	Bx of cervix w/scope, leep	Y		P3		$130.95
57461	Conz of cervix w/scope, leep	Y		P3		$139.76
57500	Biopsy of cervix	Y		P3		$60.22
57505	Endocervical curettage	Y		P3		$39.20
57510	Cauterization of cervix	Y		P3		$40.05
57511	Cryocautery of cervix	Y	CH	P3		$48.57
57513	Laser surgery of cervix	Y		A2	16.9305	$708.93
57520	Conization of cervix	Y		A2	16.9305	$708.93
57522	Conization of cervix	Y		A2	16.9305	$708.93
57530	Removal of cervix	Y		A2	28.2177	$1,181.56
57550	Removal of residual cervix	Y		A2	28.2177	$1,181.56
57556	Remove cervix, repair bowel	Y		A2	36.3764	$1,523.19
57558	D&c of cervical stump	Y		A2	17.2961	$724.24
57700	Revision of cervix	Y		A2	16.285	$681.90
57720	Revision of cervix	Y		A2	17.2961	$724.24
57800	Dilation of cervical canal	Y		P3		$21.02
58100	Biopsy of uterus lining	Y		P3		$34.94
58110	Bx done w/colposcopy add-on	N		N1		
58120	Dilation and curettage	Y		A2	16.9305	$708.93
58145	Myomectomy vag method	Y		A2	29.4001	$1,231.07
58301	Remove intrauterine device	Y		P3		$32.38
58321	Artificial insemination	Y		P3		$30.39
58322	Artificial insemination	Y		P3		$30.96
58323	Sperm washing	Y		P3		$6.53
58340	Catheter for hysterography	N		N1		
58345	Reopen fallopian tube	Y		R2	19.1772	$803.01

HCPCS Code	HCPCS Short Descriptor	Subject To Multiple Procedure Discounts	CY 2010 Comment Indicator	CY 2010 Payment Indicator	CY 2010 Third Year Transition. Pymt. Weight	CY 2010 Third Year Transition Payment
58346	Insert heyman uteri capsule	Y		A2	16.9305	$708.93
58350	Reopen fallopian tube	Y		A2	28.2177	$1,181.56
58353	Endometr ablate, thermal	Y		A2	30.988	$1,297.56
58356	Endometrial cryoablation	Y	CH	P3		$1,302.70
58545	Laparoscopic myomectomy	Y		A2	34.9531	$1,463.59
58546	Laparo-myomectomy, complex	Y		A2	41.2571	$1,727.56
58550	Laparo-asst vag hysterectomy	Y		A2	59.9976	$2,512.28
58552	Laparo-vag hyst incl t/o	Y		G2	44.8118	$1,876.40
58555	Hysteroscopy, dx, sep proc	Y		A2	18.1129	$758.44
58558	Hysteroscopy, biopsy	Y		A2	19.1238	$800.77
58559	Hysteroscopy, lysis	Y		A2	18.7584	$785.47
58560	Hysteroscopy, resect septum	Y		A2	29.6193	$1,240.25
58561	Hysteroscopy, remove myoma	Y		A2	29.6193	$1,240.25
58562	Hysteroscopy, remove fb	Y		A2	19.1238	$800.77
58563	Hysteroscopy, ablation	Y		A2	34.3546	$1,438.53
58565	Hysteroscopy, sterilization	Y		A2	39.9293	$1,671.96
58600	Division of fallopian tube	Y		G2	33.7396	$1,412.78
58615	Occlude fallopian tube(s)	Y		G2	19.1772	$803.01
58660	Laparoscopy, lysis	Y		A2	37.7042	$1,578.79
58661	Laparoscopy, remove adnexa	Y		A2	37.7042	$1,578.79
58662	Laparoscopy, excise lesions	Y		A2	37.7042	$1,578.79
58670	Laparoscopy, tubal cautery	Y		A2	36.5219	$1,529.28
58671	Laparoscopy, tubal block	Y		A2	36.5219	$1,529.28
58672	Laparoscopy, fimbrioplasty	Y		A2	37.7042	$1,578.79
58673	Laparoscopy, salpingostomy	Y		A2	37.7042	$1,578.79
58800	Drainage of ovarian cyst(s)	Y		A2	17.2961	$724.24
58805	Drainage of ovarian cyst(s)	Y		G2	33.7396	$1,412.78
58820	Drain ovary abscess, open	Y		A2	28.2177	$1,181.56
58900	Biopsy of ovary(s)	Y		A2	17.2961	$724.24
58970	Retrieval of oocyte	Y		A2	3.8502	$161.22
58974	Transfer of embryo	Y		A2	3.8502	$161.22
58976	Transfer of embryo	Y		A2	3.8502	$161.22
59000	Amniocentesis, diagnostic	Y		P3		$51.98
59001	Amniocentesis, therapeutic	Y		R2	6.5007	$272.20
59012	Fetal cord puncture,prenatal	Y		G2	3.2609	$136.54
59015	Chorion biopsy	Y		P3		$43.18
59020	Fetal contract stress test	Y		P3		$22.44
59025	Fetal non-stress test	Y		P3		$11.93
59070	Transabdom amnioinfus w/us	Y		G2	1.4616	$61.20
59072	Umbilical cord occlud w/us	Y		G2	3.2609	$136.54
59076	Fetal shunt placement, w/us	Y		G2	3.2609	$136.54
59100	Remove uterus lesion	Y		R2	33.7396	$1,412.78
59150	Treat ectopic pregnancy	Y		G2	44.8118	$1,876.40
59151	Treat ectopic pregnancy	Y		G2	44.8118	$1,876.40
59160	D & c after delivery	Y		A2	17.2961	$724.24
59200	Insert cervical dilator	Y		P3		$28.41
59300	Episiotomy or vaginal repair	Y		P3		$62.78
59320	Revision of cervix	Y		A2	16.285	$681.90
59412	Antepartum manipulation	Y		G2	19.1772	$803.01
59414	Deliver placenta	Y		G2	19.1772	$803.01
59812	Treatment of miscarriage	Y		A2	18.4785	$773.75

HCPCS Code	HCPCS Short Descriptor	Subject To Multiple Procedure Discounts	CY 2010 Comment Indicator	CY 2010 Payment Indicator	CY 2010 Third Year Transition. Pymt. Weight	CY 2010 Third Year Transition Payment
59820	Care of miscarriage	Y		A2	18.4785	$773.75
59821	Treatment of miscarriage	Y		A2	18.4785	$773.75
59840	Abortion	Y		A2	18.4785	$773.75
59841	Abortion	Y		A2	18.4785	$773.75
59866	Abortion (mpr)	Y		G2	3.2609	$136.54
59870	Evacuate mole of uterus	Y		A2	18.4785	$773.75
59871	Remove cerclage suture	Y		A2	18.4785	$773.75
60000	Drain thyroid/tongue cyst	Y		A2	7.3694	$308.58
60100	Biopsy of thyroid	Y		P3		$38.63
60200	Remove thyroid lesion	Y		A2	37.5311	$1,571.54
60210	Partial thyroid excision	Y	CH	G2	46.645	$1,953.17
60212	Partial thyroid excision	Y	CH	G2	46.645	$1,953.17
60220	Partial removal of thyroid	Y	CH	G2	46.645	$1,953.17
60225	Partial removal of thyroid	Y	CH	G2	46.645	$1,953.17
60280	Remove thyroid duct lesion	Y		A2	38.5821	$1,615.55
60281	Remove thyroid duct lesion	Y		A2	38.5821	$1,615.55
60300	Aspir/inj thyroid cyst	Y		P3		$51.98
61000	Remove cranial cavity fluid	Y		R2	6.8884	$288.44
61001	Remove cranial cavity fluid	Y		R2	6.8884	$288.44
61020	Remove brain cavity fluid	Y		A2	6.2164	$260.30
61026	Injection into brain canal	Y		A2	6.2164	$260.30
61050	Remove brain canal fluid	Y		A2	6.2164	$260.30
61055	Injection into brain canal	Y		A2	6.2164	$260.30
61070	Brain canal shunt procedure	Y		A2	5.6237	$235.48
61215	Insert brain-fluid device	Y		A2	32.3524	$1,354.69
61330	Decompress eye socket	Y		G2	41.1215	$1,721.88
61334	Explore orbit/remove object	Y		G2	41.1215	$1,721.88
61770	Incise skull for treatment	Y	CH	G2	35.6664	$1,493.46
61790	Treat trigeminal nerve	Y		A2	16.3451	$684.42
61791	Treat trigeminal tract	Y		A2	11.5129	$482.08
61795	Brain surgery using computer	N		N1		
61880	Revise/remove neuroelectrode	Y		G2	18.7878	$786.70
61885	Insrt/redo neurostim 1 array	N		H8	307.5302	$12,877.21
61886	Implant neurostim arrays	N		H8	416.231	$17,428.84
61888	Revise/remove neuroreceiver	Y		A2	22.4689	$940.84
62160	Neuroendoscopy add-on	N		N1		
62194	Replace/irrigate catheter	Y		A2	7.0685	$295.98
62225	Replace/irrigate catheter	Y		A2	12.8875	$539.64
62230	Replace/revise brain shunt	Y		A2	31.9867	$1,339.38
62252	Csf shunt reprogram	N		P3		$39.48
62263	Epidural lysis mult sessions	Y		A2	7.0685	$295.98
62264	Epidural lysis on single day	Y		A2	11.405	$477.56
62267	Interdiscal perq aspir, dx	Y		G2	4.4	$184.24
62268	Drain spinal cord cyst	Y		A2	6.2164	$260.30
62269	Needle biopsy, spinal cord	Y		A2	8.8382	$370.08
62270	Spinal fluid tap, diagnostic	Y		A2	3.4648	$145.08
62272	Drain cerebro spinal fluid	Y		A2	3.4648	$145.08
62273	Inject epidural patch	Y		A2	4.5729	$191.48
62280	Treat spinal cord lesion	Y		A2	7.0685	$295.98
62281	Treat spinal cord lesion	Y		A2	7.0685	$295.98
62282	Treat spinal canal lesion	Y		A2	7.0685	$295.98

HCPCS Code	HCPCS Short Descriptor	Subject To Multiple Procedure Discounts	CY 2010 Comment Indicator	CY 2010 Payment Indicator	CY 2010 Third Year Transition. Pymt. Weight	CY 2010 Third Year Transition Payment
62284	Injection for myelogram	N		N1		
62287	Percutaneous diskectomy	Y		A2	34.3981	$1,440.35
62290	Inject for spine disk x-ray	N		N1		
62291	Inject for spine disk x-ray	N		N1		
62292	Injection into disk lesion	Y		R2	6.8884	$288.44
62294	Injection into spinal artery	Y		A2	6.2164	$260.30
62310	Inject spine c/t	Y		A2	7.0685	$295.98
62311	Inject spine l/s (cd)	Y		A2	7.0685	$295.98
62318	Inject spine w/cath, c/t	Y		A2	7.0685	$295.98
62319	Inject spine w/cath l/s (cd)	Y		A2	7.0685	$295.98
62350	Implant spinal canal cath	Y		A2	31.9867	$1,339.38
62355	Remove spinal canal catheter	Y		A2	12.0502	$504.58
62360	Insert spine infusion device	Y		A2	31.9867	$1,339.38
62361	Implant spine infusion pump	Y		H8	291.6404	$12,211.86
62362	Implant spine infusion pump	Y		H8	291.6404	$12,211.86
62365	Remove spine infusion device	Y		A2	29.2974	$1,226.77
62367	Analyze spine infusion pump	N		P3		$14.77
62368	Analyze spine infusion pump	N		P3		$19.32
63600	Remove spinal cord lesion	Y		A2	15.9795	$669.11
63610	Stimulation of spinal cord	Y		A2	15.3342	$642.09
63615	Remove lesion of spinal cord	Y		R2	17.9094	$749.92
63650	Implant neuroelectrodes	N		H8	83.4896	$3,495.96
63655	Implant neuroelectrodes	N		J8	118.6891	$4,969.87
63660	Revise/remove neuroelectrode	N	CH	D5		
63661	Remove spine eltrd perq aray	Y	NI	G2	18.7878	$786.70
63662	Remove spine eltrd plate	Y	NI	G2	18.7878	$786.70
63663	Revise spine eltrd perq aray	Y	NI	G2	18.7878	$786.70
63664	Revise spine eltrd plate	Y	NI	G2	18.7878	$786.70
63685	Insrt/redo spine n generator	N		H8	307.5302	$12,877.21
63688	Revise/remove neuroreceiver	Y		A2	22.4689	$940.84
63744	Revision of spinal shunt	Y		A2	32.3524	$1,354.69
63746	Removal of spinal shunt	Y		A2	12.0502	$504.58
64400	N block inj, trigeminal	Y		P3		$46.59
64402	N block inj, facial	Y		P3		$44.03
64405	N block inj, occipital	Y		P3		$38.35
64408	N block inj, vagus	Y		P3		$46.02
64410	N block inj, phrenic	Y		A2	7.0685	$295.98
64412	N block inj, spinal accessor	Y		P3		$69.03
64413	N block inj, cervical plexus	Y		P3		$42.89
64415	N block inj, brachial plexus	Y		A2	3.4648	$145.08
64416	N block cont infuse, b plex	Y		G2	6.8884	$288.44
64417	N block inj, axillary	Y		A2	3.4648	$145.08
64418	N block inj, suprascapular	Y		P3		$59.94
64420	N block inj, intercost, sng	Y		A2	3.4648	$145.08
64421	N block inj, intercost, mlt	Y		A2	7.0685	$295.98
64425	N block inj, ilio-ing/hypogi	Y		P3		$42.61
64430	N block inj, pudendal	Y		A2	5.9604	$249.58
64435	N block inj, paracervical	Y		P3		$59.65
64445	N block inj, sciatic, sng	Y		P3		$54.26
64446	N blk inj, sciatic, cont inf	Y		G2	6.8884	$288.44
64447	N block inj fem, single	Y		R2	3.5609	$149.11

HCPCS Code	HCPCS Short Descriptor	Subject To Multiple Procedure Discounts	CY 2010 Comment Indicator	CY 2010 Payment Indicator	CY 2010 Third Year Transition. Pymt. Weight	CY 2010 Third Year Transition Payment
64448	N block inj fem, cont inf	Y		G2	6.8884	$288.44
64449	N block inj, lumbar plexus	Y		G2	6.8884	$288.44
64450	N block, other peripheral	Y		P3		$37.50
64455*	N block inj, plantar digit	Y		P3		$15.62
64470	Inj paravertebral c/t	N	CH	D5		
64472	Inj paravertebral c/t add-on	N	CH	D5		
64475	Inj paravertebral l/s	N	CH	D5		
64476	Inj paravertebral l/s add-on	N	CH	D5		
64479	Inj foramen epidural c/t	Y		A2	7.0685	$295.98
64480	Inj foramen epidural add-on	Y		A2	4.5729	$191.48
64483	Inj foramen epidural l/s	Y		A2	7.0685	$295.98
64484	Inj foramen epidural add-on	Y		A2	4.5729	$191.48
64490	Inj paravert f jnt c/t 1 lev	Y	NI	G2	6.8884	$288.44
64491	Inj paravert f jnt c/t 2 lev	Y	NI	G2	2.4451	$102.38
64492	Inj paravert f jnt c/t 3 lev	Y	NI	G2	2.4451	$102.38
64493	Inj paravert f jnt l/s 1 lev	Y	NI	G2	6.8884	$288.44
64494	Inj paravert f jnt l/s 2 lev	Y	NI	G2	2.4451	$102.38
64495	Inj paravert f jnt l/s 3 lev	Y	NI	G2	2.4451	$102.38
64505	N block, spenopalatine gangl	Y		P3		$32.95
64508	N block, carotid sinus s/p	Y		P3		$74.71
64510	N block, stellate ganglion	Y		A2	7.0685	$295.98
64517	N block inj, hypogas plxs	Y		A2	5.9604	$249.58
64520	N block, lumbar/thoracic	Y		A2	7.0685	$295.98
64530	N block inj, celiac pelus	Y		A2	7.0685	$295.98
64553	Implant neuroelectrodes	N		H8	82.8441	$3,468.93
64555	Implant neuroelectrodes	N		J8	87.5994	$3,668.05
64560	Implant neuroelectrodes	N		J8	87.5994	$3,668.05
64561	Implant neuroelectrodes	N		H8	83.8552	$3,511.27
64565	Implant neuroelectrodes	N		J8	87.5994	$3,668.05
64573	Implant neuroelectrodes	N		H8	218.1981	$9,136.61
64575	Implant neuroelectrodes	N		H8	113.0528	$4,733.86
64577	Implant neuroelectrodes	N		H8	113.0528	$4,733.86
64580	Implant neuroelectrodes	N		H8	113.0528	$4,733.86
64581	Implant neuroelectrodes	N		H8	114.064	$4,776.20
64585	Revise/remove neuroelectrode	Y		A2	15.9929	$669.67
64590	Insrt/redo pn/gastr stimul	N		H8	307.5302	$12,877.21
64595	Revise/rmv pn/gastr stimul	Y		A2	22.4689	$940.84
64600	Injection treatment of nerve	Y		A2	11.405	$477.56
64605	Injection treatment of nerve	Y		A2	15.3342	$642.09
64610	Injection treatment of nerve	Y		A2	15.3342	$642.09
64612	Destroy nerve, face muscle	Y		P3		$54.82
64613	Destroy nerve, neck muscle	Y		P3		$51.98
64614	Destroy nerve, extrem musc	Y		P3		$59.08
64620	Injection treatment of nerve	Y		A2	7.0685	$295.98
64622	Destr paravertebrl nerve l/s	Y		A2	11.405	$477.56
64623	Destr paravertebral n add-on	Y		A2	7.0685	$295.98
64626	Destr paravertebrl nerve c/t	Y		A2	7.0685	$295.98
64627	Destr paravertebral n add-on	Y		A2	3.7361	$156.44
64630	Injection treatment of nerve	Y		A2	7.1765	$300.50
64632*	N block inj, common digit	Y		P3		$28.41
64640	Injection treatment of nerve	Y		P3		$80.67

HCPCS Code	HCPCS Short Descriptor	Subject To Multiple Procedure Discounts	CY 2010 Comment Indicator	CY 2010 Payment Indicator	CY 2010 Third Year Transition. Pymt. Weight	CY 2010 Third Year Transition Payment
64650	Chemodenerv eccrine glands	Y		P3		$28.69
64653	Chemodenerv eccrine glands	Y		P3		$31.53
64680	Injection treatment of nerve	Y		A2	7.3995	$309.84
64681	Injection treatment of nerve	Y		A2	12.0502	$504.58
64702	Revise finger/toe nerve	Y		A2	15.3342	$642.09
64704	Revise hand/foot nerve	Y		A2	15.3342	$642.09
64708	Revise arm/leg nerve	Y		A2	15.9795	$669.11
64712	Revision of sciatic nerve	Y		A2	15.9795	$669.11
64713	Revision of arm nerve(s)	Y		A2	15.9795	$669.11
64714	Revise low back nerve(s)	Y		A2	15.9795	$669.11
64716	Revision of cranial nerve	Y		A2	16.3451	$684.42
64718	Revise ulnar nerve at elbow	Y		A2	15.9795	$669.11
64719	Revise ulnar nerve at wrist	Y		A2	15.9795	$669.11
64721	Carpal tunnel surgery	Y		A2	15.9795	$669.11
64722	Relieve pressure on nerve(s)	Y		A2	15.3342	$642.09
64726	Release foot/toe nerve	Y		A2	15.3342	$642.09
64727	Internal nerve revision	Y		A2	15.3342	$642.09
64732	Incision of brow nerve	Y		A2	15.9795	$669.11
64734	Incision of cheek nerve	Y		A2	15.9795	$669.11
64736	Incision of chin nerve	Y		A2	15.9795	$669.11
64738	Incision of jaw nerve	Y		A2	15.9795	$669.11
64740	Incision of tongue nerve	Y		A2	15.9795	$669.11
64742	Incision of facial nerve	Y		A2	15.9795	$669.11
64744	Incise nerve, back of head	Y		A2	15.9795	$669.11
64746	Incise diaphragm nerve	Y		A2	15.9795	$669.11
64761	Incision of pelvis nerve	Y		G2	17.9094	$749.92
64763	Incise hip/thigh nerve	Y		G2	17.9094	$749.92
64766	Incise hip/thigh nerve	Y		G2	35.6664	$1,493.46
64771	Sever cranial nerve	Y		A2	15.9795	$669.11
64772	Incision of spinal nerve	Y		A2	15.9795	$669.11
64774	Remove skin nerve lesion	Y		A2	15.9795	$669.11
64776	Remove digit nerve lesion	Y		A2	16.3451	$684.42
64778	Digit nerve surgery add-on	Y		A2	15.9795	$669.11
64782	Remove limb nerve lesion	Y		A2	16.3451	$684.42
64783	Limb nerve surgery add-on	Y		A2	15.9795	$669.11
64784	Remove nerve lesion	Y		A2	16.3451	$684.42
64786	Remove sciatic nerve lesion	Y		A2	29.6628	$1,242.07
64787	Implant nerve end	Y		A2	15.9795	$669.11
64788	Remove skin nerve lesion	Y		A2	16.3451	$684.42
64790	Removal of nerve lesion	Y		A2	16.3451	$684.42
64792	Removal of nerve lesion	Y		A2	29.6628	$1,242.07
64795	Biopsy of nerve	Y		A2	15.9795	$669.11
64802	Remove sympathetic nerves	Y		A2	15.9795	$669.11
64820	Remove sympathetic nerves	Y		G2	17.9094	$749.92
64821	Remove sympathetic nerves	Y		A2	23.8595	$999.07
64822	Remove sympathetic nerves	Y		G2	27.0149	$1,131.19
64823	Remove sympathetic nerves	Y		G2	27.0149	$1,131.19
64831	Repair of digit nerve	Y		A2	30.3484	$1,270.78
64832	Repair nerve add-on	Y		A2	28.6519	$1,199.74
64834	Repair of hand or foot nerve	Y		A2	29.2974	$1,226.77
64835	Repair of hand or foot nerve	Y		A2	29.6628	$1,242.07

HCPCS Code	HCPCS Short Descriptor	Subject To Multiple Procedure Discounts	CY 2010 Comment Indicator	CY 2010 Payment Indicator	CY 2010 Third Year Transition. Pymt. Weight	CY 2010 Third Year Transition Payment
64836	Repair of hand or foot nerve	Y		A2	29.6628	$1,242.07
64837	Repair nerve add-on	Y		A2	28.6519	$1,199.74
64840	Repair of leg nerve	Y		A2	29.2974	$1,226.77
64856	Repair/transpose nerve	Y		A2	29.2974	$1,226.77
64857	Repair arm/leg nerve	Y		A2	29.2974	$1,226.77
64858	Repair sciatic nerve	Y		A2	29.2974	$1,226.77
64859	Nerve surgery	Y		A2	28.6519	$1,199.74
64861	Repair of arm nerves	Y		A2	29.6628	$1,242.07
64862	Repair of low back nerves	Y		A2	29.6628	$1,242.07
64864	Repair of facial nerve	Y		A2	29.6628	$1,242.07
64865	Repair of facial nerve	Y		A2	30.3484	$1,270.78
64870	Fusion of facial/other nerve	Y		A2	30.3484	$1,270.78
64872	Subsequent repair of nerve	Y		A2	29.2974	$1,226.77
64874	Repair & revise nerve add-on	Y		A2	29.6628	$1,242.07
64876	Repair nerve/shorten bone	Y		A2	29.6628	$1,242.07
64885	Nerve graft, head or neck	Y		A2	29.2974	$1,226.77
64886	Nerve graft, head or neck	Y		A2	29.2974	$1,226.77
64890	Nerve graft, hand or foot	Y		A2	29.2974	$1,226.77
64891	Nerve graft, hand or foot	Y		A2	29.2974	$1,226.77
64892	Nerve graft, arm or leg	Y		A2	29.2974	$1,226.77
64893	Nerve graft, arm or leg	Y		A2	29.2974	$1,226.77
64895	Nerve graft, hand or foot	Y		A2	29.6628	$1,242.07
64896	Nerve graft, hand or foot	Y		A2	29.6628	$1,242.07
64897	Nerve graft, arm or leg	Y		A2	29.6628	$1,242.07
64898	Nerve graft, arm or leg	Y		A2	29.6628	$1,242.07
64901	Nerve graft add-on	Y		A2	29.2974	$1,226.77
64902	Nerve graft add-on	Y		A2	29.2974	$1,226.77
64905	Nerve pedicle transfer	Y		A2	29.2974	$1,226.77
64907	Nerve pedicle transfer	Y		A2	28.6519	$1,199.74
64910	Nerve repair w/allograft	Y		G2	35.6664	$1,493.46
65091	Revise eye	Y		A2	30.9049	$1,294.08
65093	Revise eye with implant	Y		A2	30.9049	$1,294.08
65101	Removal of eye	Y		A2	30.9049	$1,294.08
65103	Remove eye/insert implant	Y		A2	30.9049	$1,294.08
65105	Remove eye/attach implant	Y		A2	31.5903	$1,322.78
65110	Removal of eye	Y		A2	32.0873	$1,343.59
65112	Remove eye/revise socket	Y		A2	33.6752	$1,410.08
65114	Remove eye/revise socket	Y		A2	33.6752	$1,410.08
65125	Revise ocular implant	Y		G2	25.6774	$1,075.19
65130	Insert ocular implant	Y		A2	22.1711	$928.37
65135	Insert ocular implant	Y		A2	21.8055	$913.06
65140	Attach ocular implant	Y		A2	30.9049	$1,294.08
65150	Revise ocular implant	Y		A2	21.8055	$913.06
65155	Reinsert ocular implant	Y		A2	30.9049	$1,294.08
65175	Removal of ocular implant	Y		A2	14.9309	$625.20
65205	Remove foreign body from eye	N		P3		$17.90
65210	Remove foreign body from eye	N		P3		$23.01
65220	Remove foreign body from eye	N		G2	0.9139	$38.27
65222	Remove foreign body from eye	N		P3		$25.00
65235	Remove foreign body from eye	Y		A2	14.2061	$594.85
65260	Remove foreign body from eye	Y		A2	7.1103	$297.73

HCPCS Code	HCPCS Short Descriptor	Subject To Multiple Procedure Discounts	CY 2010 Comment Indicator	CY 2010 Payment Indicator	CY 2010 Third Year Transition. Pymt. Weight	CY 2010 Third Year Transition Payment
65265	Remove foreign body from eye	Y		A2	18.4618	$773.05
65270	Repair of eye wound	Y		A2	15.5764	$652.23
65272	Repair of eye wound	Y		A2	20.0566	$839.83
65275	Repair of eye wound	Y		A2	21.1076	$883.84
65280	Repair of eye wound	Y		A2	18.4618	$773.05
65285	Repair of eye wound	Y		A2	32.274	$1,351.41
65286	Repair of eye wound	Y		P2	4.3122	$180.56
65290	Repair of eye socket wound	Y		A2	19.7528	$827.11
65400	Removal of eye lesion	Y		A2	13.5608	$567.83
65410	Biopsy of cornea	Y		A2	14.2061	$594.85
65420	Removal of eye lesion	Y		A2	14.2061	$594.85
65426	Removal of eye lesion	Y		A2	21.6046	$904.65
65430	Corneal smear	N	CH	P3		$35.79
65435	Curette/treat cornea	Y		P3		$27.55
65436	Curette/treat cornea	Y		P3		$122.43
65450	Treatment of corneal lesion	N		G2	1.8727	$78.42
65600	Revision of cornea	Y		P3		$142.31
65710	Corneal transplant	Y		A2	32.6184	$1,365.83
65730	Corneal transplant	Y		A2	32.6184	$1,365.83
65750	Corneal transplant	Y		A2	32.6184	$1,365.83
65755	Corneal transplant	Y		A2	32.6184	$1,365.83
65756	Corneal trnspl, endothelial	Y		G2	35.9134	$1,503.80
65757	Prep corneal endo allograft	N		N1		
65770	Revise cornea with implant	Y		H8	134.3348	$5,625.00
65772	Correction of astigmatism	Y		A2	15.2571	$638.86
65775	Correction of astigmatism	Y		A2	15.2571	$638.86
65780	Ocular reconst, transplant	Y		A2	31.0305	$1,299.34
65781	Ocular reconst, transplant	Y		A2	31.0305	$1,299.34
65782	Ocular reconst, transplant	Y		A2	31.0305	$1,299.34
65800	Drainage of eye	Y		A2	13.5608	$567.83
65805	Drainage of eye	Y		A2	13.5608	$567.83
65810	Drainage of eye	Y		A2	20.4222	$855.14
65815	Drainage of eye	Y		A2	20.0566	$839.83
65820	Relieve inner eye pressure	Y		A2	5.1362	$215.07
65850	Incision of eye	Y		A2	21.1076	$883.84
65855	Laser surgery of eye	Y		P3		$115.33
65860	Incise inner eye adhesions	Y		P3		$107.38
65865	Incise inner eye adhesions	Y		A2	13.5608	$567.83
65870	Incise inner eye adhesions	Y		A2	21.1076	$883.84
65875	Incise inner eye adhesions	Y		A2	21.1076	$883.84
65880	Incise inner eye adhesions	Y		A2	15.2571	$638.86
65900	Remove eye lesion	Y		A2	15.7541	$659.67
65920	Remove implant of eye	Y		A2	23.1925	$971.14
65930	Remove blood clot from eye	Y		A2	21.6046	$904.65
66020	Injection treatment of eye	Y		A2	13.5608	$567.83
66030	Injection treatment of eye	Y		A2	5.1362	$215.07
66130	Remove eye lesion	Y		A2	23.1925	$971.14
66150	Glaucoma surgery	Y		A2	21.1076	$883.84
66155	Glaucoma surgery	Y		A2	21.1076	$883.84
66160	Glaucoma surgery	Y		A2	20.0566	$839.83
66165	Glaucoma surgery	Y		A2	21.1076	$883.84

HCPCS Code	HCPCS Short Descriptor	Subject To Multiple Procedure Discounts	CY 2010 Comment Indicator	CY 2010 Payment Indicator	CY 2010 Third Year Transition. Pymt. Weight	CY 2010 Third Year Transition Payment
66170	Glaucoma surgery	Y		A2	21.1076	$883.84
66172	Incision of eye	Y		A2	21.1076	$883.84
66180	Implant eye shunt	Y		A2	34.1483	$1,429.89
66185	Revise eye shunt	Y		A2	20.0566	$839.83
66220	Repair eye lesion	Y		A2	31.5886	$1,322.71
66225	Repair/graft eye lesion	Y		A2	33.6513	$1,409.08
66250	Follow-up surgery of eye	Y		A2	14.2061	$594.85
66500	Incision of iris	Y		A2	5.1362	$215.07
66505	Incision of iris	Y		A2	5.1362	$215.07
66600	Remove iris and lesion	Y		A2	20.4222	$855.14
66605	Removal of iris	Y		A2	20.4222	$855.14
66625	Removal of iris	Y		A2	13.7888	$577.38
66630	Removal of iris	Y		A2	20.4222	$855.14
66635	Removal of iris	Y		A2	20.4222	$855.14
66680	Repair iris & ciliary body	Y		A2	20.4222	$855.14
66682	Repair iris & ciliary body	Y		A2	20.0566	$839.83
66700	Destruction, ciliary body	Y		A2	14.2061	$594.85
66710	Ciliary transsleral therapy	Y		A2	14.2061	$594.85
66711	Ciliary endoscopic ablation	Y		A2	14.2061	$594.85
66720	Destruction, ciliary body	Y		A2	14.2061	$594.85
66740	Destruction, ciliary body	Y		A2	20.0566	$839.83
66761	Revision of iris	Y		P3		$161.06
66762	Revision of iris	Y		P3		$164.19
66770	Removal of inner eye lesion	Y	CH	P3		$178.39
66820	Incision, secondary cataract	Y		G2	4.3122	$180.56
66821	After cataract laser surgery	Y		A2	5.589	$234.03
66825	Reposition intraocular lens	Y		A2	21.1076	$883.84
66830	Removal of lens lesion	Y		A2	5.3646	$224.63
66840	Removal of lens material	Y		A2	14.9416	$625.65
66850	Removal of lens material	Y		A2	27.4454	$1,149.22
66852	Removal of lens material	Y		A2	25.3605	$1,061.92
66920	Extraction of lens	Y		A2	25.3605	$1,061.92
66930	Extraction of lens	Y		A2	25.8575	$1,082.73
66940	Extraction of lens	Y		A2	15.4386	$646.46
66982	Cataract surgery, complex	Y		A2	22.9847	$962.44
66983	Cataract surg w/iol, 1 stage	Y		A2	22.9847	$962.44
66984	Cataract surg w/iol, 1 stage	Y		A2	22.9847	$962.44
66985	Insert lens prosthesis	Y		A2	22.1453	$927.29
66986	Exchange lens prosthesis	Y		A2	22.1453	$927.29
66990	Ophthalmic endoscope add-on	N		N1		
67005	Partial removal of eye fluid	Y		A2	18.4618	$773.05
67010	Partial removal of eye fluid	Y		A2	32.274	$1,351.41
67015	Release of eye fluid	Y		A2	30.5775	$1,280.37
67025	Replace eye fluid	Y		A2	16.7652	$702.01
67027	Implant eye drug system	Y		A2	32.274	$1,351.41
67028	Injection eye drug	Y		P3		$71.58
67030	Incise inner eye strands	Y		A2	16.7652	$702.01
67031	Laser surgery, eye strands	Y		A2	5.589	$234.03
67036	Removal of inner eye fluid	Y		A2	32.274	$1,351.41
67039	Laser treatment of retina	Y		A2	34.3589	$1,438.71
67040	Laser treatment of retina	Y		A2	34.3589	$1,438.71

HCPCS Code	HCPCS Short Descriptor	Subject To Multiple Procedure Discounts	CY 2010 Comment Indicator	CY 2010 Payment Indicator	CY 2010 Third Year Transition. Pymt. Weight	CY 2010 Third Year Transition Payment
67041	Vit for macular pucker	Y		G2	38.2338	$1,600.96
67042	Vit for macular hole	Y		G2	38.2338	$1,600.96
67043	Vit for membrane dissect	Y		G2	38.2338	$1,600.96
67101	Repair detached retina	Y	CH	P3		$271.28
67105	Repair detached retina	Y		P2	5.0718	$212.37
67107	Repair detached retina	Y		A2	32.771	$1,372.22
67108	Repair detached retina	Y		A2	34.3589	$1,438.71
67110	Repair detached retina	Y		P3		$290.88
67112	Rerepair detached retina	Y		A2	34.3589	$1,438.71
67113	Repair retinal detach, cplx	Y		G2	38.2338	$1,600.96
67115	Release encircling material	Y		A2	17.4107	$729.04
67120	Remove eye implant material	Y		A2	17.4107	$729.04
67121	Remove eye implant material	Y		A2	17.4107	$729.04
67141	Treatment of retina	Y		A2	5.5783	$233.58
67145	Treatment of retina	Y		P3		$172.14
67208	Treatment of retinal lesion	Y		P3		$184.64
67210	Treatment of retinal lesion	Y	CH	P3		$197.14
67218	Treatment of retinal lesion	Y		A2	18.9585	$793.85
67220	Treatment of choroid lesion	Y		P2	5.5965	$234.34
67221	Ocular photodynamic ther	Y		P3		$100.56
67225	Eye photodynamic ther add-on	Y		P3		$7.39
67227	Treatment of retinal lesion	Y		A2	16.7652	$702.01
67228	Treatment of retinal lesion	Y		P2	5.0718	$212.37
67229*	Tr retinal les preterm inf	Y		R2	5.0718	$212.37
67250	Reinforce eye wall	Y		A2	15.942	$667.54
67255	Reinforce/graft eye wall	Y		A2	17.7761	$744.34
67311	Revise eye muscle	Y		A2	19.7528	$827.11
67312	Revise two eye muscles	Y		A2	20.4385	$855.82
67314	Revise eye muscle	Y		A2	20.4385	$855.82
67316	Revise two eye muscles	Y		A2	20.4385	$855.82
67318	Revise eye muscle(s)	Y		A2	20.4385	$855.82
67320	Revise eye muscle(s) add-on	Y		A2	20.4385	$855.82
67331	Eye surgery follow-up add-on	Y		A2	20.4385	$855.82
67332	Rerevise eye muscles add-on	Y		A2	20.4385	$855.82
67334	Revise eye muscle w/suture	Y		A2	20.4385	$855.82
67335	Eye suture during surgery	Y		A2	20.4385	$855.82
67340	Revise eye muscle add-on	Y		A2	20.4385	$855.82
67343	Release eye tissue	Y		A2	22.5231	$943.11
67345	Destroy nerve of eye muscle	Y		P3		$71.58
67346	Biopsy, eye muscle	Y		A2	13.053	$546.57
67400	Explore/biopsy eye socket	Y		A2	15.942	$667.54
67405	Explore/drain eye socket	Y		A2	22.8565	$957.07
67412	Explore/treat eye socket	Y		A2	17.1244	$717.05
67413	Explore/treat eye socket	Y		A2	23.3535	$977.88
67414	Explr/decompress eye socket	Y		G2	37.3223	$1,562.80
67415	Aspiration, orbital contents	Y		A2	14.9309	$625.20
67420	Explore/treat eye socket	Y		A2	32.0873	$1,343.59
67430	Explore/treat eye socket	Y		A2	32.0873	$1,343.59
67440	Explore/drain eye socket	Y		A2	32.0873	$1,343.59
67445	Explr/decompress eye socket	Y		A2	32.0873	$1,343.59
67450	Explore/biopsy eye socket	Y		A2	32.0873	$1,343.59

HCPCS Code	HCPCS Short Descriptor	Subject To Multiple Procedure Discounts	CY 2010 Comment Indicator	CY 2010 Payment Indicator	CY 2010 Third Year Transition. Pymt. Weight	CY 2010 Third Year Transition Payment
67500	Inject/treat eye socket	N		G2	1.8727	$78.42
67505	Inject/treat eye socket	Y		P3		$23.86
67515	Inject/treat eye socket	Y		P3		$24.43
67550	Insert eye socket implant	Y		A2	31.5903	$1,322.78
67560	Revise eye socket implant	Y		A2	21.8055	$913.06
67570	Decompress optic nerve	Y		A2	31.5903	$1,322.78
67700	Drainage of eyelid abscess	Y		P2	3.087	$129.26
67710	Incision of eyelid	Y		P3		$119.87
67715	Incision of eyelid fold	Y		A2	14.9309	$625.20
67800	Remove eyelid lesion	Y		P3		$45.17
67801	Remove eyelid lesions	Y		P3		$54.82
67805	Remove eyelid lesions	Y		P3		$70.73
67808	Remove eyelid lesion(s)	Y		A2	15.5764	$652.23
67810	Biopsy of eyelid	Y	CH	P3		$108.80
67820	Revise eyelashes	N		P3		$14.77
67825	Revise eyelashes	Y		P3		$45.73
67830	Revise eyelashes	Y		A2	8.031	$336.28
67835	Revise eyelashes	Y		A2	15.5764	$652.23
67840	Remove eyelid lesion	Y		P3		$126.98
67850	Treat eyelid lesion	Y		P3		$99.99
67875	Closure of eyelid by suture	Y		G2	7.3112	$306.14
67880	Revision of eyelid	Y		A2	14.5717	$610.16
67882	Revision of eyelid	Y		A2	15.942	$667.54
67900	Repair brow defect	Y		A2	22.8565	$957.07
67901	Repair eyelid defect	Y		A2	17.1244	$717.05
67902	Repair eyelid defect	Y		A2	23.3535	$977.88
67903	Repair eyelid defect	Y		A2	16.6274	$696.24
67904	Repair eyelid defect	Y		A2	16.6274	$696.24
67906	Repair eyelid defect	Y		A2	17.1244	$717.05
67908	Repair eyelid defect	Y		A2	16.6274	$696.24
67909	Revise eyelid defect	Y		A2	16.6274	$696.24
67911	Revise eyelid defect	Y		A2	15.942	$667.54
67912	Correction eyelid w/implant	Y		A2	15.942	$667.54
67914	Repair eyelid defect	Y		A2	15.942	$667.54
67915	Repair eyelid defect	Y		P3		$142.03
67916	Repair eyelid defect	Y		A2	16.6274	$696.24
67917	Repair eyelid defect	Y		A2	16.6274	$696.24
67921	Repair eyelid defect	Y		A2	15.942	$667.54
67922	Repair eyelid defect	Y		P3		$138.05
67923	Repair eyelid defect	Y		A2	16.6274	$696.24
67924	Repair eyelid defect	Y		A2	16.6274	$696.24
67930	Repair eyelid wound	Y		P3		$143.17
67935	Repair eyelid wound	Y		A2	15.5764	$652.23
67938	Remove eyelid foreign body	N		P2	1.8727	$78.42
67950	Revision of eyelid	Y		A2	15.5764	$652.23
67961	Revision of eyelid	Y		A2	15.942	$667.54
67966	Revision of eyelid	Y		A2	15.942	$667.54
67971	Reconstruction of eyelid	Y		A2	15.942	$667.54
67973	Reconstruction of eyelid	Y		A2	22.1711	$928.37
67974	Reconstruction of eyelid	Y		A2	15.942	$667.54
67975	Reconstruction of eyelid	Y		A2	15.942	$667.54

HCPCS Code	HCPCS Short Descriptor	Subject To Multiple Procedure Discounts	CY 2010 Comment Indicator	CY 2010 Payment Indicator	CY 2010 Third Year Transition. Pymt. Weight	CY 2010 Third Year Transition Payment
68020	Incise/drain eyelid lining	Y		P3		$40.05
68040	Treatment of eyelid lesions	N		P3		$19.88
68100	Biopsy of eyelid lining	Y		P3		$76.41
68110	Remove eyelid lining lesion	Y		P3		$99.42
68115	Remove eyelid lining lesion	Y		A2	15.5764	$652.23
68130	Remove eyelid lining lesion	Y		A2	14.2061	$594.85
68135	Remove eyelid lining lesion	Y		P3		$51.70
68200	Treat eyelid by injection	N		P3		$14.49
68320	Revise/graft eyelid lining	Y		A2	22.8565	$957.07
68325	Revise/graft eyelid lining	Y		A2	22.8565	$957.07
68326	Revise/graft eyelid lining	Y		A2	16.6274	$696.24
68328	Revise/graft eyelid lining	Y		A2	22.8565	$957.07
68330	Revise eyelid lining	Y		A2	21.1076	$883.84
68335	Revise/graft eyelid lining	Y		A2	22.8565	$957.07
68340	Separate eyelid adhesions	Y		A2	16.6274	$696.24
68360	Revise eyelid lining	Y		A2	20.0566	$839.83
68362	Revise eyelid lining	Y		A2	20.0566	$839.83
68371	Harvest eye tissue, alograft	Y		A2	14.2061	$594.85
68400	Incise/drain tear gland	Y		P2	3.087	$129.26
68420	Incise/drain tear sac	Y		P3		$148.28
68440	Incise tear duct opening	Y		P3		$43.18
68500	Removal of tear gland	Y		A2	22.1711	$928.37
68505	Partial removal, tear gland	Y		A2	22.1711	$928.37
68510	Biopsy of tear gland	Y		A2	14.9309	$625.20
68520	Removal of tear sac	Y		A2	22.1711	$928.37
68525	Biopsy of tear sac	Y		A2	14.9309	$625.20
68530	Clearance of tear duct	Y		P2	3.087	$129.26
68540	Remove tear gland lesion	Y		A2	15.942	$667.54
68550	Remove tear gland lesion	Y		A2	22.1711	$928.37
68700	Repair tear ducts	Y		A2	15.5764	$652.23
68705	Revise tear duct opening	Y		P3		$99.42
68720	Create tear sac drain	Y		A2	22.8565	$957.07
68745	Create tear duct drain	Y		A2	22.8565	$957.07
68750	Create tear duct drain	Y		A2	22.8565	$957.07
68760	Close tear duct opening	Y		P3		$84.65
68761	Close tear duct opening	Y		P3		$59.08
68770	Close tear system fistula	Y		A2	22.8565	$957.07
68801	Dilate tear duct opening	N		P2	0.9139	$38.27
68810	Probe nasolacrimal duct	Y		A2	3.0683	$128.48
68811	Probe nasolacrimal duct	Y		A2	15.5764	$652.23
68815	Probe nasolacrimal duct	Y		A2	15.5764	$652.23
68816	Probe nl duct w/balloon	Y		G2	17.3718	$727.41
68840	Explore/irrigate tear ducts	N		P3		$47.44
68850	Injection for tear sac x-ray	N		N1		
69000	Drain external ear lesion	Y		P2	1.3927	$58.32
69005	Drain external ear lesion	Y		P3		$88.91
69020	Drain outer ear canal lesion	Y		P2	1.3927	$58.32
69100	Biopsy of external ear	Y		P3		$51.13
69105	Biopsy of external ear canal	Y		P3		$74.99
69110	Remove external ear, partial	Y		A2	14.457	$605.36
69120	Removal of external ear	Y		A2	20.4597	$856.71

HCPCS Code	HCPCS Short Descriptor	Subject To Multiple Procedure Discounts	CY 2010 Comment Indicator	CY 2010 Payment Indicator	CY 2010 Third Year Transition. Pymt. Weight	CY 2010 Third Year Transition Payment
69140	Remove ear canal lesion(s)	Y		A2	20.4597	$856.71
69145	Remove ear canal lesion(s)	Y		A2	15.1023	$632.38
69150	Extensive ear canal surgery	Y		A2	8.1184	$339.94
69200	Clear outer ear canal	N		P2	0.6403	$26.81
69205	Clear outer ear canal	Y		A2	18.6836	$782.34
69210	Remove impacted ear wax	N		P3		$17.90
69220	Clean out mastoid cavity	Y		P2	0.8408	$35.21
69222	Clean out mastoid cavity	Y		P3		$114.76
69300	Revise external ear	Y		A2	20.8254	$872.02
69310	Rebuild outer ear canal	Y		A2	33.7542	$1,413.39
69320	Rebuild outer ear canal	Y		A2	36.5245	$1,529.39
69400	Inflate middle ear canal	Y		P3		$77.83
69401	Inflate middle ear canal	Y		P3		$41.47
69405	Catheterize middle ear canal	Y		P3		$108.23
69420	Incision of eardrum	Y		P3		$96.01
69421	Incision of eardrum	Y		A2	15.2459	$638.39
69424	Remove ventilating tube	Y		P3		$67.04
69433	Create eardrum opening	Y		P3		$96.01
69436	Create eardrum opening	Y		A2	15.2459	$638.39
69440	Exploration of middle ear	Y		A2	20.8254	$872.02
69450	Eardrum revision	Y		A2	32.7433	$1,371.06
69501	Mastoidectomy	Y		A2	36.5245	$1,529.39
69502	Mastoidectomy	Y		A2	23.5956	$988.02
69505	Remove mastoid structures	Y		A2	36.5245	$1,529.39
69511	Extensive mastoid surgery	Y		A2	36.5245	$1,529.39
69530	Extensive mastoid surgery	Y		A2	36.5245	$1,529.39
69540	Remove ear lesion	Y		P3		$112.20
69550	Remove ear lesion	Y		A2	34.9366	$1,462.90
69552	Remove ear lesion	Y		A2	36.5245	$1,529.39
69601	Mastoid surgery revision	Y		A2	36.5245	$1,529.39
69602	Mastoid surgery revision	Y		A2	36.5245	$1,529.39
69603	Mastoid surgery revision	Y		A2	36.5245	$1,529.39
69604	Mastoid surgery revision	Y		A2	36.5245	$1,529.39
69605	Mastoid surgery revision	Y		A2	36.5245	$1,529.39
69610	Repair of eardrum	Y		P3		$150.84
69620	Repair of eardrum	Y		A2	20.4597	$856.71
69631	Repair eardrum structures	Y		A2	34.9366	$1,462.90
69632	Rebuild eardrum structures	Y		A2	34.9366	$1,462.90
69633	Rebuild eardrum structures	Y		A2	34.9366	$1,462.90
69635	Repair eardrum structures	Y		A2	36.5245	$1,529.39
69636	Rebuild eardrum structures	Y		A2	36.5245	$1,529.39
69637	Rebuild eardrum structures	Y		A2	36.5245	$1,529.39
69641	Revise middle ear & mastoid	Y		A2	36.5245	$1,529.39
69642	Revise middle ear & mastoid	Y		A2	36.5245	$1,529.39
69643	Revise middle ear & mastoid	Y		A2	36.5245	$1,529.39
69644	Revise middle ear & mastoid	Y		A2	36.5245	$1,529.39
69645	Revise middle ear & mastoid	Y		A2	36.5245	$1,529.39
69646	Revise middle ear & mastoid	Y		A2	36.5245	$1,529.39
69650	Release middle ear bone	Y		A2	23.5956	$988.02
69660	Revise middle ear bone	Y		A2	34.9366	$1,462.90
69661	Revise middle ear bone	Y		A2	34.9366	$1,462.90

HCPCS Code	HCPCS Short Descriptor	Subject To Multiple Procedure Discounts	CY 2010 Comment Indicator	CY 2010 Payment Indicator	CY 2010 Third Year Transition. Pymt. Weight	CY 2010 Third Year Transition Payment
69662	Revise middle ear bone	Y		A2	34.9366	$1,462.90
69666	Repair middle ear structures	Y		A2	34.4396	$1,442.09
69667	Repair middle ear structures	Y		A2	34.4396	$1,442.09
69670	Remove mastoid air cells	Y		A2	33.7542	$1,413.39
69676	Remove middle ear nerve	Y		A2	33.7542	$1,413.39
69700	Close mastoid fistula	Y		A2	33.7542	$1,413.39
69711	Remove/repair hearing aid	Y		A2	32.7433	$1,371.06
69714	Implant temple bone w/stimul	Y		H8	153.8521	$6,442.25
69715	Temple bne implnt w/stimulat	Y		H8	153.8521	$6,442.25
69717	Temple bone implant revision	Y		H8	153.8521	$6,442.25
69718	Revise temple bone implant	Y		H8	153.8521	$6,442.25
69720	Release facial nerve	Y		A2	34.9366	$1,462.90
69740	Repair facial nerve	Y		A2	34.9366	$1,462.90
69745	Repair facial nerve	Y		A2	34.9366	$1,462.90
69801	Incise inner ear	Y		A2	22.0077	$921.53
69802	Incise inner ear	Y		A2	23.5956	$988.02
69805	Explore inner ear	Y		A2	36.5245	$1,529.39
69806	Explore inner ear	Y		A2	36.5245	$1,529.39
69820	Establish inner ear window	Y		A2	34.9366	$1,462.90
69840	Revise inner ear window	Y		A2	34.9366	$1,462.90
69905	Remove inner ear	Y		A2	36.5245	$1,529.39
69910	Remove inner ear & mastoid	Y		A2	36.5245	$1,529.39
69915	Incise inner ear nerve	Y		A2	36.5245	$1,529.39
69930	Implant cochlear device	Y		H8	636.8197	$26,665.55
69990	Microsurgery add-on	N		N1		
C9716	Radiofrequency energy to anu	Y		G2	30.7878	$1,289.18
C9724	EPS gast cardia plic	Y		G2	23.2194	$972.27
C9725	Place endorectal app	Y		G2	5.1327	$214.92
C9726	Rxt breast appl place/remov	Y		G2	23.6799	$991.55
C9727	Insert palate implants	Y		G2	7.2897	$305.24
C9728	Place device/marker, non pro	N		R2	13.1619	$551.13
G0104	CA screen;flexi sigmoidscope	N		P3		$70.16
G0105	Colorectal scrn; hi risk ind	Y		A2	8.3531	$349.77
G0121	Colon ca scrn not hi rsk ind	Y		A2	8.3531	$349.77
G0127	Trim nail(s)	Y		P3		$10.23
G0186	Dstry eye lesn,fdr vssl tech	Y		R2	5.5965	$234.34
G0247	Routine footcare pt w lops	Y		P3		$18.75
G0259	Inject for sacroiliac joint	N		N1		
G0260	Inj for sacroiliac jt anesth	Y		A2	7.0685	$295.98
G0268	Removal of impacted wax md	N		N1		
G0269	Occlusive device in vein art	N		N1		
G0289	Arthro, loose body + chondro	N		N1		
G0364	Bone marrow aspirate &biopsy	N		P3		$4.54
G0392	AV fistula or graft arterial	N	CH	D5		
G0393	AV fistula or graft venous	N	CH	D5		

HCPCS Code	HCPCS Short Descriptor	Subject To Multiple Procedure Discounts	CY 2010 Comment Indicator	CY 2010 Payment Indicator	CY 2010 Third Year Transition. Pymt. Weight	CY 2010 Third Year Transition Payment

Addendum BB

Addendum BB -- Final ASC Covered Ancillary Services Integral to Covered Surgical Procedures for CY 2010 (Including Ancillary Services for Which Payment is Packaged)

NOTE 1: *The Medicare program payment is 80 percent of the total payment amount and beneficiary coinsurance is 20 percent of the total payment amount, except for screening flexible sigmoidoscopies and screening colonoscopies for which the program payment is 75 percent and the beneficiary coinsurance is 25 percent.*

NOTE 2: *Payment indicators for radiology services (Z2, Z3) are based on a comparison of the final rates according to the ASC standard ratesetting methodology and the MPFS. Under current law, the MPFS payment rates will have a negative update for CY 2010. For a discussion of those rates, we refer readers to the CY 2010 MPFS final rule.*

HCPCS Code	HCPCS Descriptor	CY 2010 Comment Indicator	CY 2010 Payment Indicator	CY 2010 Third Year Pymt. Weight	CY 2010 Third Year Transition Weight
0042T	Ct perfusion w/contrast, cbf		N1		
0067T	Ct colonography;dx	CH	D5		
0073T	Delivery, comp imrt		Z2	5.9784	$250.33
0126T	Chd risk imt study		N1		
0144T	CT heart wo dye; qual calc	CH	D5		
0145T	CT heart w/wo dye funct	CH	D5		
0146T	CCTA w/wo dye	CH	D5		
0147T	CCTA w/wo, quan calcium	CH	D5		
0148T	CCTA w/wo, strxr	CH	D5		
0149T	CCTA w/wo, strxr quan calc	CH	D5		
0150T	CCTA w/wo, disease strxr	CH	D5		
0151T	CT heart funct add-on	CH	D5		
0159T	Cad breast mri		N1		
0174T	Cad cxr with interp		N1		
0175T	Cad cxr remote		N1		
0182T	Hdr elect brachytherapy		Z2	11.0358	$462.10
0185T	Comptr probability analysis		N1		
70010	Contrast x-ray of brain		N1		
70015	Contrast x-ray of brain		N1		
70030	X-ray eye for foreign body		Z3		$14.49
70100	X-ray exam of jaw		Z3		$16.19
70110	X-ray exam of jaw		Z3		$19.60
70120	X-ray exam of mastoids		Z3		$18.18
70130	X-ray exam of mastoids		Z2	0.6373	$26.69
70134	X-ray exam of middle ear		Z3		$21.30
70140	X-ray exam of facial bones		Z3		$14.77
70150	X-ray exam of facial bones	CH	Z3		$21.59
70160	X-ray exam of nasal bones		Z3		$17.33
70170	X-ray exam of tear duct		N1		
70190	X-ray exam of eye sockets		Z3		$18.18
70200	X-ray exam of eye sockets	CH	Z3		$21.87
70210	X-ray exam of sinuses		Z3		$15.62
70220	X-ray exam of sinuses		Z3		$19.32
70240	X-ray exam, pituitary saddle		Z3		$14.49
70250	X-ray exam of skull		Z3		$17.61
70260	X-ray exam of skull		Z3		$22.16
70300	X-ray exam of teeth		Z3		$6.25

HCPCS Code	HCPCS Descriptor	CY 2010 Comment Indicator	CY 2010 Payment Indicator	CY 2010 Third Year Pymt. Weight	CY 2010 Third Year Transition Weight
70310	X-ray exam of teeth		Z2	0.4275	$17.90
70320	Full mouth x-ray of teeth		Z2	0.4275	$17.90
70328	X-ray exam of jaw joint		Z3		$15.62
70330	X-ray exam of jaw joints	CH	Z3		$25.57
70332	X-ray exam of jaw joint		N1		
70336	Magnetic image, jaw joint		Z2	4.961	$207.73
70350	X-ray head for orthodontia		Z3		$8.52
70355	Panoramic x-ray of jaws		Z3		$8.24
70360	X-ray exam of neck		Z3		$13.63
70370	Throat x-ray & fluoroscopy	CH	Z3		$44.88
70371	Speech evaluation, complex	CH	Z3		$39.48
70373	Contrast x-ray of larynx		N1		
70380	X-ray exam of salivary gland		Z3		$21.02
70390	X-ray exam of salivary duct		N1		
70450	Ct head/brain w/o dye		Z2	2.7687	$115.93
70460	Ct head/brain w/dye	CH	Z3		$152.26
70470	Ct head/brain w/o & w/dye	CH	Z3		$187.48
70480	Ct orbit/ear/fossa w/o dye		Z2	2.7687	$115.93
70481	Ct orbit/ear/fossa w/dye		Z2	4.2158	$176.53
70482	Ct orbit/ear/fossa w/o&w/dye		Z2	4.7337	$198.21
70486	Ct maxillofacial w/o dye		Z2	2.7687	$115.93
70487	Ct maxillofacial w/dye		Z2	4.2158	$176.53
70488	Ct maxillofacial w/o & w/dye		Z2	4.7337	$198.21
70490	Ct soft tissue neck w/o dye		Z2	2.7687	$115.93
70491	Ct soft tissue neck w/dye		Z2	4.2158	$176.53
70492	Ct sft tsue nck w/o & w/dye		Z2	4.7337	$198.21
70496	Ct angiography, head		Z2	4.8324	$202.35
70498	Ct angiography, neck		Z2	4.8324	$202.35
70540	Mri orbit/face/neck w/o dye		Z2	4.961	$207.73
70542	Mri orbit/face/neck w/dye		Z2	6.0177	$251.98
70543	Mri orbt/fac/nck w/o & w/dye		Z2	7.5993	$318.21
70544	Mr angiography head w/o dye		Z2	4.961	$207.73
70545	Mr angiography head w/dye		Z2	6.0177	$251.98
70546	Mr angiograph head w/o&w/dye		Z2	7.5993	$318.21
70547	Mr angiography neck w/o dye		Z2	4.961	$207.73
70548	Mr angiography neck w/dye		Z2	6.0177	$251.98
70549	Mr angiograph neck w/o&w/dye		Z2	7.5993	$318.21
70551	Mri brain w/o dye		Z2	4.961	$207.73
70552	Mri brain w/dye		Z2	6.0177	$251.98
70553	Mri brain w/o & w/dye		Z2	7.5993	$318.21
70554	Fmri brain by tech		Z2	4.961	$207.73
70555	Fmri brain by phys/psych		Z2	4.961	$207.73
70557	Mri brain w/o dye		Z2	4.961	$207.73
70558	Mri brain w/dye		Z2	6.0177	$251.98
70559	Mri brain w/o & w/dye		Z2	7.5993	$318.21
71010	Chest x-ray		Z3		$10.79
71015	Chest x-ray		Z3		$14.20
71020	Chest x-ray		Z3		$14.77
71021	Chest x-ray		Z3		$17.90
71022	Chest x-ray	CH	Z3		$22.44
71023	Chest x-ray and fluoroscopy		Z3		$35.79
71030	Chest x-ray	CH	Z3		$22.44

HCPCS Code	HCPCS Descriptor	CY 2010 Comment Indicator	CY 2010 Payment Indicator	CY 2010 Third Year Pymt. Weight	CY 2010 Third Year Transition Weight
71034	Chest x-ray and fluoroscopy	CH	Z3		$48.57
71035	Chest x-ray		Z3		$18.75
71040	Contrast x-ray of bronchi		N1		
71060	Contrast x-ray of bronchi		N1		
71090	X-ray & pacemaker insertion		N1		
71100	X-ray exam of ribs		Z3		$15.62
71101	X-ray exam of ribs/chest		Z3		$19.03
71110	X-ray exam of ribs		Z3		$19.88
71111	X-ray exam of ribs/chest		Z3		$26.42
71120	X-ray exam of breastbone		Z3		$16.19
71130	X-ray exam of breastbone		Z3		$19.32
71250	Ct thorax w/o dye		Z2	2.7687	$115.93
71260	Ct thorax w/dye		Z2	4.2158	$176.53
71270	Ct thorax w/o & w/dye		Z2	4.7337	$198.21
71275	Ct angiography, chest		Z2	4.8324	$202.35
71550	Mri chest w/o dye		Z2	4.961	$207.73
71551	Mri chest w/dye		Z2	6.0177	$251.98
71552	Mri chest w/o & w/dye		Z2	7.5993	$318.21
72010	X-ray exam of spine	CH	Z3		$35.79
72020	X-ray exam of spine		Z3		$11.65
72040	X-ray exam of neck spine		Z3		$19.03
72050	X-ray exam of neck spine		Z3		$26.70
72052	X-ray exam of neck spine	CH	Z3		$34.94
72069	X-ray exam of trunk spine		Z3		$17.90
72070	X-ray exam of thoracic spine		Z3		$16.48
72072	X-ray exam of thoracic spine		Z3		$19.60
72074	X-ray exam of thoracic spine	CH	Z3		$24.43
72080	X-ray exam of trunk spine		Z3		$17.61
72090	X-ray exam of trunk spine		Z3		$24.15
72100	X-ray exam of lower spine		Z3		$20.45
72110	X-ray exam of lower spine		Z3		$28.41
72114	X-ray exam of lower spine	CH	Z3		$39.48
72120	X-ray exam of lower spine		Z3		$27.84
72125	Ct neck spine w/o dye		Z2	2.7687	$115.93
72126	Ct neck spine w/dye		Z2	4.2158	$176.53
72127	Ct neck spine w/o & w/dye		Z2	4.7337	$198.21
72128	Ct chest spine w/o dye		Z2	2.7687	$115.93
72129	Ct chest spine w/dye		Z2	4.2158	$176.53
72130	Ct chest spine w/o & w/dye		Z2	4.7337	$198.21
72131	Ct lumbar spine w/o dye		Z2	2.7687	$115.93
72132	Ct lumbar spine w/dye		Z2	4.2158	$176.53
72133	Ct lumbar spine w/o & w/dye		Z2	4.7337	$198.21
72141	Mri neck spine w/o dye		Z2	4.961	$207.73
72142	Mri neck spine w/dye		Z2	6.0177	$251.98
72146	Mri chest spine w/o dye		Z2	4.961	$207.73
72147	Mri chest spine w/dye		Z2	6.0177	$251.98
72148	Mri lumbar spine w/o dye		Z2	4.961	$207.73
72149	Mri lumbar spine w/dye		Z2	6.0177	$251.98
72156	Mri neck spine w/o & w/dye		Z2	7.5993	$318.21
72157	Mri chest spine w/o & w/dye		Z2	7.5993	$318.21
72158	Mri lumbar spine w/o & w/dye		Z2	7.5993	$318.21
72170	X-ray exam of pelvis		Z3		$12.78

HCPCS Code	HCPCS Descriptor	CY 2010 Comment Indicator	CY 2010 Payment Indicator	CY 2010 Third Year Pymt. Weight	CY 2010 Third Year Transition Weight
72190	X-ray exam of pelvis	CH	Z3		$21.30
72191	Ct angiograph pelv w/o&w/dye		Z2	4.8324	$202.35
72192	Ct pelvis w/o dye		Z2	2.7687	$115.93
72193	Ct pelvis w/dye		Z2	4.2158	$176.53
72194	Ct pelvis w/o & w/dye		Z2	4.7337	$198.21
72195	Mri pelvis w/o dye		Z2	4.961	$207.73
72196	Mri pelvis w/dye		Z2	6.0177	$251.98
72197	Mri pelvis w/o & w/dye		Z2	7.5993	$318.21
72200	X-ray exam sacroiliac joints		Z3		$15.06
72202	X-ray exam sacroiliac joints		Z3		$18.18
72220	X-ray exam of tailbone		Z3		$15.06
72240	Contrast x-ray of neck spine		N1		
72255	Contrast x-ray, thorax spine		N1		
72265	Contrast x-ray, lower spine		N1		
72270	Contrast x-ray, spine		N1		
72275	Epidurography		N1		
72285	X-ray c/t spine disk		N1		
72291	Perq verte/sacroplsty, fluor		N1		
72292	Perq verte/sacroplsty, ct		N1		
72295	X-ray of lower spine disk		N1		
73000	X-ray exam of collar bone		Z3		$14.49
73010	X-ray exam of shoulder blade		Z3		$14.77
73020	X-ray exam of shoulder		Z3		$11.65
73030	X-ray exam of shoulder		Z3		$14.77
73040	Contrast x-ray of shoulder		N1		
73050	X-ray exam of shoulders		Z3		$19.03
73060	X-ray exam of humerus		Z3		$14.77
73070	X-ray exam of elbow		Z3		$14.49
73080	X-ray exam of elbow		Z3		$19.03
73085	Contrast x-ray of elbow		N1		
73090	X-ray exam of forearm		Z3		$14.20
73092	X-ray exam of arm, infant		Z3		$15.06
73100	X-ray exam of wrist		Z3		$15.34
73110	X-ray exam of wrist		Z3		$19.32
73115	Contrast x-ray of wrist		N1		
73120	X-ray exam of hand		Z3		$13.92
73130	X-ray exam of hand		Z3		$16.76
73140	X-ray exam of finger(s)		Z3		$17.04
73200	Ct upper extremity w/o dye		Z2	2.7687	$115.93
73201	Ct upper extremity w/dye		Z2	4.2158	$176.53
73202	Ct uppr extremity w/o&w/dye		Z2	4.7337	$198.21
73206	Ct angio upr extrm w/o&w/dye		Z2	4.8324	$202.35
73218	Mri upper extremity w/o dye		Z2	4.961	$207.73
73219	Mri upper extremity w/dye		Z2	6.0177	$251.98
73220	Mri uppr extremity w/o&w/dye		Z2	7.5993	$318.21
73221	Mri joint upr extrem w/o dye		Z2	4.961	$207.73
73222	Mri joint upr extrem w/dye		Z2	6.0177	$251.98
73223	Mri joint upr extr w/o&w/dye		Z2	7.5993	$318.21
73500	X-ray exam of hip		Z3		$12.21
73510	X-ray exam of hip		Z3		$19.03
73520	X-ray exam of hips		Z3		$19.32
73525	Contrast x-ray of hip		N1		

HCPCS Code	HCPCS Descriptor	CY 2010 Comment Indicator	CY 2010 Payment Indicator	CY 2010 Third Year Pymt. Weight	CY 2010 Third Year TransitionWeight
73530	X-ray exam of hip		N1		
73540	X-ray exam of pelvis & hips		Z3		$20.45
73542	X-ray exam, sacroiliac joint		N1		
73550	X-ray exam of thigh		Z3		$14.20
73560	X-ray exam of knee, 1 or 2		Z3		$14.77
73562	X-ray exam of knee, 3		Z3		$18.46
73564	X-ray exam, knee, 4 or more		Z3		$21.30
73565	X-ray exam of knees		Z3		$16.48
73580	Contrast x-ray of knee joint		N1		
73590	X-ray exam of lower leg		Z3		$13.63
73592	X-ray exam of leg, infant		Z3		$15.34
73600	X-ray exam of ankle		Z3		$14.20
73610	X-ray exam of ankle		Z3		$16.76
73615	Contrast x-ray of ankle		N1		
73620	X-ray exam of foot		Z3		$13.63
73630	X-ray exam of foot		Z3		$16.48
73650	X-ray exam of heel		Z3		$13.92
73660	X-ray exam of toe(s)		Z3		$15.91
73700	Ct lower extremity w/o dye		Z2	2.7687	$115.93
73701	Ct lower extremity w/dye		Z2	4.2158	$176.53
73702	Ct lwr extremity w/o&w/dye		Z2	4.7337	$198.21
73706	Ct angio lwr extr w/o&w/dye		Z2	4.8324	$202.35
73718	Mri lower extremity w/o dye		Z2	4.961	$207.73
73719	Mri lower extremity w/dye		Z2	6.0177	$251.98
73720	Mri lwr extremity w/o&w/dye		Z2	7.5993	$318.21
73721	Mri jnt of lwr extre w/o dye		Z2	4.961	$207.73
73722	Mri joint of lwr extr w/dye		Z2	6.0177	$251.98
73723	Mri joint lwr extr w/o&w/dye		Z2	7.5993	$318.21
74000	X-ray exam of abdomen		Z3		$11.93
74010	X-ray exam of abdomen		Z3		$19.03
74020	X-ray exam of abdomen		Z3		$19.32
74022	X-ray exam series, abdomen		Z3		$23.58
74150	Ct abdomen w/o dye		Z2	2.7687	$115.93
74160	Ct abdomen w/dye		Z2	4.2158	$176.53
74170	Ct abdomen w/o & w/dye		Z2	4.7337	$198.21
74175	Ct angio abdom w/o & w/dye		Z2	4.8324	$202.35
74181	Mri abdomen w/o dye		Z2	4.961	$207.73
74182	Mri abdomen w/dye		Z2	6.0177	$251.98
74183	Mri abdomen w/o & w/dye		Z2	7.5993	$318.21
74190	X-ray exam of peritoneum		N1		
74210	Contrst x-ray exam of throat	CH	Z3		$43.18
74220	Contrast x-ray, esophagus	CH	Z3		$48.01
74230	Cine/vid x-ray, throat/esoph	CH	Z3		$46.59
74235	Remove esophagus obstruction		N1		
74240	X-ray exam, upper gi tract		Z2	1.2423	$52.02
74241	X-ray exam, upper gi tract		Z2	1.2423	$52.02
74245	X-ray exam, upper gi tract		Z2	2.0092	$84.13
74246	Contrst x-ray uppr gi tract		Z2	1.2423	$52.02
74247	Contrst x-ray uppr gi tract		Z2	1.2423	$52.02
74249	Contrst x-ray uppr gi tract		Z2	2.0092	$84.13
74250	X-ray exam of small bowel		Z2	1.2423	$52.02
74251	X-ray exam of small bowel		Z2	2.0092	$84.13
74260	X-ray exam of small bowel		Z2	1.2423	$52.02

HCPCS Code	HCPCS Descriptor	CY 2010 Comment Indicator	CY 2010 Payment Indicator	CY 2010 Third Year Pymt. Weight	CY 2010 Third Year TransitionWeight
74261	Ct colonography, w/o dye	NI	Z2	2.7687	$115.93
74262	Ct colonography, w/dye	NI	Z2	4.2158	$176.53
74270	Contrast x-ray exam of colon		Z2	1.2423	$52.02
74280	Contrast x-ray exam of colon		Z2	2.0092	$84.13
74283	Contrast x-ray exam of colon		Z2	1.2423	$52.02
74290	Contrast x-ray, gallbladder		Z3		$36.93
74291	Contrast x-rays, gallbladder		Z3		$36.64
74300	X-ray bile ducts/pancreas		N1		
74301	X-rays at surgery add-on		N1		
74305	X-ray bile ducts/pancreas		N1		
74320	Contrast x-ray of bile ducts		N1		
74327	X-ray bile stone removal		N1		
74328	X-ray bile duct endoscopy		N1		
74329	X-ray for pancreas endoscopy		N1		
74330	X-ray bile/panc endoscopy		N1		
74340	X-ray guide for GI tube		N1		
74355	X-ray guide, intestinal tube		N1		
74360	X-ray guide, GI dilation		N1		
74363	X-ray, bile duct dilation		N1		
74400	Contrst x-ray, urinary tract		Z3		$62.78
74410	Contrst x-ray, urinary tract		Z3		$66.19
74415	Contrst x-ray, urinary tract		Z3		$80.39
74420	Contrst x-ray, urinary tract		Z2	2.4358	$101.99
74425	Contrst x-ray, urinary tract		N1		
74430	Contrast x-ray, bladder		N1		
74440	X-ray, male genital tract		N1		
74445	X-ray exam of penis		N1		
74450	X-ray, urethra/bladder		N1		
74455	X-ray, urethra/bladder		N1		
74470	X-ray exam of kidney lesion		N1		
74475	X-ray control, cath insert		N1		
74480	X-ray control, cath insert		N1		
74485	X-ray guide, GU dilation		N1		
74710	X-ray measurement of pelvis		Z3		$17.61
74740	X-ray, female genital tract		N1		
74742	X-ray, fallopian tube		N1		
74775	X-ray exam of perineum		Z2	2.4358	$101.99
75557	Cardiac mri for morph		Z2	4.961	$207.73
75559	Cardiac mri w/stress img		Z2	4.961	$207.73
75561	Cardiac mri for morph w/dye		Z2	7.5993	$318.21
75563	Card mri w/stress img & dye		Z2	7.5993	$318.21
75565	Card mri vel flw map add-on	NI	N1		
75571	Ct hrt w/o dye w/ca test	NI	Z2	0.6403	$26.81
75572	Ct hrt w/3d image	NI	Z3		$40.62
75573	Ct hrt w/3d image, congen	NI	Z3		$48.57
75574	Ct angio hrt w/3d image	NI	Z2	3.82	$159.95
75600	Contrast x-ray exam of aorta		N1		
75605	Contrast x-ray exam of aorta		N1		
75625	Contrast x-ray exam of aorta		N1		
75630	X-ray aorta, leg arteries		N1		
75635	Ct angio abdominal arteries		N1		
75650	Artery x-rays, head & neck		N1		

HCPCS Code	HCPCS Descriptor	CY 2010 Comment Indicator	CY 2010 Payment Indicator	CY 2010 Third Year Pymt. Weight	CY 2010 Third Year TransitionWeight
75658	Artery x-rays, arm		N1		
75660	Artery x-rays, head & neck		N1		
75662	Artery x-rays, head & neck		N1		
75665	Artery x-rays, head & neck		N1		
75671	Artery x-rays, head & neck		N1		
75676	Artery x-rays, neck		N1		
75680	Artery x-rays, neck		N1		
75685	Artery x-rays, spine		N1		
75705	Artery x-rays, spine		N1		
75710	Artery x-rays, arm/leg		N1		
75716	Artery x-rays, arms/legs		N1		
75722	Artery x-rays, kidney		N1		
75724	Artery x-rays, kidneys		N1		
75726	Artery x-rays, abdomen		N1		
75731	Artery x-rays, adrenal gland		N1		
75733	Artery x-rays, adrenals		N1		
75736	Artery x-rays, pelvis		N1		
75741	Artery x-rays, lung		N1		
75743	Artery x-rays, lungs		N1		
75746	Artery x-rays, lung		N1		
75756	Artery x-rays, chest		N1		
75774	Artery x-ray, each vessel		N1		
75790	Visualize A-V shunt	CH	D5		
75791	Av dialysis shunt imaging	NI	N1		
75801	Lymph vessel x-ray, arm/leg		N1		
75803	Lymph vessel x-ray,arms/legs		N1		
75805	Lymph vessel x-ray, trunk		N1		
75807	Lymph vessel x-ray, trunk		N1		
75809	Nonvascular shunt, x-ray		N1		
75810	Vein x-ray, spleen/liver		N1		
75820	Vein x-ray, arm/leg		N1		
75822	Vein x-ray, arms/legs		N1		
75825	Vein x-ray, trunk		N1		
75827	Vein x-ray, chest		N1		
75831	Vein x-ray, kidney		N1		
75833	Vein x-ray, kidneys		N1		
75840	Vein x-ray, adrenal gland		N1		
75842	Vein x-ray, adrenal glands		N1		
75860	Vein x-ray, neck		N1		
75870	Vein x-ray, skull		N1		
75872	Vein x-ray, skull		N1		
75880	Vein x-ray, eye socket		N1		
75885	Vein x-ray, liver		N1		
75887	Vein x-ray, liver		N1		
75889	Vein x-ray, liver		N1		
75891	Vein x-ray, liver		N1		
75893	Venous sampling by catheter		N1		
75894	X-rays, transcath therapy		N1		
75896	X-rays, transcath therapy		N1		
75898	Follow-up angiography		N1		
75901	Remove cva device obstruct		N1		
75902	Remove cva lumen obstruct		N1		

HCPCS Code	HCPCS Descriptor	CY 2010 Comment Indicator	CY 2010 Payment Indicator	CY 2010 Third Year Pymt. Weight	CY 2010 Third Year TransitionWeight
75940	X-ray placement, vein filter		N1		
75945	Intravascular us		N1		
75946	Intravascular us add-on		N1		
75960	Transcath iv stent rs&i		N1		
75961	Retrieval, broken catheter		N1		
75962	Repair arterial blockage		N1		
75964	Repair artery blockage, each		N1		
75966	Repair arterial blockage		N1		
75968	Repair artery blockage, each		N1		
75970	Vascular biopsy		N1		
75978	Repair venous blockage		N1		
75980	Contrast xray exam bile duct		N1		
75982	Contrast xray exam bile duct		N1		
75984	Xray control catheter change		N1		
75989	Abscess drainage under x-ray		N1		
75992	Atherectomy, x-ray exam		N1		
75993	Atherectomy, x-ray exam		N1		
75994	Atherectomy, x-ray exam		N1		
75995	Atherectomy, x-ray exam		N1		
75996	Atherectomy, x-ray exam		N1		
76000	Fluoroscope examination		N1		
76001	Fluoroscope exam, extensive		N1		
76010	X-ray, nose to rectum		Z3		$13.63
76080	X-ray exam of fistula		N1		
76098	X-ray exam, breast specimen	CH	N1		
76100	X-ray exam of body section		Z2	1.0678	$44.71
76101	Complex body section x-ray	CH	Z3		$111.07
76102	Complex body section x-rays		Z2	2.9841	$124.95
76120	Cine/video x-rays	CH	Z3		$42.04
76125	Cine/video x-rays add-on		N1		
76150	X-ray exam, dry process		Z3		$14.49
76350	Special x-ray contrast study		N1		
76376	3d render w/o postprocess		N1		
76377	3d rendering w/postprocess		N1		
76380	CAT scan follow-up study		Z2	1.5586	$65.26
76496	Fluoroscopic procedure		Z2	1.2143	$50.85
76497	Ct procedure		Z2	1.5586	$65.26
76498	Mri procedure		Z2	4.961	$207.73
76499	Radiographic procedure		Z2	0.6373	$26.69
76506	Echo exam of head		Z2	0.8866	$37.12
76510	Ophth us, b & quant a		Z3		$52.55
76511	Ophth us, quant a only		Z3		$35.22
76512	Ophth us, b w/non-quant a		Z3		$29.83
76513	Echo exam of eye, water bath		Z3		$38.06
76514	Echo exam of eye, thickness		Z3		$2.84
76516	Echo exam of eye		Z3		$29.83
76519	Echo exam of eye		Z3		$33.24
76529	Echo exam of eye		Z3		$28.97
76536	Us exam of head and neck		Z2	1.3809	$57.82
76604	Us exam, chest		Z2	0.8866	$37.12
76645	Us exam, breast(s)		Z2	0.8866	$37.12
76700	Us exam, abdom, complete		Z2	1.3809	$57.82

HCPCS Code	HCPCS Descriptor	CY 2010 Comment Indicator	CY 2010 Payment Indicator	CY 2010 Third Year Pymt. Weight	CY 2010 Third Year TransitionWeight
76705	Echo exam of abdomen	CH	Z3		$55.68
76770	Us exam abdo back wall, comp		Z2	1.3809	$57.82
76775	Us exam abdo back wall, lim		Z2	1.3809	$57.82
76776	Us exam k transpl w/doppler		Z2	1.3809	$57.82
76800	Us exam, spinal canal	CH	Z3		$53.40
76801	Ob us < 14 wks, single fetus		Z2	1.3809	$57.82
76802	Ob us < 14 wks, addl fetus		Z3		$21.59
76805	Ob us >/= 14 wks, sngl fetus		Z2	1.3809	$57.82
76810	Ob us >/= 14 wks, addl fetus		Z3		$35.51
76811	Ob us, detailed, sngl fetus	CH	Z3		$74.71
76812	Ob us, detailed, addl fetus		Z2	0.8866	$37.12
76813	Ob us nuchal meas, 1 gest		Z2	0.8866	$37.12
76814	Ob us nuchal meas, add-on		Z3		$23.58
76815	Ob us, limited, fetus(s)		Z2	0.8866	$37.12
76816	Ob us, follow-up, per fetus		Z2	0.8866	$37.12
76817	Transvaginal us, obstetric		Z2	0.8866	$37.12
76818	Fetal biophys profile w/nst	CH	Z3		$51.13
76819	Fetal biophys profil w/o nst		Z3		$39.77
76820	Umbilical artery echo		Z3		$18.18
76821	Middle cerebral artery echo		Z2	0.8866	$37.12
76825	Echo exam of fetal heart		Z3		$96.58
76826	Echo exam of fetal heart		Z3		$58.80
76827	Echo exam of fetal heart	CH	Z3		$29.26
76828	Echo exam of fetal heart		Z3		$16.76
76830	Transvaginal us, non-ob		Z2	1.3809	$57.82
76831	Echo exam, uterus		Z3		$64.20
76856	Us exam, pelvic, complete		Z2	1.3809	$57.82
76857	Us exam, pelvic, limited		Z2	0.8866	$37.12
76870	Us exam, scrotum		Z2	1.3809	$57.82
76872	Us, transrectal		Z2	1.3809	$57.82
76873	Echograp trans r, pros study		Z2	1.3809	$57.82
76880	Us exam, extremity		Z2	1.3809	$57.82
76885	Us exam infant hips, dynamic		Z2	0.8866	$37.12
76886	Us exam infant hips, static		Z2	0.8866	$37.12
76930	Echo guide, cardiocentesis		N1		
76932	Echo guide for heart biopsy		N1		
76936	Echo guide for artery repair		Z2	1.5379	$64.40
76937	Us guide, vascular access		N1		
76940	Us guide, tissue ablation		N1		
76941	Echo guide for transfusion		N1		
76942	Echo guide for biopsy		N1		
76945	Echo guide, villus sampling		N1		
76946	Echo guide for amniocentesis		N1		
76948	Echo guide, ova aspiration		N1		
76950	Echo guidance radiotherapy		N1		
76965	Echo guidance radiotherapy		N1		
76970	Ultrasound exam follow-up		Z2	0.8866	$37.12
76975	GI endoscopic ultrasound		N1		
76977	Us bone density measure		Z3		$6.53
76998	Us guide, intraop		N1		
76999	Echo examination procedure		Z2	0.8866	$37.12
77001	Fluoroguide for vein device		N1		

HCPCS Code	HCPCS Descriptor	CY 2010 Comment Indicator	CY 2010 Payment Indicator	CY 2010 Third Year Pymt. Weight	CY 2010 Third Year Transition Weight
77002	Needle localization by xray		N1		
77003	Fluoroguide for spine inject		N1		
77011	Ct scan for localization		N1		
77012	Ct scan for needle biopsy		N1		
77013	Ct guide for tissue ablation		N1		
77014	Ct scan for therapy guide		N1		
77021	Mr guidance for needle place		N1		
77022	Mri for tissue ablation		N1		
77031	Stereotact guide for brst bx		N1		
77032	Guidance for needle, breast		N1		
77053	X-ray of mammary duct		N1		
77054	X-ray of mammary ducts		N1		
77071	X-ray stress view		Z3		$19.60
77072	X-rays for bone age		Z3		$9.94
77073	X-rays, bone length studies		Z3		$17.33
77074	X-rays, bone survey, limited		Z3		$34.09
77075	X-rays, bone survey complete		Z2	1.0678	$44.71
77076	X-rays, bone survey, infant		Z2	1.0678	$44.71
77077	Joint survey, single view		Z3		$18.75
77078	Ct bone density, axial		Z2	1.0289	$43.08
77079	Ct bone density, peripheral		Z3		$32.10
77080	Dxa bone density, axial	CH	Z3		$40.34
77081	Dxa bone density/peripheral		Z3		$13.35
77082	Dxa bone density, vert fx		Z3		$14.77
77083	Radiographic absorptiometry		Z3		$11.36
77084	Magnetic image, bone marrow		Z2	4.961	$207.73
77280	Set radiation therapy field		Z2	1.461	$61.18
77285	Set radiation therapy field		Z2	3.7799	$158.28
77290	Set radiation therapy field		Z2	3.7799	$158.28
77295	Set radiation therapy field		Z3		$284.91
77299	Radiation therapy planning		Z2	1.461	$61.18
77300	Radiation therapy dose plan		Z3		$29.26
77301	Radiotherapy dose plan, imrt		Z2	13.1619	$551.13
77305	Teletx isodose plan simple		Z3		$25.28
77310	Teletx isodose plan intermed		Z3		$32.95
77315	Teletx isodose plan complex		Z3		$49.71
77321	Special teletx port plan		Z3		$48.86
77326	Brachytx isodose calc simp		Z2	1.461	$61.18
77327	Brachytx isodose calc interm		Z3		$100.27
77328	Brachytx isodose plan compl	CH	Z3		$128.96
77331	Special radiation dosimetry		Z3		$14.20
77332	Radiation treatment aid(s)		Z3		$38.06
77333	Radiation treatment aid(s)		Z3		$15.62
77334	Radiation treatment aid(s)		Z3		$69.59
77336	Radiation physics consult		Z3		$41.76
77338	Design mlc device for imrt	NI	Z2	2.7055	$113.29
77370	Radiation physics consult		Z2	1.461	$61.18
77371	Srs, multisource		Z2	104.238	$4,364.76
77399	External radiation dosimetry		Z2	1.461	$61.18
77401	Radiation treatment delivery		Z3		$20.17
77402	Radiation treatment delivery		Z2	1.3168	$55.14
77403	Radiation treatment delivery		Z2	1.3168	$55.14

HCPCS Code	HCPCS Descriptor	CY 2010 Comment Indicator	CY 2010 Payment Indicator	CY 2010 Third Year Pymt. Weight	CY 2010 Third Year Transition Weight
77404	Radiation treatment delivery		Z2	1.3168	$55.14
77406	Radiation treatment delivery		Z2	2.2033	$92.26
77407	Radiation treatment delivery		Z2	1.3168	$55.14
77408	Radiation treatment delivery		Z2	1.3168	$55.14
77409	Radiation treatment delivery		Z2	1.3168	$55.14
77411	Radiation treatment delivery		Z2	2.2033	$92.26
77412	Radiation treatment delivery		Z2	2.2033	$92.26
77413	Radiation treatment delivery		Z2	2.2033	$92.26
77414	Radiation treatment delivery		Z2	2.2033	$92.26
77416	Radiation treatment delivery		Z2	2.2033	$92.26
77417	Radiology port film(s)		N1		
77418	Radiation tx delivery, imrt		Z2	5.9784	$250.33
77421	Stereoscopic x-ray guidance		N1		
77422	Neutron beam tx, simple		Z2	2.2033	$92.26
77423	Neutron beam tx, complex		Z2	2.2033	$92.26
77435	Sbrt management		N1		
77470	Special radiation treatment		Z3		$88.34
77520	Proton trmt, simple w/o comp		Z2	13.3743	$560.02
77522	Proton trmt, simple w/comp		Z2	13.3743	$560.02
77523	Proton trmt, intermediate		Z2	17.4955	$732.59
77525	Proton treatment, complex		Z2	17.4955	$732.59
77600	Hyperthermia treatment		Z2	5.4016	$226.18
77605	Hyperthermia treatment		Z2	5.4016	$226.18
77610	Hyperthermia treatment		Z2	5.4016	$226.18
77615	Hyperthermia treatment		Z2	5.4016	$226.18
77620	Hyperthermia treatment		Z2	5.4016	$226.18
77750	Infuse radioactive materials		Z3		$72.44
77761	Apply intrcav radiat simple		Z3		$126.98
77762	Apply intrcav radiat interm		Z3		$149.13
77763	Apply intrcav radiat compl	CH	Z2	4.2904	$179.65
77776	Apply interstit radiat simpl		Z3		$136.63
77777	Apply interstit radiat inter		Z3		$147.43
77778	Apply interstit radiat compl		Z3		$198.56
77785	Hdr brachytx, 1 channel		Z3		$86.64
77786	Hdr brachytx, 2-12 channel		Z3		$279.80
77787	Hdr brachytx over 12 chan	CH	Z3		$426.09
77789	Apply surface radiation		Z3		$38.35
77790	Radiation handling		N1		
77799	Radium/radioisotope therapy		Z2	4.2904	$179.65
78000	Thyroid, single uptake		Z3		$44.31
78001	Thyroid, multiple uptakes	CH	Z3		$55.96
78003	Thyroid suppress/stimul		Z3		$45.17
78006	Thyroid imaging with uptake		Z2	3.147	$131.77
78007	Thyroid image, mult uptakes		Z3		$77.55
78010	Thyroid imaging		Z2	2.066	$86.51
78011	Thyroid imaging with flow		Z2	2.066	$86.51
78015	Thyroid met imaging		Z3		$128.40
78016	Thyroid met imaging/studies		Z2	4.1171	$172.40
78018	Thyroid met imaging, body		Z2	4.1171	$172.40
78020	Thyroid met uptake		N1		
78070	Parathyroid nuclear imaging		Z3		$93.74
78075	Adrenal nuclear imaging		Z3		$278.66

HCPCS Code	HCPCS Descriptor	CY 2010 Comment Indicator	CY 2010 Payment Indicator	CY 2010 Third Year Pymt. Weight	CY 2010 Third Year TransitionWeight
78099	Endocrine nuclear procedure		Z2	2.066	$86.51
78102	Bone marrow imaging, ltd		Z3		$99.42
78103	Bone marrow imaging, mult	CH	Z3		$132.37
78104	Bone marrow imaging, body		Z2	3.6682	$153.60
78110	Plasma volume, single		Z3		$51.13
78111	Plasma volume, multiple		Z3		$59.37
78120	Red cell mass, single		Z3		$53.97
78121	Red cell mass, multiple		Z3		$60.22
78122	Blood volume		Z3		$71.30
78130	Red cell survival study		Z3		$89.48
78135	Red cell survival kinetics	CH	Z3		$218.44
78140	Red cell sequestration		Z3		$81.24
78185	Spleen imaging	CH	Z3		$126.69
78190	Platelet survival, kinetics		Z2	2.5656	$107.43
78191	Platelet survival		Z2	2.5656	$107.43
78195	Lymph system imaging		Z2	3.6682	$153.60
78199	Blood/lymph nuclear exam		Z2	3.6682	$153.60
78201	Liver imaging		Z3		$115.33
78202	Liver imaging with flow	CH	Z3		$129.25
78205	Liver imaging (3D)	CH	Z3		$143.45
78206	Liver image (3d) with flow		Z2	4.1271	$172.81
78215	Liver and spleen imaging		Z3		$119.31
78216	Liver & spleen image/flow		Z3		$77.26
78220	Liver function study		Z3		$84.37
78223	Hepatobiliary imaging		Z2	4.1271	$172.81
78230	Salivary gland imaging		Z3		$101.13
78231	Serial salivary imaging		Z3		$76.13
78232	Salivary gland function exam		Z3		$75.28
78258	Esophageal motility study	CH	Z3		$138.05
78261	Gastric mucosa imaging		Z2	3.5113	$147.03
78262	Gastroesophageal reflux exam		Z2	3.5113	$147.03
78264	Gastric emptying study		Z2	3.5113	$147.03
78270	Vit B-12 absorption exam		Z3		$50.85
78271	Vit b-12 absrp exam, int fac		Z3		$53.40
78272	Vit B-12 absorp, combined		Z3		$56.24
78278	Acute GI blood loss imaging		Z2	3.5113	$147.03
78282	GI protein loss exam		Z2	3.5113	$147.03
78290	Meckels divert exam		Z2	3.5113	$147.03
78291	Leveen/shunt patency exam		Z2	3.5113	$147.03
78299	GI nuclear procedure		Z2	3.5113	$147.03
78300	Bone imaging, limited area		Z3		$102.83
78305	Bone imaging, multiple areas	CH	Z3		$136.07
78306	Bone imaging, whole body		Z2	3.5118	$147.05
78315	Bone imaging, 3 phase		Z2	3.5118	$147.05
78320	Bone imaging (3D)	CH	Z3		$143.17
78399	Musculoskeletal nuclear exam		Z2	3.5118	$147.05
78414	Non-imaging heart function		Z2	4.3402	$181.74
78428	Cardiac shunt imaging		Z3		$114.76
78445	Vascular flow imaging	CH	Z3		$105.10
78451	Ht muscle image spect, sing	NI	Z3		$122.15
78452	Ht muscle image spect, mult	NI	Z3		$236.34
78453	Ht muscle image,planar,sing	NI	Z3		$113.91

HCPCS Code	HCPCS Descriptor	CY 2010 Comment Indicator	CY 2010 Payment Indicator	CY 2010 Third Year Pymt. Weight	CY 2010 Third Year TransitionWeight
78454	Ht musc image, planar, mult	NI	Z3		$95.73
78456	Acute venous thrombus image		Z2	2.8394	$118.89
78457	Venous thrombosis imaging	CH	Z3		$112.49
78458	Ven thrombosis images, bilat	CH	Z3		$115.61
78459	Heart muscle imaging (PET)		Z2	20.3369	$851.57
78460	Heart muscle blood, single	CH	D5		
78461	Heart muscle blood, multiple	CH	D5		
78464	Heart image (3d), single	CH	D5		
78465	Heart image (3d), multiple	CH	D5		
78466	Heart infarct image		Z3		$105.67
78468	Heart infarct image (ef)		Z3		$132.94
78469	Heart infarct image (3D)	CH	Z3		$151.69
78472	Gated heart, planar, single	CH	Z3		$150.55
78473	Gated heart, multiple		Z2	4.3402	$181.74
78478	Heart wall motion add-on	CH	D5		
78480	Heart function add-on	CH	D5		
78481	Heart first pass, single		Z3		$122.71
78483	Heart first pass, multiple	CH	Z3		$167.31
78491	Heart image (pet), single		Z2	20.3369	$851.57
78492	Heart image (pet), multiple		Z2	20.3369	$851.57
78494	Heart image, spect	CH	Z3		$157.37
78496	Heart first pass add-on		N1		
78499	Cardiovascular nuclear exam		Z2	4.3402	$181.74
78580	Lung perfusion imaging		Z2	2.9299	$122.68
78584	Lung V/Q image single breath		Z3		$76.13
78585	Lung V/Q imaging		Z2	4.5952	$192.41
78586	Aerosol lung image, single	CH	Z3		$103.68
78587	Aerosol lung image, multiple		Z2	2.9299	$122.68
78588	Perfusion lung image		Z2	4.5952	$192.41
78591	Vent image, 1 breath, 1 proj	CH	Z3		$105.10
78593	Vent image, 1 proj, gas		Z2	2.9299	$122.68
78594	Vent image, mult proj, gas		Z2	2.9299	$122.68
78596	Lung differential function		Z2	4.5952	$192.41
78599	Respiratory nuclear exam		Z2	2.9299	$122.68
78600	Brain image < 4 views	CH	Z3		$112.49
78601	Brain image w/flow < 4 views	CH	Z3		$134.08
78605	Brain image 4+ views		Z2	2.7917	$116.90
78606	Brain image w/flow 4 + views		Z3		$206.80
78607	Brain imaging (3D)		Z3		$219.01
78608	Brain imaging (PET)		Z2	14.7231	$616.50
78610	Brain flow imaging only	CH	Z2	2.7917	$116.90
78630	Cerebrospinal fluid scan		Z3		$214.75
78635	CSF ventriculography		Z3		$202.25
78645	CSF shunt evaluation		Z2	2.7917	$116.90
78647	Cerebrospinal fluid scan		Z3		$207.36
78650	CSF leakage imaging		Z3		$211.34
78660	Nuclear exam of tear flow	CH	Z3		$103.40
78699	Nervous system nuclear exam		Z2	2.7917	$116.90
78700	Kidney imaging, morphol		Z3		$109.65
78701	Kidney imaging with flow		Z3		$134.93
78707	K flow/funct image w/o drug		Z3		$138.62
78708	K flow/funct image w/drug		Z3		$91.47

HCPCS Code	HCPCS Descriptor	CY 2010 Comment Indicator	CY 2010 Payment Indicator	CY 2010 Third Year Pymt. Weight	CY 2010 Third Year Transition Weight
78709	K flow/funct image, multiple		Z2	4.6133	$193.17
78710	Kidney imaging (3D)		Z3		$142.03
78725	Kidney function study		Z3		$59.65
78730	Urinary bladder retention		Z3		$48.86
78740	Ureteral reflux study		Z3		$134.08
78761	Testicular imaging w/flow		Z3		$125.55
78799	Genitourinary nuclear exam		Z2	4.6133	$193.17
78800	Tumor imaging, limited area		Z3		$111.35
78801	Tumor imaging, mult areas		Z3		$151.69
78802	Tumor imaging, whole body		Z3		$204.81
78803	Tumor imaging (3D)		Z3		$217.59
78804	Tumor imaging, whole body		Z3		$382.63
78805	Abscess imaging, ltd area		Z3		$107.09
78806	Abscess imaging, whole body		Z3		$214.47
78807	Nuclear localization/abscess	CH	Z2	4.1171	$172.40
78808	Iv inj ra drug dx study		N1		
78811	Pet image, ltd area		Z2	14.7231	$616.50
78812	Pet image, skull-thigh		Z2	14.7231	$616.50
78813	Pet image, full body		Z2	14.7231	$616.50
78814	Pet image w/ct, lmtd		Z2	14.7231	$616.50
78815	Pet image w/ct, skull-thigh		Z2	14.7231	$616.50
78816	Pet image w/ct, full body		Z2	14.7231	$616.50
78999	Nuclear diagnostic exam		Z2	1.5972	$66.88
79005	Nuclear rx, oral admin		Z3		$42.33
79101	Nuclear rx, iv admin		Z3		$46.02
79200	Nuclear rx, intracav admin		Z3		$51.13
79300	Nuclr rx, interstit colloid		Z2	3.0955	$129.62
79403	Hematopoietic nuclear tx		Z3		$71.87
79440	Nuclear rx, intra-articular		Z3		$40.34
79445	Nuclear rx, intra-arterial		Z2	3.0955	$129.62
79999	Nuclear medicine therapy		Z2	3.0955	$129.62
90371	Hep b ig, im		K2		$111.20
90375	Rabies ig, im/sc		K2		$142.79
90376	Rabies ig, heat treated		K2		$130.16
90378	Rsv, mab, im, 50mg		K2		$937.29
90385	Rh ig, minidose, im		N1		
90396	Varicella-zoster ig, im		K2		$130.49
90476	Adenovirus vaccine, type 4	CH	K2		$72.17
90585	Bcg vaccine, percut		K2		$111.66
90632	Hep a vaccine, adult im		N1		
90633	Hep a vacc, ped/adol, 2 dose		N1		
90634	Hep a vacc, ped/adol, 3 dose		N1		
90636	Hep a/hep b vacc, adult im		N1		
90645	Hib vaccine, hboc, im		N1		
90646	Hib vaccine, prp-d, im		N1		
90647	Hib vaccine, prp-omp, im		N1		
90648	Hib vaccine, prp-t, im		N1		
90655	Flu vaccine no preserv 6-35m		L1		
90656	Flu vaccine no preserv 3 & >		L1		
90657	Flu vaccine, 3 yrs, im		L1		
90658	Flu vaccine, 3 yrs & >, im		L1		
90660	Flu vaccine, nasal		L1		

HCPCS Code	HCPCS Descriptor	CY 2010 Comment Indicator	CY 2010 Payment Indicator	CY 2010 Third Year Pymt. Weight	CY 2010 Third Year TransitionWeight
90665	Lyme disease vaccine, im		K2		$0.93
90669	Pneumococcal vacc, 7 val im		L1		
90675	Rabies vaccine, im		K2		$151.97
90676	Rabies vaccine, id		K2		$96.27
90680	Rotovirus vacc 3 dose, oral	CH	K2		$72.37
90681	Rotavirus vacc 2 dose oral		K2		$106.60
90690	Typhoid vaccine, oral		N1		
90691	Typhoid vaccine, im		N1		
90692	Typhoid vaccine, h-p, sc/id		N1		
90696	Dtap-ipv vacc 4-6 yr im	CH	N1		
90698	Dtap-hib-ip vaccine, im		N1		
90700	Dtap vaccine, < 7 yrs, im		N1		
90701	Dtp vaccine, im		N1		
90702	Dt vaccine < 7, im		N1		
90703	Tetanus vaccine, im		N1		
90704	Mumps vaccine, sc		N1		
90705	Measles vaccine, sc		N1		
90706	Rubella vaccine, sc		N1		
90707	Mmr vaccine, sc		N1		
90708	Measles-rubella vaccine, sc		N1		
90710	Mmrv vaccine, sc		N1		
90712	Oral poliovirus vaccine		N1		
90713	Poliovirus, ipv, sc/im		N1		
90714	Td vaccine no prsrv >/= 7 im		N1		
90715	Tdap vaccine >7 im		N1		
90717	Yellow fever vaccine, sc		N1		
90718	Td vaccine > 7, im		N1		
90719	Diphtheria vaccine, im		N1		
90720	Dtp/hib vaccine, im		N1		
90721	Dtap/hib vaccine, im		N1		
90725	Cholera vaccine, injectable	CH	K2		$0.16
90732	Pneumococcal vaccine		L1		
90733	Meningococcal vaccine, sc		K2		$96.66
90734	Meningococcal vaccine, im		K2		$102.46
90735	Encephalitis vaccine, sc	CH	K2		$100.15
90740	Hepb vacc, ill pat 3 dose im		F4		
90743	Hep b vacc, adol, 2 dose, im		F4		
90744	Hepb vacc ped/adol 3 dose im		F4		
90746	Hep b vaccine, adult, im		F4		
90747	Hepb vacc, ill pat 4 dose im		F4		
90749	Vaccine toxoid		N1		
A4218	Sterile saline or water		N1		
A4220	Infusion pump refill kit		N1		
A4248	Chlorhexidine antisept		N1		
A4262	Temporary tear duct plug		N1		
A4263	Permanent tear duct plug		N1		
A4270	Disposable endoscope sheath		N1		
A4300	Cath impl vasc access portal		N1		
A4301	Implantable access syst perc		N1		
A4305	Drug delivery system >=50 ML		N1		
A4306	Drug delivery system <=50 ml		N1		
A4641	Radiopharm dx agent noc		N1		

HCPCS Code	HCPCS Descriptor	CY 2010 Comment Indicator	CY 2010 Payment Indicator	CY 2010 Third Year Pymt. Weight	CY 2010 Third Year TransitionWeight
A4642	In111 satumomab		N1		
A4648	Implantable tissue marker		N1		
A4650	Implant radiation dosimeter		N1		
A9500	Tc99m sestamibi		N1		
A9501	Technetium TC-99m teboroxime		N1		
A9502	Tc99m tetrofosmin		N1		
A9503	Tc99m medronate		N1		
A9504	Tc99m apcitide		N1		
A9505	TL201 thallium		N1		
A9507	In111 capromab		N1		
A9508	I131 iodobenguate, dx		N1		
A9509	Iodine I-123 sod iodide mil		N1		
A9510	Tc99m disofenin		N1		
A9512	Tc99m pertechnetate		N1		
A9516	Iodine I-123 sod iodide mic		N1		
A9521	Tc99m exametazime		N1		
A9524	I131 serum albumin, dx		N1		
A9526	Nitrogen N-13 ammonia		N1		
A9527	Iodine I-125 sodium iodide	CH	H2		$37.92
A9528	Iodine I-131 iodide cap, dx		N1		
A9529	I131 iodide sol, dx		N1		
A9531	I131 max 100uCi		N1		
A9532	I125 serum albumin, dx		N1		
A9535	Injection, methylene blue	CH	D5		
A9536	Tc99m depreotide		N1		
A9537	Tc99m mebrofenin		N1		
A9538	Tc99m pyrophosphate		N1		
A9539	Tc99m pentetate		N1		
A9540	Tc99m MAA		N1		
A9541	Tc99m sulfur colloid		N1		
A9542	In111 ibritumomab, dx		N1		
A9544	I131 tositumomab, dx		N1		
A9546	Co57/58		N1		
A9547	In111 oxyquinoline		N1		
A9548	In111 pentetate		N1		
A9550	Tc99m gluceptate		N1		
A9551	Tc99m succimer		N1		
A9552	F18 fdg		N1		
A9553	Cr51 chromate		N1		
A9554	I125 iothalamate, dx		N1		
A9555	Rb82 rubidium		N1		
A9556	Ga67 gallium		N1		
A9557	Tc99m bicisate		N1		
A9558	Xe133 xenon 10mci		N1		
A9559	Co57 cyano		N1		
A9560	Tc99m labeled rbc		N1		
A9561	Tc99m oxidronate		N1		
A9562	Tc99m mertiatide		N1		
A9566	Tc99m fanolesomab		N1		
A9567	Technetium TC-99m aerosol		N1		
A9568	Technetium tc99m arcitumomab		N1		
A9569	Technetium TC-99m auto WBC		N1		

HCPCS Code	HCPCS Descriptor	CY 2010 Comment Indicator	CY 2010 Payment Indicator	CY 2010 Third Year Pymt. Weight	CY 2010 Third Year TransitionWeight
A9570	Indium In-111 auto WBC		N1		
A9571	Indium IN-111 auto platelet		N1		
A9572	Indium In-111 pentetreotide		N1		
A9576	Inj prohance multipack		N1		
A9577	Inj multihance		N1		
A9578	Inj multihance multipack		N1		
A9579	Gad-base MR contrast NOS,1ml		N1		
A9580	Sodium fluoride F-18		N1		
A9581	Gadoxetate disodium inj	NI	K2		$13.50
A9582	Iodine I-123 iobenguane	NI	K2		$2,329.83
A9583	Gadofosveset trisodium inj	NI	K2		$1.29
A9698	Non-rad contrast materialNOC		N1		
C1713	Anchor/screw bn/bn,tis/bn		N1		
C1714	Cath, trans atherectomy, dir		N1		
C1715	Brachytherapy needle		N1		
C1716	Brachytx, non-str, Gold-198	CH	H2		$42.85
C1717	Brachytx, non-str,HDR Ir-192	CH	H2		$231.38
C1719	Brachytx, NS, Non-HDRIr-192	CH	H2		$64.02
C1721	AICD, dual chamber		N1		
C1722	AICD, single chamber		N1		
C1724	Cath, trans atherec,rotation		N1		
C1725	Cath, translumin non-laser		N1		
C1726	Cath, bal dil, non-vascular		N1		
C1727	Cath, bal tis dis, non-vas		N1		
C1728	Cath, brachytx seed adm		N1		
C1729	Cath, drainage		N1		
C1730	Cath, EP, 19 or few elect		N1		
C1731	Cath, EP, 20 or more elec		N1		
C1732	Cath, EP, diag/abl, 3D/vect		N1		
C1733	Cath, EP, othr than cool-tip		N1		
C1750	Cath, hemodialysis,long-term		N1		
C1751	Cath, inf, per/cent/midline		N1		
C1752	Cath,hemodialysis,short-term		N1		
C1753	Cath, intravas ultrasound		N1		
C1754	Catheter, intradiscal		N1		
C1755	Catheter, intraspinal		N1		
C1756	Cath, pacing, transesoph		N1		
C1757	Cath, thrombectomy/embolect		N1		
C1758	Catheter, ureteral		N1		
C1759	Cath, intra echocardiography		N1		
C1760	Closure dev, vasc		N1		
C1762	Conn tiss, human(inc fascia)		N1		
C1763	Conn tiss, non-human		N1		
C1764	Event recorder, cardiac		N1		
C1765	Adhesion barrier		N1		
C1766	Intro/sheath,strble,non-peel		N1		
C1767	Generator, neuro non-recharg		N1		
C1768	Graft, vascular		N1		
C1769	Guide wire		N1		
C1770	Imaging coil, MR, insertable		N1		
C1771	Rep dev, urinary, w/sling		N1		
C1772	Infusion pump, programmable		N1		

HCPCS Code	HCPCS Descriptor	CY 2010 Comment Indicator	CY 2010 Payment Indicator	CY 2010 Third Year Pymt. Weight	CY 2010 Third Year Transition Weight
C1773	Ret dev, insertable		N1		
C1776	Joint device (implantable)		N1		
C1777	Lead, AICD, endo single coil		N1		
C1778	Lead, neurostimulator		N1		
C1779	Lead, pmkr, transvenous VDD		N1		
C1780	Lens, intraocular (new tech)		N1		
C1781	Mesh (implantable)		N1		
C1782	Morcellator		N1		
C1783	Ocular imp, aqueous drain de		N1		
C1784	Ocular dev, intraop, det ret		N1		
C1785	Pmkr, dual, rate-resp		N1		
C1786	Pmkr, single, rate-resp		N1		
C1787	Patient progr, neurostim		N1		
C1788	Port, indwelling, imp		N1		
C1789	Prosthesis, breast, imp		N1		
C1813	Prosthesis, penile, inflatab		N1		
C1814	Retinal tamp, silicone oil		N1		
C1815	Pros, urinary sph, imp		N1		
C1816	Receiver/transmitter, neuro		N1		
C1817	Septal defect imp sys		N1		
C1818	Integrated keratoprosthesis		N1		
C1819	Tissue localization-excision		N1		
C1820	Generator neuro rechg bat sy		N1		
C1821	Interspinous implant		N1		
C1874	Stent, coated/cov w/del sys		N1		
C1875	Stent, coated/cov w/o del sy		N1		
C1876	Stent, non-coa/non-cov w/del		N1		
C1877	Stent, non-coat/cov w/o del		N1		
C1878	Matrl for vocal cord		N1		
C1879	Tissue marker, implantable		N1		
C1880	Vena cava filter		N1		
C1881	Dialysis access system		N1		
C1882	AICD, other than sing/dual		N1		
C1883	Adapt/ext, pacing/neuro lead		N1		
C1884	Embolization Protect syst		N1		
C1885	Cath, translumin angio laser		N1		
C1887	Catheter, guiding		N1		
C1888	Endovas non-cardiac abl cath		N1		
C1891	Infusion pump,non-prog, perm		N1		
C1892	Intro/sheath,fixed,peel-away		N1		
C1893	Intro/sheath, fixed,non-peel		N1		
C1894	Intro/sheath, non-laser		N1		
C1895	Lead, AICD, endo dual coil		N1		
C1896	Lead, AICD, non sing/dual		N1		
C1897	Lead, neurostim test kit		N1		
C1898	Lead, pmkr, other than trans		N1		
C1899	Lead, pmkr/AICD combination		N1		
C1900	Lead, coronary venous		N1		
C2614	Probe, perc lumb disc		N1		
C2615	Sealant, pulmonary, liquid		N1		
C2616	Brachytx, non-str,Yttrium-90	CH	H2		$15,779.35
C2617	Stent, non-cor, tem w/o del		N1		

HCPCS Code	HCPCS Descriptor	CY 2010 Comment Indicator	CY 2010 Payment Indicator	CY 2010 Third Year Pymt. Weight	CY 2010 Third Year Transition Weight
C2618	Probe, cryoablation		N1		
C2619	Pmkr, dual, non rate-resp		N1		
C2620	Pmkr, single, non rate-resp		N1		
C2621	Pmkr, other than sing/dual		N1		
C2622	Prosthesis, penile, non-inf		N1		
C2625	Stent, non-cor, tem w/del sy		N1		
C2626	Infusion pump, non-prog,temp		N1		
C2627	Cath, suprapubic/cystoscopic		N1		
C2628	Catheter, occlusion		N1		
C2629	Intro/sheath, laser		N1		
C2630	Cath, EP, cool-tip		N1		
C2631	Rep dev, urinary, w/o sling		N1		
C2634	Brachytx, non-str, HA, I-125	CH	H2		$59.80
C2635	Brachytx, non-str, HA, P-103	CH	H2		$28.59
C2636	Brachy linear, non-str,P-103	CH	H2		$19.37
C2638	Brachytx, stranded, I-125	CH	H2		$42.48
C2639	Brachytx, non-stranded,I-125	CH	H2		$36.18
C2640	Brachytx, stranded, P-103	CH	H2		$60.36
C2641	Brachytx, non-stranded,P-103	CH	H2		$57.12
C2642	Brachytx, stranded, C-131	CH	H2		$109.84
C2643	Brachytx, non-stranded,C-131	CH	H2		$66.09
C2698	Brachytx, stranded, NOS	CH	H2		$42.48
C2699	Brachytx, non-stranded, NOS	CH	H2		$28.59
C8900	MRA w/cont, abd		Z2	6.0177	$251.98
C8901	MRA w/o cont, abd		Z2	4.961	$207.73
C8902	MRA w/o fol w/cont, abd		Z2	7.5993	$318.21
C8903	MRI w/cont, breast, uni		Z2	6.0177	$251.98
C8904	MRI w/o cont, breast, uni		Z2	4.961	$207.73
C8905	MRI w/o fol w/cont, brst, un		Z2	7.5993	$318.21
C8906	MRI w/cont, breast, bi		Z2	6.0177	$251.98
C8907	MRI w/o cont, breast, bi		Z2	4.961	$207.73
C8908	MRI w/o fol w/cont, breast,		Z2	7.5993	$318.21
C8909	MRA w/cont, chest		Z2	6.0177	$251.98
C8910	MRA w/o cont, chest		Z2	4.961	$207.73
C8911	MRA w/o fol w/cont, chest		Z2	7.5993	$318.21
C8912	MRA w/cont, lwr ext		Z2	6.0177	$251.98
C8913	MRA w/o cont, lwr ext		Z2	4.961	$207.73
C8914	MRA w/o fol w/cont, lwr ext		Z2	7.5993	$318.21
C8918	MRA w/cont, pelvis		Z2	6.0177	$251.98
C8919	MRA w/o cont, pelvis		Z2	4.961	$207.73
C8920	MRA w/o fol w/cont, pelvis		Z2	7.5993	$318.21
C9113	Inj pantoprazole sodium, via		N1		
C9121	Injection, argatroban		K2		$18.10
C9245	Injection, romiplostim	CH	D5		
C9246	Inj, gadoxetate disodium	CH	D5		
C9247	Inj, iobenguane, I-123, dx	CH	D5		
C9248	Inj, clevidipine butyrate		K2		$3.39
C9249	Inj, certolizumab pegol	CH	D5		
C9250	Artiss fibrin sealant		K2		$138.20
C9251	Inj, C1 esterase inhibitor	CH	D5		
C9252	Injection, plerixafor	CH	D5		
C9253	Injection, temozolomide	CH	D5		

HCPCS Code	HCPCS Descriptor	CY 2010 Comment Indicator	CY 2010 Payment Indicator	CY 2010 Third Year Pymt. Weight	CY 2010 Third Year TransitionWeight
C9254	Injection, lacosamide	NI	K2		$0.18
C9255	Paliperidone palmitate inj	NI	K2		$6.71
C9256	Dexamethasone intravitreal	NI	K2		$196.10
C9257	Bevacizumab injection	NI	K2		$1.41
C9352	Neuragen nerve guide, per cm		N1		
C9353	Neurawrap nerve protector,cm		N1		
C9354	Veritas collagen matrix, cm2	CH	N1		
C9355	Neuromatrix nerve cuff, cm	CH	N1		
C9356	TenoGlide tendon prot, cm2		K2		$24.86
C9358	SurgiMend, fetal		K2		$10.76
C9359	Implnt,bon void filler-putty		K2		$63.54
C9360	SurgiMend, neonatal		K2		$10.67
C9361	NeuroMend nerve wrap		K2		$247.29
C9362	Implnt,bon void filler-strip		K2		$63.60
C9363	Integra Meshed Bil Wound Mat		K2		$25.62
C9364	Porcine implant, Permacol		K2		$17.21
C9399	Unclassified drugs or biolog		K7		
E0616	Cardiac event recorder		N1		
E0749	Elec osteogen stim implanted		N1		
E0782	Non-programble infusion pump		N1		
E0783	Programmable infusion pump		N1		
E0785	Replacement impl pump cathet		N1		
E0786	Implantable pump replacement		N1		
G0130	Single energy x-ray study		Z3		$15.91
G0173	Linear acc stereo radsur com		Z2	50.6947	$2,122.74
G0251	Linear acc based stero radio		Z2	13.6624	$572.09
G0288	Recon, CTA for surg plan		N1		
G0339	Robot lin-radsurg com, first		Z2	50.6947	$2,122.74
G0340	Robt lin-radsurg fractx 2-5		Z2	35.3136	$1,478.69
J0120	Tetracyclin injection		N1		
J0129	Abatacept injection		K2		$18.98
J0130	Abciximab injection		K2		$459.36
J0132	Acetylcysteine injection		K2		$2.29
J0133	Acyclovir injection		N1		
J0135	Adalimumab injection		K2		$357.53
J0150	Injection adenosine 6 MG		K2		$9.50
J0152	Adenosine injection		K2		$76.42
J0170	Adrenalin epinephrin inject		N1		
J0180	Agalsidase beta injection		K2		$133.69
J0190	Inj biperiden lactate/5 mg		N1		
J0200	Alatrofloxacin mesylate		N1		
J0205	Alglucerase injection		K2		$41.19
J0207	Amifostine		K2		$350.07
J0210	Methyldopate hcl injection		K2		$27.64
J0215	Alefacept		K2		$30.02
J0220	Alglucosidase alfa injection		K2		$124.69
J0256	Alpha 1 proteinase inhibitor		K2		$3.63
J0278	Amikacin sulfate injection		N1		
J0280	Aminophyllin 250 MG inj		N1		
J0282	Amiodarone HCl		N1		
J0285	Amphotericin B		N1		
J0287	Amphotericin b lipid complex		K2		$9.66

HCPCS Code	HCPCS Descriptor	CY 2010 Comment Indicator	CY 2010 Payment Indicator	CY 2010 Third Year Pymt. Weight	CY 2010 Third Year TransitionWeight
J0288	Ampho b cholesteryl sulfate		K2		$13.74
J0289	Amphotericin b liposome inj		K2		$14.96
J0290	Ampicillin 500 MG inj		N1		
J0295	Ampicillin sodium per 1.5 gm		N1		
J0300	Amobarbital 125 MG inj		N1		
J0330	Succinycholine chloride inj		N1		
J0348	Anidulafungin injection		K2		$1.21
J0360	Hydralazine hcl injection		N1		
J0364	Apomorphine hydrochloride		N1		
J0365	Aprotonin, 10,000 kiu		K2		$2.60
J0380	Inj metaraminol bitartrate		N1		
J0390	Chloroquine injection		N1		
J0400	Aripiprazole injection		N1		
J0456	Azithromycin		N1		
J0460	Atropine sulfate injection	CH	D5		
J0461	Atropine sulfate injection	NI	N1		
J0470	Dimecaprol injection		K2		$26.81
J0475	Baclofen 10 MG injection		K2		$195.31
J0476	Baclofen intrathecal trial		K2		$71.24
J0480	Basiliximab		K2		$1,624.44
J0500	Dicyclomine injection		N1		
J0515	Inj benztropine mesylate		N1		
J0520	Bethanechol chloride inject		N1		
J0530	Penicillin g benzathine inj	CH	D5		
J0540	Penicillin g benzathine inj	CH	D5		
J0550	Penicillin g benzathine inj	CH	D5		
J0559	PenG benzathine/procaine inj	NI	N1		
J0560	Penicillin g benzathine inj		N1		
J0570	Penicillin g benzathine inj		N1		
J0580	Penicillin g benzathine inj		N1		
J0583	Bivalirudin		K2		$2.40
J0585	Injection,onabotulinumtoxinA		K2		$5.40
J0586	AbobotulinumtoxintypeA	NI	K2		$8.23
J0587	Inj, rimabotulinumtoxinB		K2		$10.38
J0592	Buprenorphine hydrochloride		N1		
J0594	Busulfan injection		K2		$14.18
J0595	Butorphanol tartrate 1 mg		N1		
J0598	C1 esterase inhibitor inj	NI	K2		$41.34
J0600	Edetate calcium disodium inj		K2		$78.86
J0610	Calcium gluconate injection		N1		
J0620	Calcium glycer & lact/10 ML		N1		
J0630	Calcitonin salmon injection		K2		$48.37
J0636	Inj calcitriol per 0.1 mcg		N1		
J0637	Caspofungin acetate		K2		$11.52
J0640	Leucovorin calcium injection		N1		
J0641	Levoleucovorin injection		K2		$0.99
J0670	Inj mepivacaine HCL/10 ml		N1		
J0690	Cefazolin sodium injection		N1		
J0692	Cefepime HCl for injection		N1		
J0694	Cefoxitin sodium injection		N1		
J0696	Ceftriaxone sodium injection		N1		
J0697	Sterile cefuroxime injection		N1		

HCPCS Code	HCPCS Descriptor	CY 2010 Comment Indicator	CY 2010 Payment Indicator	CY 2010 Third Year Pymt. Weight	CY 2010 Third Year TransitionWeight
J0698	Cefotaxime sodium injection		N1		
J0702	Betamethasone acet&sod phosp		N1		
J0704	Betamethasone sod phosp/4 MG		N1		
J0706	Caffeine citrate injection		N1		
J0710	Cephapirin sodium injection		N1		
J0713	Inj ceftazidime per 500 mg		N1		
J0715	Ceftizoxime sodium / 500 MG		N1		
J0718	Certolizumab pegol inj	NI	K2		$3.80
J0720	Chloramphenicol sodium injec		N1		
J0725	Chorionic gonadotropin/1000u		N1		
J0735	Clonidine hydrochloride		K2		$109.75
J0740	Cidofovir injection		K2		$746.46
J0743	Cilastatin sodium injection		N1		
J0744	Ciprofloxacin iv		N1		
J0745	Inj codeine phosphate /30 MG		N1		
J0760	Colchicine injection		N1		
J0770	Colistimethate sodium inj		N1		
J0780	Prochlorperazine injection		N1		
J0795	Corticorelin ovine triflutal		K2		$4.24
J0800	Corticotropin injection		K2		$2,394.93
J0833	Cosyntropin injection NOS	NI	K2		$91.84
J0834	Cosyntropin cortrosyn inj	NI	K2		$91.84
J0835	Inj cosyntropin per 0.25 MG	CH	D5		
J0850	Cytomegalovirus imm IV /vial		K2		$862.24
J0878	Daptomycin injection		K2		$0.40
J0881	Darbepoetin alfa, non-esrd		K2		$2.76
J0885	Epoetin alfa, non-esrd		K2		$9.40
J0894	Decitabine injection		K2		$28.42
J0895	Deferoxamine mesylate inj		N1		
J0900	Testosterone enanthate inj		N1		
J0945	Brompheniramine maleate inj	CH	K2		$0.75
J0970	Estradiol valerate injection		N1		
J1000	Depo-estradiol cypionate inj		N1		
J1020	Methylprednisolone 20 MG inj		N1		
J1030	Methylprednisolone 40 MG inj		N1		
J1040	Methylprednisolone 80 MG inj		N1		
J1051	Medroxyprogesterone inj		N1		
J1060	Testosterone cypionate 1 ML		N1		
J1070	Testosterone cypionat 100 MG		N1		
J1080	Testosterone cypionat 200 MG		N1		
J1094	Inj dexamethasone acetate		N1		
J1100	Dexamethasone sodium phos		N1		
J1110	Inj dihydroergotamine mesylt		N1		
J1120	Acetazolamid sodium injectio		N1		
J1160	Digoxin injection		N1		
J1162	Digoxin immune fab (ovine)		K2		$474.73
J1165	Phenytoin sodium injection		N1		
J1170	Hydromorphone injection		N1		
J1180	Dyphylline injection		N1		
J1190	Dexrazoxane HCl injection		K2		$340.03
J1200	Diphenhydramine hcl injectio		N1		
J1205	Chlorothiazide sodium inj		K2		$292.02

HCPCS Code	HCPCS Descriptor	CY 2010 Comment Indicator	CY 2010 Payment Indicator	CY 2010 Third Year Pymt. Weight	CY 2010 Third Year TransitionWeight
J1212	Dimethyl sulfoxide 50% 50 ML		K2		$67.46
J1230	Methadone injection		N1		
J1240	Dimenhydrinate injection		N1		
J1245	Dipyridamole injection		N1		
J1250	Inj dobutamine HCL/250 mg		N1		
J1260	Dolasetron mesylate	CH	N1		
J1265	Dopamine injection		N1		
J1267	Doripenem injection		K2		$0.57
J1270	Injection, doxercalciferol		N1		
J1300	Eculizumab injection		K2		$177.57
J1320	Amitriptyline injection		N1		
J1324	Enfuvirtide injection	CH	K2		$0.47
J1325	Epoprostenol injection		N1		
J1327	Eptifibatide injection		K2		$18.57
J1330	Ergonovine maleate injection		N1		
J1335	Ertapenem injection		N1		
J1364	Erythro lactobionate /500 MG		N1		
J1380	Estradiol valerate 10 MG inj		N1		
J1390	Estradiol valerate 20 MG inj		N1		
J1410	Inj estrogen conjugate 25 MG		K2		$83.21
J1430	Ethanolamine oleate 100 mg		K2		$147.14
J1435	Injection estrone per 1 MG		N1		
J1436	Etidronate disodium inj		K2		$70.06
J1438	Etanercept injection		K2		$183.61
J1440	Filgrastim 300 mcg injection		K2		$208.54
J1441	Filgrastim 480 mcg injection		K2		$324.44
J1450	Fluconazole		N1		
J1451	Fomepizole, 15 mg		K2		$7.99
J1453	Fosaprepitant injection		K2		$1.58
J1455	Foscarnet sodium injection	CH	N1		
J1457	Gallium nitrate injection		K2		$1.71
J1458	Galsulfase injection		K2		$339.04
J1459	Inj IVIG privigen 500 mg		K2		$35.05
J1460	Gamma globulin 1 CC inj		K2		$15.05
J1470	Gamma globulin 2 CC inj		K2		$30.10
J1480	Gamma globulin 3 CC inj		K2		$45.14
J1490	Gamma globulin 4 CC inj		K2		$60.20
J1500	Gamma globulin 5 CC inj		K2		$75.26
J1510	Gamma globulin 6 CC inj		K2		$90.35
J1520	Gamma globulin 7 CC inj		K2		$105.27
J1530	Gamma globulin 8 CC inj		K2		$120.40
J1540	Gamma globulin 9 CC inj		K2		$150.50
J1550	Gamma globulin 10 CC inj		K2		$150.50
J1560	Gamma globulin > 10 CC inj		K2		$150.50
J1561	Gamunex injection		K2		$36.71
J1562	Vivaglobin, inj		K2		$7.05
J1565	RSV-ivig	CH	D5		
J1566	Immune globulin, powder		K2		$29.83
J1568	Octagam injection		K2		$37.03
J1569	Gammagard liquid injection		K2		$37.85
J1570	Ganciclovir sodium injection		N1		
J1571	Hepagam b im injection		K2		$50.04

HCPCS Code	HCPCS Descriptor	CY 2010 Comment Indicator	CY 2010 Payment Indicator	CY 2010 Third Year Pymt. Weight	CY 2010 Third Year TransitionWeight
J1572	Flebogamma injection		K2		$36.51
J1573	Hepagam b intravenous, inj		K2		$50.04
J1580	Garamycin gentamicin inj		N1		
J1590	Gatifloxacin injection		N1		
J1595	Injection glatiramer acetate		K2		$81.23
J1600	Gold sodium thiomaleate inj		N1		
J1610	Glucagon hydrochloride/1 MG		K2		$79.20
J1620	Gonadorelin hydroch/ 100 mcg		K2		$176.89
J1626	Granisetron hcl injection	CH	N1		
J1630	Haloperidol injection		N1		
J1631	Haloperidol decanoate inj		N1		
J1640	Hemin, 1 mg		K2		$7.73
J1642	Inj heparin sodium per 10 u		N1		
J1644	Inj heparin sodium per 1000u		N1		
J1645	Dalteparin sodium		N1		
J1650	Inj enoxaparin sodium		N1		
J1652	Fondaparinux sodium		K2		$5.98
J1655	Tinzaparin sodium injection		N1		
J1670	Tetanus immune globulin inj		K2		$199.91
J1680	Human fibrinogen conc inj	NI	K2		$96.46
J1700	Hydrocortisone acetate inj		N1		
J1710	Hydrocortisone sodium ph inj		N1		
J1720	Hydrocortisone sodium succ i		N1		
J1730	Diazoxide injection		K2		$112.16
J1740	Ibandronate sodium injection		K2		$139.22
J1742	Ibutilide fumarate injection		K2		$404.01
J1743	Idursulfase injection		K2		$446.44
J1745	Infliximab injection		K2		$57.60
J1750	Inj iron dextran		K2		$14.11
J1756	Iron sucrose injection		K2		$0.37
J1785	Injection imiglucerase /unit		K2		$4.12
J1790	Droperidol injection		N1		
J1800	Propranolol injection		N1		
J1815	Insulin injection		N1		
J1817	Insulin for insulin pump use	CH	K2		$3.34
J1830	Interferon beta-1b / .25 MG		K2		$168.90
J1835	Itraconazole injection	CH	N1		
J1840	Kanamycin sulfate 500 MG inj		N1		
J1850	Kanamycin sulfate 75 MG inj		N1		
J1885	Ketorolac tromethamine inj		N1		
J1890	Cephalothin sodium injection		N1		
J1930	Lanreotide injection		K2		$28.65
J1931	Laronidase injection		K2		$25.08
J1940	Furosemide injection		N1		
J1945	Lepirudin		K2		$174.51
J1950	Leuprolide acetate /3.75 MG		K2		$480.20
J1953	Levetiracetam injection		K2		$0.75
J1956	Levofloxacin injection		N1		
J1960	Levorphanol tartrate inj		N1		
J1980	Hyoscyamine sulfate inj		N1		
J1990	Chlordiazepoxide injection		N1		
J2001	Lidocaine injection		N1		

HCPCS Code	HCPCS Descriptor	CY 2010 Comment Indicator	CY 2010 Payment Indicator	CY 2010 Third Year Pymt. Weight	CY 2010 Third Year Transition Weight
J2010	Lincomycin injection		N1		
J2020	Linezolid injection		K2		$29.37
J2060	Lorazepam injection		N1		
J2150	Mannitol injection		N1		
J2170	Mecasermin injection		N1		
J2175	Meperidine hydrochl /100 MG		N1		
J2180	Meperidine/promethazine inj		N1		
J2185	Meropenem		N1		
J2210	Methylergonovin maleate inj		N1		
J2248	Micafungin sodium injection		K2		$1.08
J2250	Inj midazolam hydrochloride		N1		
J2260	Inj milrinone lactate / 5 MG		N1		
J2270	Morphine sulfate injection		N1		
J2271	Morphine so4 injection 100mg		N1		
J2275	Morphine sulfate injection		N1		
J2278	Ziconotide injection		K2		$6.65
J2280	Inj, moxifloxacin 100 mg		N1		
J2300	Inj nalbuphine hydrochloride		N1		
J2310	Inj naloxone hydrochloride		N1		
J2315	Naltrexone, depot form		K2		$2.14
J2320	Nandrolone decanoate 50 MG	CH	K2		$7.00
J2321	Nandrolone decanoate 100 MG	CH	K2		$7.00
J2322	Nandrolone decanoate 200 MG	CH	K2		$14.74
J2323	Natalizumab injection		K2		$8.32
J2325	Nesiritide injection		K2		$36.07
J2353	Octreotide injection, depot		K2		$105.27
J2354	Octreotide inj, non-depot		N1		
J2355	Oprelvekin injection		K2		$242.16
J2357	Omalizumab injection		K2		$18.86
J2360	Orphenadrine injection		N1		
J2370	Phenylephrine hcl injection		N1		
J2400	Chloroprocaine hcl injection		N1		
J2405	Ondansetron hcl injection	CH	N1		
J2410	Oxymorphone hcl injection		N1		
J2425	Palifermin injection		K2		$11.06
J2430	Pamidronate disodium /30 MG		K2		$18.42
J2440	Papaverin hcl injection		N1		
J2469	Palonosetron hcl		K2		$17.19
J2501	Paricalcitol		N1		
J2503	Pegaptanib sodium injection		K2		$1,014.11
J2504	Pegademase bovine, 25 iu		K2		$242.67
J2505	Injection, pegfilgrastim 6mg		K2		$2,222.07
J2510	Penicillin g procaine inj		N1		
J2513	Pentastarch 10% solution		K2		$1,270.88
J2515	Pentobarbital sodium inj	CH	N1		
J2540	Penicillin g potassium inj		N1		
J2543	Piperacillin/tazobactam		N1		
J2550	Promethazine hcl injection		N1		
J2560	Phenobarbital sodium inj		N1		
J2562	Plerixafor injection	NI	K2		$268.51
J2590	Oxytocin injection		N1		
J2597	Inj desmopressin acetate		N1		

HCPCS Code	HCPCS Descriptor	CY 2010 Comment Indicator	CY 2010 Payment Indicator	CY 2010 Third Year Pymt. Weight	CY 2010 Third Year Transition Weight
J2650	Prednisolone acetate inj		N1		
J2670	Totazoline hcl injection		N1		
J2675	Inj progesterone per 50 MG		N1		
J2680	Fluphenazine decanoate 25 MG		N1		
J2690	Procainamide hcl injection		N1		
J2700	Oxacillin sodium injeciton		N1		
J2710	Neostigmine methylslfte inj		N1		
J2720	Inj protamine sulfate/10 MG		N1		
J2724	Protein c concentrate		K2		$11.96
J2725	Inj protirelin per 250 mcg		N1		
J2730	Pralidoxime chloride inj		K2		$85.83
J2760	Phentolaine mesylate inj		N1		
J2765	Metoclopramide hcl injection		N1		
J2770	Quinupristin/dalfopristin		K2		$144.08
J2778	Ranibizumab injection		K2		$398.11
J2780	Ranitidine hydrochloride inj		N1		
J2783	Rasburicase		K2		$164.00
J2785	Regadenoson injection		K2		$50.78
J2788	Rho d immune globulin 50 mcg		K2		$25.76
J2790	Rho d immune globulin inj		K2		$84.39
J2791	Rhophylac injection		K2		$5.13
J2792	Rho(D) immune globulin h, sd		K2		$18.39
J2793	Rilonacept injection	NI	K2		$23.64
J2794	Risperidone, long acting		K2		$4.93
J2795	Ropivacaine HCl injection		N1		
J2796	Romiplostim injection	NI	K2		$43.75
J2800	Methocarbamol injection		N1		
J2805	Sincalide injection	CH	N1		
J2810	Inj theophylline per 40 MG		N1		
J2820	Sargramostim injection		K2		$23.31
J2850	Inj secretin synthetic human		K2		$19.93
J2910	Aurothioglucose injeciton		N1		
J2916	Na ferric gluconate complex		N1		
J2920	Methylprednisolone injection		N1		
J2930	Methylprednisolone injection		N1		
J2940	Somatrem injection		K2		$43.99
J2941	Somatropin injection		K2		$53.47
J2950	Promazine hcl injection		N1		
J2993	Reteplase injection		K2		$1,230.80
J2995	Inj streptokinase /250000 IU		K2		$78.00
J2997	Alteplase recombinant		K2		$35.03
J3000	Streptomycin injection		N1		
J3010	Fentanyl citrate injeciton		N1		
J3030	Sumatriptan succinate / 6 MG		K2		$55.49
J3070	Pentazocine injection		N1		
J3101	Tenecteplase injection		K2		$40.10
J3105	Terbutaline sulfate inj		N1		
J3120	Testosterone enanthate inj		N1		
J3130	Testosterone enanthate inj		N1		
J3140	Testosterone suspension inj		N1		
J3150	Testosteron propionate inj		N1		
J3230	Chlorpromazine hcl injection		N1		

HCPCS Code	HCPCS Descriptor	CY 2010 Comment Indicator	CY 2010 Payment Indicator	CY 2010 Third Year Pymt. Weight	CY 2010 Third Year TransitionWeight
J3240	Thyrotropin injection		K2		$948.38
J3243	Tigecycline injection		K2		$1.15
J3246	Tirofiban HCl		K2		$7.83
J3250	Trimethobenzamide hcl inj		N1		
J3260	Tobramycin sulfate injection		N1		
J3265	Injection torsemide 10 mg/ml		N1		
J3280	Thiethylperazine maleate inj		N1		
J3285	Treprostinil injection		K2		$54.83
J3300	Triamcinolone A inj PRS-free		K2		$3.20
J3301	Triamcinolone acet inj NOS		N1		
J3302	Triamcinolone diacetate inj		N1		
J3303	Triamcinolone hexacetonl inj		N1		
J3305	Inj trimetrexate glucoronate		K2		$124.80
J3310	Perphenazine injeciton		N1		
J3315	Triptorelin pamoate		K2		$160.83
J3320	Spectinomycn di-hcl inj		N1		
J3350	Urea injection	CH	N1		
J3355	Urofollitropin, 75 iu		K2		$59.26
J3360	Diazepam injection		N1		
J3364	Urokinase 5000 IU injection		N1		
J3365	Urokinase 250,000 IU inj		K2		$449.09
J3370	Vancomycin hcl injection		N1		
J3396	Verteporfin injection		K2		$9.31
J3400	Triflupromazine hcl inj	CH	N1		
J3410	Hydroxyzine hcl injection		N1		
J3411	Thiamine hcl 100 mg		N1		
J3415	Pyridoxine hcl 100 mg		N1		
J3420	Vitamin b12 injection		N1		
J3430	Vitamin k phytonadione inj		N1		
J3465	Injection, voriconazole		K2		$5.26
J3470	Hyaluronidase injection		N1		
J3471	Ovine, up to 999 USP units		N1		
J3472	Ovine, 1000 USP units	CH	N1		
J3473	Hyaluronidase recombinant	CH	N1		
J3475	Inj magnesium sulfate		N1		
J3480	Inj potassium chloride		N1		
J3485	Zidovudine		N1		
J3486	Ziprasidone mesylate		N1		
J3487	Zoledronic acid		K2		$214.94
J3488	Reclast injection		K2		$218.59
J3490	Drugs unclassified injection		N1		
J3530	Nasal vaccine inhalation		N1		
J3590	Unclassified biologics		N1		
J7030	Normal saline solution infus		N1		
J7040	Normal saline solution infus		N1		
J7042	5% dextrose/normal saline		N1		
J7050	Normal saline solution infus		N1		
J7060	5% dextrose/water		N1		
J7070	D5w infusion		N1		
J7100	Dextran 40 infusion		N1		
J7110	Dextran 75 infusion		N1		
J7120	Ringers lactate infusion		N1		

HCPCS Code	HCPCS Descriptor	CY 2010 Comment Indicator	CY 2010 Payment Indicator	CY 2010 Third Year Pymt. Weight	CY 2010 Third Year TransitionWeight
J7130	Hypertonic saline solution		N1		
J7185	Xyntha inj	NI	K2		$1.06
J7186	Antihemophilic viii/vwf comp		K2		$0.84
J7187	Humate-P, inj		K2		$0.87
J7189	Factor viia		K2		$1.29
J7190	Factor viii		K2		$0.84
J7191	Factor VIII (porcine)		K2		$2.00
J7192	Factor viii recombinant NOS		K2		$1.08
J7193	Factor IX non-recombinant		K2		$0.88
J7194	Factor ix complex		K2		$0.85
J7195	Factor IX recombinant		K2		$1.06
J7197	Antithrombin iii injection	CH	K2		$2.28
J7198	Anti-inhibitor		K2		$1.53
J7308	Aminolevulinic acid hcl top		K2		$127.60
J7310	Ganciclovir long act implant		K2		$16,640.00
J7311	Fluocinolone acetonide implt		K2		$18,980.00
J7321	Hyalgan/supartz inj per dose		K2		$91.87
J7322	Synvisc inj per dose	CH	D5		
J7323	Euflexxa inj per dose		K2		$113.96
J7324	Orthovisc inj per dose		K2		$177.68
J7325	Synvisc or Synvisc-One	NI	K2		$11.47
J7500	Azathioprine oral 50mg		N1		
J7501	Azathioprine parenteral		K2		$90.64
J7502	Cyclosporine oral 100 mg		K2		$3.22
J7504	Lymphocyte immune globulin		K2		$453.67
J7505	Monoclonal antibodies		K2		$1,109.45
J7506	Prednisone oral		N1		
J7507	Tacrolimus oral per 1 MG		K2		$3.96
J7509	Methylprednisolone oral		N1		
J7510	Prednisolone oral per 5 mg		N1		
J7511	Antithymocyte globuln rabbit		K2		$414.44
J7513	Daclizumab, parenteral		K2		$378.20
J7515	Cyclosporine oral 25 mg	CH	K2		$0.82
J7516	Cyclosporin parenteral 250mg		K2		$21.24
J7517	Mycophenolate mofetil oral		K2		$2.45
J7518	Mycophenolic acid	CH	N1		
J7520	Sirolimus, oral		K2		$9.44
J7525	Tacrolimus injection		K2		$136.82
J7599	Immunosuppressive drug noc		N1		
J7674	Methacholine chloride, neb		N1		
J7799	Non-inhalation drug for DME		N1		
J8501	Oral aprepitant		K2		$5.42
J8510	Oral busulfan	CH	N1		
J8520	Capecitabine, oral, 150 mg		K2		$5.68
J8521	Capecitabine, oral, 500 mg		K2		$18.73
J8530	Cyclophosphamide oral 25 MG		N1		
J8540	Oral dexamethasone		N1		
J8560	Etoposide oral 50 MG		K2		$0.45
J8597	Antiemetic drug oral NOS		N1		
J8600	Melphalan oral 2 MG		N1		
J8610	Methotrexate oral 2.5 MG		N1		
J8650	Nabilone oral	CH	N1		

HCPCS Code	HCPCS Descriptor	CY 2010 Comment Indicator	CY 2010 Payment Indicator	CY 2010 Third Year Pymt. Weight	CY 2010 Third Year TransitionWeight
J8700	Temozolomide		K2		$8.59
J8705	Topotecan oral		K2		$71.35
J9000	Doxorubicin hcl injection		N1		
J9001	Doxorubicin hcl liposome inj		K2		$450.51
J9010	Alemtuzumab injection		K2		$559.46
J9015	Aldesleukin injection		K2		$831.49
J9017	Arsenic trioxide injection		K2		$36.73
J9020	Asparaginase injection		K2		$56.92
J9025	Azacitidine injection		K2		$4.78
J9027	Clofarabine injection		K2		$114.21
J9031	Bcg live intravesical vac		K2		$111.08
J9033	Bendamustine injection		K2		$18.53
J9035	Bevacizumab injection		K2		$56.39
J9040	Bleomycin sulfate injection		N1		
J9041	Bortezomib injection		K2		$36.54
J9045	Carboplatin injection		N1		
J9050	Carmustine injection		K2		$173.73
J9055	Cetuximab injection		K2		$48.79
J9060	Cisplatin 10 MG injection		N1		
J9062	Cisplatin 50 MG injection		N1		
J9065	Inj cladribine per 1 MG		K2		$25.15
J9070	Cyclophosphamide 100 MG inj		N1		
J9080	Cyclophosphamide 200 MG inj		N1		
J9090	Cyclophosphamide 500 MG inj		N1		
J9091	Cyclophosphamide 1.0 grm inj		N1		
J9092	Cyclophosphamide 2.0 grm inj		N1		
J9093	Cyclophosphamide lyophilized		N1		
J9094	Cyclophosphamide lyophilized		N1		
J9095	Cyclophosphamide lyophilized		N1		
J9096	Cyclophosphamide lyophilized		N1		
J9097	Cyclophosphamide lyophilized		N1		
J9098	Cytarabine liposome inj		K2		$480.19
J9100	Cytarabine hcl 100 MG inj		N1		
J9110	Cytarabine hcl 500 MG inj		N1		
J9120	Dactinomycin injection		K2		$533.21
J9130	Dacarbazine 100 mg inj		N1		
J9140	Dacarbazine 200 MG inj		N1		
J9150	Daunorubicin injection		K2		$14.95
J9151	Daunorubicin citrate inj		K2		$55.27
J9155	Degarelix injection	NI	K2		$2.23
J9160	Denileukin diftitox inj		K2		$1,448.32
J9165	Diethylstilbestrol injection		K2		$1,257.36
J9170	Docetaxel injection	CH	D5		
J9171	Docetaxel injection	NI	K2		$16.95
J9175	Elliotts b solution per ml		N1		
J9178	Inj, epirubicin hcl, 2 mg		K2		$2.55
J9181	Etoposide injection		N1		
J9185	Fludarabine phosphate inj		K2		$151.36
J9190	Fluorouracil injection		N1		
J9200	Floxuridine injection		K2		$46.60
J9201	Gemcitabine hcl injection		K2		$139.10
J9202	Goserelin acetate implant		K2		$193.02

HCPCS Code	HCPCS Descriptor	CY 2010 Comment Indicator	CY 2010 Payment Indicator	CY 2010 Third Year Pymt. Weight	CY 2010 Third Year Transition Weight
J9206	Irinotecan injection		K2		$13.18
J9207	Ixabepilone injection		K2		$63.74
J9208	Ifosfomide injection		K2		$29.39
J9209	Mesna injection		K2		$4.34
J9211	Idarubicin hcl injection		K2		$96.70
J9212	Interferon alfacon-1 inj	CH	K2		$6.75
J9213	Interferon alfa-2a inj		K2		$10.60
J9214	Interferon alfa-2b inj		K2		$15.54
J9215	Interferon alfa-n3 inj		K2		$17.89
J9216	Interferon gamma 1-b inj		K2		$294.03
J9217	Leuprolide acetate suspnsion		K2		$210.52
J9218	Leuprolide acetate injeciton		K2		$5.29
J9219	Leuprolide acetate implant		K2		$4,728.88
J9225	Vantas implant		K2		$1,473.60
J9226	Supprelin LA implant		K2		$14,875.43
J9230	Mechlorethamine hcl inj		K2		$144.56
J9245	Inj melphalan hydrochl 50 MG		K2		$1,622.81
J9250	Methotrexate sodium inj		N1		
J9260	Methotrexate sodium inj		N1		
J9261	Nelarabine injection		K2		$101.28
J9263	Oxaliplatin		K2		$9.55
J9264	Paclitaxel protein bound		K2		$9.09
J9265	Paclitaxel injection	CH	N1		
J9266	Pegaspargase injection		K2		$2,695.67
J9268	Pentostatin injection		K2		$1,399.56
J9270	Plicamycin (mithramycin) inj	CH	N1		
J9280	Mitomycin 5 MG inj		K2		$17.74
J9290	Mitomycin 20 MG inj		K2		$70.98
J9291	Mitomycin 40 MG inj		K2		$141.95
J9293	Mitoxantrone hydrochl / 5 MG		K2		$65.51
J9300	Gemtuzumab ozogamicin inj		K2		$2,572.82
J9303	Panitumumab injection		K2		$85.21
J9305	Pemetrexed injection		K2		$48.50
J9310	Rituximab injection		K2		$552.70
J9320	Streptozocin injection		K2		$278.35
J9328	Temozolomide injection	NI	K2		$4.90
J9330	Temsirolimus injection		K2		$47.93
J9340	Thiotepa injection		K2		$97.69
J9350	Topotecan injection		K2		$988.88
J9355	Trastuzumab injection		K2		$63.51
J9357	Valrubicin injection		K2		$953.16
J9360	Vinblastine sulfate inj		N1		
J9370	Vincristine sulfate 1 MG inj		N1		
J9375	Vincristine sulfate 2 MG inj		N1		
J9380	Vincristine sulfate 5 MG inj		N1		
J9390	Vinorelbine tartrate inj	CH	N1		
J9395	Injection, Fulvestrant		K2		$80.63
J9600	Porfimer sodium injection		K2		$2,745.46
J9999	Chemotherapy drug		N1		
L8600	Implant breast silicone/eq		N1		
L8603	Collagen imp urinary 2.5 ml		N1		
L8604	Dextranomer/hyaluronic acid		N1		

HCPCS Code	HCPCS Descriptor	CY 2010 Comment Indicator	CY 2010 Payment Indicator	CY 2010 Third Year Pymt. Weight	CY 2010 Third Year TransitionWeight
L8606	Synthetic implnt urinary 1ml		N1		
L8609	Artificial cornea		N1		
L8610	Ocular implant		N1		
L8612	Aqueous shunt prosthesis		N1		
L8613	Ossicular implant		N1		
L8614	Cochlear device		N1		
L8630	Metacarpophalangeal implant		N1		
L8631	MCP joint repl 2 pc or more		N1		
L8641	Metatarsal joint implant		N1		
L8642	Hallux implant		N1		
L8658	Interphalangeal joint spacer		N1		
L8659	Interphalangeal joint repl		N1		
L8670	Vascular graft, synthetic		N1		
L8682	Implt neurostim radiofq rec		N1		
L8690	Aud osseo dev, int/ext comp		N1		
L8699	Prosthetic implant NOS		N1		
P9041	Albumin (human),5%, 50ml		K2		$16.89
P9045	Albumin (human), 5%, 250 ml		K2		$60.58
P9046	Albumin (human), 25%, 20 ml		K2		$25.67
P9047	Albumin (human), 25%, 50ml		K2		$62.05
Q0138	Ferumoxytol, non-esrd	NI	K2		$0.82
Q0163	Diphenhydramine HCl 50mg		N1		
Q0164	Prochlorperazine maleate 5mg		N1		
Q0166	Granisetron hcl 1 mg oral	CH	N1		
Q0167	Dronabinol 2.5mg oral		N1		
Q0169	Promethazine HCl 12.5mg oral		N1		
Q0171	Chlorpromazine HCl 10mg oral		N1		
Q0173	Trimethobenzamide HCl 250mg		N1		
Q0174	Thiethylperazine maleate10mg		N1		
Q0175	Perphenazine 4mg oral		N1		
Q0177	Hydroxyzine pamoate 25mg		N1		
Q0179	Ondansetron hcl 8 mg oral	CH	N1		
Q0180	Dolasetron mesylate oral	CH	N1		
Q0515	Sermorelin acetate injection		K2		$1.77
Q1003	Ntiol category 3		L6		$50.00
Q2004	Bladder calculi irrig sol	CH	K2		$29.28
Q2009	Fosphenytoin inj PE		N1		
Q2017	Teniposide, 50 mg		K2		$319.43
Q2023	Xyntha, inj	CH	D5		
Q2024	Bevacizumab injection	CH	D5		
Q3025	IM inj interferon beta 1-a		K2		$187.24
Q4100	Skin substitute, NOS		N1		
Q4101	Apligraf skin sub		K2		$32.16
Q4102	Oasis wound matrix skin sub		K2		$4.12
Q4103	Oasis burn matrix skin sub		K2		$4.12
Q4104	Integra BMWD skin sub		K2		$11.77
Q4105	Integra DRT skin sub		K2		$11.77
Q4106	Dermagraft skin sub		K2		$39.25
Q4107	Graftjacket skin sub		K2		$89.23
Q4108	Integra matrix skin sub		K2		$17.98
Q4109	Tissuemend skin sub		N1		
Q4110	Primatrix skin sub		K2		$33.99

HCPCS Code	HCPCS Descriptor	CY 2010 Comment Indicator	CY 2010 Payment Indicator	CY 2010 Third Year Pymt. Weight	CY 2010 Third Year TransitionWeight
Q4111	Gammagraft skin sub		K2		$7.13
Q4112	Cymetra allograft		K2		$327.47
Q4113	Graftjacket express allograf		K2		$327.47
Q4114	Integra flowable wound matri		K2		$907.36
Q4115	Alloskin skin sub		K2		$9.36
Q4116	Alloderm skin sub		K2		$31.72
Q9951	LOCM >= 400 mg/ml iodine,1ml		N1		
Q9953	Inj Fe-based MR contrast,1ml		N1		
Q9954	Oral MR contrast, 100 ml		N1		
Q9955	Inj perflexane lip micros,ml		N1		
Q9956	Inj octafluoropropane mic,ml		N1		
Q9957	Inj perflutren lip micros,ml		N1		
Q9958	HOCM <=149 mg/ml iodine, 1ml		N1		
Q9959	HOCM 150-199mg/ml iodine,1ml		N1		
Q9960	HOCM 200-249mg/ml iodine,1ml		N1		
Q9961	HOCM 250-299mg/ml iodine,1ml		N1		
Q9962	HOCM 300-349mg/ml iodine,1ml		N1		
Q9963	HOCM 350-399mg/ml iodine,1ml		N1		
Q9964	HOCM>= 400mg/ml iodine, 1ml		N1		
Q9965	LOCM 100-199mg/ml iodine,1ml		N1		
Q9966	LOCM 200-299mg/ml iodine,1ml		N1		
Q9967	LOCM 300-399mg/ml iodine,1ml		N1		
Q9968	Visualization adjunct	NI	K2		$4.11
V2630	Anter chamber intraocul lens		N1		
V2631	Iris support intraoclr lens		N1		
V2632	Post chmbr intraocular lens		N1		
V2785	Corneal tissue processing		F4		
V2790	Amniotic membrane		N1		

Addendum DD-1
ASC Payment Indicators for CY 2010

Indicator	**Payment Indicator Definition**
A2	Surgical procedure on ASC list in CY 2007; payment based on OPPS relative payment weight.
D5	Deleted/discontinued code; no payment made.
F4	Corneal tissue acquisition, hepatitis B vaccine; paid at reasonable cost.
G2	Non office-based surgical procedure added in CY 2008 or later; payment based on OPPS relative payment weight.
H2	Brachytherapy source paid separately when provided integral to a surgical procedure on ASC list; payment based on OPPS rate.
H8	Device-intensive procedure on ASC list in CY 2007; paid at adjusted rate.
J7	OPPS pass-through device paid separately when provided integral to a surgical procedure on ASC list; payment contractor-priced.
J8	Device-intensive procedure added to ASC list in CY 2008 or later; paid at adjusted rate.
K2	Drugs and biologicals paid separately when provided integral to a surgical procedure on ASC list; payment based on OPPS rate.
K7	Unclassified drugs and biologicals; payment contractor-priced.
L1	Influenza vaccine; pneumococcal vaccine. Packaged item/service; no separate payment made.
L6	New Technology Intraocular Lens (NTIOL); special payment.
N1	Packaged service/item; no separate payment made.
P2	Office-based surgical procedure added to ASC list in CY 2008 or later with MPFS nonfacility PE RVUs; payment based on OPPS relative payment weight.
P3	Office-based surgical procedure added to ASC list in CY 2008 or later with MPFS nonfacility PE RVUs; payment based on MPFS nonfacility PE RVUs.
R2	Office-based surgical procedure added to ASC list in CY 2008 or later without MPFS nonfacility PE RVUs; payment based on OPPS relative payment weight.
Z2	Radiology service paid separately when provided integral to a surgical procedure on ASC list; payment based on OPPS relative payment weight.
Z3	Radiology service paid separately when provided integral to a surgical procedure on ASC list; payment based on MPFS nonfacility PE RVUs.

Addendum DD-2
Final ASC Comment Indicators for CY 2010

<u>CI</u>   <u>Comment Indicator Meanings</u>

CH   Active HCPCS code in current year and next calendar year, payment indicator assignment has changed; or active HCPCS code that is newly recognized as payable in ASC; or
active HCPCS code that is discontinued at the end of the current calendar year.

NI   New code for the next calendar year or existing code with substantial revision to its code
descriptor in the next calendar year, interim payment indicator assignment; comments
will be accepted on the interim payment indicator for the new code.

Addendum EE
Final ASC Surgical Procedures Excluded from Payment in ASCs for CY 2010

HCPCS Code	Short Description	HCPCS Code	Short Description
11004	Debride genitalia & perineum	21049	Excis uppr jaw cyst w/repair
11005	Debride abdom wall	21089	Prepare face/oral prosthesis
11006	Debride genit/per/abdom wall	21141	Reconstruct midface, lefort
11008	Remove mesh from abd wall	21142	Reconstruct midface, lefort
11975	Insert contraceptive cap	21143	Reconstruct midface, lefort
11977	Removal/reinsert contra cap	21145	Reconstruct midface, lefort
15756	Free myo/skin flap microvasc	21146	Reconstruct midface, lefort
15757	Free skin flap, microvasc	21147	Reconstruct midface, lefort
15758	Free fascial flap, microvasc	21151	Reconstruct midface, lefort
15999	Removal of pressure sore	21154	Reconstruct midface, lefort
16036	Escharotomy; add'l incision	21155	Reconstruct midface, lefort
17999	Skin tissue procedure	21159	Reconstruct midface, lefort
19260	Removal of chest wall lesion	21160	Reconstruct midface, lefort
19271	Revision of chest wall	21172	Reconstruct orbit/forehead
19272	Extensive chest wall surgery	21175	Reconstruct orbit/forehead
19305	Mast, radical	21179	Reconstruct entire forehead
19306	Mast, rad, urban type	21180	Reconstruct entire forehead
19307	Mast, mod rad	21182	Reconstruct cranial bone
19361	Breast reconstr w/lat flap	21183	Reconstruct cranial bone
19364	Breast reconstruction	21184	Reconstruct cranial bone
19367	Breast reconstruction	21188	Reconstruction of midface
19368	Breast reconstruction	21193	Reconst lwr jaw w/o graft
19369	Breast reconstruction	21194	Reconst lwr jaw w/graft
19499	Breast surgery procedure	21195	Reconst lwr jaw w/o fixation
20100	Explore wound, neck	21196	Reconst lwr jaw w/fixation
20101	Explore wound, chest	21247	Reconstruct lower jaw bone
20102	Explore wound, abdomen	21255	Reconstruct lower jaw bone
20660	Apply, rem fixation device	21256	Reconstruction of orbit
20661	Application of head brace	21261	Revise eye sockets
20664	Halo brace application	21263	Revise eye sockets
20802	Replantation, arm, complete	21268	Revise eye sockets
20805	Replant forearm, complete	21299	Cranio/maxillofacial surgery
20808	Replantation hand, complete	21343	Treatment of sinus fracture
20816	Replantation digit, complete	21344	Treatment of sinus fracture
20824	Replantation thumb, complete	21346	Treat nose/jaw fracture
20827	Replantation thumb, complete	21347	Treat nose/jaw fracture
20838	Replantation foot, complete	21348	Treat nose/jaw fracture
20930	Sp bone algrft morsel add-on	21365	Treat cheek bone fracture
20931	Sp bone algrft struct add-on	21366	Treat cheek bone fracture
20936	Sp bone agrft local add-on	21385	Treat eye socket fracture
20937	Sp bone agrft morsel add-on	21386	Treat eye socket fracture
20938	Sp bone agrft struct add-on	21387	Treat eye socket fracture
20955	Fibula bone graft, microvasc	21395	Treat eye socket fracture
20956	Iliac bone graft, microvasc	21408	Treat eye socket fracture
20957	Mt bone graft, microvasc	21422	Treat mouth roof fracture
20962	Other bone graft, microvasc	21423	Treat mouth roof fracture
20969	Bone/skin graft, microvasc	21431	Treat craniofacial fracture
20970	Bone/skin graft, iliac crest	21432	Treat craniofacial fracture
20999	Musculoskeletal surgery	21433	Treat craniofacial fracture
21045	Extensive jaw surgery	21435	Treat craniofacial fracture

HCPCS Code	Short Description	HCPCS Code	Short Description
21436	Treat craniofacial fracture	22610	Thorax spine fusion
21470	Treat lower jaw fracture	22612	Lumbar spine fusion
21499	Head surgery procedure	22614	Spine fusion, extra segment
21510	Drainage of bone lesion	22630	Lumbar spine fusion
21615	Removal of rib	22632	Spine fusion, extra segment
21616	Removal of rib and nerves	22800	Fusion of spine
21620	Partial removal of sternum	22802	Fusion of spine
21627	Sternal debridement	22804	Fusion of spine
21630	Extensive sternum surgery	22808	Fusion of spine
21632	Extensive sternum surgery	22810	Fusion of spine
21705	Revision of neck muscle/rib	22812	Fusion of spine
21740	Reconstruction of sternum	22818	Kyphectomy, 1-2 segments
21742	Repair stern/nuss w/o scope	22819	Kyphectomy, 3 or more
21743	Repair sternum/nuss w/scope	22830	Exploration of spinal fusion
21750	Repair of sternum separation	22840	Insert spine fixation device
21810	Treatment of rib fracture(s)	22841	Insert spine fixation device
21825	Treat sternum fracture	22842	Insert spine fixation device
21899	Neck/chest surgery procedure	22843	Insert spine fixation device
22010	I&d, p-spine, c/t/cerv-thor	22844	Insert spine fixation device
22015	I&d, p-spine, l/s/ls	22845	Insert spine fixation device
22100	Remove part of neck vertebra	22846	Insert spine fixation device
22101	Remove part, thorax vertebra	22847	Insert spine fixation device
22110	Remove part of neck vertebra	22848	Insert pelv fixation device
22112	Remove part, thorax vertebra	22849	Reinsert spinal fixation
22114	Remove part, lumbar vertebra	22850	Remove spine fixation device
22116	Remove extra spine segment	22851	Apply spine prosth device
22206	Cut spine 3 col, thor	22852	Remove spine fixation device
22207	Cut spine 3 col, lumb	22855	Remove spine fixation device
22208	Cut spine 3 col, addl seg	22856	Cerv artific diskectomy
22210	Revision of neck spine	22857	Lumbar artif diskectomy
22212	Revision of thorax spine	22861	Revise cerv artific disc
22214	Revision of lumbar spine	22862	Revise lumbar artif disc
22216	Revise, extra spine segment	22864	Remove cerv artif disc
22220	Revision of neck spine	22865	Remove lumb artif disc
22222	Revision of thorax spine	22899	Spine surgery procedure
22224	Revision of lumbar spine	22999	Abdomen surgery procedure
22226	Revise, extra spine segment	23200	Removal of collar bone
22318	Treat odontoid fx w/o graft	23210	Removal of shoulder blade
22319	Treat odontoid fx w/graft	23220	Partial removal of humerus
22325	Treat spine fracture	23332	Remove shoulder foreign body
22326	Treat neck spine fracture	23470	Reconstruct shoulder joint
22327	Treat thorax spine fracture	23472	Reconstruct shoulder joint
22328	Treat each add spine fx	23900	Amputation of arm & girdle
22526	Idet, single level	23920	Amputation at shoulder joint
22527	Idet, 1 or more levels	23929	Shoulder surgery procedure
22532	Lat thorax spine fusion	24150	Extensive humerus surgery
22533	Lat lumbar spine fusion	24900	Amputation of upper arm
22534	Lat thor/lumb, add'l seg	24920	Amputation of upper arm
22548	Neck spine fusion	24930	Amputation follow-up surgery
22554	Neck spine fusion	24931	Amputate upper arm & implant
22556	Thorax spine fusion	24935	Revision of amputation
22558	Lumbar spine fusion	24940	Revision of upper arm
22585	Additional spinal fusion	24999	Upper arm/elbow surgery
22590	Spine & skull spinal fusion	25170	Extensive forearm surgery
22595	Neck spinal fusion	25900	Amputation of forearm
22600	Neck spine fusion	25905	Amputation of forearm

HCPCS Code	Short Description	HCPCS Code	Short Description
25909	Amputation follow-up surgery	27218	Treat pelvic ring fracture
25915	Amputation of forearm	27222	Treat hip socket fracture
25920	Amputate hand at wrist	27226	Treat hip wall fracture
25924	Amputation follow-up surgery	27227	Treat hip fracture(s)
25927	Amputation of hand	27228	Treat hip fracture(s)
25999	Forearm or wrist surgery	27232	Treat thigh fracture
26551	Great toe-hand transfer	27235	Treat thigh fracture
26553	Single transfer, toe-hand	27236	Treat thigh fracture
26554	Double transfer, toe-hand	27240	Treat thigh fracture
26556	Toe joint transfer	27244	Treat thigh fracture
26989	Hand/finger surgery	27245	Treat thigh fracture
26992	Drainage of bone lesion	27248	Treat thigh fracture
27005	Incision of hip tendon	27253	Treat hip dislocation
27006	Incision of hip tendons	27254	Treat hip dislocation
27025	Incision of hip/thigh fascia	27258	Treat hip dislocation
27027	Buttock fasciotomy	27259	Treat hip dislocation
27030	Drainage of hip joint	27268	Cltx thigh fx w/mnpj
27036	Excision of hip joint/muscle	27269	Optx thigh fx
27054	Removal of hip joint lining	27280	Fusion of sacroiliac joint
27057	Buttock fasciotomy w/dbrdmt	27282	Fusion of pubic bones
27070	Partial removal of hip bone	27284	Fusion of hip joint
27071	Partial removal of hip bone	27286	Fusion of hip joint
27075	Extensive hip surgery	27290	Amputation of leg at hip
27076	Extensive hip surgery	27295	Amputation of leg at hip
27077	Extensive hip surgery	27299	Pelvis/hip joint surgery
27078	Extensive hip surgery	27303	Drainage of bone lesion
27090	Removal of hip prosthesis	27365	Extensive leg surgery
27091	Removal of hip prosthesis	27412	Autochondrocyte implant knee
27120	Reconstruction of hip socket	27415	Osteochondral knee allograft
27122	Reconstruction of hip socket	27445	Revision of knee joint
27125	Partial hip replacement	27447	Total knee arthroplasty
27130	Total hip arthroplasty	27448	Incision of thigh
27132	Total hip arthroplasty	27450	Incision of thigh
27134	Revise hip joint replacement	27454	Realignment of thigh bone
27137	Revise hip joint replacement	27455	Realignment of knee
27138	Revise hip joint replacement	27457	Realignment of knee
27140	Transplant femur ridge	27465	Shortening of thigh bone
27146	Incision of hip bone	27466	Lengthening of thigh bone
27147	Revision of hip bone	27468	Shorten/lengthen thighs
27151	Incision of hip bones	27470	Repair of thigh
27156	Revision of hip bones	27472	Repair/graft of thigh
27158	Revision of pelvis	27477	Surgery to stop leg growth
27161	Incision of neck of femur	27485	Surgery to stop leg growth
27165	Incision/fixation of femur	27486	Revise/replace knee joint
27170	Repair/graft femur head/neck	27487	Revise/replace knee joint
27175	Treat slipped epiphysis	27488	Removal of knee prosthesis
27176	Treat slipped epiphysis	27495	Reinforce thigh
27177	Treat slipped epiphysis	27506	Treatment of thigh fracture
27178	Treat slipped epiphysis	27507	Treatment of thigh fracture
27179	Revise head/neck of femur	27511	Treatment of thigh fracture
27181	Treat slipped epiphysis	27513	Treatment of thigh fracture
27185	Revision of femur epiphysis	27514	Treatment of thigh fracture
27187	Reinforce hip bones	27519	Treat thigh fx growth plate
27215	Treat pelvic fracture(s)	27524	Treat kneecap fracture
27216	Treat pelvic ring fracture	27535	Treat knee fracture
27217	Treat pelvic ring fracture	27536	Treat knee fracture

HCPCS Code	Short Description	HCPCS Code	Short Description
27540	Treat knee fracture	31599	Larynx surgery procedure
27556	Treat knee dislocation	31600	Incision of windpipe
27557	Treat knee dislocation	31601	Incision of windpipe
27558	Treat knee dislocation	31610	Incision of windpipe
27580	Fusion of knee	31725	Clearance of airways
27590	Amputate leg at thigh	31760	Repair of windpipe
27591	Amputate leg at thigh	31766	Reconstruction of windpipe
27592	Amputate leg at thigh	31770	Repair/graft of bronchus
27596	Amputation follow-up surgery	31775	Reconstruct bronchus
27598	Amputate lower leg at knee	31780	Reconstruct windpipe
27599	Leg surgery procedure	31781	Reconstruct windpipe
27645	Extensive lower leg surgery	31785	Remove windpipe lesion
27646	Extensive lower leg surgery	31786	Remove windpipe lesion
27702	Reconstruct ankle joint	31800	Repair of windpipe injury
27703	Reconstruction, ankle joint	31805	Repair of windpipe injury
27712	Realignment of lower leg	31899	Airways surgical procedure
27715	Revision of lower leg	32035	Exploration of chest
27722	Repair/graft of tibia	32036	Exploration of chest
27724	Repair/graft of tibia	32095	Biopsy through chest wall
27725	Repair of lower leg	32100	Exploration/biopsy of chest
27727	Repair of lower leg	32110	Explore/repair chest
27880	Amputation of lower leg	32120	Re-exploration of chest
27881	Amputation of lower leg	32124	Explore chest free adhesions
27882	Amputation of lower leg	32140	Removal of lung lesion(s)
27886	Amputation follow-up surgery	32141	Remove/treat lung lesions
27888	Amputation of foot at ankle	32150	Removal of lung lesion(s)
27899	Leg/ankle surgery procedure	32151	Remove lung foreign body
28360	Reconstruct cleft foot	32160	Open chest heart massage
28800	Amputation of midfoot	32200	Drain, open, lung lesion
28805	Amputation thru metatarsal	32201	Drain, percut, lung lesion
28899	Foot/toes surgery procedure	32215	Treat chest lining
29799	Casting/strapping procedure	32220	Release of lung
29867	Allgrft implnt, knee w/scope	32225	Partial release of lung
29868	Meniscal trnspl, knee w/scpe	32310	Removal of chest lining
29999	Arthroscopy of joint	32320	Free/remove chest lining
30999	Nasal surgery procedure	32402	Open biopsy chest lining
31225	Removal of upper jaw	32440	Removal of lung
31230	Removal of upper jaw	32442	Sleeve pneumonectomy
31290	Nasal/sinus endoscopy, surg	32445	Removal of lung
31291	Nasal/sinus endoscopy, surg	32480	Partial removal of lung
31292	Nasal/sinus endoscopy, surg	32482	Bilobectomy
31293	Nasal/sinus endoscopy, surg	32484	Segmentectomy
31294	Nasal/sinus endoscopy, surg	32486	Sleeve lobectomy
31299	Sinus surgery procedure	32488	Completion pneumonectomy
31360	Removal of larynx	32491	Lung volume reduction
31365	Removal of larynx	32500	Partial removal of lung
31367	Partial removal of larynx	32501	Repair bronchus add-on
31368	Partial removal of larynx	32503	Resect apical lung tumor
31370	Partial removal of larynx	32504	Resect apical lung tum/chest
31375	Partial removal of larynx	32540	Removal of lung lesion
31380	Partial removal of larynx	32551	Insertion of chest tube
31382	Partial removal of larynx	32560	Treat lung lining chemically
31390	Removal of larynx & pharynx	32561	Lyse chest fibrin init day
31395	Reconstruct larynx & pharynx	32562	Lyse chest fibrin subq day
31584	Treat larynx fracture	32601	Thoracoscopy, diagnostic
31587	Revision of larynx	32602	Thoracoscopy, diagnostic

HCPCS Code	Short Description	HCPCS Code	Short Description
32603	Thoracoscopy, diagnostic	33254	Ablate atria, lmtd
32604	Thoracoscopy, diagnostic	33255	Ablate atria w/o bypass, ext
32605	Thoracoscopy, diagnostic	33256	Ablate atria w/bypass, exten
32606	Thoracoscopy, diagnostic	33257	Ablate atria, lmtd, add-on
32650	Thoracoscopy, surgical	33258	Ablate atria, x10sv, add-on
32651	Thoracoscopy, surgical	33259	Ablate atria w/bypass add-on
32652	Thoracoscopy, surgical	33261	Ablate heart dysrhythm focus
32653	Thoracoscopy, surgical	33265	Ablate atria, lmtd, endo
32654	Thoracoscopy, surgical	33266	Ablate atria, x10sv, endo
32655	Thoracoscopy, surgical	33300	Repair of heart wound
32656	Thoracoscopy, surgical	33305	Repair of heart wound
32657	Thoracoscopy, surgical	33310	Exploratory heart surgery
32658	Thoracoscopy, surgical	33315	Exploratory heart surgery
32659	Thoracoscopy, surgical	33320	Repair major blood vessel(s)
32660	Thoracoscopy, surgical	33321	Repair major vessel
32661	Thoracoscopy, surgical	33322	Repair major blood vessel(s)
32662	Thoracoscopy, surgical	33330	Insert major vessel graft
32663	Thoracoscopy, surgical	33332	Insert major vessel graft
32664	Thoracoscopy, surgical	33335	Insert major vessel graft
32665	Thoracoscopy, surgical	33400	Repair of aortic valve
32800	Repair lung hernia	33401	Valvuloplasty, open
32810	Close chest after drainage	33403	Valvuloplasty, w/cp bypass
32815	Close bronchial fistula	33404	Prepare heart-aorta conduit
32820	Reconstruct injured chest	33405	Replacement of aortic valve
32850	Donor pneumonectomy	33406	Replacement of aortic valve
32851	Lung transplant, single	33410	Replacement of aortic valve
32852	Lung transplant with bypass	33411	Replacement of aortic valve
32853	Lung transplant, double	33412	Replacement of aortic valve
32854	Lung transplant with bypass	33413	Replacement of aortic valve
32855	Prepare donor lung, single	33414	Repair of aortic valve
32856	Prepare donor lung, double	33415	Revision, subvalvular tissue
32900	Removal of rib(s)	33416	Revise ventricle muscle
32905	Revise & repair chest wall	33417	Repair of aortic valve
32906	Revise & repair chest wall	33420	Revision of mitral valve
32940	Revision of lung	33422	Revision of mitral valve
32997	Total lung lavage	33425	Repair of mitral valve
32999	Chest surgery procedure	33426	Repair of mitral valve
33015	Incision of heart sac	33427	Repair of mitral valve
33020	Incision of heart sac	33430	Replacement of mitral valve
33025	Incision of heart sac	33460	Revision of tricuspid valve
33030	Partial removal of heart sac	33463	Valvuloplasty, tricuspid
33031	Partial removal of heart sac	33464	Valvuloplasty, tricuspid
33050	Removal of heart sac lesion	33465	Replace tricuspid valve
33120	Removal of heart lesion	33468	Revision of tricuspid valve
33130	Removal of heart lesion	33470	Revision of pulmonary valve
33140	Heart revascularize (tmr)	33471	Valvotomy, pulmonary valve
33141	Heart tmr w/other procedure	33472	Revision of pulmonary valve
33202	Insert epicard eltrd, open	33474	Revision of pulmonary valve
33203	Insert epicard eltrd, endo	33475	Replacement, pulmonary valve
33236	Remove electrode/thoracotomy	33476	Revision of heart chamber
33237	Remove electrode/thoracotomy	33478	Revision of heart chamber
33238	Remove electrode/thoracotomy	33496	Repair, prosth valve clot
33243	Remove eltrd/thoracotomy	33500	Repair heart vessel fistula
33244	Remove eltrd, transven	33501	Repair heart vessel fistula
33250	Ablate heart dysrhythm focus	33502	Coronary artery correction
33251	Ablate heart dysrhythm focus	33503	Coronary artery graft

HCPCS Code	Short Description	HCPCS Code	Short Description
33504	Coronary artery graft	33726	Repair pul venous stenosis
33505	Repair artery w/tunnel	33730	Repair heart-vein defect(s)
33506	Repair artery, translocation	33732	Repair heart-vein defect
33507	Repair art, intramural	33735	Revision of heart chamber
33510	Cabg, vein, single	33736	Revision of heart chamber
33511	Cabg, vein, two	33737	Revision of heart chamber
33512	Cabg, vein, three	33750	Major vessel shunt
33513	Cabg, vein, four	33755	Major vessel shunt
33514	Cabg, vein, five	33762	Major vessel shunt
33516	Cabg, vein, six or more	33764	Major vessel shunt & graft
33517	Cabg, artery-vein, single	33766	Major vessel shunt
33518	Cabg, artery-vein, two	33767	Major vessel shunt
33519	Cabg, artery-vein, three	33768	Cavopulmonary shunting
33521	Cabg, artery-vein, four	33770	Repair great vessels defect
33522	Cabg, artery-vein, five	33771	Repair great vessels defect
33523	Cabg, art-vein, six or more	33774	Repair great vessels defect
33530	Coronary artery, bypass/reop	33775	Repair great vessels defect
33533	Cabg, arterial, single	33776	Repair great vessels defect
33534	Cabg, arterial, two	33777	Repair great vessels defect
33535	Cabg, arterial, three	33778	Repair great vessels defect
33536	Cabg, arterial, four or more	33779	Repair great vessels defect
33542	Removal of heart lesion	33780	Repair great vessels defect
33545	Repair of heart damage	33781	Repair great vessels defect
33548	Restore/remodel, ventricle	33782	Nikaidoh proc
33572	Open coronary endarterectomy	33783	Nikaidoh proc w/ostia implt
33600	Closure of valve	33786	Repair arterial trunk
33602	Closure of valve	33788	Revision of pulmonary artery
33606	Anastomosis/artery-aorta	33800	Aortic suspension
33608	Repair anomaly w/conduit	33802	Repair vessel defect
33610	Repair by enlargement	33803	Repair vessel defect
33611	Repair double ventricle	33813	Repair septal defect
33612	Repair double ventricle	33814	Repair septal defect
33615	Repair, modified fontan	33820	Revise major vessel
33617	Repair single ventricle	33822	Revise major vessel
33619	Repair single ventricle	33824	Revise major vessel
33641	Repair heart septum defect	33840	Remove aorta constriction
33645	Revision of heart veins	33845	Remove aorta constriction
33647	Repair heart septum defects	33851	Remove aorta constriction
33660	Repair of heart defects	33852	Repair septal defect
33665	Repair of heart defects	33853	Repair septal defect
33670	Repair of heart chambers	33860	Ascending aortic graft
33675	Close mult vsd	33861	Ascending aortic graft
33676	Close mult vsd w/resection	33863	Ascending aortic graft
33677	Cl mult vsd w/rem pul band	33864	Ascending aortic graft
33681	Repair heart septum defect	33870	Transverse aortic arch graft
33684	Repair heart septum defect	33875	Thoracic aortic graft
33688	Repair heart septum defect	33877	Thoracoabdominal graft
33690	Reinforce pulmonary artery	33880	Endovasc taa repr incl subcl
33692	Repair of heart defects	33881	Endovasc taa repr w/o subcl
33694	Repair of heart defects	33883	Insert endovasc prosth, taa
33697	Repair of heart defects	33884	Endovasc prosth, taa, add-on
33702	Repair of heart defects	33886	Endovasc prosth, delayed
33710	Repair of heart defects	33889	Artery transpose/endovas taa
33720	Repair of heart defect	33891	Car-car bp grft/endovas taa
33722	Repair of heart defect	33910	Remove lung artery emboli
33724	Repair venous anomaly	33915	Remove lung artery emboli

HCPCS Code	Short Description	HCPCS Code	Short Description
33916	Surgery of great vessel	34820	Xpose for endoprosth, iliac
33917	Repair pulmonary artery	34825	Endovasc extend prosth, init
33920	Repair pulmonary atresia	34826	Endovasc exten prosth, add'l
33922	Transect pulmonary artery	34830	Open aortic tube prosth repr
33924	Remove pulmonary shunt	34831	Open aortoiliac prosth repr
33925	Rpr pul art unifocal w/o cpb	34832	Open aortofemor prosth repr
33926	Repr pul art, unifocal w/cpb	34833	Xpose for endoprosth, iliac
33930	Removal of donor heart/lung	34834	Xpose, endoprosth, brachial
33933	Prepare donor heart/lung	34900	Endovasc iliac repr w/graft
33935	Transplantation, heart/lung	35001	Repair defect of artery
33940	Removal of donor heart	35002	Repair artery rupture, neck
33944	Prepare donor heart	35005	Repair defect of artery
33945	Transplantation of heart	35011	Repair defect of artery
33960	External circulation assist	35013	Repair artery rupture, arm
33961	External circulation assist	35021	Repair defect of artery
33967	Insert ia percut device	35022	Repair artery rupture, chest
33968	Remove aortic assist device	35045	Repair defect of arm artery
33970	Aortic circulation assist	35081	Repair defect of artery
33971	Aortic circulation assist	35082	Repair artery rupture, aorta
33973	Insert balloon device	35091	Repair defect of artery
33974	Remove intra-aortic balloon	35092	Repair artery rupture, aorta
33975	Implant ventricular device	35102	Repair defect of artery
33976	Implant ventricular device	35103	Repair artery rupture, groin
33977	Remove ventricular device	35111	Repair defect of artery
33978	Remove ventricular device	35112	Repair artery rupture,spleen
33979	Insert intracorporeal device	35121	Repair defect of artery
33980	Remove intracorporeal device	35122	Repair artery rupture, belly
33981	Replace vad pump ext	35131	Repair defect of artery
33982	Replace vad intra w/o bp	35132	Repair artery rupture, groin
33983	Replace vad intra w/bp	35141	Repair defect of artery
33999	Cardiac surgery procedure	35142	Repair artery rupture, thigh
34001	Removal of artery clot	35151	Repair defect of artery
34051	Removal of artery clot	35152	Repair artery rupture, knee
34101	Removal of artery clot	35180	Repair blood vessel lesion
34111	Removal of arm artery clot	35182	Repair blood vessel lesion
34151	Removal of artery clot	35184	Repair blood vessel lesion
34201	Removal of artery clot	35189	Repair blood vessel lesion
34203	Removal of leg artery clot	35190	Repair blood vessel lesion
34401	Removal of vein clot	35201	Repair blood vessel lesion
34421	Removal of vein clot	35206	Repair blood vessel lesion
34451	Removal of vein clot	35211	Repair blood vessel lesion
34471	Removal of vein clot	35216	Repair blood vessel lesion
34501	Repair valve, femoral vein	35221	Repair blood vessel lesion
34502	Reconstruct vena cava	35226	Repair blood vessel lesion
34510	Transposition of vein valve	35231	Repair blood vessel lesion
34520	Cross-over vein graft	35236	Repair blood vessel lesion
34530	Leg vein fusion	35241	Repair blood vessel lesion
34800	Endovas aaa repr w/sm tube	35246	Repair blood vessel lesion
34802	Endovas aaa repr w/2-p part	35251	Repair blood vessel lesion
34803	Endovas aaa repr w/3-p part	35256	Repair blood vessel lesion
34804	Endovas aaa repr w/1-p part	35261	Repair blood vessel lesion
34805	Endovas aaa repr w/long tube	35266	Repair blood vessel lesion
34806	Aneurysm press sensor add-on	35271	Repair blood vessel lesion
34808	Endovas iliac a device addon	35276	Repair blood vessel lesion
34812	Xpose for endoprosth, femorl	35281	Repair blood vessel lesion
34813	Femoral endovas graft add-on	35286	Repair blood vessel lesion

HCPCS Code	Short Description	HCPCS Code	Short Description
35301	Rechanneling of artery	35533	Artery bypass graft
35302	Rechanneling of artery	35535	Artery bypass graft
35303	Rechanneling of artery	35536	Artery bypass graft
35304	Rechanneling of artery	35537	Artery bypass graft
35305	Rechanneling of artery	35538	Artery bypass graft
35306	Rechanneling of artery	35539	Artery bypass graft
35311	Rechanneling of artery	35540	Artery bypass graft
35321	Rechanneling of artery	35548	Artery bypass graft
35331	Rechanneling of artery	35549	Artery bypass graft
35341	Rechanneling of artery	35551	Artery bypass graft
35351	Rechanneling of artery	35556	Artery bypass graft
35355	Rechanneling of artery	35558	Artery bypass graft
35361	Rechanneling of artery	35560	Artery bypass graft
35363	Rechanneling of artery	35563	Artery bypass graft
35371	Rechanneling of artery	35565	Artery bypass graft
35372	Rechanneling of artery	35566	Artery bypass graft
35390	Reoperation, carotid add-on	35570	Artery bypass graft
35400	Angioscopy	35571	Artery bypass graft
35450	Repair arterial blockage	35583	Vein bypass graft
35452	Repair arterial blockage	35585	Vein bypass graft
35454	Repair arterial blockage	35587	Vein bypass graft
35456	Repair arterial blockage	35600	Harvest art for cabg add-on
35458	Repair arterial blockage	35601	Artery bypass graft
35459	Repair arterial blockage	35606	Artery bypass graft
35470	Repair arterial blockage	35612	Artery bypass graft
35471	Repair arterial blockage	35616	Artery bypass graft
35472	Repair arterial blockage	35621	Artery bypass graft
35474	Repair arterial blockage	35623	Bypass graft, not vein
35480	Atherectomy, open	35626	Artery bypass graft
35481	Atherectomy, open	35631	Artery bypass graft
35482	Atherectomy, open	35632	Artery bypass graft
35483	Atherectomy, open	35633	Artery bypass graft
35484	Atherectomy, open	35634	Artery bypass graft
35485	Atherectomy, open	35636	Artery bypass graft
35490	Atherectomy, percutaneous	35637	Artery bypass graft
35491	Atherectomy, percutaneous	35638	Artery bypass graft
35493	Atherectomy, percutaneous	35642	Artery bypass graft
35494	Atherectomy, percutaneous	35645	Artery bypass graft
35495	Atherectomy, percutaneous	35646	Artery bypass graft
35500	Harvest vein for bypass	35647	Artery bypass graft
35501	Artery bypass graft	35650	Artery bypass graft
35506	Artery bypass graft	35651	Artery bypass graft
35508	Artery bypass graft	35654	Artery bypass graft
35509	Artery bypass graft	35656	Artery bypass graft
35510	Artery bypass graft	35661	Artery bypass graft
35511	Artery bypass graft	35663	Artery bypass graft
35512	Artery bypass graft	35665	Artery bypass graft
35515	Artery bypass graft	35666	Artery bypass graft
35516	Artery bypass graft	35671	Artery bypass graft
35518	Artery bypass graft	35681	Composite bypass graft
35521	Artery bypass graft	35682	Composite bypass graft
35522	Artery bypass graft	35683	Composite bypass graft
35523	Artery bypass graft	35685	Bypass graft patency/patch
35525	Artery bypass graft	35686	Bypass graft/av fist patency
35526	Artery bypass graft	35691	Arterial transposition
35531	Artery bypass graft	35693	Arterial transposition

HCPCS Code	Short Description	HCPCS Code	Short Description
35694	Arterial transposition	37788	Revascularization, penis
35695	Arterial transposition	37799	Vascular surgery procedure
35697	Reimplant artery each	38100	Removal of spleen, total
35700	Reoperation, bypass graft	38101	Removal of spleen, partial
35701	Exploration, carotid artery	38102	Removal of spleen, total
35721	Exploration, femoral artery	38115	Repair of ruptured spleen
35741	Exploration popliteal artery	38120	Laparoscopy, splenectomy
35800	Explore neck vessels	38129	Laparoscope proc, spleen
35820	Explore chest vessels	38207	Cryopreserve stem cells
35840	Explore abdominal vessels	38208	Thaw preserved stem cells
35860	Explore limb vessels	38209	Wash harvest stem cells
35870	Repair vessel graft defect	38210	T-cell depletion of harvest
35879	Revise graft w/vein	38211	Tumor cell deplete of harvst
35881	Revise graft w/vein	38212	Rbc depletion of harvest
35883	Revise graft w/nonauto graft	38213	Platelet deplete of harvest
35884	Revise graft w/vein	38214	Volume deplete of harvest
35901	Excision, graft, neck	38215	Harvest stem cell concentrte
35903	Excision, graft, extremity	38240	Bone marrow/stem transplant
35905	Excision, graft, thorax	38380	Thoracic duct procedure
35907	Excision, graft, abdomen	38381	Thoracic duct procedure
36299	Vessel injection procedure	38382	Thoracic duct procedure
36460	Transfusion service, fetal	38562	Removal, pelvic lymph nodes
36660	Insertion catheter, artery	38564	Removal, abdomen lymph nodes
36822	Insertion of cannula(s)	38589	Laparoscope proc, lymphatic
36823	Insertion of cannula(s)	38720	Removal of lymph nodes, neck
36838	Dist revas ligation, hemo	38724	Removal of lymph nodes, neck
37140	Revision of circulation	38746	Remove thoracic lymph nodes
37145	Revision of circulation	38747	Remove abdominal lymph nodes
37160	Revision of circulation	38765	Remove groin lymph nodes
37180	Revision of circulation	38770	Remove pelvis lymph nodes
37181	Splice spleen/kidney veins	38780	Remove abdomen lymph nodes
37182	Insert hepatic shunt (tips)	38999	Blood/lymph system procedure
37183	Remove hepatic shunt (tips)	39000	Exploration of chest
37195	Thrombolytic therapy, stroke	39010	Exploration of chest
37201	Transcatheter therapy infuse	39200	Removal chest lesion
37202	Transcatheter therapy infuse	39220	Removal chest lesion
37204	Transcatheter occlusion	39400	Visualization of chest
37205	Transcath iv stent, percut	39499	Chest procedure
37206	Transcath iv stent/perc addl	39501	Repair diaphragm laceration
37207	Transcath iv stent, open	39502	Repair paraesophageal hernia
37208	Transcath iv stent/open addl	39503	Repair of diaphragm hernia
37209	Change iv cath at thromb tx	39520	Repair of diaphragm hernia
37210	Embolization uterine fibroid	39530	Repair of diaphragm hernia
37215	Transcath stent, cca w/eps	39531	Repair of diaphragm hernia
37216	Transcath stent, cca w/o eps	39540	Repair of diaphragm hernia
37501	Vascular endoscopy procedure	39541	Repair of diaphragm hernia
37565	Ligation of neck vein	39545	Revision of diaphragm
37600	Ligation of neck artery	39560	Resect diaphragm, simple
37605	Ligation of neck artery	39561	Resect diaphragm, complex
37606	Ligation of neck artery	39599	Diaphragm surgery procedure
37615	Ligation of neck artery	40799	Lip surgery procedure
37616	Ligation of chest artery	40899	Mouth surgery procedure
37617	Ligation of abdomen artery	41130	Partial removal of tongue
37618	Ligation of extremity artery	41135	Tongue and neck surgery
37620	Revision of major vein	41140	Removal of tongue
37660	Revision of major vein	41145	Tongue removal, neck surgery

Addendum EE

HCPCS Code	Short Description	HCPCS Code	Short Description
41150	Tongue, mouth, jaw surgery	43400	Ligate esophagus veins
41153	Tongue, mouth, neck surgery	43401	Esophagus surgery for veins
41155	Tongue, jaw, & neck surgery	43405	Ligate/staple esophagus
41599	Tongue and mouth surgery	43410	Repair esophagus wound
41899	Dental surgery procedure	43415	Repair esophagus wound
42299	Palate/uvula surgery	43420	Repair esophagus opening
42426	Excise parotid gland/lesion	43425	Repair esophagus opening
42699	Salivary surgery procedure	43460	Pressure treatment esophagus
42842	Extensive surgery of throat	43496	Free jejunum flap, microvasc
42844	Extensive surgery of throat	43499	Esophagus surgery procedure
42845	Extensive surgery of throat	43500	Surgical opening of stomach
42894	Revision of pharyngeal walls	43501	Surgical repair of stomach
42953	Repair throat, esophagus	43502	Surgical repair of stomach
42961	Control throat bleeding	43510	Surgical opening of stomach
42971	Control nose/throat bleeding	43520	Incision of pyloric muscle
42999	Throat surgery procedure	43605	Biopsy of stomach
43020	Incision of esophagus	43610	Excision of stomach lesion
43045	Incision of esophagus	43611	Excision of stomach lesion
43100	Excision of esophagus lesion	43620	Removal of stomach
43101	Excision of esophagus lesion	43621	Removal of stomach
43107	Removal of esophagus	43622	Removal of stomach
43108	Removal of esophagus	43631	Removal of stomach, partial
43112	Removal of esophagus	43632	Removal of stomach, partial
43113	Removal of esophagus	43633	Removal of stomach, partial
43116	Partial removal of esophagus	43634	Removal of stomach, partial
43117	Partial removal of esophagus	43635	Removal of stomach, partial
43118	Partial removal of esophagus	43640	Vagotomy & pylorus repair
43121	Partial removal of esophagus	43641	Vagotomy & pylorus repair
43122	Partial removal of esophagus	43644	Lap gastric bypass/roux-en-y
43123	Partial removal of esophagus	43645	Lap gastr bypass incl smll i
43124	Removal of esophagus	43647	Lap impl electrode, antrum
43135	Removal of esophagus pouch	43648	Lap revise/remv eltrd antrum
43279	Lap myotomy, heller	43651	Laparoscopy, vagus nerve
43280	Laparoscopy, fundoplasty	43652	Laparoscopy, vagus nerve
43281	Lap paraesophag hern repair	43659	Laparoscope proc, stom
43282	Lap paraesoph her rpr w/mesh	43770	Lap place gastr adj device
43289	Laparoscope proc, esoph	43771	Lap revise gastr adj device
43300	Repair of esophagus	43772	Lap rmvl gastr adj device
43305	Repair esophagus and fistula	43773	Lap replace gastr adj device
43310	Repair of esophagus	43774	Lap rmvl gastr adj all parts
43312	Repair esophagus and fistula	43775	Lap sleeve gastrectomy
43313	Esophagoplasty congenital	43800	Reconstruction of pylorus
43314	Tracheo-esophagoplasty cong	43810	Fusion of stomach and bowel
43320	Fuse esophagus & stomach	43820	Fusion of stomach and bowel
43324	Revise esophagus & stomach	43825	Fusion of stomach and bowel
43325	Revise esophagus & stomach	43830	Place gastrostomy tube
43326	Revise esophagus & stomach	43831	Place gastrostomy tube
43330	Repair of esophagus	43832	Place gastrostomy tube
43331	Repair of esophagus	43840	Repair of stomach lesion
43340	Fuse esophagus & intestine	43842	V-band gastroplasty
43341	Fuse esophagus & intestine	43843	Gastroplasty w/o v-band
43350	Surgical opening, esophagus	43845	Gastroplasty duodenal switch
43351	Surgical opening, esophagus	43846	Gastric bypass for obesity
43352	Surgical opening, esophagus	43847	Gastric bypass incl small i
43360	Gastrointestinal repair	43848	Revision gastroplasty
43361	Gastrointestinal repair	43850	Revise stomach-bowel fusion

HCPCS Code	Short Description	HCPCS Code	Short Description
43855	Revise stomach-bowel fusion	44211	Lap colectomy w/proctectomy
43860	Revise stomach-bowel fusion	44212	Laparo total proctocolectomy
43865	Revise stomach-bowel fusion	44213	Lap, mobil splenic fl add-on
43880	Repair stomach-bowel fistula	44227	Lap, close enterostomy
43881	Impl/redo electrd, antrum	44238	Laparoscope proc, intestine
43882	Revise/remove electrd antrum	44300	Open bowel to skin
43999	Stomach surgery procedure	44310	Ileostomy/jejunostomy
44005	Freeing of bowel adhesion	44314	Revision of ileostomy
44010	Incision of small bowel	44316	Devise bowel pouch
44015	Insert needle cath bowel	44320	Colostomy
44020	Explore small intestine	44322	Colostomy with biopsies
44021	Decompress small bowel	44345	Revision of colostomy
44025	Incision of large bowel	44346	Revision of colostomy
44050	Reduce bowel obstruction	44602	Suture, small intestine
44055	Correct malrotation of bowel	44603	Suture, small intestine
44110	Excise intestine lesion(s)	44604	Suture, large intestine
44111	Excision of bowel lesion(s)	44605	Repair of bowel lesion
44120	Removal of small intestine	44615	Intestinal stricturoplasty
44121	Removal of small intestine	44620	Repair bowel opening
44125	Removal of small intestine	44625	Repair bowel opening
44126	Enterectomy w/o taper, cong	44626	Repair bowel opening
44127	Enterectomy w/taper, cong	44640	Repair bowel-skin fistula
44128	Enterectomy cong, add-on	44650	Repair bowel fistula
44130	Bowel to bowel fusion	44660	Repair bowel-bladder fistula
44132	Enterectomy, cadaver donor	44661	Repair bowel-bladder fistula
44133	Enterectomy, live donor	44680	Surgical revision, intestine
44135	Intestine transplnt, cadaver	44700	Suspend bowel w/prosthesis
44136	Intestine transplant, live	44715	Prepare donor intestine
44137	Remove intestinal allograft	44720	Prep donor intestine/venous
44139	Mobilization of colon	44721	Prep donor intestine/artery
44140	Partial removal of colon	44799	Unlisted procedure intestine
44141	Partial removal of colon	44800	Excision of bowel pouch
44143	Partial removal of colon	44820	Excision of mesentery lesion
44144	Partial removal of colon	44850	Repair of mesentery
44145	Partial removal of colon	44899	Bowel surgery procedure
44146	Partial removal of colon	44900	Drain app abscess, open
44147	Partial removal of colon	44901	Drain app abscess, percut
44150	Removal of colon	44950	Appendectomy
44151	Removal of colon/ileostomy	44955	Appendectomy add-on
44155	Removal of colon/ileostomy	44960	Appendectomy
44156	Removal of colon/ileostomy	44970	Laparoscopy, appendectomy
44157	Colectomy w/ileoanal anast	44979	Laparoscope proc, app
44158	Colectomy w/neo-rectum pouch	45110	Removal of rectum
44160	Removal of colon	45111	Partial removal of rectum
44180	Lap, enterolysis	45112	Removal of rectum
44186	Lap, jejunostomy	45113	Partial proctectomy
44187	Lap, ileo/jejuno-stomy	45114	Partial removal of rectum
44188	Lap, colostomy	45116	Partial removal of rectum
44202	Lap, enterectomy	45119	Remove rectum w/reservoir
44203	Lap resect s/intestine, addl	45120	Removal of rectum
44204	Laparo partial colectomy	45121	Removal of rectum and colon
44205	Lap colectomy part w/ileum	45123	Partial proctectomy
44206	Lap part colectomy w/stoma	45126	Pelvic exenteration
44207	L colectomy/coloproctostomy	45130	Excision of rectal prolapse
44208	L colectomy/coloproctostomy	45135	Excision of rectal prolapse
44210	Laparo total proctocolectomy	45136	Excise ileoanal reservoir

HCPCS Code	Short Description	HCPCS Code	Short Description
45395	Lap, removal of rectum	47381	Open ablate liver tumor cryo
45397	Lap, remove rectum w/pouch	47399	Liver surgery procedure
45400	Laparoscopic proc	47400	Incision of liver duct
45402	Lap proctopexy w/sig resect	47420	Incision of bile duct
45499	Laparoscope proc, rectum	47425	Incision of bile duct
45540	Correct rectal prolapse	47460	Incise bile duct sphincter
45550	Repair rectum/remove sigmoid	47480	Incision of gallbladder
45562	Exploration/repair of rectum	47490	Incision of gallbladder
45563	Exploration/repair of rectum	47550	Bile duct endoscopy add-on
45800	Repair rect/bladder fistula	47570	Laparo cholecystoenterostomy
45805	Repair fistula w/colostomy	47579	Laparoscope proc, biliary
45820	Repair rectourethral fistula	47600	Removal of gallbladder
45825	Repair fistula w/colostomy	47605	Removal of gallbladder
45999	Rectum surgery procedure	47610	Removal of gallbladder
46705	Repair of anal stricture	47612	Removal of gallbladder
46710	Repr per/vag pouch sngl proc	47620	Removal of gallbladder
46712	Repr per/vag pouch dbl proc	47700	Exploration of bile ducts
46715	Rep perf anoper fistu	47701	Bile duct revision
46716	Rep perf anoper/vestib fistu	47711	Excision of bile duct tumor
46730	Construction of absent anus	47712	Excision of bile duct tumor
46735	Construction of absent anus	47715	Excision of bile duct cyst
46740	Construction of absent anus	47720	Fuse gallbladder & bowel
46742	Repair of imperforated anus	47721	Fuse upper gi structures
46744	Repair of cloacal anomaly	47740	Fuse gallbladder & bowel
46746	Repair of cloacal anomaly	47741	Fuse gallbladder & bowel
46748	Repair of cloacal anomaly	47760	Fuse bile ducts and bowel
46751	Repair of anal sphincter	47765	Fuse liver ducts & bowel
46999	Anus surgery procedure	47780	Fuse bile ducts and bowel
47010	Open drainage, liver lesion	47785	Fuse bile ducts and bowel
47011	Percut drain, liver lesion	47800	Reconstruction of bile ducts
47015	Inject/aspirate liver cyst	47801	Placement, bile duct support
47100	Wedge biopsy of liver	47802	Fuse liver duct & intestine
47120	Partial removal of liver	47900	Suture bile duct injury
47122	Extensive removal of liver	47999	Bile tract surgery procedure
47125	Partial removal of liver	48000	Drainage of abdomen
47130	Partial removal of liver	48001	Placement of drain, pancreas
47133	Removal of donor liver	48020	Removal of pancreatic stone
47135	Transplantation of liver	48100	Biopsy of pancreas, open
47136	Transplantation of liver	48105	Resect/debride pancreas
47140	Partial removal, donor liver	48120	Removal of pancreas lesion
47141	Partial removal, donor liver	48140	Partial removal of pancreas
47142	Partial removal, donor liver	48145	Partial removal of pancreas
47143	Prep donor liver, whole	48146	Pancreatectomy
47144	Prep donor liver, 3-segment	48148	Removal of pancreatic duct
47145	Prep donor liver, lobe split	48150	Partial removal of pancreas
47146	Prep donor liver/venous	48152	Pancreatectomy
47147	Prep donor liver/arterial	48153	Pancreatectomy
47300	Surgery for liver lesion	48154	Pancreatectomy
47350	Repair liver wound	48155	Removal of pancreas
47360	Repair liver wound	48160	Pancreas removal/transplant
47361	Repair liver wound	48400	Injection, intraop add-on
47362	Repair liver wound	48500	Surgery of pancreatic cyst
47370	Laparo ablate liver tumor rf	48510	Drain pancreatic pseudocyst
47371	Laparo ablate liver cryosurg	48511	Drain pancreatic pseudocyst
47379	Laparoscope procedure, liver	48520	Fuse pancreas cyst and bowel
47380	Open ablate liver tumor rf	48540	Fuse pancreas cyst and bowel

HCPCS Code	Short Description	HCPCS Code	Short Description
48545	Pancreatorrhaphy	50220	Remove kidney, open
48547	Duodenal exclusion	50225	Removal kidney open, complex
48548	Fuse pancreas and bowel	50230	Removal kidney open, radical
48550	Donor pancreatectomy	50234	Removal of kidney & ureter
48551	Prep donor pancreas	50236	Removal of kidney & ureter
48552	Prep donor pancreas/venous	50240	Partial removal of kidney
48554	Transpl allograft pancreas	50250	Cryoablate renal mass open
48556	Removal, allograft pancreas	50280	Removal of kidney lesion
48999	Pancreas surgery procedure	50290	Removal of kidney lesion
49000	Exploration of abdomen	50300	Remove cadaver donor kidney
49002	Reopening of abdomen	50320	Remove kidney, living donor
49010	Exploration behind abdomen	50323	Prep cadaver renal allograft
49020	Drain abdominal abscess	50325	Prep donor renal graft
49021	Drain abdominal abscess	50327	Prep renal graft/venous
49040	Drain, open, abdom abscess	50328	Prep renal graft/arterial
49041	Drain, percut, abdom abscess	50329	Prep renal graft/ureteral
49060	Drain, open, retrop abscess	50340	Removal of kidney
49061	Drain, percut, retroper absc	50360	Transplantation of kidney
49062	Drain to peritoneal cavity	50365	Transplantation of kidney
49203	Exc abd tum 5 cm or less	50370	Remove transplanted kidney
49204	Exc abd tum over 5 cm	50380	Reimplantation of kidney
49205	Exc abd tum over 10 cm	50400	Revision of kidney/ureter
49215	Excise sacral spine tumor	50405	Revision of kidney/ureter
49220	Multiple surgery, abdomen	50500	Repair of kidney wound
49255	Removal of omentum	50520	Close kidney-skin fistula
49323	Laparo drain lymphocele	50525	Repair renal-abdomen fistula
49329	Laparo proc, abdm/per/oment	50526	Repair renal-abdomen fistula
49425	Insert abdomen-venous drain	50540	Revision of horseshoe kidney
49428	Ligation of shunt	50541	Laparo ablate renal cyst
49491	Rpr hern preemie reduc	50542	Laparo ablate renal mass
49492	Rpr ing hern premie, blocked	50543	Laparo partial nephrectomy
49605	Repair umbilical lesion	50544	Laparoscopy, pyeloplasty
49606	Repair umbilical lesion	50545	Laparo radical nephrectomy
49610	Repair umbilical lesion	50546	Laparoscopic nephrectomy
49611	Repair umbilical lesion	50547	Laparo removal donor kidney
49659	Laparo proc, hernia repair	50548	Laparo remove w/ureter
49900	Repair of abdominal wall	50549	Laparoscope proc, renal
49904	Omental flap, extra-abdom	50593	Perc cryo ablate renal tum
49905	Omental flap, intra-abdom	50600	Exploration of ureter
49906	Free omental flap, microvasc	50605	Insert ureteral support
49999	Abdomen surgery procedure	50610	Removal of ureter stone
50010	Exploration of kidney	50620	Removal of ureter stone
50020	Renal abscess, open drain	50630	Removal of ureter stone
50021	Renal abscess, percut drain	50650	Removal of ureter
50040	Drainage of kidney	50660	Removal of ureter
50045	Exploration of kidney	50700	Revision of ureter
50060	Removal of kidney stone	50715	Release of ureter
50065	Incision of kidney	50722	Release of ureter
50070	Incision of kidney	50725	Release/revise ureter
50075	Removal of kidney stone	50728	Revise ureter
50100	Revise kidney blood vessels	50740	Fusion of ureter & kidney
50120	Exploration of kidney	50750	Fusion of ureter & kidney
50125	Explore and drain kidney	50760	Fusion of ureters
50130	Removal of kidney stone	50770	Splicing of ureters
50135	Exploration of kidney	50780	Reimplant ureter in bladder
50205	Biopsy of kidney	50782	Reimplant ureter in bladder

HCPCS Code	Short Description	HCPCS Code	Short Description
50783	Reimplant ureter in bladder	54390	Repair penis and bladder
50785	Reimplant ureter in bladder	54411	Remov/replc penis pros, comp
50800	Implant ureter in bowel	54417	Remv/replc penis pros, compl
50810	Fusion of ureter & bowel	54430	Revision of penis
50815	Urine shunt to intestine	54535	Extensive testis surgery
50820	Construct bowel bladder	54650	Orchiopexy (fowler-stephens)
50825	Construct bowel bladder	54699	Laparoscope proc, testis
50830	Revise urine flow	55559	Laparo proc, spermatic cord
50840	Replace ureter by bowel	55605	Incise sperm duct pouch
50845	Appendico-vesicostomy	55650	Remove sperm duct pouch
50860	Transplant ureter to skin	55801	Removal of prostate
50900	Repair of ureter	55810	Extensive prostate surgery
50920	Closure ureter/skin fistula	55812	Extensive prostate surgery
50930	Closure ureter/bowel fistula	55815	Extensive prostate surgery
50940	Release of ureter	55821	Removal of prostate
50945	Laparoscopy ureterolithotomy	55831	Removal of prostate
50949	Laparoscope proc, ureter	55840	Extensive prostate surgery
51060	Removal of ureter stone	55842	Extensive prostate surgery
51525	Removal of bladder lesion	55845	Extensive prostate surgery
51530	Removal of bladder lesion	55862	Extensive prostate surgery
51550	Partial removal of bladder	55865	Extensive prostate surgery
51555	Partial removal of bladder	55866	Laparo radical prostatectomy
51565	Revise bladder & ureter(s)	55899	Genital surgery procedure
51570	Removal of bladder	55970	Sex transformation, m to f
51575	Removal of bladder & nodes	55980	Sex transformation, f to m
51580	Remove bladder/revise tract	56630	Extensive vulva surgery
51585	Removal of bladder & nodes	56631	Extensive vulva surgery
51590	Remove bladder/revise tract	56632	Extensive vulva surgery
51595	Remove bladder/revise tract	56633	Extensive vulva surgery
51596	Remove bladder/create pouch	56634	Extensive vulva surgery
51597	Removal of pelvic structures	56637	Extensive vulva surgery
51800	Revision of bladder/urethra	56640	Extensive vulva surgery
51820	Revision of urinary tract	57106	Remove vagina wall, partial
51840	Attach bladder/urethra	57107	Remove vagina tissue, part
51841	Attach bladder/urethra	57109	Vaginectomy partial w/nodes
51845	Repair bladder neck	57110	Remove vagina wall, complete
51860	Repair of bladder wound	57111	Remove vagina tissue, compl
51865	Repair of bladder wound	57112	Vaginectomy w/nodes, compl
51900	Repair bladder/vagina lesion	57120	Closure of vagina
51920	Close bladder-uterus fistula	57270	Repair of bowel pouch
51925	Hysterectomy/bladder repair	57280	Suspension of vagina
51940	Correction of bladder defect	57282	Colpopexy, extraperitoneal
51960	Revision of bladder & bowel	57283	Colpopexy, intraperitoneal
51980	Construct bladder opening	57284	Repair paravag defect, open
51990	Laparo urethral suspension	57285	Repair paravag defect, vag
51999	Laparoscope proc, bla	57292	Construct vagina with graft
52649	Prostate laser enucleation	57296	Revise vag graft, open abd
53415	Reconstruction of urethra	57305	Repair rectum-vagina fistula
53448	Remov/replc ur sphinctr comp	57307	Fistula repair & colostomy
53500	Urethrlys, transvag w/ scope	57308	Fistula repair, transperine
53899	Urology surgery procedure	57310	Repair urethrovaginal lesion
54125	Removal of penis	57311	Repair urethrovaginal lesion
54130	Remove penis & nodes	57330	Repair bladder-vagina lesion
54135	Remove penis & nodes	57335	Repair vagina
54332	Revise penis/urethra	57423	Repair paravag defect, lap
54336	Revise penis/urethra	57425	Laparoscopy, surg, colpopexy

HCPCS Code	Short Description	HCPCS Code	Short Description
57531	Removal of cervix, radical	58920	Partial removal of ovary(s)
57540	Removal of residual cervix	58925	Removal of ovarian cyst(s)
57545	Remove cervix/repair pelvis	58940	Removal of ovary(s)
57555	Remove cervix/repair vagina	58943	Removal of ovary(s)
58140	Myomectomy abdom method	58950	Resect ovarian malignancy
58146	Myomectomy abdom complex	58951	Resect ovarian malignancy
58150	Total hysterectomy	58952	Resect ovarian malignancy
58152	Total hysterectomy	58953	Tah, rad dissect for debulk
58180	Partial hysterectomy	58954	Tah rad debulk/lymph remove
58200	Extensive hysterectomy	58956	Bso, omentectomy w/tah
58210	Extensive hysterectomy	58957	Resect recurrent gyn mal
58240	Removal of pelvis contents	58958	Resect recur gyn mal w/lym
58260	Vaginal hysterectomy	58960	Exploration of abdomen
58262	Vag hyst including t/o	58999	Genital surgery procedure
58263	Vag hyst w/t/o & vag repair	59030	Fetal scalp blood sample
58267	Vag hyst w/urinary repair	59074	Fetal fluid drainage w/us
58270	Vag hyst w/enterocele repair	59120	Treat ectopic pregnancy
58275	Hysterectomy/revise vagina	59121	Treat ectopic pregnancy
58280	Hysterectomy/revise vagina	59130	Treat ectopic pregnancy
58285	Extensive hysterectomy	59135	Treat ectopic pregnancy
58290	Vag hyst complex	59136	Treat ectopic pregnancy
58291	Vag hyst incl t/o, complex	59140	Treat ectopic pregnancy
58292	Vag hyst t/o & repair, compl	59325	Revision of cervix
58293	Vag hyst w/uro repair, compl	59350	Repair of uterus
58294	Vag hyst w/enterocele, compl	59409	Obstetrical care
58300	Insert intrauterine device	59514	Cesarean delivery only
58400	Suspension of uterus	59525	Remove uterus after cesarean
58410	Suspension of uterus	59612	Vbac delivery only
58520	Repair of ruptured uterus	59620	Attempted vbac delivery only
58540	Revision of uterus	59830	Treat uterus infection
58541	Lsh, uterus 250 g or less	59850	Abortion
58542	Lsh w/t/o ut 250 g or less	59851	Abortion
58543	Lsh uterus above 250 g	59852	Abortion
58544	Lsh w/t/o uterus above 250 g	59855	Abortion
58548	Lap radical hyst	59856	Abortion
58553	Laparo-vag hyst, complex	59857	Abortion
58554	Laparo-vag hyst w/t/o, compl	59897	Fetal invas px w/us
58570	Tlh, uterus 250 g or less	59898	Laparo proc, ob care/deliver
58571	Tlh w/t/o 250 g or less	59899	Maternity care procedure
58572	Tlh, uterus over 250 g	60240	Removal of thyroid
58573	Tlh w/t/o uterus over 250 g	60252	Removal of thyroid
58578	Laparo proc, uterus	60254	Extensive thyroid surgery
58579	Hysteroscope procedure	60260	Repeat thyroid surgery
58605	Division of fallopian tube	60270	Removal of thyroid
58611	Ligate oviduct(s) add-on	60271	Removal of thyroid
58679	Laparo proc, oviduct-ovary	60500	Explore parathyroid glands
58700	Removal of fallopian tube	60502	Re-explore parathyroids
58720	Removal of ovary/tube(s)	60505	Explore parathyroid glands
58740	Adhesiolysis tube, ovary	60512	Autotransplant parathyroid
58750	Repair oviduct	60520	Removal of thymus gland
58752	Revise ovarian tube(s)	60521	Removal of thymus gland
58760	Fimbrioplasty	60522	Removal of thymus gland
58770	Create new tubal opening	60540	Explore adrenal gland
58822	Drain ovary abscess, percut	60545	Explore adrenal gland
58823	Drain pelvic abscess, percut	60600	Remove carotid body lesion
58825	Transposition, ovary(s)	60605	Remove carotid body lesion

HCPCS Code	Short Description	HCPCS Code	Short Description
60650	Laparoscopy adrenalectomy	61535	Remove brain electrodes
60659	Laparo proc, endocrine	61536	Removal of brain lesion
60699	Endocrine surgery procedure	61537	Removal of brain tissue
61105	Twist drill hole	61538	Removal of brain tissue
61107	Drill skull for implantation	61539	Removal of brain tissue
61108	Drill skull for drainage	61540	Removal of brain tissue
61120	Burr hole for puncture	61541	Incision of brain tissue
61140	Pierce skull for biopsy	61542	Removal of brain tissue
61150	Pierce skull for drainage	61543	Removal of brain tissue
61151	Pierce skull for drainage	61544	Remove & treat brain lesion
61154	Pierce skull & remove clot	61545	Excision of brain tumor
61156	Pierce skull for drainage	61546	Removal of pituitary gland
61210	Pierce skull, implant device	61548	Removal of pituitary gland
61250	Pierce skull & explore	61550	Release of skull seams
61253	Pierce skull & explore	61552	Release of skull seams
61304	Open skull for exploration	61556	Incise skull/sutures
61305	Open skull for exploration	61557	Incise skull/sutures
61312	Open skull for drainage	61558	Excision of skull/sutures
61313	Open skull for drainage	61559	Excision of skull/sutures
61314	Open skull for drainage	61563	Excision of skull tumor
61315	Open skull for drainage	61564	Excision of skull tumor
61316	Implt cran bone flap to abdo	61566	Removal of brain tissue
61320	Open skull for drainage	61567	Incision of brain tissue
61321	Open skull for drainage	61570	Remove foreign body, brain
61322	Decompressive craniotomy	61571	Incise skull for brain wound
61323	Decompressive lobectomy	61575	Skull base/brainstem surgery
61332	Explore/biopsy eye socket	61576	Skull base/brainstem surgery
61333	Explore orbit/remove lesion	61580	Craniofacial approach, skull
61340	Subtemporal decompression	61581	Craniofacial approach, skull
61343	Incise skull (press relief)	61582	Craniofacial approach, skull
61345	Relieve cranial pressure	61583	Craniofacial approach, skull
61440	Incise skull for surgery	61584	Orbitocranial approach/skull
61450	Incise skull for surgery	61585	Orbitocranial approach/skull
61458	Incise skull for brain wound	61586	Resect nasopharynx, skull
61460	Incise skull for surgery	61590	Infratemporal approach/skull
61470	Incise skull for surgery	61591	Infratemporal approach/skull
61480	Incise skull for surgery	61592	Orbitocranial approach/skull
61490	Incise skull for surgery	61595	Transtemporal approach/skull
61500	Removal of skull lesion	61596	Transcochlear approach/skull
61501	Remove infected skull bone	61597	Transcondylar approach/skull
61510	Removal of brain lesion	61598	Transpetrosal approach/skull
61512	Remove brain lining lesion	61600	Resect/excise cranial lesion
61514	Removal of brain abscess	61601	Resect/excise cranial lesion
61516	Removal of brain lesion	61605	Resect/excise cranial lesion
61517	Implt brain chemotx add-on	61606	Resect/excise cranial lesion
61518	Removal of brain lesion	61607	Resect/excise cranial lesion
61519	Remove brain lining lesion	61608	Resect/excise cranial lesion
61520	Removal of brain lesion	61609	Transect artery, sinus
61521	Removal of brain lesion	61610	Transect artery, sinus
61522	Removal of brain abscess	61611	Transect artery, sinus
61524	Removal of brain lesion	61612	Transect artery, sinus
61526	Removal of brain lesion	61613	Remove aneurysm, sinus
61530	Removal of brain lesion	61615	Resect/excise lesion, skull
61531	Implant brain electrodes	61616	Resect/excise lesion, skull
61533	Implant brain electrodes	61618	Repair dura
61534	Removal of brain lesion	61619	Repair dura

HCPCS Code	Short Description	HCPCS Code	Short Description
61623	Endovasc tempory vessel occl	62164	Remove brain tumor w/scope
61624	Transcath occlusion, cns	62165	Remove pituit tumor w/scope
61626	Transcath occlusion, non-cns	62180	Establish brain cavity shunt
61630	Intracranial angioplasty	62190	Establish brain cavity shunt
61635	Intracran angioplsty w/stent	62192	Establish brain cavity shunt
61640	Dilate ic vasospasm, init	62200	Establish brain cavity shunt
61641	Dilate ic vasospasm add-on	62201	Brain cavity shunt w/scope
61642	Dilate ic vasospasm add-on	62220	Establish brain cavity shunt
61680	Intracranial vessel surgery	62223	Establish brain cavity shunt
61682	Intracranial vessel surgery	62256	Remove brain cavity shunt
61684	Intracranial vessel surgery	62258	Replace brain cavity shunt
61686	Intracranial vessel surgery	62351	Implant spinal canal cath
61690	Intracranial vessel surgery	63001	Removal of spinal lamina
61692	Intracranial vessel surgery	63003	Removal of spinal lamina
61697	Brain aneurysm repr, complx	63005	Removal of spinal lamina
61698	Brain aneurysm repr, complx	63011	Removal of spinal lamina
61700	Brain aneurysm repr, simple	63012	Removal of spinal lamina
61702	Inner skull vessel surgery	63015	Removal of spinal lamina
61703	Clamp neck artery	63016	Removal of spinal lamina
61705	Revise circulation to head	63017	Removal of spinal lamina
61708	Revise circulation to head	63020	Neck spine disk surgery
61710	Revise circulation to head	63030	Low back disk surgery
61711	Fusion of skull arteries	63035	Spinal disk surgery add-on
61720	Incise skull/brain surgery	63040	Laminotomy, single cervical
61735	Incise skull/brain surgery	63042	Laminotomy, single lumbar
61750	Incise skull/brain biopsy	63043	Laminotomy, add'l cervical
61751	Brain biopsy w/ct/mr guide	63044	Laminotomy, add'l lumbar
61760	Implant brain electrodes	63045	Removal of spinal lamina
61850	Implant neuroelectrodes	63046	Removal of spinal lamina
61860	Implant neuroelectrodes	63047	Removal of spinal lamina
61863	Implant neuroelectrode	63048	Remove spinal lamina add-on
61864	Implant neuroelectrde, addl	63050	Cervical laminoplasty
61867	Implant neuroelectrode	63051	C-laminoplasty w/graft/plate
61868	Implant neuroelectrde, add'l	63055	Decompress spinal cord
61870	Implant neuroelectrodes	63056	Decompress spinal cord
61875	Implant neuroelectrodes	63057	Decompress spine cord add-on
62000	Treat skull fracture	63064	Decompress spinal cord
62005	Treat skull fracture	63066	Decompress spine cord add-on
62010	Treatment of head injury	63075	Neck spine disk surgery
62100	Repair brain fluid leakage	63076	Neck spine disk surgery
62115	Reduction of skull defect	63077	Spine disk surgery, thorax
62116	Reduction of skull defect	63078	Spine disk surgery, thorax
62117	Reduction of skull defect	63081	Removal of vertebral body
62120	Repair skull cavity lesion	63082	Remove vertebral body add-on
62121	Incise skull repair	63085	Removal of vertebral body
62140	Repair of skull defect	63086	Remove vertebral body add-on
62141	Repair of skull defect	63087	Removal of vertebral body
62142	Remove skull plate/flap	63088	Remove vertebral body add-on
62143	Replace skull plate/flap	63090	Removal of vertebral body
62145	Repair of skull & brain	63091	Remove vertebral body add-on
62146	Repair of skull with graft	63101	Removal of vertebral body
62147	Repair of skull with graft	63102	Removal of vertebral body
62148	Retr bone flap to fix skull	63103	Remove vertebral body add-on
62161	Dissect brain w/scope	63170	Incise spinal cord tract(s)
62162	Remove colloid cyst w/scope	63172	Drainage of spinal cyst
62163	Neuroendoscopy w/fb removal	63173	Drainage of spinal cyst

HCPCS Code	Short Description	HCPCS Code	Short Description
63180	Revise spinal cord ligaments	64760	Incision of vagus nerve
63182	Revise spinal cord ligaments	64804	Remove sympathetic nerves
63185	Incise spinal column/nerves	64809	Remove sympathetic nerves
63190	Incise spinal column/nerves	64818	Remove sympathetic nerves
63191	Incise spinal column/nerves	64866	Fusion of facial/other nerve
63194	Incise spinal column & cord	64868	Fusion of facial/other nerve
63195	Incise spinal column & cord	64911	Neurorraphy w/vein autograft
63196	Incise spinal column & cord	64999	Nervous system surgery
63197	Incise spinal column & cord	65273	Repair of eye wound
63198	Incise spinal column & cord	65760	Revision of cornea
63199	Incise spinal column & cord	65765	Revision of cornea
63200	Release of spinal cord	65767	Corneal tissue transplant
63250	Revise spinal cord vessels	65771	Radial keratotomy
63251	Revise spinal cord vessels	66999	Eye surgery procedure
63252	Revise spinal cord vessels	67299	Eye surgery procedure
63265	Excise intraspinal lesion	67399	Eye muscle surgery procedure
63266	Excise intraspinal lesion	67599	Orbit surgery procedure
63267	Excise intraspinal lesion	67999	Revision of eyelid
63268	Excise intraspinal lesion	68399	Eyelid lining surgery
63270	Excise intraspinal lesion	68899	Tear duct system surgery
63271	Excise intraspinal lesion	69090	Pierce earlobes
63272	Excise intraspinal lesion	69155	Extensive ear/neck surgery
63273	Excise intraspinal lesion	69399	Outer ear surgery procedure
63275	Biopsy/excise spinal tumor	69535	Remove part of temporal bone
63276	Biopsy/excise spinal tumor	69554	Remove ear lesion
63277	Biopsy/excise spinal tumor	69710	Implant/replace hearing aid
63278	Biopsy/excise spinal tumor	69725	Release facial nerve
63280	Biopsy/excise spinal tumor	69799	Middle ear surgery procedure
63281	Biopsy/excise spinal tumor	69949	Inner ear surgery procedure
63282	Biopsy/excise spinal tumor	69950	Incise inner ear nerve
63283	Biopsy/excise spinal tumor	69955	Release facial nerve
63285	Biopsy/excise spinal tumor	69960	Release inner ear canal
63286	Biopsy/excise spinal tumor	69970	Remove inner ear lesion
63287	Biopsy/excise spinal tumor	69979	Temporal bone surgery
63290	Biopsy/excise spinal tumor		
63295	Repair of laminectomy defect		
63300	Removal of vertebral body		
63301	Removal of vertebral body		
63302	Removal of vertebral body		
63303	Removal of vertebral body		
63304	Removal of vertebral body		
63305	Removal of vertebral body		
63306	Removal of vertebral body		
63307	Removal of vertebral body		
63308	Remove vertebral body add-on		
63700	Repair of spinal herniation		
63702	Repair of spinal herniation		
63704	Repair of spinal herniation		
63706	Repair of spinal herniation		
63707	Repair spinal fluid leakage		
63709	Repair spinal fluid leakage		
63710	Graft repair of spine defect		
63740	Install spinal shunt		
63741	Install spinal shunt		
64752	Incision of vagus nerve		
64755	Incision of stomach nerves		

Processing Notes
Processing Notes for CY 2010

| **Number** | **Description** |

0001   THIS PROCESSING NOTE DELETED 1/1/97.

0002   THESE CODES (82585, 82595) PERTAIN TO PERFORMING THE ANALYSIS FOR THE ANALYTE AS OPPOSED TO AD-MINISTRATION OF THE ANALYTE.

0003   THIS PROCEDURE (85029, 85030) IS USUALLY PART OF THE AUTOMATED PROFILES FOR CBC AND CONSIDER-ATION SHOULD BE GIVEN TO NOT PAYING SEPARATELY FOR THESE INDICES.

0004   THIS PROCESSING NOTE DELETED 1/1/97.

0005   THE CERTIFICATION CATEGORY WILL DEPEND ON THE TYPE OF TEST/OR ORGANISM IDENTIFIED AND THERE MUST BE AN IDENTIFIER TO INDICATE THE SPECIFIC TESTING PERFORMED (87082-87085, 89100, 89130, 89132, 86403).

0006   THIS IS NOT A LAB TEST AND IS NOT CERTIFIED.

0007   THIS PROCESSING NOTE DELETED 1/1/97.

0008   THIS PROCESSING NOTE DELETED 1/1/97.

0009   THIS PROCESSING NOTE DELETED 1/1/97.

0010   THIS PROCESSING NOTE DELETED 1/1/97.

0011   THIS PROCESSING NOTE DELETED 1/1/97.

0012   THIS PROCESSING NOTE DELETED 1/1/97.

0013   THIS DEVICE (E0194) SHOULD NOT BE CONFUSED WITH E0193 POWERED FLOTATION THERAPY BED (LOW AIR LOSS BED). SEE CIM TRANS. NO. 44, JULY 1990.

0014   CLAIMS SUBMITTED WITH THIS CODE (J9218) WITH OR WITHOUT A MULTIPLIER IN IN THE UNITS FIELD SHOULD BE REVIEWED IN TERMS OF THE POLICY PERTAINING TO SELF ADMINISTERED DRUG

0015   REIMBURSEMENT IS INCLUDED IN THE BASIC ALLOWANCE OF ANOTHER PROCEDURE.

0016   DEVICE IS SUITABLE FOR VISUALLY IMPAIRED (E0609).

0017   SEE INTERMEDIARY MANUAL SECTION 3170.5 FOR COVERAGE INSTRUCTIONS PERTAINING TO E1510-E1600, E1620, E1630-E1699, A4650-A4663, A4690, A4712, A4730-A4870, A4890-A4927.

0018   CODE J2545 TO BE REPORTED WITH 94642 WHERE APPROPRIATE.

0019   SERVICE REPRESENTED BY D4211 CAN BE CODED USING CPT 41820 WITH -52 MODIFIER.

0020   SERVICES REPRESENTED BY D7410 AND D7420 CAN BE CODED FROM CPT-4 USING CODES 21015 FF AND 40810 FF.

0021   SERVICES REPRESENTED BY D7430-D7461 CAN BE CODED FROM CPT-4 USING CODES 21029-21045 AND 41820-41827.

0022   SERVICE REPRESENTED BY D7610 CAN BE CODED USING CPT 21346 WITH -52 MODIFIER.

0023   SERVICE REPRESENTED BY D7620 CAN BE CODED USING CPT 21345 WITH -52 MODIFIER.

0024   SERVICE REPRESENTED BY D7630 CAN BE CODED USING CPT 21461 OR CPT 21462 WITH -52 MODIFIER.

0025--SERVICE REPRESENTED BY D7620 CAN BE CODED USING CPT 21455 WITH -52 MODIFIER.

0026   SERVICE REPRESENTED BY D7650 CAN BE CODED USING CPT 21360 WITH -52 MODIFIER OR 21365 WITH -52 MODIFIER.

<u>Number</u>	<u>Description</u>

0027   SERVICE REPRESENTED BY D7660 CAN BE CODED USING 21355 WITH -52 MODIFIER.

0028   SERVICE REPRESENTED BY D7670 CAN BE CODED USING CPT 21422 WITH -52 MODIFIER.

0029   SERVICE REPRESENTED BY D7680 CAN BE CODED USING CPT 21433 WITH -52 MODIFIER OR 21435 WITH -52 MODIFIER.

0030   SERVICE REPRESENTED BY D7920 CAN BE REPORTED USING A MORE SPECIFIC CPT CODE.

0031   SERVICE REPRESENTED BY D7949 CAN BE CODED USING CPT 21151, OR CODES 21154-21160.

0032   SERVICE REPRESENTED BY D7970 CAN BE CODED USING CPT 41828 WITH -52 MODIFIER.

0033   THIS PROCESSING NOTE DELETED 1/1/96.

0034   SERVICE REPRESENTED BY D9220 CAN BE CODED FROM CPT-4 USING 00170-00192.

0035   SERVICE REPRESENTED BY D9310 CAN BE CODED USING CPT CODES 90600-90643.

0036   SERVICE REPRESENTED BY D9410 CAN BE CODED USING CPT CODES 90100-90170.

0037   SERVICE REPRESENTED BY D9420 CAN BE CODED USING CPT CODES 90200-90282.

0038   SERVICE REPRESENTED BY D9430 CAN BE CODED USING CPT CODES 90000-90080.

0039   SEE MEDICARE INTERMEDIARY MANUAL, PART 3 CLAIMS PROCESS SECTION 3628.F FOR PAYMENT GUIDELINES (P9610, P9615, G0001).

0040   SEE MEDICARE INTERMEDIARY MANUAL 3628.E FOR PAYMENT GUIDELINES (P9610, P9615, G0001).

0041   SEE MEDICARE INTERMEDIARY MANUAL SECTION 3112.4 (Q0081, Q0083, Q0084, Q0085).

0042   SERVICES REPRESENTED BY 92392 SHOULD BE RECODED WITH SPECIFIC SYSTEMS FROM A-N V2600-V2615.

0043   SERVICES REPRESENTED BY 92395 SHOULD BE RECODED WITH SPECIFIC LENS TYPE FROM A-N V2100-V2499.

0044   SERVICES REPRESENTED BY 92396 SHOULD BE RECODED WITH SPECIFIC LENS TYPE FROM V2500-V2599.

0045   SEE INTERMEDIARY MANUAL 3628.1A FOR PAYMENT INSTRUCTIONS. (P3000,P3001 G0123, G0124, G0141, G0143, G0144, G0145, G0147, G0148). PROGRAM MEMORANDUM AB-98-71.60.

0046   THIS MODIFIER (Q2) IS AUTHORIZED FOR USE BY THE HCFA OFFICE OF RESEARCH AND DEMONSTRATIONS ONLY; FOR CLAIMS SUBMITTED TO ORD FOR PAYMENT IN CONNECTION WITH DEMONSTRATION PROJECTS.

0047   THIS PROCESSING NOTE DELETED 1/1/97.

0048   SEE MEDICARE INTERMEDIARY MANUAL, SECTION 3112.7D1.E (Q0082).

0049   SEE MEDICARE INTERMEDIARY MANUAL, SECTION 3148 (CPT 97001, 97002).

0050   THIS CODE MUST INCLUDE NON-CORING NEEDLES, PRESSURE MONITOR WITH STOPCOCK AND TEMPLATES. CARRIERS SHOULD NOT ALLOW SEPARATE PAYMENT FOR THIS CODE AND FOR A4212.

0051   SPECIAL PAYMENT RULES APPLY. SEE MCM SECTION 15022.F (A4644, A4645, A4646).

0052   PAYMENT BUNDLED INTO PROCEDURE CODE (A4262, A4647, 99141, 99142).

0053   THIS MODIFIER CODE CROSSWALKS TO A0999 UNLISTED AMBULANCE SERVICE.

0054   CODE Q0144 ESTABLISHED AS A NATIONAL CODE FOR MEDICAID USE.

0055   NONCOVERED BY MEDICARE STATUTE, 1862a1a (G0061).

0056   PAYMENT FOR THIS SERVICE IS INCLUDED IN THE APPROPRIATE E/M SERVICE (99371, 99374, 99377, 99379, 99380).

Number   **Description**

0057   SEE CPT (YY, ZZ).

0058   THIS PROCEDURE (A2000) CROSSWALKS TO CPT.

0059   SEE COVERAGE ISSUES MANUAL, SECTION 50-26 (D0120, D0415, D0425).

0060   SEE MCM 2136 (D2385) XXXXXXX.

0061   IN 1997, PAYMENT FOR R0076 IS BUNDLED INTO THE PAYMENT FOR THE REPORTED EKG SERVICE. IN 1998, PER BALANCED BUDGET ACT OF 1997, SEPARATE PAYMENT FOR R0076 IS MANDATED.

0062   CPT 32491 - PAYMENT RESTRICTED TO CERTAIN BENEFICIARIES ENROLLED IN THE HCFA/NHLBI STUDY.

0063   GO100 - SEE PROGRAM MEMO AB-97-9.60 TO INTERMEDIARIES/CARRIERS

0064   COVERAGE AND PAYMENT BASED ON BALANCED BUDGET ACT OF 1997 (G0101 -   SEC 4102; G0104, G0105, G0106, G0107, G0120, G0121, G0122 - SEC 4104).

0065   THESE CODES CAN BE REPORTED ONLY FOR THOSE MEDICARE BENEFICIARIES ENROLLED IN THE NATIONAL EMPHYSEMA TREATMENT TRIALS, DEMONSTRATION #30.

0066   EFFECTIVE 1/1/98, 76076 AND 76078 ARE BENEFITS UNDER THE BALANCED BUDGET ACT OF 1997, SECTION 4106.

0067   BENEFIT PER BALANCED BUDGET ACT OF 1997 SECTION 4101 (76092).

0068   CODES 76070, 76075, 78350, 82523 WERE REINSTATED IN 1998. BENEFIT UNDER BALANCED BUDGET ACT OF 1997 SECTION 4106. SEE G0131 AND G0132.

0069   FOR ASSISTANT SURGEON SERVICES MODIFIERS 80, 81, 82, AK, AL, AM, AN, AS, AU, AV, AW, AY, QB, QU SEE MCM SECTION 15044.

0070   G0128 MAY BE BILLED BY A COMPREHENSIVE OUTPATIENT REHABILITATION FACILITY ONLY. G0128 ESTABLISHED TO IMPLEMENT BBA (97) SECTION 4541(a)(2).

0071   G0108, G0109, SEE PROGRAM MEMORANDUM AB-99-30, MAY 1999, PROGRAM MEMORANDUM AB-98-36.

0072   COMPRESSION LEVELS FOR PRODUCTS IDENTIFIED BY THESE CODES (L8100 - L8200) HAVE BEEN VALIDATED BY A ASTM/NAHM SANCTIONED INDEPENDENT TEST FACILITY.

0073   SEE SECTION 4206(a)(b) OF THE BALANCED BUDGET ACT (BBA) OF 1997. PROGRAM MEMORANDOM B-99-2, JANUARY 1999.

0074   PER BBA 1997, SECTION 44105, EXPANDED COVERAGE OF SUPPLIES FOR DIABETIC BENEFICIARIES.

0075   PER BBA 1997, SECTION 4541, OUTPATIENT REHABILITATION THERAPY PAYMENT LIMITATION APPLIES.

0076   THE EXISTING LEVEL II CODES ARE J1460 THROUGH J1560.

0077   CR#259, AB-97-23 DATED 12-97 IMPLEMENTATION OF 1998 CLINICAL DIAGNOSTIC LABORATORY FEE SCHEDULE AND MAPPING FOR 1998 LABORATORY CODING CHANGES.

0078   PROGRAM MEMORANDUM AB-99-51, JULY 1999.

0079   ESTABLISHED PER BBA `97, SEC 4103.

0080   SEE CR#855, TRANSMITTAL NO. AB-99-22, DATED APRIL 1999.

0081   WHEN ACUITY IS MEASURED AS PART OF A GENERAL OPHTHALMOLOGICAL SERVICE OR OF AN E/M SERVICE OF THE EYE, IT IS A DIAGNOSTIC EXAMINATION AND NOT A SCREENING TEST, AND PAYMENT IS THEREFORE INCLUDED IN THE PAYMENT FOR THE E/M SERVICE.

0082   G0151-G0156 MAY BE BILLED ONLY FOR HOME HEALTH CARE SERVICES PROVIDED UNDER A PLAN OF CARE. SEE CR#588.

<u>Number</u>	<u>Description</u>

0083   MODIFIER G8 FOR USE WITH THE FOLLOWING SIX ANESTHESIA CODES; 00100, 00300, 00400, 00160, 00532 AND 00920.

0084   MODIFIER G7 FOR USE WITH CPT CODES FOR MEDICAL ABORTIONS: 59840, 59841, 59850, 59851, 59852, 59855, 59856, 59857 AND 59866.

0085   CODE Q0186 ESTABLISHED PER THE AUTHORITY PROVIDED UNDER SECTION 4531 OF THE BALANCED BUDGET ACT OF 1997.

0086   Q1001, Q1002, Q1003, Q1004, AND Q1005 MUST BE BILLED WITH ONE OF THE FOLLOWING PROCEDURE CODES - 66983, 66984, 66985 OR 66986 BY ASC.

0087   SERVICES REPRESENTED BY G0129 IS DEFINED IN SSA 1861(ff)(2)(B) BBA 1997 SECTION 4523 (d)(3) AMENDS SSA 1833(a)(2).

0088   S" CODES ARE UNIQUE TEMPORARY CODES ESTABLISHED BY BCBSA AND HIAA FOR PRIVATE PAYOR USE. THEY ARE NOT VALID NOR PAYABLE BY MEDICARE.

0089   REFER TO AB-99-52 SUSPENDING NON-COVERAGE PER CIM 35-98.

0090   THIS SERVICE IS BUNDLED WITH THE VISIT SERVICE.

0091   AS OF 10/1/1999, THIS VACCINE HAS NOT RECEIVED FDA APPROVAL.

0092   SEE NPRN FOR THE MEDICARE PHYSICIANS' FEE SCHEDULE FOR 2000, PUBLISHED IN THE FEDERAL REGISTER ON JULY 22, 1999.

0093   "C" CODES ARE UNIQUE TEMPORARY PRICING CODES THAT WERE INITIALLY ESTABLISHED BY CMS FOR THE HOSPITAL OUTPATIENT PROSPECTIVE PAYMENT SYSTEM (OPPS). THE "C" CODES ARE USED ON MEDICARE OPPS CLAIMS BUT MAY ALSO BE RECOGNIZED ON CLAIMS FROM OTHER PROVIDERS OR BY OTHER PAYMENT SYSTEMS.

0094   CODES G0173 AND G0174 REPLACE CPT 61793 ON THE OPPS PAYMENT METHODOLOGY. CODES MAY NOT BE USED IN MEDICARE PHYSICIAN FEE SCHEDULE SYSTEM.

0095   AS REQUIRED BY BBRA SECTION 201.

0096   SERVICE REPRESENTED BY G9106 IS REPORTABLE ONLY BY PARTICIPANTS IN THE SMOKING CESSATION COUN-SELING DEMONSTRATION PROJECT.

0097   FOR INSTRUCTIONS RELATED TO THE MEDICARE COORDINATED CARE DEMONSTRATION (MCCD) SEF CR1050, 1116 AND 1118.

0098   G0188 IS THE COMPREHENSIVE CODE FOR ANY COMBINATION OF XRAYS OF HIP, KNEE AND ANKLE (E.G. 73500, 73510, 73550, 73560, 73590, 73600).

0099   SEE NPRM SPING 2000.

0100   SERVICE REPRESENTED BY G0180 PERTAINS TO SSA 1814(A)(2)(C) AND 1835(A)(2)(A).

0101   G0175 REPRESENTS A SERVICE PAYABLE BY THE OPPS. IT MAY NOT BE USED IN THE MEDICARE PHYSICIAN FEE SCHEDULE SYSTEM.

0102   SERVICES REPRESENTED BY G0176 AND G0177 MAY BE REPORTED BY HOPD AND PARTIAL HOSPITALIZATION PROGRAMS ONLY (1861FF).

0103   G0172 WAS ESTABLISHED TO BE USED FOR PARTIAL HOSPITALIZATION PROGRAM REPORTING. EFFECTIVE 1/1/2001, IT HAS BEEN REPLACED BY G0177. (1861(FF)).

0104   CODE 92525 IS NOT RECOGNIZED BY MEDICARE. REFER TO CODE G0195.

0105   MODIFIER 60 IS NOT USED FOR MEDICARE PURPOSES.

0106   FOR MEDICARE CLAIMS - CODE A9270 ONLY FOR USE ON BILLS SUBMITTED BY DMEPOS SUPPLIERS.

0107   PAYMENT IS FOR HOSPITAL OUTPATIENT ONLY. NOT PAYABLE UNDER THE PHYSICIAN FEE SCHEDULE; IN AC-CORDANCE WITH FR DATE 8/9/2002 (HOPPS), PAGE 52105.

| **Number** | **Description** |

0108--NOT PAYABLE AS A SEPARATE PROCEDURE; SERVICE CONSIDERED BUNDLED INTO PRIMARY PROCEDURE.

0109--PAYMENT IS FOR HOSPITAL OUTPATIENT ONLY; NOT PAYABLE UNDER THE PHYSICIAN FEE SCHEDULE.

0110   SEE TRANSMITTAL AB-02-065. CIM 50-36 WILL GIVE COVERAGE INDICATIONS. 78459 SHOULD BE USED FOR DE-TERMINATION OF MYOCARDIAL VIABILITY AS A PRIMARY OR INITIAL DIAGNOSTIC STUDY PRIOR TO REVASCU-LARIZATION.

0111--IN ACCORDANCE WITH 42 CFR 411.4 (B).

0112   THE BASIS FOR THE PASRR LEVEL I SCREEN IS IN REGULATIONS ONLY AT 42 CFR 483.128(a).

0113   THE BASIS FOR THE PASRR LEVEL II SCREEN IS IN STATUTE AT SECTION 1919(b)(3)(F) AND SECTION 1919(e)(7) OF THE SOCIAL SECURITY ACT.

0114   FOR MEDICARE PURPOSES, MODIFIERS UN-US WOULD BE REPORTED WITH R0075.

0115   PHOTODYNAMIC THERAPY (INCLUDES INTRAVENOUS INFUSION) COVERAGE LIMITED TO AGE RELATED MAC-ULAR DEGENERATION (AMD) WITH OCCULT LESIONS WITH NO CLASSIC CHOROIDAL NEOVASCULARIZATION.

0116   FOR MEDICARE, FOR CAH METHOD II BILLING ONLY.

0117   SEE G CODES FOR REPORTING.

0118   INITIAL PREVENTIVE PHYSICAL EXAM CONSISTS OF MEASUREMENT OF HEIGHT, WEIGHT AND BLOOD PRES-SURE; MUST INCLUDE AN ELECTROCARDIOGRAM OR THIS CODE IS NOT BILLABLE.

0119   SEE NCDM REFERENCE 110.17.

0120   SEE BPM (BENEFIT POLICY MANUAL) 7/50.4.3.

0121   SECTION 303(e)(2) OF THE MMA IMPLEMENTS A SUPPLYING FEE FOR IMMUNOSUPPRESSIVE DRUGS, ORAL ANTI-CANCER CHEMOTHERAPEUTIC DRUGS, AND ANTI-EMETIC DRUGS USED AS PART OF AN ANTI-CANCER CHEMO-THERAPEUTIC REGIMEN.

0122   THE CONCEPT OF "COVERAGE UNDER PROTOCOL (CUP)" REFERS TO A COVERAGE CONDITION THAT REQUIRES MEDICARE BENEFICIARIES AND PROVIDERS TO PARTICIPATE IN RESEARCH STUDIES CONCERNING THE ITEM OR SERVICE TO BE COVERED.

0123   PUBLICATION 100.2, CHAPTER 15, SS 502.

0124   PUBLICATION 100.2, CHAPTER 15, SS 120.

0125   NCD MANUAL 280.1.

0126   NCD MANUAL 180.2.

0127   PUBLICATION 100.2, CHAPTER 15, 50.1.

0128   THIS CODE IS AN ADD ON CODE USED IN ADDITION TO E/M CODE ONLY. INFORMATION CAN BE FOUND IN 42 CFR PART 410 PAGE 50941.

0129   MMA section 303(e).

0130   MEDICARE RECOGNIZED CODE 1/1/2006. PRIOR TO THIS DATE, SERVICES BILLED WITH UNLISTED CODE.

0131   PUBLICATION 100.2, CHAPTER 16, SECTION 20 - SERVICES NOT REASONABLE AND NECESSARY.

0132   CARRIER PROCESSING MANUAL, CHAPTER 17.

0133   SEE ONLINE MANUAL 100-02.9.

0134   SECTION 5112 OF THE DRA.

0135   MEDICARE BENEFIT POLICY MANUAL, PUB 100.2, CHAPTER 15, SECTION 110.3 (100.02,15,110.3).

<u>Number</u>	<u>Description</u>

0136   PAID ON THE OPPS FEE SCHEDULE FOR USE WITH REV CODE 068X.

0137   PUBLICATION 100-03, CHAPTER 1, SECTION 280.1 (100.03, 1, 280.1).

0138   MEDICARE RECOGNIZED ANOTHER CODE FOR PAYMENT.

0139   COVERAGE IS LIMITED TO PERSONS WITH DYSPLASTIC NEVUS SYNDROME ONLY; NO PAYMENT FOR MONITOR-ING OF HIGH RISK PATIENTS WITH A FAMILY HISTORY.

0140   CLAIMS PROCESSING MANUAL PUBLICATION 100-04, CHAPTER 13, SECTION 140.

0141   SEE NATIONAL COVERAGE DETERMINATION MANUAL FOR TRANSCATHETER STENT PLACEMENT.

0142   SERVICES ARE CONSIDERED INCLUSIVE OF ANOTHER CODE. PAYMENT FOR SERVICE IS NOT MADE SEPARATE-LY.

0143   INTERNET ONLY MANUAL 100.4, CHAPTER 4, SECTION 61.3.

0144   SERVICES CONSIDERED PART OF THE CORRESPONDING E & M VISIT.

0145   MEDICARE CLAIMS PROCESSING MANUAL PUB 100-4, CHAPTER 8, SECTION 60.4.

0146   NCD MANUAL, SECTION 310.1, 42 CFR 405.205, SUBPART B SECTION 1862(A) OF THE ACT.

0147   CLAIMS PROCESSING MANUAL PUB 100-04, CHAPTER 17, SECTION 80.9.

0148   NCD MANUAL 220.6.

0149   THIS DEVICE WAS ONLY APPROVED BY THE FDA TO OBTAIN, MONITOR AND ANALYZE PRESSURES AT THE TIME AN ENDOVASCULAR PROCEDURE IS PERFORMED. THE FDA HAS NOT APPROVED THE DEVICE FOR FOLLOW-UP EVALUATION OF ENDOVASCULAR GRAFT PRESSURES IN THE OUTPATIENT SETTING.

0150   SEE NEW 2008 CPT CODES.

0151   SERVICES ARE CONSIDERED UNDER G CODES G0396 AND G0397.

0152   NCD 100-3, 160.12.

0153   PURSUANT TO SECTION 101 (B) OF THE MEDICARE IMPROVEMENT FOR PATIENTS AND PROVIDERS ACT OF 2008 (MIPPA) EFFECTIVE JANUARY 1, 2009, WE EXPANDED COVERAGE FOR THE WELCOME TO MEDICARE BENEFIT; IT IS SUBJECT TO CERTAIN ELIGIBILITY AND OTHER LIMITATIONS THAT ALLOW PAYMENT FOR AN INITIAL PRE-VENTIVE PHYSICAL EXAMINATION (IPPE), NOT LATER THAN 12 MONTHS AFTER THE DATE THE INDIVIDUAL'S FIRST COVERAGE PERIOD BEGIN UNDER MEDICARE PART B.

0154   MEDICARE RECOGNIZES THE FOLLOWING CODES G0412-G0415 FOR THIS SERVICE.

0155   MEDICARE DOES NOT RECOGNIZE CODES 27215, 27216, 27217 AND 27218 FOR 2009.

0156   1833(+)(2)(B) OF THE ACT; CY 2008 OPPS/ASC FINAL RULE (DATED NOVEMBER 22, 2007), P. 66611.

0157   MEDICARE BENEFIT POLICY MANUAL, PUB 100.02, CHAPTER 15, SECTION 110.2.

0158   SEE NEW OR ESTABLISHED VISIT CODES.

0159   THIS DENTAL SERVICE IS NOT PAYABLE OR PROCESSED UNDER THE PHYSICIAN FEE SCHEDULE.

0160   THIS SERVICE IS ONLY PAYABLE FOR RESTRICTIVE USE ONLY.

0161   MEDICARE ALLOWS PAYMENT FOR COLON SCREENING WITH ANOTHER CODE.

0162   THIS CODE IS NOT PAYABLE UNDER THE MEDICARE PROGRAM.

2010 HCPCS
Alpha-Numeric Index

A

B

Brompheniramine maleate, J0945
Budesonide inhalation solution, J7626, J7627, J7633, J7634
Bulking agent, L8604
Buprenorphine hydrochloride, J0592
Bus, nonemergency transportation, A0110
Busulfan, J0594, J8510
Butorphanol tartrate, J0595

C

C-1 Esterase Inhibitor, J0598
Cabergoline, oral, J8515
Caffeine citrate, J0706
Calcitriol, J0636
Calcitonin-salmon, J0630
Calcium disodium edetate, J0600
Calcium gluconate, J0610
Calcium glycerophosphate and calcium lactate, J0620
Calcium lactate and calcium glycerophosphate, J0620
Calcium leucovorin, J0640
Calibrator solution, A4256
Cane, E0100, E0105
        accessory, A4636, A4637
Canister, disposable, used with suction pump, A7000
Canister, non-disposable, used with suction pump, A7001
Cannula, nasal, A4615
Capecitabine, oral, J8520, J8521
Carbon filter, A4680
Carboplatin, J9045
Cardia Event, recorder, implantable, E0616
Cardiokymography, Q0035
Cardiovascular services, M0300-M0301
Carmustine, J9050
Caries susceptibility test, D0425
Case management, T1016, T1017
Caspofungin acetate, J0637
Cast
        diagnostic, dental, D0470
        hand restoration, L6900-L6915
        materials, special, A4590
        supplies, A4580, A4590, Q4001-Q4051
        thermoplastic, L2106, L2126
Caster, front, for power wheelchair, K0099
Caster, wheelchair, E0997, E0998
Catheter, A4300-A4355
        anchoring device, A5200, A4333, A4334
        cap, disposable (dialysis), A4860
        external collection device, A4327-A4330, A4347
        implanted, A7042, A7043
        indwelling, A4338-A4346
        insertion tray, A4354
        intermittent with insertion supplies, A4353

D

DMSO, J1212
Dobutamine HCl, J1250
Docetaxel, J9171
Dolasetron mesylate, J1260
Dome and mouthpiece (for nebulizer), A7016
Dopamine HCl, J1265
Doripenem, J1267
Dornase alpha, inhalation solution, unit dose form, J7639
Doxercalciferol, J1270
Doxil, J9001
Doxorubicin HCl, J9000, J9001
Drainage
        bag, A4357, A4358
        board, postural, E0606
        bottle, A5102
Dressing (see also Bandage), A6020-A6406
        alginate, A6196-A6199
        collagen, A6020-A6024
        composite, A6200-A6205
        contact layer, A6206-A6208
        foam, A6209-A6215
        gauze, A6216-A6230, A6402-A6406
        holder/binder, A4462
        hydrocolloid, A6234-A6241
        hydrogel, A6242-A6248
        specialty absorptive, A6251-A6256
        transparent film, A6257-A6259
        tubular, A6457
Droperidol, J1790
        and fentanyl citrate, J1810
Dropper, A4649
Drugs (see also Table of Drugs)
        administered through a metered dose inhaler, J3535
        chemotherapy, J8500-J9999
        disposable delivery system, 5 ml or less per hour, A4306
        disposable delivery system, 50 ml or greater per hour, A4305
        immunosuppressive, J7500-J7599
        infusion supplies, A4230-A4232, A4221, A4222
        inhalation solutions, J7608-J7699
        not otherwise classified, J3490, J7599, J7699, J7799, J8499, J8999, J9999
        prescription, oral, J8499, J8999
Dry pressure pad/mattress, E0179, E0184, E0199
Durable medical equipment (DME), E0100-E1830, K Codes
Duraclon, see Clonidine
Dyphylline, J1180

E

Ear mold, V5264
Echocardiography injectable contrast material, A9700
Eculizumab, J1300
Edetate calcium disodium, J0600

F

Heel
   elevator, air, E0370
   protector, E0191
   shoe, L3430-L3485
   stabilizer, L3170
Helicopter, ambulance (see also Ambulance)
Helmet, cervical, L0100, L0110
Helmet, head, A8000-A8004
Hemin, J1640
Hemi-wheelchair, E1083-E1086
Hemipelvectomy prosthesis, L5280
Hemodialysis
   machine, E1590
Hemodialyzer, portable, E1635
Hemofil M, J7190
Hemophilia clotting factor, J7190-J7198
Hemophilia clotting factor, NOC, J7199
Hemostats, A4850
Hemostix, A4773
Hepagam B IM, J1571
Hepagam B IV, J1573
Heparin infusion pump, dialysis, E1520
Heparin lock flush, J1642
Heparin sodium, J1644
Hep-Lock (U/P), J1642
Hexalite, A4590
High osmolar contrast material, Q9958-Q9964
Hip
   disarticulation prosthesis, L5250, L5270
   orthosis (HO), L1600-L1690
Hip-knee-ankle-foot orthosis (HKAFO), L2040-L2090
Histrelin acetate, J1675
Histrelin implant, J9225
HKAFO, L2040-L2090
Home Health Agency Services, T0221
Hot water bottle, E0220
Human fibrinogen concentrate, J1680
Humidifier, A7046, E0550-E0563
Hyalgan, J7321
Hyaluronate, sodium, J7317
Hyaluronidase, J3470
Hyaluronidase, ovine, J3471-J3473
Hydralazine HCl, J0360
Hydraulic patient lift, E0630
Hydrocollator, E0225, E0239
Hydrocolloid dressing, A6234-A6241
Hydrocortisone
   acetate, J1700
   sodium phosphate, J1710
   sodium succinate, J1720
Hydrogel dressing, A6242-A6248, A6231-A6233
Hydromorphone, J1170

J

K

Kits
       enteral feeding supply (syringe) (pump) (gravity), B4034-B4036
       fistula cannulation (set), A4730
       parenteral nutrition, B4220-B4224
       surgical dressing (tray), A4550
       tracheostomy, A4625
Knee
       disarticulation, prosthesis, L5150, L5160
       joint, miniature, L5826
       orthosis (KO), E1810, L1800-L1885
Knee-ankle-foot orthosis (KAFO), L2000-L2039, L2126-L2136
Knee-ankle-foot orthosis (KAFO) addition, high strength, lightweight material, L2755
Kyphosis pad, L1020, L1025

L

Laboratory tests
       chemistry, P2028-P2038
       microbiology, P7001
       miscellaneous, P9010-P9615, Q0111-Q0115
       toxicology, P3000-P3001, Q0091
Lacrimal duct implant
       permanent, A4263
       temporary, A4262
Lactated Ringer's infusion, J7120
Laetrile, J3570
Lancet, A4258, A4259
Lanreotide, J1930
Laronidase, J1931
Larynx, artificial, L8500
Laser blood collection device and accessory, E0620, A4257
Lead investigation, T1029
Lead wires, per pair, A4557
Leg
       bag, A4358, A5105, A5112
       extensions for walker, E0158
       rest, elevating, K0195
       rest, wheelchair, E0990
       strap, replacement, A5113-A5114
Legg Perthes orthosis, L1700-L1755
Lens
       aniseikonic, V2118, V2318
       contact, V2500-V2599
       eye, V2100-V2615, V2700-V2799
       intraocular, V2630-V2632
       low vision, V2600-V2615
       progressive, V2781
Lepirudin, J1945
Leucovorin calcium, J0640
Leukocyte poor blood, each unit, P9016
Leuprolide acetate, J9217, J9218, J9219, J1950
Levalbuterol, all formulations, inhalation solution, concentrated, J7607, J7612

M

O

P

Surgical
    boot, L3208-L3211
    brush, dialysis, A4910
    dressing, A6196-A6406
    stocking, A4490-A4510
    supplies, A4649
    tray, A4550
Swabs, betadine or iodine, A4247
Syringe, A4213
    with needle, A4206-A4209
Synvisc and Synvisc-One, J7325

T

Tables, bed, E0274, E0315
Tacrolimus, oral, J7507
Tacrolimus, parenteral, J7525
Taxi, non emergency transportation, A0100
Technetium TC 99M Arcitumomab, A9568
Technetium TC 99M Bicisate, A9557
Technetium TC 99M Depreotide, A9536
Technetium TC 99M Disofenin, A9510
Technetium TC 99M Exametazine, A9521
Technetium TC 99M Exametazine labeled autologous white blood cells, A9569
Technetium TC 99M Fanolesomab, A9566
Technetium TC 99M Glucepatate, A9550
Technetium TC 99M - Labeled red blood cells, A9560
Technetium TC 99M Macroaggregated albumin, A9540
Technetium TC 99M Mebrofenin, A9537
Technetium TC 99M Mertiatide, A9562
Technetium TC 99M Oxidronate, A9561
Technetium TC 99M Pentetate, A9539, A9567
Technetium TC 99M Pertechnetate, A9512
Technetium TC 99M Pyrophosphate, A9538
Technetium TC 99M Sestamibi, A9500
Technetium TC 99M Succimer, A9551
Technetium TC 99M Sulfur colloid, A9541
Technetium TC 99M Teboroxime, A9501
Technetium TC 99M Tetrofosmin, A9502
TEEV, J0900
Telehealth, Q3014
Telehealth transmission, T1014
Temozolomide, injection, J9328
Temozolomide, oral, J8700
Temporomandibular joint, D0320, D0321
Temsirolimus, J9330
Tenecteplase, J3101
Teniposide, Q2017
TENS, A4595, E0720-E0749
Tent, oxygen, E0455
Terbutaline sulfate, J3105
Terbutaline sulfate, inhalation solution, concentrated, J7680